10
D1549621

Pain in Infants, Children, and Adolescents

Second Edition

Pain in Infants, Children, and Adolescents

Second Edition

Editors

Neil L. Schechter, M.D.
Professor
Department of Pediatrics
University of Connecticut School of Medicine
Director, Pain Relief Program
Connecticut Children's Medical Center
Director, Section of Developmental and Behavioral Pediatrics
St. Francis Hospital and Medical Center
Hartford, Connecticut

Charles B. Berde, Ph.D., M.D.
Professor
Departments of Anesthesia and Pediatrics
Harvard Medical School
Director, Pain Treatment Service
Department of Anesthesia
The Children's Hospital
Boston, Massachusetts

Myron Yaster, M.D.
Professor
Departments of Anesthesiology/Critical Care Medicine and Pediatrics
The Johns Hopkins University School of Medicine
Clinical Director, Anesthesiology and Pain Management
The Johns Hopkins Hospital
Baltimore, Maryland

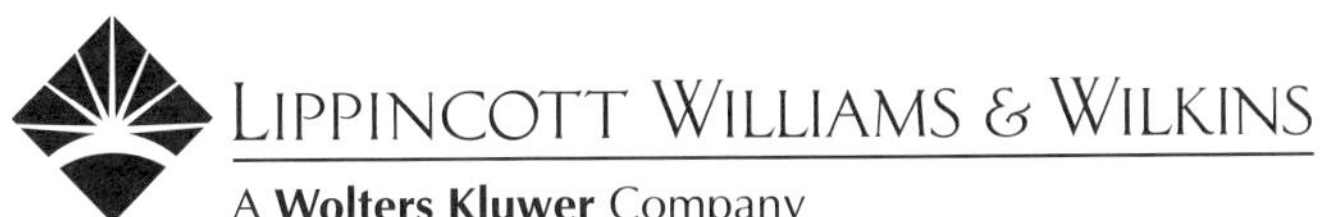

Philadelphia • Baltimore • New York • London
Buenos Aires • Hong Kong • Sydney • Tokyo

Acquisitions Editor: R. Craig Percy
Developmental Editor: Lisa Consoli
Production Editor: Jonathan Geffner
Manufacturing Manager: Colin Warnock
Cover Designer: Mark Lerner
Compositor: Lippincott Williams & Wilkins Desktop Division
Printer: Edwards Brothers

530 Walnut Street
Philadelphia, PA 19106 USA
LWW.com

Printed in the USA

Library of Congress Cataloging-in-Publication Data

Pain in infants, children, and adolescents / editors, Neil L. Schechter, Charles B. Berde, Myron Yaster.--2nd ed.
p. cm.
Includes bibliographical references and index.
ISBN 0-7817-2644-1
1. Pain in children. 2. Pain in adolescence. 3. Pain in infants. I. Schechter, Neil L. II. Berde, Charles B. III. Yaster, Myron.

RJ365 .P35 2002
618.92--dc21

2002016224

Care has been taken to confirm the accuracy of the information presented and to describe generally accepted practices. However, the authors, editors, and publisher are not responsible for errors or omissions or for any consequences from application of the information in this book and make no warranty, expressed or implied, with respect to the currency, completeness, or accuracy of the contents of the publication. Application of this information in a particular situation remains the professional responsibility of the practitioner.

The authors, editors, and publisher have exerted every effort to ensure that drug selection and dosage set forth in this text are in accordance with current recommendations and practice at the time of publication. However, in view of ongoing research, changes in government regulations, and the constant flow of information relating to drug therapy and drug reactions, the reader is urged to check the package insert for each drug for any change in indications and dosage and for added warnings and precautions. This is particularly important when the recommended agent is a new or infrequently employed drug.

Some drugs and medical devices presented in this publication have Food and Drug Administration (FDA) clearance for limited use in restricted research settings. It is the responsibility of the health care provider to ascertain the FDA status of each drug or device planned for use in their clinical practice.

10 9 8 7 6 5 4 3 2 1

Contents

Part III: Specific Pain Problems

Contributing Authors

Kanwaljeet S. Anand, M.B.B.S., D. Phil.
Professor
Department of Pediatrics
University of Arkansas for Medical Sciences
Section Chief
Pediatric Critical Care Medicine
Arkansas Children's Hospital
Little Rock, Arkansas

Katharine A. Andrews, Ph.D., M.Sc.
Postdoctoral Research Fellow
Department of Anatomy and Developmental Biology
University College London
Children Nationwide Pain Research Centre
Institute of Child Health
London, England
United Kingdom

Ronald G. Barr, M.D.C.M.
Professor
Department of Pediatrics and Psychiatry
McGill University
Head, Child Development Program
Montreal Children's Hospital
Montreal, Quebec
Canada

Charles B. Berde, M.D., Ph.D.
Professor
Departments of Anesthesia and Pediatrics
Harvard Medical School
Director, Pain Treatment Service
Department of Anesthesia
The Children's Hospital
Boston, Massachusetts

Bruce A. Bernstein, Ph.D.
Assistant Professor
Departments of Pediatrics and Surgery
University of Connecticut School of Medicine
Farmington, Connecticut
Department of Anthropology
University of Connecticut
Storrs, Connecticut
Director, Research and Performance Improvement
St. Francis Hospital and Medical Center
Hartford, Connecticut

Kristina Boyer, M.Sc.(A)
Graduate Student
School of Nursing
McGill University
Montreal, Quebec
Canada

Marion E. Broome, Ph.D., R.N., F.A.N.N.
Associate Dean and Professor
School of Nursing
University of Alabama at Birmingham
Birmingham, Alabama

Jeffrey P. Burns, M.D., M.P.H.
Assistant Professor
Department of Anesthesia
Harvard Medical School
Associate Director
Multidisciplinary Intensive Care Unit
Children's Hospital
Boston, Massachusetts

Brenda Bursch, Ph.D.
Assistant Professor
Departments of Psychiatry and Biobehavioral Sciences, and Pediatrics
University of California at Los Angeles School of Medicine
Associate Director, Pediatric Pain Program
University of California at Los Angeles Mattel Children's Hospital
Los Angeles, California

Robert C. Cassidy, Ph.D.
Assistant Professor
Department of Pediatrics
Albert Einstein College of Medicine
Bronx, New York
Director of Bioethics and Social Policy
Schneider Children's Hospital
Long Island Jewish Medical Center
North Shore–Long Island Jewish Health System
New Hyde Park, New York

John J. Collins, M.B.B.S., Ph.D.
Head, Pain and Palliative Care Service
The Children's Hospital at Westmead
Sydney, New South Wales
Australia

Kenneth D. Craig, Ph.D.
Professor
Department of Psychology
University of British Columbia
Vancouver, British Columbia
Canada

Bernard Dalens, M.D.
Head, Pediatric Anesthesia Unit
Department on Anesthesiology
University Hospital Hotel-Dieu
Clermont-Ferrand
France

Carlton Dampier, M.D.
Professor
Department of Pediatrics
MCP Hahnemann University School of Medicine
Director, Marian Anderson Sickle Cell Center
St. Christopher's Hospital for Children
Philadelphia, Pennsylvania

Joëlle F. Desparmet, M.D.
Associate Professor
Department of Anesthesia
McGill University
Director, Pain Management Centre
Department of Anesthesia
Montreal Children's Hospital
Montreal, Quebec
Canada

Bruce Dick, Ph.D. Candidate
Department of Psychology
Dalhousie University
Psychology Intern
Department of Psychology
IWK Health Centre
Halifax, Nova Scotia
Canada

Nalton F. Ferraro, D.M.D., M.D.
Instructor
Department of Oral and Maxillofacial Surgery
Harvard School of Dental Medicine
Senior Associate
Department of Oral and Maxillofacial Surgery
Children's Hospital
Boston, Massachusetts

G. Allen Finley, M.D.
Professor
Departments of Anesthesia and Psychology
Dalhousie University
Medical Director, Pediatric Pain Management
Department of Pediatric Anesthesia
IWK Health Centre
Halifax, Nova Scotia
Canada

Maria Fitzgerald, Ph.D.
Professor of Developmental Neurobiology and Scientific Director of Pediatric Pain Research Group
Department of Anatomy and Developmental Biology
University College London
London, England
United Kingdom

Gerri Frager, R.N., M.D.
Assistant Professor
Department of Pediatrics
Dalhousie University
Medical Director
Department of Pediatric Palliative Care
IWK Health Centre
Halifax, Nova Scotia
Canada

Linda S. Franck, Ph.D., R.N., R.G.N., R.S.C.N.
Professor of Children's Nursing Research
School of Nursing and Midwifery
King's College London
Directorate of Nursing
Great Ormond Street Hospital
London, England
United Kingdom

Anne Gaffney, Ph.D.
College Lecturer
Department of Pediatrics and Child Health
National University of Ireland
University of Cork
Cork, Ireland

Paula Gardiner, M.D.
Research Associate
Center for Holistic Education and Research
Children's Hospital
Boston, Massachusetts
Tufts Family Practice Residency
Hallmark Health
Malden, Massachusetts

M. Alex Geertsma, M.D.
Clinical Associate Professor
Department of Pediatrics
Connecticut Children's Medical Center
University of Connecticut School of Medicine
Hartford, Connecticut
Chairman
Department of Pediatrics
St. Mary's Hospital
Waterbury, Connecticut

Ann Goldman, M.B.
Honorary Senior Lecturer
Institute of Child Health
Consultant in Pediatric Palliative Care
Department of Hematology and Oncology
Great Ormond Street Hospital
London, England
United Kingdom

Kenneth R. Goldschneider, M.D.
Assistant Professor
University of Cincinnati College of Medicine
Director, Division of Pain Management
Department of Anesthesia
Children's Hospital Medical Center
Cincinnati, Ohio

Brenda Golianu, M.D.
Assistant Professor
Department of Anesthesia
Stanford University School of Medicine
Stanford, California

Mirja Hämäläinen, M.D., Ph.D.
Specialist in Pediatric Neurology
Department of Pediatric Neurology
University of Helsinki
Pediatric Neurologist
Hospital for Children and Adolescents
Helsinki University Central Hospital
Helsinki, Finland

Richard A. Hardart, M.D.
Instructor
Departments of Anesthesiology and Critical Care Medicine
The Johns Hopkins University School of Medicine
Attending Anesthesiologist
Departments of Anesthesiology and Critical Care Medicine
The Johns Hopkins Hospital
Baltimore, Maryland

Loretta M. Hillier, M.A.
Research Associate
Pain Innovations, Inc.
London, Ontario
Canada

Richard F. Howard, B.Sc., M.B., Ch.B.
Honorary Senior Lecturer
Department ofAnesthesia
Institute of Child Health
University College London
Consultant in Anesthesia and Pain Management
Department of Anesthesia
Great Ormond Street Children's Hospital
London, England
United Kingdom

Myra M. Huth, Ph.D., R.N.
Assistant Adjunct Professor
Department of Anesthesiology
Medical College of Wisconsin
Research Associate
Jane B. Pettit Pain Management and Palliative Care Center
Children's Hospital of Wisconsin
Milwaukee, Wisconsin

C. Celeste Johnston, R.N., D.Ed.
James McGill Professor
School of Nursing
McGill University
Consultant
Department of Nursing
Montreal Children's Hospital
Montreal, Quebec
Canada

Michael H. Joseph, M.D.
Assistant Clinical Professor
Departments of Anesthesiology and Pediatrics
University of Southern California, Keck School of Medicine
Director of Pain Services
Departments of Anesthesiology and Pediatrics
Chldren's Hospital Los Angeles
Los Angeles, California

Madelyn D. Kahana, M.D.
Professor
Departments of Anesthesia and Critical Care
University of Chicago
Medical Director
Pediatric Intensive Care Unit
University of Chicago Children's Hospital
Chicago, Illinois

Kathi J. Kemper, M.D., M.P.H.
Professor
Department of Pediatrics
Wake Forest University School of Medicine
Winston-Salem, North Carolina

Stephen R. King, Ph.D.
Assistant Professor of Clinical Pediatrics
Department of Pediatrics
University of Connecticut School of Medicine
Farmington, Connecticut
Co-Director
Jaycee Center for the Evaluation of Children's Development
Center for Children's Health and Development
St. Francis Hospital and Medical Center
Hartford, Connecticut

Sabine Kost-Byerly, M.D.
Assistant Professor
Department of Pediatric Anesthesiology and Critical Care Medicine
The Johns Hopkins University
Baltimore, Maryland

Elliot J. Krane, M.D.
Professor
Departments of Pediatrics and Anesthesia
Stanford University
Chief, Department of Anesthesia
Packard Children's Hospital
Department of Anesthesia
Stanford University Hospital
Stanford, California

Donald T. Kulas, M.D.
Division of Pediatric Rheumatology
Duke Children's Hospital and Health Center
Duke University Medical Center
Durham, North Carolina

Leora Kuttner, Ph.D. (Clin Psyc)
Clinical Professor and Clinical Psychologist
Department of Pediatrics
University of British Columbia
British Columbia Children's Hospital
Vancouver, British Columbia
Canada

Fran Lang Porter, Ph.D.
Assistant Professor
Departments of Pediatrics and Psychology
Washington University
St. Louis, Missouri

Alyssa A. Lebel, M.D.
Instructor
Department of Anesthesiology
Harvard Medical School
Assistant Professor in Anesthesia
Department of Anesthesia
Children's Hospital
Boston, Massachusetts

Alan M. Leichtner, M.D.
Associate Professor
Department of Pediatrics
Harvard Medical School
Chief, Division of Gastroenterology and Nutrition
Children's Hospital
Boston, Massachusetts

Michael S. Leong, M.D.
Assistant Professor
Department of Anesthesia
Stanford University
Stanford, California

Yvonne Y. Leong, Pharm.D.
Clinical Pharmacist
Department of Pharmacy
Lucile Packard Children's Hospital at Stanford
Palo Alto, California

Yuan-Chi Lin, M.D., M.P.H.
Associate in Anesthesia
Department of Anesthesia
Children's Hospital Boston
Boston, Massachusetts

Joseph R. Madsen, M.D.
Associate Professor
Department of Surgery
Harvard Medical School
Neurosurgeon
Department of Neurosurgery
Children's Hospital
Boston, Massachusetts

Bruce J. Masek, Ph.D.
Associate Professor
Department of Psychiatry
Harvard Medical School
Clinical Director
Department of Child Psychology
Massachusetts General Hospital
Boston, Massachusetts

Eeva-Liisa Maunuksela, M.D., Ph.D.
Associate Professor
Department of Anesthesia and Intensive Care
University of Kuopio
Kuopio, Finland
Conultant Anesthesiologist
Helsinki University Eye and ENT Hospital
Helsinki, Finland

Lynne G. Maxwell, M.D.
Associate Professor
Departments of Anesthesiology and Pediatrics
University of Pennsylvania
Attending Anesthesiologist
Departments of Anesthesiology and Critical Care Medicine and Pediatrics
The Children's Hospital of Philadelphia
Philadelphia, Pennsylvania

Claire F. McCarthy, P.T., M.S.
Clinical Associate Professor
Graduate Programs in Physical Therapy
MGH Institute of Health Professions
Charlestown, Massachusetts
Director Emeritus
Department of Physical and Occupational Therapy
Children's Hospital
Boston, Massachusetts

Patricia A. McGrath, Ph.D.
Professor
Department of Anesthesia
University of Toronto
Scientific Director
Chronic Pain Program
Department of Anesthesia
The Hospital for Sick Children
Toronto, Ontario
Canada

Patrick J. McGrath, Ph.D.
Professor and Canada Research Chair
Department of Psychology
Dalhousie University
Psychologist
Pain Service
IWK Health Centre
Halifax, Nova Scotia
Canada

Neil McIntosh, M.B., D.Sc.(Med.)
Professor
Department of Child Life and Health
University of Edinburgh
Consultant Neonatologist
Neonatal Unit
New Royal Infirmary
Edinburgh, Scotland
United Kingdom

Gopi Menon, M.B.B.Chir.
Honorary Senior Lecturer
Department of Child Life and Health
University of Edinburgh
Consultant Neonatologist
Department of Neonatology
Royal Infirmary of Edinburgh
Edinburgh, Scotland
United Kingdom

Tim F. Oberlander, M.D.
Associate Professor
Department of Pediatrics
University of British Columbia
Developmental Pediatrician
Division of Developmental Pediatrics
Children's and Women's Health Centre of British Columbia
Vancouver, British Columbia
Canada

Klaus T. Olkkola, M.D., Ph.D.
Associate Professor
Department of Anesthesia and Intensive Care Medicine
University of Helsinki
Medical Director
Department of Anesthesia and Intensive Care Medicine
Helsinki University Central Hospital
Helsinki, Finland

Gunnar Olsson, M.D., Ph.D.
Department of Pediatric Anesthesia
Astrid Lindgren Children's Hospital
Stockholm
Sweden

Lee M. Pachter, D.O.
Associate Professor
Departments of Pediatrics and Anthropology
University of Connecticut School of Medicine
Farmington, Connecticut
Department of Pediatrics
St. Francis Hospital and Medical Center
Hartford, Connecticut

Maureen Pomietto, R.N., M.N.
Clinical Faculty
Department of Family and Child Nursing
University of Washington School of Nursing
Clinical Nurse Specialist
Children's Hospital & Regional Medical Centre
Seattle, Washington

Leonard A. Rappaport, M.D., M.S.
Associate Professor
Department of Pediatrics
Harvard Medical School
Director, Developmental Medicine Center
Department of Medicine
Children's Hospital Boston
Boston, Massachusetts

Laura E. Schanberg, M.D.
Assistant Professor
Department of Pediatrics
Division of Pediatric Rheumatology
Medical Director
Pediatric Pain Clinic
Duke University Medical Center
Durham, North Carolina

Lisa Scharff, Ph.D.
Assistant Professor
Department of Psychiatry
Harvard Medical School
Cambridge, Massachusetts
Associate Director
Pain Treatment Service
Department of Psychiatry
Children's Hospital
Boston, Massachusetts

Neil L. Schechter, M.D.
Professor
Department of Pediatrics
University of Connecticut School of Medicine
Director, Pain Relief Program
Connecticut Children's Medical Center
Director, Section of Developmental and Behavioral Pediatrics
St. Francis Hospital and Medical Center
Hartford, Connecticut

Steven M. Selbst, M.D.
Professor
Department of Pediatrics
Jefferson Medical College
Thomas Jefferson University
Philadelphia, Pennsylvania
Vice Chair for Education
Pediatrics Residency Director
Department of Pediatrics
A. I. DuPont Hospital for Children
Wilmington, Delaware

Barbara S. Shapiro, M.D.
Associate Clinical Professor
Departments of Pediatrics and Psychiatry
University of Pennsylvania School of Medicine
Philadelphia, Pennsylvania

Alice M. Shea, P.T., M.P.H., Sc.D.
Associate for Research and Education
Department of Physical Therapy and Occupational Therapy Services
Children's Hospital Boston
Boston, Massachusetts

Lu Ann Sifford, M.D.
Senior Associate Consultant
Department of Psychiatry and Psychology
Mayo Clinic
Rochester, Minnesota

Jodi L. Smith, M.D., Ph.D.
Assistant Professor
Department of Surgery
Division of Neurological Surgery
Indiana University School of Medicine
Assistant Professor
Department of Pediatric Neurosurgery
Riley Hospital for Children
Indianapolis, Indiana

Jean Solodiuk, R.N., P.N.P.
Advanced Practice Nurse
Pain Treatment Service
Children's Hospital
Boston, Massachusetts

Richard Solomon, M.D.
Clinical Associate Professor
Department of Pediatrics and Communicable Diseases
University of Michigan
Ann Arbor, Michigan

Bonnie J. Stevens, R.N., Ph.D.
Professor
Faculties of Nursing and Medicine
University of Toronto
Signy Hildur Eaton Chair in Pediatric Nursing Research
The Hospital for Sick Children
Toronto, Ontario
Canada

Maureen Strafford, M.D.
Associate Professor of Anesthesiology and Pediatrics
Department of Anesthesiology
Tufts University School of Medicine
Associate Anesthesiologist
Department of Anesthesiology
New England Medical Center
Boston, Massachusetts

Penny Sullivan, P.T., P.C.S.
Consulant, Pain Treatment Service
Department of Physical and Occupational Therapy
Children's Hospital Boston
Boston, Massachusetts

Joseph D. Tobias, M.D.
Professor of Anesthesiology and Pediatrics
Russell D. Sheldon Chair of Pediatric Anesthesiology
The University of Missouri
Vice Chairman
Department of Anesthesiology
Chief, Pediatric Anesthesiology of Clinical Care
The University of Missouri Hospital
Columbia, Missouri

Joseph R. Tobin, M.D.
Professor
Departments of Anesthesiology and Pediatrics
Wake Forest University School of Medicine
Section Head
Pediatric Anesthesia and Critical Care
Brenner Children's Hospital
Winston-Salem, North Carolina

Anita Unruh, Ph.D., OT(C)RegNS
Associate Professor
School of Occupational Therapy
Dalhousie University
Halifax, Nova Scotia
Canada

Gary A. Walco, Ph.D.
Associate Professor
Department of Pediatrics
University of Medicine and Dentistry of New Jersey
New Jersey Medical School
Newark, New Jersey
Director, The David Center for Children's Pain and Palliative Care
Department of Pediatrics
Hackensack University Medical Center
Hackensack, New Jersey

Steven J. Weisman, M.D.
Professor
Departments of Anesthesiology and Pediatrics
Medical College of Wisconsin
Jane B. Pettit Chair in Pain Management
Jane B. Pettit Pain and Palliative Care Center
Children's Hospital of Wisconsin
Milwaukee, Wisconsin

Robert T. Wilder, M.D., Ph.D.
Assistant Professor
Department of Anesthesiology
Mayo Medical School
Senior Associate Consultant
Department of Anesthesiology
Mayo Clinic
Rochester, Minnesota

C. Mae Wong, B.M.B.S.
Rivendell Research Fellow in Neonatology
Department of Child Life and Health
University of Edinburgh
Rivendell Research Fellow in Neonatology
Neonatal Unit
Royal Infirmary of Edinburgh
Edinburgh, Scotland
United Kingdom

Myron Yaster, M.D.
Professor
Departments of Anesthesiology/CriticalCare Medicine and Pediatrics
The Johns Hopkins University School of Medicine
Clinical Director, Pediatric Anesthesiology and Pain Management
The Johns Hopkins Hospital
Baltimore, Maryland

Lonnie K. Zeltzer, M.D.
Professor of Pediatrics, Anesthesiology, Psychiatry, and Biobehavioral Sciences
Department of Pediatrics
Director, Pediatric Pain Program
UCLA, Mattel Children's Center
University of California at Los Angeles
Los Angeles, California

William T. Zempsky, M.D.
Associate Professor
Department of Pediatrics
University of Connecticut School of Medicine
Associate Director
Pain Relief Program
Connecticut Children's Medical Center
Emergency Center
Hartford, Connecticut

Preface

Although work on this volume has been in progress for over 3 years, this preface is being written shortly after the tragic circumstances of September 11, 2001, in which so many died in the wreckage of the World Trade Center in New York, at the Pentagon, and in the fields of Pennsylvania. This sorry episode, as so many others that have occurred throughout history, highlighted the complex tension implicit in human nature with the capacity for enormous destruction coexisting with that for almost limitless generosity and heroism. It also reminded us that simple acts of kindness take place all around us all of the time, often without our recognition. This volume summarizes the collective efforts of hundreds of clinicians and scientists who have devoted their energies to one visible manifestation of that spirit—harnessing science and technology to address the physical suffering of those with the softest voices, children.

Since the first edition of this text was published almost 10 years ago, we have made enormous progress in alleviating pain and providing comfort to those in need. Our understanding of the nature of pain has deepened, and we have unlocked some of the mysteries of the nervous system that create and sustain pain. The critical role of psychologic factors in pain has been amplified by new research. Significantly, we also have become aware of the devastating consequences of inadequate treatment and the unchecked persistence of pain. The importance of pain control during medical procedures has been definitively established, and sedation is now routine for many procedures for which it was not even considered when the earlier edition of this volume was written. We also have many new tools available to us. Our improved understanding of how existing anesthetics and analgesics work has yielded not only improvement of their efficacy but new agents as well. The role of adjuvants has expanded greatly. Cognitive, behavioral, and psychologic strategies have been refined and now play a role in all pain problems. Multidisciplinary teams have become commonplace, bringing expertise from various streams simultaneously to the child. Expert guidelines have been developed to help direct clinical practice, legislative and regulatory efforts mandate attention to pain, and educational programs regarding pain management exist in essentially all clinical domains. We have come very far, and it is our goal to present these extraordinary developments in as comprehensive a way as possible.

The format of this book remains unchanged. The first section discusses the theoretical underpinnings of pain treatment—transmission and interpretation of pain, cultural and psychological factors involved, the manifestations of pain and how they can be used to assess it, and the ethical decision-making associated with pain treatment. The second section describes the wide assortment of treatment strategies we have available to us—pharmacologic, physical, and psychologic. In the third section, unique pain problems are described comprehensively. These chapters are intended to present a state-of-the-art comprehensive review and to serve as an independent resource on the subject. As a result, if one reads this volume cover to cover (as we are sure you will), there will be some redundancy because so many of the general principles and specific treatment strategies are similar among the problems described. We ask your indulgence.

It is our hope, in this book, to document the remarkable changes in attitude and practice that have occurred in the area of pain and its control in children and to offer clinicians the rationale and tools to promote further growth. The management of pain is a cornerstone of the compassionate practice of medicine. The knowledge exists to ameliorate pain in most of our patients. We now require the will to do so.

Neil L. Schechter, M.D.
Charles B. Berde, Ph.D., M.D.
Myron Yaster, M.D.

Acknowledgments

This volume is a composite of the hard work of many individuals. When compared to its predecessor, it demonstrates the enormous growth of our knowledge in the past ten years and is a testimony to the vitality and creativity of this new discipline. The contributing authors are among the most talented investigators and clinicians in this young field and we are highly indebted to them for their willingness to participate in this endeavor. We especially appreciate their cheerful (most of the time) acceptance of the inefficiency and disorganization of the editors. It is our hope that they are as proud of this volume as we are. We are indebted as well to Lippincott Williams & Wilkins for their recognition of the importance of pain management in children and their unwavering support of this project. Without the commitment and efforts of their editorial team, Craig Percy and Lisa Consoli, this book would never have come to fruition.

As in the first edition of this text, each editor would like to independently thank those who have supported him in this process:

I am indebted to friends and colleagues at St. Francis Hospital and Medical Center and at the Connecticut Children's Medical Center for their continuing support and for providing the stimulating intellectual environment in which this work could be pursued. In particular, I appreciate the friendship and advice of Nancy Bright, the nursing coordinator of the Pain Relief Program; William Zempsky, my pediatric pain partner; and Paul Dworkin, my colleague and confidante of many years. I also greatly value the loyalty and support of Tamara Pezzente, who graciously provided secretarial support for this volume above and beyond the call. I remain indebted to three pediatric mentors who shaped my thinking about the world and my caring for my patients: Milton Markowitz, the late and much missed Joseph Cullina, and Melvin Levine. Finally, the continuous love and support of my wife, Carlota; children, Ben and Anna; and parents, Sylvia and Stanley, has enriched my life beyond measure.

N.L.S.

I am honored to work with a superb group of friends and colleagues at the Pain Treatment Service at Children's Hospital, including Navil Sethna, Lisa Scharff, Christine Greco, Alyssa Lebel, Yuan-Chi Lin, Tom Mancuso, Hyun Kee Chung, Nancy Rotter, Jean Solodiuk, Lori McDonald-Nolan, Mary Drew, and Penny Sullivan. I have had the good fortune to collaborate in research with other current and former colleagues at Children's Hospital, at other Harvard hospitals, and at Massachusetts Institute of Technology, most notably Bruce Masek, Bob Langer, Dan Kohane, Brian Cairns, Bob Truog, Claire McCarthy, Alice Shea, David Zurakowski, Mary Ellen McCann, Gary Strichartz, Bob Wilder, John Collins, Tim Oberlander, Greta Palmer, Ken Goldschneider, and Holcombe Grier. Most of all, I would like to thank my family for their love and patience: my children, David and Anna, who inspire me daily as they travel the sometimes bumpy road of adolescence; my father, Sydney, who instilled in me a love of learning and a commitment to serve others; and my wife, Evelyn, for her love and courage and her amazing capacity to infuse beauty into the lives of everyone around her.

C.B.B.

I would like to express my thanks to my mentors, Dr. John J. Downes, Dr. Mark C. Rogers, and Dr. Richard Traystman; whose leadership, commitment to excellence, wisdom, and dedication to the welfare of children have made my career possible. I am also indebted to my colleagues and friends at the Johns Hopkins Hospital, particularly Dr. David G. Nichols and Dr. Lynne G. Maxwell; and to my family, Ben, Jake, Suzy, and Pam for their unconditional love and support.

M.Y.

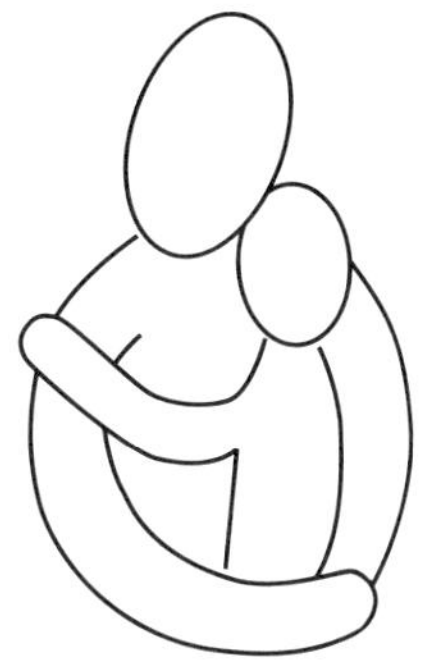

PART I

Theoretic Perspectives

1

Pain in Infants, Children, and Adolescents

An Overview

Neil L. Schechter, Charles B. Berde, and Myron Yaster

Although the world is full of suffering, it is also full of the overcoming of it. —*Helen Keller*

The field of pediatric pain has changed dramatically since the first edition of this textbook. An outpouring of research has altered societal and professional attitudes as well as clinical practice in this area. New information about the basic mechanism of pain transmission and the consequences of inadequate treatment has deepened our understanding of the phenomena of pain. Research on pain assessment, analgesic pharmacology, and behavioral and cognitive strategies have given us the tools to significantly reduce the historic undertreatment of pain in children. Although new research continues to illuminate existing controversies, at this juncture, the uniform application of available knowledge and technology would significantly reduce the burden of illness and medical treatment for many children and their families.

This chapter reviews the evolution of pain treatment in children from nearly universal undertreatment to its present level. The barriers that militated against adequate treatment are reviewed and strategies to eliminate existing barriers are discussed. Finally, the broad conceptual framework with which pain is currently understood is examined.

THE UNDERTREATMENT OF PAIN IN CHILDREN

Before the 1970s, the medical literature is essentially devoid of any formal reviews or research specifically addressing the management of pain in children. The limited discussion of this subject tended to be anecdotal and revealed the underlying bias of the era that minimized the experience of pain in children. For example, Swafford and Allen (1) reported that only two of the 60 postoperative patients on their pediatric service required any analgesia. They also reported that 26 of 180 children admitted to their intensive care unit in a 4-month period received opioid analgesics. By way of explanation, they stated that "pediatric patients seldom need medication for the relief of pain. They tolerate discomfort well. The child will say he does not feel well or that he is uncomfortable, that he wants his parents but often he will not relate this unhappiness to pain." Such a statement reveals the lens with which pain in children was viewed. Children neither responded to nor remembered painful experiences to the same degree that adults did. To appreciate the clinical manifestations of this philosophy, one needs only to examine the evolution of pain management in three sentinel pain problems: postoperative pain, pain in newborns, and pain in chronic disease.

Postoperative Pain

In her classic studies in the mid-1970s of postoperative pain management in children, Eland (2) identified both significant undertreatment and enormous discrepancies in child and adult prescribing practices. She examined the charts of 25 children who had various types of surgery (nephrectomies, palate repairs, traumatic amputations) at a large teaching hospital and found that 13 children received no analgesics during their hospital stay. For the group of 12 who received analgesia, a total of 24 analgesic doses (half opioid, half nonopioid) was administered. She compared the care of that group with a convenience sample of 18 adult surgical patients who had received 372 opioid and 299 nonopioid doses of analgesics during their hospital stay.

Unfortunately, Eland's study had limited clinical impact. Several investigators surveyed postoperative pain management in children during the subsequent decade and found it to be persistently inadequate, particularly in contrast with adult pain management. For example, Mather and Mackie (3) almost 10 years later examined the incidence of pain and analgesic administration in 170 postoperative children. They found that although most children experienced severe pain, no analgesics were ordered for 16%. They were not even administered to almost 40% of the group for whom they were ordered. Finally, they found that only 25% of children were pain free on the day of their surgery, whereas 40% complained of moderate to severe pain. In aggregate, their data suggested that almost 75% of children had insufficient analgesia. Mather and Mackie explained this phenomenon by citing educational inadequacies in both the medical and nursing staff regarding analgesics and by attitudes that denigrated the importance of adequate pain relief. They stated that nurses interpreted p.r.n., the most common format by which analgesics were ordered, to mean "as little as possible," and when given a choice of drugs and range of doses, nurses would select the least potent drug at the lowest dose.

Beyer et al. (4) studied the administration of analgesics to adults and children after cardiac surgery and found that children had fewer opioids ordered for and administered to them. When all the opioid doses administered to the 50 children and 50 adults in their sample for the first 3 postoperative days were combined, 70% of the opioids ordered were for adults. By the fifth postoperative day, children received only ten of the 136 doses of analgesics administered. In 1986, Schechter et al. (5) reviewed the charts of 90 children and 90 adults with identical diagnoses: hernia repairs, appendectomies, body burns of less than 20%, and fractured femurs. In general, adults received twice the number of opioid doses per hospital day that children received. In addition, there was a clear relationship between length of hospital stay and opioid dosing patterns. The longer the hospital stay, the greater the discrepancy between child and adult prescribing practices. Finally, they noted institutional differences regarding analgesic administration with some institutions prescribing opioids more liberally than others.

By the late 1980s, however, a perceptible change in postoperative pain management began to occur. Several streams of information coalesced to allow this change. Data about the inadequacies of adult pain treatment had become commonplace and entered the popular press. This information filtered down to pediatric clinicians. In response, consensus statements that emphasized the critical importance of adequate pain management began to emerge (6), and evidence-based reviews began to seep into the literature (7). A pediatric literature had also begun to develop independently, fostered by the evolution of adequate assessment techniques that allowed even preverbal children to report their discomfort. Pediatric pain services began to appear at major children's hospitals paralleling the development of such programs for adults. These multidisciplinary teams not only offered clinical care but also served as a catalyst for education and research in this area. The seminal work of Anand et al. (8–10), which is discussed later in this chapter, also cast an enormous shadow. In a series of papers, they demonstrated that premature infants undergoing surgery with minimal anesthesia, which was the standard practice of the era, exhibited a significant stress response to surgery that negatively influenced their morbidity and mortality. These studies were interpreted as "pain kills," in particular by parents whose children had undergone surgery with minimal anesthesia. Their public anguish coupled with the elegance of the research of Anand et al. culminated in a spate of editorials in the late 1980s in the major medical journals decrying the practice of minimal anesthesia during surgery in infants (11–14). These editorials stimulated broader interest in the general area of pediatric postoperative pain management, and the impact of this research was almost immediately evident. Asprey (15), working at the same institution as Eland et al., replicated her landmark 1974 study in 1991. She found that 968 doses of analgesics were administered to the same population who had had only 24 doses administered 16 years earlier. This study demonstrated that, at least in that institution, significant progress in the treatment of postoperative pain had been made. Other more recent studies (16,17) also point to an improvement in the management of postoperative pain in children. More morphine and less meperidine are used. Less noxious routes (intravenous and oral instead of intramuscular) and more scheduled analgesics are typical. The use of regional techniques for certain surgeries also assures more attention to pain control. Other broader surveys also suggest improvement in postoperative pain management, if only by comparison with other aspects of pediatric pain. Johnston and colleagues (17) surveyed children in every other bed at the Children's Hospital of Montreal admitted to the hospital for any reason. They found that children who had undergone surgery were three to four times more likely to have received opioid analgesics than nonsurgical patients, although similar proportions in both groups reported moderate to severe pain. Likewise, Broome and colleagues (18) surveyed residency directors regarding pain management in their institutions. Respondents endorsed a significant improvement in pain management in school-aged and adolescent children but continued to believe that pain assessment and management were suboptimal in younger children.

In summary, it appears that the predictable pain that occurs postoperatively for school-aged children is better treated than it was historically. Clearly, advances in the field have filtered down to clinical practice with more scheduled opioids, less noxious routes, and more regional anesthetic approaches. For children who are younger and for those who are discharged immediately from the hospital ("day case") (19), problems still persist.

Pain Management in the Newborn

Adequate management of pain in the newborn had been handicapped by a number of factors. These included the lack of basic information on the developmental neurobiology of nociception and the pharmacokinetics of analgesics in the newborn period coupled with the complexities of pain assessment in a population that is unable to communicate verbally (infant from *infans* meaning not speaking or voiceless). As a result, newborns were often treated as though they did not experience pain. In a 1986 paper on attitudes toward pain in children (20), 40% of a sample of pediatricians, surgeons, and family practitioners suggested that newborns did not experience pain in the first month of life. Such attitudes were clearly reflected in clinical practice.

It was typical before the 1990s for newborns to undergo surgery with minimal anesthesia, to receive essentially no postoperative pain management, and to be subjected to painful procedures such as lumbar punctures, circumcisions, chest tube insertions, and arterial blood gas sampling without consideration of their discomfort or potential long-term negative consequences. The thoughtful work of Anand et al., previously mentioned, and Fitzgerald et al. (21,22), who not only helped to define pain transmission in the neonate but also identified negative consequences from its undertreatment, had a dramatic impact on changing practices toward pain relief in the newborn period. Surveys of clinicians in the late 1980s in England by Purcell-Jones and colleagues (23) revealed that 80% of neonatologists believed that newborns experienced pain. More recently, McLaughlin et al. (24) found that

99% of nurses who work with newborns believe that they experience pain. Despite this recognition, however, only 50% of the sample believed that postoperative analgesia was necessary. Similarly, Tohill and McMorrow (25) in the mid-1990s found that 70% of neonatal intensive care nurses believed that analgesia was underprescribed by physicians in their units. Similar attitudes prevailed in the United States as identified in the survey by Broome et al. (18), who found that pediatric residency directors suggested that pain assessment and management were less than adequate in infants and toddlers.

This importance of adequate pain management during this vulnerable period has been reinforced by the emerging information on the negative consequences for the developing infant nervous system of repeated painful procedures as well as ventilation without adequate sedation.

In summary, then, it is clear that although change in attitude and practice is evident, pain in infants continues to be harder to assess and less likely to be adequately managed than pain in older children or adults.

Pain Associated with Chronic Disease

Pain is often, unfortunately, an aspect of chronic disease, either related to the disease itself or to its diagnosis and treatment. Chronic disease–associated pain has typically been poorly addressed for a variety of reasons. Because pain in chronic disease is less predicable and often cannot be anticipated in the same way that postoperative pain can, increased staff awareness and vigilance is necessary to address it. Adequate treatment also depends on the development of a trusting and continuous relationship between the child and his or her family and the medical staff. Unfortunately, in some chronic diseases such as sickle cell disease and human immunodeficiency virus/acquired immunodeficiency syndrome, there is often a socioeconomic and ethnic disparity between the provider and the patient, and as a result, such relationships are more difficult to establish.

There are multiple potential sources of pain associated with chronic disease. In some, such as cancer, the major sources of discomfort are the necessary frequent diagnostic procedures and treatment interventions. In multiple studies exploring the epidemiology of pain in childhood cancer (26–28), procedural pain and treatment-related pain dominated. In other chronic diseases, however, such as sickle cell disease, procedural pain does not play as prominent a role as does the pain associated the disease itself.

Although treatment of pain associated with chronic disease continues to be less adequate than that of postoperative pain, advances have been made on this front as well. The area of procedural pain has been one that has been well investigated and has witnessed a marked improvement in practice. Surveys performed in the mid-1980s suggest that most cancer centers did not routinely sedate children for painful procedures such as bone marrow aspirations or biopsies (29,30). One study (29) found that only 30% of centers routinely premedicated children undergoing bone marrow aspirations. The sedation regimen most commonly used was an intramuscularly administered concoction developed in the mid-1950s that consisted of an opioid and two phenothiazines [meperidine (Demerol), promethazine (Phenergan), chlorpromazine (Thorazine)] and had a relatively high incidence of side effects and caused prolonged sedation. By the early 1990s, 75% of children were sedated before bone marrow aspiration (A. Homan, personal communication, 1995) and opioid-benzodiazepine combinations, which were intravenously administered, achieved prominence.

Although there are no recent surveys of sedation practices in children with cancer available, anecdotal experience suggests that very few children undergo these procedures without adequate sedation.

Disease-related pain, however, which is less predictable, continues to be problematic. According to surveys by Ljungman et al. (31,32), 49% of children experience cancer-related pain, and 72% of physicians and nurses in Sweden who work with children with cancer believed that pain could be more effectively treated.

The pain associated with other chronic diseases continues to be problematic as well. Consensus statements on pain in sickle cell disease and human immunodeficiency virus/acquired immunodeficiency syndrome have dictated appropriate analgesic dosing guidelines and alternative pain-relieving strategies, but implementation is not uniform and socioeconomic factors continue to limit the effectiveness of pain management in children with these diseases.

It is evident that overall pain management has improved dramatically in children. New research has been translated to the bedside, especially for the predictable pain problems that require less vigilance and for which protocols can be devised and implemented. At this point, although there is certainly room for improvement, most children receive adequate postoperative pain control while in the hospital. Pain management in chronic diseases, postoperative pain associated with day case surgery, and in young preverbal children remain problem areas and require further research. We still have obstacles to overcome. As a result, children continue to suffer needlessly, despite the availability of adequate pain control for most clinical conditions.

CAUSES OF UNDERTREATMENT

Although many of the reasons for undertreatment have been previously mentioned, it is helpful to examine them methodically as they may offer insight into the elimination of residual barriers to the provision of adequate pain control in children.

Limited Clinical Information

In the past, even if one were interested in pain control in children, there were few easily accessible sources of information available. Rana (33) documented this fact when he surveyed ten leading pediatric textbooks in 1987 regarding their general and specific information on pain control and analgesic usage. Of 12,000 combined pages in those volumes, he identified only one page in total on pain management. This lack of information stemmed from multiple sources. Pain is an extremely personal and multifactorial phenomenon. Its complex nature with both physiologic and psychologic components transcends traditional disciplinary boundaries, and, as a result, it fell under the purview of no single discipline. The available knowledge base was divided among many fields including neurologists, anesthesiologists, nurses, psychologists, surgeons, pediatricians, and physical therapists who all deal with children in pain but traditionally had information limited to specific pain types and situations. Articles relating to pain were published therefore in discipline-specific journals that had a narrow readership and were not read by the provider community as a whole, which limited the access of the practicing community to pain information. The lack of information reflected a lack of research interest. Research in the area of pain management in children was quite difficult. Difficulties in pain assessment in children were handicapped by the lack of reliable and valid instruments. Ethical constraints limited pain research to the bedside and prevented the use of laboratory-induced pain, which is a mainstay of adult pain research. There were limited financial incentives for pharmaceutical companies to perform research on children because of the small market that they represent, and, as a result, a significant source of research funding was eliminated.

Persistence of Misinformation

The limited available research and limited access to information allowed the persistence of a number of myths regarding children's pain and its treatment (34). The most pervasive and most noxious of these myths suggested that because children's nervous systems are immature, children are unable to perceive and experience pain. This unfortunate misinterpretation of anatomic data and behavioral observation allowed care providers to rationalize inadequate pain treatment. Because young children's discomfort is different from that of adults, they reasoned that attention to painful procedures such as circumcision, suturing, and debridement and to postoperative and disease-related pain was of limited importance. As outlined in this volume, all available neuroanatomic, neurochemical, and behavioral data suggest that these theories are fallacious. Children clearly are capable of experiencing discomfort, have memory of it, and, as a result, may anticipate it from early on.

Attitudes That Denigrate Adequate Pain Management

The lack of interest in pain management was further fostered by a number of individual and societal attitudes about children and about pain. Unlike the misinformation previously described that could be countered by research, these attitudes represented sociocultural trends and could not be proven or disproven.

McGrath and Unruh (35) examined historic attitudes about pain in children. Their summary of child-rearing practices disputes the traditional notion that, until this century, the treatment of children was brutal and indifferent. Throughout all eras, humane and compassionate child rearing has existed alongside cold and inhumane practices. It is generally clear, however, that during eras when disease or circumstance have devalued individual life, concerns with the quality-of-life issues such as pain control and comfort are less likely to be emphasized. Given the relatively recent changes in childhood mortality in industrialized nations, one might predict that historically little importance was placed on child comfort when child survival was in question. In addition to these societal attitudes toward children, there are strong societal biases against pain expression. As described in detail elsewhere in this volume (Chapter 9), different cultures have different attitudes regarding the expression and response to pain. In some cultures, pain is thought to be a private phenomenon and endurance of pain is promoted as character building. Although it is hard to appreciate how much character is actually enhanced by enduring unanesthetized circumcision or the pain after surgery or during medical illness, this remains a point of view held by some individuals and groups. Pain also has spiritual and religious implications in some faiths. Several groups clearly believe that suffering itself has cleansing role. Obviously, for such individuals, discussion about pain treatment is essential before aggressive interventions are considered.

There are professional disciplinary biases that determine practice patterns. Attitudes and beliefs regarding pain in children were surveyed among a group of surgeons, pediatricians, and family practitioners (20). Pediatricians tended to assume that children experienced pain at a younger age than did the other medical specialists. They were also more likely to use analgesics to treat it. Interestingly, however, this survey suggested that individual disciplines were more likely to assign pain to the procedures of other disciplines and less likely to see their own as causing pain. For example, pediatricians tended to regard postoperative pain, which is traditionally controlled by surgeons, as a significant source of distress in children, whereas they associated less pain with the procedures for which they were responsible (e.g., lumbar punctures). However, surgeons tended to view postoperative pain as a less significant problem than lumbar punctures and other procedures that pediatricians perform. Both groups thought that circumcisions, which were primarily performed by obstetricians when this survey was completed, were major stresses for infants and required the use of anesthesia, which was rarely used at that time. In another study, the impact of patient age on analgesic prescribing was surveyed (36). When pediatricians, family practice physicians, and emergency department physicians were presented with a typical case of otitis media complicated by pain so severe that it limited the patient's sleep, as a group, they were less likely to prescribe opioid analgesics if patients were

2 years old than if they were 22 (22% versus 41%). Emergency department physicians were more generous than family physicians or pediatricians, prescribing opioids almost half the time, whereas the other groups prescribed opioids only 22% of the time.

Parental attitudes also handicap adequate pain treatment because, unlike adult patients, pain management in children is often dependent on the ability of parents to recognize and assess pain and on their decision to treat or not treat it (37–44). Parental attitudes concerning pain assessment and pain management may therefore result in inadequate pain treatment. This is particularly true in patients who are too young or too developmentally handicapped to report their pain. Even in hospitalized patients, most of the pain that children experience is managed by the patient's parents. Parents may fail to report pain either because they are unable to assess it or are afraid of the consequences of pain therapy. In one study, beliefs about addiction and the proper use of acetaminophen and other analgesics resulted in the failure to provide analgesia to children (43). In another, the belief that pain was useful or that repeated doses of analgesics lead to medication ineffectiveness resulted in the failure of the parents to provide or ask for prescribed analgesics to treat their child's pain (40).

Undertreatment of pain in children stemmed from multiple sources. The intricacies of conducting adequate research on pain in general and more specifically on children's pain created a situation in which there was limited available information. Such limitations in the database allowed some myths about pain to persist, which dampened enthusiasm to treat it adequately. Societal, personal, and disciplinary biases often denigrated the importance of providing adequate pain relief, and, as a result, children often suffered needlessly.

BREAKING THE CYCLE

This cycle persisted until the late 1980s when a number of changes occurred simultaneously that altered the course of pediatric pain management. Multidisciplinary pain teams became increasingly prominent and could address the transdisciplinary nature of pain and develop theoretical models that were not limited by discipline. Numerous investigators developed assessment techniques for children of all ages that allowed interventions to be more effectively measured. Data began to emerge that suggested that inadequate pain management was not only inhumane but had potentially long-term negative consequences for the child. The public awareness of this information created consumer pressure for more adequate pain control. Finally, legislation in the United States was passed that promoted pediatric drug development by lengthening the patent exclusivity for those companies that performed pediatric trials. This decreased some of the financial disincentive for doing this research in children. Slowly but surely, practice patterns began to change.

FOSTERING FURTHER CHANGE IN PRACTICE

Given the dramatic outpouring of new information on pediatric pain and the improved accessibility to this information, it remains striking that undertreatment of pain still persists in some settings and for some problems (45,46). Changing long-established practice patterns in the treatment of pain is quite complex, however. Although it seems intuitive that the mere presentation of this new information to clinicians who care for children would significantly alter their practice, this is not the case in pain management or in any other aspect of medicine. Eliciting behavioral change in medical providers, especially in the area of pain management, presents unique challenges (47). For many clinicians, the new information on pain management necessitates a conceptual shift in their practice. Practitioners must generally confront the possibility that in the past they may have caused unnecessary discomfort and begin to use approaches and medications that were previously available but rejected. As a result, passive educational approaches are less likely to incite change and need to be coupled with various other interventions. Alternative educational efforts, multidisciplinary approaches, and regulatory interventions all offer unique opportunities.

Educational Efforts

For health care professionals, various educational opportunities exist to acquire new information about pain and its management and to integrate it into practice. At the undergraduate professional level, the International Association of for the Study of Pain and several other professional organizations have developed specific curricular materials to be inserted in the educational programs of medical, dental, nursing, pharmacy, physical and occupational therapy, and psychology graduate programs. Unfortunately, given the vast amount of material and concomitant time limitations in the education of health care professionals, this information has not been inculcated into undergraduate education at the level that was anticipated and it is unlikely that it will be. At the postgraduate training level and in continuing professional education, however, lectures on pain management have become relatively commonplace. Most physician training programs, for example, incorporate pain management into their core lecture series, and lectures on pain management are frequently offered at professional educational meetings. Since 1988, the American Academy of Pediatrics has had a workshop or plenary talk concerning pediatric pain at every one of its national meetings. Such educational efforts represent a positive step. Unfortunately, studies have suggested that the efficacy of passive didactic teaching in promoting practice change is limited (48,49). The lack of immediate applicability, coupled with the potential for misinterpretation, has a role in diminishing the value of this traditional educational strategy. The information offered must be meaningful within the unique scope of the individual's practice. For example, Francke and colleagues (50) reported on an intensive course on pain documentation for Dutch nurses in five hospitals. The educational program consisted of 3 hours of didactic material weekly for 8 weeks. At the end of the course, although nurses clearly had more information, there was no significant change in their clinical behavior regarding the use of quantitative pain ratings. The investigators speculate that, at least in part, the behavioral change was hampered by the lack of response by physicians to their documentation efforts. As a result, these efforts were seen as meaningless, and even such an extensive course yielded no improved documentation of pain. The emerging literature suggests that continuing education that includes interactive interventions such as small group discussion and is problem based is more effective in changing health care provider behavior, at least in the short term (51,52).

The development of clinical practice guidelines and consensus statements by professional organizations have attempted to address the belief that accessible, detailed, and usable evidence based information might be more likely to change behaviors than didactic presentations. Many professional groups and nongovernmental agencies have developed consensus statements regarding pediatric pain (53,54). In general, these guidelines are developed by a group of experts who review available literature in a given area, evaluate the quality of the supporting evidence, and develop a consensus based on scientific credibility of the available information. Such guidelines allow clinicians easy access to a carefully developed algorithm that is endorsed by national authorities to address a clinical problem. Unfortunately, guideline creation, publication, and dissemination have not appeared to significantly alter clinical care (55–57). Clinicians often think that guidelines are too esoteric and have limited applicability to their own setting.

As a result, another educational strategy that has been attempted is the education of local "opinion leaders." Such individuals either volunteer or are designated as local experts who will be called about policy or clinical matters for a specific type of problem. In the pain arena, opinion leaders are often nurses, pharmacists, or physicians from any number of disciplines who function as local experts. The Wisconsin Cancer Pain Initiative developed a training program for opinion leaders, and there are preliminary data that such a program can have an impact on practice patterns (58).

In addition to professional education, education of health care consumers can create pressure on health care providers to change traditional practice patterns and emphasize more appropriate treatment of pain. In some communities, nongovernmental agencies and support groups have created billboards that inform consumers of their right to adequate pain management and urge them to request it. Articles in the lay press and parenting magazines also have been very effective at informing consumers about options regarding pain control. Significant consumer requests for change may create financial imperatives for institutions and cause them to critically evaluate their practices.

Multidisciplinary Approaches

Because of the multidisciplinary nature of pain, no one discipline historically has been responsible for its treatment. Over the past 15 years, multidisciplinary and institutional approaches have attempted to address this problem. Multidisciplinary pain services have evolved and often contain clinical, educational, and research arms. They are responsible for caring for the pain of patients with a particularly complex or unique set of pain problems (Chapter 27). For example, in many settings, the pain management of all children who have undergone surgery will be addressed by a pain service. Pain services often also function as clearinghouses for pain information and have ongoing teaching programs through which new advances in pain management are brought to the bedside. Many pain services also engage in active research, and it is through their efforts that many of the new advances in the treatment of pain have emerged. It is quite clear that there are benefits to the patients seen by the pain service. In a study of 23 hospitals, Miaskowski et al. (59) examined the pain control of almost 6,000 patients, half of whom had been on a pain service and half of whom had not. They found that the group who had been cared for by the pain service had decreased pain intensity, nausea, itching, and sedation, had less pain than they had expected, and were more likely to receive education regarding pain. As a group, they were discharged more rapidly than the group who had not been on a pain service.

Pain services do bring some disadvantages with them, however. Because pain information is often centralized to this group of experts, the knowledge base and practice patterns of practitioners who are not on the pain service may not improve and, in fact, may deteriorate. The pain service will often only care for a select group of patients (e.g., postoperative patients), and groups for which they are not responsible (e.g., ambulatory patients) may continue to receive less than optimal care. In addition, some institutions such as community hospitals are too small to support pain services. To address these concerns, pain committees or pain interest groups have emerged that assume some but not all the responsibilities of the pain service. These committees are not necessarily responsible for the ongoing management of patients in pain but instead function to increase awareness of pain, develop educational programs, and develop protocols that can be used by all practitioners to provide a uniform standard of care throughout the institution. In a number of settings, such committees have developed systemwide approaches to pain management that are sensitive to the available personnel and logistics at a given institution (60). These programs typically include the following components: bringing new information about the importance of pain management to all settings within the hospital, both inpatient and outpatient; development of educational materials for parents informing them of their child's right to adequate pain management and requesting their help in decision making;

the standardization of pain assessment and pain management protocols throughout the institution; ensuring the routine use of local anesthetics; and the incorporation of distraction and hypnotic techniques into care. These multidisciplinary efforts when incorporated into the fabric of an institution can have a significant impact on decreasing pain for all patients who enter its doors.

Regulatory Interventions

Efforts to change practice through education and multidisciplinary teams are far more effective if there are consequences for inadequate pain treatment. Regulatory activities to mandate change and monitor practice therefore have an important role in promoting changes in practice and attitude regarding pain.

At the local level, quality improvement programs are extremely important. Model programs to monitor adequacy of pain management have been developed by professional societies and can be modified to fit the unique aspects of an institution. Such programs identify gaps in documentation and treatment and alert practitioners to their variation from current standards of care. Although quality audits are critical, several investigators (61,62) have reported on failures of this type of monitoring. It is imperative that identification and documentation of persistent pain mandate a predictable response. Audits of one aspect of care (documentation) without evaluating the appropriateness of the response by medical staff does not reinforce subsequent documentation. Therefore, there must be a seamless link between documentation and intervention as well as the authority to mandate change if audits are to be meaningful.

At the level beyond the institution, laws that describe medical practice can have a positive or negative role in the appropriate treatment of pain. In the United States, for example, several state medical practice acts tend to discourage adequate pain treatment. The influence of the Drug Enforcement Agency in the United States and other similar agencies internationally has also had a dampening effect on the legitimate prescription of opioids for people in pain by highly scrutinizing physicians who prescribe larger than expected doses of opioids (63). Other programs that have focused on attempting to decrease diversion of opioids such as triplicate prescription have had the simultaneous effect of decreasing legitimate opioid use in patients who need them by making physicians and patients feel like criminals. The negative impact of such programs needs to be addressed.

Finally, at the national level, policies can be put in place that reinforce the importance of adequate pain treatment. In the United States, the Joint Commission on Accreditation of Healthcare Organizations has recently mandated that institutions must promote the availability of pain management as a patient right, demonstrate that pain assessment is documented in a predictable way, and have in place educational programs and protocols to ensure that clinicians have available information to adequately reduce pain in the hospital. Institutions that cannot demonstrate such policies run the risk of losing their accreditation. It is hoped that these new regulations will have a significant impact on the treatment of pain in hospitals in the United States and may well generalize to other countries that do not have such policies in place.

In summary, the treatment of pain has undergone enormous change over the past 20 years. Predictable pain problems are now more reliably treated. Gaps still remain, particularly in the pain associated with chronic disease and in infants and young children. Further change can occur not only through focused educational efforts but also through collaborative institutional approaches and regulatory reform.

WHY TREAT PAIN?

After elaborate discussion of the evolution of pain relief in childhood and ways to promote its improvement, the seminal question needs to be asked: "Why treat pain?" The editors of this book believe strongly that the treatment and alleviation of pain are a basic human right that exists regardless of age and mandates treatment for this reason alone. This philosophic belief, however, is buttressed by recent research that reveals that not only do children experience pain but that they are particularly vulnerable to the consequences of its undertreatment.

As is evident throughout this volume, the conventional "wisdom" that children neither respond to nor remember painful experiences to the same degree that adults do is simply untrue (64). Indeed, all the nerve pathways essential for the transmission and perception of pain are present and functioning by 24 weeks of gestation. Recent research in newborn animals has revealed that the failure to provide analgesia for pain results in "rewiring" the nerve pathways responsible for pain transmission in the dorsal horn of the spinal cord and results in increased pain perception for future painful insults (65–68). This confirms human newborn research in which the failure to provide anesthesia or analgesia for newborn circumcision resulted not only in short-term physiologic perturbations but also in longer term behavioral changes, particularly during immunization (69).

Many well-controlled clinical studies have documented the deleterious effects that acute pain and the failure to treat it have on patient outcome (70–74). Regardless of etiologic factors, tissue injury, ischemia, and destruction will cause the local release of prostaglandins, serotonin, bradykinin, norepinephrine, hydrogen ion, potassium ion, and substance P, a peripheral pain transmitter. These substances increase the responsiveness of the peripheral nociceptors to painful stimuli, thereby producing the sensation of pain and a systemic "fight-or-flight" response by evoking the release of systemic stress hormones. Additionally, these substances affect the mechanisms that have been identified as playing important roles in the altered central processing of afferent inputs that intensify pain and include expansion of receptive fields and a decrease in thresholds of dorsal horn neurons, enhancement of responses of dorsal horn neurons elicited by repetitive C-fiber stimuli (windup), and an increase in dynorphin gene expression (75–77).

Stress hormones, which include epinephrine, norepinephrine, glucagon, cortisol, aldosterone, thyroid-stimulating hormone, and growth hormone, promote the breakdown of body tissues and water retention. They increase blood glucose, prevent its utilization, and increase the body's metabolic rate. They increase heart rate, blood pressure, cardiac output, and the inotropic state of the heart and impair normal gastric and bowel function and motility. Finally, they also impair immune function and increase the ability of blood to clot. Indeed, in the perioperative period, untreated pain or pain that has not been prevented preemptively is associated with a state of immunosuppression, which has been shown in animal studies to underlie the promotion of tumor metastasis by surgery (78–80). Immunosuppressive effects of surgery have also been reported in children, and the degree of surgical trauma and the maturity of infants undergoing surgery have an influence on susceptibility to postoperative sepsis (81–84).

Therefore, the consequences of not treating or ameliorating acute pain can be catastrophic. The unchecked release of stress hormones by untreated pain may exacerbate injury, prevent wound healing, lead to infection, prolong hospitalization, and even lead to death. These deleterious effects are greatest in the sickest and frailest of patients. Indeed, a landmark study by Anand and Hickey (74) demonstrated that postoperative infant cardiac patients who were not treated with high-dose systemic opioids during the postoperative period actually experienced a significantly increased risk of death compared with infants who received high-dose opioids. Thus, the concept that a critically ill child or newborn is too sick to be treated with analgesics may need to be changed completely. Indeed, these patients may be too sick not to be treated.

There are also other reasons that mandate attention to pain control. In older children, adequate analgesia postoperatively may allow earlier ambulation and prevention of the atelectasis that often accompanies splinting and failure to breathe deeply. There are psychologic consequences to undertreatment as well, especially in children with chronic or life-threatening diseases. For example, the long-term negative consequences of inadequately treated procedure pain have become increasingly clear (85). Children who are subjected to painful procedures without adequate anesthesia develop increased anxiety about the next procedure and often will experience increased pain despite adequate analgesia compared with a group who had adequate pain control initially. Their anxiety about upcoming procedures may be so overwhelming that it can dominate and color their relationship with their health care providers and even with their parents.

For humanitarian, physiologic, and psychologic reasons, pain control should be considered an integral part of the compassionate medical care of children.

THE NATURE OF PAIN

Pain has been defined by the International Association for the Study of Pain as an unpleasant sensory and emotional experience associated with actual or potential tissue damage or described in terms of such damage (86). This definition emphasizes the essential bipartite nature of pain: the amount of pain that an individual experiences is the composite of physiologic and psychologic variables and is not predetermined by the extent of tissue damage. In fact, the term nociception refers to the noxious sensation per se, without regard to its emotional significance. Others have suggested that pain is whatever the individual experiencing it says that it is and it exists whenever he or she says that it does (87). These definitions have had an important impact on framing the concept of "pain" and have helped explain the variability of the pain experience. Clinicians have long recognized the lack of one-to-one correspondence between the extent of injury and the intensity of pain experience. Context, biologic variation, previous pain experience, and various psychologic factors modify the experience of pain. These concepts are discussed further in Chapter 6.

Although these definitions have been extremely valuable in the evolution of the understanding of pain, several concerns have recently been raised regarding their applicability to all situations. The International Association for the Study of Pain definition states that pain needs to be learned through experiences early in life. This would make it impossible for the newborn or very young child to experience pain. There is enormous human and laboratory evidence demonstrating that sensation of pain does not require prior experience (88–93). Likewise, the McCaffery definition implies a level of communication that may not exist for infants, preverbal children, mentally retarded, or comatose individuals. The distress expressed by human newborns to a heel stick is obvious to observers (94), even though infants cannot formally report it. This led Anand and Craig (88) to propose that the "behavioral alterations caused by pain are the infantile forms of self-report and are not 'surrogate measures' of pain." Clearly, infants, children, and the cognitively impaired do not have to know (or be able to express) the meaning of an experience to have the experience.

A major function of the pain experience is to signal ongoing or potential tissue injury. Patients who lack pain sensation, such as those with certain hereditary sensory neuropathies or with acquired neurologic injury, are at risk of harm because they do not adequately respond to impending tissue injury. Much of the subject of this book and the focus of pain treatment is on the forms of pain that are not protective and can be ameliorated without risk to the patient. The anatomy and physiology underlying pain sensation are outlined in Chapters 2 and 3 as well in other sources (95).

Acute pain is the term generally ascribed to pain associated with a brief episode of tissue injury or inflammation, such as that caused by surgery, burns, or a fracture. In most cases, the intensity of pain diminishes steadily with time over a period of days to weeks. There are exceptions to this monotonic improving trend, however. Analgesia may occur secondary to the stress of major trauma with increased pain the next day as the stress-induced analgesia subsides (96). Even though acute pain resolves, it produces long-lasting changes in both the peripheral and central nervous system that can be ameliorated with proper treatment (97,98).

The term *chronic persistent pain* generally describes conditions of persistent or nearly constant pain over a period of 3 months or longer. Chronic persistent pain is distinguished from recurrent pain for which repetitive painful episodes alternate with pain-free intervals. Pain may persist or recur for a variety of reasons. In a patient with arthritis or during a sickle-cell pain episode, pain recurs either from repeated joint inflammation (arthritis) or repeated episodes of vaso-occlusion with distal ischemia or infarction. These types of persistent pain are mechanistically similar to repetitive acute pain, although their persistence may generate psychologic sequelae and plastic changes in the central nervous system may follow repetitive injury or inflammation.

Pain may also persist not only secondary to ongoing injury but rather from persistent or abnormal excitability in the peripheral or central nervous system in the absence of ongoing tissue injury; this form of pain is known as neuropathic. In recent years in adults, it has been appreciated that neuropathic pains are common and underrecognized. Treatment of neuropathic pain poses unique problems. Neuropathic pain, not rare among children, is discussed in detail in Chapter 34.

A relatively small subgroup of patients experience persistent pain as a manifestation of psychiatric disease, what was formerly known as psychogenic pain or hypochondriasis and now is known as somatoform pain disorder. As discussed in Chapters 15 and 16, this is relatively uncommon; a diagnosis of somatoform pain disorder should not be invoked simply as a diagnosis of exclusion but rather based on positive psychiatric findings.

Although some children and adolescents experience chronic persistent pain of great severity, recurrent pain is much more common. Common types of recurrent pain, including headache, abdominal pain, chest pain, and limb pains, may occur in 5% to 10% of unselected school children and are reviewed in Chapters 32, 39, 40, and 41. A considerable number of children with recurrent pains has neither evidence of psychopathology nor signs of a specific organic disease. For example, most patients with recurrent abdominal pain fall into this intermediate category. It is important to reinforce that these patients are not necessarily psychologically distinct from control populations. For some patients with chronic pain, reinforcement of a sick or disabled role appears to amplify or perpetuate both pain behaviors and the intensity of the pain experience. Fordyce (99) emphasized viewing certain aspects of chronic pain as learned behavior.

Chronic pain is a major economic and social problem among adults. In the United States, estimates are that low back pain alone produces economic losses in excess of 80 billion dollars annually (100). Although chronic and recurrent pain in children produces less direct economic loss, it exacts an enormous toll in suffering and produces school absenteeism, a disability syndrome with some analogies to adult work avoidance (see Chapter 45) (101). It is an important topic of future research to determine whether appropriate interventions in children and adolescents with chronic pain and disability will diminish the likelihood of their becoming disabled or dysfunctional adults.

SUMMARY

Pain is a complex, multidimensional phenomenon. Its historic undertreatment in children is a reflection of its nature and of attitudes and values that surround both pain and children. Unfortunately, this lack of treatment has allowed the persistence of unnecessary suffering in children, particularly in those most vulnerable (infants and chronically and critically ill children) and is responsible for short- and long-term changes in their physiologic and psychologic functioning.

Our goal for this book is to provide children's health care professionals with the tools to comfortably assess and manage the pain that children might encounter in essentially any situation. In the process, we hope to catalog available information about children's pain, dispel the remaining myths about the child's experience of pain, provide a foundation for future research, and change attitudes that foster undertreatment. It continues to be our hope that once this information is easily accessible, compassion, which has always been a hallmark of those who care for ill children, and not misinformation will dictate the course of treatment.

REFERENCES

1. Swafford L, Allen D. Relief in pediatric patients. *Med Clin North Am* 1968;52:131–136.
2. Eland JM. Children's communication of pain (thesis). Iowa City, IA: University of Iowa, 1974.
3. Mather L, Mackie J. The incidence of postoperative pain in children. *Pain* 1983;15:271–282.
4. Beyer JE, DeGood DE, Ashley LC, et al. Patterns of postoperative analgesic use with adults and children following cardiac surgery. *Pain* 1983;17:71–81.
5. Schechter NL, Allen DA, Hanson K. Status of pediatric pain control: a comparison of hospital analgesic usage in children and adults. *Pediatrics* 1986;77: 11–15.
6. Schechter NL, Altman A, Weisman SJ, eds. Report of the consensus conference on the management of pain in childhood cancer. *Pediatrics* 1990;86[Suppl]: 813–834.
7. Acute Pain Management Guideline. *Acute pain management: operative or medical procedures and trauma. Clinical practice guideline* (publication 92-0032). Rockville, MD: Agency for Health Care Policy and Research, Public Health Service, U.S. Department of Health and Human Services, 1992.
8. Anand KJS, Sippell WG, Aynsley Green A. Randomized trial of fentanyl anesthesia in preterm babies undergoing surgery: effects on stress response. *Lancet* 1987;8524:62–67.
9. Anand KJS, Aynsley Green A. Measuring the severity of surgical stress in newborn infants. *J Pediatr Surg* 1988;23:297–305
10. Anand KJ, Hansen DD, Hickey PR. Hormonal metabolic stress response in neonates undergoing cardiac surgery. *Anesthesiology* 1990;73:661–670.
11. Berry FA, Gregory GA. Do premature infants require anesthesia for surgery? *Anesthesiology* 1987;67: 291–293.
12. Booker PD. Postoperative analgesia for neonates. *Anesthesia* 1987;42:343–345.
13. Fletcher AB. Pain in the neonate. *N Engl J Med* 1987;317:1347–1348.
14. Hatch DJ. Analgesia in the neonate. *BMJ* 1987;294: 920.
15. Asprey JR. Postoperative analgesic prescription and administration in a pediatric population. *J Pediatr Nurs* 1994;9:150–157.
16. Tesler MD, Wilkie DJ, Holzemer WL, et al. Postoperative analgesics for children and adolescents: prescription and administration. *J Pain Symptom Manage* 1994;9:85–94.
17. Johnston CC, Abbott FV, Gray-Donald K, et al. A survey of pain in hospitalized patients aged 4–14 years. *Clin J Pain* 1992;8:154–163.
18. Broome ME, Richtsmeier A, Maikler V, et al. Pediatric pain practices: a national survey of health professionals. *J Pain Symptom Manage* 1996;11:312–320.
19. Nikanne E, Kokki H, Tuovinen K. Postoperative pain after adenoidectomy in children. *Br J Anaesth* 1999; 82:886–889.
20. Schechter NL, Allen DA. Physicians' attitudes towards pain in children. *J Dev Behav Pediatr* 1986;7:350–354.
21. Fitzgerald M, Millard C, McIntosh N. Cutaneous hypersensitivity following peripheral tissue damage in newborn infants and its reversal with topical anaesthesia. *Pain* 1989;39:31–36.
22. Reynolds M, Fitzgerald M. Longterm sensory hyperinnervation following neonatal skin wounds. *J Comp Neurol* 1995;358:487–498.
23. Purcell-Jones G, Dorman F, Sumner E. Paediatric anaesthetists' perception of neonatal pain and infant pain. *Pain* 1988;33:181–187.
24. McLaughlin CR, Hull JG, Edwards WH, et al. Neonatal pain: a comprehensive survey of attitudes and practices. *J Pain Symptom Manage* 1993;8:7–16.
25. Tohill J, McMorrow O. Pain relief in neonatal intensive care. *Lancet* 1996;336:569.
26. Miser AW, Dothage JA, Wesley RA, et al. The prevalence of pain in a pediatric and young adult cancer population. *Pain* 1987;29:73–83.
27. McGrath PJ, Hsu E, Cappelli M, et al. Pain from pediatric cancer: a survey of an outpatient oncology clinic. *J Psychosoc Oncol* 1990;8:109–124.
28. Ljungman G, Kreuger A, Gordh T, et al. Treatment of pain in pediatric oncology: a Swedish nationwide survey. *Pain* 1996:68:385–394.
29. Bernstein B, Schechter NL, Hickman T, et al. Premedication for painful procedures in children: a national survey. *J Pain Symptom Manage* 1991;6:190(abst).
30. Hockenberry MJ, Bologna-Vaughn S. Preparation for intrusive procedures using non-invasive techniques in children with cancer: state of the art vs. new trends. *Cancer Nurs* 1985:8:97–102.
31. Ljungman G, Gordh T, Sorensen S, et al. Pain in pediatric oncology: interviews with children, adolescents and their parents. *Acta Paediatr* 1999;88:623–630.
32. Ljungman G, Gordh T, Sorensen S, et al. Pain variations during cancer treatment in children: a descriptive study. *Pediatr Hematol Oncol* 2000:17:211–221.
33. Rana S. Pain: a subject ignored [Letter]. *Pediatrics* 1987;79:309–310.
34. Eland JM, Anderson JE. The experience of pain in children. In: Jacox A, ed. *Pain: a source book for nurses and other health professionals*. Boston: Little, Brown, 1977.
35. McGrath PJ, Unruh A. *Pain children and adolescents*. Amsterdam: Elsevier, 1987.

36. Hauswald M, Anison C. Prescribing analgesics: the effect of patient age and physician specialty. *Pediatr Emerg Care* 1997;13:262–263.
37. Reid GJ, Hebb JP, McGrath PJ, et al. Cues parents use to assess postoperative pain in their children. *Clin J Pain* 1995;11:229–235.
38. McGrath PJ, Finley GA. Attitudes and beliefs about medication and pain management in children. *J Palliat Care* 1996;12:46–50.
39. Gedaly-Duff V, Ziebarth D. Mothers' management of adenoid-tonsillectomy pain in 4- to 8- year-olds: a preliminary study. *Pain* 1994;57:293–299.
40. Finley GA, McGrath PJ, Forward SP, et al. Parents' management of children's pain following 'minor' surgery. *Pain* 1996;64:83–87.
41. Sutters KA, Miaskowski C. Inadequate pain management and associated morbidity in children at home after tonsillectomy. *J Pediatr Nurs* 1997;12: 178–185.
42. Romsing J, Walther-Larsen S. Postoperative pain in children: a survey of parents' expectations and perceptions of their children's experiences. *Paediatr Anaesth* 1996;6:215–218.
43. Forward SP, Brown TL, McGrath PJ. Mothers' attitudes and behavior toward medicating children's pain. *Pain* 1996;67:469–474.
44. Greenberg RS, Billett C, Zahurak M, et al. Videotape increases parental knowledge about pediatric pain management. *Anesth Analg* 1999;89:899–903.
45. Hamers JPH, Abu-Saad HH, van den Hout MA, et al. Are children given insufficient pain relieving medication postoperatively. *J Adv Nurs* 1998;27:37–44.
46. Clarke EB, French B, Bilodeau ML, et al. Pain management knowledge, attitudes, and clinical practice: the impact of nurses characteristics and education. *J Pain Symptom Manage* 1996;11:18–31.
47. Bauchner H, Simpson L, Chessare J. Changing physician behaviour. *Arch Dis Child* 2001;84:459–462.
48. Davis D, Thomson MA, Oxman A, et al. Changing physician performance: a systematic review of the effect of continuing medical education strategies. *JAMA* 1995;274:700–705.
49. Davis D, Thomson MA, Oxman AD, et al. Evidence for the effectiveness of CME: a review of 50 randomized controlled trials. *JAMA* 1992;268:1111–1117.
50. Francke AL, Luiken JB, deSchepper AM, et al. Effects of a continuing education program on nurses pain assessment practices. *J Pain Symptom Manage* 1997;13: 90–97.
51. David TJ, Patel L. Adult learning theory, problem based learning and paediatrics. *Arch Dis Child* 1995; 73:357–363.
52. Ozuah P, Curtis J, Stein RE. Impact of problem based learning on residents self-directed learning. *Arch Pediatr Adolesc Med* 2001;155:669–672.
53. American Pain Society. *Principles of analgesic use in the treatment of acute pain and chronic cancer pain*. Skokie, IL: American Pain Society, 1989.
54. World Health Organization Expert Committee. *Cancer pain relief and palliative care*. Geneva: World Health Organization, 1990.
55. Audet A-M, Greenfield S, Field M. Medical practice guidelines: current activities and future directions. *Ann Intern Med* 1990;113:709–714.
56. Lomas J, Anderson GM, Dominick-Pierre K, et al. Do practice guidelines guide practice? *N Engl J Med* 1989;321:1306–1311.
57. Devine EC, Bevsek SA, Brubakken K, et al. AHCPR clinical practice guideline on surgical pain management: adoption and outcomes. *Res Nurs Health* 1999;22:119–130.
58. Weissman DE, Dahl HL, Beasley JW. The cancer pain role model program of the Wisconsin Cancer Pain Initiative. *J Pain Symptom Manage* 1993;8:29–35.
59. Miaskowski C, Crews J, Ready LB, et al. Anesthesia-based pain services improve the quality of postoperative pain management. *Pain* 1999;80:23–29.
60. Schechter NL, Sullivan C, Pachter L, et al. The ouchless place: no pain, children's gain. *Pediatrics* 1997; 99:890–894.
61. Joyce BD, Keck JF, Gerkensmeyer JE. Evaluating the implementation of a pain management flow sheet. *J Pediatr Nurs* 1999;14:304–312.
62. Miaskowski C, Donovan M. Implementation of the American Pain Society Quality Assurance Standards for Relief of Acute and Cancer Pain in oncology nursing practice. *Oncol Nurs Forum* 1992;19:411–415.
63. Morrison RS, Wallenstein C, Natale DK, et al. "We don't carry that"—failure of pharmacies in predominantly nonwhite neighborhoods to stock opioids. *N Engl J Med* 2000;342:1023–1026.
64. Fitzgerald M. Neurobiology of fetal and neonatal pain. In: Wall PD, Melzack R, eds. *Textbook of pain*. Edinburgh: Churchill-Livingstone, 1994:153–164.
65. Coggeshall RE, Jennings EA, Fitzgerald M. Evidence that large myelinated primary afferent fibers make synaptic contacts in lamina II of neonatal rats. *Brain Res Dev Brain Res* 1996;92:81–90.
66. Fitzgerald M, Shaw A, MacIntosh N. Postnatal development of the cutaneous flexor reflex: comparative study of preterm infants and newborn rat pups. *Dev Med Child Neurol* 1988;30:520–526.
67. Porter FL, Grunau RE, Anand KJ. Long-term effects of pain in infants. *J Dev Behav Pediatr* 1999;20: 253–261.
68. Porter FL, Wolf CM, Miller JP. Procedural pain in newborn infants: the influence of intensity and development. *Pediatrics* 1999;104:e13.
69. Taddio A, Katz J, Ilersich AL, et al. Effect of neonatal circumcision on pain response during subsequent routine vaccination. *Lancet* 1997;349:599–603.
70. McQuay HJ. Pre-emptive analgesia: a systematic review of clinical studies. *Ann Med* 1995;27:249–256.
71. Kissin I. Preemptive analgesia. Why its effect is not always obvious. *Anesthesiology* 1996;84:1015–1019.
72. Kehlet H. Effect of pain relief on the surgical stress response. *Reg Anesth* 1996;21[Suppl 6]:35–37.
73. Rockemann MG, Seeling W, Bischof C, et al. Prophylactic use of epidural mepivacaine/morphine, systemic diclofenac, and metamizole reduces postoperative morphine consumption after major abdominal surgery. *Anesthesiology* 1996;84:1027–1034.
74. Anand KJ, Hickey PR. Halothane-morphine compared with high-dose sufentanil for anesthesia and postoperative analgesia in neonatal cardiac surgery. *N Engl J Med* 1992;326:1–9.
75. Mannion RJ, Woolf CJ. Pain mechanisms and management: a central perspective. *Clin J Pain* 2000;16[Suppl 3]:S144–S156.
76. Woolf CJ, Mannion RJ. Neuropathic pain: aetiology,

symptoms, mechanisms, and management. *Lancet* 1999;353:1959–1964.
77. Woolf CJ, Chong MS. Preemptive analgesia—treating postoperative pain by preventing the establishment of central sensitization. *Anesth Analg* 1993;77:362–379.
78. Bar-Yosef S, Melamed R, Page GG, et al. Attenuation of the tumor-promoting effect of surgery by spinal blockade in rats. *Anesthesiology* 2001;94:1066–1073.
79. Page GG, Ben Eliyahu S. The immune-suppressive nature of pain. *Semin Oncol Nurs* 1997;13:10–15.
80. Page GG, Ben Eliyahu S, Yirmiya R, et al. Morphine attenuates surgery-induced enhancement of metastatic colonization in rats. *Pain* 1993;54:21–28.
81. Mattila-Vuori A, Salo M, Iisalo E, et al. Local and systemic immune response to surgery under balanced anaesthesia in children. *Paediatr Anaesth* 2000;10: 381–388.
82. Salo M. Effects of anaesthesia and surgery on the immune response. *Acta Anaesthesiol Scand* 1992;36: 201–220.
83. Kurz R, Pfeiffer KP, Sauer H. Immunologic status in infants and children following surgery. *Infection* 1983;11:104–113.
84. Madden NP, Levinsky RJ, Bayston R, et al. Surgery, sepsis, and nonspecific immune function in neonates. *J Pediatr Surg* 1989;24:562–566.
85. Weisman SJ, Bernstein B, Schechter NL. The consequences of inadequate analgesia during painful procedures in children. *Arch Pediatr Adolesc Med* 1998;152: 147–149.
86. International Association for the Study of Pain, Subcommittee on Taxonomy. Pain terms: a list with definitions and notes on usage. *Pain* 1979;6:249–252.
87. McCaffery M, Beebe A. *Pain: clinical manual for nursing practice*. St. Louis: Mosby, 1989.
88. Anand KJ, Craig KD. New perspectives on the definition of pain [Editorial]. *Pain* 1996;67:3–6; discussion 209–211.
89. Craig KD, Whitfield MF, Grunau RV, et al. Pain in the preterm neonate: behavioural and physiological indices [published erratum appears in *Pain* 1993;54: 111]. *Pain* 1993;52:287–299.
90. Grunau RV, Johnston CC, Craig KD. Neonatal facial and cry responses to invasive and non-invasive procedures. *Pain* 1990;42:295–305.
91. Johnston CC, Stevens B, Craig KD, et al. Developmental changes in pain expression in premature, full-term, two- and four-month-old infants. *Pain* 1993;52: 201–208.
92. Andrews K, Fitzgerald M. Biological barriers to paediatric pain management. *Clin J Pain* 1997;13: 138–143.
93. Hadjistavropoulos HD, Craig KD, Grunau RV, et al. Judging pain in newborns: facial and cry determinants. *J Pediatr Psychol* 1994;19:485–491.
94. Wall PD, Melzack R. *Textbook of pain*, 4th ed. New York: Churchill-Livingstone, 1999.
95. Loeser JD, Butler SH, Chapman CR, et al., eds. *Bonica's management of pain*, 3rd ed. Philadelphia: Lippincott Williams & Wilkins, 2001.
96. Beecher HK. Relationship of significance to wound to the pain experience. *JAMA* 1956;161:1609–1613.
97. Wall PD. The prevention of postoperative pain. *Pain* 1988;33:289–290.
98. Woolf CJ. Evidence for a central component of post-injury pain hypersensitivity. *Nature* 1983;306: 686–688.
99. Fordyce WE. Learned pain: pain as a behavior. In: Loeser JD, Butler SH, Chapman CR, et al., eds. *Bonica's management of pain*, 3rd ed. Philadelphia: Lippincott Williams & Wilkins, 2001:478–482.
100. Bigos SJ, Muller G. Primary care approach to acute and chronic back problem: definitions and care. In: Loeser JD, Butler SH, Chapman CR, et al., eds. *Bonica's management of pain*, 3rd ed. Philadelphia: Lippincott Williams & Wilkins, 2001.
101. Bursch B, Walco GA, Zeltzer L. Clinical assessment and management of chronic pain and pain associated disability syndrome. *J Dev Behav Pediatr* 1998;19: 45–53.

2

The Neurobiologic Basis of Pediatric Pain

Maria Fitzgerald and Richard F. Howard

The past 30 years have brought a revolution in pain research using powerful new techniques in cellular, molecular, and systems neuroscience. As a result, our understanding of peripheral transduction, central plasticity, and cortical activation leading to the perception of pain has considerably increased, and research into these underlying mechanisms is now a focus of many laboratories around the world. Yet with every advance, the gulf between the basic science and the experience of the patient with pain becomes wider, and the need to make a bridge between pain mechanisms and pain management becomes stronger (1).

Nowhere is this more evident than in the treatment of pediatric pain. The developing nervous system and its functional and structural plasticity lie at the heart of sensory and pain processing in the infant and child. Appreciation of the emerging physiologic and pharmacologic processes in the maturing nervous system is the key to effective pain measurement and management in children. Despite this, contemporary pediatric pain management is often empirical, based on tradition and routine with little awareness of the increasing scientific knowledge in the field.

In this chapter, we attempt to bridge this gap by focusing on four clinical situations in which a child experiences pain. In each, we selectively review current aspects of the cellular and developmental biology underlying the pain and discuss how this knowledge may relate to pediatric pain and its management. Other background material may be obtained from several earlier reviews in this field (2,3).

PAIN ASSOCIATED WITH A SINGLE BRIEF PROCEDURE

Many diagnostic and therapeutic interventions involve brief but painful procedures that can cause considerable distress. The pain and dread of needles are frequently cited as an important cause of suffering in children undergoing medical care (4). Typical examples include venipuncture, arterial puncture, heel or finger lance, lumbar puncture, and vaccination. Venipuncture to draw blood for diagnostic testing is common practice at all ages, e.g., most newborns undergo diagnostic screening for a number of important inherited metabolic and endocrine disorders such as phenylketonuria and hypothyroidism. In a normal infant, a single venipuncture, although painful at the time, would not be expected to induce significant local inflammation or ongoing pain.

The Pain Response

The application of the needle or lance triggers an immediate pain response, which is a strong warning of injury that can be observed in the youngest infant (Fig. 2.1). The response has been measured as crying, changes in facial expression, heart rate, respiration, sweating, body movement, hormonal responses (5), and flexion reflex responses (6,7). Spinal reflex responses to mechanical skin stimulation are exaggerated in young infants compared with those of the adult, with lower thresholds and more synchronized, longer lasting reflex muscle contractions. Thresholds for withdrawal from heat stimuli are also lower in younger animals (8–10). The exaggerated

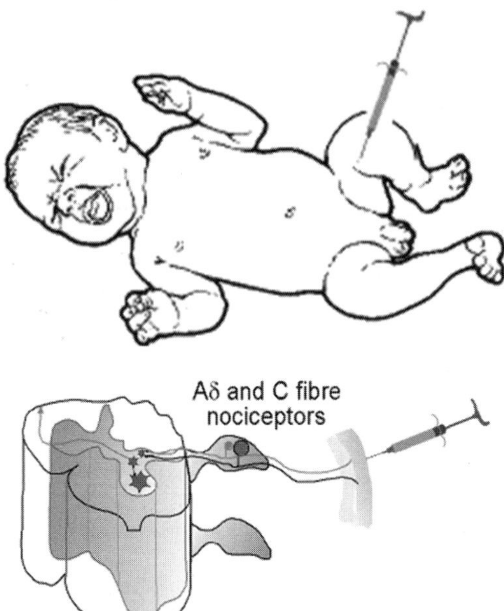

FIG. 2.1. Pain associated with a single brief noxious procedure is nociception. Peripheral Aδ- and C-fiber nociceptors in the skin activate central pathways that produce nociceptive reflexes at both the spinal and brainstem levels and transmit information to higher cortical centers.

spinal responses are in contrast to the facial expression response, which is weaker in younger infants and increases with postnatal age (11,12). This may reflect a slower maturation of facial motor responses or onset of the affective or emotional response to pain compared with the sensory motor response. Little is known about the maturation of central pain processes in the brainstem, thalamus, and cortex and their contribution to these responses (see below).

Activation of Nociceptors

The needle or lance penetrates the skin and activates sensory nerve terminals. In addition to low threshold Aβ fibers that are sensitive to mechanical skin stimulation, nociceptive Aδ and C fibers are activated. Nociceptors are those primary afferents that can be activated by harmful or potentially harmful stimuli. The transduction of these stimuli into neural signals is the beginning of a sequence of events that finally initiate pain sensation. Among the many chemical and physical stimuli that excite nociceptors, low extracellular pH, noxious heat, and capsaicin (the active ingredient of chili peppers) have attracted particular interest because of their persistent and specific activation of these receptors. The recent molecular cloning of membrane receptors for capsaicin, protons, and heat has greatly advanced our knowledge of nociceptive signal transduction (13,14). As yet, very little is known about the developmental regulation of these receptors (15), but in the following sections we review relevant information on the general anatomic and physiologic development of nociceptors.

The Development of Nociceptors

Sensory nerve fibers terminating in nociceptive or low-threshold mechanoreceptive endings grow out from the dorsal root ganglion prenatally and innervate the skin in an organized proximodistal manner. By birth in the rat and by the second trimester in the human, they have reached the most distal skin of the foot (16,17). The large-diameter A cells are born first, and their nerve fibers reach the skin and form the initial cutaneous nerve plexus before the C fibers, which follow soon after (18). C nociceptors fall into two groups: those that contain neuropeptides (e.g., substance P (SP) and calcitonin gene–related peptide) and express the neurotrophin receptor for nerve growth factor (NGF) trkA (see below) and those that do not express any of the above but bind the lectin IB4 and express receptors for the neurotrophin GDNF. The functional roles of these two groups of nociceptors are not clear, but it is of particular interest that the latter IB4+ve group only mature postnatally in the rat, so that in early life, most C nociceptors express trkA (19). The onset of production of neuropeptides by these neurons appears to be triggered by peripheral innervation (18).

The process of terminal elaboration of sensory nerves in the skin is a prolonged one, but all the main functional cutaneous afferent types found in the adult rat hindlimb can be found at birth, maturity depending on receptor type (20,21). C-fiber polymodal nociceptors, responding to mechanical, thermal, and chemical noxious stimuli, are fully mature in their thresholds, pattern, and frequency of firing at birth. High-threshold Aδ mechanoreceptors, responding maximally to noxious mechanical rather than chemical and thermal stimulation, can also be distinguished, but their peak firing frequencies are lower than in adults. Low-threshold Aβ mechanoreceptors responding to touch or brush with brief, rapidly adapting bursts of spikes are, relatively, the most immature at birth, with low frequencies of firing and amplitude of response.

The Role of Neurotrophins in Nociceptor Development

The final number of sensory afferents responding to the needle prick and their pattern and amplitude of the response depends on the level of neurotrophic factors in the skin or other target tissue (22,23). While sensory neurons are being born and innervating the skin, they are also dying as a result of programmed cell death (24), and their survival depends on access to neurotrophic factors. NGF produced in the skin and other target cells, for example, is critically important for the survival of trkA-expressing, peptidergic C nociceptor neurons (25). Humans who have deletions, mutations, or aberrations of the gene encoding the trkA receptor have a rare sensory and autonomic neuropathy with congenital insensitivity to pain (26). In addition, neurotrophic factors play an important role in the development of normal receptor properties independent of their effect on survival. NGF and neurotrophin 3 regulate the differentiation of myelinated and C-fiber nociceptors and their mechanical thresholds and brain-derived neurotrophic factor (BDNF) regulates mechanoreceptor properties (27). Last, neurotrophin levels determine the innervation density of the skin, and access to excess NGF and BDNF leads to skin hyperinnervation (28,29).

Activation of Central Nociceptive Pathways

The needle or lance may activate nociceptors, but the production of a sensory response and ultimately perception will depend critically on their ability to excite neurons within the central nervous system (CNS). The first important central synapses are in the spinal cord and effective postsynaptic dorsal horn cell activation requires considerable summation and integration of the primary nociceptor and mechanoreceptor input. This only occurs if the afferent terminals have formed appropriate synapses in the correct spinal cord areas. The activation of afferent A and C fibers leads to rapid excitation of dorsal horn cells by release of the neurotransmitter glutamate acting on postsynaptic receptors. The activity of many dorsal horn cells converges onto flexor motor neurons in the ventral horn of the spinal cord, which, in turn, result in withdrawal of the limb. In addition, these dorsal horn cells send information up the long projecting axons in the ascending tracts of the spinal cord to nuclei within the brainstem and thalamus and higher brain centers. Effective responses to the needle prick therefore depend on the developmental stage of all these components.

Development of the Spinal Cord: Structural Aspects

Spinal cord neurogenesis takes place in a ventrodorsal direction beginning with motor neurons and ending with the local interneurons in the superficial dorsal horn or substantia gelatinosa (SG) (30,31). In the rat, both A and C fibers have grown into the spinal cord by birth, but C-fiber terminals are very immature and many C-fiber specific chemical markers are not apparent in the spinal cord until the perinatal period (18). C-type afferent terminals within synaptic glomeruli are not observed at electron microscope level until P5

(32). Synaptogenesis in the rat dorsal horn is at its maximum in the first postnatal weeks. The pattern is similar in the primate, but maturation occurs earlier so that by embryonic day 40 (of a 165-day gestation), all types of primary afferent terminal and postsynaptic specialization can be observed in the SG (33). The growth of both A and C fibers into the rat cord is somatotopically precise (34,35), such that the pattern of skin innervation by individual peripheral nerves is preserved as an interlocking pattern of terminal fields within the spinal cord. This is not true of the laminar organization, however. Whereas in the adult, Aβ afferents are restricted to laminae III and IV, in the fetus and neonate, their terminals extend dorsally right up into laminae II and I to reach the surface of the gray matter. This is followed by a gradual withdrawal from the superficial laminae over the first 3 postnatal weeks (36). C fibers, conversely, grow specifically to laminae I and II (37), and so for a considerable postnatal period, these laminae are occupied by both A- and C-fiber terminals. During their occupation of the SG, A-fiber terminals can be seen to form synaptic connections at the electron microscope level (38). C fibers play an important role in the withdrawal of A fibers from laminae I and II because administration of neonatal capsaicin, which destroys most C fibers, leaves A-fiber terminals located more superficially than in normal animals (39,40).

Development of Spinal Cord: Functional Aspects

In the newborn rat, the synaptic linkage between afferents and dorsal horn cells is still weak, and electrical stimulation often evokes only a few spikes at long and variable latencies (35,41). Despite this, the needle puncture produces intense afferent activation of dorsal horn cells that outlasts the stimulus and leads to the rapid, transient central response. In immature rats, excitatory postsynaptic currents can be elicited by Aβ afferents in the majority of SG neurons, whereas in adults, this is only possible with Aδ or C afferents (42). Expression of c-fos in SG neurons, which in adults is evoked by noxious and Aδ and C fiber inputs only, can also be evoked by innocuous inputs and A-fiber activation in the newborn (43). Furthermore, receptive fields of the dorsal horn cells are larger in the newborn, occupying a relatively larger area of the body surface and gradually diminish over the first 2 postnatal weeks (35,44) (Fig. 2.2). The large receptive fields and dominant A-fiber input in-

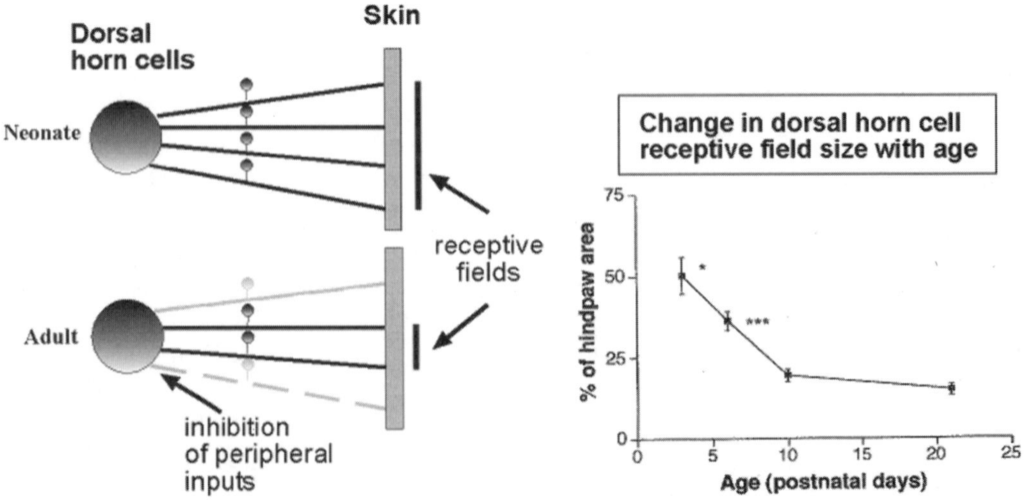

FIG. 2.2. Dorsal horn sensory neuron receptive fields are larger in young rat pups. This increases the chance of activation of these cells by peripheral stimulation and thus increases central nervous system excitability.

crease the chance of central cells being excited by peripheral sensory simulation and act to increase the sensitivity of infant sensory reflexes.

The postnatal maturation of synaptic connections between afferent C fibers and SG cells takes place over a prolonged period. C-fiber activation is unable to evoke spike activity in the rat spinal cord until the second postnatal week and is unlikely to be involved in the immediate reaction to the heel stick in young infants (44–46). C fibers are apparently able to produce subthreshold activation of central neurons before that time (47) and are therefore likely to trigger the more persistent responses described in the following sections.

Development of Fast Transmitter Responses in the Spinal Cord

The rapid excitation of dorsal horn cells by the venipuncture is the result of release of the neurotransmitter glutamate from the activated afferent fibers acting on postsynaptic receptors. The pattern of postsynaptic activity produced in the dorsal horn neurons codes the onset, duration, intensity, and location of the stimulus. Fast excitatory synaptic transmission in adult pain pathways is mediated by glutamate acting on amino-3-hydroxy-5-methyl-4-isoxazoleproprionic acid (AMPA) and kainate ligand gated ion channels (48). AMPA and kainate receptors are expressed early in the developing spinal cord and are evident in the first trimester of human development (49). Expression in the neonatal rat spinal cord shows a wider distribution than in the adult and decreases over the first postnatal 3 weeks (50,51). The glutamate receptor subunits GluR1, 2, and 4 are generally more abundant in the neonatal spinal cord compared with the adult spinal cord, although the ratio of GluR2 to GluR1, 3, and 4 is lower. Different combinations of subunits affect desensitization, ionic permeability, and current/voltage relationships. There are also changes in the distribution of the flip-flop variants with postnatal age; the flip variants are generally more sensitive to agonists than the flop, resulting in higher levels of depolarization from glutamate release (52). The implications of these findings with regard to immature sensory processing the spinal cord are not yet known.

Development of Activity in Higher Brain Centers

The brief experience of unpleasantness that accompanies the venipuncture depends on activity in higher brain centers. The sensory, autonomic, arousal, and motor responses to pain all contribute to the unpleasantness, but all in relation to the meanings of the pain and the context in which it presents itself (53). The emotions evoked, such as fear and distress, relate to the understanding of the current situation and the short-term future, which is inevitably limited in small infants. Several ascending pathways and brain regions are activated by noxious inputs, but there is considerable controversy as to the extent and degree of activation of these areas in the adult, and no information is available in infants (54). Some pathways project directly from the spinal cord dorsal horn to the brainstem and limbic system and cortical areas such as the cingulate cortex and the insula. Others project via multiple thalamic nuclei to the somatosensory cortices (53). Very little is known about the development and maturation of these pathways, and this area is in great need of investigation.

In the rat, dorsal horn projection cells begin to grow axons prenatally (31) and spinothalamic afferents reach the thalamus at E19. The earliest thalamic axons also reach the cortical plate at E19, and by postnatal day 0 (P0), there is a plexus of growth cone–tipped axons in the cortical plate and a few thalamic axons have reached the marginal zone (55). At P2 to P5, many thalamocortical synapses do not have functional AMPA receptors and are incapable of rapid excitatory transmission (silent synapses, see below). They appear to be converted to functional synapses by activity-dependent mechanisms at P8 to P9 (56). Thcsc findings are consistent with the observation that somatosensory cortical evoked potentials from the forepaw acquire an adult pattern at P12 (57). Electrophysiologic analysis of cortical cells at P7 shows them to be organized in columns as in the adult but to have larger receptive fields, suggesting a lack of inhibition, as discussed above for the spinal cord (58). The rodent cortex remains immature for as long as 6 weeks after birth.

The human cortex takes many years to develop, and indeed recent reports have shown that there is still considerable maturation during adolescence. Thalamocortical axons are first observed in the human cortex at 22 to 34 weeks in the human (59), but synaptogenesis continues on for many years (60). The earliest that somatosensory evoked potentials can be recorded in humans is 29 weeks of gestation, but, again, this is an area that requires more investigation (61). The complex developmental processes that contribute to the onset of affective dimensions of pain leading to feelings of unpleasantness are beyond the scope of this chapter but are a subject of considerable importance.

Analgesia

The pain of venipuncture is generally abolished or reduced by the use of topical local anesthetics such as lidocaine-prilocaine cream (EMLA) or amethocaine gel. These surface analgesics prevent the transmission of painful stimuli by nociceptors largely by their action on sodium channels (62). Developmental aspects of local anesthetic activity have not been studied in detail, but there is evidence that important developmental changes may exist in their properties. Susceptibility of rabbit vagus to neural blockade by lidocaine has been shown to be age dependent (63). The duration of intrathecal local anesthesia is shorter in human neonates than in adults (64) as is the duration of sciatic nerve block in the rat (9). Recently, developmentally regulated sensitivity to antinociceptive effects of epidural analgesia in rat has also been described (65). The pharmacokinetics and toxicity of amide local anesthetics may also be a function of age and maturity; reduced doses are often recommended in the neonatal period, and further study is warranted (66).

Topical local anesthetic use in neonates is controversial for some procedures because studies of efficacy have been inconclusive (67). Lidocaine-prilocaine cream (EMLA) and amethocaine gel are clearly effective local anesthetics from 29 to 42 weeks after gestation (68), and repeated application reduces the hypersensitivity that follows repeated heel-lance injury in the neonatal period (128). However, it does not block the direct response to heel lance itself or to a number of other painful procedures (67,69). This may be a reflection of the nature of the particular injury and the depth of nerve terminals involved in a heel lance compared with a very brief noxious stimulus such as venipuncture.

PAIN ASSOCIATED WITH MINOR SURGERY OR INFLAMMATION

The pain of surgery is not confined to the duration of the procedure itself but persists for some time afterward. Normally, after minor surgery, not only is there persisting pain for hours, days, or weeks depending on the location and severity of injury but changes in sensitivity at the operation site itself and the surrounding area.

Inguinal hernia repair, for example, is a common surgical operation that is performed across the age spectrum including premature neonates, infants, children, and adults. It is generally regarded as relatively minor surgery with a well-defined postoperative course and low rate of short- or long-term sequelae. Superficially, the pain response and its time course may appear to be similar at all ages. In fact, there are important differences in pain processing in early life that influence the biologic events after surgery and hence the management of pain and any possible long-term consequences.

The trauma, manipulation, and damage at the wound site after surgery result in local inflammation. Inflammation is characterized by an altered perception of pain (hypersensitivity) that includes an enhanced pain sensation to a noxious stimulus (hyperalgesia) and an abnormal sensation of pain to previously nonnoxious stimuli (allodynia) (Figs. 2.3 and 2.4). In addition, there may be spontaneous or ongoing pain (70). The hyperalgesia that follows tissue injury can be divided into primary and secondary hyperalgesia. Primary hyperalgesia develops at the site of an injury and appears to arise largely from peripheral nociceptor sensitization. Surrounding this is a zone of secondary mechanical hyperalgesia, which is proposed to arise from central plastic changes in spinal cord connectivity modifying CNS responsiveness to future stimuli.

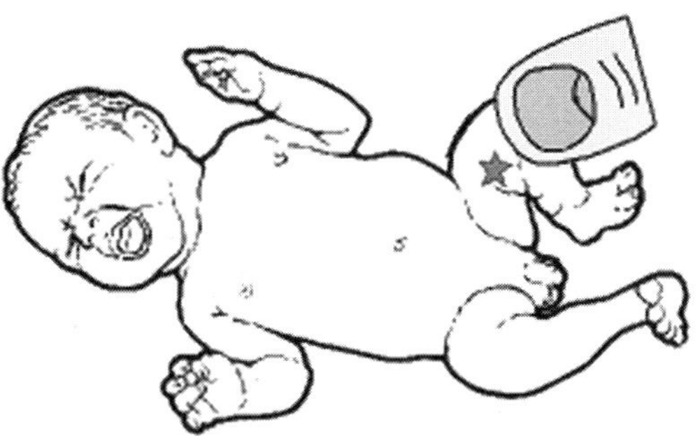

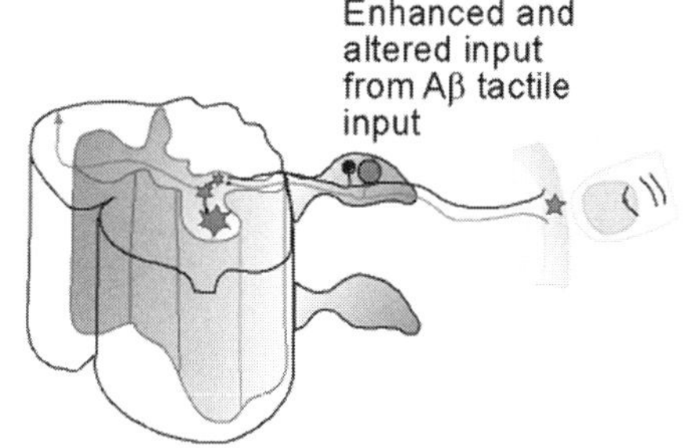

FIG. 2.4. More severe or repeated injury may lead to allodynia, a delayed appearance of tenderness, or pain evoked by a previously nonnoxious stimulus owing to (a) central sensitization that increases the input from Aβ fibers or (b) change in A-fiber properties (altered gene expression).

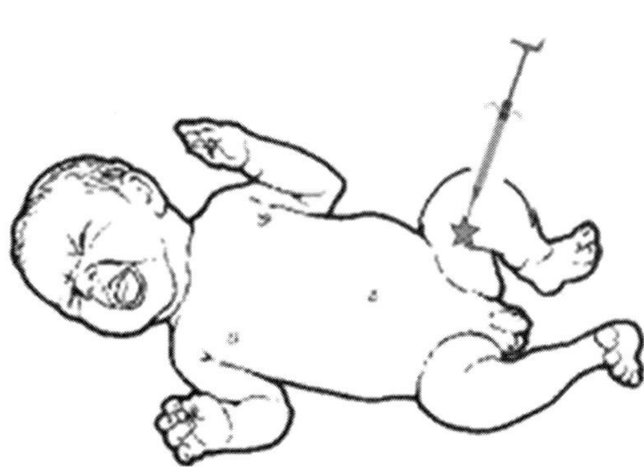

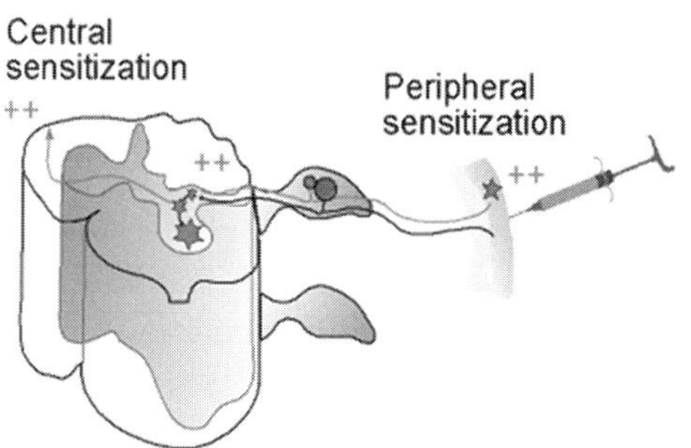

FIG. 2.3. More severe or repeated injury may lead to hyperalgesia, which is an enhancement of pain response to subsequent noxious stimuli owing to (a) sensitization of Aδ- and C-fiber nociceptors or (b) central sensitization that increases the central neuronal response to Aδ and C fibers.

The Pain Response

In very young infants, cutaneous reflex responses become sensitized with repeated mechanical stimulation, even in the innocuous range. The response magnitude increases and the threshold decreases after repeated innocuous mechanical stimulation at 10-second intervals. This effect is greatest in the 28 to 33 week postconceptional age group and is lost by 42 weeks (6,7). A striking hypersensitivity has also been observed in preliminary studies in infants after surgery. Tissue injury after pyeloplasty in infants results in a decrease in the sensory reflex thresholds in the wound area and surrounding hyperalgesia (71) (Chapter 3). Although postoperative pain in children is well described, sensory examination of their hyperalgesia and allodynia has not been undertaken.

Animal models of postoperative pain involve the induction of a persistent inflammation that lasts for hours (subcutaneous formalin), days (local carrageenan injection), or weeks (complete Freund adjuvant injection). The responses to some of these agents have been examined in young rat pups. Until day 10, the behavioral responses after application of inflammatory agents are predominantly nonspecific, whole-body movements, whereas the specific flexion reflex and shaking and licking the paw predominate from then on (72). As with surgery, there is a need for clarification about the development of pain responses to inflammatory agents. The response to formalin was found to have a tenfold higher sensitivity in neonatal rats compared with weanlings (73), although the classic biphasic behavioral response to formalin is not apparent in the rat pup until P15, coinciding with the overall depression in the response. In contrast, the hyperalgesia or drop in mechanical threshold that follows carrageenan injection (74) and mustard oil application (75) is smaller in amplitude at P3 in neonates than at P21. This may be a reflection of the high level of background sensitivity of young rats that limits the degree of hypersensitivity that they can display. Nevertheless, it is possible to demonstrate a clear enhancement of amplitude and duration of the flexion reflex (76) and of dorsal horn cell responses (77) after carrageenan injection after P3.

Peripheral Sensitization

The pain arising from the surgical wound differs from the pain from the hypodermic needle described in previously because it activates a number of new mechanisms within the nervous system. Local consequences of inflammation include the release of algogenic substances from damaged cells, recruitment of inflammatory cells, and release of further mediators from cells in the vicinity. These include H^+ and K^+, serotonin, histamine, bradykinin, prostaglandins, nitric oxide, cytokines, and growth factors (78). These may directly activate peripheral nociceptors to cause pain, but more often they act indirectly to sensitize nociceptors and alter their response properties to subsequent stimuli (79). This occurs by modification of receptor molecules or voltage-gated sodium channels by transcriptional and posttranslational events to reduce the activation threshold and thus allow lower intensity stimuli to evoke pain and a greater response to be evoked. Other proposals include the recruitment of formerly "silent" nociceptors by the release of active factors. Neutralization of endogenous NGF prevents the sensitization of nociceptors supplying inflamed skin (80).

Central Sensitization

The region of secondary hyperalgesia and allodynia that surrounds an area of tissue damage results from central synaptic rather than peripheral receptor alterations. The hyperexcitability of sensory neurons in the dorsal horn of the spinal cord and brainstem that follow inflammation is termed central sensitization (81). Activation of these central cells by repetitive Aδ- and C-fiber inputs initiates sensitization such that they respond to normal inputs in an exaggerated and extended manner (82). This mechanism is likely to account for hyperalgesia and allodynia because the resultant prolonged depolarization allows inputs that were previously ineffective to activate the neuron and previously effective inputs to become even more so.

There is a large body of evidence implicating the glutamate *N*-methyl-D-aspartate receptor system as the primary candidate for this form of plasticity (82–84). As discussed above, normal spinal nociceptive processing is mediated via the ionotropic AMPA and kainate glutamate receptors. However, repetitive activation of nociceptors associated with tissue injury results in the activation of the NMDA glutamate receptor (Fig. 2.5). This involvement of NMDA receptors is a consequence of two mechanisms:

1. The removal of the Mg^{2+} ions, which normally block the channel at resting mem-

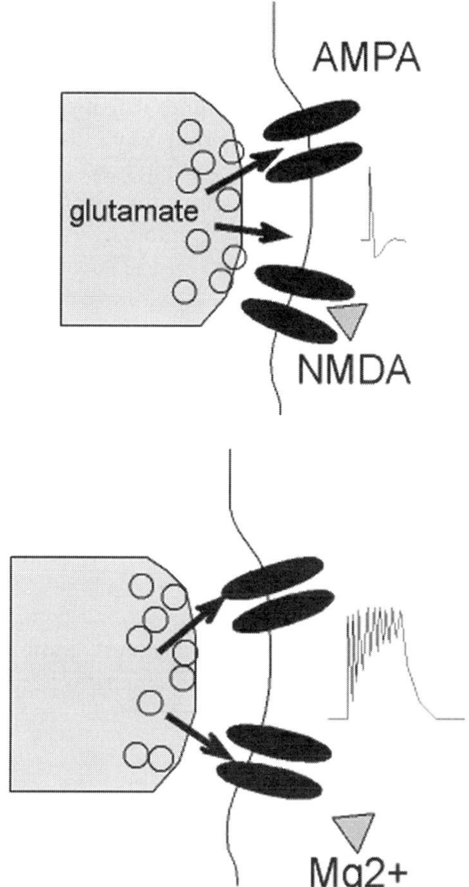

FIG. 2.5. Activation of the *N*-methyl-D-aspartate (NMDA) receptor is the principal mechanism by which neuronal activity alters synaptic strength. It is the basis of learning, memory, and conditioning closely involved in altered sensory processing and pathologic pain states. This diagram shows how, under normal conditions, sensory input from the periphery would activate amino-3-hydroxy-5-methyl-4-isoxazoleproprionic acid (AMPA) receptors only and the NMDA receptor would be blocked with Mg^{2+} ions (*triangle*) **(top)**. **Bottom:** In the presence of increased sensory input after injury, the Mg^{2+} is removed from the NMDA receptor, the postsynaptic response is increased, and increased calcium enters the cell.

brane potential, by the cumulative depolarization arising from summation of nociceptor-evoked slow synaptic potentials.

2. The release of the excitatory neuropeptide SP. The role of SP and NK1 receptors in pain processing is well established (85,86). Neuropeptides such as CGRP and SP (acting on NK1 receptors) and growth factors such as BDNF (acting on trkB receptors) released by the C fibers may potentiate the release of glutamate and its actions on the NMDA receptor. G protein–coupled receptors such as NK1 and mGlu receptors and receptor tyrosine kinases such as the trkB receptors may also enhance NMDA currents via activation of protein kinase C (87).

An important additional mechanism of central sensitization is the induction of novel genes. After inflammation, A-fiber neurons, which do not normally express neuropeptides, begin to express SP and BDNF, which may contribute to the allodynic response (88,89).

The effect of this enhanced neurotransmission and hyperexcitability includes enlargement of receptive fields; increased spontaneous activity; greater discharges to mechanical, thermal, and electrical stimulation; and sometimes decreased thresholds (90). All these lead to increased neuronal activity transmitted to supraspinal sites and therefore the onset of persistent pain.

The persistent pain response of the pediatric patient after surgery depends on the ability of the developing sensory nervous system to activate these mechanisms of peripheral and central sensitization.

Development of Central Sensitization

Central sensitization as described in adult spinal cord results from repetitive C-fiber input. However, C-fiber evoked activity is not observed in dorsal horn cells in the first postnatal week and repetitive peripheral stimulation at C fiber strength also has no observable effects on dorsal horn cell spike responses. From P10, repetitive C-fiber stimulation at three times the C-fiber threshold produces a classic windup as reported in the adult dorsal horn (31–37) in 18% of cells. This has increased to 40% of cells by P21 (44). The role of immature C terminals before P10 requires further investigation.

In contrast to the lack of C-fiber influence, stimulation of the peripheral receptive field on the hindlimb at twice the A-fiber threshold at a frequency of 0.5 Hz can produce considerable sensitization of the dorsal horn cells in the neonate (41). This sensitization takes the form of a buildup of background activity in the cells during repetitive stimulation that outlasts the stimulation period, thereby producing a prolonged afterdischarge of as long as 138 seconds. It is particularly apparent in younger animals. At P6, 33% of cells display background firing during stimulation followed by a prolonged afterdischarge of 70.6 ± 18 seconds after repetitive A-fiber stimulation, at P10 only 6%, and by P21, it was absent (41).

In the adult, the glutamate NMDA receptor is important in the generation of central sensitization (Fig. 2.5), but the developmental regulation of NMDA receptor function in relation to central sensitization has not been directly investigated. NMDA-dependent C-fiber evoked depolarization of spinal cord cells and windup of cells to repeated C-fiber stimulation has been demonstrated in the young (8 to 14 days) spinal cord *in vitro* (91), but the effects on A fiber sensitization are not known. Preliminary results show that the ability of dorsal horn cells to display enlargement of receptive fields; increased spontaneous activity; and enhanced responses to mechanical, thermal, and electrical stimulation differs in the newborn cord (77). A feature of the neonatal dorsal horn is the presence of synapses with NMDA receptors only, i.e., no functional AMPA receptors. These are called silent synapses because of their inability to function at resting membrane potentials. These silent synapses disappear with age with the onset of colocalization of AMPA and NMDA receptors (92,93). However, there is evidence that in lamina II of the postnatal rat dorsal horn, the NMDA receptors' silence is limited and that they can significantly affect neuron excitability even in the absence of coactivation of AMPA receptors (94). The neonatal spinal cord has a higher concentration of NMDA receptors in the gray matter than that observed in older animals (95). All laminae in the dorsal horn are uniformly labeled with NMDA-sensitive [^{3}H]glutamate until P10 to P12, when higher densities gradually appear in the SG, so that by P30, binding is similar to that in the adult. Furthermore, the affinity of the receptors for NMDA decreases with postnatal age. NMDA-evoked calcium efflux in neonatal rat SG is very high in the first postnatal week and then declines (96). This is delayed by neonatal capsaicin treatment, suggesting that C-fiber afferent activity regulates the postnatal maturation of NMDA receptors (96). The different NMDA receptor channel subunits are independently regulated. Of particular interest are the NR2 subunits, which are modulatory because their expression alters properties such as voltage-dependent Mg^{2+} block and deactivation kinetics of NMDA receptors. The subunit composition of the NMDA channel complex undergoes considerable rearrangement during spinal cord development (52), which appears to be activity dependent (97).

SP release from the activated C fibers causes slow depolarization via NK1 receptors, which contributes to central sensitization. NK1 receptor density is maximal in the first 2 postnatal weeks; at P60, the cord has one-sixth of the binding sites present at P11. Furthermore, in the newborn, the receptor distribution is the inverse of that in the adult, i.e., the superficial laminae have very few receptors, and the high density observed in the adult SG is not apparent until the second week of life (98). In contrast to receptor levels, SP levels are low at birth in the rat. This immaturity of the SP/NK1 system undoubtedly affects central sensitization in the infant nervous system, but it is not known how. Stimulation of central C-fiber terminals in isolated newborn rat cord produces a long-lasting ventral root potential that is blocked by SP antagonists (46). At P12, both NK1 and NK2 receptors are involved in C-fiber evoked slow potentials (99).

The developmental pharmacology of other excitatory and inhibitory systems are also important and have been reviewed elsewhere

(15,100). As in the adult, inflammation results in the expression of new genes in the neonate, but the pattern of change is somewhat different. CGRP (which is coexpressed with SP) expression is switched on in both A cells and IB4+ C neurons in the dorsal root ganglion for 7 days after carrageenan inflammation of the hindpaw at birth and only returns to normal after the inflammation has subsided (101). This suggests that the nonpeptidergic A and C fibers have the ability to express peptides under some circumstances in the postnatal period.

Activation of Descending Inhibition

It is well established that descending pathways originating in higher centers can modulate the output of spinal nociceptive neurons. In addition, it appears that these pathways are activated in the presence of persistent pain (102). Descending inhibitory controls are immature at birth (103). Animals given a midthoracic spinal cord transection before P15 are markedly less affected than those transected at older ages (104). In spinalized rats younger than 15 days of age, tactile and noxious stimuli continue to evoke withdrawal responses that are similar to those observed in intact rats. Older animals show severely depressed responses for several days and then recover flexor responses to cutaneous stimuli with decreased duration. The slow maturation of descending inhibitory pathways traveling from the brainstem via the dorsolateral funiculus of the spinal cord to the dorsal horn is particularly relevant to pain processing. Although descending axons from brainstem projection neurons grow down the spinal cord early in fetal life, they do not extend collateral branches into the dorsal horn for some time and do not become functionally effective until P10 in the rat (105,106). This may in part be owing to low levels of neurotransmitters, in this case serotonin and norepinephrine, but may also be owing to delayed maturation of crucial interneurons.

It has been suggested that the maturation of descending inhibition depends on afferent C-fiber activity. Rats treated with capsaicin as adults have reduced inhibitory controls (107), and mutant mice lacking the NK1 receptor gene (and consequently altered C-fiber activity) have high dorsal horn cell firing rates (85). The lack of descending inhibition in the neonatal dorsal horn means that an important endogenous analgesic system that might dampen noxious inputs as they enter the CNS is lacking, and their effects may therefore be more profound than in the adult. It also explains why stimulus-produced analgesia from the periaqueductal gray is not effective until P21 in rats (108).

Analgesia

The mechanisms of postoperative pain and hypersensitivity reveal important peripheral and central targets for analgesics forming the basis of a balanced or multimodal analgesic strategy (109). Local anesthesia, acetaminophen, nonsteroidal analgesics, and opioids are generally used in combination during the perioperative and postoperative period in children. The effects of these agents in early development have still not been fully characterized, and several newer approaches are potentially interesting.

Local anesthetic management of inguinal hernia repair might include local anesthetic wound infiltration, ilioinguinal peripheral nerve block, or caudal epidural block. There is evidence that local anesthetics have a specific antinociceptive effect after inflammation separate from the direct nerve conduction blocking effect. This has been demonstrated in both laboratory animals and humans and is also developmentally regulated (65,110,111), suggesting there may be differences in the effects in infancy.

The importance of the NMDA receptor in the generation of central hypersensitivity and its developmental regulation have been discussed above. Our own preliminary data show that sensitivity to the NMDA antagonist ketamine in reversing inflammatory hyperalgesia is greatly increased in young rats (76). Ketamine has been used in postoperative analgesia in children. Caudal epidural ketamine is as effective as local anesthetic (bupivacaine) for postoperative analgesia after hernia repair (112) and has also been shown to enhance caudal local anesthesia after other similar operations (113,114). Increase in the duration of pain relief is also a feature of augmented analgesia by ketamine, although the mechanisms of this effect are not established (113).

Clonidine, an α-adrenergic agonist, has also been used both systemically and centrally for acute pain in children, although systematic study is lacking (115).

The inflammatory response is developmentally regulated, but we know little of the specific effects in early life of nonsteroidal analgesics acting principally on prostaglandin synthesis by inhibition of cyclooxygenase. Nonsteroidal anti-inflammatory drugs have an established place in pediatric postoperative pain management (116), although they are not usually used in the neonatal period for fear of toxicity. Newer, more specific and less toxic agents are now available and deserve further study, particularly in the neonatal period.

Acetaminophen is widely used for postoperative analgesia in children, but many fundamental questions remain unanswered (117). Although the pharmacokinetics and toxicity of acetaminophen have been studied (118–121), there are few investigations of analgesic efficacy in young children particularly neonates (122).

Opioid use after minor surgery is limited because of troublesome side effects, particularly nausea, vomiting, and respiratory depression. The moderate potency opioid codeine, which is sometimes considered to have a lower incidence of such effects, is traditionally used in children (123,124). Codeine analgesia is largely owing to metabolism to morphine by a genetically and developmentally regulated cytochrome enzyme system that may limit its efficacy and suitability in early life (125). The development of opioid analgesia is discussed in the next section.

PAIN ASSOCIATED WITH REPEATED PAINFUL INTERVENTIONS OR CHRONIC INFLAMMATION: INTENSIVE CARE, REPEATED SURGERY, AND JUVENILE RHEUMATOID ARTHRITIS

Although minor surgery produces tissue damage and inflammation, the pain is normally of limited duration and subsides as the wound heals. Major surgery, conversely, may result in a prolonged and painful postoperative course. It may also be accompanied by a period of intensive care, requiring further potentially painful procedures or even reoperation before the effects of the initial injury have resolved. Thoracoabdominal, cardiothoracic, and spinal surgeries are frequently in this category. Insertion or removal of chest tubes, invasive monitoring devices, peritoneal or intravascular dialysis, central venous lines, and diagnostic procedures are all potentially painful. These may have a compounding effect, so that repeated procedures become more and more painful.

Juvenile rheumatoid arthritis and other chronic inflammatory diseases are obviously a completely separate group clinically, but their pain may also be viewed as repetitive over a period of years. An important aspect of this repetitive pain is that there is the possibility that such repeated injuries in infancy and childhood cause long-lasting sensitization, changing the response to future painful interventions months or years later (126).

The Pain Response

There is evidence that repeated intensive care procedures do affect sensory processing in even the youngest infants. One demonstration of this is that the mechanical sensory reflex threshold of preterm infants in an area of local tissue damage created by repeated heel lances is half the value of that on the intact contralateral heel (127). The tenderness is established for days and weeks in the presence of tissue damage but can be alleviated by repeated application of lidocaine-prilocaine cream (128). This response can spread outside the immediate area of injury. Preterm infants with established unilateral leg injuries from repeated procedures in intensive care show significantly lower sensory thresholds even on the unaffected, contralateral foot (7). The low thresholds were similar in value to those of much younger, preterm infants. Consistent with this is the report that infants who spend weeks 28 to 32 in neonatal intensive care and undergo frequent invasive procedures have delayed maturation of the facial action response to heel lance (129).

The sensitization may last even longer than the period of clinical care. Circumcised infants have been shown to display a stronger pain response to subsequent routine vaccination at 4 and 6 months than uncircumcised infants. Preoperative treatment with lidocaine-prilocaine cream attenuates the pain response to subsequent vaccination (130).

In addition, it is also clear that the existence of background recurrent pain alters acute pain thresholds. In children aged 6 to 17 years with juvenile chronic arthritis, both the inflamed joints and noninflamed paraspinal areas show reduced pressure thresholds (131, 132). The increased sensitivity of paraspinal sites suggests a central site of inflammatory sensitization. Furthermore, this sensitization remains even when the primary inflammation has subsided.

The effect of repeated neonatal noxious stimulation has been modeled in rat pups by stimulation four times each day from P0 to P7 with either needle prick or cotton tip rub. Testing for defensive withdrawal, alcohol preference, air-puff startle, and social discrimination was carried out when they had reached adulthood. As adults, the repeated needle prick group displayed decreased latencies to intense heat, increased preference for alcohol, increased latency in exploratory and defensive withdrawal behavior, and a prolonged chemosensory memory in the social discrimination tests. These data suggest that repetitive noxious stimulation in neonatal rat pups may lead to an altered ability to cope with stress and pain in adulthood (133).

Possible Peripheral Causes for Sensitization on Repeated Injury

Repeated noxious stimulation before the effects of the previous injury has subsided results in a Aδ- and C-fiber input that is enhanced by the sensitizing effects of the inflammatory injury, as described previously. The critical question here is whether neonatal injury can result in peripheral changes that outlast the period of injury itself. Tissue damage in the early postnatal period in rats has been shown to cause a profound and lasting sprouting response of the local sensory nerve terminals leaving an area of hyperinnervation in the wounded area that lasts into adulthood (134,135) (Fig. 2.6). Behavioral studies show long-lasting hypersensitivity and lowered mechanical threshold in the injured region (134,136). This phenomenon, if it occurs in humans, could well account for any long-term sensitization to repeated in-

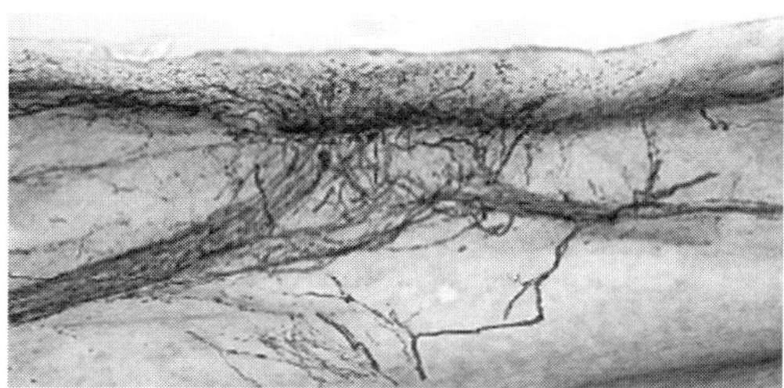

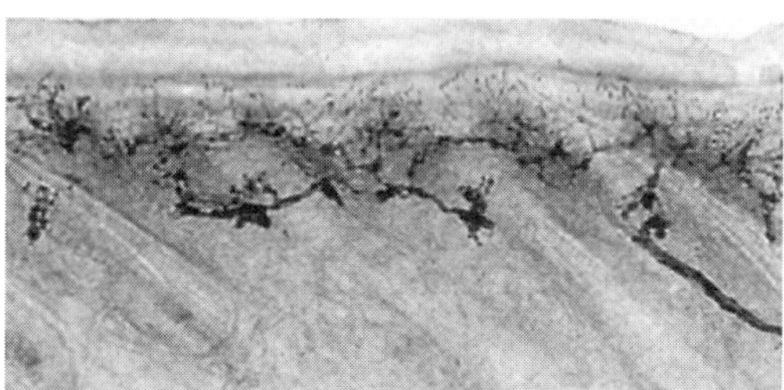

FIG. 2.6. Hyperinnervation of mouse skin after neonatal skin wounding **(top)** compared with normal contralateral side **(bottom)**. Sections of postnatal day 6 mouse dorsal foot skin with nerve endings immunostained with PGP 9.5.

jury to the same area. The sprouting response is clearly greatest when the wound is performed at birth and declines with age at wounding. The response to adult wounds is weak and transient in comparison, resulting in a temporary hyperinnervation that recovers after a few weeks. Both myelinated A fibers and unmyelinated C fibers, but not sympathetic fibers, contribute to the sprouting response (16), and it is unaffected by local anesthetic block of the sensory nerve during wounding (136).

A feature of this wound-induced sprouting is that all the sprouts are oriented toward the wound margin exactly as if attracted to the wound site by a specific signal. It therefore seems likely that the sprouting results from the release of neurotrophic factors from the damaged region. Skin wounding at birth results in a substantial upregulation of NGF (137), which decreases with increasing age, but this is unlikely to be the main cause of sprouting because systemic anti-NGF treatment fails to prevent it (135) or the neurite outgrowth toward injured skin in an *in vitro* coculture model (138). Nevertheless, upregulation of NGF at the site of injury may lead to changes in receptor function (as discussed previously). BDNF, neurotrophin 3, and neurotrophin 4 are also all expressed in the skin during development (139) and may be upregulated after skin wounds along with other growth factors (15,140).

Possible Central Causes for Sensitization on Repeated Injury

The central hypersensitivity state after tissue injury was described earlier. However, the critical question here is whether such central hypersensitivity can really explain the prolonged alterations in sensory processing that can occur over months and possibly years (130,141,142). At present, it is not clear whether central sensitization persists only as long as the afferent barrage is maintained, i.e., when the injury subsides, so does the hypersensitivity state (143,144), or whether it can persist beyond that time (145).

There is considerable evidence that alterations in normal activity patterns during development can permanently alter the future pattern of connections within the CNS. Normal sensory experience during the postnatal period is essential to ensure that appropriate connections are strengthened and inappropriate ones eliminated. This has been most intensively studied in the visual system, particularly in the patterning of connections within the retinogeniculocortical pathway where physiologic activity (i.e., light-evoked retinal activity) becomes necessary to fine-tune connections and allow correct functioning of the system (146,147). Competition for target neurons in the cortex between axons receiving input from either eye drives the segregation, probably via a Hebbian mechanism, such that some synapses are strengthened at the cost of others that are weakened and eliminated (148). A similar developmental process exists in the somatosensory cortex where diffuse thalamocortical projections that relay sensory information from the vibrissae to the whisker barrels of the somatosensory cortex are refined by postnatal sensory experience to create appropriate somatotopic projections of sensory stimuli to the relevant cortical area (149). This period of plasticity exists for a strictly defined critical period and can be disrupted by changing activity patterns either by surgical or pharmacologic means (149,150). More recently, we demonstrated the activity dependence of the postnatal laminar organization of primary afferent terminals in the spinal cord dorsal horn (151).

The molecular mechanisms responsible for these changes have been the subject of considerable recent research. Mechanisms analogous to long-term potentiation and long-term depression in the hippocampus and elsewhere have been proposed to mediate activity-dependent development where synapse stabilization and elimination refine dendritic connections (152,153). Three basic possibilities exist for functional alterations in synaptic efficacy: changing the probability of presynaptic neurotransmitter release, the size of the postsynaptic quantal response to the transmitter, and the number of functional synapses at a given synaptic connection. The third of these three possible mechanisms of plasticity has received much attention recently with the concept of silent synapse conversion to functionality proposed as a mechanism for activity-dependent plasticity. Electrophysiologic studies of developing spinal cord and hippocampus have revealed synapses that appear to contain only functional NMDA receptors with no AMPA component (56,154). Cells containing these synapses when at or near normal resting potential remain functionally silent to presynaptic transmitter release. Synaptic transmission only occurs with previous postsynaptic depolarization and the activation of NMDA receptors. Strong afferent input would provide this depolarization, activating the NMDA receptors and effectively switching on the cell.

The tantalizing questions remain as to whether these and other examples of activity-dependent plasticity are triggered by early tissue damage and pain and whether connections within pain pathways can be altered by alterations in nociceptive input at a critical stage of development.

Analgesia

Very little is known about the optimal analgesic management of persistent and ongoing pain. In the neonatal period, there is controversy regarding thresholds for analgesic administration and concern about the possible long- and short-term adverse effects of both pain and analgesia (155). Opioids are the most important group of drugs used after major surgery and in intensive care. They are usually infused systemically, often for prolonged periods. The developmental biology of opioids was reviewed recently (156). Morphine pharmacokinetics has also been studied at most ages and recommendations for the safe clinical use of morphine (in terms of short-term complications) are available for neonates, infants, and children (157,158). The opioid receptor is developmentally regulated, and the number and distribution of receptor subtypes in the CNS undergo considerable reorganization in early life. Receptor function may also change during this period (159). Despite the fact that opioids are now widely used in neonates and infants (160), there is still a lack of knowledge of their specific effects in this population of patients (156). Animal studies indicate that the analgesic effectiveness of opioid agonists is likely to be different in human neonates compared with adults (10,159,161). Although opioid agonists specifically depress nociceptive C and Aδ inputs in the adult, *in vitro* and *in vivo* studies suggest an effect on nonnociceptive Aβ-mediated stimuli in neonatal rats (10,161, 162). Differences in opioid pharmacology compared with that in the adult may arise from changes in drug metabolism and transport and receptor expression and function. Most spinal opioid receptors are located presynaptically on central terminals of small nociceptive primary afferents (163), but μ- and δ-opioid receptor immunoreactivities are also found in large primary sensory neurons of neonatal rats and are downregulated postnatally (164) (Fig. 2.7). Both NMDA antagonists such as ketamine and α_2 adrenergic agonists such as clonidine potentiate the antinociceptive effects of opioids; in addition, the NMDA receptor that is important in the development of central hypersensitivity is also implicated in the phenomenon of morphine tolerance (165–167). The influence of early injury and exposure to opioids and other agents on these processes, including the development of long-term hypersensitivity, may be important but have not been studied.

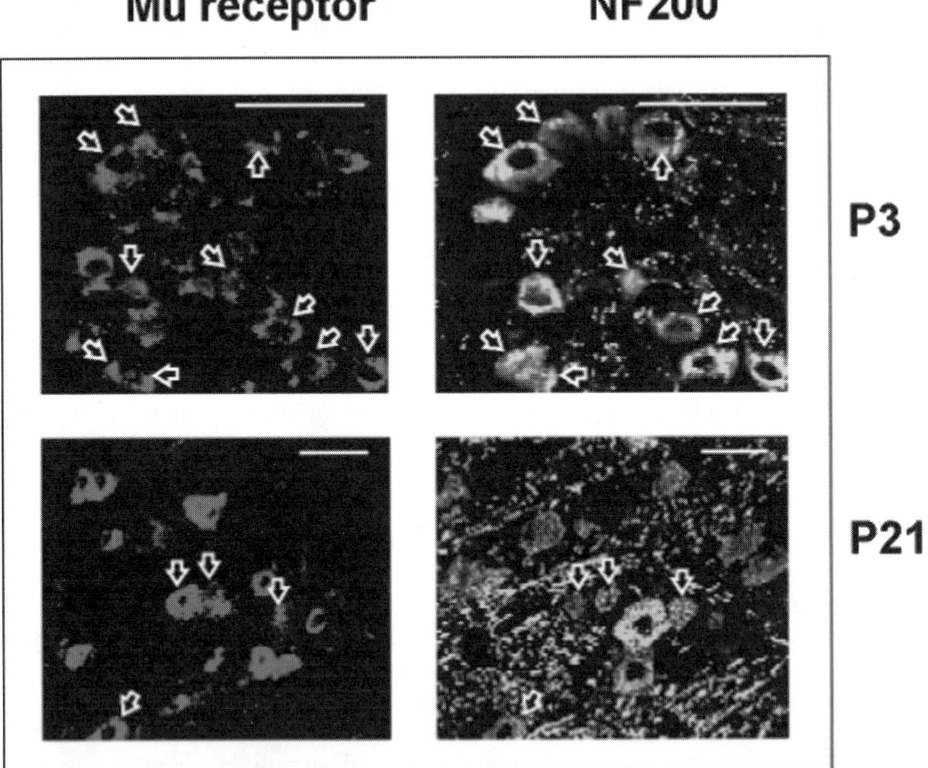

FIG. 2.7. Double immunostaining of rat dorsal root ganglion cells at postnatal days 3 and 21 with the μ-opiate receptor **(left)** and NF200 **(right)**, a selective marker of nonnociceptive A-fiber neurons. *Arrows* help to identify the same neurons on the left and right sides viewed through two different filters. At postnatal day 3, many μ-receptor +ve neurons also stain positively for NF200. At postnatal day 21, μ-receptor expression is restricted to NF200–ve neurons. [Courtesy of B. Beland (See ref. 164.)]

NEUROPATHIC PAIN

Pain from nerve injury or neuropathic pain is a common source of suffering in chronic disease in children. It is estimated that neuropathic syndromes comprise 50% of chronic pain referrals in children and can result from surgery, traumatic injury, malignancy, and many metabolic disorders (168). Children also frequently report phantom sensations after amputation and the majority also experience phantom pain (169).

A typical patient presents in the pain clinic, often many months or years after the initial insult, complaining of spontaneous pain, a bizarre or abnormal sensation, and possibly numbness. These symptoms occur usually in a limited area that may or may not correspond with the distribution of a peripheral nerve or dermatome but may be related to the site of surgery or injury.

The Pain Response

The neuropathic pain reported by the child in the clinic is characterized by allodynia (touch-evoked pain), spontaneous pain, hyperalgesia (enhanced pain to a given noxious stimulus), and sensory deficits with some sympathetic involvement. There are several animal models that demonstrate some or all of these symptoms ranging from the classic methods of complete nerve section to recent models based on a restricted partial denervation of the hindlimb after sciatic nerve injury (170–173). Examples of the latter are loose ligation of the entire nerve (chronic constriction injury), selective tight ligation of two (L5 and L6) of the three spinal nerves that form the sciatic nerve (171), and, more recently, a model of spared nerve injury involving ligation of two of the three distal branches of the sciatic nerve (174). To date, only the selective spinal ligation model has been tested to a limited degree in rat pups (175,176). Young rats were found to display much more vigorous behavioral signs of mechanical allodynia and ongoing pain than mature rats, but mechanical allodynia lasted for a shorter period of time in animals younger than 3 weeks of age.

Mechanisms of Chronic Pain: Peripheral Mechanisms

In the adult, it is clear that the mechanisms of chronic inflammatory and neuropathic pain are very different from acute pain, and there is evidence for plasticity in both the transmission and modulating systems in these prolonged pain states (82,177). This is of great importance when considering a rational basis for the treatment of neuropathic pain in which the pathology leads to alterations in both peripheral and central pain pathways. With respect to infants and children, this plasticity is superimposed on a nervous system that is still immature and in which sensory pathways are still undergoing synaptogenesis and fine-tuning of connections.

Some of the plasticity arises from altered peripheral input (144). Axon damage in adults causes a considerable alteration in the structure, function, and phenotypic expression of cell bodies in the dorsal root ganglion including altered neurotrophin, neurotrophin receptor, neuropoietic cytokine, neuropeptide, opioid peptide, and glutamate receptor expression (15,82). Many of these changes are thought to be as a result of the loss of neurotrophic influences from the periphery, and some can be reversed by exogenous application of NGF or GDNF (23). Adult nerve section also triggers the generation of ectopic discharges within the neuroma and the dorsal root ganglia (178), and after partial denervation, high-frequency spontaneous activity originating in the dorsal root ganglion targets the spinal neurons via injured A fibers. Sodium channels are known to accumulate at the site of axotomy or nerve (179) and may contribute to the membrane achieving a hyperexcitable state, associated with hyperalgesia and other chronic pain states.

It is clear from numerous studies that peripheral nerve injury has far more dramatic consequences if it occurs during a critical neonatal period when extensive death of axotomized dorsal root ganglion cells occurs (180–184). In the adult, axotomy-induced cell death does not begin until approximately 3 months after the lesion and is limited to the unmyelinated axons (185). However, in the neonate, death occurs rapidly and involves many populations (181). Approximately 50% of neonatal motor and sensory neurons die 1 week after peripheral nerve injury (182). Both application of exogenous NGF and GDNF and decreasing p75 expression with antisense oligos in axotomized sensory neurons can temporarily prevent the loss of dorsal root ganglion neurons occurring after neonatal axotomy (23,183), and recently this cell loss has been linked with low levels of heat-shock proteins, such as hsp27 (185), which are induced after stress in tissues, perhaps with a protective role.

Mechanisms of Chronic Pain: Central Mechanisms

The substantial cell loss after neonatal nerve injury has central consequences within the spinal cord, and plastic changes result from this deafferentation. An initial consequence of the cell death is a transganglionic degeneration and subsequent withdrawal of central terminals of those cells (186,187). A further consequence is the sprouting of adjacent, intact axon collaterals into the denervated region (39,188,189) disrupting the somatotopic organization of central terminals within the dorsal horn. Both intact A (189) and C fibers (39) sprout and grow arbors outside their normal central terminal field, making functional synaptic connections within new areas of the cord (190). The resulting rearrangement of connections in the developing rat nervous system is not confined to dorsal horn cells but is found in higher levels of the nervous system including the cortex (191,192). Although in the short term, this could be a useful compensatory device to restore sensory input from an area of the body surface in which it has been lost, the effects may be detrimental and trigger chronic pain.

The few surviving axotomized neurons also undergo a sprouting response (39) similar to that seen in the adult. Adult axotomy causes Aβ afferents, which are normally restricted to laminae III and IV, to sprout and extend right up into laminae I and II (193) and form synaptic connections with lamina II cells (194). This is thought to allow low-threshold inputs to excite nociceptive circuits and therefore contribute to allodynia (82). Interestingly, this mimics the normal situation in the neonate in which Aβ afferents extend dorsally right up into laminae I and II to reach the surface of the gray matter (37), followed by a gradual withdrawal from the superficial laminae over the first 3 postnatal weeks. C fibers, conversely, grow specifically to laminae I and II, and for a considerable postnatal period, these laminae are occupied by both A- and C-fiber terminals (37). During their occupation of superficial laminae, A-fiber terminals form synaptic connections at EM level (38) and are functional (42,43). It is likely that they form the pure NMDA receptor–mediated excitatory postsynaptic currents or silent synapses transiently present in the neonatal dorsal horn (93,195), although interestingly, these silent synapses do not reappear in the adult after nerve damage.

The effects of nerve damage in infancy on synaptic transmission and sensory neuron activity in the CNS have not been examined. A striking feature of central dorsal horn cells after adult nerve damage is an increase in neuronal excitability (82,83). In the adult chronic constriction injury model, a high percentage of spinal neurons exhibit abnormal levels of spontaneous activity despite the absence of somatic receptive fields and are sensitive to tapping of the nerve injury site (196). After selective spinal nerve ligation, neurons with increased spontaneous activity, lowered thresholds to thermal and mechanical stimuli, and enlarged mechanical receptive fields accompanied by decreased response magnitudes have been reported (197).

Analgesia

The NMDA receptor plays a key role in the induction and maintenance of spinal nociceptive events leading to hyperalgesia after nerve damage (82,177,198). Thus, it is likely that aberrant peripheral activity is amplified and enhanced by NMDA receptor–mediated spinal mechanisms in neuropathic pain, and there is evidence for effectiveness of agents acting at the NMDA receptor complex, especially ketamine in humans (199–201). The use of ketamine in neuropathic pain in children is still not fully documented, but there are reasons to suspect that it is used differently in children than in adults because there is considerable developmental regulation of NMDA receptors (see above).

Opioids are also used to treat neuropathic pain with mixed success (199). One problem with assessment of opioids in both the animal studies and in the clinic is that the type of neuropathy and the extent, duration, and intensity of the symptoms may well be critical factors as may be the route of administration and type of opioid used. A similar series of discrepant results can be found in the animal literature (202). Resolution of the efficacy of opioids in pediatric neuropathic pain would be extremely important.

The current mainstays of treatments of neuropathic pain in adults are anticonvulsants (e.g., carbamazepine, lamotrigine, and gabapentin) and tricyclic antidepressants (e.g., imipramine and desipramine). Controlled studies using tricyclic antidepressants have shown that these agents are effective against neuropathic pain states such as diabetic neuropathy and postherpetic neuralgia in a manner that is independent of their antidepressant effects (200). Because these drugs act on the descending monoamine systems, linking the brain to the spinal cord, a system that has been shown to develop slowly over the postnatal period (44), it is likely that their efficacy changes with age. Recently, attention has focused on the novel anticonvulsant gabapentin, which has established efficacy in patients with diabetic neuropathy and postherpetic neuralgia (203). These drugs have been used in children, but, again, systematic investigations have not been carried out (204,205).

CONCLUSION

Significant progress in the effective control of pain in children after surgery or trauma or as a result of underlying disease processes can only take place if treatments are closely related to the underlying neurobiology. Furthermore, understanding the development of pain processing by the maturing nervous system is crucial if we are to appreciate the perception and consequences of pain in early life. Progress is being made in this important field, but there is still a need for more research, especially in the areas of developmental neurophysiology, pharmacology, and synaptic plasticity in response to early pain.

ACKNOWLEDGMENT

Support from the Medical Research Council, Children Nationwide, Great Ormond Street Children's Charity, and Portex Industries is gratefully acknowledged.

REFERENCES

1. Woolf CJ, Decosterd I. Implications of recent advances in the understanding of pain pathophysiology for the assessment of pain in patients. *Pain* 1999;6[Suppl]: S141–S147.
2. Fitzgerald M. The neurobiology of fetal and infant pain. In: Wall PD, Melzack R, eds. *Textbook of pain*, 4th ed. London: Churchill-Livingstone 1999:235–252.
3. Fitzgerald M. Development of the peripheral and spinal pain system. In: Anand KJS, Stevens BJ, McGrath PJ, eds. *Pain in neonates*, 2nd ed. Amsterdam: Elsevier, 2000:9–22.
4. Fassler D. The fear of needles in children. *Am J Orthopsychiatry* 1985;55:371–377.
5. Franck LS, Miaskowski C. Measurement of neonatal responses to painful stimuli: a research review. *J Pain Symptom Manage* 1997;14:343–378.
6. Fitzgerald M, Shaw A, MacIntosh N. Postnatal development of the cutaneous flexor reflex: comparative study of preterm infants and newborn rat pups. *Dev Med Child Neurol* 1988;30:520–526.
7. Andrews K, Fitzgerald M. The cutaneous withdrawal reflex in human neonates: sensitization, receptive fields, and the effects of contralateral stimulation. *Pain* 1994;56:95–101.
8. Falcon M, Guendellman D, Stolberg A, et al. Development of thermal nociception in rats. *Pain* 1996;67: 203–208.
9. Hu D, Hu R, Berde CB. Neurologic evaluation of infant and adult rats before and after sciatic nerve blockade. *Anesthesiology* 1997;86:957–965.
10. Marsh D, Dickenson A, Hatch D, et al. Epidural opioid analgesia in infant rats I: mechanical and heat responses. *Pain* 1999;82:23–32.
11. Johnston CC, Stevens B, Craig KD, et al. Developmental changes in pain expression in premature, full-term, two- and four-month-old infants. *Pain* 1993;52: 201–208.
12. Johnston CC, Stevens BJ, Yang F, et al. Differential response to pain by very premature neonates. *Pain* 1995; 61:471–479.
13. Kress M, Zeilhofer HU. Capsaicin, protons and heat: new excitement about nociceptors. *Trends Pharmacol Sci* 1999;20:112–118.
14. McCleskey EW, Gold MS. Ion channels of nociception. *Annu Rev Physiol* 1999;61:835–856.
15. Alvares D, Fitzgerald M. Building blocks of pain: the regulation of key molecules in spinal sensory neurones during development and following peripheral axotomy. *Pain* 1999;6[Suppl]:S71–S85.
16. Reynolds ML, Fitzgerald M, Benowitz LI. GAP-43 expression in developing cutaneous and muscle nerves in the rat hindlimb. *Neuroscience* 1991;41: 201–211.
17. Payne J, Middleton J, Fitzgerald M. The pattern and timing of cutaneous hair follicle innervation in the rat pup and human fetus. *Brain Res Dev Brain Res* 1991; 61:173–182.
18. Jackman A, Fitzgerald M. Development of peripheral hindlimb and central spinal cord innervation by subpopulations of dorsal root ganglion cells in the embryonic rat. *J Comp Neurol* 2000;418:281–298.
19. Bennett DL, Averill S, Clary DO, et al. Postnatal changes in the expression of the trkA high-affinity NGF receptor in primary sensory neurons. *Eur J Neurosci* 1996;8:2204–2208.
20. Fitzgerald M. Cutaneous primary afferent properties in the hindlimb of the neonatal rat. *J Physiol* 1987;383: 79–92.
21. Fitzgerald M, Fulton B P. The physiological properties of developing sensory neurons. In: Scott, ed. *Sensory*

neurons: diversity, development and plasticity. Oxford: Oxford University Press, 1992:287–306.
22. Snider WD. Functions of neurotrophins during nervous system development: what the knockouts are teaching us. *Cell* 1994;77:627–638.
23. McMahon SB. Neurotrophins and sensory neurons: role in development, maintenance and injury. *Philos Trans R Soc Lond B Biol Sci* 1996;351:405–411.
24. Coggeshall RE, Pover CM, Fitzgerald M. Dorsal root ganglion cell death and surviving cell numbers in relation to the development of sensory innervation in the rat hindlimb. *Brain Res Dev Brain Res* 1994;82: 193–212.
25. Ruit KG, Elliott JL, Osborne PA, et al. Selective dependence of mammalian dorsal root ganglion neurons on nerve growth factor during embryonic development. *Neuron* 1992;8:573–587.
26. Indo Y, Tsuruta M, Hayashida Y, et al. Mutations in the TRKA/NGF receptor gene in patients with congenital insensitivity to pain with anhidrosis. *Nat Genet* 1996; 13:485–488.
27. Koltzenburg M. The changing sensitivity in the life of the nociceptor. *Pain* 1999;6[Suppl]:S93–S102.
28. Albers KM, Wright DE, Davis BM. Overexpression of nerve growth factor in epidermis of transgenic mice causes hypertrophy of the peripheral nervous system. *J Neurosci* 1994;14:1422–1432.
29. LeMaster AM, Krimm RF, Davis BM, et al. Overexpression of brain-derived neurotrophic factor enhances sensory innervation and selectively increases neuron number. *J Neurosci* 1999;19:5919–5931.
30. Altman J, Bayer SA. The development of the rat spinal cord. *Adv Anat Embryol Cell Biol* 1984;85:1–164.
31. Bicknell HRJ, Beal JA. Axonal and dendritic development of substantia gelatinosa neurons in the lumbosacral spinal cord of the rat. *J Comp Neurol* 1984; 226:508–522.
32. Pignatelli D, Ribeiro-da-Silva A, Coimbra A. Postnatal maturation of primary afferent terminations in the substantia gelatinosa of the rat spinal cord. An electron microscopic study. *Brain Res* 1989;491:33–44.
33. Knyihar-Csillik E, Rakic P, Csillik B. Development of glomerular synaptic complexes and immunohistochemical differentiation in the superficial dorsal horn of the embryonic primate spinal cord. *Anat Embryol* 1999;199:125–148.
34. Fitzgerald M, Swett J. The termination pattern of sciatic nerve afferents in the substantia gelatinosa of neonatal rats. *Neurosci Lett* 1983;43:149–154.
35. Fitzgerald M. The post-natal development of cutaneous afferent fibre input and receptive field organization in the rat dorsal horn. *J Physiol* 1985;364:1–18.
36. Fitzgerald M, Butcher T, Shortland P. Developmental changes in the laminar termination of A fibre cutaneous sensory afferents in the rat spinal cord dorsal horn. *J Comp Neurol* 1994;348:225–233.
37. Fitzgerald M. The prenatal growth of fine diameter afferents into the rat spinal cord—a transganglionic study. *J Comp Neurol* 1987;261:98–104.
38. Coggeshall RE, Jennings EA, Fitzgerald M. Evidence that large myelinated primary afferent fibers make synaptic contacts in lamina II of neonatal rats. *Brain Res Dev Brain Res* 1996;92:81–90.
39. Shortland P, Fitzgerald M. Neonatal sciatic nerve section results in a rearrangement of the central terminals of saphenous and axotomized sciatic nerve afferents in the dorsal horn of the spinal cord of the adult rat. *Eur J Neurosci* 1994;6:75–86.
40. Torsney C, Meredith-Middleton J, Fitzgerald M. Neonatal capsaicin treatment prevents the normal postnatal withdrawal of A fibres from lamina II without affecting Fos responses to innocuous peripheral stimulation. *Brain Res Dev Brain Res* 2000;121:55–65.
41. Jennings E, Fitzgerald M. Postnatal changes in responses of rat dorsal horn cells to afferent stimulation: a fibre-induced sensitization. *J Physiol (Lond)* 1998; 509:859–868.
42. Park JS, Nakatsuka T, Nagata K, et al. Reorganization of the primary afferent termination in the rat spinal dorsal horn during post-natal development. *Brain Res Dev Brain Res* 1999;113:29–36.
43. Jennings E, Fitzgerald M. C-fos can be induced in the neonatal rat spinal cord by both noxious and innocuous peripheral stimulation. *Pain* 1996;68:301–306.
44. Fitzgerald M, Jennings E. The postnatal development of spinal sensory processing. *Proc Natl Acad Sci U S A* 1999;96:7719–7722.
45. Fitzgerald M. The development of activity evoked by fine diameter cutaneous fibres in the spinal cord of the newborn rat. *Neurosci Lett* 1988;86:161–166.
46. Nakatsuka T, Ataka T, Kumamoto E, et al. Alteration in synaptic inputs through C afferent fibers to substantia gelatinosa neurons of the rat spinal dorsal horn during postnatal development. *Neuroscience* 2000;99: 549–556.
47. Akagi H, Konishi S, Yanagisawa M, et al. Effects of capsaicin and a substance P antagonist on a slow reflex in the isolated rat spinal cord. *Neurochem Res* 1983;8: 795–796.
48. Li P, Wilding TJ, Kim SJ, et al. Kainate-receptor-mediated sensory synaptic transmission in mammalian spinal cord. *Nature* 1999;397:161–164.
49. Akesson E, Kjaeldgaard A, Samuelsson EB, et al. Ionotropic glutamate receptor expression in human spinal cord during first trimester development. *Brain Res Dev Brain Res* 2000;119:55–63.
50. Jakowec MW, Fox AJ, Martin LJ, et al. Quantitative and qualitative changes in AMPA receptor expression during spinal cord development. *Neuroscience* 1995; 67:893–907.
51. Jakowec MW, Yen L, Kalb RG. In situ hybridization analysis of AMPA receptor subunit gene expression in the developing rat spinal cord. *Neuroscience* 1995;67: 909–920.
52. Watanabe M, Mishina M, Inoue Y. Distinct spatiotemporal expressions of five NMDA receptor channel subunit mRNAs in the cerebellum. *J Comp Neurol* 1994; 343:513–519.
53. Price DD. Psychological and neural mechanisms of the affective dimension of pain. *Science* 2000;288: 1769–1772.
54. Davis KD, Kwan CL, Crawley AP, et al. Functional MRI study of thalamic and cortical activations evoked by cutaneous heat, cold, and tactile stimuli. *Journal of Neurophysiology* 1998;80:1533–1546.
55. Erzurumlu RS, Jhaveri S. Thalamic axons confer a blueprint of the sensory periphery onto the developing rat somatosensory cortex. *Brain Res Dev Brain Res* 1990;56:229–234.
56. Isaac JT, Nicoll RA, Malenka RC. Silent glutamatergic

synapses in the mammalian brain. *Can J Physiol Pharmacol* 1999;77:735–737.
57. Thairu BK. Post-natal changes in the somaesthetic evoked potentials in the albino rat. *Nat New Biol* 1971; 231:30–31.
58. Armstrong-James M. The functional status and columnar organization of single cells responding to cutaneous stimulation in neonatal rat somatosensory cortex S1. *J Physiol* 1975;246:501–538.
59. Mrzljak L, Uylings HB, Kostovic I, et al. Prenatal development of neurons in the human prefrontal cortex: I. A qualitative Golgi study. *J Comp Neurol* 1988;271: 355–386.
60. Huttenlocher PR, de Courten C, Garey LJ, et al. Synaptogenesis in the human visual cortex—evidence for synapse elimination during normal development. *Neurosci Lett* 1982;33:247–252.
61. Klimach VJ, Cooke RW. Maturation of the neonatal somatosensory evoked response in preterm infants. *Dev Med Child Neurol* 1988;30:208–214.
62. Butterworth JFT, Strichartz GR. Molecular mechanisms of local anesthesia: a review. *Anesthesiology* 1990;72:711–734.
63. Benzon HT, Strichartz GR, Gissen AJ, et al. Developmental neurophysiology of mammalian peripheral nerves and age-related differential sensitivity to local anaesthetic. *Br J Anaesth* 1988;61:754–760.
64. Abajian JC, Mellish RW, Browne AF, et al. Spinal anesthesia for surgery in the high-risk infant. *Anesth Analg* 1984;63:359–362.
65. Howard RF, Hatch DJ, Cole TJ, et al. Inflammatory pain and hypersensitivity are selectively reversed by epidural bupivacaine and are developmentally regulated. *Anesthesiology* 2001;95:421–427.
66. Berde CB. Toxicity of local anesthetics in infants and children. *J Pediatr* 1993;122:S14–S20.
67. Taddio A, Ohlsson A, Einarson TR, et al. A systematic review of lidocaine-prilocaine cream (EMLA) in the treatment of acute pain in neonates. *Pediatrics* 1998; 101:E1.
68. Jain A, Rutter N. Local anaesthetic effect of topical amethocaine gel in neonates: randomised controlled trial. *Arch Dis Child Fetal Neonatal Ed* 2000;82: F42–F45.
69. Larsson BA, Jylli L, Lagercrantz H, et al. Does a local anaesthetic cream (EMLA) alleviate pain from heel-lancing in neonates? *Acta Anaesthesiol Scand* 1995; 39:1028–1031.
70. Cervero F, Laird JM. From acute to chronic pain: mechanisms and hypotheses. *Prog Brain Res* 1996; 110:3–15.
71. Andrews K, Fitzgerald M. Wound sensitivity as a measure of analgesic effects following surgery in human neonates and infants. *Pain* 2002, *in press*.
72. Guy ER, Abbott FV. The behavioral response to formalin in preweanling rats. *Pain* 1992;51:81–90.
73. Teng CJ, Abbott FV. The formalin test: a dose-response analysis at three developmental stages. *Pain* 1998;76: 337–347.
74. Marsh D, Dickenson A, Hatch D, et al. Epidural opioid analgesia in infant rats II: responses to carrageenan and capsaicin. *Pain* 1999;82:33–38.
75. Jiang MC, Gebhart GF. Development of mustard oil-induced hyperalgesia in rats. *Pain* 1998;77:305–313.
76. De Lima J, Hatch D, Fitzgerald M. The postnatal development of ketamine analgesia—an electrophysiological study in rat pups. *Proceedings of the IXth World Congress on Pain*. Seattle: IASP Press, 2000:411.
77. Torsney C, Fitzgerald M. Electrophysiological properties of neonatal dorsal horn neurons following peripheral inflammation. *Eur J Neurosci* 2000;12:S11.
78. Woolf CJ, Costigan M. Transcriptional and posttranslational plasticity and the generation of inflammatory pain. *Proc Natl Acad Sci U S A* 1999;96:7723–7730.
79. Yaksh TL. Spinal systems and pain processing: development of novel analgesic drugs with mechanistically defined models. *Trends Pharmacol Sci* 1999;20: 329–337.
80. Koltzenburg M, Bennett DL, Shelton DL, et al. Neutralization of endogenous NGF prevents the sensitization of nociceptors supplying inflamed skin. *Eur J Neurosci* 1999;11:1698–1704.
81. Woolf CJ, Shortland P, Sivilotti LG. Sensitization of high mechanothreshold superficial dorsal horn and flexor motor neurones following chemosensitive primary afferent activation. *Pain* 1994;58:141–155.
82. Woolf CJ, Mannion RJ. Neuropathic pain: aetiology, symptoms, mechanisms, and management. *Lancet* 1999; 353:1959–1964.
83. Dubner R, Ruda MA. Activity-dependent neuronal plasticity following tissue injury and inflammation. *Trends Neurosci* 1992;15:96–103.
84. Dickenson AH. Mechanisms of central hypersensitivity. In: Besson J-M, Dickenson AH eds. *Handbook of experimental pharmacology*. Berlin: Springer-Verlag, 1997:168–210.
85. De Felipe C, Herrero JF, O'Brien JA, et al. Altered nociception, analgesia and aggression in mice lacking the receptor for substance P. *Nature* 1998;392:394–397.
86. Cao YQ, Mantyh PW, Carlson EJ, et al. Primary afferent tachykinins are required to experience moderate to intense pain. *Nature* 1998;392:390–394.
87. Woolf CJ, Salter MW. Neuronal plasticity: increasing the gain in pain. *Science* 2000;288:1765–1769.
88. Neumann S, Doubell TP, Leslie T, et al. Inflammatory pain hypersensitivity mediated by phenotypic switch in myelinated primary sensory neurons. *Nature* 1996; 384:360–364.
89. Ji RR, Baba H, Brenner GJ, et al. Nociceptive-specific activation of ERK in spinal neurons contributes to pain hypersensitivity. *Nat Neurosci* 1999;2:1114–1119.
90. Ren K, Dubner R. Enhanced descending modulation of nociception in rats with persistent hindpaw inflammation. *J Neurophysiol* 1996;76:3025–3037.
91. Sivilotti LG, Gerber G, Rawat B, et al. Morphine selectively depresses the slowest, NMDA-independent component of C-fibre-evoked synaptic activity in the rat spinal cord in vitro. *Eur J Neurosci* 1995;7:12–18.
92. Petralia RS, Esteban JA, Wang YX, et al. Selective acquisition of AMPA receptors over postnatal development suggests a molecular basis for silent synapses. *Nat Neurosci* 1999;2:31–36.
93. Baba H, Doubell TP, Moore KA, et al. Silent NMDA receptor-mediated synapses are developmentally regulated in the dorsal horn of the rat spinal cord. *J Neurophysiol* 2000;83:955–962.
94. Bardoni R, Magherini PC, MacDermott AB. Activation of NMDA receptors drives action potentials in superficial dorsal horn from neonatal rats. *Neuroreport* 2000;11:1721–1727.

95. Gonzalez DL, Fuchs JL, Droge MH. Distribution of NMDA receptor binding in developing mouse spinal cord. *Neurosci Lett* 1993;151:134–137.
96. Hori Y, Kanda K. Developmental alterations in NMDA receptor-mediated [Ca2+]i elevation in substantia gelatinosa neurons of neonatal rat spinal cord. *Brain Res Dev Brain Res* 1994;80:141–148.
97. Audinat E, Lambolez B, Rossier J, et al. Activity-dependent regulation of N-methyl-D-aspartate receptor subunit expression in rat cerebellar granule cells. *Eur J Neurosci* 1994;6:1792–1800.
98. Kar S, Quirion R. Neuropeptide receptors in developing and adult rat spinal cord: an in vitro quantitative autoradiography study of calcitonin gene-related peptide, neurokinins, mu-opioid, galanin, somatostatin, neurotensin and vasoactive intestinal polypeptide receptors. *J Comp Neurol* 1995;354:253–281.
99. Nagy I, Miller BA, Woolf CJ. NK1 and NK2 receptors contribute to C-fibre evoked slow potentials in the spinal cord. *Neuroreport* 1994;5:2105–2108.
100. Fitzgerald M. Neonatal pharmacology of pain. In: J-M B, AH D, eds. *The pharmacology of pain*. Berlin: Springer-Verlag, 1997:447–465.
101. Beland B, Fitzgerald M. Influence of peripheral inflammation on the postnatal maturation of primary sensory neuron phenotype in rats. *J Pain* 2000;2:36–45.
102. Dubner R, Ren K. Endogenous mechanisms of sensory modulation. *Pain* 1999;6[Suppl]:S45–S54.
103. Fitzgerald M. The development of descending brainstem control of spinal cord sensory processing. In: Hanson MA, ed. *The fetal and neonatal brainstem*. Cambridge: Cambridge University Press, 1991:127–136.
104. Weber ED, Stelzner DJ. Behavioural effects of spinal cord transection in the developing rat. *Brain Res* 1977; 125:241–255.
105. Fitzgerald M, Koltzenburg M. The functional development of descending inhibitory pathways in the dorsolateral funiculus of the newborn rat spinal cord. *Brain Res* 1986;389:261–270.
106. Boucher T, Jennings E, Fitzgerald M. The onset of diffuse noxious inhibitory controls in postnatal rat pups: a C-Fos study. *Neurosci Lett* 1998;257:9–12.
107. Cervero F, Plenderleith MB. C-fibre excitation and tonic descending inhibition of dorsal horn neurones in adult rats treated at birth with capsaicin. *J Physiol* 1985;365:223–237.
108. van Praag H, Frenk H. The development of stimulation-produced analgesia (SPA) in the rat. *Brain Res Dev Brain Res* 1991;64:71–76.
109. Kehlet H, Werner M, Perkins F. Balanced analgesia: what is it and what are its advantages in postoperative pain? *Drugs* 1999;58:793–797.
110. Nagy I, Rang HP. Similarities and differences between the responses of rat sensory neurons to noxious heat and capsaicin. *J Neurosci* 1999;19:10647–10655.
111. Koppert W, Ostermeier N, Sittl R, et al. Low-dose lidocaine reduces secondary hyperalgesia by a central mode of action. *Pain* 2000;85:217–224.
112. Marhofer P, Krenn CG, Plochl W, et al. S(+)-ketamine for caudal block in pediatric anaesthesia. *Br J Anaesth* 2000;84:341–345.
113. Cook B, Grubb DJ, Aldridge LA, et al. Comparison of the effects of adrenaline, clonidine and ketamine on the duration of caudal analgesia produced by bupivacaine in children. *Br J Anaesth* 1995;75:698–701.
114. Johnston P, Findlow D, Aldridge LM, et al. The effect of ketamine on 0.25% and 0.125% bupivacaine for caudal epidural blockade in children. *Paediatr Anaesth* 1999;9:31–34.
115. Nishina K, Mikawa K, Shiga M, et al. Clonidine in paediatric anaesthesia. *Paediatr Anaesth* 1999;9:187–202.
116. Walson PD, Mortensen ME. Pharmacokinetics of common analgesics, anti-inflammatories and antipyretics in children. *Clin Pharmacokinet* 1989;17 [Suppl 1]:116–137.
117. Anderson BJ. What we don't know about paracetamol in children. *Paediatr Anaesth* 1998;8:451–460.
118. Hansen TG, O'Brien K, Morton NS, et al. Plasma paracetamol concentrations and pharmacokinetics following rectal administration in neonates and young infants. *Acta Anaesthesiol Scand* 1999;43:855–859.
119. van Lingen RA, Deinum JT, Quak JM, et al. Pharmacokinetics and metabolism of rectally administered paracetamol in preterm neonates. *Arch Dis Child Fetal Neonatal Ed* 1999;80:F59–F63.
120. van Lingen RA, Deinum HT, Quak CM, et al. Multiple-dose pharmacokinetics of rectally administered acetaminophen in term infants. *Clin Pharmacol Ther* 1999;66:509–515.
121. Hynson JL, South M. Childhood hepatotoxicity with paracetamol doses less than 150 mg/kg per day. *Med J Aust* 1999;171:497.
122. Shah V, Taddio A, Ohlsson A. Randomised controlled trial of paracetamol for heel prick pain in neonates. *Arch Dis Child Fetal Neonatal Ed* 1998;79:F209–F211.
123. Tobias JD, Lowe S, Hersey S, et al. Analgesia after bilateral myringotomy and placement of pressure equalization tubes in children: acetaminophen versus acetaminophen with codeine. *Anesth Analg* 1995;81: 496–500.
124. Semple D, Russell S, Doyle E, et al. Comparison of morphine sulphate and codeine phosphate in children undergoing adenotonsillectomy. *Paediatr Anaesth* 1999;9:135–138.
125. William DG, Hatch DJ, Howard RF. Codeine phosphate in paediatric medicine. *Br J Anaesth* 2001;86: 413–421.
126. Porter FL, Grunau RE, Anand KJ. Long-term effects of pain in infants. *J Dev Behav Pediatr* 1999;20: 253–261.
127. Fitzgerald M, Millard C, MacIntosh N. Hyperalgesia in premature infants. *Lancet* 1988;1:292.
128. Fitzgerald M, Millard C, McIntosh N. Cutaneous hypersensitivity following peripheral tissue damage in newborn infants and its reversal with topical anaesthesia. *Pain* 1989;39:31–36.
129. Johnston CC, Stevens BJ. Experience in a neonatal intensive care unit affects pain response. *Pediatrics* 1996;98:925–930.
130. Taddio A, Katz J, Ilersich AL, et al. Effect of neonatal circumcision on pain response during subsequent routine vaccination. *Lancet* 1997;349:599–603.
131. Walco GA, Dampier CD, Harstein G, et al. The relationship between recurrent clinical pain and pain threshold in children. In: Tyler DC, Krane EJ, eds. *Advances in pain research and therapy: volume 15: pediatric pain*. New York: Raven Press, 1990:333–340.
132. Hogeweg JA, Kuis W, Oostendorp RA, et al. General and segmental reduced pain thresholds in juvenile chronic arthritis. *Pain* 1995;62:11–17.

133. Anand KJ, Coskun V, Thrivikraman KV, et al. Long-term behavioral effects of repetitive pain in neonatal rat pups. *Physiol Behav* 1999;66:627–637.
134. Reynolds ML, Fitzgerald M. Long-term sensory hyperinnervation following neonatal skin wounds. *J Comp Neurol* 1995;358:487–498.
135. Alvares D, Torsney C, Beland B, et al. Modelling the prolonged effects of neonatal pain. *Prog Brain Res* 2000;129;365–373.
136. De Lima J, Alvares D, Hatch DJ, et al. Sensory hyperinnervation after neonatal skin wounding: effect of bupivacaine sciatic nerve block. *Br J Anaesth* 1999;83: 662–664.
137. Constantinou J, Reynolds ML, Woolf CJ, et al. Nerve growth factor levels in developing rat skin: upregulation following skin wounding. *Neuroreport* 1994;5: 2281–2284.
138. Reynolds M, Alvares D, Middleton J, et al. Neonatally wounded skin induces NGF-independent sensory neurite outgrowth in vitro. *Brain Res Dev Brain Res* 1997; 102:275–283.
139. Ernfors P, Wetmore C, Olson L, et al. Cells expressing mRNA for neurotrophins and their receptors during embryonic rat development. *Eur J Neurosci* 1992;4: 1140–1158.
140. Whitby DJ, Ferguson MW. Immunohistochemical localization of growth factors in fetal wound healing. *Dev Biol* 1991;147:207–215.
141. Grunau RV, Whitfield MF, Petrie JH, et al. Early pain experience, child and family factors, as precursors of somatization: a prospective study of extremely premature and fullterm children. *Pain* 1994;56:353–359.
142. Grunau RV, Whitfield MF, Petrie JH. Pain sensitivity and temperament in extremely low-birth-weight premature toddlers and preterm and full-term controls. *Pain* 1994;58:341–346.
143. Dickenson AH, Sullivan AF. Peripheral origins and central modulation of subcutaneous formalin-induced activity of rat dorsal horn neurons following peripheral inflammation. *Neurosci Lett* 1987;83:207–211.
144. Gracely RH, Lynch SA, Bennett GJ. Painful neuropathy: altered central processing maintained dynamically by peripheral input [published erratum appears in *Pain* 1993;52:251–3]. *Pain* 1992;51:175–194.
145. Coderre TJ, Melzack R. The role of NMDA receptor-operated calcium channels in persistent nociception after formalin induced tissue injury. *J Neurosci* 1992; 12:3671–3675.
146. Cellerino A, Maffei L. The action of neurotrophins in the development and plasticity of the visual cortex. *Prog Neurobiol* 1996;49:53–71.
147. Fox K, Daw NW. Do NMDA receptors have a critical function in visual cortical plasticity? *Trends Neurosci* 1993;16:116–122.
148. Miller KD, Keller JB, Stryker MP. Ocular dominance column development: analysis and simulation. *Science* 1989;245:605–615.
149. Schlaggar BL, Fox K, O'Leary DD. Postsynaptic control of plasticity in developing somatosensory cortex. *Nature* 1993;364:623–626.
150. Gu GA, Bear MF, Singer W. Blockade of NMDA receptors prevents ocularity changes in kitten visual cortex after reversed monocular deprivation. *Brain Res Dev Brain Res* 1989;47:281–288.
151. Beggs SA, Aynsley-Green A, Wood JN, et al. Withdrawal of A fibres from substantia gelatinosa during normal postnatal development is an activity-dependent process. *Soc Neurosci* 1999;25:222.
152. Bear MF, Cooper LN, Ebner FF. A physiological basis for a theory of synapse modification. *Science* 1987; 237:42–48.
153. Katz LC, Shatz CJ. Synaptic activity and the construction of cortical circuits. *Science* 1996;274:1133–1138.
154. Durand GM, Kovalchuk Y, Konnerth A. Long-term potentiation and functional synapse induction in developing hippocampus. *Nature* 1996;381:71–75.
155. Ambalavanan N, Carlo WA. Analgesia for ventilated neonates: where do we stand? *J Pediatr* 1999;135: 403–404.
156. Marsh DF, Hatch DJ, Fitzgerald M. Opioid systems and the newborn. *Br J Anaesth* 1997;79:787–795.
157. Kart T, Christrup LL, Rasmussen M. Recommended use of morphine in neonates, infants and children based on a literature review: part 1—pharmacokinetics. *Paediatr Anaesth* 1997;7:5–11.
158. Kart T, Christrup LL, Rasmussen M. Recommended use of morphine in neonates, infants and children based on a literature review: part 2—clinical use. *Paediatr Anaesth* 1997;7:93–101.
159. Rahman W, Dashwood MR, Fitzgerald M, et al. Postnatal development of multiple opioid receptors in the spinal cord and development of spinal morphine analgesia. *Brain Res Dev Brain Res* 1998;108:239–254.
160. De Lima J, Lloyd-Thomas A, Howard RF, et al. Infant and neonatal pain: anaesthetists' perceptions and prescribing patterns. *BMJ* 1996;313:787.
161. Marsh D, Dickenson A, Hatch D, et al. Epidural opioid analgesia in infant rats II: responses to carrageenan and capsaicin. *Pain* 1999;82:33 38.
162. Faber ES, Chambers JP, Brugger F, et al. Depression of A and C fibre-evoked segmental reflexes by morphine and clonidine in the in vitro spinal cord of the neonatal rat. *Br J Pharmacol* 1997;120:1390–1396.
163. Besse D, Lombard MC, Zajac JM. Pre- and postsynaptic distribution of mu, delta and kappa opioid receptors in the superficial layers of the cervical dorsal horn of the rat spinal cord. *Brain Res* 1990;521: 15–22.
164. Beland B, Fitzgerald M. Postnatal development of mu-opioid receptor expression in rat primary sensory neurons. *Pain* 2001;90:143–150.
165. Mao J, Price DD, Mayer DJ. Mechanisms of hyperalgesia and morphine tolerance: a current view of their possible interactions. *Pain* 1995;62:259–274.
166. Advokat C, Rhein FQ. Potentiation of morphine-induced antinociception in acute spinal rats by the NMDA antagonist dextrorphan. *Brain Res* 1995;699: 157–160.
167. Meert TF, De Kock M. Potentiation of the analgesic properties of fentanyl-like opioids with alpha 2-adrenoceptor agonists in rats. *Anesthesiology* 1994;81: 677–688.
168. Olsson G, Berde CB. Neuropathic pain in children and adolescents. In: Schechter N, Berde CB, Yaster M, eds. *Pain in infants, children and adolescents*. Baltimore: Williams & Wilkins: 1993:473–494
169. Wilkins KL, McGrath PJ, Finley GA, et al. Phantom limb sensations and phantom limb pain in child and adolescent amputees. *Pain* 1998;78:7–12.
170. Bennett GJ, Xie YK. A peripheral mononeuropathy in

rat that produces disorders of pain sensation like those seen in man. *Pain* 1988;33:87–107.
171. Seltzer Z, Dubner R, Shir Y. A novel behavioral model of neuropathic pain disorders produced in rats by partial sciatic nerve injury. *Pain* 1990;43:205–218.
172. Kim SH, Chung JM. An experimental model for peripheral neuropathy produced by segmental spinal nerve ligation in the rat. *Pain* 1992;50:355–363.
173. DeLeo JA, Coombs DW, Willenbring S, et al. Characterization of a neuropathic pain model: sciatic cryoneurolysis in the rat. *Pain* 1994;56:9–16.
174. Decosterd I, Woolf CJ. Spared nerve injury: an animal model of persistent peripheral neuropathic pain. *Pain* 2000;87:149–158.
175. Chung JM, Choi Y, Yoon YW, et al. Effects of age on behavioral signs of neuropathic pain in an experimental rat model. *Neurosci Lett* 1995;183:54–57.
176. Lee DH, Chung JM. Neuropathic pain in neonatal rats. *Neurosci Lett* 1996;209:140–142.
177. Bennett GJ. Update on the neurophysiology of pain transmission and modulation: focus on the NMDA-receptor. *J Pain Symptom Manage* 2000;19:S2–S6.
178. Hee HC, Lee DH, Chung JM. Characteristics of ectopic discharges in a rat neuropathic pain model. *Pain* 2000;84:253–261.
179. Cummins TR, Waxman SG. Downregulation of tetrodotoxin-resistant sodium currents and upregulation of a rapidly repriming tetrodotoxin-sensitive sodium current in small spinal sensory neurons after nerve injury. *J Neurosci* 1997;17:3503–3514.
180. Bondock AA, Sansone FM. Quantitative ultrastructural stereology of synapses in nucleus dorsalis after a peripheral nerve injury at birth. *Exp Neurol* 1984;86:331–341.
181. Yip HK, Rich KM, Lampe PA, et al. The effects of nerve growth factor and its antiserum on the postnatal development and survival after injury of sensory neurons in rat dorsal root ganglia. *J Neurosci* 1984;4: 2986–2992.
182. Himes BT, Tessler A. Death of some dorsal root ganglion neurons and plasticity of others following sciatic nerve section in adult and neonatal rats. *J Comp Neurol* 1989;284:215–230.
183. Cheema SS. Reducing p75 nerve growth factor receptor levels using antisense oligonucleotides prevents the loss of axotomized sensory neurons in the dorsal root ganglia of newborn rats. *J Neurosci Res* 1996;46:239–245.
184. Lewis SE, Mannion RJ, White FA, et al. A role for HSP27 in sensory neuron survival. *J Neurosci* 1999; 19:8945–8953.
185. Costigan M, Mannion RJ, Kendall G, et al. Heat shock protein 27: developmental regulation and expression after peripheral nerve injury. *J Neurosci* 1998;18: 5891–5900.
186. Aldskogius H, Risling M. Preferential loss of unmyelinated L7 dorsal root axons following sciatic nerve resection in kittens. *Brain Res* 1983;289:358–361.
187. Bondok AA, Sansone FM. Retrograde and transganglionic degeneration of sensory neurons after a peripheral nerve lesion at birth. *Exp Neurol* 1984;86: 322–330.
188. Fitzgerald M. The sprouting of saphenous nerve terminals in the spinal cord following early postnatal sciatic nerve section in the rat. *J Comp Neurol* 1985;240: 407–413.
189. Fitzgerald M, Woolf CJ, Shortland P. Collateral sprouting of the central terminals of cutaneous primary afferent neurons in the rat spinal cord: pattern, morphology, and influence of targets. *J Comp Neurol* 1990; 300:370–385.
190. Shortland P, Molander C, Woolf CJ, Fitzgerald M. Neonatal capsaicin treatment induces invasion of the substantia gelatinosa by the terminal arborizations of hair follicle afferents in the rat dorsal horn. *J Comp Neurol* 1990;296:23–31.
191. Kaas JH, Merzenich MM, Killackey HP. The reorganization of somatosensory cortex following peripheral nerve damage in adult and developing mammals. *Annu Rev Neurosci* 1983;6:325–356.
192. Killackey HP, Dawson DR. Expansion of the central hindpaw representation following fetal forelimb removal in the rat. *Eur J Neurosci* 1989;1:210–221.
193. Woolf CJ, Shortland P, Coggeshall RE. Peripheral nerve injury triggers central sprouting of myelinated afferents. *Nature* 1992;355:75–77.
194. Woolf CJ, Shortland P, Reynolds M. Reorganization of central terminals of myelinated primary afferents in the rat dorsal horn following peripheral axotomy. *J Comp Neurol* 1995;360:121–134.
195. Bardoni R, Magherini PC, MacDermott AB. NMDA EPSCs at glutamatergic synapses in the spinal cord dorsal horn of the postnatal rat. *J Neurosci* 1998;18: 6558–6567.
196. Laird JM, Bennett GJ. An electrophysiological study of dorsal horn neurons in the spinal cord of rats with experimental neuropathy. *J Neurophysiol* 1993;69: 2072–2085.
197. Chapman V, Suzuki R, Chamarette HL. Effects of systemic carbamazepine and gabapentin on spinal neuronal responses in spinal nerve ligated rats. *Pain* 1998; 75:261–272.
198. Eide K, Stubhaug A, Oye I, et al. Continuous subcutaneous administration of the N-methyl-D-aspartic acid receptor antagonist ketamine in the treatment of postherpetic neuralgia. *Pain* 1995;61:221–228.
199. Fields H, Rowbotham M. Multiple mechanisms of neuropathic pain: a clinical perspective. In: Gebhart G, et al., eds. *Progress in pain research and management*. Seattle: IASP Press, 1994:437–454.
200. Kingery WS. A critical review of controlled clinical trials for peripheral neuropathic pain and complex regional pain syndromes. *Pain* 1997;73:123–139.
201. Klepstad P, Borchgrevink PC. Four years treatment with ketamine and a trial of dextromethorphan in a patient with severe postherpetic neuralgia. *Acta Anesth Scand* 1997;41:422–426.
202. Suzuki R, Chapman V, Dickenson AH. The effectiveness of spinal and systemic morphine on rat dorsal horn neuronal responses in the spinal nerve ligation model of neuropathic pain. *Pain* 1999;80:215–228.
203. Rowbotham M, Harden N, Stacey B, et al. Gabapentin for the treatment of postherpetic neuralgia: a randomized controlled trial. *JAMA* 1998;280:1837–1842.
204. Collins JJ, Kerner J, Sentivany S, et al. Intravenous amitriptyline in pediatrics. *J Pain Symptom Manage* 1995;10:471–475.
205. McGraw T, Stacey BR. Gabapentin for treatment of neuropathic pain in a 12-year-old girl. *Clin J Pain* 1998;14:354–356.

3

The Human Developmental Neurophysiology of Pain

Katharine A. Andrews

There is still much to be discovered about the structural and functional development of the components of the nervous system concerned with pain processing in the human. Although there have been elegant studies on developing animals that have elucidated some of the elements underlying pain mechanisms, particularly at the level of the spinal cord (1–14), very little is known about how signals from painful stimuli are processed at higher levels, up to and including the cerebral cortex, in either animals or humans when they are very young. Neurophysiologic studies on human neonates and infants are technically difficult to perform, and ethically it is totally unacceptable to give children painful stimuli of any kind except through clinical necessity, such as a heel lance for required blood sampling (15). Therefore, as in the studies from our research group, inference has to be drawn by recording responses that are modulated by the presence of ongoing pain but that can be elicited using nonpainful stimuli, such as the flexion withdrawal reflex (15–19), and the abdominal skin reflex (ASR) (20,21).

Another problem is that evoked responses in neonates and infants, whether behavioral or more specifically neurophysiologic, are sometimes inconsistent and may fail altogether (22), the reliability of responses to stimuli being dependent on the type of response examined, the age of the subject, and the level of the nervous system from which that response emanates. For example, studies of changes in facial expression in human neonates in response to painful stimuli have demonstrated that the more preterm the infants being studied are, the less robust their responses are (23,24). This is because a fully developed facial response probably requires the presence of functional connections at higher levels of the nervous system than the spinal cord, and these connections may not be fully developed in the most preterm infants (25). It has been demonstrated in studies of motor cortex development in newborn human infants of less than 1 month postnatal age that the region for the face is the least differentiated (26,27). Furthermore, the outgrowth of corticospinal fibers caudally in the human fetus occurs latest for those fibers supplying innervation for face musculature (28).

Nevertheless, the development of neural function has been studied extensively in children using neurophysiologic approaches, and reflex studies have been particularly useful in gaining information in preverbal children (15–17,19,29–33). However, the emphasis in the greater proportion of published literature has been on the development of sensorimotor control (29–40), and less work has been published on the assessment of sensory function in children, using neurophysiologic methods (15–20,41–45).

WHAT REFLEXES TELL US ABOUT THE DEVELOPING NERVOUS SYSTEM

The study of reflexes has proved valuable in observing the development of pain mechanisms because it is possible to obtain objective, quantitative measurements of threshold (15–21) and other reflex parameters through electromyography (EMG) recordings (15,19). These measurements change according to stimulus type and intensity (15,19) and in the presence of tissue injury (15,17). Threshold changes also reflect alterations in cutaneous sensitivity owing to the application of topical local anaesthesia (46,47).

In addition, there are features common to cutaneous and proprioceptive reflexes in preverbal children that indicate how the nervous system behaves at this stage of development and therefore point to how painful inputs are processed. For example, studies in normal human infants have demonstrated exaggerated reflex responses (15,16,18,31,32), indicative of increased excitability in the developing nervous system. In the neonate, cutaneous reflexes elicited using individual nonnoxious electrical stimuli applied to the fingers produce such a strong reflex response that a synchronous muscle action potential is seen in both forearm flexor and extensor muscles, a response not seen in normal adults and older children (30,34).

Studies of the stretch reflex during development have revealed similar developmental changes. The threshold for eliciting the reflex is low in the newborn but increases over the first 6 years when it reaches adult values (32). The amplitude of the stretch reflex is also higher in the newborn than in adults (31). However, the most striking feature of the stretch reflex in the newborn (31,32,48) is that a tendon tap also causes excitation of both agonist and antagonist muscles in an almost synchronous EMG burst. In addition, stretch-evoked EMG responses are elicited in neonates from tapping sites not normally thought to excite muscle spindle afferents (31).

One reason for this may be that, at the level of the spinal cord, the connections necessary for the presence of these reflexes are fully functional but lack input from descending inhibitory fibers (8,30). Other reasons are discussed in the section on the flexion reflex. The fact that studies of reflex responses in the human neonate and infant indicate a higher level of excitability in the developing human nervous system has implications for the study of pain processing in this population. For example, the threshold for the flexion withdrawal reflex is much lower than that of the older child and adult (15,19), reflexes being evoked by nonnoxious and noxious stimuli. Therefore, it is sometimes difficult to separate neonatal and infant responses to pain from those to other stimuli.

Nevertheless, the advantage of using reflexes such as the cutaneous withdrawal reflex and the ASR is that they are relatively unaffected by factors such as hunger or stress and can be elicited equally well during regular sleep or quiet wakefulness (49). Both reflexes have been used successfully in the neonatal intensive care environment and postoperatively to yield information on human somatosensory development, with and without the presence of tissue injury consequent to intensive care or abdominal surgery (15–21).

THE FLEXION WITHDRAWAL REFLEX

In both preterm and full-term human neonates, the flexion withdrawal reflex can be evoked using low-intensity mechanical stimuli to the foot (16–18) and has a much lower threshold than the nociceptive flexion reflex in the adult human (RIII) (50). A low threshold reflex response to tactile stimulation has been reported in the adult (RII) (50), but it cannot be elicited with mechanical stimuli, only with a brief train of electrical stimuli (50,51). The threshold of the withdrawal reflex in the neonate rises with increasing postconceptional age (PCA) (15–18) and reflects the change from the predominant low-threshold A-fiber influence in the spinal cord dorsal horn early in development to increasing Aδ- and C-fiber convergence on dorsal horn neurons in the superficial laminae as development proceeds (52).

The threshold of the reflex in humans is significantly lowered in the presence of tissue injury of the type received during neonatal intensive care (15,17). It is also interesting to note that there is a large difference in threshold between those infants who receive intensive care and those who do not (18). In addition, the normal increase in flexion reflex threshold with postconceptional age does not occur in infants with substantial contralateral leg injury (Fig. 3.1) (15). Therefore, it seems possible to use withdrawal reflex threshold changes to monitor the effects of trauma on the developing somatosensory system.

Another feature of the cutaneous withdrawal reflex in human neonates less than 30 to 35 weeks PCA is the sensitization that occurs with repeated innocuous stimulation. This has been measured both by an increase in the amplitude and number of responses with decreasing PCA (Fig. 3.2) (15–18), and by a significant drop in threshold after repeated stimulation of 10% to 20% (18). Beyond approximately 35 weeks PCA, habituation to repeated innocuous stimulation occurs, characterized by a decrease in the number of responses and no drop in threshold on repeated stimulation (15,16,18). This is more akin to the habituation of withdrawal reflex responses seen in adults after repeated stimulation at regular intervals (53,54), although Hugon (50) reported that sensitization occurs in adults but only in response to noxious stimulation. The point of interest here is that, in the human neonate, nonnoxious stimulation produces sensitization. The sensitization of neonatal rat dorsal horn cells to repeated cutaneous A-fiber stimulation (13) is likely to be the mechanism underlying the sensitization of the flexion reflex in younger infants.

The receptive field for the withdrawal reflex in the human neonate occupies the same area as that of the flexor reflex in the adult cat and rat, extending from the toes to the top of the thigh and buttock (18,55,56). In the human neonate, as in the adult cat (55) and rat (56), there is also a graded distribution of thresholds within the receptive field, with a "hot spot" of maximum sensitivity on the plantar surface of the foot and a decrease in sensitivity progressing up the leg toward the knee (18). However, there is far more uniformity of threshold within the receptive field in the younger neonates (less than 35 weeks PCA), and, overall, the thresholds within the receptive field are lower in this age group (18).

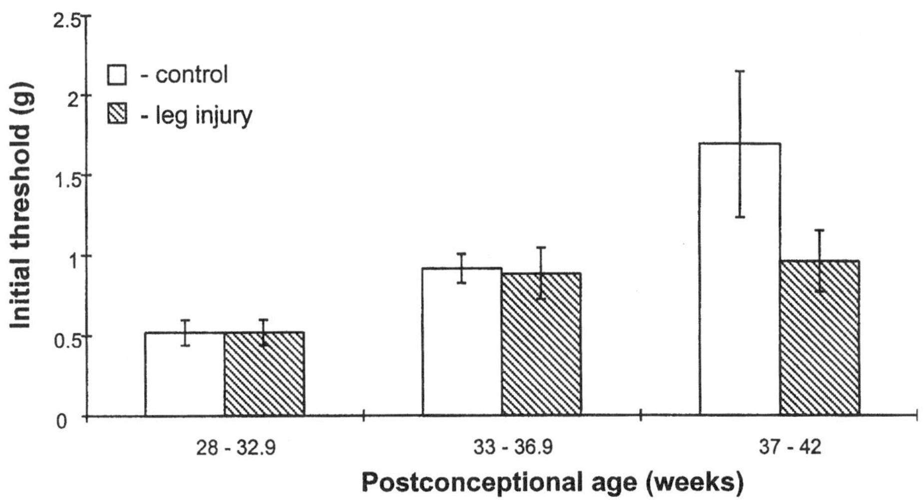

FIG. 3.1. Mean initial threshold for the mechanically evoked flexion reflex rises with postconceptional age in the control group (*plain bars*) (*p* = 0.027, one-way analysis of variance (ANOVA), n = 3, 24, and 9 for three age bands, respectively) but less markedly in the leg injury group (*hatched bars*) (*p* = 0.022, one-way ANOVA, n = 6, 7, and 6 for three age bands, respectively). Error bars denote standard error of the mean.

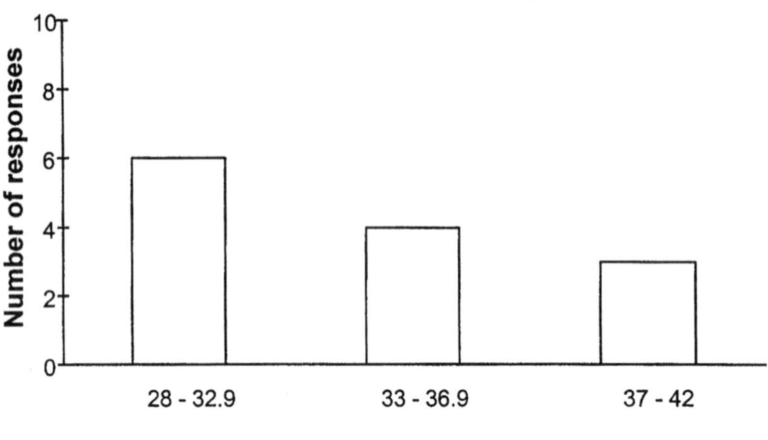

FIG. 3.2. Median number of responses to repeated mechanical stimulation at 2.8 × threshold decreases significantly relative to postconceptional age (p = 0.044, Kruskal–Wallis test, n = 8, 27, and 12 for three age groups, respectively).

In common with other reflexes in human neonates and infants, the spread of excitation of the flexion reflex is greater in the neonate than in the adult, an EMG response being seen in the tibialis anterior muscle as well as in biceps femoris muscle, the site at which it is usually recorded in the adult (19). The response in tibialis anterior muscle occurs at a shorter latency, and its area is larger than that observed in the biceps femoris muscle (Fig. 3.3) (19). This spread of excitation seems to underlie the positive Babinski response that is observed in the neonate (57) and in patients with paraparesis (53) or cerebral palsy (48). In all three instances, this may be because of incomplete descending inhibitory connections, particularly those of the corticospinal tract (14,58).

Despite all these indications of a higher level of excitability in the neonatal spinal cord, there is evidence that segmental, as opposed to descending, inhibitory mechanisms are well established. The withdrawal reflex in the human neonate is clearly inhibited by nonnoxious contralateral stimulation, even in infants from as young as 27.5 weeks PCA and onward (18). The responses are similar across all PCAs and up to full term. Contralateral inhibition has been clearly observed in spinal adult rats in response to both noxious stimuli involving Aδ and C fibers and nonnoxious stimuli involving Aβ fibers (59). The former type of inhibition appears to be more powerful in the adult (59), but this seems not to be the case in the neonate (18).

THE ABDOMINAL SKIN REFLEX

The use of reflexes to elucidate mechanisms of pain processing in neonates and infants has been extended to the study of abdominal sensitivity in infants after surgery, using the ASR (20,21). Postsurgical pain in children continues to be an issue because it remains undertreated despite improvements in pain treatment over the past decade (60).

Studies of pain and wound sensitivity after surgery in adults have determined sensory thresholds using von Frey hairs (61–63), pressure algometry (64–66), and electrical stimulation (67–71). Both decreased and increased sensory thresholds have been reported after surgery, which have been interpreted as indications of central sensitization (61,62, 64–66,68) or inhibition by analgesic agents and supraspinal inhibitory mechanism, respectively (67,69,70). Such studies in adults rely on verbal report, not possible in infant

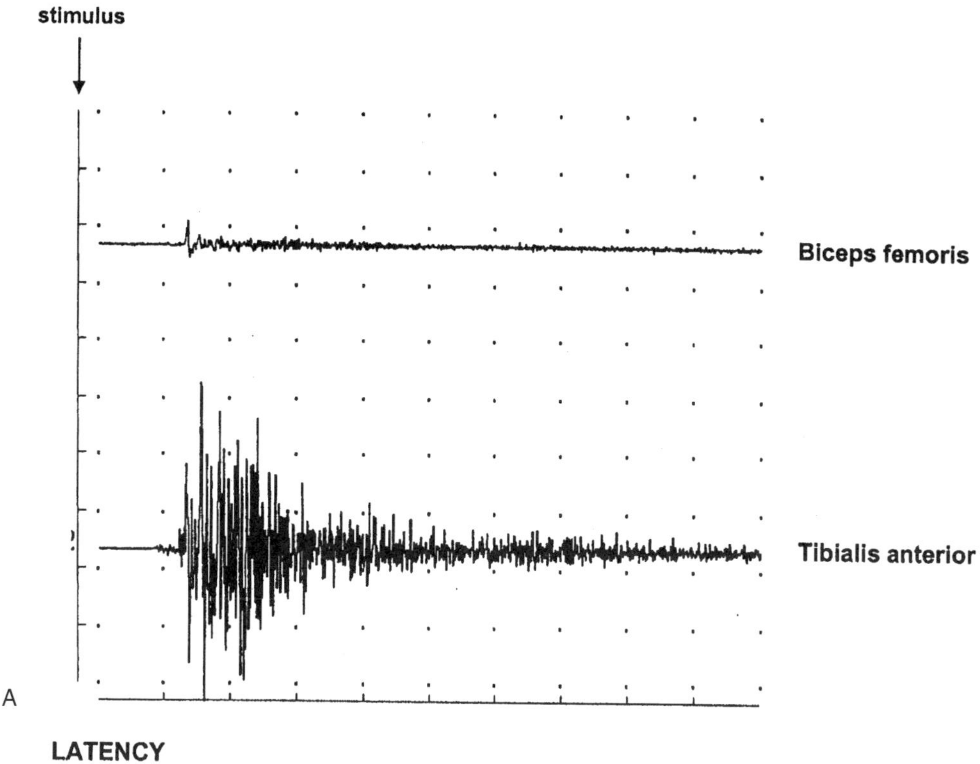

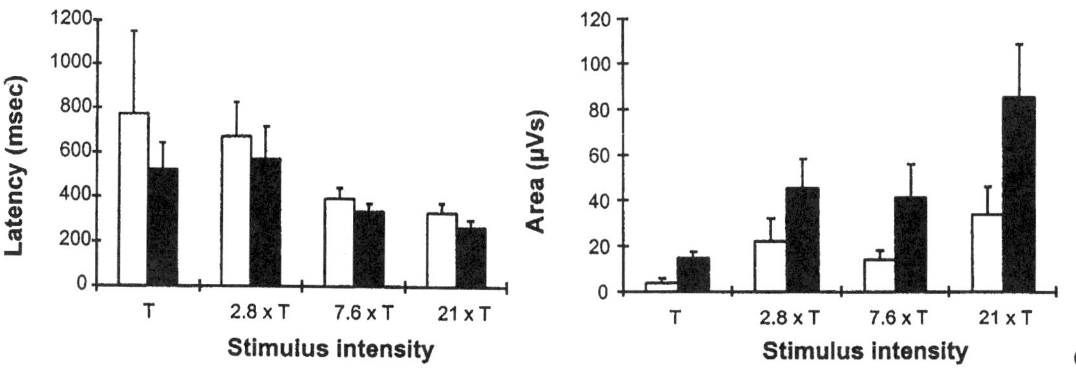

FIG. 3.3. A: Earlier and larger flexion reflex response in the tibialis anterior muscle (TA) (*bottom trace*) than in the biceps femoris muscle (BF) (*top trace*) to mechanical stimulation at 7.6 × threshold in an infant of 36.86 weeks postconceptional age. The increased amplitude and duration of the response in tibialis anterior muscle are not owing to movement artifact but to greater electromyographic activity. Vertical calibration per division 100 µV, horizontal calibration per division 500 milliseconds, sweep speed 5 seconds. The stimulus occurred at the beginning of the sweep. **B and C:** Flexion reflex stimulus–response characteristics in BF and TA over four levels of mechanical stimulation. There was a tendency for the latency of the response to be shorter in the TA than in the BF, although this did not reach statistical significance [p = 0.097, three-factor analysis of variance (ANOVA) allowing for repeated measures]. However, the area of the response was significantly larger in the TA than in the BF (p = 0.001, three-factor ANOVA allowing for repeated measures). *Plain bars* indicate mean responses in the BF; *filled bars* indicate mean responses in the TA; error bars denote standard error of the mean; n = 8.

populations, which is why the ASR has been developed as a quantitative measure of abdominal skin wound sensitivity.

Studies on this reflex in adults have shown it to be a protective reflex of the trunk that protects the abdominal organs from impact (72). It shares a number of features with the flexion withdrawal reflex, the first being that, although more reliably evoked by painful stimulation of the abdomen, it can also be elicited by innocuous stimuli such as touch (72,73). Before our recent studies (20,21), the ASR threshold had never been quantified in infants, but previous work suggested that it might be lower in neonates and infants, again possibly because of the lack of descending inhibitory connections from the brain in infancy (74,75). Also, in common with other reflexes at this age (32,48), reflex radiation to the flexor muscles of the thigh has been observed, whereby a contraction of the abdominal muscles is accompanied by either bilateral or unilateral hip flexion, not seen in adults except those with transverse lesions of the spinal cord (74).

The ASR threshold is clearly developmentally regulated (21), there being a rise in threshold with increasing PCA, similar to that seen in the cutaneous flexion reflex of the leg over a similar time period (Fig. 3.4) (15,16,18), particularly the sharp rise in threshold occurring at approximately 37 weeks (18). As observed by previous investigators, a decrease in ASR radiation with increasing PCA was shown (74), bilateral hip flexion being replaced by unilateral hip flexion, and subsequently no hip flexion, with the progression from neonatal period to infancy (Fig. 3.5) (21).

These developmental changes in ASR properties are likely to reflect alterations in spinal cord connectivity during this period. Studies in the newborn rat have shown that low-threshold Aβ afferent fibers terminate

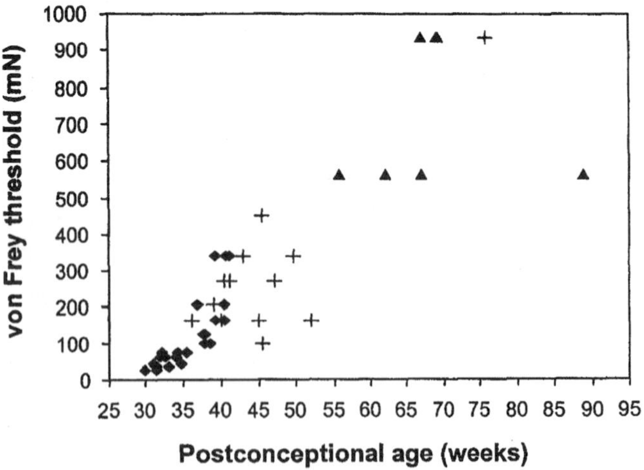

FIG. 3.4. Abdominal skin reflex (ASR) threshold rises with increasing postconceptional age (PCA). ASR thresholds in response to punctate von Frey hair stimulation in infants of 30 to 42 weeks PCA not undergoing surgery (n = 25) (*diamonds*, mean of both sides), infants of 36 to 75.86 weeks PCA before undergoing herniotomy (n = 13) (+, mean of both sides), and infants of 55.71 to 89 weeks PCA before undergoing pyeloplasty (n = 7) (*triangles*, naïve side). There is a significant rise in ASR threshold with increasing age ($p = 0.00$, F = 144.31, df = 1, regression analysis). The average of the two sides was taken for the infants not undergoing surgery and infants before undergoing herniotomy because there was no significant difference between sides for these two groups ($p = 0.82$, t = 0.22 and $p = 0.84$, t = 0.21, respectively, two-sample *t* test). There are some overlapping data points in this figure, which is why the full number of thresholds appears not to be visible.

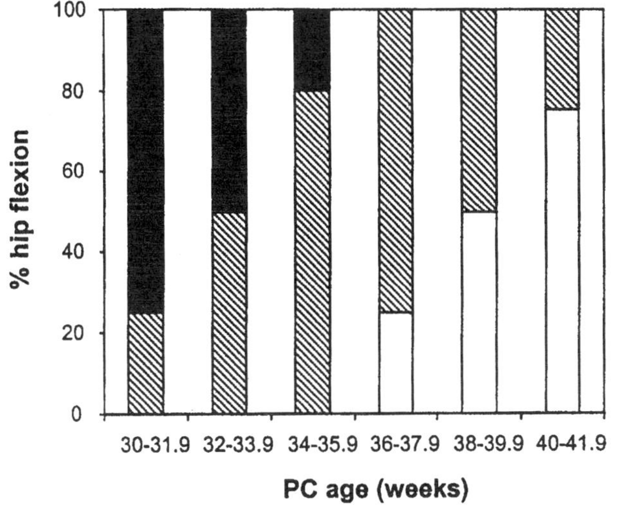

FIG. 3.5. The incidence of hip flexion decreases with increasing postconceptional age (PCA) in infants not undergoing surgery. The percentage of incidence of either bilateral (*solid bars*), unilateral (*hatched bars*), or no (*plain bars*) hip flexion, accompanying the abdominal skin reflex in infants not undergoing surgery grouped into 2-week age bands from 30 to 42 weeks PCA (n = 25). There is a significant decrease in bilateral hip flexion and then in unilateral hip flexion and a significant increase in no hip flexion with age ($p = 0.00$, df = 1, ordinal logistic regression).

more superficially in the substantia gelatinosa of the neonatal dorsal horn (9), which may allow them to activate cells that only have a high-threshold input in the adult (12,13). Cutaneous mechanical receptive fields for neonatal flexion reflexes (10,18) and dorsal horn cells (2,52) are also larger and less organized than in the adult. There is also evidence in the embryonic rat (75) and chick (76,77) of exuberant monosynaptic projections of muscle afferents to motor neurons innervating synergistic and even antagonistic muscle groups, which may also contribute to reflex radiation in infancy. Immaturity of descending inhibitory pathways is also likely to play an important part (8,57,74) because radiation of the ASR to the flexor muscles of the thigh reappears in adults with transverse lesions of the spinal cord (74).

A large postsurgical drop in threshold was also observed in both operation groups studied, herniotomy and pyeloplasty (as much as 78%) (Fig. 3.6) (21), which was maximal 1 to 3 hours after surgery, indicating that infants are clearly more sensitive in the wound area. This is similar to the lowering of flexion withdrawal reflex thresholds observed in human infants after repeated heel lancing (17) and with tissue damage to the leg after long-term intensive care (15) and reflects the sensitivity of damaged skin. It is also analogous to the sensory changes, including tenderness and pain, seen in adult human subjects after experimental tissue injury (78,79). Perhaps surprisingly, sensitivity in the wound area in the surgical infants in this study occurred even in the presence of intra- and postoperative analgesia (21). Several studies in adults also reported a drop in von Frey pricking pain threshold (61–63) and pressure pain threshold (64,66) around surgical wounds and also showed that various analgesic regimes are insufficient to prevent the initial postsurgical drop in threshold. In the ASR study, a significant increase in threshold 6 to 8 hours after herniotomy was seen only if analgesia had been given within the previous 2 hours and in infants who underwent pyeloplasty who were receiving ongoing intravenous analgesia with morphine.

A significant drop in ASR threshold is seen at the same segmental level on the contralateral side of the abdomen 1 to 3 hours after surgery and also 6 to 8 hours after surgery in infants who underwent herniotomy to whom no recent analgesia has been given (21). This is further evidence of changes in sensory processing at the spinal cord level because the threshold drop was remote from the site of injury (80) and indicates that the tenderness

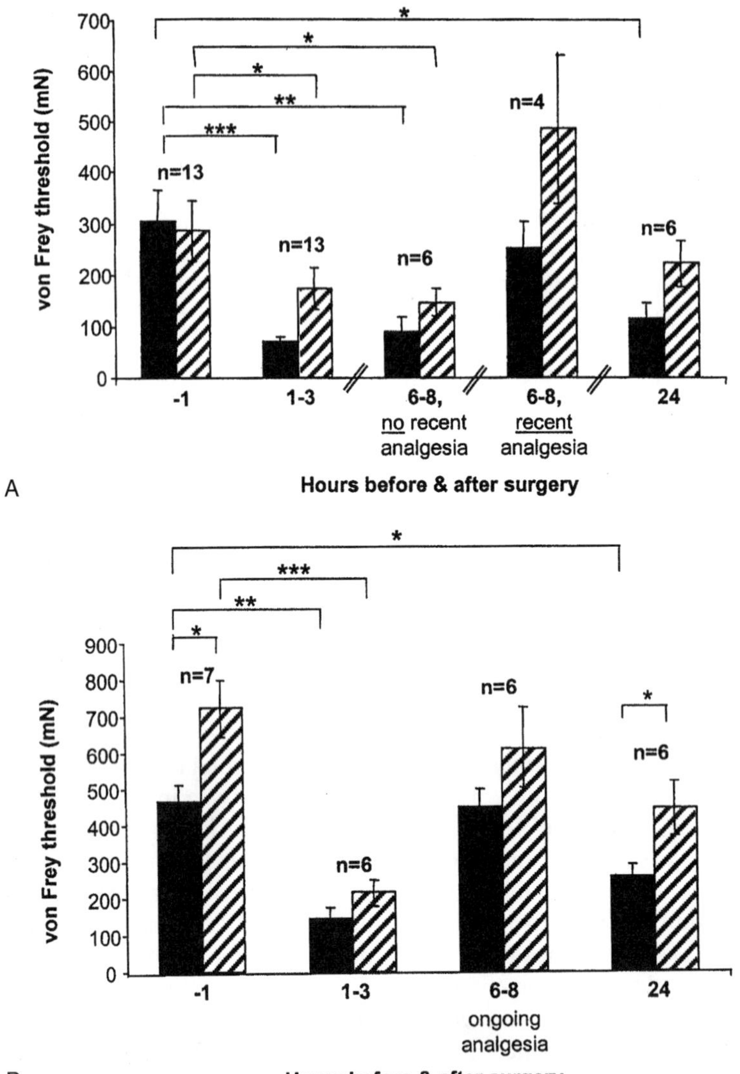

FIG. 3.6. Significant drop in abdominal skin reflex (ASR) threshold after surgery. Mean ASR thresholds from the surgical side (*solid bars*) and the contralateral naïve side (*hatched bars*) of the abdomen in infants who underwent unilateral herniotomy, aged 36 to 75.86 weeks PCA **(A)** and unilateral pyeloplasty, aged 55.71 to 89 weeks PCA **(B)**. Error bars denote standard error of the mean. *Asterisks* denote levels of significance as follows: $*p \leq 0.05$, $**p \leq 0.01$, $***p \leq 0.001$. All *post hoc* comparisons were made using the Bonferroni correction after three-factor, repeated measures analysis of variance. Both groups of infants showed a significant drop in threshold 1 to 3 hours after surgery on both surgical and naïve sides of the abdomen (**A:** infants who underwent herniotomy, surgical side, $p = 0.0002$; naïve side, $p = 0.05$; n = 13; **B:** infants who underwent pyeloplasty, surgical side, $p = 0.01$; naïve side, $p = 0.0003$; n = 6). In infants who underwent herniotomy **(A)**, the threshold on both sides remained significantly lower than that of the control 6 to 8 hours after surgery if no analgesia had been given since then (surgical side, $p = 0.01$; naïve side, $p = 0.05$; n = 6), a complete reversal only being seen in infants who had had analgesia within the previous 2 hours (surgical side, $p = 0.4$; naïve side, $p = 0.19$; n = 4). For those infants who remained in the hospital 24 hours after surgery, the threshold on the surgical side was still significantly lower than before surgery (surgical side, $p = 0.05$; n = 6). In infants who underwent pyeloplasty **(B)**, the threshold was significantly lower on the surgical side than on the naïve side before surgery ($p = 0.017$, n = 7). Six to 8 hours after surgery, with ongoing analgesia, thresholds on both sides were not significantly different from preoperative values (surgical side, $p = 0.5$; naïve side, $p = 0.2$; n = 6). However, the threshold on the surgical side was significantly lower than that of the control 24 hours after surgery, when, in all cases, the morphine infusion had either been reduced or discontinued ($p = 0.05$, n = 6).

surrounding the wound had spread from the incision site. In adult studies, no changes in pressure pain threshold either consequent to surgery or as a result of analgesia could be demonstrated on the contralateral side of the abdomen (64) or on the thigh (66). The contralateral effects seen in infants are again likely to be owing to increased excitability in the infant spinal cord, which would increase the extent of central sensitization.

Evidence of more long-lasting postsurgical wound sensitivity in infants in the ASR study is reflected in lower than preoperative thresholds on the surgical side of the abdomen 24 hours after surgery (21). Studies in adults have also shown a significant reduction in electrical pain threshold on the day after gynecologic laparotomy (68) and 4 days after abdominal hysterectomy after cessation of morphine infusions (71). In the latter study, this rebound sensitization after discontinuation of morphine was thought to be owing to convergent visceral inputs, which may also have been a factor in the ASR study, particularly in the pyeloplasty group.

Another interesting finding in this study was that infants who underwent pyeloplasty displayed significantly lower thresholds on the affected side compared with the contralateral side before surgery. Therefore, in addition to being a measure of wound sensitivity, ASR threshold may also indicate the existence of more chronic disease–related pain. These infants had been diagnosed prenatally on ultrasonographic scan as having a pelviureteric junction obstruction with accompanying dilation of the renal pelvis, and months of varying degrees of hydronephrosis, accompanied in some cases by episodes of infection, had preceded surgery. In adult humans after renal/ureteral calculosis, decreased pain thresholds to electrical stimulation in the affected dermatome have been reported (81) and in adult rats with artificial ureteral calculosis (82,83). This phenomenon, described as referred visceral hyperalgesia, has never been demonstrated in infants before. In both humans (81) and rats (82,83), the severity of referred hyperalgesia depends on the number of episodes of renal colic and appears to arise from central sensitization of spinal sensory neurons but not motor neurons (83).

The changes in ASR threshold after surgery seen in this study and with visceral pathology were accompanied by alterations in reflex radiation, as denoted by the degree of hip flexion. Again, central sensitization of spinal cord neurons in these infants would increase the size of dorsal horn cell and reflex receptive fields (84), leading to reflex spread to adjacent muscle groups.

SECONDARY HYPERSENSITIVITY AROUND A WOUND IN NEONATES AND INFANTS

The phenomenon of increased sensitivity to touch in the area around a skin wound or skin irritation, but not directly over the wound itself (termed secondary allodynia), has been extensively studied in adults (79,85,86). These studies demonstrated that increases in spinal cord excitability caused by prolonged input from C fibers are responsible for the maintenance of the area of hypersensitivity (Fig. 3.7). This phenomenon has hardly been investigated in neonates and infants, although repeated heel lancing in neonates receiving intensive care has been shown to produce an area of reddening and inflammation that extends beyond the immediate puncture sites (17). Furthermore, lowering of flexion withdrawal reflex thresholds on the limb contralateral to substantial leg injury received during intensive care has been demonstrated in infants of 38 to 42 weeks PCA (15), and a drop in the ASR threshold on the opposite side of the abdomen to a surgical wound has been shown in infants younger than 1 year old (21). Both of these phenomena provide evidence of central changes in nervous system excitability because they occur remote from the site of injury.

Therefore, we studied this phenomenon in neonates and infants (20) to observe how it differs in this population and as a means of gaining hitherto unobtained information on sensory processing. Unlike studies on older children and adults, it is impossible to exam-

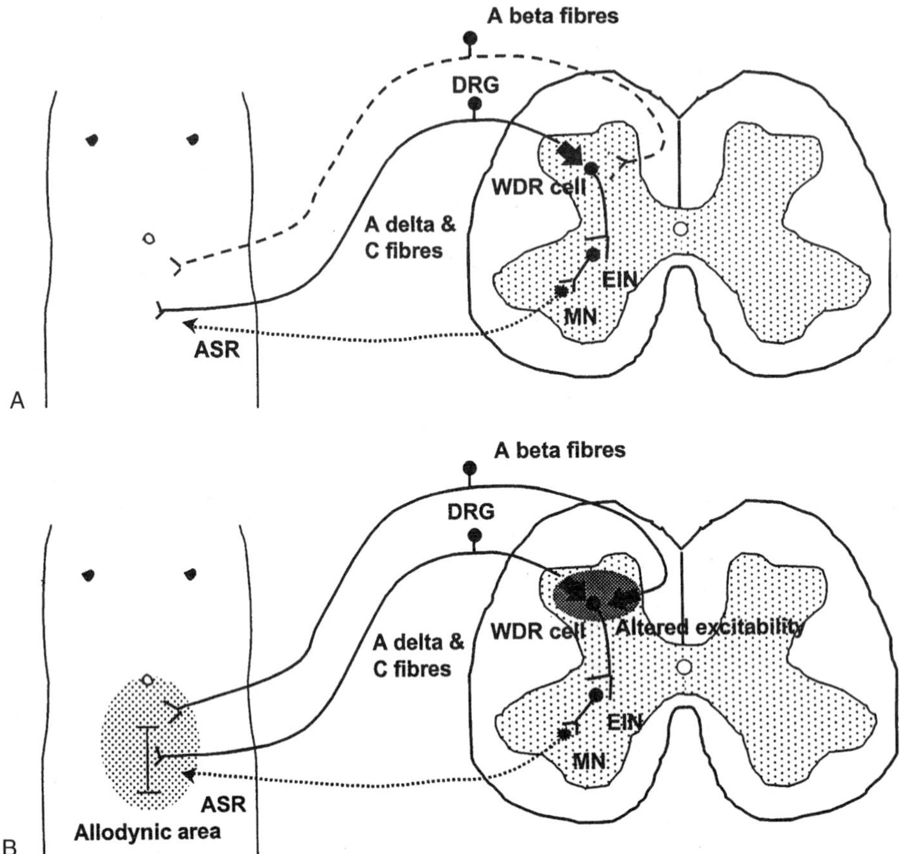

FIG. 3.7. Diagrammatic representation of possible changes in neuronal circuitry underlying mechanisms of secondary allodynia as they relate to abdominal skin reflex (*ASR*) threshold changes in infants after surgery. In the normal state **(A)**, wide dynamic range (*WDR*) neurons in the dorsal horn of the spinal cord receive input predominantly from Aδ and C fibers via small-diameter primary sensory neurons in the dorsal root ganglion (*DRG*) and a lesser input from Aβ fibers. After a stimulus, information to these cells is conveyed via excitatory interneurons (*EIN*) to motor neurons (*MN*), thus producing an ASR. However, in an allodynic state, such as may occur after an abdominal surgical wound **(B)**, peripheral sensitization and greatly increased C-fiber input to the dorsal horn lead to an increase in spinal cord excitability, termed central sensitization. The balance of inputs to WDR cells is altered in favor of Aβ fibers, causing increased abdominal sensitivity and consequent lowering of the ASR threshold.

ine this phenomenon using a verbal report; therefore, changes in ASR thresholds were used to map an area of secondary hypersensitivity around an abdominal surgical wound (20). Rostral measurements were made to observe intersegmental changes and medial thresholds to give information on intrasegmental changes, including those involving the midline of the abdomen.

An area of secondary hypersensitivity surrounding the surgical incision was reflected in significantly lowered ASR thresholds rostral and medial to the wound to a distance of 4 cm, although thresholds were lowest closest to the incision (20). The drops in threshold were significantly greater medially (intrasegmentally) than rostrally (extrasegmentally) and were present from 1 hour after surgery. These changes were attenuated by postoperative analgesia, particularly 6 to 8 hours after surgery with ongoing intravenous opioids but were not abolished by it except in the case of continuous epidural anesthesia. The threshold gradient with distance from the wound was significantly steeper rostrally than medially. The control group of infants not having surgery did not display significant intra- or extrasegmental changes in threshold over time (20).

A zone of secondary hypersensitivity around a surgical wound displaying similar features has been demonstrated in human adult studies using verbal report (as opposed to reflex thresholds) (63,66). In the first study of wound tenderness and subjective pain ratings after hysterectomy, pressure pain thresholds 15 cm from the incision were significantly higher than at 5 cm and 10 cm (66). In the latter study, von Frey hair pain detection thresholds after herniotomy were lower caudal to the incision than rostral to it (63). These features may be owing to incision-induced changes in the receptive field properties of individual dorsal horn neurons, which contribute to postsurgical central sensitization (87). Study of these cells has demonstrated that thresholds of individual neurons are greater distant to the incision than close to it, and receptive fields to pinch are enlarged after surgery in both wide dynamic range and high-threshold cells (87).

INVESTIGATION OF SENSORY PROCESSING AT HIGHER LEVELS IN THE CENTRAL NERVOUS SYSTEM IN INFANTS

Although the study of reflexes has provided useful insights into developmental aspects of sensory processing in preverbal children, this information only tells us about how neonates and infants process sensory input at the level of the spinal cord. Very little is known about the development of functional connections at higher levels in the central nervous system, up to and including the cerebral cortex (22). The use of somatosensory evoked potentials (SEPs) is one possible means by which the functional development of sensory connectivity in the brain could be examined.

SEPs can be reliably elicited from 27 weeks PCA (88,89). They have been used to investigate the integrity of somatosensory pathways during the neonatal period and in infancy (38,88,90–92) and as prognostic indicators of neurologic impairment in infants at high-risk (38,90,92). The median nerve is the most usual site for stimulation (38,88,90–92), although the posterior tibial nerve has been used also (89,93,94). The median nerve SEP waveform in the neonate has a large negative deflection (N1), the latency of which has been shown to decrease with increasing PCA from 27 to 47 weeks (88,92). The latency of N1 is often lengthened in infants with intracranial pathology owing to hypoxic-ischemic injury (90,92), although infants can still develop severe neurologic impairment despite an N1 latency within the normal range (90,92). The posterior tibial SEP exhibits a triphasic waveform (89,94), comprising two low-amplitude positive deflections (P1 and P2) followed by a larger negative deflection (N2). The appearance of the waveform does not alter from 27 to 40 weeks PCA (89). The maturation of the SEP in the human neonate occurs according to PCA, independent of gestational age at birth (91).

Despite information already gained concerning SEP maturation in infants and children, studies so far have only been performed using electrical stimulation, which activates mixed-modality nerve fibers, the greater proportion of which are presumably putative Aβ afferents (95). Nothing is known about small fiber connectivity in infants and young children. However, studies in adults have shown that it is possible to gain information concerning the contributions of Aβ, Aδ, and C sensory nerve fibers and the functional integrity of the pathways in which they are involved using mechanical, electrical, and laser stimulation to elicit SEPs (96–104).

Both cutaneous mechanical stimulation and low-intensity electrical nerve stimulation activate mixed modality, mainly Aβ fibers carrying tactile and proprioceptive information, and the SEPs thus generated are correlates of mechanosensitivity and proprioception (98,102). Conversely, cutaneous thermal stimuli generated by a laser activate the most superficial cutaneous afferent fibers of Aδ and C types, which subserve temperature sensations and project in the spinothalamic tract (98,105).

In addition, studies in adult humans using surface (101) and intracortical recordings of laser evoked potentials (100) and magnetoencephalography after laser stimulation (106) have shown that the specificity of laser stimulation in activating Aδ fibers (96,97,101, 105,107) enables observation of the sequence of Aδ fiber activation of primary (SI) and secondary (SII) somatosensory cortices. All three studies demonstrated that contralateral SII has a substantial role in the processing of small-diameter afferent input, possibly through direct thalamocortical projections (100,101,106). Two of the studies (100,106) showed that ipsilateral SII is activated 12 to 15 milliseconds after contralateral SII, indicating callosal transmission of small fiber inputs between the two SII areas (100). The second study also showed parallel activation of SI and SII in adulthood, unlike the activation pattern seen in higher primates (106). It would be interesting to observe activation sequences of the somatosensory cortices during development and functional development of thalamocortical connections in infants and young children.

CONCLUSIONS

It is evident that the study of neurophysiologic phenomena can provide direct and quantitative information concerning processing of sensory information on the developing nervous system. It is also true that there are structural and functional features of this immature system that have a profound influence on pain processing in the neonate and infant. Nevertheless, understanding of central effects of ongoing pain and tissue damage in this age group is still rudimentary, even though preliminary investigation of secondary hypersensitivity in infants indicates that, despite the slow maturation of C-fiber central connections, features of central sensitization seen in adults are present at this time.

Furthermore, laboratory and clinical investigations of both mechanisms and behavior have provided information about pain processing at the spinal cord level, but the challenge is to unravel the mystery of how much of a painful stimulus reaches and is processed in the brain in the neonate and infant and how this can be investigated. In the mean time, the information that we already have is sufficient to tell us that the management of pain in infancy requires not only limiting procedures performed as much as possible but also careful and creative analgesic management.

ACKNOWLEDGMENT

The author thanks Professor Maria Fitzgerald for her ongoing support and encouragement, Dr. Stewart Boyd for kindly reading and commenting on this manuscript, and the Wellcome Trust and Children Nationwide for financial support.

REFERENCES

1. Ekholm J. Postnatal changes in cutaneous reflexes and in the discharge pattern of cutaneous and articular sense organs. *Acta Physiol Scand Suppl* 1967;297: 1–130.
2. Fitzgerald M. The postnatal development of cutaneous afferent fibre input and receptive field organization in the rat dorsal horn. *J Physiol* 1985;364:1–18.
3. Fitzgerald M. Cutaneous primary afferent properties in the hind limb of the neonatal rat. *J Physiol* 1987;383: 79–92.
4. Fitzgerald M. Spontaneous and evoked activity of fetal primary afferents in vivo. *Nature* 1987;326:603–604.
5. Fitzgerald M. The development of activity evoked by fine diameter cutaneous fibres in the spinal cord of the newborn rat. *Neurosci Lett* 1988;86:161–166.
6. Fitzgerald M. A physiological study of the prenatal development of cutaneous sensory inputs to dorsal horn cells in the rat. *J Physiol* 1991;432:473–482.
7. Fitzgerald M, Gibson S. The postnatal physiological and neurochemical development of peripheral sensory C fibres. *Neuroscience* 1984;13:933–944.
8. Fitzgerald M, Koltzenburg M. The functional development of descending inhibitory pathways in the dorsolateral funiculus of the newborn rat spinal cord. *Dev Brain Res* 1986;24:261–270.

9. Fitzgerald M, Butcher T, Shortland P. Developmental changes in the laminar termination of A fibre cutaneous sensory afferents in the rat spinal cord dorsal horn. *J Comp Neurol* 1994;348:225–233.
10. Holmberg H, Schouenborg J. Postnatal development of the nociceptive withdrawal reflexes in the rat: a behavioural and electromyographic study. *J Physiol* 1996; 493:239–252.
11. Coggeshall RE, Jennings EA, Fitzgerald M. Evidence that large myelinated primary afferent fibres make synaptic contacts in lamina II of neonatal rats. *Dev Brain Res* 1996;92:81–90.
12. Jennings E, Fitzgerald M. C-Fos can be induced in the neonatal rat spinal cord by both noxious and innocuous peripheral stimulation. *Pain* 1996;68: 301–306.
13. Jennings EA, Fitzgerald M. Postnatal changes in responses of rat dorsal horn cells to afferent stimulation: a fibre induced sensitization. *J Physiol* 1998;509: 859–867.
14. Levinsson A, Luo XL, Holmberg H, et al. Developmental tuning in a spinal nociceptive system: effects of neonatal spinalization. *J Neurosci* 1999;19: 10397–10403.
15. Andrews KA, Fitzgerald M. The cutaneous flexion reflex in human neonates: a quantitative study of threshold and stimulus/response characteristics, following single and repeated stimuli. *Dev Med Child Neurol* 1999;41:696–703.
16. Fitzgerald M, Shaw A, MacIntosh N. The postnatal development of the cutaneous flexor reflex: comparative study of preterm infants and newborn rat pups. *Dev Med Child Neurol* 1988;30:520–526.
17. Fitzgerald M, Millard C, MacIntosh N. Cutaneous hypersensitivity following peripheral tissue damage in newborn infants and its reversal with topical anaesthesia. *Pain* 1989;39:31–36.
18. Andrews KA, Fitzgerald M. The cutaneous withdrawal reflex in human neonates: sensitization, receptive fields, and the effects of contralateral stimulation. *Pain* 1994;56:95–101.
19. Andrews KA, Fitzgerald M. Flexion reflex responses in biceps femoris and tibialis anterior in human neonates. *Early Hum Dev* 2000;57:105–110.
20. Andrews KA, Fitzgerald M. Mapping of the area of secondary hypersensitivity around a surgical wound in human infants using the abdominal skin reflex threshold. *Eur J Neurosci* 2000;12[Suppl 11]:71.
21. Andrews KA, Fitzgerald M. Wound sensitivity as a measure of analgesic effects following surgery in human neonates and infants. Submitted to *Pain* 2002, *in press*.
22. Andrews KA, Fitzgerald M. Biological barriers to paediatric pain management. *Clin J Pain* 1997;3: 138–143.
23. Craig KD, Whitfield MF, Grunau R-VE, et al. Pain in the preterm neonate: behavioural and physiological indices. *Pain* 1993;52:287–299.
24. Johnston CC, Stevens BJ, Yang F, et al. Differential response to pain by very premature neonates. *Pain* 1995; 61:3:471–480.
25. Fitzgerald M. The neurobiology of fetal and neonatal pain. In: Wall PD, Melzack R, eds. *A textbook of pain*, 3rd ed. London: Churchill-Livingstone, 1993.
26. Conel JL. *The postnatal development of the human cerebral cortex, vol I, the cortex of the newborn*. Cambridge, MA: Harvard University Press, 1939.
27. Conel JL. *The postnatal development of the human cerebral cortex, vol II, the cortex of the one-month infant*. Cambridge, MA: Harvard University Press, 1941.
28. Humphrey T. The development of the pyramidal tracts in human fetuses, correlated with cortical differentiation. In: Tower DB, Schadé JP, eds. *Structure and function of the cerebral cortex*. Amsterdam: Elsevier, 1960: 93–103.
29. Jenner JR, Stephens JA. Cutaneous reflex responses and their central nervous pathways studied in man. *J Physiol* 1982;333:405–419.
30. Issler H, Stephens JA. The maturation of cutaneous reflexes studied in the upper limb in man. *J Physiol* 1983;335:643–654.
31. Myklebust BM, Gottlieb GL, Agrawal GC. Stretch reflexes of the normal infant. *Dev Med Child Neurol* 1986;28:440–449.
32. O'Sullivan MC, Eyre JA, Miller S. Radiation of phasic stretch reflex in biceps brachii to muscles of the arm in man and its restriction during development. *J Physiol* 1991;439:529–543.
33. Leonard CT, Matsumoto T, Diedrich P. Human myotatic reflex development of the lower extremities. *Early Hum Dev* 1995;43:75–93.
34. Crum JE, Stephens JA. Cutaneous reflex responses recorded in the lower limb of the newborn infant. *J Physiol* 1982;332:30P–31P.
35. Mayer RF, Mosser RS. Maturation of human reflexes. In: Desmedt JE, ed. *New developments in electromyography and clinical neurophysiology, vol. 3*. Basel: Karger, 1973:294–307.
36. Berger W, Quintern J, Dietz V. Afferent and efferent control of stance and gait: developmental changes in children. *Electroencephalogr Clin Neurophysiol* 1987; 66:244–252.
37. Eyre JA, Gibson M, Koh THHG, et al. Corticospinal transmission excited by electromagnetic stimulation of the brain is impaired in children with spastic hemiparesis but normal in those with quadriparesis. *J Physiol* 1989;414:9P.
38. Eyre JA, Miller S, Ramesh V. Constancy of central conduction delays during development in man: investigation of motor and somatosensory pathways. *J Physiol* 1991;434:441–452.
39. Leonard CT, Hirschfeld H, Forssberg H. The development of independent walking in children with cerebral palsy. *Dev Med Child Neurol* 1991;33:567–577.
40. Eyre JA, Miller S, Clowry GJ, et al. Functional corticospinal projections are established prenatally in the human foetus permitting involvement in the development of spinal motor centres. *Brain* 2000;123:51–64.
41. Hogeweg JA, Kuis W, Oostendorp RAB, et al. General and segmental reduced pain thresholds in juvenile chronic arthritis. *Pain* 1995;62:11–17.
42. Hogeweg JA, Kuis W, Huygen ACJ, et al. The pain threshold in juvenile chronic arthritis. *Br J Rheumatol* 1995;34:61–67.
43. Hilz MJ, Glorius S, Beric A. Thermal perception thresholds: influence of determination paradigm and reference temperature. *J Neurol Sci* 1995;129:135–140.
44. Hilz MJ, Glorius SE, Schweibold G, et al. Quantitative thermal perception testing in preschool children. *Muscle Nerve* 1996;19:381–383.

45. Meier P, Berde C, DiCanzio J, et al. Thermal and vibratory perception and pain thresholds in children. 9th World Congress on Pain, Vienna, Austria. 1999: 406(abst).
46. Barker DP, Rutter N. Lignocaine ointment and local anaesthesia in preterm infants. *Arch Dis Child Fetal Neonatal Ed* 1995;72:F203–F204.
47. Jain A, Rutter N. Local anaesthetic effect of topical amethocaine gel in neonates: randomised controlled trial. *Arch Dis Child Fetal Neonatal Ed* 2000;82: F42–F45.
48. Myklebust BM, Gottlieb GL. Development of the stretch reflex in the newborn: reciprocal excitation and reflex irradiation. *Child Dev* 1993;64:1036–1045.
49. Prechtl HFR, Vlach V, Lenard HG, et al. Exteroceptive and tendon reflexes in various behavioural states in the newborn infant. *Biol Neonate* 1967;11:159–175.
50. Hugon M. Exteroceptive reflexes to stimulation of the sural nerve in normal man. In: Desmedt JE, ed. *New developments in electromyography and clinical neurophysiology, vol. 3.* Basel: Karger, 1973:713–729.
51. Willer JC. Comparative study of perceived pain and nociceptive flexion reflex in man. *Pain* 1977;3:69–80.
52. Fitzgerald M, Jennings E. The postnatal development of spinal sensory processing. *Proc Natl Acad Sci USA* 1999;96:7719–7722.
53. Dimitrijevic MR, Nathan PW. Studies of spasticity in man. 4. Changes in flexion reflex with repetitive cutaneous stimulation in spinal man. *Brain* 1970;93: 743–768.
54. Dimitrijevic MR, Faganel J, Gregoric M, et al. Habituation: effects of regular and stochastic stimulation. *J Neurol Neurosurg Psychiatry* 1972;35:234–242.
55. Sherrington CS. Flexion reflex of the limb, crossed extension reflex, and reflex stepping and standing. *J Physiol* 1910;40:28–121.
56. Woolf CJ, Swett J. The cutaneous contribution to the hamstring flexor reflex in the rat. An electrophysiological and anatomical study. *Brain Res* 1984;303: 299–312.
57. Lenard H-G, von Bernuth H, Prechtl HFR. Reflexes and their relationship to behavioural state in the newborn. *Acta Paediatr Scand* 1968;57:177–185.
58. Kugelberg E. Polysynaptic reflexes of clinical importance. *Electroencephalogr Clin Neurophysiol Suppl* 1962;22:103–111.
59. Fitzgerald M. The contralateral input to the dorsal horn of the spinal cord in the decerebrate spinal rat. *Brain Res* 1982;236:275–287.
60. Cummings EA, Reid GJ, Finley GA, et al. Prevalence and source of pain in pediatric inpatients. *Pain* 1996; 68:1:25–31.
61. Richmond CE, Bromley LM, Woolf CJ. Preoperative morphine pre-empts postoperative pain. *Lancet* 1993; 342:73–75.
62. Collis R, Brandner B, Bromley LM, et al. Is there any clinical advantage of increasing the pre-emptive dose of morphine or combining pre-incisional with postoperative morphine administration? *Br J Anaesth* 1995; 74:396–399.
63. Callesen T, Bech K, Thorup J, et al. Cryoanalgesia: effect on postherniorrhaphy pain. *Anesth Analg* 1998;87: 896–899.
64. Dahl JB, Rosenberg J, Molke Jensen F, et al. Pressure pain thresholds in volunteers and herniorrhaphy patients. *Acta Anaesthesiol Scand* 1990;34:673–676.
65. Erichsen CJ, Vibits H, Dahl JB, et al. Wound infiltration with ropivacaine and bupivacaine for pain after inguinal herniotomy. *Acta Anaesthesiol Scand* 1995;39: 67–70.
66. Möiniche S, Dahl JB, Erichsen CJ, et al. Time course of subjective pain ratings, and wound and leg tenderness after hysterectomy. *Acta Anaesthesiol Scand* 1997;41:785–789.
67. Lund C, Hansen OB, Kehlet H. Effect of surgery on sensory threshold and somatosensory evoked potentials after skin stimulation. *Br J Anaesth* 1990;65: 173–176.
68. Dahl JB, Erichsen CJ, Fuglsang-Frederiksen A, et al. Pain sensation and nociceptive reflex excitability in surgical patients and human volunteers. *Br J Anaesth* 1992;69:117–121.
69. Wilder-Smith OHG, Tassonyi E, Senly C, et al. Surgical pain is followed not only by spinal sensitization but also by supraspinal antinociception. *Br J Anaesth* 1996;76:816–821.
70. Wilder-Smith OHG, Arendt-Nielsen L, Gäumann D, et al. Sensory changes and pain after abdominal hysterectomy: a comparison of anesthetic supplementation with fentanyl versus magnesium or ketamine. *Anesth Analg* 1998;86:95–101.
71. Wilder-Smith CH, Hill L, Wilkins J, et al. Effects of morphine and tramadol on şomatic and visceral sensory function and gastrointestinal motility after abdominal surgery. *Anesthesiology* 1999;91:639–647.
72. Kugelberg E, Hagbarth KE. Spinal mechanism of the abdominal and erector spinae skin reflexes. *Brain* 1958;81:290–304.
73. Magladery JW, Teasdall RD, French JH, et al. Cutaneous reflex changes in development and aging. *Arch Neurol* 1960;3:1–9.
74. Harlem OK, Lönnum A. A clinical study of the abdominal skin reflexes in newborn infants. *Arch Dis Child* 1957;32:127–130.
75. Seebach B, Ziskind-Conhaim L. Formation of transient inappropriate sensorimotor synapses in developing rat spinal cords. *J Neurosci* 1994;14:4520–4528.
76. Mendelson B, Frank E. Specific monosynaptic sensory-motor connections form in the absence of patterned neural activity and motoneuronal cell death. *J Neurosci* 1991;11:1390–1403.
77. Lee MT, O'Donovan MJ. Organization of hindlimb muscle afferent projections to lumbosacral motoneurons in the chick embryo. *J Neurosci* 1991;11: 2564–2573.
78. Lewis T. Experiments relating to cutaneous hyperalgesia and its spread through somatic nerves. *Clin Sci* 1936;2:373–421.
79. Hardy JD, Wolff HG, Goodell H. *Pain sensations and reactions*. Baltimore: Williams & Wilkins, 1952: 73–215.
80. LaMotte RH, Shain CN, Simone DA, et al. Neurogenic hyperalgesia: psychophysical studies of underlying mechanisms. *J Neurophysiol* 1991;66:190–211.
81. Vecchiet L, Giamberardino MA, Dragani L, et al. Pain from renal/ureteral calculosis: evaluation of sensory thresholds in the lumbar area. *Pain* 1989;36:289–295.
82. Giamberardino MA, Valente R, de Bigontina P, et al.

Artificial ureteral calculosis in rats: behavioural characterization of visceral pain episodes and their relationship with referred lumbar muscle hyperalgesia. *Pain* 1995;61:459–469.
83. Giamberardino MA, Dalal A, Valente R, et al. Changes in activity of spinal cells with muscular input in rats with referred muscular hyperalgesia from ureteral calculosis. *Neurosci Lett* 1996;203:89–92.
84. Dubner R. Hyperalgesia and expanded receptive fields, editorial comment. *Pain* 1992;48:3–4.
85. Torebjörk HE, Lundberg LER, LaMotte RH. Central changes in processing of mechanoreceptive input in capsaicin-induced secondary hyperalgesia in humans. *J Physiol* 1992;448:765–780.
86. Koltzenburg M, Torebjörk HE, Wahren LK. Nociceptor modulated central sensitization causes mechanical hyperalgesia in acute chemogenic and chronic neuropathic pain. *Brain* 1994;117:579–591.
87. Zahn PK, Brennan TJ. Incision-induced changes in receptive field properties of rat dorsal horn neurons. *Anesthesiology* 1999;91:772–785.
88. Klimach VJ, Cooke RWI. Maturation of the neonatal somatosensory evoked response in preterm infants. *Dev Med Child Neurol* 1988;30:208–214.
89. Pike AA, Marlow N, Dawson C. Posterior tibial somatosensory evoked potentials in very preterm infants. *Early Hum Dev* 1997;47:71–84.
90. Majnemer A, Rosenblatt B, Riley P, et al. Somatosensory evoked response abnormalities in high-risk newborns. *Pediatr Neurol* 1987;3:350–355.
91. Majnemer A, Rosenblatt B, Willis D, et al. The effect of gestational age at birth on somatosensory-evoked potentials performed at term. *J Child Neurol* 1990;5: 329–335.
92. Pierrat V, Eken P, Duquennoy C, et al. Prognostic value of early somatosensory evoked potentials in neonates with cystic leukomalacia. *Dev Med Child Neurol* 1993;35:683–690.
93. Tranier S, Chevallier B, Lemaigre D, et al. Potentiel évoqué somesthésique du membre inférieur chez le nouveau-né prématuré. *Neurophysiol Clin* 1990;20: 463–479.
94. White CP, Cooke RWI. Maturation of the cortical evoked response to posterior tibial nerve stimulation in the preterm neonate. *Dev Med Child Neurol* 1989;31: 657–664.
95. Handwerker HG, Kobal G. Psychophysiology of experimentally induced pain. *Physiol Rev* 1993;73: 639–671.
96. Bromm B, Jahnke MT, Treede R-D. Responses of human cutaneous afferents to CO2 laser stimuli causing pain. *Exp Brain Res* 1984;55:158–166.
97. Bromm B, Treede R-D. Human cerebral potentials evoked by CO2 laser stimuli causing pain. *Exp Brain Res* 1987;67:153–162.
98. Bromm B, Treede R-D. Laser-evoked cerebral potentials in the assessment of cutaneous pain sensitivity in normal subjects and patients. *Rev Neurol (Paris)* 1991; 147:625–643.
99. Bromm B, Lorenz J. Neurophysiological evaluation of pain. *Electroencephalogr Clin Neurophysiol* 1998; 107:227–253.
100. Frot M, Rambaud L, Guénot M, et al. Intracortical recordings of early pain-related CO2-laser evoked potentials in the human second somatosensory (SII) area. *Clin Neurophysiol* 1999;110:133–145.
101. Spiegel J, Hansen C, Treede R-D. Laser-evoked potentials after painful hand and foot stimulation in humans: evidence for generation of the middle-latency component in the secondary somatosensory cortex. *Neurosci Lett* 1996;216:179–182.
102. Spitzer A, Claus D. The influence of the shape of mechanical stimuli on muscle stretch reflexes and SEP. *Electroencephalogr Clin Neurophysiol* 1992;85: 331–336.
103. Towell AD, Boyd SG. Sensory and cognitive components of the CO2 laser evoked cerebral potential. *Electroencephalogr Clin Neurophysiol* 1993;88:237–239.
104. Towell AD, Purves AM, Boyd SG. CO2 laser activation of nociceptive and non-nociceptive thermal afferents from hairy and glabrous skin. *Pain* 1996;66: 79–86.
105. Treede R-D, Magerl W, Baumgärtner U. Laser-evoked potentials for assessment of nociceptive pathways in humans. *Pain Forum* 1998;7:191–195.
106. Ploner M, Schmitz F, Freund H-J, et al. Parallel activation of primary and secondary somatosensory cortices in human pain processing. *J Neurophysiol* 1999;81: 3100–3104.
107. Kakigi R, Endo C, Neshige R, et al. Estimation of conduction velocity of Aδ fibres in humans. *Muscle Nerve* 1991;14:1193–1196.

4

Long-Term Consequences of Pain in Neonates

Kenneth R. Goldschneider and Kanwaljeet S. Anand

Pain in infants has historically been an area lacking in both study and clinical attention. As we have moved past the point of accepting the fact that infants feels pain, attention has been drawn to the possible consequences of untreated pain in this age group.

Over the past decade, pain in preterm neonates has come under increasing investigation. Although there is no doubt that even the smallest neonate feels pain and displays some range of pain behavior, assessment continues to bedevil caregivers and researchers. Space does not permit a discussion of assessment issues here; the reader is referred to Chapter 1 and to other excellent reviews (1–3). For reasons beyond solely assessment difficulties, pain treatment for neonates remains poorly utilized in neonatal intensive care units (NICUs) across the United States and Canada (4–6). Whether pain is treated or not, invasive procedures abound in the NICU setting (7). Understanding the outcomes of untreated pain in this patient population should help to improve the care that we can provide these young patients.

For both ethical and practical reasons, pain and its outcomes are difficult to study in human infants. Pain is only one component of a multifaceted experience that ill neonates undergo. In addition to pain, factors affecting outcome include not only severity of illness but also an overlay of social, cultural, parental, and school-related influences on the subsequent neurobehavioral development of ex-preterm or ex-term neonates. These confounding factors make it difficult to isolate the long-term effects of neonatal pain in long-term follow-up studies. Therefore, animal models have been developed that have greatly contributed to our understanding of neonatal pain processing and the long-term consequences of pain. Any attempts to extrapolate data from animal studies to human neonates should be tempered with caution because of the enormous differences in complexity and in the regulation of developmental processes between the rodent and human brains. These differences endow the human brain with a great deal of redundancy, adaptability, and resilience, which may allow much greater compensation for early adverse life events. Conversely, the complex behavioral and cognitive repertoire required for human life, as well as the complex role of specific developmental epochs, suggests that damage or deranged development occurring in particular critical windows may exert a "permissive" effect on subsequent development. With this cautionary proviso, we can proceed to correlate some of the data from animal investigations and human studies on the long-term effects of pain.

THE NEWBORN RAT PUP AS A MODEL FOR PAIN IN HUMAN NEONATES

Similarities in the pain pathways of human infants and neonatal rat pups have made the neonatal rat pup a useful model for understanding the development of pain pathways and associated mechanisms (8). Development of the rat brain at birth [postnatal day 0 (P0)] is similar to that of a 24-week-old premature neonate; at P7, rat pups have the maturity of full-term neonates, and P14 rats correspond to 1-year-old human infants (8,9). Similarities in the pain system of newborn rodents and humans include exaggerated cutaneous reflexes (10), functional polymodal nociceptors (11), sensitization caused by repeated noxious stimulation (12), relatively large receptive fields of dorsal horn cells (13), and immaturity of the descending inhibitory systems (14). Pain-related neurotransmitters in the spinal cord including substance P, galanin, met-enkephalin, somatostatin, calcitonin gene–related peptide, vasoactive intestinal polypeptide, and other ligands seem to follow similar developmental patterns of expression in newborn rats and human neonates (8,15).

Behavioral Responses to Pain in Newborn Rats

Newborn rat pups subjected to noxious stimuli or tissue damage will manifest identical and stereotypic behavioral responses as those observed in adult animals (16). This holds true for classic tests of nociception, such as the formalin test (17), hot-plate test (18), the tail-flick test (19), and after stimulation with von Frey filaments (20). Formalin injection into the hindlimb elicits a pattern of acute response, followed by paw lifting, paw licking, and other recuperative behaviors in rats at P3, P7, and P10 (17,21,22). These studies have noted uniphasic behavioral response to formalin injection in neonatal rats (P0 to P14), which lasts as long as 60 minutes in the younger rats and 30 minutes in the older rats (21,22). The combination of paw flexion, shaking, and licking as well as kicking movements were specifically related to increases in formalin concentration (23). Guy and Abbott (22) noted that the expression of specific pain behaviors increases and nonspecific behaviors decrease in newborn rat pups subjected to painful stimulation during the first 2 weeks of postnatal life.

Further studies noted that treatment with morphine (1 mg/kg) suppresses both specific and nonspecific indicators of pain and produces mild sedation relative to handled control pups. Pentobarbital (10 mg/kg) produces sedation and suppression of nonspecific measures but has poor effects on specific pain behaviors, whereas amphetamine (2 mg/kg) decreases both specific and nonspecific pain measures in the second week of life without any sedation (24). Thus, the effects of analgesic agents can be objectively evaluated in neonatal rats and showed that the analgesic effects of morphine were qualitatively different from a sedative dose of pentobarbital.

Cardiovascular Responses to Pain in Newborn Rats

Examination of cardiovascular changes and their correlation with pain behaviors in immature animals has been used to provide some insight into the development of autonomic control. These studies suggest that both tonic and phasic controls of the heart rate and other hemodynamic parameters develop during the weaning period in rats (25). Neonatal rats subjected to the formalin test at P7, P14, and P21 showed significant increases in heart rate compared with saline-injected controls but did not develop the typical adult biphasic response until P35 (21).

Cellular Responses to Pain in Newborn Rats

Several studies have mapped the neuroanatomic patterns of neuronal activity after painful stimulation by the transcription of immediate early genes (e.g., *c-fos*, *c-jun*) and immunocytochemical localization of their protein products, most commonly the Fos protein, in the nucleus of activated neurons. Thus, when mechanical (paw pinch), thermal (hot water immersion), or inflammatory stimuli (formalin injection) were applied to the hindpaw to newborn rats on the day of birth, all stimuli elicited Fos expression in dorsal horn cells, indicating that nociceptive primary afferents are functional at this age (13). Cellular Fos expression increased linearly with the intensity of stimulation and age of the neonatal rat (at P0, P1, P2, and P3) and was greater than in rats at P14 (13). Thermal or chemical stimuli showed similar neuronal activation in the superficial dorsal horn at 2 hours, but thermal stimulation was associated with a second wave of Fos-positive neurons located bilaterally and in deeper laminae (26,27). To confirm the specificity of these cellular responses, neuronal Fos expression was reduced by endogenous mechanisms in the cervical spinal cord (28) or by the local injection of morphine (29) after inflammatory pain.

Similar data for Fos expression in the supraspinal areas associated with pain processing were reported from our laboratory (30). Specific patterns of neuronal activation were noted at different postnatal ages (P1, P7, and P14), highlighting the ontogeny of supraspinal pain processing in newborn rat pups. Nuclear Fos expression mostly occurred in the subcortical areas (thalamus, limbic system) in neonatal rats (P1, P7), with marked activation of the somatosensory, piriform, and other cortical areas in rats at P14. Formalin injections causing an inflammatory response in the right forepaw were associated with bilateral patterns of Fos expression at all ages. In rats at P14, robust neuronal activation occurred in areas/nuclei associated with emotional regulation (amygdaloid complex, hippocampus, piriform cortex), sensory processing (somatosensory cortex, other cortical areas), and neuroendocrine regulation (hypothalamus, hippocampus). These data describe the ontogeny of the cellular responses to pain in neonatal rats.

Evidence for Increased Pain Sensitivity in Neonates

More than a decade ago (31), the traditional view that neonates are insensitive to pain was refuted by presenting a physiologic rationale for the development and function of the pain system. Since then, comparative studies of human infants and rat pups have reported that the thresholds for the dorsal cutaneous withdrawal reflex increase progressively in preterm neonates and postnatal rat pups, suggesting lower pain thresholds during early development (10). Multiple other studies have demonstrated that the intensity and duration of pain responses are developmentally regulated (21,22,30). Teng and Abbott (23) found that the thresholds for formalin-induced inflammatory pain increased 2.5-fold from 3 to 15 days of age and 11-fold from the newborn to the adult rat (23). Thermal stimulation using withdrawal latencies to a hot plate (32) or tail flick (19) also reported lower pain thresholds in the younger rats. Mechanisms underlying the increased pain sensitivity of neonatal rat pups and human infants may augment their vulnerability to the long-term effects of pain.

Prolonged or Repetitive Pain Alters Development of the Pain System

Pain associated with or without tissue injury causes the activation of widely distributed and highly variable elements in the peripheral and central nervous systems, depending on the noxious stimulus, the context in which pain occurs, and characteristics of the subject (e.g., age, gender, disease states, previous experiences of pain). The three types of pain [i.e., physiologic (related to tissue injury), inflammatory, and neuropathic] stimulate distinct but related mechanisms of neuroplasticity that will alter the structure and function of different elements within the pain system via activation, modulation, or modification, often leading to increases in pain sensitivity (33). In this section, we can only provide a brief overview of the available data on the long-term, often permanent alterations in the developing pain system after exposure to acute, repetitive, or prolonged pain.

Changes in the Peripheral Pain System

Neurotrophic factors play a crucial role in the survival and maintenance of primary afferent neurons, and the terminal density of cutaneous fibers is regulated by release of nerve growth factor (NGF), brain-derived neurotrophic factor, and other trophic factors (34). The onset of NGF synthesis is correlated with onset of innervation. During normal development, skin NGF levels remain steady from P0 to P7 and increase progressively from P7 to P21 before decreasing to adult levels. By P14, high-threshold mechanoceptors mature with significant increases in their firing frequencies and stimulation thresholds (33,35,36).

In the developing dorsal root ganglia, cell death occurs from embryonic day 15 (E15), peaks at E17 to E19, and correlates with innervation of the cord by central sensory axons. Despite this, surviving cell numbers increase steadily until birth, and then decrease by 16% from P0 to P5, which correlates with the development of the peripheral innervation (37). Peripheral sensory axons grow into proximal parts of the hindlimb by E15 and finally arrive at their distal peripheral targets at birth (11,37). Thus, prenatal cell death in DRGs is controlled by local or central factors, whereas postnatal cell death depends on peripheral targets. There is a loss of nearly 50% of afferent axons from birth to adulthood, which cannot be explained by neuronal cell death (38).

Skin injury at birth causes an increased expression of NGF and other neurotrophic factors (34), leading to a marked degree of hyperinnervation with exuberant sprouting of cutaneous nerve fibers after neonatal skin wounds (39). This nerve sprouting was sixfold greater than the responses after skin injury in the adult rat and withdrawal reflex thresholds in that area of skin were reduced for as long as 12 weeks after the injury (40). Nerve sprouting was inhibited by anti-NGF antibody in adult rats, but not in neonatal rats, indicating a role for other neurotrophic factors (40) that are not altered by sciatic nerve blockade (41). During maturation of these peripheral nociceptors, the central terminals of primary afferent neurons continue to express the mRNA of axonal growth cone proteins (e.g., GAP-43) until the second postnatal week, thus allowing peripheral injury or inflammation to permanently alter spinal patterns of primary afferent innervation (42).

Changes in the Spinal Pain System

During development, thickly myelinated Aβ fibers are the first to penetrate the dorsal horn at E15, whereas the central terminals of C fibers penetrate the dorsal horn at E19 and synaptogenesis with neurons in the substantia gelatinosa is noted at P5 in a somatotopically precise manner (43,44). In the adult spinal cord, Aβ fibers form connections with deep neurons in laminae III and IV of the dorsal horn, but in the developing cord, their collateral terminals extend up to superficial neurons in the substantia gelatinosa (45). After synaptogenesis between C-fiber terminals and substantia gelatinosa neurons is completed, these unique superficial terminals from the Aβ fibers disappear (45). Thus, in the neonatal rat, it appears that the same high-velocity Aβ axons transmit tactile and noxious impulses, thus explaining the similar patterns of neuronal activation noted by *c-fos* expression after innocuous and noxious stimuli (13,46).

In the immature spinal cord, synaptic connections between the C fibers and dorsal horn neurons cause prolonged excitation after a single stimulus, and repetitive stimulation leads to *temporal summation* or windup, associated with considerable background activity and lowered thresholds to subsequent stimuli. In addition, the receptive fields of adjacent dorsal horn neurons are large and overlapping, allowing *spatial summation*, whereby weak peripheral stimuli produce exaggerated withdrawal reflexes in the newborn rats, associated with reflex radiation and facilitated transmission to supraspinal centers (8,35). Thus, acute pain or inflammation produces robust and specific pain behaviors, neuronal

Fos expression in the dorsal horn (13), leading to Aβ fiber–mediated sensitization and C fiber–mediated windup, as the putative mechanisms underlying primary and secondary hyperalgesia (12,33,47). Because of the delayed development of C-fiber synapses within the dorsal horn, pure C-fiber stimulation remains subthreshold until the second postnatal week (47).

Descending axons from brainstem grow down from the periaqueductal gray matter, pontine reticular nuclei, locus ceruleus, and other foci in the brainstem into the spinal cord in early fetal life, but they do not extend collateral branches into the dorsal horn until around birth (14). Boucher and colleagues (48) demonstrated that the development of diffuse noxious inhibitory controls was functionally mature by P21 but not effective at P12. The development of diffuse noxious inhibitory controls follows a rostrocaudal pattern, leading to higher pain thresholds in the forelimbs compared with the hindlimbs of 10-day-old rats (28). This delayed maturation of descending inhibition may be owing to a deficiency of neurotransmitters (dopamine, serotonin, and norepinephrine) in the axon terminals or lack of specific receptors (α_2-adrenergic, 5-HT_{1A}) in their spinal targets. Alternately, a delayed maturation of interneurons (49) or the excitatory role of neurotransmitters such as γ-aminobutyric acid and glycine in the dorsal horn may contribute to the delayed maturation of inhibitory mechanisms in spinal cord. Although γ-aminobutyric acid and glycine are inhibitory neurotransmitters in the adult, in the neonatal dorsal horn, they mediate increased calcium influx into immature neurons and enhance the action potential duration from these neurons (50). Because of these immature gating mechanisms, we propose that newborns may be incapable of filtering out sensory stimulation from the periphery. Given the plasticity of the supraspinal foci involved in sensory processing, repetitive pain during infancy may therefore cause widespread changes in the developing brain.

The long-term effects of prolonged or repetitive pain in the neonatal period have been investigated using different experimental paradigms. For example, neonatal rats exposed to four daily needle sticks from P0 to P7 subsequently developed lower pain thresholds at P16 and P22 (18). Localized inflammation for 5 to 7 days, caused by injecting complete Freund adjuvant into the left hindpaw of neonatal rat pups, led to striking increases in the number of primary sensory fibers forming connections with superficial layers of the dorsal horn in adult rats (51). These abnormal nerve fibers also extended into caudal segments of the spinal cord (L6, S1) that do not normally receive sensory input from the sciatic nerve. Hyperexcitability of the dorsal horn neurons was noted by increased activity at rest and increased responses to tactile or noxious stimuli and was correlated with increased pain behaviors in adult rats (51). Localized inflammation for 48 hours, caused by injecting carrageenan into the hindpaws of 1-day-old rats, also led to marked reductions (33%) in the receptive field size of dorsal neurons to subsequent noxious stimulation (pinch) (52). In summary, neonatal interventions lead to permanent alterations in the structure and function of the adult pain system, with hyperinnervation in areas of wounded skin (39), an increased sprouting of primary afferent fibers and hyperexcitability of dorsal horn neurons (51), leading to adaptive changes within the dorsal horn that decrease the receptive field size of these afferent neurons (52). Putative mechanisms for such adaptive changes await further investigation and may include reduced dendritic arborization of dorsal horn neurons, increased connections with inhibitory interneurons, upregulation of inhibitory receptors or ion channels, or enhanced activity of the diffuse noxious inhibitory controls from supraspinal centers. The long-term effects of peripheral nerve damage in neonatal rats were reviewed recently (53) and are beyond the scope of this chapter.

Changes in the Supraspinal Pain System

Given the plasticity of supraspinal foci involved in sensory processing, repetitive pain during infancy may cause widespread changes in the immature brain leading to abnormal behaviors in adulthood. Exposure of neonatal rat pups to daily needle-stick pain led to decreased pain thresholds during later infancy (18), thus demonstrating a prolonged secondary hyperalgesia that lasted until P22 in infant rats. During adulthood, these same rats manifested an increased alcohol preference, anxiety-mediated behaviors, defensive withdrawal, and hypervigilance behaviors associated with diminished expression of neuronal Fos in the somatosensory cortex after exposure to a hot plate (18). Some of these behavioral changes are reminiscent of the behaviors seen in older children who were born prematurely and exposed to multiple painful procedures in the neonatal ICU (see below).

Further experiments suggest differential long-term effects of repetitive pain depending on whether the neonatal rats were exposed to acute pain (needle sticks) or inflammatory pain (formalin injection). Adult rats exposed to repetitive inflammatory pain during the neonatal period exhibited longer hot-plate latencies than controls, and this long-term effect was ameliorated, at least partially, by morphine pretreatment. Adult male rats had longer hot-plate latencies compared with female rats. Responsiveness to morphine analgesia was tested by measuring inhibition of the tail-flick response after cumulative morphine doses. Adult female rats exposed to neonatal inflammatory pain were significantly more responsive to morphine analgesia compared with the control group or with those that received morphine treatment alone in the absence of pain. Both neonatal morphine treatment and exposure to neonatal inflammatory pain seemed to decrease ethanol preference during adulthood. Adult rats exposed to neonatal inflammatory pain exhibited less locomotor activity than untreated controls. These data suggest that neonatal inflammation and neonatal morphine treatment have distinct patterns of long-term behavioral effects in adulthood, and both these patterns are attenuated when the two treatments are combined (54).

CONSEQUENCES OF PAIN IN HUMAN NEONATES

The rodent model has much to offer our understanding of neonatal pain. However, in evaluating the clinical relevance of these findings, we must consider several things. There are large differences between humans and rodents regarding the complexity and adaptability of their brains, their developmental differences, their behavioral repertoires, and the various coping strategies initiated by the infants and their caregivers.

The great strides in understanding the developmental physiology and anatomy are discussed in Chapters 2 and 3, and the animal data enhance similar studies of human infants. New clinically relevant questions have arisen. Are there long-term implications for neonatal pain? Do preterm and term human infants differ in their pain responses or in the immediate and long-term outcomes of untreated pain? What can be done to minimize effects of necessary but noxious treatments on long-term outcome?

The types of painful stimuli seen most commonly in premature and full-term infants are somewhat different. The preterm infants who spend weeks and months in the intensive care environment are subjected to repetitive noxious stimulation (mechanical ventilation, blood draws, and surgical interventions). In contrast to the "chronically instrumented" state of many extremely-low-birth-weight (ELBW) infants, full-term infants deal with more isolated stimuli (circumcision, immunizations, surgical interventions). Outcome ramifications of both differences in physiologic maturity and differences in acute versus chronic stimulation are likely. We now turn our attention to pain-related outcome in preterm infants and then that in full-term in-

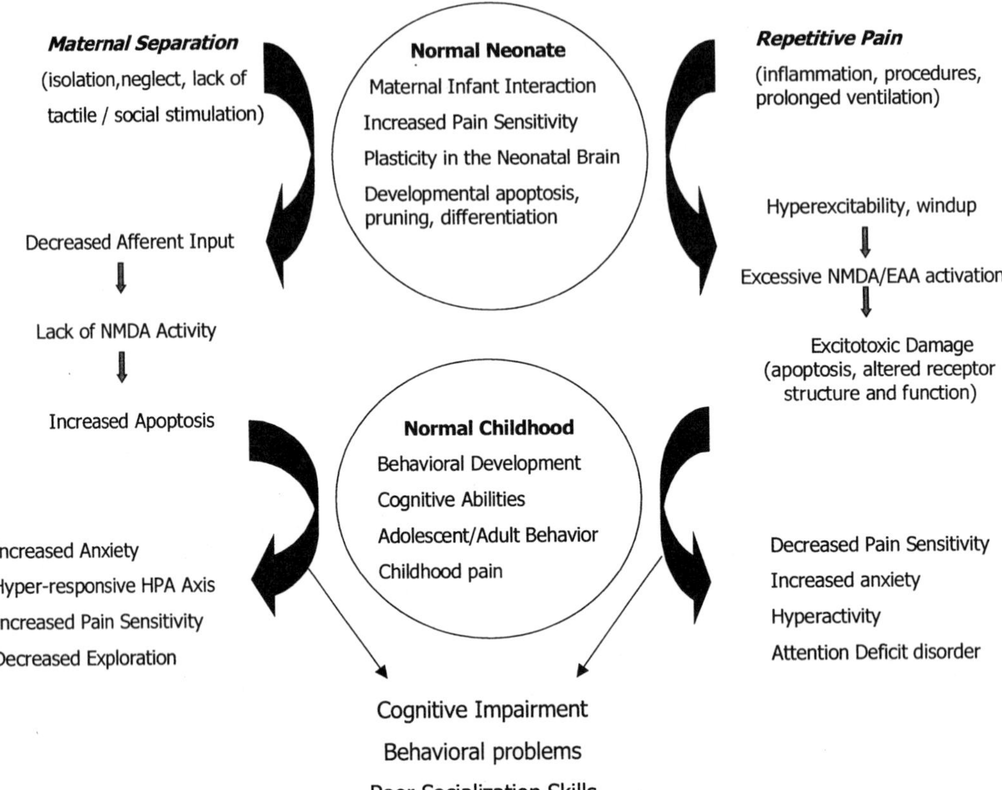

FIG. 4.1. The interplay of factors affecting long-term outcome of pain in neonates.

fants. A summary timeline of both short- and long-term effects of pain in the neonatal period is displayed in Figure 4.1.

Short-Term Outcomes of Pain in Preterm Neonates

There are few outcome measures more concrete than survival. Several studies have shown that patients who receive opioids, in either the operating room or the NICU, have improved survival compared with control subjects. Anand and Hickey (55) found that high-dose sufentanil cardiac anesthesia followed by sufentanil infusion in the postoperative period reduced mortality and morbidity and hormonal responses. An elegant pilot study recently demonstrated that there were fewer deaths and fewer intracranial hemorrhages in ventilated premature infants who received morphine infusion for 2 weeks than either placebo controls or subjects receiving midazolam infusions. During the study period, patients receiving either of the pharmacologically active interventions showed less response to endotracheal tube suctioning than did controls (56). Interestingly, the midazolam group had significantly more deaths than either the morphine or placebo group; the reasons for this surprising result are not yet clear.

These often critically ill neonates have been shown to be able to mount a stress response (57) proportionate to their level of illness (58) and in response to noxious stimuli (59). Premature infants have little physiologic or metabolic reserves and may tolerate autonomic instability, pulmonary dysfunction, or physical agitation poorly. Opioids (58,60,61) and phenobarbital (62) have been shown to reduce the hormonal stress response to routine NICU procedures. Fentanyl was shown to reduce the hormonal stress response to surgical ligation of patent ductus arteriosus (63) as well as to reduce growth hormone levels and behavioral indices of pain (64). Meperidine has been shown to be effective in reducing the duration of hypoxia stemming from endotracheal tube suctioning (65).

Respiratory disease is common in premature infants. Endotracheal intubation, ventilator support, chest physiotherapy, endotracheal suctioning, and blood gas sampling are common sourced of noxious stimulation. Reducing morbidity of respiratory treatment and enhancing the effects of pulmonary therapy would be valuable. Ventilated premature infants have reduced fluctuations in blood pressure after opioid administration than do those simply paralyzed and have lower peak inspiratory pressures as well (66). Ventilated premature infants breathe more synchronously with the ventilator when morphine is administered. Infants treated with opioids continue to contribute to respiratory effort, so ventilator contributions remain modest, as opposed to paralyzed patients, for whom the ventilator support is complete (66–68). Specific effects on the development of bronchopulmonary dysplasia have not been found (69). High-pressure ventilation has long-term effects on the pulmonary system (70), and circulatory fluctuations are seen in sick neonates (71,72), which may have a role in the cause of intraventricular hemorrhage (73). Reducing the effects of cardiopulmonary instability would be of great benefit to the patients.

Long-Term Outcomes of Pain in Preterm Neonates

Premature infants endure a variety of repeated noxious procedures. It is of relevance that repeated stimulation via heel lancing leads to increased withdrawal response in human premature neonates (74). Furthermore, comparison studies have been done that suggest that human premature infants may show the same long-term changes seen in rat pups. For example, Fitzgerald et al. (10) showed that flexor reflexes in response to noxious stimuli were exaggerated in the younger premature infants and directly mirrored the findings in rat pups of equivalent ages, as discussed earlier. In another study, the equivalent to secondary hyperalgesia was generated in young infants by repeated heel lancing. In this study, lidocaine-prilocaine (EMLA) cream was used to raise the response thresholds (12). These studies indicate that changes analogous to those seen in pathologic pain in adults can be induced in premature infants. A history of repeated procedures in premature infants appears to increase the stress response in response to heel stick compared with the responses of infants of equal postconceptional age. At 32 weeks postconceptional age, neonates maintained their oxygenation above 90% and had lower heart rates and more complex behavioral responses than infants 32 weeks postconceptional age who had been born several weeks earlier and subjected to a longer NICU course (75). We have begun to see that the underlying changes in sensory processing and neuroanatomy result in behavioral abnormalities for those premature infants exposed to repeated painful procedures. Once the infants have "graduated" from the NICU, their experiences may portend altered behaviors compared with their peers.

The number of clinics devoted to following the progress of former premature infants has multiplied greatly as the survival rate of these infants has risen. Many of the patients do well relative to their peers. However, some of them develop social, educational, and intellectual deficits (76–78), often inversely related to weight at delivery (79). Patients have been followed as long as their teenage years (80). Grunau et al. (81) followed former premature infants for varying lengths of time and found persistent differences in several areas of behavior relevant to early pain experience. At 18 months, former ELBW infants (weighing less than 1,000 g at birth) were judged to be less sensitive to pain by their parents than were full-term infants (81). The response to pain was not related to the children's temperament as it was for full-term toddlers. Direct correlation was not made to the pain experiences of the subjects, and subtle neurologic differences may have caused the differences. Conversely, early experience of repeated noxious stimulation without possibility for escape may have led to a situation of learned helplessness (82), which might be reflected in the toddlers' lack of pain expression.

At age 4.5 years, former ELBW children tended to have higher somatization scores and to derive less gratification from maternal contact than their full-term counterparts (81). By age 8 to 10 years, children can ascribe pain intensity ratings to drawings of painful situations. Former premature infants of this age were found to rate medically related pain higher than psychosocial pain. Controls made no such distinction. Duration of NICU stay was related to higher pain affect or intensity scores for some subsets of painful situation (83). Overall, former ELBW infants judged painful situations similarly to their peers, with some differences. Little is known about this cohort of patients when they reach adolescence. One study suggested that a subgroup of former ELBW infants saw themselves with limitations in pain, cognition, self-care, and sensation (80). Fortunately, most former premature infants reported a high quality of life.

Short-Term Outcomes of Pain in Full-Term Neonates

In contrast to the "chronically instrumented" state of many ELBW infants, healthy full-term infants undergo fewer noxious stimuli. Blood draws for metabolic screening, circumcision, and the occasional surgical procedure comprise the majority of painful interventions for normal neonates. Despite the isolated nature of each intervention, autonomic perturbations occur, and pain can be expressed clearly by the infants. Circumcision has been studied most comprehensively and presents an elegant model for the effects of pain control for discreet noxious events. The basic principles can be extrapolated to similar, one-time painful procedures.

Transcutaneously measured oxygen pressure decreases during circumcision. Dorsal penile nerve blocks can preserve oxygenation (84,85), as can a eutectic mixture of local anesthetics (lidocaine-prilocaine cream) (86). Relatively early on, Emde et al. (87) found that sleep stages were disturbed in newborn boys undergoing circumcision when compared with uncircumcised controls. Others found similar changes, although interpretation of the meaning of such changes varied (88). Stress hormones, such as cortisol, have been measured after circumcision. A rise in cortisol levels has been found; little or no rise is seen if anesthesia is provided (usually in the form of a nerve block with local anesthetic) (89–91). The cortisol elevations resolved in an hour or so, but some of the behavioral changes lasted through the next day (87,92). This suggests that painful stimuli are remembered by the infant and manifest as altered attention, state control, and sleep patterns.

Long-Term Outcomes of Pain in Full-Term Neonates

Long-term effects of painful stimuli in full-term infants have only just begun to be studied. Taddio and colleagues (93,94) have examined the effects of circumcision pain on male infants. When comparing circumcised with uncircumcised infants at ages 4 and 6 months, blinded observers reported higher behavioral pain scores for the circumcised infants than for the controls. Circumcised infants also cried longer than controls. Use of lidocaine-prilocaine cream during circumcision attenuated some aspects of the subsequent pain response (94). These studies represent an initial foray into this important area, and future study should elucidate the role for true preemptive analgesia.

IMPLICATIONS FOR CLINICAL PRACTICE

Preemptive analgesia has garnered a fair amount of attention in the adult pain and

TABLE 4.1. *Timeline for the long-term consequences of neonatal pain*

Consequence	25 wk PCA	Full term	4–6 mo	1–2 yr	4 yr	10 yr	18 yr
Hyperalgesia	Yes	Yes	Probably	?	?	?	?
Sensitization/windup	Yes	Yes	?	?	?	?	?
Physiologic destabilization	Yes	Yes	?	?	?	?	?
Behavioral changes	Yes	Yes	Yes	Probably	Possibly	?	?
Personality effects	?	?	?	Probably	Possibly	Possibly	Possibly

anesthesia literature (95–97) with a few pediatric studies (98,99), although results have been mixed. Fewer situations can be imagined in which preemptive analgesia could be of longer term consequence than in infants. There is much to be learned about the use of *N*-methyl-D-aspartate antagonists, neurokinin modulators, and their role as adjuncts to opioids and neural blockade in neonates before preemptive analgesia can become a clinical reality. For now, universal use of appropriate anesthesia and analgesia is the next step. Many options are available for the multiple settings in which infants encounter pain.

For minor procedures, swaddling (100, 101), sucrose pacifiers (102), and lidocaine-prilocaine cream (103) have proven safe and effective. For more stimulating procedures, local anesthesia (with attention to local anesthetic dosing), opioids, and nonsteroidal anti-inflammatory drugs should be added. For postoperative pain, continuous epidural analgesia and opioids form the mainstay of pain therapy. Both modalities are used safely and effectively to control pain from operative interventions (104–108). Centers with experience and expertise in all these modalities use them safely for all ages of infants. Teamwork between neonatologists and anesthesiologists should merge the expertise needed to provide viable protocols and treatments for infants in all situations.

CONCLUSION

Neonatal display of pain and other related responses become more robust and recognizable during development (109). Assessment becomes easier, and the immediate results of pain treatment can be ascertained somewhat more readily. The limited repertoire of pain behaviors manifested by the smallest preterm neonates put them at risk for a greater undertreatment of their pain. The key for practitioners is not to underestimate the invasiveness of the procedures that they perform on ELBW infants. Assuming that if a given procedure is noxious to older individuals, it will also be noxious to the preterm patient seems most prudent (110) and has been given the importance of a moral emergency (111). The greater recognition of the importance of pain care for neonates is also reflected in the joint statement issued by the American Academy of Pediatrics and the Canadian Pediatric Society, highlighting the need for analgesia for circumcision (112) and for reducing pain and stress in the neonate (113). For many years, practitioners have comforted themselves with the delusion that younger infants could not feel pain or would not remember it. A growing body of data, summarized in Table 4.1, shows that sustained physiologic, anatomic, and behavioral changes can and do result from repetitive or prolonged exposure to noxious stimuli in neonates.

REFERENCES

1. Finley GA, McGrath PJ. Measurement of pain in infants and children. *Progress in pain research and management.* Seattle: IASP Press, 1998.
2. Stevens BJ, Johnston CC, Grunau RV. Issues of assessment of pain and discomfort in neonates. *J Obstet Gynecol Neonatal Nurs* 1995;24:849–855.
3. Franck LS, Miaskowski C. Measurement of neonatal responses to painful stimuli: a research review. *J Pain Symptom Manage* 1997;14:343–378.
4. Franck LS. A national survey of the assessment and treatment of pain and agitation in the neonatal intensive care unit. *J Obstet Gynecol Neonatal Nurs* 1987; 16:387–393.
5. Johnston CC, Collinge JM, Henderson SJ, et al. A

cross-sectional survey of pain and pharmacological analgesia in Canadian neonatal intensive care units. *Clin J Pain* 1997;13:308–312.

6. McLaughlin CR, Hull JG, Edwards WH, et al. Neonatal pain: a comprehensive survey of attitudes and practices. *J Pain Symptom Manage* 1993;8:7–16.
7. Barker DP, Rutter N. Exposure to invasive procedures in neonatal intensive care unit admissions. *Arch Dis Child Fetal Neonatal Ed* 1995;72:F47–F48.
8. Anand KJS. Physiology of pain in infants and children. *Ann Nestle* 1999;57:7–18.
9. Dobbing J. Nutritional growth restriction and the nervous system. In: Davison AN, Thompson RHS, eds. *The molecular basis of neuropathology*. London: Edward Arnold, 1981.
10. Fitzgerald M, Shaw A, MacIntosh N. Postnatal development of the cutaneous flexor reflex: comparative study of preterm infants and newborn rat pups. *Dev Med Child Neurol* 1988;30:520–526.
11. Fitzgerald M. Spontaneous and evoked activity of fetal primary afferents in vivo. *Nature* 1987;326:603–605.
12. Fitzgerald M, Millard C, McIntosh N. Cutaneous hypersensitivity following peripheral tissue damage in newborn infants and its reversal with topical anaesthesia. *Pain* 1989;39:31–36.
13. Yi DK, Barr GA. The induction of Fos-like immunoreactivity by noxious thermal, mechanical and chemical stimuli in the lumbar spinal cord of infant rats. *Pain* 1995;60:257–265.
14. Fitzgerald M, Koltzenburg M. The functional development of descending inhibitory pathways in the dorsolateral funiculus of the newborn rat spinal cord. *Brain Res* 1986;389:261–270.
15. Marti E, Gibson SJ, Polak JM, et al. Ontogeny of peptide- and amine-containing neurones in motor, sensory, and autonomic regions of rat and human spinal cord, dorsal root ganglia, and rat skin. *J Comp Neurol* 1987;266:332–359.
16. Abbott FV, Franklin KB, Westbrook RF. The formalin test: scoring properties of the first and second phases of the pain response in rats. *Pain* 1995;60:91–102.
17. McLaughlin CR, Lichtman AH, Fanselow MS, et al. Tonic nociception in neonatal rats. *Pharmacol Biochem Behav* 1990;36:859–862.
18. Anand KJ, Coskun V, Thrivikraman KV, et al. Long-term behavioral effects of repetitive pain in neonatal rat pups. *Physiol Behav* 1999;66:627–637.
19. Falcon M, Guendellman D, Stolberg A, et al. Development of thermal nociception in rats. *Pain* 1996;67: 203–208.
20. Fitzgerald M. The postnatal development of cutaneous afferent fibre input and receptive field organization in the rat dorsal horn. *J Physiol* 1985;364:1–18.
21. Barr GA. Maturation of the biphasic behavioral and heart rate response in the formalin test. *Pharmacol Biochem Behav* 1998;60:329–335.
22. Guy ER, Abbott FV. The behavioral response to formalin in preweanling rats. *Pain* 1992;51:81–90.
23. Teng CJ, Abbott FV. The formalin test: a dose-response analysis at three developmental stages. *Pain* 1998;76: 337–347.
24. Abbott FV, Guy ER. Effects of morphine, pentobarbital and amphetamine on formalin-induced behaviours in infant rats: sedation versus specific suppression of pain. *Pain* 1995;62:303–312.
25. Quigley KS, Shair HN, Myers MM. Parasympathetic control of heart period during early postnatal development in the rat. *J Auton Nerv Syst* 1996;59:75–82.
26. Williams S, Evan G, Hunt SP. Spinal c-fos induction by sensory stimulation in neonatal rats. *Neurosci Lett* 1990;109:309–314.
27. Williams S, Evan GI, Hunt SP. Changing patterns of c-fos induction in spinal neurons following thermal cutaneous stimulation in the rat. *Neuroscience* 1990;36: 73–81.
28. Ren K, Blass EM, Zhou Q, et al. Suckling and sucrose ingestion suppress persistent hyperalgesia and spinal Fos expression after forepaw inflammation in infant rats. *Proc Natl Acad Sci U S A* 1997;94:1471–1475.
29. Barr GA. Antinociceptive effects of locally administered morphine in infant rats. *Pain* 1999;81:155–161.
30. Newton BW, Rovnaghi CR, Golzar Y, et al. Supraspinal FOS expression in neonatal rat pups following graded inflammatory pain. *Soc Neurosci* 1999; 25:1044(abst).
31. Anand KJ, Hickey PR. Pain and its effects in the human neonate and fetus. *N Engl J Med* 1987;317: 1321–1329.
32. Hu D, Hu R, Berde CB. Neurologic evaluation of infant and adult rats before and after sciatic nerve blockade. *Anesthesiology* 1997;86:957–965.
33. Woolf CJ, Salter MW. Neuronal plasticity: increasing the gain in pain. *Science* 2000;288:1765–1769.
34. Constantinou J, Reynolds ML, Woolf CJ, et al. Nerve growth factor levels in developing rat skin: upregulation following skin wounding. *Neuroreport* 1994;5: 2281–2284.
35. Fitzgerald M, Anand KJS. The developmental neuroanatomy and neurophysiology of pain. In: Schechter N, Berde C, Yaster M, eds. *Pain management in infants, children and adolescents*. Baltimore: Williams & Wilkins; 1993:11–32.
36. McCleskey EW, Gold MS. Ion channels of nociception. *Annu Rev Physiol* 1999;61:835–856.
37. Coggeshall RE, Pover CM, Fitzgerald M. Dorsal root ganglion cell death and surviving cell numbers in relation to the development of sensory innervation in the rat hindlimb. *Brain Res Dev Brain Res* 1994;82: 193–212.
38. Jenq CB, Chung K, Coggeshall RE. Postnatal loss of axons in normal rat sciatic nerve. *J Comp Neurol* 1986;244:445–450.
39. Reynolds ML, Fitzgerald M. Long-term sensory hyperinnervation following neonatal skin wounds. *J Comp Neurol* 1995;358:487–498.
40. Reynolds M, Alvares D, Middleton J, et al. Neonatally wounded skin induces NGF-independent sensory neurite outgrowth in vitro. *Brain Res* 1997;102:275–283.
41. De Lima J, Alvares D, Hatch DJ, et al. Sensory hyperinnervation after neonatal skin wounding: effect of bupivacaine sciatic nerve block. *Br J Anaesth* 1999;83: 662–664.
42. Fitzgerald M, Reynolds ML, Benowitz LI. GAP-43 expression in the developing rat lumbar spinal cord. *Neuroscience* 1991;41:187–199.
43. Fitzgerald M. Cutaneous primary afferent properties in the hind limb of the neonatal rat. *J Physiol* 1987;383: 79–92.
44. Pignatelli D, Ribeiro-da-Silva A, Coimbra A. Postnatal maturation of primary afferent terminations in the sub-

stantia gelatinosa of the rat spinal cord. An electron microscopic study. *Brain Res* 1989;491:33–44.
45. Fitzgerald M, Butcher T, Shortland P. Developmental changes in the laminar termination of A fibre cutaneous sensory afferents in the rat spinal cord dorsal horn. *J Comp Neurol* 1994;348:225–233.
46. Jennings E, Fitzgerald M. C-fos can be induced in the neonatal rat spinal cord by both noxious and innocuous peripheral stimulation. *Pain* 1996;68:301–306.
47. Jennings E, Fitzgerald M. Postnatal changes in responses of rat dorsal horn cells to afferent stimulation: a fibre-induced sensitization. *J Physiol* 1998;509: 859–868.
48. Boucher T, Jennings E, Fitzgerald M. The onset of diffuse noxious inhibitory controls in postnatal rat pups: a C-Fos study. *Neurosci Lett* 1998;257:9–12.
49. Bicknell HR Jr, Beal JA. Axonal and dendritic development of substantia gelatinosa neurons in the lumbosacral spinal cord of the rat. *J Comp Neurol* 1984; 226:508–522.
50. Wang J, Reichling DB, Kyrozis A, et al. Developmental loss of GABA- and glycine-induced depolarization and Ca2+ transients in embryonic rat dorsal horn neurons in culture. *Eur J Neurosci* 1994;6:1275–1280.
51. Ruda MA, Ling QD, Hohmann AG, et al. Altered nociceptive neuronal circuits after neonatal peripheral inflammation. *Science* 2000;289:628–531.
52. Rahman W, Fitzgerald M, Aynsley-Green A, et al. The effects of neonatal exposure to inflammation and/or morphine on neuronal responses and morphine analgesia in adult rats. In: Jensen TS, Turner JA, Weisenfield-Hallin Z, eds. *Proceedings of the 8th World Congress on Pain*. Seattle: IASP Press, 1997:783–794.
53. Alvares D, Fitzgerald M. Building blocks of pain: the regulation of key molecules in spinal sensory neurones during development and following peripheral axotomy. *Pain* 1999;6[Suppl]:S71–S85.
54. Bhutta AT, Rovnaghi CR, Simpson PM, et al. Interactions of inflammatory pain and morphine treatment in infant rats: long-term behavioral effects. *Physiol Behav* 2001;73:51–58.
55. Anand KJ, Hickey PR. Halothane-morphine compared with high-dose sufentanil for anesthesia and postoperative analgesia in neonatal cardiac surgery. *N Engl J Med* 1992;326:1–9.
56. Anand KJ, Barton BA, McIntosh N, et al. Analgesia and sedation in preterm neonates who require ventilatory support: results from the NOPAIN trial. Neonatal Outcome and Prolonged Analgesia in Neonates [published erratum appears in *Arch Pediatr Adolesc Med* 1999;153:895]. *Arch Pediatr Adolesc Med* 1999;153: 331–338.
57. Schmeling DJ, Coran AG. Hormonal and metabolic response to operative stress in the neonate. *JPEN J Parenteral Enteral Nutr* 1991;15:215–238.
58. Barker DP, Rutter N. Stress, severity of illness, and outcome in ventilated preterm infants. *Arch Dis Child Fetal Neonatal Ed* 1996;75:F187–F190.
59. Lagercrantz H, Nilsson E, Redham I, et al. Plasma catecholamines following nursing procedures in a neonatal ward. *Early Hum Dev* 1986;14:61–65.
60. Quinn MW, Otoo F, Rushforth JA, et al. Effect of morphine and pancuronium on the stress response in ventilated preterm infants. *Early Hum Dev* 1992;30: 241–248.
61. Barker DP, Simpson J, Pawula M, et al. Randomised, double blind trial of two loading dose regimens of diamorphine in ventilated newborn infants. *Arch Dis Child Fetal Neonatal Ed* 1995;73:F22–F26.
62. Greisen G, Frederiksen P, Hertel J, et al. Catecholamine response to chest physiotherapy and endotracheal suctioning in preterm infants. *Acta Paediatr Scand* 1985;74:525–529.
63. Anand KJ, Sippell WG, Aynsley-Green A. Randomised trial of fentanyl anaesthesia in preterm babies undergoing surgery: effects on the stress response [published erratum appears in *Lancet* 1987;1:234]. *Lancet* 1987;1:62–66.
64. Guinsburg R, Kopelman BI, Anand KJ, et al. Physiological, hormonal, and behavioral responses to a single fentanyl dose in intubated and ventilated preterm neonates. *J Pediatr* 1998;132:954–959.
65. Pokela ML. Pain relief can reduce hypoxemia in distressed neonates during routine treatment procedures. *Pediatrics* 1994;93:379–383.
66. Goldstein RF, Brazy JE. Narcotic sedation stabilizes arterial blood pressure fluctuations in sick premature infants. *J Perinatol* 1991;11:365–371.
67. Dyke MP, Kohan R, Evans S. Morphine increases synchronous ventilation in preterm infants. *J Paediatr Child Health* 1995;31:176–179.
68. Shaw NJ, Cooke RW, Gill AB, et al. Randomised trial of routine versus selective paralysis during ventilation for neonatal respiratory distress syndrome. *Arch Dis Child* 1993;69:479–482.
69. Orsini AJ, Leef KH, Costarino A, et al. Routine use of fentanyl infusions for pain and stress reduction in infants with respiratory distress syndrome. *J Pediatr* 1996;129:140–145.
70. Gannon CM, Wiswell TE, Spitzer AR. Volutrauma, PaCO2 levels, and neurodevelopmental sequelae following assisted ventilation. *Clin Perinatol* 1998;25: 159–175.
71. Ramaekers VT, Casaer P, Daniels H. Cerebral hyperperfusion following episodes of bradycardia in the preterm infant. *Early Hum Dev* 1993;34:199–208.
72. Perlman J, Thach B. Respiratory origin of fluctuations in arterial blood pressure in premature infants with respiratory distress syndrome. *Pediatrics* 1988;81:399–403.
73. Abdel-Rahman AM, Rosenberg AA. Prevention of intraventricular hemorrhage in the premature infant. *Clin Perinatol* 1994;21:505–521.
74. Andrews K, Fitzgerald M. Cutaneous flexion reflex in human neonates: a quantitative study of threshold and stimulus-response characteristics after single and repeated stimuli. *Dev Med Child Neurol* 1999;41: 696–703.
75. Johnston CC, Stevens BJ. Experience in a neonatal intensive care unit affects pain response. *Pediatrics* 1996;98:925–390.
76. Sommerfelt K, Troland K, Ellertsen B, et al. Behavioral problems in low-birthweight preschoolers. *Dev Med Child Neurol* 1996;38:927–940.
77. Hack M, Taylor HG, Klein N, et al. School-age outcomes in children with birth weights under 750 g. *N Engl J Med* 1994;331:753–759.
78. Whitfield MF, Grunau RV, Holsti L. Extremely premature (< or = 800 g) schoolchildren: multiple areas of hidden disability. *Arch Dis Child Fetal Neonatal Ed* 1997;77:F85–F90.

79. McCarton CM, Brooks-Gunn J, Wallace IF, et al. Results at age 8 years of early intervention for low-birth-weight premature infants. The Infant Health and Development Program. *JAMA* 1997;277:126–132.
80. Saigal S, Feeny D, Rosenbaum P, et al. Self-perceived health status and health-related quality of life of extremely low-birth-weight infants at adolescence. *JAMA* 1996;276:453–459.
81. Grunau RV, Whitfield MF, Petrie JH, et al. Early pain experience, child and family factors, as precursors of somatization: a prospective study of extremely premature and fullterm children. *Pain* 1994;56:353–359.
82. Seligman MEP. *Helplessness: on depression, development and death.* San Francisco: Freeman, 1975.
83. Grunau RE, Whitfield MF, Petrie J. Children's judgements about pain at age 8–10 years: do extremely low birthweight (< or = 1000 g) children differ from full birthweight peers? *J Child Psychol Psychiatry* 1998; 39:587–594.
84. Williamson PS, Williamson ML. Physiologic stress reduction by a local anesthetic during newborn circumcision. *Pediatrics* 1983;71:36–40.
85. Maxwell LG, Yaster M, Wetzel RC, et al. Penile nerve block for newborn circumcision. *Obstet Gynecol* 1987;70:415–419.
86. Benini F, Johnston CC, Faucher D, et al. Topical anesthesia during circumcision in newborn infants. *JAMA* 1993;270:850–853.
87. Emde RN, Harmon RJ, Metcalf D, et al. Stress and neonatal sleep. *Psychosom Med* 1971;33:491–497.
88. Anders TF, Chalemian RJ. The effects of circumcision on sleep-wake states in human neonates. *Psychosom Med* 1974;36:174–179.
89. Gunnar M, Fisch R, Korsvik S, et al. The effects of circumcision on serum cortisol and behavior. *Psychoneuroendocrinology* 1981;6:269–275.
90. Gunnar MR, Malone S, Vance G, et al. Coping with aversive stimulation in the neonatal period: quiet sleep and plasma cortisol levels during recovery from circumcision. *Child Dev* 1985;56:824–834.
91. Stang HJ, Gunnar MR, Snellman L, et al. Local anesthesia for neonatal circumcision. Effects on distress and cortisol response. *JAMA* 1988;259:1507–1511.
92. Dixon S, Snyder J, Holve R, et al. Behavioural effects of circumcision with and without anesthesia. *J Dev Behav Pediatr* 1984;5:246–250.
93. Taddio A, Goldbach M, Ipp M, et al. Effect of neonatal circumcision on pain responses during vaccination in boys. *Lancet* 1995;345:291–292.
94. Taddio A, Katz J, Ilersich AL, et al. Effect of neonatal circumcision on pain response during subsequent routine vaccination. *Lancet* 1997;349:599–603.
95. Tverskoy M, Oz Y, Isakson A, et al. Preemptive effect of fentanyl and ketamine on postoperative pain and wound hyperalgesia. *Anesth Analg* 1994;78:205–209.
96. Ke RW, Portera SG, Bagous W, et al. A randomized, double-blinded trial of preemptive analgesia in laparoscopy. *Obstet Gynecol* 1998;92:972–975.
97. Katz J, Clairoux M, Redahan C, et al. High dose alfentanil pre-empts pain after abdominal hysterectomy. *Pain* 1996;68:109–118.
98. Altintas F, Bozkurt P, Ipek N, et al. The efficacy of pre-versus postsurgical axillary block on postoperative pain in paediatric patients. *Paediatr Anaesth* 2000;10:23–28.
99. Ho JW, Khambatta HJ, Pang LM, et al. Preemptive analgesia in children. Does it exist? *Reg Anesth* 1997; 22:125–130.
100. Fearon I, Kisilevsky BS, Hains SM, et al. Swaddling after heel lance: age-specific effects on behavioral recovery in. *J Dev Behav Pediatr* 1997;18:222–232.
101. Campos RG. Soothing pain-elicited distress in infants with swaddling and pacifiers. *Child Dev* 1989;60: 781–792.
102. Stevens B, Taddio A, Ohlsson A, et al. The efficacy of sucrose for relieving procedural pain in neonates—a systematic review and meta-analysis. *Acta Paediatr* 1997;86:837–842.
103. Taddio A, Ohlsson A, Einarson TR, et al. A systematic review of lidocaine-prilocaine cream (EMLA) in the treatment of acute pain in neonates. *Pediatrics* 1998;101:E1.
104. Tobias JD, O'Dell N. Chloroprocaine for epidural anesthesia in infants and children. *AANA J* 1995;63: 131–135.
105. Williams RK, McBride WJ, Abajian JC. Combined spinal and epidural anaesthesia for major abdominal surgery in infants. *Can J Anaesth* 1997;44:511–514.
106. Murrell D, Gibson PR, Cohen RC. Continuous epidural analgesia in newborn infants undergoing major surgery. *J Pediatr Surg* 1993;28:548–552.
107. Truog R, Anand KJ. Management of pain in the postoperative neonate. *Clin Perinatol* 1989;16:61–78.
108. Bosenberg AT. Epidural analgesia for major neonatal surgery. *Paediatr Anaesth* 1998;8:479–483.
109. Johnston CC, Stevens B, Craig KD, et al. Developmental changes in pain expression in premature, fullterm, two- and four-month-old infants. *Pain* 1993;52: 201–208.
110. Porter FL, Wolf CM, Miller JP. Procedural pain in newborn infants: the influence of intensity and development. *Pediatrics* 1999;104:e13.
111. Cunningham N. Inclusion of the nonverbal patient: a matter of moral emergency. *Pain Forum* 1999;8: 110–112.
112. Anonymous. Circumcision policy statement. American Academy of Pediatrics. Task Force on Circumcision. *Pediatrics* 1999;103:686–693.
113. Anonymous. Prevention and management of pain and stress in the neonate. American Academy of Pediatrics. Committee on Fetus and Newborn. Committee on Drugs. Section on Anesthesiology. Section on Surgery. Canadian Paediatric Society. Fetus and Newborn Committee. *Pediatrics* 2000;105:454–461.

5
Clinical Pharmacology

Myron Yaster

When physicians administer drugs to their patients, they do so with the expectation that an anticipated therapeutic effect will occur. Unfortunately, other less desired results can also occur, namely, the patient may derive inadequate or no therapeutic benefit from the administered drug, or, worse yet, he/she may develop a toxic reaction. The aim of modern clinical pharmacology is to take the guesswork out of this process and to establish the relationship between the dose of a drug given and the response elicited. To attain this goal, clinicians need a working knowledge of the principles of drug absorption, distribution, and elimination and how these processes relate to the intensity and duration of drug action.

Unfortunately, it is also important to understand that the science of clinical pharmacology is not always predictable and exact. The relationship between the concentration of drug in the blood and the clinical response to that plasma drug level is not always predictable. Individuals vary widely in their response to drugs, and this may be owing to both differences in the concentration of drug available at the drug's site of action and to differences in the individual's inherent sensitivity to the drug. Clearly, the end point of drug therapy is clinical efficacy, not simply attaining a specific blood level of drug. "Best practice" requires an attempt by the physician to define the optimal dose–response relationship in each individual patient based on history, diagnosis, and clinical judgment.

Drugs are fundamental in the treatment of pain. A thorough understanding of the history, chemical and physical properties, physiologic effects, disposition, mechanisms of action, and therapeutic uses of the drugs used in the treatment of pain is essential for clinicians who treat pain in infants, children, and adolescents. This chapter describes the relationship between dose and response in a general fashion using specific illustrative examples. The principles can then be applied in succeeding chapters. Finally, rather than citing a voluminous literature, references consist of timely reviews from which the reader can pursue more specific and detailed listings (1–12).

PHARMACOKINETICS

A dose–response curve can be constructed (Fig. 5.1) that relates therapeutic responses and adverse effects to drug concentration. Usually, therapeutic concentrations within the "therapeutic window" are those that produce a desired therapeutic effect in a large proportion of patients while producing adverse effects in few. The ratio of plasma concentrations that produce therapeutic effects to those producing adverse effects is known as the *therapeutic ratio*. Basically, toxicity is less likely to occur at usual therapeutic concentrations with drugs with higher therapeutic ratios than with drugs with lower ones. For example, warfarin, an oral anticoagulant, has a narrow therapeutic index, whereas penicillin, a commonly used antibiotic, has a large therapeutic index (Fig. 5.1) (13).

An understanding of the factors that determine drug concentrations within the body is crucial to rational drug use in patients and to achieving desirable plasma drug concentrations. *Pharmacokinetics* is the term used to

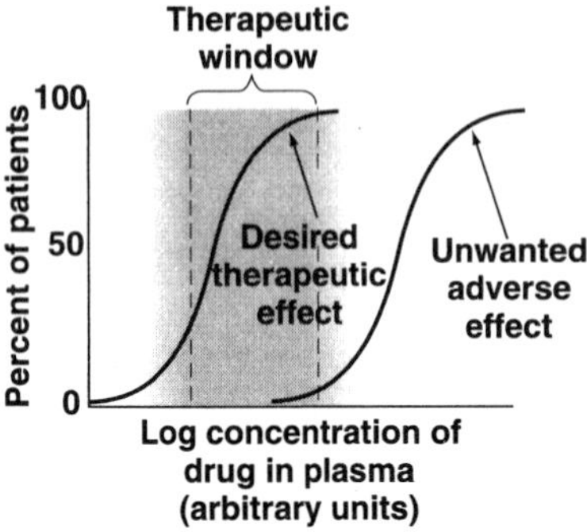

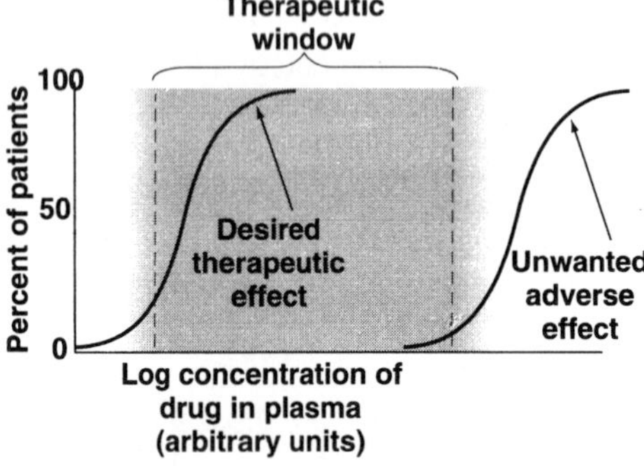

FIG. 5.1. The therapeutic index is a measure of a drug's safety. Warfarin, an oral anticoagulant, has a small therapeutic index, whereas penicillin has a large therapeutic index. The figure represents cumulative percentage of patients responding to plasma levels of drug. (From Mycek MJ, Harvey RA, Champe PC. Pharmacokinetics and drug receptors. In: Mycek MJ, Harvey RA, Champe PC, eds. *Lippincott's illustrated reviews: pharmacology*, 2nd ed. Philadelphia: Lippincott Williams & Wilkins, 2000:17–20, with permission.)

describe the study of drug disposition within the body. It includes absorption, distribution, metabolism, and elimination of drug molecules from the body. *Pharmacodynamics* is the term used to describe the study of drug action within the body. It defines the relationship between the concentration of the drug at the site of action and the physiologic response. The relationship between pharmacokinetics and pharmacodynamics provides an understanding of the dose–response curves for the onset of action, magnitude of action, and duration of action of drugs used in treating patients (8–11).

Physiologic Changes Affecting Pharmacokinetics in Infants, Children, and Adolescents

Unfortunately, very few studies have evaluated the pharmacokinetic and pharmacodynamic properties of drugs in children. Most pharmacokinetic studies are performed using healthy adult volunteers, adult patients who are only minimally ill, or adult patients in a stable phase of a chronic disease. These data are then extrapolated to infants, children, and adolescents and to the critically ill (both adult and pediatric). Drug manufacturers simply do not perform these studies in children. In fact, so little pharmacokinetic and dynamic testing has been performed in children that they are often considered "therapeutic orphans" (14). Indeed, more than 70% of all the drugs used to treat children have never been formally tested or approved for use in children. Occasionally, this has resulted in catastrophe, as in the development of gray baby syndrome in neonates treated with chloramphenicol (15,16). Why children are different is obvious. The newborn, children younger than 2 to 3 years of age, and unstable, critically ill pediatric patients of any age often present significant hemodynamic alterations and organ dysfunction that may significantly alter drug absorption, transport, metabolism, and excretion of drugs. Studies performed in healthy older children or adult patients may offer little insight into how these drugs perform in these other patient populations (17–20). To help remedy this situation, the U.S. Food and Drug Administration has mandated pediatric pharmacokinetic and dynamic studies of all new drugs that enter the American marketplace (21–23). Unfortunately, despite these new regulations, the pharmaceutical industry has, with very few exceptions, delayed, evaded, and stonewalled the process, leaving children with very little protection.

Pharmacokinetic Modeling

Mathematical models have been constructed that describe the movement of drugs in the body. Knowledge of a drug's general disposition and behavior improves the ability to optimize drug-dosing regimens and achieve therapeutic outcomes while minimizing toxicity. Compartment models are often used to describe the physiologic and mathematical distribution of a drug within the body. Compartments can be thought of as containers into which drugs are added and mixed. Compartment models may contain one or more compartments, depending on how rapidly an administered drug equilibrates between serum and tissues. In the simplest case, a single compartment model, an intravenously administered drug, is distributed instantly throughout the entire body. The whole body is considered a single container or compartment. The concentration of drug in the container or compartment (C_P) is defined by the formula:

$$C_P = \frac{\text{dose}}{\text{Vd}} \quad (1)$$

where Vd is the volume of distribution (or the volume of the container). Unfortunately, when most drugs are administered, they do not instantly distribute throughout the body and act as if they are in a single compartment or container. More commonly, the drug is rapidly distributed from the central compartment and then slowly equilibrates with one or more peripheral compartments. Although these compartments do not have anatomic correlates, it can best be thought of as follows. In a two-compartment model, the small central compartment consists of the intravascular volume and the rapidly perfused organs and tissues. The drug then circulates throughout the body and may distribute into a second peripheral compartment consisting of various organs such as the skin, muscle, bone, and fat. In both models, drug is eliminated from the central compartment, but in the two-compartment model, the drug must first return to the central compartment for elimination to occur.

After distribution, the administered drug is eliminated from the body by processes such as metabolism or renal excretion. The elimination of most drugs from the central compartment is a linear process (phenytoin and ethanol are exceptions). With linear, or *first-order*, kinetics, the body eliminates the same percentage of drug per unit of time. The amount of drug removed per unit of time will decrease as the serum concentration decreases (Fig. 5.2). In first-order kinetics, a plot of the logarithm of serum concentration versus time results in a straight line. Nonlin-

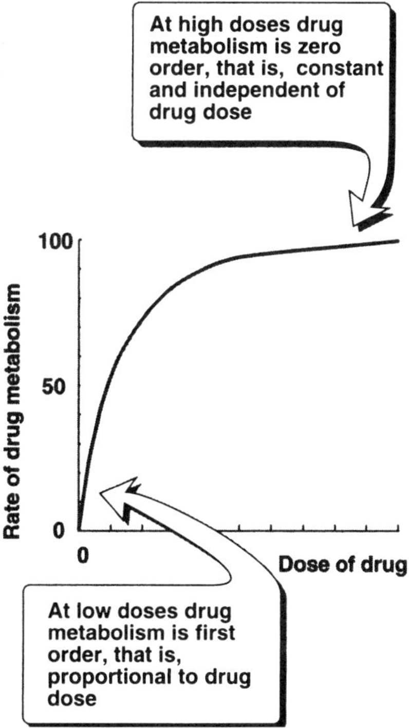

FIG. 5.2. Effect of drug on the rate of metabolism. (From Mycek MJ, Harvey RA, Champe PC. Absorption, distribution, and elimination of drugs. In: Mycek MJ, Harvey RA, Champe PC, eds. *Lippincott's illustrated reviews: pharmacology*, 2nd ed. Philadelphia: Lippincott Williams & Wilkins, 2000:1–16, with permission.)

ear, or *zero-order*, kinetics is a saturable process in which a constant amount of drug is eliminated per unit of time (Fig. 5.2). This is usually an enzyme-mediated reaction in which all available enzyme is involved. Unlike first-order kinetics, drug elimination is proportional, not to serum concentration but rather to the rate at which an enzyme can catalyze a drug reaction.

Occasionally, a first-order process changes to a zero-order process at high doses and will result in a much greater rise in plasma concentrations and a prolongation of the time needed to eliminate the drug. For example, phenytoin, salicylate, and theophylline exhibit first-order elimination at low doses and zero-order elimination at higher doses because of saturation of the process of elimination. This means that an increase in dose produces the expected and proportional increase in plasma level until saturation is reached, and plasma levels will increase rapidly with very small further increases in drug dose (Fig. 5.2).

Four main pharmacokinetic parameters are used to characterize drug disposition within the body: volume of distribution (Vd), half-life ($t_{1/2}$), elimination rate constant (Ke), and clearance (Cl). The Vd is the apparent size of the compartment into which a drug distributes. This is not necessarily a physiologic volume because the Vd often exceeds total body water as a result of tissue distribution and binding. The Vd is measured as (Equation 2) (rearranged Equation 1):

$$\mathrm{Vd} = \frac{\text{Dose administered}}{\text{Peak concentration}} \qquad (2)$$

Half-life is the time required for the serum concentration to decrease by 50% and is the most commonly used pharmacokinetic parameter. The elimination rate constant Ke is the fraction of drug removed from the body per unit time. Half-life is mathematically related to Ke by Equation 3:

$$t_{1/2} = \frac{0.693}{\mathrm{Ke}} \quad \text{or} \quad \mathrm{Ke} = \frac{0.693}{t_{1/2}} \qquad (3)$$

Clearance (Cl) is the volume of blood that is cleared of drug per unit of time. For example, a Cl = 3 L/hr means that drug is completely removed from 3 L of blood every hour. Clearance is dependent on the functions of the organs that metabolize and eliminate drug from the body. Clearance is mathematically related to Ke, $t_{1/2}$, and Vd by the Equation 4:

$$\mathrm{Cl} = (\mathrm{Ke})(\mathrm{Vd}) \qquad (4)$$

Substituting Ke from Equation 3 produces Equation 4:

$$\mathrm{Cl} = \left(\frac{0.693}{t_{1/2}}\right)(\mathrm{Vd}) \qquad (5)$$

Rearranging Equation 4 allows us to solve for $t_{1/2}$ (Equation 6):

$$t_{1/2} = 0.693\left(\frac{\mathrm{Vd}}{\mathrm{Cl}}\right) \qquad (6)$$

Equation 6 is essential in understanding the importance of half-life because it reveals that changes in both Cl and Vd independently affect $t_{1/2}$. Increasing the volume of distribution increases the elimination half-life but does not affect clearance. Similarly, increasing clearance decreases the elimination half-life and does not affect the volume of distribution. In theory, it would appear that the elimination of drug is exponential and that it would be impossible, based on half-life, to calculate how much drug remains in the body. In reality, 94% of an administered dose of drug is eliminated in four half-lives.

In multicompartment models, drug is rapidly distributed in the central compartment and then slowly equilibrates with another peripheral compartment. During the period immediately after administration, the distribution or α phase, drug is moving from the central compartment to the peripheral compartment. This results in a rapid fall in plasma levels until equilibrium is achieved between the drug in the blood and the drug in the tissues. From that point on, the tissue and blood concentrations fall in parallel owing to drug elimination. This phase is known as the elimination or β phase. A two-compartment model such as this will result in a biexponential plot when plasma drug concentrations are plotted

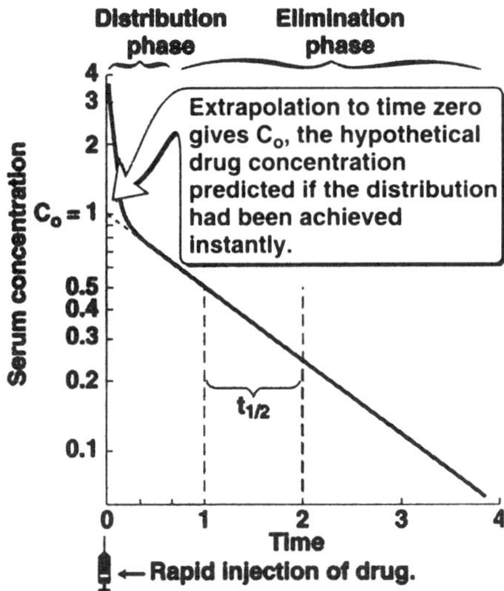

FIG. 5.3. Drug concentrations in serum after a single injection at time 0. Data are plotted on a log scale. (From Mycek MJ, Harvey RA, Champe PC. Absorption, distribution, and elimination of drugs. In: Mycek MJ, Harvey RA, Champe PC, eds. *Lippincott's illustrated reviews: pharmacology,* 2nd ed. Philadelphia: Lippincott Williams & Wilkins, 2000:1–16, with permission.)

against time. This biexponential has the form (Fig. 5.3) (Equation 7):

$$Cp = Ae^{-\alpha t} + Be^{-\beta t} \qquad (7)$$

where Cp is the drug concentration at time t. The terms α and β are both rate constants from which respective half-lives can be calculated. A and B are intercepts with the *Y* axis. The extrapolation of the β phase defines B. Generation of another line by subtracting the extrapolated β phase from the curve defines α and A. From A, B, α, and β, clearance and volume of distribution can be calculated. The importance of Equation 7 in clinical practice is best understood by using fentanyl as an example.

Fentanyl is highly lipid soluble and is rapidly distributed to tissues that are well perfused, such as the brain and heart. Normally, the effect of a single dose of fentanyl is terminated by rapid redistribution (α phase) to inactive tissue sites such as fat, skeletal muscles, and lung rather than by elimination. This rapid redistribution produces a dramatic decline in the plasma concentration of the drug to subtherapeutic levels and essentially terminates the analgesic action of the drug (Fig. 5.3). In this manner, fentanyl's very short duration of action is very much akin to other drugs whose action is terminated by redistribution rather than elimination such as thiopental. However, after multiple or large doses of fentanyl (e.g., when it is used as a primary anesthetic agent or when used in high dose or lengthy continuous infusions), prolongation of effect will occur because elimination (β phase) and not distribution will determine the duration of effect.

It is also now clear that the duration of drug action for many drugs is not solely the function of clearance or terminal elimination half-life but rather reflects the complex interaction of drug elimination, drug absorption, and rate constants for drug transfer to and from sites of action (effect sites). The term context-sensitive half-time refers to the time for drug concentration at idealized effect sites to decrease by half (24). The context-sensitive half-time for fentanyl increases dramatically when it is administered by continuous infusion (24,25). In newborns receiving fentanyl infusions for more than 36 hours, the context-sensitive half-time was greater than 9 hours after cessation of the infusion (26).

One of the most important uses of half-life is to predict how long it takes for a dosing regimen to achieve steady-state concentrations of drug in the blood. With initiation of therapy, if a loading dose is not used, it will require four to five half-lives until steady-state drug concentrations are achieved (Figs. 5.4 and 5.5). For a drug such as morphine, with a half-life of approximately 4 hours, it will take almost an entire day of therapy (assuming that the drug is given every 4 hours) to achieve steady-state plasma levels. Thus, in patients not receiving a loading dose, it will take almost an entire day before pain control is consistently adequate. Similarly, these principles come into play if a drug dose is changed, either increased or decreased. Changing a dose will require four to five half-lives to elapse before the new steady state is attained.

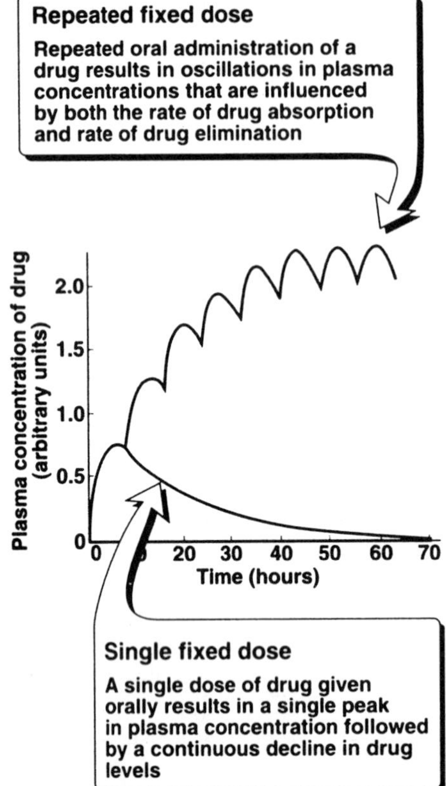

FIG. 5.4. Predicted plasma concentrations of a drug given by repeated oral administrations. Note that steady-state levels are not achieved until the fourth dose. (From Mycek MJ, Harvey RA, Champe PC. Pharmacokinetics and drug receptors. In: Mycek MJ, Harvey RA, Champe PC, eds. *Lippincott's illustrated reviews: pharmacology*, 2nd ed. Philadelphia: Lippincott Williams & Wilkins, 2000:17–20, with permission.)

When an effect is required immediately, it is impractical to wait for four to five half-lives to pass to achieve the desired effect. In these situations, a loading dose can be used to achieve a steady-state therapeutic plasma concentration. The loading dose can be achieved by using Equation 8.

loading dose =

$$\frac{\text{Usual maintenance dose}}{(\text{Usual dose interval})(\text{Ke})} \quad (8)$$

Substituting Ke from Equation 3 results in Equation 9:

Loading dose =

$$\frac{\text{Usual maintenance dose}}{(\text{Usual dose interval})\left(\frac{0.693}{t_{1/2}}\right)} \quad (9)$$

Absorption

Virtually all drugs used in current practice are delivered to their site of action by the blood. Drugs enter the bloodstream via enteral (e.g., oral and rectal) or parenteral (e.g., intravenous, intramuscular, subcutaneous, transdermal, inhalational, and transmucosal) routes. In healthy patients, the enteral route of drug administration is the most commonly used and studied. Enterally administered drugs must pass through the cells lining the mucosal surface of the gastrointestinal (GI) tract to enter the bloodstream. Although absorption can occur anywhere within the GI tract, the principal site of absorption, because of its large absorptive surface, is the small intestine. Thus, the rate at which drug leaves the stomach is the determinant of the speed of drug absorption. Anything that delays gastric emptying, such as opioid administration, will significantly affect the speed of absorption of orally administered drugs. Absorption from the GI tract may be reduced for many reasons. Obviously diarrhea, cystic fibrosis, critical illness, and celiac disease will significantly affect drug absorption from the GI tract. In many hospitalized and critically ill patients, the oral route of drug administration is so erratic that it is basically precluded until the patient recovers. In these patients, altered GI motility and peristalsis (ileus, recent GI surgery), reduced gut function and absorptive surface area (pancreatitis, recent GI surgery), reduced GI blood flow (shock), and physical removal of drug by nasogastric suctioning makes the absorption of drug erratic and unpredictable. Another pediatric patient population in whom oral drug administration is unpredictable is the newborn. In the newborn, diminished intestinal motility, delayed gastric emptying, different flora, and pH may result in a longer period for a drug to reach similar plasma concentrations than would be seen in older children or adolescents. For example, oral administration of acetaminophen has been shown to be lower in infants compared with adults. Finally, regardless of absorption issues, how drugs are manufactured may make oral administration impossible in some children. For example, many drugs are manufactured only as tablets; many children simply cannot swallow tablets. Additionally, some drugs are manufactured as sustained-release preparations, e.g., oxycodone (Oxy-Contin) and morphine (MS-Contin). These sustained-release tablets must be swallowed whole and cannot be crushed or given via a nasogastric tube. Obviously, young children and infants and the critically ill will not be able to do this. Furthermore, crushing sustained-release opioid tablets either deliberately or by biting into them will release huge amounts of opioids into the circulation with catastrophic consequences.

Once absorbed from the intestinal tract into the bloodstream, drug must reach the target organ. Drainage of intestinal blood flow into the portal system presents the drug to the liver for metabolism before the drug can be distributed throughout the body. This leads to the *first-pass* effect seen with many oral drugs. In the first pass, much of the absorbed drug is taken directly to the liver via the portal circulation and is rapidly metabolized and "lost" before it ever reaches the systemic circulation. Alteration of venous blood flow such that it bypasses the liver could result in significantly higher serum drug levels after oral absorption and lead to serious clinical catastrophes. Conversely, increased liver blood will have the opposite effect.

Parenteral (intravenous, intramuscular, and subcutaneous) drug administration is the most common method of drug administration in the hospitalized patient. Intravenous administration deposits drug directly into the bloodstream, bypassing the portal circulation and hepatic first pass, and makes drug dosing more predictable. Intramuscular, transdermal, and subcutaneous injections are dependent on blood supply and flow to and from the injected site or skin. Clinical conditions such as low cardiac output, respiratory distress, edema, and immobility may compromise blood supply and flow and decrease absorption from the injection site or skin, making these routes less predictable and useful. Fi-

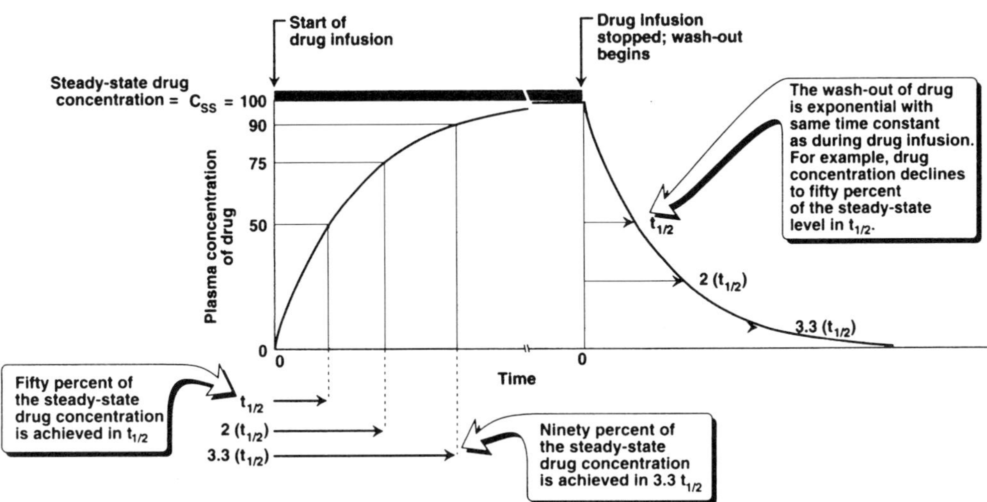

FIG. 5.5. Rate of attainment of steady-state concentrations of drug in plasma. (From Mycek MJ, Harvey RA, Champe PC. Pharmacokinetics and drug receptors. In: Mycek MJ, Harvey RA, Champe PC, eds. *Lippincott's illustrated reviews: pharmacology*, 2nd ed. Philadelphia: Lippincott Williams & Wilkins, 2000:17–20, with permission.)

nally, even if one believed that the intramuscular or subcutaneous administration was appropriate, this method of drug administration is painful and hardly makes sense as a mode of therapy in the treatment of pain. Conversely, transdermal fentanyl provides sustained plasma fentanyl concentrations and may be extremely useful in the treatment of pain in the nonacute, chronic setting. This is discussed more fully in Chapter 12.

TABLE 5.1. *Pathophysiologic states associated with increases $\alpha 1$-acid glycoprotein levels*

Burns
Infection
Inflammatory bowel disease
Malignancy
Postoperative period
Rheumatoid arthritis
Trauma

Drug Distribution and Protein Binding

Drug distribution and protein binding describe the transportation and movement of a drug throughout the body. Several factors have the potential to affect the distribution of drugs in the body. Total body water and extracellular fluid change dramatically with age. Water-soluble drugs (e.g., the aminoglycosides) are distributed throughout the extracellular water compartment. Changes in extracellular water compartment (40% of body weight in the newborn, 20% in the adult) affect how much drug reaches the receptor site. Poor perfusion is another factor that limits distribution of a drug to its target tissue. Altered receptor binding as a result of edema, malnutrition, uremic toxins, and downregulation will also change the amount of drug attached to tissue.

The newborn and the pregnant patient have decreased plasma concentrations of total proteins and albumin, which leads to decreased drug protein binding and more unbound or free drug in the plasma. It is the free drug that exerts a pharmacologic effect, and increased free drug in the blood may result in greater drug effect or even toxicity despite normal total (bound plus unbound) drug concentrations. Many analgesic drugs are transported through the body attached to the serum proteins albumin and γ-globulin. The extent of protein binding varies considerably among analgesic drugs, from 7% for codeine to 93% for sufentanil (27). Indeed, all the fentanyls are highly bound to α_1-acid glycoproteins in the plasma, which are reduced in the newborn (28,29). The fraction of free unbound sufentanil is significantly increased in neonates and children younger than 1 year of age (19.5 ± 2.7 and 11.5 ± 3.2%, respectively) compared with older children and adults (8.1 ±1.4 and 7.8 ± 1.5%, respectively), and this correlates to levels of α_1-acid glycoproteins in the blood. Conversely, several disease states, listed in Table 5.1, increase α_1-acid glycoprotein levels. An increased α_1-acid glycoprotein level will increase bound drug and decrease the free fraction of drug in the blood. In these patients, an administered dose of drug would produce less effect than expected.

Metabolism and Elimination

Metabolism is the physical and chemical alteration of drug molecules for the purposes of detoxifying parent molecules and rendering fat-soluble chemicals more water soluble. Drugs or their metabolites are then eliminated by the kidneys. Any disease that affects hepatic or renal function or causes hypoperfusion of the liver or kidneys may diminish metabolism and elimination of the drug, possibly resulting in drug accumulation and toxicity (17,20,27). It is common for newborn and critically ill patients to have some degree of either renal or hepatic function impairment. Furthermore, many critically ill children and newborns have diseases in which intra-abdominal pressure is significantly increased (necrotizing enterocolitis, severe ileus, recent GI surgery), which will impair both portal and renal blood flow (30,31). In critically ill patients with organ dysfunction, the clinician must expect unpredictable metabolism and elimination of drugs and must monitor for therapeutic outcomes and possible adverse effects.

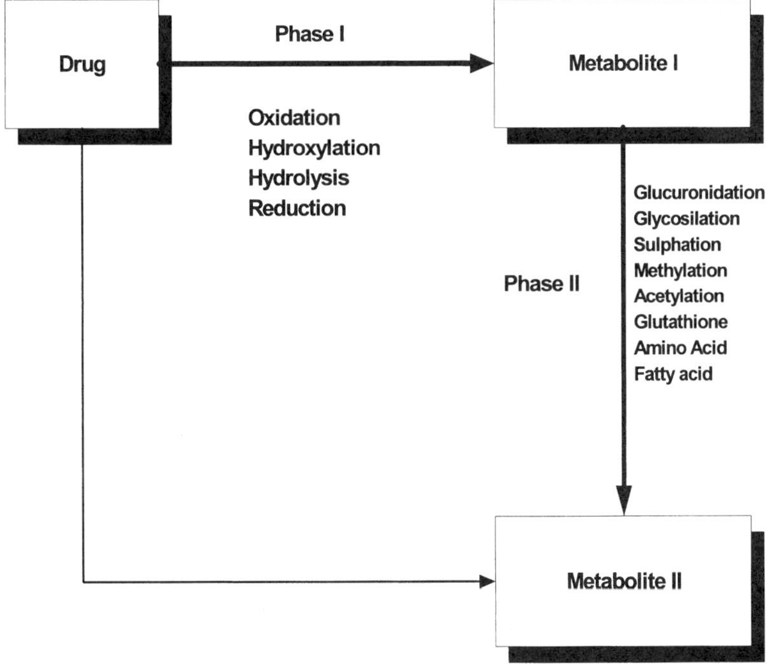

FIG. 5.6. The biotransformation of drugs.

The liver is the major route for drug metabolism and detoxification for a wide variety of analgesic drugs. Analgesic drugs are lipid-soluble compounds; this lipid solubility enhances their passage through the blood–brain barrier and also preselects the liver as the organ of elimination (because renal physiology requires drugs to be water soluble to be filtered and excreted). Some degree of hepatic dysfunction is present in many critically ill patients and may result in reduced drug clearance because of decreased hepatocellular enzyme activity or reduced hepatic blood and/or bile flow.

Most, but not all, drugs are metabolized in a two-part process, the goal of which is to change fat-soluble, active, unexcretable drugs into water-soluble, inactive drugs that can be excreted in the bile or by the kidneys (Fig. 5.6). The first part of the process, phase I metabolism, commonly involves the cytochrome P-450 system, which is a large family of hemoproteins involved in the metabolism of drugs and in the manufacture of steroids. Phase I metabolism usually involves oxidation, hydroxylation, hydrolysis, or reduction. Phase I reactions are listed in Table 5.2.

The cytochrome P-450 system is a mixed-function oxidase system that involves both reduction and oxidation and requires the presence of nicotinamide adenine dinucleotide phosphate and molecular oxygen (8–11). It is the most important of the phase I enzymes and is responsible for the metabolism of most lipophilic drugs used in pain management (e.g., opioids, acetaminophen, nonsteroidal anti-inflammatory drugs). In humans, 32 genes and five putative pseudo-

TABLE 5.2. *Enzymes performing phase I reactions*

P-450 system
Alcohol dehydrogenases
Aldehyde dehydrogenases
Amine oxidases
Xanthine oxidases
Aromatases

genes have been described to date that can be divided into two distinct classes: the steroidogenic enzymes expressed in specialized tissues, such as the adrenal glands and gonads, and the P-450s involved in metabolism of drugs, pesticides, and environmental contaminants (32–34). There is considerable inherited genetic variation in the activity of this enzyme system. This variation in drug response is often referred to as pharmacogenetics and is responsible clinically for individuals to be classified as being fast, extensive, or rapid metabolizers at one end of the spectrum and slow or poor metabolizers at the other.

Clearly, genetic factors have an important role in influencing a patient's physical characteristics such as height, weight, and eye and hair color. It is also likely that genetic constitution contributes to disease susceptibility and is an important determinant of inter- and intraindividual variability in drug disposition and response. For example, succinylcholine is a very fast-acting, short-lived muscle relaxant that can produce prolonged paralysis in patients with an inherited variation (deficiency) in plasma cholinesterase activity. Pharmacogenetics is the study of genetically determined variations in drug response. Children present unique challenges in this context because developmental changes in drug disposition and response are superimposed on a basal pharmacogenetic variability.

Newborns are phenotypically slow metabolizers for many drug-metabolizing pathways and become more consistent with their inherited genotype as they develop and grow. This process is referred to as ontogeny and has considerable implications in how the newborn metabolizes drugs (32,34). In general, the developmental pattern of drug-metabolizing enzyme activity has been viewed as being virtually absent in the fetus, limited in the newborn, and rapidly increasing in the first year or two of life to a capacity that exceeds the adult, and then declining to adult levels by puberty.

A nomenclature for the P-450 system has evolved in which the root CYP stands for cytochrome P-450 (32–34). It is followed by an Arabic numeral, e.g., CYP1, CYP 2, CYP 3, and subfamilies designated by a letter and number, e.g., CYP2D6, CYP2C19. The most important and best studied of the many enzymes is CYP2D6 (Table 5.3). This enzyme is responsible for the metabolism of more than 40 different drugs and drug families including β-receptor antagonists, antiarrhythmics, antidepressants, and morphine derivatives. Indeed, it is required for the bioactivation of codeine into morphine and of tramadol into O-desmethyl tramadol. Thus, patients who lack a functioning CYP2D6, either genetically or because of liver disease, will receive little, if any, therapeutic effect after codeine and tramadol administration (36,37). The CYP2D6 gene locus is highly polymorphic, with more than 50 allelic variants (http://www.imm.ki.se/cypalleles/cyp2d6.htm). Approximately 10% of the white population and 1% of the American-Asian and black population have little CYP2D6 activity and are poor responders to codeine administration (38–41). The newborn also has very little detectable CYP2D6 activity for the first few weeks of life and would similarly be expected to obtain little, if any, analgesia with codeine administration

TABLE 5.3. *Substrates for major cytochrome P-450 enzymes in humans*

CYP1A2	Caffeine, theophylline, R-warfarin
CYP2C9	Diclofenac, ibuprofen and other NSAIDs, phenytoin, S-warfarin, tetrahydrocannabinol
CYP2C19	Diazepam, imipramine, omeprazole
CYP2D6	Amitriptyline, codeine, dextromethorphan, haloperidol, hydrocodone, imipramine, β-blockers, tramadol
CYP3A4	Alfentanil, amiodarone, cisapride, cyclosporin, diazepam, erythromycin, fentanyl, imipramine, lidocaine, methadone, meperidine, midazolam, quinidine, triazolam, verapamil

NSAIDs, nonsteroidal anti-inflammatory drugs.

(42). Finally, CYP2D6 activity can be inhibited by some drugs such as fluoxetine and quinidine (1,43). Patients being concomitantly treated with codeine and either fluoxetine or quinidine will have little, if any, analgesia as well (Table 5.3).

The metabolites of these phase I reactions may be less active or highly reactive and even toxic. The phase I metabolite is then metabolized further by a phase II enzyme that conjugates it with either a glucuronide, a sulphide group, an amino acid, or glutathione (Fig. 5.6). The phase II enzymes include the glucuronosyl transferases, sulfotransferases, arylamine *N*-acetyl transferases (NAT1 and NAT2), glutathione S-transferases, and methyl transferases (e.g., catechol O-methyl transferase, thiopurine S-methyltransferase). The glucuronosyl transfcrascs conjugate their respective substrates into glucuronic acid. Several mutations have been reported, the most well known of which give rise to the clinical conditions of Crigler–Najjar syndrome and Gilbert syndrome (44). In these two conditions, there is a reduction in bilirubin-conjugating activity. Some drugs, such as morphine, do not require a phase I reaction and are metabolized directly by phase II enzymes. Phase II conjugation pathways such as glucuronidation may be impaired in the newborn and in critically ill patients, particularly if the liver is subjected to low blood flow, hypoxia, and/or stress. Chronic liver disease appears selectively to impair oxidative pathways while leaving glucuronidation intact. The ontogeny of phase II enzymes has not been well studied (45). However, important developmental differences between adults and children involving these enzymes, specifically the glucuronosyl transferases, were responsible for the development of gray baby syndrome in children being treated with chloramphenicol (15,16). *In vitro*, glucuronidation of morphine in fetal liver is less than 20% of that observed in adult liver (46). Morphine clearance is correlated closely with gestational age and increases fourfold between 27 weeks of gestation and term (47–50). In addition, in the newborn, the lack of activity of one enzyme system may be compensated for by an increase in another pathway. For example, glucuronidation of acetaminophen is impaired in the newborn compared with the adult but is compensated for by increased sulfation (51).

A third metabolic pathway is becoming increasingly important, namely, metabolism by blood and tissue esterases. These enzymes are ubiquitous and are found in large supply in the blood and elsewhere. Drugs that are metabolized by esterases such as remifentanil, succinylcholine, and mivacurium are unlikely to be affected by disease or duration of drug infusion.

Most pain and sedation medications are metabolized by phase I or II reactions in the liver. In general, the metabolism of opioid analgesics is very effective and limited more by blood flow to the liver than by the inherent ability of the hepatocyte enzymes. Drainage of intestinal blood flow into the portal circulation presents the drug to the liver for metabolism before it can be distributed to the body. This flow-dependent metabolism leads to the first-pass effect seen with many orally administered drugs. Alterations of venous blood flow such that it bypasses the liver could result in significantly higher serum drug levels that persist than would otherwise be expected. This effects not only orally administered drugs but intravenous administration as well. Thus, even single doses of fentanyl may have prolonged effects in the newborn, particularly those neonates with abnormal or decreased liver blood flow after acute illness or abdominal surgery (52–55). Additionally, some conditions that may raise intra-abdominal pressure may further decrease liver blood flow by shunting blood away from the liver via the still patent ductus venosus (30,31,55,56). The cytochrome P-450 microenzyme system is significantly altered in critical illness, decreasing phase I oxidative metabolism (57–60).

The kidneys are responsible for clearing both the parent drug and metabolites produced by the liver. In renal failure or in patients with reduced glomerular filtration rates, both the parent drug and metabolites may accumulate and result in toxicity. Interestingly, this is crucial in the newborn, in whom the glomerular filtration rate is 30% to 40% of the adult value. Many drugs used in the management of pain are affected. Morphine is metabolized to morphine-3-glucuronide and morphine-6-glucuronide. Morphine-3-glucuronide does not have analgesic activity, whereas morphine-6-glucuronide is an active metabolite eliminated by the kidneys. In renal failure, morphine-6-glucuronide may accumulate and has been associated with toxicity (61,62). Meperidine is also metabolized to a metabolite, normeperidine, which is renally cleared. In renal failure, normeperidine may accumulate and result in seizures. Finally, oxycodone is metabolized in the liver into oxymorphone, an active metabolite, both of which may accumulate in patients with renal failure (63).

CONCLUSION

In this chapter, we attempted to provide the fundamentals of pharmacokinetics and pharmacodynamics by describing the relationship between drug dosing and response. It is hoped that this will provide the reader with a better understanding of how the drugs used in pain management are prescribed and used.

REFERENCES

1. Kathiramalainathan K, Kaplan HL, Romach MK, et al. Inhibition of cytochrome P450 2D6 modifies codeine abuse liability. *J Clin Psychopharmacol* 2000;20: 435–444.
2. Anderson BJ, McKee AD, Holford NH. Size, myths and the clinical pharmacokinetics of analgesia in paediatric patients. *Clin Pharmacokinet* 1997;33:313–327.
3. Kart T, Christrup LL, Rasmussen M. Recommended use of morphine in neonates, infants and children based on a literature review: part 1—pharmacokinetics. *Paediatr Anaesth* 1997;7:5–11.
4. Jacqz-Aigrain E, Burtin P. Clinical pharmacokinetics of sedatives in neonates. *Clin Pharmacokinet* 1996;1: 423–443.
5. Olkkola KT, Hamunen K, Maunuksela EL. Clinical pharmacokinetics and pharmacodynamics of opioid analgesics in infants and children. *Clin Pharmacokinet* 1995;28:385–404.
6. van Hoogdalem E, de Boer AG, Breimer DD. Pharmacokinetics of rectal drug administration, part I. General considerations and clinical applications of centrally acting drugs. *Clin Pharmacokinet* 1991;21:11–26.
7. Morselli PL, Franco-Morselli R, Bossi L. Clinical pharmacokinetics in newborns and infants. Age-related differences and therapeutic implications. *Clin Pharmacokinet* 1980;5:485–527.
8. Benet LZ, Kroetz DL, Sheiner LB. Pharmacokinetics: the dynamics of drug absorption, distribution, and elimination. In: Hardman JG, Limbird LE, eds. *Goodman and Gilman's the pharmacologic basis of therapeutics*. New York: McGraw-Hill, 1996:3–28.
9. Ross EM. Pharmacodynamics: mechanisms of drug action and the relationship between drug concentration and effect. In: Hardman JG, Limbird LE, eds. *Goodman and Gilman's the pharmacologic basis of therapeutics*. New York: McGraw-Hill, 2001:29–42.
10. Stoelting RK. Pharmacokinetics and pharmacodynamics of injected and inhaled drugs. In: Stoelting RK, ed. *Pharmacology and physiology in anesthetic practice*. Philadelphia: Lippincott–Raven, 2001:3–35.
11. Wood AJ. Drug disposition and pharmacokinetics. In: Wood M, Wood AJ, eds. *Drugs and anesthesia: pharmacology for anesthesiologists*. Baltimore: Williams & Wilkins, 1990:3–42.
12. Mycek MJ, Harvey RA, Champe PC. *Lippincott's illustrated reviews: pharmacology* , 2nd ed. Philadelphia: Lippincott Williams & Wilkins, 2000.
13. Mycek MJ, Harvey RA, Champe PC. Pharmacokinetics and drug receptors. In: Mycek MJ, Harvey RA, Champe PC, eds. *Lippincott's illustrated reviews: pharmacology*, 2nd ed. Philadelphia: Lippincott Williams & Wilkins, 2000:17–20.
14. Blumer JL. The therapeutic orphan—30 years later. Proceedings of a joint conference of the Pediatric Pharmacology Research Unit Network, the European Society of Developmental Pharmacology, and the National Institute of Child Health and Human Development. Washington, DC, USA, May 2, 1997. *Pediatrics* 1999; 104:581–645.
15. Lietman PS. Chloramphenicol and the neonate—1979 view. *Clin Perinatol* 1979;6:151–162.
16. Young WS, Lietman PS. Chloramphenicol glucuronyl transferase: assay, ontogeny and inducibility. *J Pharmacol Exp Ther* 1978;204:203–211.
17. Power BM, Forbes AM, van Heerden PV, et al. Pharmacokinetics of drugs used in critically ill adults. *Clin Pharmacokinet* 1998;34:25–56.
18. Wagner BK, O'Hara DA. Pharmacokinetics and pharmacodynamics of sedatives and analgesics in the treatment of agitated critically ill patients. *Clin Pharmacokinet* 1997;33:426–453.
19. Park GR. Sedation, analgesia and muscle relaxation and the critically ill patient. *Can J Anaesth* 1997;44: R40–R51.
20. Volles DF, McGory R. Pharmacokinetic considerations. *Crit Care Clin* 1999;15:55–75.
21. Cohen SN. The Pediatric Pharmacology Research Unit (PPRU) Network and its role in meeting pediatric labeling needs. *Pediatrics* 1999;104:644–645.
22. Connor JD. A look at the future of pediatric therapeutics: an investigator's perspective of the new pediatric rule. *Pediatrics* 1999;104:610–613.
23. Wilson JT, Kearns GL, Murphy D, et al. Paediatric la-

belling requirements. Implications for pharmacokinetic studies. *Clin Pharmacokinet* 1994;26:308–325.
24. Hughes MA, Glass PS, Jacobs JR. Context-sensitive half-time in multicompartment pharmacokinetic models for intravenous anesthetic drugs. *Anesthesiology* 1992;76:334–341.
25. Scholz J, Steinfath M, Schulz M. Clinical pharmacokinetics of alfentanil, fentanyl and sufentanil. An update. *Clin Pharmacokinet* 1996;31:275–292.
26. Santeiro ML, Christie J, Stromquist C, et al. Pharmacokinetics of continuous infusion fentanyl in newborns. *J Perinatol* 1997;17:135–139.
27. Davies G, Kingswood C, Street M. Pharmacokinetics of opioids in renal dysfunction. *Clin Pharmacokinet* 1996;31:410–422.
28. Wilson AS, Stiller RL, Davis PJ, et al. Fentanyl and alfentanil plasma protein binding in preterm and term neonates. *Anesth Analg* 1997;84:315–318.
29. Wood M. Plasma drug binding: implications for anesthesiologists. *Anesth Analg* 1986;65:786–804.
30. Masey SA, Koehler RC, Buck JR, et al. Effect of abdominal distension on central and regional hemodynamics in neonatal lambs. *Pediatr Res* 1985;19:1244–1249.
31. Yaster M, Scherer TL, Stone MM, et al. Prediction of successful primary closure of congenital abdominal wall defects using intraoperative measurements. *J Pediatr Surg* 1989;24:1217–1220.
30. Leeder JS, Kearns GL. Pharmacogenetics in pediatrics. Implications for practice. *Pediatr Clin North Am* 1997;44:55–77.
33. Nelson DR, Koymans L, Kamataki T, et al. P450 superfamily: update on new sequences, gene mapping, accession numbers and nomenclature. *Pharmacogenetics* 1996;6:1–42.
34. Nelson DR, Kamataki T, Waxman DJ, et al. The P450 superfamily: update on new sequences, gene mapping, accession numbers, early trivial names of enzymes, and nomenclature. *DNA Cell Biol* 1993;12:1–51.
35. de Wildt SN, Kearns GL, Leeder JS, et al. Cytochrome P450 3A: ontogeny and drug disposition. *Clin Pharmacokinet* 1999;37:485–505.
36. Caraco Y, Sheller J, Wood AJ. Pharmacogenetic determination of the effects of codeine and prediction of drug interactions. *J Pharmacol Exp Ther* 1996;278:1165–1174.
37. Caraco Y, Sheller J, Wood AJ. Impact of ethnic origin and quinidine coadministration on codeine's disposition and pharmacodynamic effects. *J Pharmacol Exp Ther* 1999;290:413–422.
38. Bradford LD, Gaedigk A, Leeder JS. High frequency of CYP2D6 poor and "intermediate" metabolizers in black populations: a review and preliminary data. *Psychopharmacol Bull* 1998;34:797–804.
39. Evans WE, Relling MV, Rahman A, et al. Genetic basis for a lower prevalence of deficient CYP2D6 oxidative drug metabolism phenotypes in black Americans. *J Clin Invest* 1993;91:2150–2154.
40. Relling MV, Lin JS, Ayers GD, et al. Racial and gender differences in N-acetyltransferase, xanthine oxidase, and CYP1A2 activities. *Clin Pharmacol Ther* 1992;52:643–658.
41. Johnson JA, Herring VL, Wolfe MS, et al. CYP1A2 and CYP2D6 4-hydroxylate propranolol and both reactions exhibit racial differences. *J Pharmacol Exp Ther* 2000;294:1099–1105.
42. Treluyer JM, Jacqz-Aigrain E, Alvarez F, et al. Expression of CYP2D6 in developing human liver. *Eur J Biochem* 1991;202:583–588.
43. Branch RA, Adedoyin A, Frye RF, et al. In vivo modulation of CYP enzymes by quinidine and rifampin. *Clin Pharmacol Ther* 2000;68:401–411.
44. Mackenzie PI, Owens IS, Burchell B, et al. The UDP glycosyltransferase gene superfamily: recommended nomenclature update based on evolutionary divergence. *Pharmacogenetics* 1997;7:255–269.
45. de Wildt SN, Kearns GL, Leeder JS, et al. Glucuronidation in humans. Pharmacogenetic and developmental aspects. *Clin Pharmacokinet* 1999;36:439–452.
46. Pacifici GM, Sawe J, Kager L, et al. Morphine glucuronidation in human fetal and adult liver. *Eur J Clin Pharmacol* 1982;22:553–558.
47. Scott CS, Riggs KW, Ling EW, et al. Morphine pharmacokinetics and pain assessment in premature newborns. *J Pediatr* 1999;135:423–429.
48. Mikkelsen S, Feilberg VL, Christensen CB, et al. Morphine pharmacokinetics in premature and mature newborn infants. *Acta Paediatr* 1994;83:1025–1028.
49. Hartley R, Green M, Quinn MW, et al. Development of morphine glucuronidation in premature neonates. *Biol Neonate* 1994;66:1–9.
50. Lynn A, Nespeca MK, Bratton SL, et al. Clearance of morphine in postoperative infants during intravenous infusion: the influence of age and surgery. *Anesth Analg* 1998;86:958–963.
51. Miller RP, Roberts RJ, Fischer LJ. Acetaminophen elimination kinetics in neonates, children, and adults. *Clin Pharmacol Ther* 1976;19:284–294.
52. Koehntop DE, Rodman JH, Brundage DM, et al. Pharmacokinetics of fentanyl in neonates. *Anesth Analg* 1986;65:227–232.
53. Hertzka RE, Gauntlett IS, Fisher DM, et al. Fentanyl-induced ventilatory depression: effects of age. *Anesthesiology* 1989;70:213–218.
54. Gauntlett IS, Fisher DM, Hertzka RE, et al. Pharmacokinetics of fentanyl in neonatal humans and lambs: effects of age. *Anesthesiology* 1988;69:683–687.
55. Kuhls E, Gauntlett IS, Lau M, et al. Effect of increased intra-abdominal pressure on hepatic extraction and clearance of fentanyl in neonatal lambs. *J Pharmacol Exp Ther* 1995;274:115–119.
56. Yaster M, Buck JR, Dudgeon DL, et al. Hemodynamic effects of primary closure of omphalocele/gastroschisis in human newborns. *Anesthesiology* 1988;69:84–88.
57. Park GR, Pichard L, Tinel M, et al. What changes drug metabolism in critically ill patients? Two preliminary studies in isolated human hepatocytes. *Anaesthesia* 1994;49:188–189.
58. Park GR, Miller E, Navapurkar V. What changes drug metabolism in critically ill patients?—II Serum inhibits the metabolism of midazolam in human microsomes. *Anaesthesia* 1996;51:11–15.
59. Park GR, Miller E. What changes drug metabolism in critically ill patients—III? Effect of pre-existing disease on the metabolism of midazolam. *Anaesthesia* 1996;51:431–434.
60. Park GR. Molecular mechanisms of drug metabolism in the critically ill. *Br J Anaesth* 1996;77:32–49.

61. Shelly MP, Cory EP, Park GR. Pharmacokinetics of morphine in two children before and after liver transplantation. *Br J Anaesth* 1986;58:1218–1223.
62. Osborne RJ, Joel SP, Slevin ML. Morphine intoxication in renal failure: the role of morphine-6-glucuronide. *BMJ* 1986;292:1548–1549.
63. Kirvela M, Lindgren L, Seppala T, et al. The pharmacokinetics of oxycodone in uremic patients undergoing renal transplantation. *J Clin Anesth* 1996;8:13–18.
64. Mycek MJ, Harvey RA, Champe PC. Absorption, distribution, and elimination of drugs. In: Mycek MJ, Harvey RA, Champe PC, eds. *Lippincott's illustrated reviews: pharmacology*, 2nd ed. Philadelphia: Lippincott Williams & Wilkins, 2000:1–16.

6

Modifying the Psychologic Factors That Intensify Children's Pain and Prolong Disability

Patricia A. McGrath and Loretta M. Hillier

THE PLASTICITY AND COMPLEXITY OF CHILDREN'S PAIN

Unprecedented scientific and clinical attention has focused on the unique pain problems of infants, children, and adolescents during the past two decades. As a consequence of intensive research, our knowledge of how children perceive pain and how we can alleviate their suffering has dramatically improved. In particular, we now recognize that children's pain is not simply and directly related to the extent of their physical injuries or to the severity of their disease. Like adults, children's pain perception depends on complex neural interactions in which impulses generated by tissue damage are modified both by ascending systems activated by innocuous stimuli and descending pain-suppressing systems activated by various situational and psychologic factors (for reviews, see references 1–4). However, children's pain seems more plastic than that of adults, so that environmental and psychologic factors may exert a more powerful influence on children's pain perceptions.

Our increasing appreciation of the plasticity and complexity of children's pain has profound implications for pain management. We now understand that we cannot completely control a child's pain by gearing our treatment solely to the putative source of tissue damage. Instead, we must also identify the situational and psychologic factors that can cause or exacerbate a child's pain and target our interventions accordingly. Our treatment emphasis should shift from an exclusive disease-centered focus to a more child-centered focus. This chapter describes the varied psychologic aspects of children's pain, illustrating the profound impact of cognitive, behavioral, and emotional factors. Particular emphasis focuses on how to modify the common factors responsible for increasing pain, exacerbating distress, prolonging pain-related disability, and triggering pain episodes.

FACTORS THAT MODIFY CHILDREN'S PAIN

Tissue damage initiates a sequence of neural events that may lead to pain, but many factors can intervene to alter the sequence of nociceptive transmission and thereby modify children's pain, as illustrated in Figure 6.1. This model provides a framework for assessing the relevant causative and contributing factors for children, based on our knowledge of the plasticity and complexity of children's pain. Some factors are relatively stable for children, such as age, cognitive level, gender, temperament, previous pain experience, family learning, and cultural background (shown in the bottom box in the figure). These child characteristics shape how children generally interpret and experience the various sensations caused by tissue damage.

In contrast, the cognitive, behavioral, and emotional factors (shown in the shaded boxes) are not stable. These situational factors represent a unique interaction between the child and the situation in which the pain is experienced (2,5). They can vary dynamically,

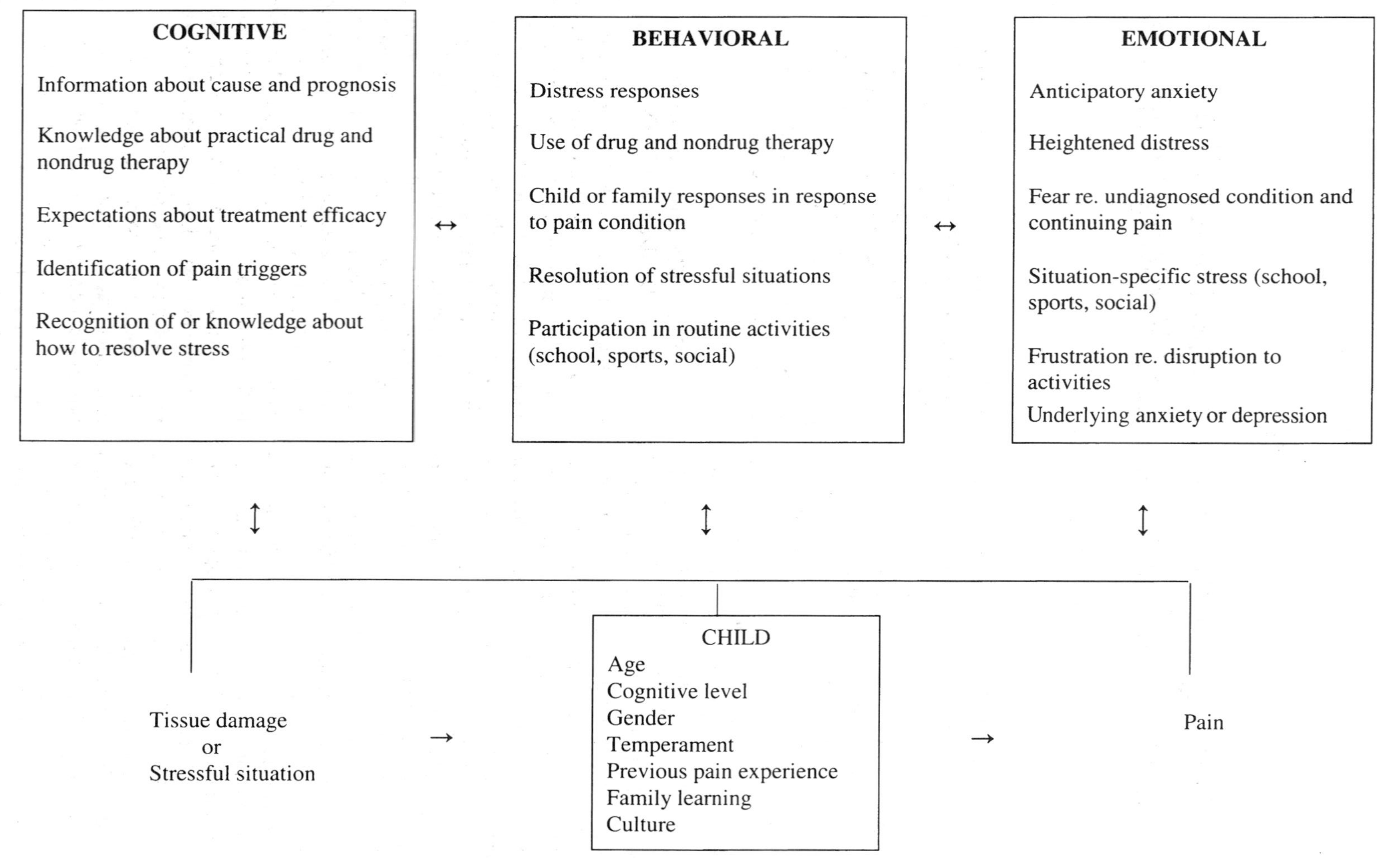
COGNITIVE
Information about cause and prognosis
Knowledge about practical drug and nondrug therapy
Expectations about treatment efficacy
Identification of pain triggers
Recognition of or knowledge about how to resolve stress
BEHAVIORAL
Distress responses
Use of drug and nondrug therapy
Child or family responses in response to pain condition
Resolution of stressful situations
Participation in routine activities (school, sports, social)
EMOTIONAL
Anticipatory anxiety
Heightened distress
Fear re. undiagnosed condition and continuing pain
Situation-specific stress (school, sports, social)
Frustration re. disruption to activities
Underlying anxiety or depression
Tissue damage or Stressful situation
CHILD
Age
Cognitive level
Gender
Temperament
Previous pain experience
Family learning
Culture
Pain

FIG. 6.1. Situational and child factors that modify pain and disability.

depending on the specific circumstances in which children experience pain. Cognitive factors include parents' and children's understanding of the pain problem, their knowledge of effective therapies, and their expectations for the future. Behavioral factors refer to the specific behaviors of children, parents, and staff during pain episodes and also encompass parents' and children's wider behaviors in response to a recurrent or chronic pain problem. Emotional factors include parents' and children's feelings about scheduled painful treatments, the subsequent impact of pain and illness on the family, and anxiety or depression that may underlie some chronic conditions.

Although the causal relationship between an injury and consequent pain seems direct and obvious, what children understand, what they do, and how they feel all affect their pain. Some situational factors can intensify pain and distress, whereas others can eventually trigger pain episodes, prolong pain-related disability, or maintain the cycle of repeated pain episodes in recurrent pain syndrome. Thus, it is essential to recognize and evaluate the mitigating impact of these factors to relieve any type of pain that children experience. Differences in situational factors may account for why the same tissue damage can evoke pains that vary in intensity and may partially explain why proven analgesics can vary in effectiveness for different children and for the same child at different times. Although parents and health care providers may be unable to change the more stable child characteristics, they can dramatically lessen children's pain and minimize their disability by modifying situational factors.

Complex and dynamic interactions occur among cognitive, behavioral, and emotional factors. Parents' understanding of the causes of pain, possible treatments, and prognosis guides their behaviors toward children and shapes children's emotional responses to the pain problem. Thus, multiple factors can affect children's pain and disability, but the extent to which each factor represents a primary underlying cause or a secondary contributing factor varies among children and may vary over time for the same child. We must ascertain which factors are relevant for which children so that we can select the most appropriate drug or nondrug therapy for each child. The model in Figure 6.1 provides a framework for evaluating and managing these myriad factors that can attenuate or exacerbate children's pain.

CHILD CHARACTERISTICS

Age and Cognitive Level

At a very early age, children recognize that pain is an unpleasant sensory and emotional experience. Their understanding and descriptions of pain naturally depend on their age, cognitive level, and previous pain experience (2,5–11). Children learn to judge the strength and unpleasantness of any pain in comparison with sensations that they have already experienced. Like adults, the nature and diversity of children's pain experience form their frame of reference for perceiving any new pain. Yet, unlike adults who have generally a wide frame of reference of pain experience, children's frames of reference change considerably as they mature and sustain more diverse types of tissue damage (12).

The changing frames of reference are illustrated by children's responses to the questions "What is the least pain that you have experienced . . . and the most pain?" As shown in Table 6.1, the nature and diversity of responses change with children's ages (2). Younger children usually report acute pains caused by common childhood injuries for both their least and most pains; these children typically cite pains of almost comparable tissue damage. As children mature, they naturally experience different types of pain and report more unusual acute, recurrent, and chronic pain experiences. Older children typically cite examples of least and most pains that are caused by injuries that differ greatly with respect to severity and duration of tissue damage. Despite their changing frames of reference, children learn to describe the diverse features of their pain sensations in the same

TABLE 6.1. *Children's least and most pain experiences*

Age (yr)	Gender	Minimum	Maximum
6	Girl	"Fell down running"	"Fell off bike . . . had great big scab on knee . . . bled a lot and hurt"
7	Girl	"Cut my knee"	"Really bad stomach ache and headache"
6	Boy	"Bashed my elbow, it tickles when you touch your fingers"	"Fell down the stairs at school and hurt my knees, elbows, and head"
10	Boy	"Stubbed my toe"	"Got hit by a hardball by a fast pitch on my thigh"
11	Girl	"Scraped my knee"	"When I fell out of a truck, it was moving"
13	Boy	"Cut finger with paring knife"	"Migraine"
15	Boy	"Pulling one hair out for science project"	"Finger jammed in car door"
17	Boy	"Paper cut"	"Being beaten up"
17	Girl	"Scratch from my kitten, not deep"	"Breaking my elbow, really badly, I had an operation on it"

manner that they learn specific words to describe the different sounds, tastes, smells, and colors that they experience.

When they hurt, most children communicate their pain quickly to their parents through their words or behaviors. However, their ability to describe specific pain features—the quality (aching, burning, pounding, sharp), intensity (mild to severe), duration and frequency (a few seconds to years), location (diffuse location on surface of the skin to more precise localization internally), and unpleasantness (mild annoyance to an intolerable discomfort)—develops as they mature. Children naturally differ in the words that they use to describe their pains because of differences in their backgrounds, previous pain experiences, and learning. Their understanding of pain and the pain language that they learn develops through their culture from the words and expressions used by their families and peers and from characters depicted in books, videos, and movies.

Yet, all children seem to understand both the intrinsic physical and emotional aspects of hurting. Children begin to understand pain by their own experiences and describe pain in the language that represents those experiences. Table 6.2 lists the definitions of pain for the same nine children whose least and most pain responses were shown in Table 6.1. The sophistication of their definitions parallels their chronologic age. Younger children use concrete examples in response to "What is pain?" As children mature, they rely less frequently on analogies drawn from their personal experience and convey their understanding of pain in more abstract concepts, composed of both physical and psychologic components (8,9, 13–15).

Children's level of cognitive development determines how they are able to understand pain and helps us to select age-appropriate psychologic therapies. Research on the impact of children's age and cognitive level on children's pain perception includes interview studies that examined children's understanding and attitudes about pain (8,9,13,14, 16–20), observational studies that described children's distress during invasive medical procedures (21–26), and experimental pain studies that evaluated differences in children's thresholds for reporting pain or tolerating painful stimulation (27–29). Most of these studies reported some developmental trends. Children's understanding of pain, pain coping strategies, and the impact of pain increased with age.

For example, we interviewed 187 children, 5 to 16 years of age, to evaluate differences in their understanding of pain and in their pain experiences according to their age, sex, and health status (9). To ensure that children would have had distinct pain experiences, they were drawn from five health groups: healthy, recurrent headache, cancer, enuresis, and arthritis.

TABLE 6.2. *Children's definitions of pain*

Age	Gender	Definition
6	Girl	"When you fell, did you have a big scab or a little scab?"
7	Girl	"Not too bad, hurts, not too much but sometimes a lot."
6	Boy	"Hurt. Sometimes you get a little cut . . . it's like twisting your ankle . . . that hurts bad, very bad and unuseful."
10	Boy	"An uncomfortable feeling when something is injured."
11	Girl	"Something that hurts very much."
13	Boy	"Something hurts you, makes you sad, upset."
15	Boy	"Reaction of nerves telling your brain that some damage is being caused to your body."
17	Boy	"Either physical or emotional. The physical is self-explanatory and is healed naturally, while the emotional is attained by life circumstances which sadden, anger, and disturb."
17	Girl	"The sensation completely opposite to comfort. It can be physical or emotional. When my father died, I felt deep emotional pain that was stronger than any physical discomfort I had ever experienced."

The interview included questions to capture their knowledge of the word pain, its varied sensory aspects, their understanding of the variations in pain experiences, the emotional impact, the different causes, the positive aspect as a warning signal to prevent further injury, the varied possible interventions, and the associated disability component. Almost all children (99%) understood the hurting aspect of pain. However, children's understanding of the word pain increased with age from 66% for the youngest children (5- to 7-year-old group) to 95% for the oldest children (14- to 16-year-old group). Most children indicated that pain could vary in location, duration, intensity, quality, and affect. However, children's understanding that pain could vary in all these sensory attributes increased with age, as did their recognition that pain provides an important warning signal, that pain interferes with activities, and that there are several pain control interventions.

Most studies of children's acute pain caused by invasive medical procedures (e.g., venipunctures) reveal age-related differences in pain intensity (2,23,30–32) and behavioral distress (2,27,30,33–35). Children's pain ratings and overt distress (e.g., crying, resisting) during invasive medical procedures generally decrease with age. However, the effect of age probably varies depending on the type of pain children experience and the nature of their previous pain experiences (i.e., positive experiences with similar painful situations). Bennett-Branson and Craig (36) reported that postoperative pain (minor surgery) increased with age (60 children, 7 to 16 years old), whereas Palermo and Drotar (37) reported age-related decreases in postoperative pain (inpatient surgery) for 28 children (7 to 17 years old) and Gidron et al. (38) reported no age-related differences in pain after oral surgery in a study of 67 children and young adults, ages 13 to 20 years old. (The impact of previous pain experience is described later in this chapter.)

Sex and Gender

Dramatic attention is now focused on the roles of sex (the physiologic male and female makeup) and gender (the psychologic male and female traits) in influencing pain sensitivity, pain vulnerability, and treatment efficacy. The results of studies evaluating sex- and gender-related trends in children's pain perception yield equivocal results. Some studies report differences in pain expression, pain behaviors, and coping strategies (19,22,25,36, 39), whereas other studies have not found significant differences (18,30,32,34,35,40). Such inconsistent findings are understandable because studies differ widely with respect to the number of children sampled, their ages and health status, the type of pain studied, and the specific outcome measures evaluated. The extent to which sex- and gender-related differences are present may vary according to the type of pain children experience and the particular pain features evaluated.

As an example, the lifetime prevalence of acute headache was 87.7% for a sample of 187 children, ages 5 to 16 years old; this rate did not vary by sex (12). However, the point prevalence did vary by sex; more females (67.4%) than males (48.3%) reported that they had a headache within the previous month. The number of headaches that children experienced each month was comparable for females and males. Yet, exploratory analyses revealed that children's pain intensity and pain affect ratings did differ significantly by sex; females reported stronger and more unpleasant pain than males.

There is likely a complex relationship among age, sex, gender, temperament, and learning in shaping children's pain perceptions. Familial, cultural, and societal expectations may gradually teach boys and girls to react differently. Boys generally may be encouraged to suppress their verbal pain complaints and to develop active pain coping methods such as sports and physical activities. Girls may be subtly reinforced for their pain complaints, especially if they develop pains similar to those experienced by a mother, as is often the case for girls who develop migraine headache (41). Girls may also be encouraged to rely on more passive pain control methods or be disabled for a longer period. As a result, boys may appear more stoic when they experience pain, whereas girls may express pain more openly. In addition, boys may be expected to tolerate stronger levels of pain than girls.

At present, our observations of sex- and gender-related differences in children's pain—sensitivity, experience, expression, and coping—reveal a complex interplay among many of the child and situational factors listed in Table 6.1.

Temperament

A child's temperament undoubtedly influences how he or she responds to new stimuli, including threatening or potentially harmful events. A child's tendency to withdraw or approach, to cope independently or seek support, and to appraise what may happen or depend on his or her parents' appraisal underlies how they cope in these situations. The primary focus of research has been on children's reactivity to pain, as defined by whether they tend to augment (sensitizers) or blunt (reducers) sensory input, and on their preferred coping style, the extent to which they attend to (approachers) or distract themselves away from (avoiders) pain (25,27,42–50).

Most studies report that children who approach new situations well or who seek information about the situation have less distress. As an example, children who have difficulty adapting to new situations showed greater distress during immunization injections (25). Higher sensitivity, as assessed by the Sensitivity Treatment Inventory for Pain (51), was associated with greater anticipatory distress, procedural anxiety, and pain during lumbar punctures (45).

Studies evaluating the relationship between the type of effective psychologic intervention and children's coping style (i.e., distraction for children who are repressors) yield mixed results. Smith and colleagues (52) reported that children had better pain control when they were taught methods that contrasted with their preferred style (i.e., distraction for sensitizers), whereas Fanurik and colleagues (27) found that children had better pain control when interventions were matched to their coping style. The discrepant results from these two studies are likely owing to differences between study samples: children with cancer versus health children, specific interventions (conversation versus imagery training), and type of pain (bone marrow aspirations versus cold pressor stimulation). However, the different results may also reflect the contribution of many of the factors outlined in Figure 6.1. Like other child characteristics, temperament and children's general coping style are probably not the sole determinants of what children should do to cope effectively in a particular pain situation. Children's motivation to cope is likely a key component that should be considered (48).

In their review of the influence of environmental factors and coping style on children's coping, Blount and colleagues (43) emphasize the need for future research with creative approaches from different perspectives because the issues are multifaceted. In our clinical experience (based on objective evaluation of children treated in the Pain Clinic), health care providers should assess children's preferred style (particularly for children who require prolonged medical treatment). However, they should have a variety of simple coping strategies to teach children because children may need different strategies for different types of pain or for different stages of their treatment.

Previous Pain Experience

As described previously, children evaluate any new pain—the sensory features, its meaning or relevance, and their possible responses in accordance with their previous pain experiences. Previous pain experience encompasses several aspects: the number of pains, the type of pain, the strength of pain, and the quality of the experience (e.g., positive or negative). Each aspect may have a different, but equally important, impact on children's pain perception. As children mature, they experience a wider variety of pains that differ in quality, intensity, location, and duration (2,12). They also learn new methods for lessening pain and gradually develop a flexible repertoire of strategies to cope with different types of pain. Thus, children's previous pain experiences shape their understanding, influence their perceptions, and affect their emotional reactions.

Initial studies evaluated whether children's distress and pain during invasive procedures differed according to whether children have already experienced these procedures (2,23, 24,53). The findings are inconsistent, suggesting that the critical feature is the nature of children's experience rather than only previous exposure to the painful procedure (2,54,55). Negative experiences increase children's anxiety and distress, and subsequently their pain. Bijttebier and Vertommen (56) studied 47 children (2 to 13 years old) during a routine blood test before hospitalization for elective surgery to evaluate differences in anxiety and distress related to the quality of children's previous venipuncture experiences and to children's coping style (sensitizer or repressor). Children with a history of negative experiences, regardless of their coping style, had higher anxiety before blood sampling and exhibited more distress during the procedure than children with previous positive or neutral experiences.

The nature of children's previous pain experiences shapes generally what they understand, do, and feel when encountering any new pain. However, the similarity of a previous experience (i.e., the particular type of pain, the sensory attributes, or the external circumstances) to their current pain is probably the most salient feature in signaling the aversive significance of the pain. Children with negative previous experiences will undoubtedly expect a continuing negative experience, display more anxiety and distress, and be at risk for heightened pain.

Family and Learning

Although hereditary factors can contribute to the onset of some painful diseases in childhood and may account for a familial predisposition to some recurrent pains, the family's influence on children's pain is not limited solely to genetic factors. Parents and siblings shape what children learn about pain, how they express pain, and how they cope with different types of pain. Children first learn to evaluate the significance or relevance of a pain from their parents' reactions, as readily evidenced when toddlers fall during play and experience a mild pain. Children quickly look at their parents to see how their parents are reacting. Some parents remain calm, reassure children, and encourage them to get up and continue playing, and other parents are visibly distressed, smother children with attention, focus on the hurt area, and encourage them to be comforted and stop their play.

Parents may respond differently when children sustain mild injuries, depending on the age, sex, or birth order of children. They may provide more attention to younger children but encourage older children to cope more independently. They may encourage boys to be stoic, suppress overt distress behaviors, and develop active behavioral responses. In contrast, parents may subtly reinforce girls to express their discomfort, exhibit more sick behaviors, and rely on passive pain coping methods. Parents may be more anxious, overtly protective, and concerned about the routine bumps and scrapes of childhood for their first-born child than for later children. Differences in parental responses may account for the higher pain sensitivity reported for first-born children (57).

Diverse family and cultural beliefs lead to significant variations in how children are raised, so that there are many differences in what children learn about pain and how to behave when in pain. The family and society, in addition to being the primary models for the development of children's pain attitudes and behaviors, may also influence children's actual pain experiences. Edwards and colleagues (58,59) demonstrated a positive relationship between the number of familial pain models and the frequency of an individual's pain complaints and nature of his or her coping strategies. More recently, Schanberg et al. (60) demonstrated that parental pain history and family environment were related to the functional status and pain complaints of children with juvenile primary fibromyalgia. Parents who reported multiple chronic pain conditions were more likely to have children with higher impairment and disability. Children's chronic pain problems should be viewed within the broader context of their family (61–65). Specific examples of the impact of parents, family, and learning are presented later in this chapter according to the type of pain children experience. (Cultural aspects of childhood pain are reviewed in detail in Chapter 9.)

SITUATIONAL FACTORS

Like adults, children can experience many different types of pain throughout their lives: acute pain owing to disease or trauma; acute pain and heightened emotional distress owing to repeated invasive medical procedures, recurrent episodes of headache, stomach ache, or limb pain unrelated to disease; and chronic pain owing to injury, disease, psychologic factors, or of unknown cause. A child's perception of these different types of pain, regardless of the specific etiologic factors, is modified by many situational factors. To control pain, we must target our interventions to the primary pain source and to the situational factors that intensify pain and distress and prolong disability.

Although each child has a unique set of factors that influence his or her pain experience, some factors have been identified as consistently relevant for certain types of acute pain, whereas others have been identified for recurrent pain and chronic pain.

Situational Factors That Intensify Acute Pain

There is a dynamic interplay among the situational factors that affect acute pain for children. Children's understanding, expectations, knowledge of simple pain control interventions, and the aversive significance of the pain (and/or responsible disease) affect their behaviors and shape their emotional responses. The common cognitive, behavioral, and emotional factors that can intensify acute pain are listed in Table 6.3.

Acute pain, relatively brief pain caused by tissue damage, provides a warning signal to children about physical injury so that the pain has an adaptive biologic significance. Acute pains caused by trauma/disease are the most common types of pain that children report (2,12,17). Children typically do not experience any prolonged emotional distress because the pain lessens progressively as the injury heals. They perceive acute pains more as the occasionally inevitable result of daily ac-

TABLE 6.3. *Situational factors that increase children's acute pain*

Cognitive
Lack of age-appropriate information about pain source
Inaccurate expectation of uncontrolled pain
Lack of knowledge about practical nondrug therapies
Lack of choice and little perceived control during treatment
Inaccurate information about child's prognosis
Behavioral
Overt physical distress
Inconsistent or inappropriate responses from staff or parents during treatments
Altered parental and sibling behaviors toward child within the family
Emotional
Anticipatory anxiety toward treatments
Heightened distress during treatment
Fear about continuing pain, increasing disability, or death
Frustration about disruption to activities
Depression about condition or treatments

tivities than as something to fear. They quickly learn that the cause of their pain is physical damage, often easily visible, that their pain is relatively brief, and that many interventions can alleviate their discomfort. As a consequence, children usually have accurate age-appropriate information about the pain source and positive expectations for pain relief. They perceive that they have some control and have developed some pain-reducing strategies, such as seeking a parent for a special hug, cleansing and bandaging an injured area, or swallowing medication. The aversive significance is determined more by the actual pain intensity and by any disruption in children's normal activities than by fears of continued pain and disability.

In contrast, a very different set of cognitive factors is typically present when children experience acute pain during invasive medical and dental procedures. (Procedural pain is covered in detail in Chapter 33.) Children often feel that they have no control in the situation; they may be uncertain about what to expect; they may not understand the need for a treatment that will hurt, particularly if they do not feel sick, and they may not know any simple pain-reducing strategies that they can use during the procedure. In fact, children may be told how to cope during a painful procedure in a manner that makes it easier for the adult administering the procedure but does not necessarily make it better for the child. These factors can intensify children's pain and distress, even when children receive anxiolytics and analgesics.

Children who receive multiple invasive procedures throughout a prolonged time period are at risk for developing increasing anxiety about these procedures (66). Some inconsistencies in how procedures are conducted are common in clinical practice. The more procedures that children undergo, the more likely that they will experience a difficult procedure (i.e., more pain, more nausea). Children then become fearful and expect that another difficult procedure is inevitable. Because the dynamics within a family change when a child is diagnosed with a major disease, the broader impact of the disease on the lives of the entire family can affect a child's pain. Parents, siblings, and extended family members must adjust to an altered life wherein the family schedule is determined by the schedule of medical treatments and their impact on the ill child. Parents are distressed by the disease and its implications: the life-threatening potential (if any), pain, physical symptoms, and accompanying disability. Parents' heightened anxiety may affect how they behave towards the ill child (67–69). They may become too protective, inadvertently encouraging the child to become overly dependent on them and to become passive sufferers during procedures rather than active copers. Physical disability, inaccurate expectations, social isolation, and loss of control over events will heighten a child's distress and can exacerbate his or her pain.

Many cognitive-behavioral interventions have been designed to lessen children's anxiety and pain during invasive treatments. These interventions share a common theme in that they reduce fear and anxiety and improve children's control by providing them with a concrete physical pain control technique such as deep breathing, counting slowly and regularly, or progressive muscle relaxation (2, 70–83). Children's treatment-related pain will increase when they have an inaccurate understanding of their disease, misperceptions of their parents' reactions to their diagnosis and treatments, uncertainty about treatment schedules, inconsistency in treatment administration, lack of control, few coping strategies, and fears about the effects of the disease or side effects of treatment.

Although drug and nondrug therapies are reviewed in other chapters, even the simple provision of information about what is happening, why the procedure is conducted in a certain manner, what equipment will be used, who will be present, the nature of the child's sensations during different phases of the procedure, and some straightforward instructions about what the child can do to help lessen pain will dramatically reduce the pain caused by any invasive procedure. For planned hospital admissions, children should attend relevant preparation programs to learn about what will happen during their stay, including the type of medical procedures they will receive. Most parents benefit from written guidelines for how they should respond to children's questions, such as those summarized in Table 6.4 for parents of children with cancer.

The cognitive, behavioral, and emotional factors that modify children's acute pain are dynamic and vary over time. Thus, children who require multiple invasive treatments throughout a prolonged time period will undoubtedly experience some changes in their understanding, parental and health staff behaviors, and their emotions. Few, if any, children can always achieve the same level of pain relief throughout a lengthy treatment protocol form the same medications or the same cognitive-behavioral interventions. Reg-

TABLE 6.4. *Guidelines for preparing children for invasive procedures*

Be honest with your child about what will happen.

Explain the procedure in age-appropriate language so your child can understand the whys, whats, and whos with respect to the rationale for the procedure, the equipment that will be used, and who will be present. (For young children, analogies with a pet are often beneficial. If your child has a pet and can understand that it needs injections and examinations, he/she may be less frightened when you explain what will happen as if the pet needed it. Ask your child how he/she could make it easier for the pet. In this way, your child may focus more on actively coping than on being frightened.

Emphasize the qualitative sensations that he/she may experience such as cold, tingling, and pressure so that your child focuses on what he/she is feeling, not just on a hurting aspect.

If the procedure will cause some pain, describe the pain that your child may feel in familiar terms that he/she will understand. Use examples of pain that your child has experienced already during play or pain that he/she may have observed other family members experience without distress.

Focus on what you and your child can do to make the procedure less distressing and less painful. Have a game plan of simple things that he/she can do such as taking slow deep breaths while you pace the rhythm, becoming immersed in a distracting image, or attending to the various stages of the procedure (depending on his/her preference for being involved or being distracted).

Choice, control, and predictability are very important for children receiving invasive treatments. Allow your child as much choice as possible such as which arm (for injections), whether to watch or look away, and which pain-reducing tool to use.

Remember that you and your child may have different preferences for coping with invasive procedures. You might prefer to be distracted, whereas your child might prefer to be involved. It is important to follow your child's preferences rather than unintentionally require him/her to follow your preferences. You should know which is your child's preference from his/her past experiences, for example, does he/she watch or look away if you remove a sliver from his/her finger, does he/she like to remove bandages independently or prefer that you do it.

After the procedure is over, praise your child for coping and following the plan that you both chose. Even if your child showed some distress, praise him/her for trying and explain that you will work on the plan to make it better. Your child may need practice as with any other activity that he/she has tried (e.g., riding a bike, rollerblading, skating). Be careful to not praise your child for just getting through it because you might be rewarding him/her for enduring it as a victim and inadvertently make him/her more frightened or distressed for future procedures.

ular assessments, including an appraisal of the factors listed in Table 6.3, are essential to understand the factors that affect their distress and pain.

Situational Factors That Can Intensify Recurrent Pain and Prolong Disability

Many otherwise healthy children and adolescents experience frequent debilitating episodes of migraine or tension-type headache, abdominal pain, or limb pain. These recurrent pains are not symptoms of an underlying physical disorder. Instead, the pain syndrome is the disorder and the situational factors responsible for triggering painful episodes must be identified and managed. Although the specific prevalence rates for recurrent pains vary widely from 1.4% to 37% depending on the age and gender of the study population, the country of origin, and the sampling methodology used (84), recurrent pains are a significant health problem in many countries. In this section, we describe the common factors that can intensify children's pain and prolong their pain-related disability, using recurrent migraine and tension-type headache as an example. (For a comprehensive review of the cause, diagnosis, and treatment of recurrent pain syndromes, see references 2,5,64,85–95.)

Several cognitive, behavioral, and emotional factors are important for children who develop recurrent headaches. Although hereditary factors may predispose some children to develop the condition, other situational factors trigger recurrent attacks, increase pain, prolong disability, or maintain the cycle of repeated attacks. The most common cause is stress associated with normal childhood activities, especially related to schoolwork, sports participation, or peer relationships. Often children do not recognize that they are stressed or are unable to fully deal with their stress and anxiety, which eventually trigger a headache. However, several interrelated factors are evident for children. The extent to which they represent a trigger, the primary underlying cause, or a secondary contributing factor, however, varies for individual children (41).

The common cognitive factors noted in children with recurrent pain are listed in Table 6.5. Parents often hold inaccurate beliefs about headache etiology, effective drug and nondrug therapies, and the role of environmental versus stress triggers. Parents usually try to understand recurrent pain from an acute pain perspective, in which pain is owing to a single cause and treatment. They do not understand that the pain, unlike most acute disease- or trauma-related pains that their children have already experienced, may have several interrelated causes. Parents expect that they will eventually find one treatment that will immediately stop recurrent attacks or immediately relieve chronic pain complaints. Thus, they may reject potentially effective treatments after only one attempt, even though the treatment might address some of the causes and might help to lessen pain over time. The lack of understanding about the many causes of pain, especially recurrent pain, leads some parents to continue to search for specific environmental triggers that chil-

TABLE 6.5. *Common cognitive factors for children with recurrent or chronic pain*

Beliefs about cause
Belief in single, as yet undiagnosed, cause
Inaccurate understanding of the primary and secondary causes
Belief in presumed environmental triggers[a]
Expectation of pain and related disability continuing for years
Beliefs about pain control
Poor knowledge about using and evaluating drug therapies
Little knowledge about effective nondrug therapies
Belief that children should rest and sleep during all attacks[a]
Reliance on a particular, but ineffective, method[a]
Belief that no treatment will be effective
Beliefs about the role of stress
Limited understanding that stress can cause pain (especially headache)[a]
Little knowledge about the situations that are continuing stressors for children[a]
Little understanding of the impact of children's high expectations for achievement[a]

[a]Particularly relevant for children with recurrent headache.

dren could avoid to prevent future attacks. Their children are then at risk for developing various learned pain triggers.

Almost all parents have used some nondrug methods with children during their headache attacks. Parents' attitudes and beliefs about nondrug therapies exert a powerful influence on children. Some parents, especially those whose own headache attacks are relieved only by potent medication, doubt the efficacy of any nondrug therapies. Even if they attempt to use them with their children, they often communicate their attitudes to children. Children's negative expectations will counteract any potential benefits. Other parents may select only passive nondrug methods that increase children's dependency and lack of control. Parents may not know how to assist children to use active and independent pain coping strategies that they could incorporate into their regular activities. These methods could improve children's control, lessen pain, and minimize any maladaptive disability behaviors.

Parents' and children's beliefs guide what they do to relieve pain during headache attacks and shape their broader efforts to resolve the cause of headache. Several behaviors are critical for the development of recurrent headache, as listed in Table 6.6.

TABLE 6.6. *Behavioral factors for children with recurrent or chronic pain*

Child and parental behaviors during pain episodes
Inconsistent parental responses[a]
Ineffective use of analgesic drugs and independent nondrug therapies
Children withdrawn from school, sports, or social activities
Children relieved from routine family responsibilities
Parental responses that reinforce illness and disability
Parental modeling of pain behaviors
Parental behaviors in response to a painful condition
Primary focus on additional medical consultations and diagnostic investigations
Persistent search for environmental triggers[a]
Failure to resolve continuing sources of stress[a]

[a]Particularly relevant for children with recurrent headache.

Typically, several of these behaviors are present for a child, with all equally contributing to the pain syndrome. Parents' uncertainty about how to control pain can lead them to respond to a child's headache complaints in a manner that inadvertently increases the child's distress, pain, and disability. Moreover, when parents seek additional diagnostic tests, attribute headaches solely to environmental triggers, and fail to identify and resolve relevant stress triggers, their behaviors directly maintain the cycle of repeat headache attacks.

Parents' behaviors (as well as those of care providers, teachers, coaches, and instructors) shape how children respond during headache attacks. Parents may reinforce headache-related disability when they allow children to stay at home instead of attending school, encourage them to withdraw from potentially stressful sports or social situations, and relieve them of routine family responsibilities, without helping children to address the underlying causes for headache attacks. Children, whose headaches are triggered by their high expectations for achievement, feel relieved of some pressure to excel (either self-imposed pressure or parents'/coach's pressure). Some children may begin to complain about a headache at the first sign of any muscle tightness, so that they have a legitimate excuse if their performance fails to meet their standards. Other children, whose headaches are triggered by their anxiety about coping in particular situations (gym class, social interactions at lunch, team games), begin to develop more frequent headaches in association with those situations. They initially miss a few classes, for example, on an intermittent basis because of their headache attacks, but children then avoid these situations on a more consistent basis. Stress reduction, inadvertently reinforced by parents, is a major secondary gain that prolongs headache episodes or contributes to the development of new attacks when children are stressed.

In addition to anxiety related to situation-specific stress, children's recurrent headaches may be influenced by several emotional factors, as listed in Table 6.7. When parents do not understand a child's diagnosis, they become anxious and frightened that the child has an underlying medical condition. Despite reassurance, some parents are concerned that their child has a malignant tumor. Even when reassured that the headaches are not life threatening, many parents and almost all children remain anxious about the likelihood of increasing pain and disability. Some children, particularly those who do not receive adequate pain control during headache attacks, become progressively distressed at headache onset. Parents are equally distressed that their child is suffering. When parents are unable to provide consistent pain relief, they become increasingly frustrated by the headache problem. Some children interpret that they, rather than their headaches, are the source of frustration. As headache attacks continue, families are also frustrated by the constant and unpredictable disruptions to their lives. Parents often miss work and cancel planned social activities to care for the child, and siblings are upset that they have to be quiet and that life again revolves around their brother (or sister) with a headache. Some parents eventually become angry at the health care system because no one has been able to help their children and stop the headache attacks.

TABLE 6.7. *Emotional factors for children with recurrent or chronic pain*

Situation-specific stress[a]
Emotional suppression or denial[a]
Anxiety about high expectations for achievement[a]
Fear of an undiagnosed condition
Fear of life-threatening potential
Fear of the likelihood of increasing pain and disability
Frustration about the unpredictability of painful episodes
Frustration about the interruption of activities life for child and family
Anger toward health care providers for failing to cure the pain
Underlying depression or anxiety

[a]Particularly relevant for children with recurrent headache.

Effective management of recurrent pain syndromes requires a multimodal approach to modify both the factors that trigger attacks and the conditions that exacerbate pain and disability, as demonstrated in the following case illustration (96). An 8-year-old girl was referred to the pain clinic for assessment and management. The purposes of the assessment were to evaluate the sensory characteristics of her headaches, to identify the primary and secondary factors responsible, to determine whether her headaches were characteristic of recurrent headache, and to recommend appropriate treatment. The assessment included structured interviews with the girl and her mother standardized pain questionnaires.

Headache Characteristics

Onset: Gradual onset, 5 years ago
Frequency: Approximately two headaches per week
Location: Unilateral, left or right eye and temporal region
Duration: Approximately 2 hours
Intensity: Described as a strong pain, numerical rating usually 8 (on the 0 to 10 Colored Analog Scale)
Quality: "Pushing" and aching
Accompanying symptoms: Nausea, lethargy, photophobia, and phonophobia
Seasonal/temporal variation: Headache attacks usually begin at school
Pain control: Lacks effective methods; for mild headaches, she puts her head down on her desk for a few minutes; for severe headaches, she sleeps and intermittently uses acetaminophen
Perceived control: None
Level of disability: Moderate; she misses class time and is bedridden at least twice a week
Triggers: Exclusive focus on external factors: various foods and drinks, weather (humidity, bright sun, change of weather, low or high barometric pressure)
Other pains: No other recurrent pains
Family history: Strong positive history; her mother has debilitating migraine headaches; her father has chronic back pain

The patient's pain assessment revealed that several factors maintained her headaches. The primary cause was underlying emotional distress. She had difficulty maintaining peer relationships and in resolving conflicts with classmates and teammates. The family's beliefs that her headaches were caused only by environmental triggers, combined with the patient's tendency to deny the existence of any familial stress (considerable owing to her father's disability) and school-related stress, prevented her from resolving her true headache triggers. In addition, her mother inadvertently served as a salient role model for headache disability and suffering. The therapist recommended a cognitive-behavioral program in which she would assist the patient and her family to identify and resolve the true headache triggers, develop more effective stress management and problem-solving skills, learn some active and independent pain control methods, and assist the girls's mother to differentiate her own headaches from those of her daughter so that she could respond to her daughter's pain complaints in a manner that encouraged her to relieve her headache and minimize her disability. The patient's headaches and disability improved significantly throughout the program, with headache frequency reduced to one mild attack per month.

Situational Factors That Increase Chronic Pain and Prolong Children's Disability

Children can experience a diverse array of chronic pain related to disease, trauma, and psychologic factors (2,5,93,97–101). Irrespective of the primary cause, many situational factors can affect children's pain, distress, and disability. The common cognitive, behavioral, and emotional factors are listed in Tables 6.5 to 6.7. Although many of these factors were described previously in the section on recurrent pain syndromes, the most salient situational factor for children is probably the aversive significance or relevance of the persistent pain and any accompanying disability.

The pain adversely affects all aspects of children's lives. Children may endure a prolonged period of physical disability, continuing pain, and varied medical treatments. Parents are distressed by the pain itself, its implications for their children's future, its life-threatening potential (if any), and the prospect of continuing pain and progressive disability. Parents and adolescents tend to emphasize and fear the future consequences of children's physical condition, whereas young children are more preoccupied by the immediate consequences and disruption of their daily activities. The dynamics within the family (both for siblings and extended family members) inevitably change as chronic pain prevents the child from pursuing normal activities and as family schedules adjust accordingly to the health care needs of the child with pain.

Although most families receive accurate information about their children's disease or condition and required medical treatments, few receive concrete information about the pain, the environmental factors that intensify it, and effective nondrug therapies to complement the primary analgesic or anesthetic treatment regimen. Thus, most children do not know simple pain control methods that they can incorporate practically into their daily activities. Of paramount importance, most families do not receive any information about the plasticity and complexity of pain so that they try to understand their children's chronic pain from an erroneous acute pain model, wherein there is a single cause and a single treatment. Because children with chronic pain typically have multiple sources of pain, affecting both peripheral and central nervous systems, with nociceptive and neuropathic components, parents and children become confused, anxious, and frustrated by the apparent failure of the health care system to find and treat the cause. Families become fearful that the children will continue to have pain or that they must rely on potent opioid analgesics to obtain even partial pain relief. Children's persistent pain is further complicated by decreased independence, reduced control, and an uncertain prognosis.

Children's usual behaviors are restricted by the disability caused by their condition or injury. They may gradually withdraw from social activities with peers and from most physical sports. As children's normal activities decrease, abnormal sensory input may increase, producing concomitant increases in pain. This problem can be confounded by the responses of parents, siblings, and health care providers. They may inadvertently encourage children to adopt passive patient roles, to behave differently from other children, and to depend primarily on others for pain control. These situational factors can intensify pain, distress, and prolong disability. Parents who encourage children to resume as many of their normal activities as possible create a situation wherein children's pain should be minimized.

Children with chronic pain typically are anxious and distressed by their prolonged suffering. Medications may cause various adverse physical effects, such as hair loss, itching, bloating, and constipation. Children may become overly self-conscious about their physical appearance and about their inability to participate in daily activities, so that they become ill at ease with their peers. They may withdraw socially because they anticipate negative reactions from their friends. Increased withdrawal and social isolation can exacerbate their pain. When their prognosis is uncertain, they may feel extremely anxious and frightened. Some children may become increasingly irritable and may act out by provoking arguments, disobeying parents, and not fulfilling routine responsibilities. Other children may outwardly cope with the pain and accept required treatments but may actually suppress their true emotional reactions—anger, anxiety, or depression. These children are at risk for developing progressively more somatic complaints as other outlets for their emotional expression diminish.

The following case illustrates how a cognitive-behavioral approach addresses the myriad cognitive, behavioral, and emotional factors that can intensify chronic pain. A 16-year-old girl with cerebral palsy was hospitalized for assessment and management of persistent pain.

Pain characteristics

Onset: Abrupt onset, 9 months ago
Frequency: Constant pain, with episodic exacerbations
Location: Shooting pain extending from her groin and abdomen to her back
Intensity: Described as intense pain; she was unable to use numerical rating scales
Affect: Affective rating 0.97 on the (0 to 1) Facial Affective Scale
Quality: Stabbing
Accompanying symptoms: Intermittent nausea and vomiting, increased bladder spasms, and constipation
Pain control: Opioid analgesics lessen, but do not fully relieve pain; the patient does not use any nondrug therapies
Perceived control: None
Level of disability: Despite significant physical disability (motor, visual) owing to cerebral palsy, the patient reports major pain-related disability so that she is often bedridden and has been unable to sit in her wheelchair, attend school, or perform her part-time work
Other pains: The patient has experienced intermittent bladder spasms for several years, has recent onset of abdominal pain from opioid-related constipation, and has tolerated intermittent back pain postsurgery; despite a history of chronic or intermittent pain, she has participated (with assistance) in school and typical childhood social activities with peers
Family history: No family history of chronic pain

The patient's assessment revealed that her pain was caused primarily by nerve compression but that several secondary factors contributed to her pain, distress, and increased disability. In particular, staff had been concerned about the relatively frequent opioid dosing that she required so they tried to delay drug administration. The patient had become extremely concerned about receiving her medication because she felt that delays meant stronger pain for a longer period. She had coped with much pain in her life and did not display the usual type of pain behaviors to staff, often only quietly saying she hurt and asking for medication. Some staff, concerned by the apparent disparity between her words and her behaviors, did not believe her. She felt that she needed to begin to act like it hurt and not try to fight the pain by getting in her wheelchair and interacting as normally as possible. She was extremely frightened that her pain would not be controlled and felt that she should show some disability or otherwise she would not be believed.

The patient needed to know that she would receive appropriate doses of medication at regular intervals and that staff would ensure that she receive them. The pain team would decide the type of medication to address both neuropathic and nociceptive causes, and she would learn some nondrug methods to complement (not as a substitute for) her drug therapy. As she began to trust that she would receive adequate pain control, that staff would listen to her (she felt that many people talked down to her because she was visibly handicapped or trivialized her descriptions of what she experienced), and that we would monitor her pain relief so that she could more actively try to resume some activities, her distress (and her parents' distress) decreased and her pain-related disability lessened.

RECOMMENDATIONS FOR OPTIMAL PAIN CONTROL

Children's pain is plastic and complex. The neural responses initiated by tissue damage can be modified by a diverse array of physical and psychologic factors, so that children can experience very different pains from the same injury or condition. Thus, we cannot adequately treat children by gearing our interventions solely to the responsible disease or condition. Instead, we must also control the situational factors that affect children's nociceptive processing and pain. We must ascertain which factors are relevant for which children. Treatment emphasis should shift accordingly from an exclusively disease-centered focus to a more child-centered focus.

The challenge for the future is to integrate this child-centered approach more efficiently into clinical practice. To lessen acute pain from invasive procedures, children require basic information about what is happening, why it is necessary, and what it may feel like. They should know what equipment will be used and be prepared for the sights, sounds, and physical sensations that they will experience. If the procedure will hurt, then children should be told that it might hurt. Because the pain probably varies, with some children experiencing slight pain (assuming that appropriate analgesics or anesthetics are used), the most accurate preparation is "It sometimes hurts a little, but not always." Emphasis should be placed on what sensations that children will feel: the warmth, coolness, or pressure associated with the procedure rather than the frightening label hurt.

For example, before an injection, children can be told "I am not sure exactly what you will feel, some children your age describe it as a tickling jab, a prick like a mosquito's bite, or like a sharp sting. It doesn't always hurt. Also, we can do things to make it hurt less. You can choose which finger (or arm), help to get the area ready, and then deeply rub the area to close your pain gate. Do you want to look or do you want to look away?" Some children prefer to watch intently, and others prefer to look away, watch something interesting, and use other forms of distraction. A practical form of distraction for children who choose to watch is asking them to describe the sensations that they feel. The amount of information that children require depends on their interest and their needs. Most children will state when they have heard enough or ask more in-depth questions if needed. All children require some control; that can be provided by allowing them to have as much choice as possible during invasive treatments, by teaching them some simple pain control methods, and by motivating children to select and routinely use them during procedures. Procedures should be conducted as consistently as possible. So that staff members do not inadvertently reinforce distress behaviors, they should set clear limits for children and encourage them to actively use independent pain control methods.

Children with recurrent pains require accurate information about the syndrome and its unique nature as a specific health problem rather than as a symptom of some undiagnosed condition. Children should understand the multiple causative and contributing factors and the difference between true and learned pain triggers and learn the impact of unresolved stress. All children should learn some simple and versatile methods for pain control during painful attacks rather than relying exclusively on medication or parents for pain relief. Some children require assistance to learn how to recognize and cope effectively with stressful situations and to set reasonable expectations for achievement. Other children may require structured behavioral programs to encourage them to resume normal activities and to reduce disability behaviors.

In contrast to the primary cognitive-behavioral approach for recurrent pain, children with chronic pain require a drug or physical approach to address the primary source(s) of noxious stimulation complemented by a cognitive-behavioral approach to address the secondary contributing factors. Childhood chronic pain must be viewed from a multidimensional perspective because multiple sensory, environmental, and psychologic factors are responsible for the pain, no matter how seemingly clear-cut the cause. Children require accurate information about the cause of their pain, presented in a calm, reassuring manner. Children should be encouraged to live as normally as possible and should resume as many activities as possible. A normal predictable routine provides them with a sense of reassurance and enhances their feelings of control. Parents should discipline children in the same manner as before they were diagnosed; rules should not be altered because they have pain. No matter how much children may be reassured that all is normal, any changes in parents' behaviors toward them signify a different and stronger message that the child is ill and all is not well. Thus, the aversive significance is increased. Children should receive supportive counseling as necessary to ameliorate their emotional distress. Individual differences among children and their families, as well as among relevant situational factors, necessitates that we treat children's pain problems in a creative and flexible manner so as to adapt our treatments to the needs of each child and family.

REFERENCES

1. Loeser JD, ed. *Bonica's management of pain*. Philadelphia: Lippincott Williams & Wilkins, 2001.
2. McGrath PA. *Pain in children: nature, assessment and treatment*. New York: Guilford Publications, 1990.
3. Price DD. *Psychological mechanisms of pain and analgesia*. Seattle: IASP Press, 1999.
4. Wall PD, Melzack R, eds. *Textbook of pain*. London: Churchill-Livingstone, 1994.
5. Ross DM, Ross SA. *Childhood pain: current issues, research, and management*. Baltimore: Urban & Schwarzenberg, 1988.
6. Brown JM, O'Keeffe J, Sanders SH, et al. Developmental changes in children's cognition to stressful and painful situations. *J Pediatr Psychol* 1986;11: 343–357.
7. Gaffney A. Cognitive developmental aspects of pain in school-age children. In: Schechter NL, Berde CB, Yaster M, eds. *Pain in infants, children, and adolescents*. Baltimore: Williams & Wilkins, 1993:75–85.
8. Gaffney A, Dunne EA. Developmental aspects of children's definitions of pain. *Pain* 1986;26:105–117.
9. McGrath PA, Speechley KN, Seifert CE, et al. A survey of children's pain experience and knowledge—phase 1. In: Jensen TS, Turner JA, Wiesenfeld-Hallin Z, eds. *Proceedings of the 8th World Congress on Pain: Progress in Pain Research and Management*. Seattle: IASP Press, 1997:903–916.
10. McGrath PJ, Unruh A. *Pain in children and adolescents*. Amsterdam: Elsevier, 1987.
11. Peterson L, Harbeck C, Farmer J, et al. Developmental contributions to the assessment of children's pain: conceptual and methodological implications. In: Bush JP, Harkins SW, eds. *Children in pain: clinical and research issues from a developmental perspective*. New York: Springer-Verlag, 1991:33–58.
12. McGrath PA, Speechley KN, Seifert CE, et al. A survey of children's acute, recurrent, and chronic pain: validation of the Pain Experience Interview. *Pain* 2000;87:59–73.
13. Gaffney A. How children describe pain: a study of words and analogies used by 5–14 year-olds. In: Dubner R, Gebhart GF, Bond MR, eds. *Pain research and clinical management (vol. 3)*. Amsterdam: Elsevier, 1988:341–347.

14. Gaffney A, Dunne EA. Children's understanding of the causality of pain. *Pain* 1987;29:91–104.
15. Harbeck C, Peterson L. Elephants dancing in my head: a developmental approach to children's concepts of specific pains. *Child Dev* 1992;63:138–149.
16. Lollar DJ, Smits SJ, Patterson DL. Assessment of pediatric pain: an empirical perspective. *J Pediatr Psychol* 1982;7:267–277.
17. Ross DM, Ross SA. *A study of the pain experience in children* (final report, ref. no. 1 RO1 HD13672-01). Bethesda, MD: National Institute of Child Health and Human Development, 1982.
18. Ross DM, Ross SA. Childhood pain: the school-aged child's viewpoint. *Pain* 1984;20:179–191.
19. Savedra MC, Gibbons PT, Tesler MD, et al. How do children describe pain? A tentative assessment. *Pain* 1982;14:95–104.
20. Schultz NV. How children perceive pain. *Nurs Outlook* 1971;19:670–673.
21. Craig KD, McMahon RJ, Morison JD, et al. Developmental changes in infant pain expression during immunization injections. *Soc Sci Med* 1984;19: 1331–1337.
22. Grunau RVE, Craig KD. Pain expression in neonates: facial action and cry. *Pain* 1987;28:395–410.
23. Jay SM, Ozolins M, Elliott CH, et al. Assessment of children's distress during painful medical procedures. *Health Psychol* 1983;2:133–147.
24. Katz ER, Kellerman J, Siegel SE. Behavioral distress in children with cancer undergoing medical procedures: developmental considerations. *J Consult Clin Psychol* 1980;48:356–365.
25. Schechter NL, Bernstein BA, Beck A, et al. Individual differences in children's response to pain: role of temperament and parental characteristics. *Pediatrics* 1991; 87:171–177.
26. Tesler MD, Holzemer WL, Savedra MC. Pain behaviors: postsurgical responses of children and adolescents. *J Pediatr Nurs* 1998;13:41–47.
27. Fanurik D, Zeltzer LK, Roberts MC, et al. The relationship between children's coping styles and psychological interventions for cold pressor pain. *Pain* 199353;:213–222.
28. LeBaron S, Zeltzer L, Fanurik D. An investigation of cold pressor pain in children (part I). *Pain* 1989;37: 161–171.
29. Zeltzer L, Fanurik D, LeBaron S. The cold pressor pain paradigm in children: feasibility of an intervention model (part II). *Pain* 1989;37:305–313.
30. Fradet C, McGrath PJ, Kay J, et al. A prospective survey of reactions to blood tests by children and adolescents. *Pain*1990;40:53–60.
31. Lander J, Fowler-Kerry S. Age differences in children's pain. *Percept Mot Skills* 1991;73:415–418.
32. Manne SL, Jacobsen PB, Redd WH. Assessment of acute pediatric pain: do child self-report, parent ratings, and nurse ratings measure the same phenomenon? *Pain* 1992;48:45–52.
33. Bournaki MC. Correlates of pain-related responses to venipunctures in school-age children. *Nurs Res* 1997; 46:147–154.
34. Jacobsen PB, Manne SL, Gorfinkle K, et al. Analysis of child and parent behavior during painful medical procedures. *Health Psychol* 1990;9:559–576.
35. Humphrey GB, Boon CM, van Linden van den Heuvell GF, et al. The occurrence of high levels of acute behavioral distress in children and adolescents undergoing routine venipunctures. *Pediatrics* 1992;90: 87–91.
36. Bennett-Branson SM, Craig KD. Post-operative pain in children: developmental and family influences on spontaneous coping strategies. *Can J Behav Sci* 1993; 25:355–383.
37. Palermo TM, Drotar D. Prediction of children's postoperative pain: the role of presurgical expectations and anticipatory emotions. *J Pediatr Psychol* 1996;21: 683–698.
38. Gidron Y, McGrath PJ, Goodday R. The physical and psychosocial predictors of adolescents' recovery from oral surgery. *J Behav Med* 1995;18:385–399.
39. Wallace MR. Temperament: a variable in children's pain management. *Pediatr Nurs* 1989;15:118–121.
40. Fowler-Kerry S, Lander J. Assessment of sex differences in children's and adolescents' self-reported pain from venipuncture. *J Pediatr Psychol* 1991;16: 783–793.
41. McGrath PA, Hillier LM. Recurrent headache: triggers, causes, and contributing factors. In: McGrath PA, Hillier LM, eds. *The child with headache: diagnosis and treatment*. Seattle: IASP Press, 2001:77–107.
42. Blount RL, Landolf-Fritsche B, Powers SW, et al. Differences between high and low coping children and between parent and staff behaviors during painful medical procedures. *J Pediatr Psychol* 1991;16:795–809.
43. Blount RL, Davis N, Powers SW, et al. The influence of environmental factors and coping style on children's coping and distress. *Clin Psychol Rev* 1991;11: 93–116.
44. Burnstein S, Meichenbaum D. The work of worrying in children undergoing surgery. J Abnorm Child Psychol 1979;7:121–132.
45. Chen E, Craske MG, Katz ER, et al. Pain-sensitive temperament: does it predict procedural distress and response to psychological treatment among children with cancer? *J Pediatr Psychol* 2000;25:269–278.
46. Field T, Alpert B, Vega-Lahr N, et al. Hospitalization stress in children: Sensitizer and repressor coping styles. *Health Psychol* 1988;7:433–445.
47. Peterson L, Crowson J, Saldana L, et al. Of needles and skinned knees: children's coping with medical procedures and minor injuries for self and other. *Health Psychol* 1999;18:197–200.
48. Peterson L, Toler SM. An information seeking disposition in child surgery patients. *Health Psychol* 1986;5: 343–358.
49. Thastum M, Zachariae R, Scholer M, et al. A Danish adaptation of the Pain Coping Questionnaire for children: preliminary data concerning reliability and validity. *Acta Paediatr* 1999;88:132–138.
50. Young MR, Fu VR. Influence of play and temperament on the young child's response to pain. *Child Health Care* 1988;18:209–217.
51. Baum LD. The Sensitivity Temperament Inventory for Pain (STIP): a new method for identifying the pain-vulnerable child. 55-02B-University Microfilms no. 94-18966, 1994.
52. Smith KE, Ackerson JD, Blotcky AD. Reducing distress during invasive medical procedures: Relating behavioral interventions to preferred coping style in pediatric cancer patients. *J Pediatr Psychol* 1989;14:405–419.

53. Klorman R, Michael R, Hilpert PL, et al. A further assessment of predictors of the child's behavior in dental treatment. J Dentistry Res 1979;58:2338–2343.
54. Dahlquist LM, Gil KM, Armstrong D, et al. Preparing children for medical examinations: the importance of previous medical experience. *Health Psychol* 1986;5: 249–259.
55. Siegel LJ, Smith KE. Coping and adaptation in children's pain. In: Bush JP, Harkins SW, eds. *Children in pain: clinical and research issues from a developmental perspective*. New York: Springer-Verlag, 1991: 149–170.
56. Bijttebier P, Vertommen H. The impact of previous experience on children's reactions to venepunctures. *J Health Psychol* 1998;3:39–46.
57. Vernon DTA. Modeling and birth order in responses to painful stimuli. *J Pers Soc Psychol* 1974;29:794–799.
58. Edwards PW, O'Neill GW, Zeichner A, et al. Effects of familial pain models on pain complaints and coping strategies. *Percept Mot Skills* 1985;61:1053–1054.
59. Edwards PW, Zeichner A, Kuczmierczyk AR, et al. Familial pain models: the relationship between family history of pain and current pain experience. *Pain* 1985; 21:379–384.
60. Schanberg LE, Keefe FJ, Lefebvre JC, et al. Social context of pain in children with juvenile primary fibromyalgia syndrome: parental pain history and family environment. *Clin J Pain* 1998;14:107–115.
61. Covelman K, Scott S, Buchanan B, et al. Pediatric pain control: a family systems model. In: Tyler DC, Krane EJ, eds. *Pediatric pain: advances in pain research therapy*. New York: Raven Press, 1990:225–236.
62. Ehde DM, Holm JE, Metzger DL. The role of family structure, functioning, and pain modeling in headache. *Headache* 1991;31:35–40.
63. Gulhati A, Minty B. Parental health attitudes, illnesses and supports and the referral of children to medical specialists. *Child Care Health Dev* 1998;24:295–313.
64. Walker LS. The evolution of research on recurrent abdominal pain: history, assumptions, and a conceptual model. In: McGrath PJ, Finley GA, eds. *Chronic and recurrent pain in children and adolescents*. Seattle: IASP Press, 1999:141–172.
65. Walker LS, Garber J, Greene JW. Psychosocial correlates of recurrent childhood pain: A comparison of pediatric patients with recurrent abdominal pain, organic illness, and psychiatric disorders. *J Abnorm Psychol* 1993;102:248–258.
66. Kellerman J, Zeltzer L, Ellenberg L, et al. Adolescents with cancer: hypnosis for the reduction of the acute pain and anxiety associated with medical procedures. *J Adolesc Health Care* 1983;4:85–90.
67. Bush JP, Melamed BG, Sheras PL, et al. Mother-child patterns of coping with anticipatory medical stress. *Health Psychol* 1986;5:137–157.
68. Blount RL, Corbin SM, Sturges JW, et al. The relationship between adults' behavior and child coping and distress during BMA/LP Procedures: a sequential analysis. *Behav Ther* 1989;20:585–601.
69. Blount RL, Sturges JW, Powers SW. Analysis of child and adult behavioral variations by phase of medical procedure. *Behav Ther* 1990; 21:33–48.
70. Barrera M. Brief clinical report: procedural pain and anxiety management with mother and sibling as cotherapists. *J Pediatr Psychol* 2000;25:117–121.
71. Ellis JA, Spanos NP. Cognitive-behavioral interventions for children's distress during bone marrow aspirations and lumbar punctures: a critical review. *J Pain Symptom Manage* 1994;9:96–108.
72. Jay SM, Elliot CH. A stress inoculation program for parents whose children are undergoing painful medical procedures. *J Consult Clin Psychol* 1990;58:799–804.
73. Jay SM, Elliott CH, Ozolins M, et al. Behavioural management of children's distress during painful medical procedures. *Behav Res Ther* 1985;23:513–552.
74. Jay S, Elliott CH, Fitzgibbons I, et al. A comparative study of cognitive behavior therapy versus general anesthesia for painful medical procedures in children. *Pain* 1995;62:3–9.
75. Katz ER, Kellerman J, Ellenberg L. Hypnosis in the reduction of acute pain and distress in children with cancer. *J Pediatr Psychol* 1987;12:379–394.
76. Kazak AE, Penati B, Brophy P, et al. Pharmacologic and psychologic interventions for procedural pain. *Pediatrics* 1998;102:59–66.
77. McGrath PA. Pain control in paediatric palliative care. In: Doyle D, Hanks GW, MacDonald N, eds. *Oxford textbook of palliative medicine*. Oxford: Oxford University Press, 1996.
78. Manne SL, Andersen BL. Pain and pain-related distress in children with cancer. In: Bush JP, Harkins SW, eds. *Children in pain: clinical and research issues from a developmental perspective*. New York: Springer-Verlag, 1991:337–372.
79. Maron M, Bush JP. Burn injury and treatment pain. In: Bush JP, Harkins SW, eds. *Children in pain: clinical and research issues from a developmental perspective*. New York: Springer-Verlag, 1991:275–296.
80. Powers SW, Blount RL, Bachanas PJ, et al. Helping preschool leukemia patients and their parents cope during injections. *J Pediatr Psychol* 1993;18:681–695.
81. Routh DK, Sanfilippo MD. Helping children cope with painful medical procedures. In: Bush JP, Harkins SW, eds. *Children in pain: clinical and research issues from a developmental perspective*. New York: Springer-Verlag, 1991:397–424.
82. Siegel LJ, Peterson L. Maintenance effects of coping skills and sensory information on young children's response to repeated dental procedures. *Behav Ther* 1981;12:530–535.
83. Zeltzer L, LeBaron S. Hypnosis and nonhypnotic techniques for reduction of pain and anxiety during painful procedures in children and adolescents with cancer. *J Pediatr* 1982;101:1032–1035.
84. McGrath PA. Chronic pain in children. In: Crombie IK, ed. *The epidemiology of chronic pain*. Seattle: IASP Press, 1999:81–101.
85. Apley J. *The child with abdominal pains*. Oxford: Blackwell Scientific, 1975.
86. Apley J, MacKeith R, Meadow R. *The child and his symptoms: a comprehensive approach*. Oxford: Blackwell Scientific, 1978.
87. Barr RG. Pain experience in children: developmental and clinical characteristics. In: Wall PD, Melzack R, eds. *Textbook of pain*. London: Churchill-Livingstone, 1994:739–765.
88. Barr RG, Rappaport L. Infant colic and childhood recurrent abdominal pain syndromes: is there a relationship? *J Dev Behav Pediatr* 1999;20:315–317.
89. Hodges K, Burbach DJ. Recurrent abdominal pain. In:

Bush JP, Harkins SW, eds. *Children in pain: clinical and research issues from a developmental perspective*. New York: Springer-Verlag, 1991:251–273.

90. Holden EW, Deichmann MM, Levy JD. Empirically supported treatments in pediatric psychology: recurrent pediatric headache. *J Pediatr Psychol* 1999;24:91–109.
91. Larsson B. Recurrent headaches in children and adolescents. In: McGrath PJ, Finley GA, eds. *Chronic and recurrent pain in children and adolescents*. Seattle: IASP Press, 1999:115–140.
92. McGrath PA, Hillier LM, eds. *The child with headache: diagnosis and treatment*. Seattle: IASP Press, 2001.
93. McGrath PJ, Unruh A. *Pain in children and adolescents*. Amsterdam: Elsevier, 1987.
94. Oster J. Growing pain: a symptom and its significance. *Danish Med Bull* 1972;19:72–79.
95. Scharff L. Recurrent abdominal pain in children: a review of psychological factors and treatment. *Clin Psychol Rev* 1997;17:145–166.
96. Hillier LM, McGrath PA. A cognitive-behavioral program for treating recurrent headache. In: McGrath PA, Hillier LM, eds. *The child with headache: diagnosis and treatment*. Seattle: IASP Press, 2001:183–220.
97. Bush JP, Harkins SW. *Children in pain: clinical and research issues from a developmental perspective*. New York: Springer-Verlag, 1991.
98. McGrath, PJ, Finley, AG, eds. *Chronic and recurrent pain in children and adolescents*. Seattle: IASP Press, 1999.
99. Pichard-Leandri E, Gauvain-Piquard A, eds. *La douleur chez l'enfant*. Paris: Medsi/McGraw-Hill, 1989.
100. Schechter NL, Berde CB, Yaster M, eds. *Pain in infants, children and adolescents*. Baltimore: Williams & Wilkins, 1993.
101. Tyler DC, Krane EJ, eds. *Advances in pain research and therapy*. New York: Raven Press, 1990.

7

Development of Psychologic Responses to Pain and Assessment of Pain in Infants and Toddlers

C. Celeste Johnston, Bonnie J. Stevens, Kristina Boyer, and Fran Lang Porter

The purpose of this chapter is to give an overview of pain in infants, with an emphasis on pain in hospitalized preterm infants who are more likely to need pain relief from health care professionals. The initial portion of the chapter includes evidence of the infant's ability to experience and express pain as well as data on the immediate, short-term, and long-term consequences of pain. Specific indicators of pain are presented. That section is followed by a brief discussion of pain as an emotional experience, the evidence of memory of pain, and a possible redefinition of memory of pain. The subsequent sections of the chapter are more clinically applicable, with presentation of options for assessment of pain in infants and assessment challenges that remain.

EVIDENCE OF EARLY RESPONSE TO PAIN

There is growing evidence that both the fetus and the newborn infant are capable of experiencing pain. Initial research into this question focused on differential response of stress hormones to surgery under opiate- and nonopiate-based anesthesia or analgesia (1,2). Although controlling for the surgical procedures in these two landmark studies, but not controlling for type and amount of anesthesia or analgesia, there was a clinically detrimental outpouring of stress hormones in those infants who had received minimal or no pain control. In subsequent studies of actual tissue damage from painful procedures compared with handling in preterm neonates, a significant increase in heart rate (3–5), heart rate variability (6), and a decrease in vagal tone (7) and oxygen saturation (4,5) have been reported. Facial actions, which in combination create a grimace interpreted as an expression of pain, have consistently been reported to reflect a greater proportionate disparity between painful and nonpainful situations than physiologic parameters (4,5,8). Furthermore, the newborn can localize the site of pain, which was formerly thought to be beyond their capabilities. Franck (9) documented that full-term newborns swiped the foot that had been subjected to heel lancing with the unaffected foot. Thus, it is now evident that infants born at term or much before term can distinguish pain from other tactile experiences.

There is also evidence that, as an infant matures, the response to pain becomes more *differentiated*. This differentiation is reflected in both autonomic and central parameters with increasing changes to pain but decreasing changes to other stimuli, for example, heart rate (10), facial actions (10–12), and body movements (12). In another approach to determining the effect of maturity, infants who showed no changes in either physiologic or behavioral response to heel stick were younger, both postconceptionally and postnatally, than those who responded (13). Although the lack of response was confounded by less recovery time between painful events, age was the factor that accounted for most of the difference between infants who did and did not show a reaction to the heel stick.

There have been some reports that severely ill infants show less benefit from nonnutritive sucking intervention for heel stick in terms of heart rate accelerations (14) and that sicker infants have a higher cry pitch in response to a painful stimulus (15). Severity of illness has not been an influencing factor for heart rate, oxygen saturation, or facial actions in response to untreated heel sticks in other reports (4,5,16).

Not only can preterm infants respond in a different way to pain versus other stimuli and therefore presumably experience pain, they can distinguish *degrees of invasiveness* or the *amount of pain* (17). One hundred thirty-five infants ranging from 26 to 41 weeks of gestational age were studied from birth throughout their hospitalizations during at least two of 12 procedures commonly performed in neonatal intensive care. In general, infants at all ages showed graded increases in heart rate and arterial pressure and graded decreases in oxygen saturation in response to procedures ranging from mild to moderate to high painfulness, as rated by health care professionals (17). Consistent with the above studies that showed increased distinguishing responses with maturity, the older infants in this study showed greater gradations of response between the categories of painful procedures.

Although it now seems clear that preterm infants can experience pain, pain is possibly experienced at *greater intensities* by these very young humans than by full-term infants, children, or adults. This possibility should not be surprising because the mechanisms for nociception begin shortly after conception, whereas inhibitory mechanisms appear later in fetal development. Researchers studying spinal cord processing have clearly demonstrated the hyperexcitability and wider receptive fields in infants born before their expected birth date (18,19). Because inhibitory mechanisms develop higher up in the central nervous system than the spinal cord and are thus more complex, their functionality is not operative until later along the developmental trajectory. The flexor reflex, which in adults is a nociceptive reflex, is elicited in infants with only mild mechanical stimulation. The threshold of this reflex increases over the last trimester of gestation (18). The receptive field where this reflex can be elicited decreases with age. In infants younger than 33 weeks postconceptional age and older than 37 weeks postconceptional age, there were clear differences in the receptive fields, with a supposed transition period between those two ages. The amount of tissue damage to the leg or foot from intravenous lines or repeated lancing was reflected in changes in the threshold (2, 20,21).

Finally, because of the high plasticity of the developing fetus or preterm neonate, there may be permanent neurologic structural changes with frequent or extreme exposure to pain during this vulnerable period (22,23). Evidence is beginning to accumulate that suggests that this phenomenon may be occurring (24). The influence of repeated painful procedures in preterm neonates on clinical and developmental outcomes is a priority area for research in the future.

IMMEDIATE PHYSIOLOGIC RESPONSE TO PAIN

There have been numerous studies on the immediate physiologic response in neonates to tissue-damaging procedures such as heel stick, intravenous starts, injections, circumcision, and lumbar punctures. *Heart rate* typically increases in response to an acute painful stimulus (4,10,12,15,25–33). The range of increase varies but is usually at least ten beats per minute, with reports of as many as 20 to 25 beats per minute (15,34). Not all studies, however, have reported an increase in heart rate (6). Although reported infrequently (13), bradycardia has been reported as a response by preterm infants to acute pain. For example, intubation (35), besides being painful, also stimulates visceral tissue, which may influence heart rate. Some infants exhibit neither increases nor decreases in heart rate and do not respond at all to painful procedures or respond minimally (13). Heart rate may thus not be the most consistent indicator of response to acute pain, despite its common use.

Other cardiovascular indicators used in the assessment of pain in infants have been *heart rate variability*, which increased in response to heel stick (14,36) or heel squeeze after the lancing of the heel (37). *Vagal tone*, a more precise indicator of cardiac and respiratory sympathetic response to pain, decreased in response to heel stick (37), circumcision (7), and injection (2,20,38). *Oxygen saturation*, usually measured transcutaneously, has been reported as a response to procedural pain less often, but when reported, it had decreased (15,31,32,35,39,40). Some researchers report a decrease to a level of 80%, in both full-term (31) and preterm newborns in response to acute painful stimuli (34,41). In studies in which the transcutaneous oxygenation level did not drop so precipitously, there is the possibility that the infants were on assisted ventilation and the percentage of inhaled oxygen was increased by the health professional caring for the infant during the procedure to compensate for the desaturation (42). This adjustment may not have been reflected in the measured indicator.

Skin conductivity, measured in infants via palmar or plantar sweat, is a reflection of stimulation of the sympathetic nervous system and is thus an indicator of arousal and stress (43–45). When used with infants, Harpin and Rutter (46) found that it was unreliable in infants younger than 37 weeks postconceptional age owing to immature sweat production patterns. Thus, there seems to be an important developmental factor in differential emotional sweating.

Intracranial pressure or cerebral blood flow can be measured in infants noninvasively, with sensors placed on the anterior fontanel. Intracranial pressure is an indirect measure of cerebral blood flow and wide fluctuations or dramatic drops or increases in either can result in neurologic sequelae of varying duration (46a). Both measures have been used infrequently as indicators of response to invasive procedures. Increases were reported in response to intubation (47), suctioning (48), and heel stick (47). However, many other factors influence intracranial pressure and cerebral blood flow, including crying (49) or even routine nursing care as seemingly benign as opening isolette doors (50). The measurement of either intracranial pressure with a fiberoptic pressure sensor or cerebral blood flow with either an ultrasonographic Doppler or near-infrared spectroscopy requires equipment not typically available in clinical settings, although for research purposes it can provide important insights into the infant's physiologic response to acute pain.

IMMEDIATE BEHAVIORAL RESPONSES TO PROCEDURAL PAIN

Immediate behavioral responses to pain generally reflect a tensing of the entire body, including vocal tract, body, and face. The specific behaviors that have been examined are cries, body movement, and facial actions. The *amount of crying* has often been used as an indicator of pain, with the underlying assumption that the greater the amount of crying, the greater the pain intensity (30,39,51–63). Researchers who have attempted to look at *crying characteristics* have reported that "pain cries" are high pitched and strident (7,64–66), more so than cries resulting from hunger, frustration, or being startled (67–69). However, this finding is not always consistent (5,8,31), and this inconsistency in findings is difficult to explain given that some of the same authors using the same techniques and similar situations in different samples are reporting these results. In the one study in which acoustical cry features were examined in response to analgesia (sucrose or pacifier), there were no differences in cry features, although there were differences in incidence of crying (70). At present, it can only be concluded that the amount of crying, but not cry characteristics, is reflective of acute pain in infants.

Body movements, reported infrequently, are a tensing and/or thrashing of limbs (9,11,12, 71). Grunau et al. (72), based on a study comparing body movements in preterm neonates in response to procedures of differing invasiveness (e.g., diaper change and endotracheal tube suctioning), warn that only leg extension and finger splay, as defined using the developmentally appropriate Assessment of Premature Infant Behavior of Als et al. (73), are the specific body movement indicators of pain, whereas torso squirming and twitching occur in response to milder procedures and spontaneously. There have been a few reports of protecting surgical site (74) or massaging affected area (9). With current neonatal intensive care unit (NICU) practices based on developmental care of swaddling infants, these indicators are not readily available for most preterm neonates, although they can be appropriate for older infants.

Facial actions, when taken together, compose a grimace that was described more than a century ago by Darwin (75). That original description of a squared mouth, furrowed brow, and eyes closed continues to be reliably observed using the Neonatal Facial Coding System (8,76,77). The Neonatal Facial Coding System, the most validated facial action measure, comprises ten facial actions (brow bulge, eye squeeze, nasolabial furrow, open lips, horizontal and vertical mouth stretch, taut tongue, chin quiver, lip purse, and tongue protrusion), although two of these (lip purse and tongue protrusion) are not seen in response to pain. Open lips were not discriminative of pain from other situations (4,78,79), although some researchers suggest that the action of open lips contributes to the pain response facies (8,76,80). For very preterm infants whose facial musculature is not strongly developed or who have apparatus (e.g., tubes or tape) obscuring the view of some facial actions, the three upper facial actions alone (brow bulge, eye squeeze, nasolabial furrow) have been sufficient to discriminate pain from nonpain situations (4,79).

SHORT-TERM RESPONSE TO PAIN

For infants who have undergone surgery, the response to pain reported in the literature may take place from over 30 minutes to several days. The predominant indicators in these studies are hormonal but also include behavioral state and the cutaneous flexor reflex.

Hormonal

Stress hormones, particularly cortisol and the catecholamines (most commonly epinephrine and norepinephrine), have been studied in response to postsurgical pain after cardiac, open heart, and general surgery in preterm and full-term infants and circumcision in term infants (81–83). Cortisol has also been studied in response to more minor procedures such as endotracheal suctioning or routine nursing care (35,84,85). In one study, increased levels of both cortisol and β-endorphins were found in fetuses undergoing needling for transfusion for greater than 15 minutes (86). These substances are clearly related to stress but not always to pain. For example, in response to procedures such as circumcision, heel stick, or even physical examination, there were no differences in cortisol levels (87–90). Yet these were procedures of presumably differing pain intensity to which there had been predictable differences in the behavioral state (i.e., more crying with the more invasive procedures). Similarly, there were no differences in cortisol levels for pacifier (90) or dorsal penile nerve block (91) treatments for circumcision, although there was less crying with these interventions compared with nontreated circumcision. However, when ill preterm infants were given the synthetic opiate meperidine for endotracheal suctioning, cortisol levels were less elevated (92). Furthermore, for major surgery, there were significantly fewer increases in cortisol for infants who received a high-dose intraoperative opiate (2) or an intraoperative and postoperative high-dose opiate (1). Based on findings of studies on hormonal response to pain conducted to date, it would seem that these substances are related to general arousal and/or stress, and only with major analgesic agents (i.e., opioids) do they change significantly.

State regulation is a task of newborns (93, 94), and pain disrupts the infants' ability to maintain a steady state. Infants who are able to regulate state are more likely to engage in positive interactions with their parents and learn in their environment (95), and, thus, there has been much attention given to promoting steady state and smooth transitions between states (96–105). Aside from the crying state, presumably reflective of pain (106), the ability to have long periods of quiet sleep is presumed to reflect comfort. This component, i.e., amount of time in quiet sleep, has been incorporated into composite measures of pain (107,108) or lack of pain (109). More broadly, behavioral state has been used as a contextual factor in a composite measure of infant pain in a counterbalancing fashion to account for the effect of state on pain expression (79). As an independent indicator of pain, it has been used post-procedure (110) and postoperatively (111,112).

Cutaneous Flexor Reflex

Although the studies using cutaneous flexor reflex are actually testing peripheral sensitivity, it is proposed that tissue damage (18) and thus presumably pain alter the thresholds that make the flexor reflex a candidate indicator of pain. For example, the threshold of reflex seen in the tensor flexion reflex in infant heels that had been subjected to multiple lancing was raised with the use of topical anesthetic on the lanced area (2,20,21,38,113). Similarly, the threshold of cutaneous withdrawal reflex in skin near a surgical wound was raised after the administration of opiate analgesia (114). Thus, although a measure of hypersensitivity, the changes in threshold related to analgesia make it a promising measure of relatively localized peripheral pain. More research is needed using this indicator to determine whether it correlates with other indicators of pain, particularly facial actions, which thus far appear to be sensitive to pain.

LONG-TERM CONSEQUENCES OF PAIN

There is mounting evidence that the repeated painful events as part of clinical care endured by the neonate, especially those born preterm, can have long-term effects (see Chapter 4). In one study, two groups of preterm infants of 32 weeks postconceptional age, one 4 days postnatal age (newly born), and the other 4 weeks postnatal age (early born) were compared on acute pain response to heel stick (115). The early-born infants showed a less mature, less organized response in that their heart rates were higher, their oxygen saturation was lower, and they failed to show the classic facial actions associated with pain. In a regression analysis including perinatal factors, current situational factors (e.g., severity of illness and behavioral state), and care factors, the differences in physiologic response between the age groups were Apgar scores and birth weight. Behavioral differences, however, were accounted for by the number of invasive procedures (calculated from the medical records). The infants with more previous invasive procedures showed fewer facial actions.

This finding was further corroborated by a recent study of pain reactivity, also of infants of 32 weeks postconceptional age who had spent several weeks in the NICU environment (116). Infants whose pain had been controlled by morphine during their stay demonstrated more robust responses in both facial actions and heart rate change from baseline to heel stick. Furthermore, the infants who had been exposed to steroid therapy showed the least responsiveness. The underlying assumption in interpreting these two studies is that the more robustly the infant responds to noxious stimuli, the healthier the infant is. Certainly from a survival perspective, it is important for the infant to be able to signal distress to his or her caregivers.

There are, however, seemingly conflicting reports on the long-term effects of pain in infancy. Oberlander et al. (117) compared infants, either born at a mean age of less than 26 weeks or at term, on biobehavioral responses to finger lance for serum iron testing at 4 months corrected age. There were no differences in facial actions between the groups, which was dissimilar to the above studies

(115,116). In the study of Oberlander et al., both groups demonstrated increased cardiac sympathetic and decreased parasympathetic responses to the lance, a physiologically less mature response similar to one of the earlier studies (115). Specifically, the former preterm infants showed a milder parasympathetic withdrawal during the lance and a prolonged sympathetic response than the full-term infants. In searching for explanations of the differences in the study of 4-month-old infants versus the 32-week-old infants, the most obvious one is the difference in age at the time of study. The Oberlander et al. (117) study is the first to prospectively compare pain response in infants beyond the NICU experience. It also is the first to examine response to pain inflicted at a naïve site, i.e., the earlier studies used heel lance as the painful event on heels that had experienced many lances. The peripheral changes described in animals after repeated injury (118) may also occur in preterm infants who have highly plastic nervous systems (23), so that testing pain response in a site that has been subjected to repeated pain may be measuring peripheral sensitivity, which was not the case in the Oberlander et al. study.

In a study of full-term infants undergoing routine immunization at 2 months of age, males who had undergone unanesthetized circumcision cried more and showed more facial action than uncircumcised males (63). However, those infants had been born at term, and circumcision, although painful with the pain lasting longer than most NICU procedures, only occurred once. Furthermore, although the infants who were circumcised were randomized to receive either a local anesthetic [e.g., lidocaine-prilocaine cream (EMLA)] or placebo (e.g., placebo cream) (119), they were not randomized as to whether they would be circumcised. Therefore, there may be a selection bias from parents who do or do not have their infant circumcised (see reference 120 for influence of parental response). Thus, in examining long-term responses to pain, the age at which the pain occurs, the time between painful events, and the number of times that the infant is exposed to pain need to be considered. In the study by Grunau et al. (116), 19 procedures were the cutoff point of the number of painful procedures that separated the infants in that study from being more expressive. Unfortunately, this number is reflective only of that one report in which the exact number of procedures was examined and may be different in different samples.

In reports of much longer term consequences of pain, Grunau and colleagues (121, 122) found that infants who had experienced NICU care for several weeks showed insensitivity to pain at 18 months, used somatization as a coping mechanism at 4 years, and reported higher pain affect at 8 to 10 years of age than their full-term counterparts. Important positive correlations were found between the length of stay in the NICU and somatization in the 4-year-old and greater affectivity in the 8-year-old former preterms. Those researchers assumed that these differences between infants prematurely born and infants born at term were owing to pain, although pain was not explicitly measured in any way, and very low birth weight infants who need to spend long periods in the NICU are likely to have psychomotor immaturity and have more minor injuries in childhood, which could account for these differences (123).

For ethical reasons, controlled studies of pain in humans are not possible. Controlled animal studies of pain may provide insights into mechanisms underlying pain processing, although extrapolation from animal models to humans requires some caution. With respect to the development of pain pathways, the neonatal period of the rat corresponds to the last trimester of human development (124). There were two recent studies on the long-term effects of pain in the neonatal period (125,126). In the first study, neonatal rat paws were exposed to one, two, or four needle sticks or touch with cotton swab to the separate paws daily for the first week of postnatal life. Then at 16, 22, and 65 days of age, they were tested for pain threshold using a hot-plate test. Behaviors related to stress were tested during adulthood (60 days or older) and included alcohol preference, defensive withdrawal test, corticotropin and cortisol response to air-puff startle, and social discrimination. The rats that had received pain four times daily showed a decreased pain threshold at 16 and 22 days, but as adults (65 days), there were no differences. This group was more vigilant in the social discrimination task and showed an increased preference for alcohol and increased anxiety in the open field test. However, the corticotropin and cortisol levels after the air-puff startle were not different between the groups. These results require replication before generalizing but indicate that the long-term effects of pain may be more enduring than previously thought.

In the second study (126), newborn rat pups were injected with an inflammatory agent that resulted in edema, erythema, and pain behaviors for a week. As adults, the rats that had received the inflammatory agent showed increased sensitivity to a formalin test. More important, there were structural changes of sprouting of nociceptive receptors in the dorsal root ganglia of the spinal cord, supporting the idea that prolonged neonatal inflammation and pain can result in permanent alterations of nociceptive neural circuitry. The particular model of the injection of an inflammatory agent that causes extreme pain behaviors (e.g., paw lifting, licking, shaking) for a week in the life a neonatal rat [comparable with the entire last trimester in humans (127)] is fortunately more extreme than most human neonates endure, and, thus, comparing these findings to human neonates should be tempered with some reserve.

DEVELOPMENT OF DIFFERENTIATION OF PAIN FROM OTHER NEGATIVE EMOTIONS

One major role of infant caregivers is to be able to interpret correctly the emotional state of the infant through various cues. Emotions and emotional expression have been viewed as functional (i.e., the experience of the emotion), as well as having a purpose. The purpose of mutual expression of joy in the act of smiling between an infant and its caregiver has the purpose of promoting bonding. The expression of fear by a toddler regarding another child in a day-care setting will elicit protection from the aggressor by the day-care staff; thus, that expression's purpose of safety is realized. The expression of pain in infants signals to caregivers the need to escape from the source of pain and elicits comforting strategies from them. In a study of pain response in day-care toddlers, the expression of pain behaviors elicited attention, kisses, hugs, and distractions from day-care staff (C. L. von Baeyer and P. J. McGrath, unpublished, 1997).

Basic emotions are considered to be joy, sadness, fear, anger, and interest, and these are clearly recognizable and differentiated (128,129). As the infant develops a sense of self, the social emotion of empathy evolves. Self-conscious emotions such as pride, guilt, shame, and embarrassment emerge as the child experiences social interactions and social reinforcements. None of these emotions is present at birth, yet there is a tendency by caregivers to ascribe these emotions to infants. There is an ongoing controversy over the role of cognitive development in emotional development. Izard and Ackerman (128) take the position that at the time that the *expression* of the emotion occurs, the emotion is *experienced*. Accordingly, a facial expression of guilt, which can be observed before 1 year of age (30), precedes the ability to *cognitively* understand guilt; that is, there is a distinction between emotion and cognition. Others (130,131) explain that a sense of self is needed before emotions can be experienced, such that a 10-month-old infant whose facial expression resembles a facial expression of guilt would *not actually be experiencing* guilt. Goleman (132) provides some resolution of the controversy by dividing the developmental stages of emotional response into arousal stage and cognitive appraisal. Pain qualifies as an emotion in the context of arousal, but in infants, it probably does not qualify as an emotion from the perspective of cognitive processing. Currently, this hypothesis can neither be proved nor disproved.

Pain is perhaps the *most* basic of emotions in that it is present from birth, even a premature birth, and its expression serves as a signal to caregivers of the need for safety from danger and provision of comfort (133). The infant's ability to mount an expression of pain has survival value, without which the infant is at risk of dying. The cry from pain, for example, has been labeled a "siren" for caregiver attention (133,134). Once attention is obtained and the caregiver focuses on the infant, the facial expression of pain facilitates the caregiver's appraisal of the infant's state. Once the caregiver determines that the infant is in pain, actions are taken to relieve the pain and promote comfort.

Studies that have attempted to differentiate hunger from pain have been unable to do so successfully because the cry of hunger (after a few minutes) evolves into a cry of pain. Presumably, the hunger that the infant is experiencing becomes painful. However, both removal of pain and the promotion of comfort and satiation of hunger and promotion of nutrition are necessary for survival and demand caregiver attention. Thus, attempts to differentiate hunger or even fear from pain in early infancy may be futile.

MEMORY OF PAIN

There has been a long-standing assumption that whatever pain may be experienced by infants is quickly recovered from and there is no memory of it. A lack of reporting about pain during infancy by the children as they grow older is largely the basis of this assumption. Because self-report is the main way in which we communicate our pain, the absence of this self-report was taken to reflect no memory or long-lasting effects of the pain.

Memory may be explicit (i.e., it can be recalled and reported) or implicit (i.e., unconscious) (123,135). It is explicit memory of pain in infancy that cannot be documented. Implicit memory is stored at an unconscious level, probably in the basal ganglia or cerebellum, and is not available for self-report. Converging evidence from both animal and human infant studies provides strong arguments that memories of pain may be stored in the nervous system at a level that precludes consciousness but may still influence subsequent reactions to painful experiences.

Much of our knowledge of the basic biology of pain has been obtained from studies on laboratory rats. Although rats and humans have different developmental timetables, the basic sequences of events in the maturation of sensory systems are the same. Newborn rat pups actively respond to painful stimuli immediately after birth (136,137), even before their visual (fused eyes) and hearing (poor response to ultrasonics) capacities are completely functional. The way in which these animals respond to pain later in life, however, can be shaped by environmental events occurring while they were neonates. For example, rats who were routinely handled after birth show reduced behavioral distress to painful stimuli as adults when compared with previously nonhandled pups (138,139). Rats who were routinely exposed to painful stimuli after birth show a higher rate of active avoidance learning as adults when compared with controls (140) or preference for alcohol and social anxiety (125). At the neurophysiologic level, when cutaneous sensory nerves are damaged during a critical stage of development, this can result in a cascade of events including the death of dorsal root ganglion cells (141,142), deafferentation of an area in the spinal cord, and development of synaptic connections between collateral sprouts and the deafferented area of the spinal cord (143,144). Thus, cord regions normally devoted to input from the damaged area now process information from nearby undamaged skin, totally distorting the representation of the somatotopic map in the brain (145). Although the applicability of these data to humans has not been firmly established, there is concern that these long-term consequences of injury in laboratory rats may have important implications for human infants who undergo painful tissue-damaging experiences.

Early reports from studies of infants undergoing circumcision suggested that behavioral changes could persist long after the acute pain of circumcision and that these changes appeared to disrupt newborn infants' adaptive responses to both feeding and mother–infant interactions (146,147). Persistent behavioral changes also were indicated by premature infants' hyperalgesic pain responses after tissue damage caused by frequent heel-stick procedures (21). The adverse postoperative metabolic responses of premature infants have also been cited as evidence of persistent effects of significant pain (2). These hyperalgesic and adverse metabolic responses could be reversed with anesthesia. Others have reported that the best predictor of pain response magnitude among premature infants was the number of invasive procedures that the infants had previously experienced (115). Newborn infants who have undergone mild handling and immobilization (148) or who have been circumcised (63,149) do respond more robustly to a subsequent painful heel stick.

The most obvious mechanism that could mediate these patterns is sensitization, an enhanced response to stimulation that follows an exposure to a strong noxious stimulus. Conversely, in the heel-stick study (148), the cardiac and behavioral responses of the handled and nonhandled groups could not be differentiated before the heel stick. If the handled group were simply more agitated from handling, one would expect group differences to be exhibited before pain exposure. Further, in the circumcision study (149), all circumcised infants had been anesthetized for circumcision, theoretically protecting them against much of the pain of the surgery. If their responses to pain were blocked during circumcision, one would expect little correlation between that response and responses to subsequent pain. That they responded more robustly to subsequent pain despite anesthesia suggests that either their pain was inadequately managed during circumcision or they were very aroused in response to being restrained for the procedure. The process responsible for these persistent effects, however, remains unclear.

Human infants are capable of auditory learning in the third trimester while still *in utero*. Newborns can distinguish their mother's voice from other female voices (150,151). Fifer and Moon (152) found that when presented with a choice of hearing their own mother's voice in speech or a filtered version in such a way as to mimic womb-like sounds, newborns chose to suck more often to the signal predicting the *in utero* versions of their own mother's voice. During the third trimester (27 weeks gestational age), fetuses are able to hear and respond behaviorally to sound and auditory stimuli (150,153). DeCasper and Spence (154) studied pregnant women at 7.5 months' gestation who recited a target story aloud to their fetuses twice daily until birth, at which time the target story had greater reinforcing value (measured by sucking bursts) to the novel story and was independent of who recited the story. In another study, pregnant women at 33 weeks' gestation recited a target rhyme three times daily for 4 weeks, which the fetuses differentially responded to with a brief decrease in fetal heart rate (155). These studies exemplify the neonate's memory of auditory stimulation at the same developmental stage that a preterm infant will be exposed to tissue-damaging tactile stimulation. Because the sense of touch developmentally precedes the sense of hearing, it seems that there would be tactile memory at least to the extent that there is auditory memory, so that there is reason to believe that there may well be memory of painful events in preterm neonates.

Early learning is of special importance because it lays down the foundation on which future behavior, experience, and learning will depend (156). Just as the capacity to respond to and signal the presence of pain early in life is critical for survival, so is the capacity to learn. Indeed, behaviors that are critical for survival are learned very quickly, even after only one opportunity. A classic example of early, one-trial learning is the illness-induced odor aversion demonstrated in newborn rat pups. Three-day-old rat pups (equivalent to a 25 to 26 weeks of gestation in the human infant) learn an odor aversion after a single pairing of lithium chloride toxicosis with a neutral olfactory stimulus (157). Similar conditioning has also been demonstrated in fetal rat pups by pairing a neutral taste/odor with lithium chloride injected into the amniotic fluid. In both cases, the pairing of the odor with the aversive substance elicited responses to the injection on re-exposure not shown by controls that did not receive the pairing. These studies provide evidence for associative learning in subjects whose central nervous system is undergoing rapid changes that characterize early development.

Despite the immaturity of the nervous system, these studies demonstrate that it supports learning in the young animal. There is good evidence that the human newborn is capable of one-trial learning by complex processing of olfactory information as early as the first hours of life (158). However, surprisingly little is known about how infants learn about pain (159). Because the capacity to learn and the capacity to signal pain are so critical to survival for the newborn infant, researchers in infant pain have hypothesized that the newborn learns about pain from early exposure to pain. At approximately 6 months of age, there is clear evidence that memory of pain exists because the infant shows anticipatory fear (11,160,161). An early attempt to demonstrate memory of pain in a newborn (3) may have failed because of a long delay between the conditioned and unconditioned stimuli and the conditioned stimulus (tactile stimulation) was one that has since been shown to produce variable responses (41,148).

In a small pilot study using a classic conditioning paradigm to investigate memory of pain in the newborn (F. L. Porter and W. P. Smotherman, unpublished data), eight healthy full-term 24- to 48-hour-old infants were presented with an olfactory- (citrus) conditioned stimulus (CS) that then overlapped in time with a required heel-stick procedure, the unconditioned stimulus (US). The overlap (pairing) of the olfactory CS and the heel stick US comprised the conditioning phase of the experiment (odor paired with pain). After the heel stick, the infants were returned to the nursery where they were undisturbed and sleeping. One hour later, the infants were re-exposed to the odor CS alone (the testing phase). During the conditioning and testing phases, heart rate and behavior were continuously recorded before, during, and after the odor exposure. Coded from these recordings were heart rate, behavioral state, arm movements, head turns, and mouth movements. An increase in heart rate and a decrease in the percentage of time spent in sleepy/drowsy states were found during testing compared with the conditioning phase. The frequency of occurrence of specific movements was also higher during testing compared with their first exposure to the odor CS during conditioning. For example:

	Conditioning Phase	Testing Phase	Difference	One-tailed *t* test
Arm movements (n)	22	42	2.5	0.10
Head turns (n)	4	9	0.6	0.09
Mouth movements (n)	12	27	1.9	0.05

These pilot data indicate that the infants' physiologic and behavioral responses to the odor during the test re-exposure are characteristically greater and more robust than they were when they were exposed to the odor the first time. Because these data were derived only from a pairing of CS and US, it is not clear whether the increased responsivity is owing to sensitization (from previous exposure to the odor CS) or to associative learning (from a previous pairing of the odor CS with the pain US). Appropriate control groups are necessary to make this distinction. However, this pilot study indicates that such a paradigm can be used to investigate memory of pain in the newborn infant.

The risk of having memory of pain is clearly higher for premature infants, particularly extremely low birth weight infants, because of their prolonged exposure to potentially painful hospital experiences. As we continue to explore the important issue of memory of pain, it is advisable to treat infants, whether premature or older, as if everything we do to them has both immediate and long-lasting effects and memory.

APPROACHES FOR ASSESSMENT OF PAIN IN INFANTS

Various physiologic and behavioral indicators of immediate, short-term, and long-term pain are presented above. Some of the indicators are immediately available, and others require elaborate technology or are labor intensive.

Immediately Available Indicators of Pain

The behavioral indicators of pain are the most available for caretakers of infants. Vocalizations are the most basic communication modality; the birth cry is awaited by those attending the delivery and its lustiness signals the state of the infant. For infants who are capable of crying, a high-pitched, harsh cry is most indicative of pain (67–69,162). These cry characteristics are extremely alerting to caregivers (163). However, because nonnutritive sucking appears to be beneficial in decreasing pain in infants (16,39,53,164), if this method of comfort is used, then crying is inhibited. Of course infants who are intubated are also unable to cry, although they may have a "silent cry" (165).

Facial expression of emotional state is a fundamental communication modality (77). Although in tiny infants, facial expression is less robustly displayed, the facial grimacing of pain can be seen as early as 24 weeks postconceptional age (4,12). Even with much of the face obscured with tape holding ventilation tubes in place, the facial expressions of brow bulge, eye squeeze, and nasolabial furrow usually can be seen (4). The precise quantification of facial actions is potentially desirable for research, and the precision in the development and psychometric testing of the Neonatal Facial Coding System with laboratory coding was essential. For clinical purposes, however, more gross estimates are both feasible and reliable. As mentioned above, body movements, although easily observable, are often subject to feasibility problems. Standard care of neonates, especially preterm neonates, includes swaddling or nesting, thus inhibiting limb movement.

The *physiologic* parameters of heart rate, respiratory rate, and transcutaneous oxygen saturation are typically monitored through noninvasive probes attached to the infant's hand or foot in hospitals. Some units have data acquisition facilities, so that changes or trends in these parameters can be viewed. Charting of vital signs before and after analgesic administration will allow evaluation of the effect of the analgesic on these parameters. Observation of changes can also be seen over short periods, particularly in relationship to painful procedures. Blood pressure is less commonly monitored except in cases of severely ill infants because its measurement is invasive either with an indwelling probe or inflation of a cuff. For infants who are severely ill, blood pressure can easily be included in the monitoring of pain.

Some *composite* measures that incorporate both physiologic and behavioral parameters have been tested at the bedside for (a) feasibility in terms of time, ease of scoring, and ease of understanding and (b) clinical utility that allows the clinician to use the measure to make decisions about treatment for a particular infant in the evaluation of procedural pain (Table 7.1). The Premature Infant Pain Profile has been shown to be feasible, reliable, and valid and to have clinical utility (79,166,167). In a study that compared three other composite measures, the Comfort Scale, the Neonatal Infant Pain Scale, and the Scale for Use in Newborns (168), the Comfort Scale did not show a return to baseline after a procedure and thus did not demonstrate clinical utility for procedural pain. This finding is not surprising because it was not developed for procedural pain. The Neonatal Infant Pain Scale had a large coefficient of variation; thus, it might be less specific and sensitive.

TABLE 7.1. *Composite pain measures for infants*[a]

Measure	Target population	Behavioral indicators	Physiologic indicators	Other indicators	Strengths	Limitations	Comments
Pain Assessment Tool (182)	Neonates (postoperative pain)	5 indicators: posture/tone, sleep pattern, expression, color, cry	4 indicators: respiration, heart rate, saturation, blood pressure	Rating of nurse's perception of pain	Preliminary psychometric testing was done on 20 infants in the first 24-hr postoperative period by the developers of the measure	Psychometric testing is limited in scope and to the infant in the immediate postoperative period	Tool was designed to be a clinical measure for neonatal nurses to use at the bedside
*C*rying, *r*equires O_2 for saturation >95%, *i*ncreased vital signs (heart rate and blood pressure), *e*xpression, and *s*leepless (CRIES) (183)	Neonates (postoperative pain)	3 indicators: crying, expression, sleepless	2 indicators: requires oxygen for saturation >95%, increased vital signs		The initial reliability and validity of the measure were established with a group of 24 infants (32–60 wk gestational age), after surgery; beginning clinical utility established in a comparative study with the PIPP (184)	CRIES has been used primarily for research purposes and therefore has no established feasibility; limited to use for postoperative pain assessment in neonates	Title of the measure is an acronym created to stimulate memory of the indicators; coding tips for using the measure are included to facilitate scoring
Neonatal Pain Assessment Tool (185)	Neonates (acute pain)	3 indicators: state, crying, activity	4 indicators: heart rate, blood pressure, respiratory rate, oxygen saturation		Measure developed by a group of interdisciplinary clinicians and has reported feasibility in the clinical setting	No reporting of the psychometric properties of the measure	Measure developed as part of a quality improvement project to improve pain management within the neonatal intensive care unit
Premature Infant Pain Profile (79)	Neonates (acute pain)	3 indicators: brow bulge, eye squeeze, nasolabial furrow	2 indicators: heart rate, oxygen saturation	2 indicators: gestational age, behavioral state	Developed to assess acute pain in preterm and term neonates in both research and clinical practice; psychometric properties have been established in preterm and term infants and very-low-birth	PIPP has been primarily used for assessing pain associated with heel lance in preterm neonates and for postoperative pain assessment in term and preterm neonates (40)	PIPP has been translated into several other languages including French and Swedish

					weight infants (167), and clinically validated (166); beginning clinical utility established in a comparative study with CRIES (184)		
Distress Scale for Ventilated Newborn Infants (DSVNI) (165)	Neonates (ventilated)	3 indicators: (comprising a behavioral score): facial expression, body movements, color	4 indicators: (assessing physiologic change): heart rate, blood pressure, oxygenation, temperature differential		Measure based on 5 previously developed scoring systems including the Neonatal Behavioral Assessment Scale (186), Assessment of Preterm Infant's Behavior (187), Neonatal Facial Coding System (65,76), Infant Body Coding System (11,12), and the Gustave–Roussy Child Behavior Scale (188) were validated to varying extent	Measure has no reported psychometric properties, feasibility, or clinical utility; the detailed scoring is complex and time-consuming	DSVNI is unique for neonates who are ventilated and are therefore unable to respond using some of the behavioral indicators such as crying that are usually used to assess pain; detailed instructions and diagrams are provided to assist with scoring
Scale for Use in Newborns (SUN) (168)	Neonates (acute pain)	3 indicators: movement, tone, face	4 indicators: central nervous system state, breathing, heart rate, mean blood pressure		Initial psychometric properties were determined by comparing SUN with NIPS and Comfort Scale during 4 neonatal intensive care unit procedures; clinical utility has also been reported	Clinical utility only reported in relation to clinicians' preference for the scale; more extensive clinical utility testing required	

[a]Presented in chronologic order of development.

Less Accessible Indicators of Pain

The biochemical and hormonal responses to pain require blood or saliva sampling and expensive assays either through radioimmunoassay or high-pressure liquid chromatography. Although these parameters of pain are important and the reporting of significant changes in them by Anand and colleagues (1,2) led to widespread change in practice, they are not widely available owing to practical and ethical reasons, particularly for the minute amounts of blood that would be feasible to obtain from preterm neonates.

Vagal tone, which some consider to be preferable to separate measures of heart rate and respiratory rate or oxygen saturation, requires electrocardiographic wave form and respiratory rate to be fed into a complex and relatively expensive software system. Currently, this indicator is used only for research purposes.

Although cries can be heard, the interpretation of them to health care professionals who do not know the infant well can be imprecise. Even using spectrographic analysis, which requires specialized computer software, cry is not always definitive (169). Artificial Neurological Networks, a mathematical modeling of a collection of signals, promises to be a more precise methodology (170,171); however, this methodology is highly specialized at present and the analysis of a single cry utterance requires a large amount of time and expertise, thus, making it unfeasible.

Dissociation of Responses to Pain

A difficulty that both clinicians and researchers face when assessing pain in infants is that behavioral and physiologic parameters do not always covary in response to painful events (4,79,88). This issue is even more problematic when attempting to evaluate an intervention aimed at pain relief. If facial action decreases but there is no change in heart rate, how is the efficacy of the intervention to be evaluated? There could be any number of combination of increases, decreases, or unchanged responses depending on the number of parameters measured. The infant may only have the energy or maturity resources to respond through one system. There are numerous unanswered questions that need much further study. To date, however, in terms of response to *analgesia*, i.e., degrees of pain as opposed to untreated pain versus absence of pain, behavioral parameters appear to be more sensitive (33,172). Behavioral indicators are also better able to distinguish infants with or without colic (173). Barr (174) has used the concept of "honest signaling" from evolutionary biology to understand that behavioral expressions of pain, which act as signals to caregivers, are more salient than "hidden" physiologic responses. Infants had to signal pain well before there were heart rate monitors or anyone thought to count the heart rate. Infants in settings such as intensive care units or acute care units of hospitals are more likely to be exposed to pain than infants in the home. Therefore, physiologic indicators of pain will be available so that the most valid measures should be used, and these are more often composite measures.

AVAILABLE MEASURES

There are now almost two dozen pain measures that have been developed to assess pain in infants. These measures can be labeled as unidimensional or multidimensional. Unidimensional measures assess one type of indicator (e.g., facial expression), and multidimensional measures assess either multiple types of indicators within one broad category (e.g., behavioral) or multiple indicators within several categories (e.g., behavioral and physiologic). Multidimensional measures that include multiple categories are often referred to as composite measures. Infant pain assessment measures that have been published (excluding abstracts) are summarized in Table 7.1 (composite pain measures) and Table 7.2 (unidimensional and multidimensional behavioral pain measures).

Several additional measures were not specifically developed to assess pain in infants but the broader phenomenon of comfort. The Clinical Scoring System (108,175) combines a variety of behavioral and neurologic indicators (the infant's sleep during the preceding hour, facial expression, infant cry, spontaneous motor activity, excitability, flexion of fingers and toes, sucking, tone, consolability, and sociability) for evaluating the infant's general degree of comfort in infants 1 to 7 months of age. Another example of a measure with similar behavioral categories, the Liverpool Infant Distress Scale (176) was developed to assess distress associated with postoperative pain in infants. Similarly, the Comfort Scale (109) is an eight-dimension scale that was developed for pediatric intensive care patients (newborn to 24 months) to measure distress. Distress included all behaviors of negative affect associated with pain, anxiety, and fear. The Comfort Scale was evaluated in comparison with the Neonatal Infant Pain Scale (177) and the Scale for Use in Newborns (168) for its psychometric properties and clinical utility (168). All scales demonstrated significant score changes associated with four different procedures in neonates. The Comfort Scale was reported to be most difficult to use because of its multiple gradations of scale and nonsymmetric design. More recently, the behavioral components of the Comfort Scale (calmness, alertness, crying, movement, muscle tone, facial expression) derived from structural equation modeling showed good stability and convergent validity with observer-rated visual analog scales in infants and toddlers (as old as 3 years of age) 3, 6, and 9 hours postoperatively (178), supporting the use of the Comfort Scale for this situation.

Two additional pain measures can be described as multimodal item behavioral pain scales. Within each item, several modes of behavior are included. The Pain Rating Scale (179), developed for infants 1 to 36 months of age includes six multimodal categories of behavior that increase in intensity. The no pain category (i.e., scored 0) has several behaviors that the authors suggest indicate no pain including smiling, sleeping, and no change in behavior when moved or touched. Conversely, the worst pain category (i.e., scored 5) includes sleeping with prolonged periods interrupted by jerking, continuous crying, and rapid shallow respirations. The Riley Infant Pain Scale was developed in a similar manner by the same group of investigators (180) for use with children younger than 36 months of age and children with cerebral palsy.

REMAINING CHALLENGES

Nonresponse

Infants who are extremely ill (14) or extremely immature (10,12) or who have become exhausted from the number and/or close temporal proximity of painful experiences (13,115) will show less robust response to pain than older, healthier, rested infants. Some infants will show no change that can currently be measured in response to a painful event (13). If these infants had received analgesia before the painful event [the infants in the study by Jain and Rutter (13) had not], the interpretation would be that the analgesia had been effective. Thus, there is a dilemma in interpreting nonresponse: Is it effective analgesia or some other factor related to the infant that interferes with response?

Careful consideration needs to be given to several factors when an infant appears not to respond to pain. Age is the most consistent factor affecting pain response, with younger infants showing less response (10,12,17,134). This finding is included as a weighting item in one composite measure, the Premature Infant Pain Profile (79). By knowing that motor development lags behind sensory development, it is understandable that an infant may feel pain but not have the motor capacity to demonstrate pain behaviors. Consideration needs also to be given to the amount of pain or handling that the infant has experienced and concomitant treatments (e.g., other pharmacologic interventions). In the section on long-term responses to pain in which increased amounts of early experienced pain resulted in decreased behavioral responses to

TABLE 7.2. *Unidimensional and multidimensional behavioral pain measures for infants*[a]

Measure	Target population	Type of dimension	Indicators	Strengths	Limitations	Comments
Neonatal Facial Coding System (NFCS) (65,76)	Neonates and infants	Facial actions	10 indicators: brow bulge, eye squeeze, nasolabial furrow, open lips, vertically stretched mouth, horizontally stretched mouth, taut tongue, chin quiver, tongue protrusion	Established psychometric properties; most reliable and valid *behavioral* measure for assessing pain in term and preterm neonates	Substantial individual variation occurs in these actions and the vigor of the infant's response (40); trained coders are required, making use costly and time-consuming; clinical utility has not been established	NFCS is best suited to research, although there is beginning validation for use at the bedside
Infant Body Coding System (IBCS) (11,12)	Neonates and infants	Body movements	6 indicators: movements of the hand, foot, arm, leg, head, and torso	When used with NFCS to determine the effect of gestational age on the pain response (11), IBCS was more sensitive with increasing levels of activity in term as compared to preterm infants but less specific to the painful event	Limited establishment of reliability, validity, and clinical utility	
Neonatal Infant Pain Scale (NIPS) (189)	Neonates	Facial actions, crying, breathing patterns, body movements, state of arousal	6 indicators: facial expression, crying, breathing patterns, arm movement, leg movement, state of arousal	Initial validity, reliability, and internal consistency established with term and preterm neonates procedures; further construct validity established (169) in neonates at 24–40 wk gestational age	NIPS has been used primarily for research purposes and therefore has no established feasibility or clinical utility	Each indicator has an operational definition provided on the score sheet for easy scoring reference

Behavioural Pain Score (92)	Neonates and infants	Facial expression, body movements, handling/ consolability	4 indicators: facial expression, body movements, response to handling/consolability, rigidity of limbs and body	Based on the Children's Hospital of Eastern Ontario Pain Scale (190), a validated measure for assessing postoperative pain in children 1–7 yr of age	Limited establishment of validity (construct) and no reported reliability, clinical utility, or feasibility	
Modified Behavioural Pain Scale (191)	Infants	Facial expression, crying, and body movements	3 indicators: facial expression, crying, gross body movements	Based on the Children's Hospital of Eastern Ontario Pain Scale (191); initial validity established with 96 healthy infants during routine immunization	Limited reliability and validity and no reported clinical utility or feasibility; use limited to healthy infants undergoing immunization	
Douleur Aigue du Nouveau-né (192)	Neonates	Facial expression, limb movements, vocal expression	3 indicators: facial expression, limb movements, vocal expressions	Beginning construct validity, interrater reliability, and internal consistency reported by the developers of the scale	Limited establishment of psychometric properties; no reported clinical utility or feasibility	
FLACC (face, legs, activity, crying, consolability) (193)	Infants 2 mo to children 7 yr	Face, legs, activity, crying, consolability	5 indicators: face, legs, activity, crying, consolability	Beginning interrater reliability, construct, and convergent validity established by the developers of the scale	Limited establishment of psychometric properties; no reported clinical utility or feasibility, although the measure was developed for clinical use; limited to postoperative pain	Acronym FLACC was devised to facilitate recall of the categories included in the measure

[a]Presented in chronologic order from the earliest.

pain (115,116), as well as the study on nonresponse to pain (13), it would appear that the infant can become exhausted from the stress of repeated pain with little rest and be unable to respond. This phenomenon can be understood clearly within the context of Als' (94) synactive theory of development in which it is explained that energy used to cope with the stress of NICU care can deplete energy stores needed for maintaining homeostasis and for growth and development. Although severity of illness has not often been reported from empirical data as a factor that alters pain response, it has not been adequately investigated because severely ill infants are typically excluded from studies. The same issue of energy consumption that applies to the number and timing of painful events applies to infants who are extremely ill.

Chronic Pain

There are currently no measures for chronic pain in infants. Fortunately, chronic pain, partly by definition, is probably less common in infants than in older populations. However, there are some infants who may be born with some condition that is painful and essentially are in pain from the time of their birth. Owing to both the small numbers of these infants and selection criteria that exclude infants who may not respond "normally," these infants have not been studied. The major obstacle to developing measures of chronic pain lies in knowing the stimuli that may be responsible for causing the persistent pain. In measures of procedural pain, the stimulus is clear and the timing can be controlled as can the intensity to some extent. However, the need for assessing pain in infants who are in states of prolonged pain from mechanical irritants such as intubation or disease such as necrotizing enterocolitis remains to be addressed.

Neurologically impaired infants have been excluded from studies and yet, paradoxically, may be in pain by virtue of the insults to their neurologic system and/or coexisting morbidities. To date, we have no measures that have been shown to be valid in assessing pain in infants with neurologic impairments. In older children, cues to pain are sometimes idiosyncratic and parents who have had close contact with them are the only ones who can identify the pain behaviors that a particular child demonstrates. In older children, for example, giggling was reported as a painful behavior by one parent (181). For neonates, even parents have not had the opportunity to learn how their infant expresses pain. Often health professionals will interpret behaviors that in normal infants would be considered indicative of pain (e.g., facial grimacing) as agitation as opposed to pain in neurologically compromised infants. Much challenging work is needed for this group of infants to better promote pain relief in them.

SUMMARY

The amount of recent knowledge of pain in infants has grown tremendously in the past one and a half decades. There are now more than two dozen published measures of acute pain in infants, some of which have been tested extensively. There is better understanding of the factors that influence pain response and underlying mechanisms than previously. There is a beginning understanding of the affects of pain on subsequent development. Major challenges remain for particular populations of infants.

REFERENCES

1. Anand KJS, Hickey PR. Halothane morphine compared with high dose sufentanil for anesthesia and postoperative analgesia in neonatal cardiac surgery. *N Engl J Med* 1992;326:1–9.
2. Anand KJS, Sippell WG, Aynsley-Green A. Randomised trial of fentanyl anaesthesia in preterm babies undergoing surgery: effects on the stress response. *Lancet* 1987;62–65.
3. Owens ME, Todt EH. Pain in infancy: neonatal reaction to heel lance. *Pain* 1984;20:77–86.
4. Johnston C, Stevens BJ, Yang F, et al. Differential response to pain by very premature neonates. *Pain* 1995; 61:471–479.
5. Stevens BJ, Johnston CC. Physiological responses of premature infants to a painful stimulus. *Nurs Res* 1994;43:226–231.
6. McIntosh N, Van Veen L, Brameyer H. The pain of

heel prick and its measurement in preterm infants. *Pain* 1993;52:71–74.
7. Porter FL, Porges SW, Marshall RE. Newborn pain cries and vagal tone :Parallel change in response to circumcision. *Child Dev* 1988;59:495–505.
8. Grunau RVE, Johnston CC, Craig KD. Neonatal facial and cry responses to invasive and noninvasive procedures. *Pain* 1990;42:295–305.
9. Franck LS. A new method to quantitatively describe pain behavior in infants. *Nurs Res* 1986;35:28–31.
10. Johnston CC, Stevens BJ, Yang F, et al. Developmental changes in response to heelstick by premature infants: a prospective cohort study. *Dev Med Child Neurol* 1996;38:438–445.
11. Craig KD, McMahon RJ, Morison JD, et al. Developmental changes in infant pain expression during immunization injections. *Soc Sci Med* 1984;19:1331–1337.
12. Craig KD, Whitfield MF, Grunau RV, et al. Pain in the preterm neonate: behavioural and physiological indices. *Pain* 1993;52:287–299.
13. Johnston CC, Stevens BJ, Franck LS, et al. Factors explaining lack of response to tissue damage in preterm neonates. *J Obstet Gynecol Neonat Nurs* 1999;28: 587–594.
14. Field T, Goldson E. Pacifying effects of nonnutritive sucking on term and preterm neonates during heelstick procedures. *Pediatrics* 1984;74:1012–1015.
15. Stevens BJ, Johnston CC, Horton L. Factors that influence the behavioral pain responses of premature infants. *Pain* 1994;59:101–109.
16. Stevens BJ, Johnston C, Franck L, et al. The efficacy of developmentally sensitive interventions and sucrose for relieving procedural pain in very low birth weight neonates. *Nurs Res* 1999;98:35–43.
17. Porter FL, Wolf CM, Miller JP. Procedural pain in newborn infants: the influence of intensity and development. *Pediatrics* 1999;104:e13.
18. Andrews K, Fitzgerald M. The cutaneous withdrawal reflex in human neonates: sensitization, receptive fields, and the effects of contralateral stimulation. *Pain* 1994;56:95–101.
19. Fitzgerald M, Millard C, MacIntosh N. Hyperalgesia in premature infants. *Lancet* 1988;292.
20. Andrews K, Fitzgerald M. Cutaneous flexion reflex in human neonates: a quantitative study of threshold and stimulus-response characteristics after single and repeated stimuli. *Dev Med Child Neurol* 1999;41: 696–703.
21. Fitzgerald M, Millard C, McIntosh N. Cutaneous hypersensitivity following peripheral tissue damage in newborn infants and its reversal with topical anaesthesia. *Pain* 1989;39:31–36.
22. Anand KJ, Scalzo FM. Can adverse neonatal experiences alter brain development and subsequent behavior? *Biol Neonate* 2000;77:69–82.
23. Anand KJ. Effects of perinatal pain and stress. *Prog Brain Res* 2000;122:117–129.
24. Anand KJ, Barton BA, McIntosh N, et al. Analgesia and sedation in preterm neonates who require ventilatory support: results from the NOPAIN trial. Neonatal outcome and prolonged analgesia in neonates [published erratum appears in *Arch Pediatr Adolesc Med* 1999;153:895]. *Arch Pediatr Adolesc Med* 1999;153: 331–338.
25. Barker DP, Latty BW, Rutter N. Heel blood sampling in preterm infants: which technique? *Arch Dis Child* 1994;71:F206–F208.
26. Fearon I, Kisilevsky BS, Hains SM, et al. Swaddling after heel lance: age specific effects on behavioral recovery in preterm infants. *J Dev Behav Pediatr* 1997; 18:222–232.
27. Abe JA. The developmental functions of emotions: An analysis in terms of differential emotions theory. *Cognition Emotion* 1900;13.
28. McIntosh N, Van Veen L, Brameyer H. Alleviation of the pain of heel prick in preterm infants. *Arch Dis Child* 1994;70:F177–F181.
29. Miller HD, Anderson GC. Nonnutritive sucking: effects on crying and heart rate in intubated infants requiring assisted mechanical ventilation. *Neonatal Intensive Care* 1994;46–48.
30. Izard CE, Schultz D. Independent emotions and consciousness: self-consciousness and dependent emotions. In: Singer JA, Salovey P, eds. *At play in the fields of consciousness: essays in honor of Jerome L. Singer*. Mahwah, NJ: Lawrence Erlbaum, 1999:83–102.
31. Benini F, Johnston CC, Faucher DJ, et al. Topical anesthesia during circumcision in newborn infants. *JAMA* 1993;270:850–853.
32. Franck LS, Miaskowski C. Measurement of neonatal responses to painful stimuli: a research review. J Pain Symptom Manage 1997;14:343–378.
33. Johnston CC, Stremler RL, Stevens BJ, et al. Effectiveness of oral sucrose and simulated rocking on pain response in preterm neonates. *Pain* 1997;72:193–199.
34. Stevens BJ, Johnston CC. Premature infants response to pain: a pilot study. *Nurs Que* 1991;11:90–95.
35. Pokela ML, Koivisto M. Physiological changes, plasma beta endorphin and cortisol responses to tracheal intubation in neonates. *Acta Paediatr* 1994;83: 151–156.
36. McIntosh N, Van Veen L, Brammeyer H. The use of physiological variability to evaluate pain in preterm infants. *J Pain Symptom Manage* 1991;6:205(abst).
37. Campos JJ, Kermoian R, Witherington D. An epigenetic perspective on emotional development. Kavanaugh RD, Zimmerberg B, Fein S, eds. *Emotion: interdisciplinary perspectives*. Mahwah, NJ: Lawrence Erlbaum, 1996:119–138.
38. Oberlander TF, Grunau RE, Pitfield S, et al. The developmental character of cardiac autonomic responses to an acute noxious event in 4- and 8-month-old healthy infants. *Pediatr Res* 1999;45:519–525.
39. Herschel M, Khoshnood B, Ellman C, et al. Neonatal circumcision. Randomized trial of a sucrose pacifier for pain control. *Arch Pediatr Adolesc Med* 1998;152: 279–284.
40. McNair C, Ballantyne M, Dionne K, et al. Post-operative pain assessment in the neonatal intensive care unit. *International Symposium on Pediatric Pain* 2000; 5:P102(abst).
41. Porter FL, Miller JP, Cole FS, et al. A controlled clinical trial of local anesthesia for lumbar punctures in newborns. *Pediatrics* 1991;88:663–669.
42. Cordero L, Gardner DK, O'Shaughnessy R. Analgesia versus sedation during Broviac catheter placement. *Am J Perinatol* 1991;8:284–287.
43. Dabbs JM, Johnson JE, Leventhal H. Palmar sweating: a quick and simple measure. *J Exp Psychol* 1968;78: 347–350.

44. Gedaly-Duff V. Palmar Sweat Index (PSI) used with children in pain research. *J Pediatr Nurs* 1989;4:3–8.
45. Johnson PA, Stockdale DF. Effects of puppet therapy on palmar sweating of hospitalized children. *Johns Hopkins Med J* 1975;137:1–5.
46. Harpin VA, Rutter N. Development of emotional sweating in the newborn infant. *Arch Dis Child* 1982; 57:691–695.
46a. Volpe JJ. Intraventricular hemorrhage in the premature infant. Current concepts. Part I. *Ann Neurol* 1989;25: 3–11.
47. Raju TNK, Vidjasagar D, Torres C, et al. Intracranial pressure during intubation and anesthesia in infants. *J Pediatr* 1980;96:860–862.
48. Durand M, Sangha B, Cabal LA, et al. Cardiopulmonary and intracranial pressure changes related to endotracheal suctioning in preterm infants. *Crit Care Med* 1989;17:506–510.
49. Brazy JE. Effects of crying on cerebral blood volume and cytochrome aa3. *J Pediatr* 1988;112:457–461.
50. Gagnon RE, Leung A, Macnab AJ. Variations in regional cerebral blood volume in neonates associated with nursery care events. *Am J Perinatol* 1999;16: 7–11.
51. Abad F, Diaz NM, Domenech E, et al. Oral sweet solution reduces pain related behaviour in preterm infants. *Acta Paediatr* 1996;85:854–858.
52. Barr RG, Quek VSH, Cousineau D, et al. Effects of intraoral sucrose on crying, mouthing and hand mouth contact in newborn and six week old infants. *Dev Med Child Neurol* 1994;36:608–618.
53. Blass EM, Hoffmeyer LB. Sucrose as an analgesic for newborn infants. *Pediatrics* 1991;87:215–218.
54. Bucher HU, Moser T, Von Siebenthal K, et al. Sucrose reduces pain reaction to heel lancing in preterm infants: a placebo controlled randomized and masked study. *Pediatr Res* 1995;38:332–335.
55. Graillon A, Barr RG, Young SN, et al. Differential response to intraoral sucrose, quinine and corn oil in crying human newborns. *Physiol Behav* 1997;62: 317–325.
56. Hunziker UA, Barr RG. Increased carrying reduces infant crying : a randomized controlled trial. *Pediatrics* 1986;77:641–648.
57. Lander J, Brady-Fryer B, Metcalfe JB, et al. Comparison of ring block, dorsal penile nerve block, and topical anesthesia for neonatal circumcision: a randomized controlled trial. *JAMA* 1997;278:2157–2162.
58. Larsson BA, Tannfeldt G, Lagercrantz H, et al. Venipuncture is more effective and less painful than heel lancing for blood tests in neonates. *Pediatrics* 1998;101:882–886.
59. Mohan CG, Risucci DA, Casimir M, et al. Comparison of analgesics in ameliorating the pain of circumcision. *J Perinatol* 1998;18:13–19.
60. Ramenghi LA, Griffith GC, Wood CM, et al. Effect of nonsucrose sweet tasting solution on neonatal heel prick responses. *Arch Dis Child* 1996;74:F129–F131.
61. Ramenghi LA, Wood CM, Griffith GC, et al. Reduction of pain response in premature infants using intraoral sucrose. *Arch Dis Child* 1996;74:F126–F128.
62. Stevens BJ, Taddio A, Ohlsson A, et al. The efficacy of sucrose for relieving procedural pain in neonates: a systematic review and meta-analysis. *Acta Paediatr* 1997;86:837–842.
63. Taddio A, Katz J, Ilersich AL, et al. Effect of neonatal circumcision on pain response during subsequent routine vaccination. *Lancet* 1997;349:599–603.
64. Grunau R. Neonatal responses to invasive procedures. *Nurs Times* 1991;87:53–54.
65. Grunau RVE, Craig KD. Pain expression in neonates: facial action and cry. *Pain* 1987;28:395–410.
66. Porter FL, Miller RH, Marshall RE. Neonatal pain cries: effect of circumcision on acoustic features and perceived urgency. *Child Dev* 1986; 57:790–802.
67. Fuller BF. Acoustic discrimination of three types of infant cries. *Nurs Res* 1991;40:156–160.
68. Fuller BF. Differences in acoustic cry measures and facial and body behaviors of infants experiencing severe, moderate, mild and no pain. Seventh World Congress on Pain, Paris, 1993 (abst).
69. Johnston CC, O'Shaughnessy D. Acoustical attributes of pain cries: distinguishing features. In: Dubner R, Gebbart GF, Bond MR, eds. *Advances in pain research and therapy*. Amsterdam: Elsevier, 1988:336–340.
70. Barr RG, Pantel MS, Young SN, et al. The response of crying newborns to sucrose: is it a "sweetness" effect? *Physiol Behav* 1999;66:409–417.
71. Johnston CC, Strada ME. Acute pain responses in infants: a multidimensional description. *Pain* 1986;24: 373–382.
72. Grunau RE, Holsti L, Whitfield MF, et al. Are twitches, startles, and body movements pain indicators in extremely low birth weight infants? *Clin J Pain* 2000;16:37–45.
73. Als H, Duffy FH, McAnulty G. Behavioural differences between preterm and fullterm newborns as measured with the APIB system scores: I. *Infant Behav Dev* 1988;11:305–318.
74. Taylor P. Postoperative pain in toddler and preschool age children. *Matern Child Nurs J* 1983;12:35–50.
75. Darwin CR. *The expression of emotion in man and animals*. Chicago: The University of Chicago Press, 1965 (reprint of study originally published in 1872).
76. Grunau RVE, Craig KD. Facial activity as a measure of neonatal pain expression. In: Tyler DC, Krane EJ, eds. *Advances in pain therapy and research, volume 15: pediatric pain*. New York: Raven Press, 1990:147–156.
77. Craig KD. The facial expression of pain better than a thousand words? *APSJ* 1992;1:153–162.
78. Rosmus C, Johnston CC, Chan-Yip A, et al. Pain response in Chinese and non-Chinese Canadian infants: is there a difference? *Soc Sci Med* 2000;51:175–184.
79. Stevens BJ, Johnston C, Petryshen P, et al. Premature infant pain profile: development and initial validation. *Clin J Pain* 1996;12:13–22.
80. Scott CS, Riggs KW, Ling EW, et al. Morphine pharmacokinetics and pain assessment in premature newborns. *J Pediatr* 1999;135:423–429.
81. Kurtis PS, DeSilva HN, Bernstein BA, et al. A comparison of the Mogen and Gomco clamps in combination with dorsal penile nerve block in minimizing the pain of neonatal circumcision. *Pediatrics* 1999;103:E23.
82. Anand KJS. Hormonal and metabolic functions of neonates and infants undergoing surgery. *Curr Opin Cardiol* 1986;1:681–689.
83. Schmeling DJ, Coran AG. Hormonal and metabolic response to operative stress in the neonate. *J Parenteral Enteral Nutr* 1991;15:215–238.
84. Mooncey S, Giannakoulopoulos X, Glover V, et al. The

effect of mother-infant skin-to-skin contact on plasma cortisol and beta-endorphin concentrations in preterm newborns. *Infant Behav Dev* 1997;20:553–557.
85. Peters KL. Neonatal stress reactivity and cortisol. *J Perinat Neonat Nurs* 1998;11:45–59.
86. Giannakoulopoulos X, Sepulveda W, Kourtis P, et al. Fetal plasma cortisol and beta-endorphin response to intrauterine needling. *Lancet* 1994;344:77–81.
87. Gunnar MR, Hertsgaard L, Larson M, et al. Cortisol and behavioural responses to repeated stressors in the human newborn. *Dev Psychobiol* 1992;24:487–505.
88. Gunnar MR, Fisch RO, Korsvik S, et al. The effects of circumcision on serum cortisol and behavior. *Psychoneuroendocrinology* 1981;6:269–275.
89. Gunnar MR, Connars J, Isensee J, et al. Adrenocortical activity and behavioral distress in human newborns. *Dev Psychobiol* 1988;2:297–310.
90. Gunnar MR, Fisch RO, Malone S. The effects of a pacifying stimulus on behavioral and adrenocortical responses to circumcision in the newborn. *J Am Acad Child Psychiatry* 1984;23:34–38.
91. Williamson PS, Evans ND. Neonatal cortisol response to circumcision with anesthesia. *Clin Pediatr (Phila)* 1986;25:412–415.
92. Pokela ML. Pain relief can reduce hypoxemia in distressed neonates during routine treatment procedures. *Pediatrics* 1994;3:379–383.
93. Als H, Duffy FH, McAnulty GB. The APIB, an assessment of functional competence in preterm and fullterm newborns regardless of gestational age at birth: II. *Infant Behav Dev* 1988;11:319–331.
94. Als H. Towards a synactive theory of development: promise for the assessment of infant individuality. *Infant Mental Health J* 1982;3:229–243.
95. Lawhon G. Providing developmentally supportive care in the newborn intensive care unit: an evolving challenge. *J Perinat Neonat Nurs* 1997;10:48–61.
96. Becker PT, Brazy JE, Grunwald PC. Behavioral state organization of very low birth weight infants: effects of developmental handling during caregiving. *Infant Behav Dev* 1997;20:503–514.
97. Berg WK, Berg KM. Psychophysiological development in infancy: state, startle, and attention. In: Osofsky JD, ed. *Handbook of infant development*. Toronto: John Wiley & Sons, 1987:238–317.
98. Holditch-Davis D, Edwards LJ. Modeling development of sleep-wake behaviors. II. Results of two cohorts of preterms. *Physiol Behav* 1998;63:319–328.
99. Kaminski J, Hall W. The effect of soothing music on neonatal behavioral states in the hospital newborn nursery. *Neonat Network* 1996;15:45–54.
100. Korner AF, Lane NM, Berry KL, et al. Sleep enhanced and irritability reduced in preterm infants: differential efficacy of three types of waterbeds. *J Dev Behav Pediatr* 1990;11:240–246.
101. Ludington SM. Energy conservation during skin-to-skin contact between premature infants and their mothers. *Heart Lung* 1990;19:445–451.
102. McCain GC. Facilitating inactive awake states in preterm infants: a study of three interventions. *Nurs Res* 1992;41:157–160.
103. Nijhuis J, Prechtl HFR, Martin C, et al. Are there behavioural states in the human fetus? *Early Hum Dev* 1982;6:177–195.
104. Prechtl HFR, Beintema D. The neurological examination of the full-term newborn infant. *Clin Dev Med* 1977;63.
105. Yokochi K, Shiroiwa Y, Inukai K, et al. Behavioral state distribution throughout 24h video recordings in preterm infants at term with good prognosis. *Early Hum Dev* 1989;19:183–190.
106. Anders TF, Sachar EJ, Kream J, et al. Behavioral state and plasma cortisol response in human newborn. *Pediatrics* 1970;46:532–537.
107. Attia J, Amiel-Tison C, Mayer M-N, et al. Measurement of postoperative pain and narcotic administration in infants using a new clinical scoring system. *Anesthesiology* 1987;67:A532.
108. Barrier G, Attia J, Mayer MN, et al. Measurement of postoperative pain and narcotic administration in infants using a new clinical scoring system. *Intensive Care Med* 1989;15[Suppl 1]:S37–S39.
109. Ambuel B, Hamlett KW, Marx CM, et al. Assessing distress in pediatric intensive care environments: the COMFORT scale. *J Pediatr Psychol* 1992;17:95–109.
110. Corff KE, Seideman R, Venkataraman PS, et al. Facilitated tucking: a nonpharmacologic comfort measure for pain in preterm neonates. *J Obstet Gynecol Neonat Nurs* 1995;24:143–147.
111. Gedaly-Duff V, Huff-Slankard J. Sleep as an indicator for pain relief in an infant: a case study. *J Pediatr Nurs* 1998;13:32–40.
112. Elander G, Hellstrom G, Qvarnstrom B. Care of infants after major surgery: observation of behavior and analgesic administration. *Pediatr Nurs* 1993;19:221–226.
113. Jain A, Rutter N. Topical amethocaine gel in the newborn infant—how soon does it work and how long does it last? In: *International Symposium on Pediatric Pain 5*, London, 2000:P81(abst).
114. Andrews K, Fitzgerald M. The abdominal skin reflex in human neonates and infants: threshold changes with age, surgery, and post-operative analgesia. In: *Abstracts of the 9th World Congress on Pain*. Seattle: IASP Press, 1999:398(abst).
115. Johnston CC, Stevens BJ. Experience in a neonatal intensive care unit affects pain response. *Pediatrics* 1996;98:925–930.
116. Grunau RVE, Oberlander TF, Whitfied MF, et al. Early morphine exposure and subsequent pain reactivity in preterm infants at 32 weeks post-conceptional age. *Pediatrics (in press)*.
117. Oberlander TF, Grunau RE, Whitfield MF, et al. Biobehavioral pain responses in former extremely low birth weight infants at four months' corrected age. *Pediatrics* 2000;105:e6.
118. Fitzgerald M. Development of the peripheral and spinal pain system. In: Anand KJS, Stevens BJ, McGrath PJ, eds. *Pain in neonates*. Amsterdam: Elsevier, 2000:9–21.
119. Taddio A, Stevens BJ, Craig KD, et al. Efficacy and safety of lidocaine-prilocaine cream for neonatal circumcision pain management. *N Engl J Med* 1997;336: 1197–1201.
120. Sweet SD, McGrath PJ, Symons D. The roles of child reactivity and parenting context in infant pain response. *Pain* 1999;80:655–661.
121. Grunau RVE, Whitfield MF, Petrie JH, et al. Early pain experience, child and family factors, as precursors of somatization: a prospective study of extremely premature and full-term children. *Pain* 1994;56:353–359.

122. Grunau RVE, Whitfield MF, Petrie JH, et al. Somatization at 4 1/2 years of age in preterm children and controls as a function of family factors, mother-child interactions, child temperament and pain sensitivity at 3 years of age. *J Pain Symptom Manage* 1991;6:146 (abst).
123. Grunau RE. Long-term consequences of pain in human neonates. In: Anand KJS, Stevens BJ, McGrath PJ, eds. *Pain in neonates*, 2nd ed. Amsterdam: Elsevier, 2000:55–76.
124. Fitzgerald M. Development of pain pathways and mechanisms. In: Anand KJS, McGrath PJ, eds. *Pain in neonates*. Amsterdam: Elsevier, 1993:19–37.
125. Anand KJS, Coskun V, Thrivikraman KV, et al. Long-term behavioral effects of repetitive pain in neonatal rat pups. *Physiol Behav* 1999;66:627–637.
126. Ruda MA, Ling Q-D, Hohmann AG, et al. Altered nociceptive neuronal circuits after neonatal peripheral inflammation. *Science* 2000;289:628–631.
127. Plotsky PM, Bradley CC, Anand KJS. Behavioral and neuroendocrine consequences of neonatal stress. In: Anand KJS, Stevens BJ, McGrath PJ, eds. *Pain in neonates,* 2nd ed. Amsterdam: Elsevier, 2000:77–99.
128. Izard CE, Ackerman BP. Children's emotional memories: an analysis in terms of differential emotions theory. *Imagination Cognition Pers* 1998;18:173–188.
129. Izard CE. Four systems for emotion activation: cognitive and noncognitive processes. *Psychol Rev* 1993; 100:68–90.
130. Lewis M. The role of the self in cognition and emotion. In: Dalgleish T, Power MJ, eds. *Handbook of cognition and emotion*. Chichester, UK: Wiley & Sons, 1999: 125–142.
131. Lewis M. Social cognition and the self. In: Rochat P, ed. *Early social cognition: understanding others in the first months of life*. Mahwah, NJ: Lawrence Erlbaum, 1999:81–98.
132. Goleman D. *Emotional intelligence*. New York: Bantam Books, 1995.
133. Craig KD. Implications of concepts of consciousness for understanding pain behaviour and the definition of pain. *Pain Res Manage* 1997;2:111–117.
134. Johnston CC, Stevens BJ, Craig KD, et al. Developmental changes in pain expression in premature, full-term, two, and four month old infants. *Pain* 1993;52: 201–208.
135. Willis WD. Is there a mechanism for the spinal cord to remember pain? In: Bostock H, Kirkwood PA, Pullen AH, eds. *The neurobiology of disease: contributions from neuroscience to clinical neurology* . Cambridge: Cambridge University Press, 1996:177–188.
136. Guy ER, Abbott FV. The behavioral response to formalin in preweanling rats. *Pain* 1992;51:81–90.
137. McLaughlin CR, Lichtman AH, Fanselow MS, et al. Tonic nociception in neonatal rats. *Pharmacol Biochem Behav* 1990;36:859–862.
138. d'Amore A, Mazzucchelli A, Loizzo A. Long-term changes induced by neonatal handling in the nociceptive threshold and body weight in mice. *Physiol Behav* 1995;57:1195–1197.
139. Meaney MJ, Mitchell JB, Aitken DH, et al. The effects of neonatal handling on the development of the adrenocortical response to stress: implications for neuropathology and cognitive deficits in later life. *Psychoneuroendocrinology* 1991;16:85–103.
140. Bernardi M, Genedani S, Bertolini A. Behavioral activity and active avoidance learning and retention in rats neonatally exposed to painful stimuli. *Physiol Behav* 1986;36:553–555.
141. Himes BT, Tessler A. Death of some dorsal root ganglion neurons and plasticity of others following sciatic nerve section in adult and neonatal rats. *J Comp Neurol* 1989;284:215–230.
142. Yip HK, Rich KM, Lampe PA, et al. The effects of nerve growth factor and its antiserum on the postnatal development and survival after injury of sensory neurons in rat dorsal root ganglia. *J Neurosci* 1984;4: 2986–2992.
143. Fitzgerald M, Woolf CJ, Shortland P. Collateral sprouting of the central terminals of cutaneous primary afferent neurons in the rat spinal cord: pattern, morphology, and influence of targets. *J Comp Neurol* 1990; 300:370–385.
144. Shortland P, Woolf CJ, Fitzgerald M. Morphology and somatotopic organization of the central terminals of hindlimb hair follicle afferents in the rat lumbar spinal cord. *J Comp Neurol* 1989;289:416–433.
145. Coskun V, Anand KJS. Development of supraspinal pain processing. In: Anand KJS, Stevens BJ, McGrath PJ, eds. *Pain in neonates*, 2nd ed. Amsterdam: Elsevier, 2000:23–54.
146. Marshall RE, Stratton WC, Moore JA, et al. Circumcision: effects on newborn behavior. *Infant Behav Dev* 1980;3:1–14.
147. Marshall RE, Porter FL, Rogers AG, et al. Circumcision: II. Effects upon mother-infant interaction. *Early Hum Dev* 1982;7:367–374.
148. Porter FL, Wolf CM, Miller JP. The effect of handling and immobilization on the response to acute pain in newborn infants. *Pediatrics* 1998;102:1383–1389.
149. Gunnar MR, Porter FL, Wolf CM, et al. Neonatal stress reactivity: predictions to later emotional temperament. *Child Dev* 1995;66:1–13.
150. DeCasper AJ, Fifer WP. Of human bonding: newborns prefer their mothers voices. *Science* 1980;208: 1174–1176.
151. Standley JM, Masen CK. Comparison of infant preferences and responses to auditory stimuli: music, mother, and other female voices. *J Music Ther*1990; 27:54–97.
152. Fifer WP, Moon C. The effects of fetal experience with sound. In: Lecanuet JP, Fifer WP, Krasnegor N, eds. *Fetal development, a psychobiological perspective*. Hillsdale, NJ: Lawrence Erlbaum Associates, 1995:351–366.
153. Ockleford EM, Vince MA, Layton C, et al. Response of neonates to parent's and other's voices. *Early Hum Dev* 1988;18:27–36.
154. DeCasper AJ, Spence MJ. Prenatal maternal speech influences newborn's perception of speech sounds. *Infant Behav Dev* 1986;9:133–150.
155. DeCasper AJ, Lecanuet JP, Busnel MC, et al. Fetal reactions to recurrent maternal speech. *Infant Behav Dev* 1994;17:159–164.
156. Alberts J. Early learning and ontogenetic adaptions. In: Krasnegor N, Blass EM, Hofer M, eds. *Perinatal development: a psychobiological perspective*. Orlando, FL: Academic Press, 1987:11–38.
157. Rudy JW, Cheatle MD. Odor-aversion learning in neonatal rats. *Science* 1977;198:845–846.
158. Sullivan RM, Taborsky-Barba S, Mendoza R, et al. Ol-

factory classical conditioning in neonates. *Pediatrics* 1991;87:511–518.

159. McGrath PJ, McAlpine L. Psychologic perspectives on pediatric pain. *J Pediatr* 1993;122:S2–S8.
160. Levy DM. The infant's earliest memory of inoculation: a contribution to public health procedures. *J Genet Psychol* 1960;96:3–46.
161. McGraw MB. Neural maturation as exemplified in the changing reactions of the infant to pin prick. *Child Dev* 1941;12:31–42.
162. Fuller BF, Conner DA. Distribution of cues across assessed levels of infant pain. *Clin Nurs Res* 1996;5: 167–184.
163. Zeskind PS, Lester BM. Acoustic features and auditory perception of the cries of newborns with prenatal and perinatal complications. *Child Dev* 1978;49:580–589.
164. Campos RG. Rocking and pacifiers: two comforting interventions for heelstick pain. *Res Nurs Health* 1994;17:321–331.
165. Sparshott M. The development of a clinical distress scale for ventilated newborn infants: identification of pain and distress based on validated behavioural scores. *J Neonat Nurs* 1996;2:5–11.
166. Ballantyne M, Stevens B, McAllister M, et al. Validation of the Premature Infant Pain Profile in the clinical setting. *Clin J Pain* 2000;16:297–333.
167. Stevens BJ, Johnston CC, Franck LS, et al. Validation of the Premature Infant Pain Profile (PIPP) with very low birthweight neonates. *International Pediatric Nursing Research Symposium on Clinical Care of the Child and Family*. 8. 1999(abst).
168. Blauer T, Gerstmann D. A simultaneous comparison of three neonatal pain scales during common NICU procedures. *Clin J Pain* 1998;14:39–47.
169. Johnston CC, Sherrard A, Stevens B, et al. Do cry features reflect pain intensity in preterm neonates? A preliminary study. *Biol Neonate* 1999;76:120–124.
170. Petroni M, Malowany AS, Johnston CC, et al. A new, robust vocal fundamental frequency (Fo) determination method for the analysis of infant cries. In: *Proceedings of the Seventh Annual IEEE Symposium on Computer-based Medical Systems* 1994;223–228.
171. Petroni M, Malowany AS, Johnston CC, et al. Classification of infant cries using artificial neural networks (ANNS). *Proceedings of the IEEE International Conference on Acoustics, Speech, and Signal Processing*, Detroit, MI, 1995.
172. Johnston CC, Stremler RL, Horton L, et al. Single dose vs triple dose oral sucrose for decreasing pain from heelstick in preterm neonates. *Proceedings of the 4th International Symposium on Pediatric Pain* 4, 4. 1997(abst).
173. Barr RG, Rotman A, Yaremko J, et al. The crying of infants with colic: a controlled empirical description. *Pediatrics* 1992;90:14–21.
174. Barr RG. Reflections on measuring pain in infants: dissociation in responsive systems and "honest signalling." *Arch Dis Child* 1998;79:F152–F156.
175. Attia J, Mayer M-N, Shnider SM, et al. Correlation of a clinical pain score with catecholamine and endorphin levels in small infants. *Intensive Care Med* 1987; 13:459(abst).
176. Horgan M, Choonara I. Measuring pain in neonates: an objective score. *Pediatr Nurs* 1996;8:24–27.
177. Lawerence J, Alcock D, McGrath PJ, et al. The development of a tool to assess neonatal pain. *Neonat Network* 1993;12:59–66.
178. van Dijk M, de Boer JB, Koot HM, et al. The reliability and validity of the COMFORT scale as a postoperative pain instrument in 0 to 3-year-old infants. *Pain* 2000;84:367–377.
179. Joyce BA, Schade JG, Keck JF, et al. Reliability and validity of preverbal pain assessment tools. *Issues Compr Pediatr Nurs* 1994;17:121–135.
180. Schade JG, Joyce BA, Gerkensmeyer J, et al. Comparison of three preverbal scales for postoperative pain assessment in a diverse pediatric sample. J Pain Symptom Manage 1996;12:348–359.
181. McGrath PJ, Canfield C, Campbell MA, et al. Behaviours caregivers use to determine pain in non-verbal, cognitively impaired individuals. *Dev Med Child Neurol*1998;40:340–343.
182. Hodgkinson K, Bear M, Thorn J, et al. Measuring pain in neonates: evaluating an instrument and developing a common language. *Australian Journal of Advanced Nursing* 1994;12:17–22.
183. Krechel SW, Bildner J. CRIES: A new neonatal postoperative pain measurement score. Initial testing of validity and reliability. *Paediatric Anaesthesia* 1995;5: 53–61.
184. Schiller C. Clinical utility of two neonatal pain assessment measures. Toronto: University of Toronto, 1998 (dissertation).
185. Friedrichs JB, Young S, Gallagher D, et al. Where does it hurt? An interdisciplinary approach to improving the quality of pain assessment and management in the neonatal intensive care unit. *Nurs Clin North Am* 1995; 30:143–159.
186. Brazleton TB, Nugent KN. *Neonatal behavioral assessment Scale.* 3rd ed. London: MacKeith Press, Holborn, 1995.
187. Als H, Lester BM, Tronick EZ, et al. Manual for the assessment of preterm infants' behavior (APIB). In: Fitzgerald HE, Lester BM, Yogman MW, eds. *Theory and research in behavioral pediatrics.* New York: Plenum Press, 1982:65–131.
188. Gauvain-Piquard A, Rodary C, Rezvani A, et al. Pain in children aged 2–6 years: a new observational rating scale elaborated in a pediatric oncology unit preliminary report. *Pain* 1987;31:177–188.
189. Lawrence J, Alcock D, McGrath PJ, et al. The development of a tool to assess neonatal pain. *Neonat Network* 1993;12:59–66.
190. McGrath PA, DeVeber LL, Hearn MT. Multidimensional pain assessment in children. In: Fields HL, Dubner R, Cervero F, eds. *Advances in pain research and therapy.* 4th ed. New York: Raven Press, 1985: 387–393.
191. Taddio A, Goldbach M, Ipp M, et al. Effect of neonatal circumcision on pain responses during vaccination in boys. *Lancet* 1995;345:291–292.
192. Carbajal R, Paupe A, Hoenn E, et al. APN: evaluation of behavioral scale of newborn infants [French]. *Archives de Pediatrie* 1997;4:23–28.
193. Merkel SI, Voepel-Lewis T, Shayevitz JR, et al. The FLACC: a behavioral scale for scoring postoperative pain in young children. *Pediatr Nurs* 1997;23:293–297.

8

Measuring Pain in Children: Developmental and Instrument Issues

Anne Gaffney, Patrick J. McGrath, and Bruce Dick

The experience of pain is private, subjective, and not directly accessible to others. Thus, the humane and clinical goals of pain prevention and relief present the problem of collecting and analyzing information about other individuals' experiences of pain. This general process, usually termed pain assessment, may include the biologic, personal, and social contexts in which pain occurs. Pain measurement is more specific, involving the application of some metric to a selected aspect of pain and is the basis for a scientific approach to pain. Many different aspects, including the frequency, intensity, and duration of pain, pain-related affect, and disability can be measured. Adequate pain measurement makes it possible to evaluate levels of pain to see whether or what treatment is needed and to determine its effectiveness. Finally, measurement can make important contributions to research on the origins of pain and factors that influence the expression of pain.

MEASURING PAIN IN CHILDREN

The ability to measure pain in pediatric clinical settings has improved dramatically in recent years. Several thorough reviews outline this progress (1–6). However, the measurement of different aspects of pain in children is a complex and challenging area, and further theoretic and empiric progress in extending and combining our knowledge of pain, measurement, and children will be required.

Developmental Factors

Developmental factors are clearly relevant to the measurement and assessment of pain in children and adolescents. Children's understanding of pain and their ability to describe it change with increasing age in a developmental pattern consonant with the characteristics of Piaget's preoperational, concrete operational, and early formal operational stages in cognitive development (7–9). Children of approximately 5 years of age, and even younger, understand pain as an aversive sensory experience ("it hurts and you don't like it") often linked to the themes of "tummy" and eating ("it's a thing in your tummy, it's sore"; "you get it if you eat too much"). With increasing age and cognitive development, there is a shift from the objectification (i.e., the ability to think about as opposed to the ability to simply experience) of the physical, sensory aspects of pain to inclusion of the psychologic-affective and psychosocial dimensions. In addition to the development of children's understanding of pain, developmental patterns in other cognitive competencies, for example, children's understanding of measurement and numbers, are also relevant to the measurement of pain in children.

In this chapter, we first refer briefly to the theoretic model that we consider most appropriate in the context of pain assessment and measurement. We then describe the characteristics of good pain measurement and outline the main types of measures. The developmental factors that influence the ability of children of different ages to report their pain are then discussed in sections on the measurement of pain in preschool-age children (ages 1 to 5 years), school-age children (ages 6 to 12 years), and adolescents (ages 13 to 16 years). Finally, we refer to general issues that cut across developmental levels and conclude with suggestions for future directions in clinical practice and research.

MODEL OF PAIN UNDERLYING PEDIATRIC PAIN MEASUREMENT

An important consideration in pain measurement is the theoretic model underlying a measure of pain. The World Health Organization Model of the Consequences of Disease (10) has been proposed as a model that can be adapted for this purpose (1,11). This classification system provides a model of the consequences of disease conceptualized as occurring at four levels or planes of experience: (a) a disease itself; (b) an impairment, the level at which an individual becomes aware of a symptom or abnormality; in the case of pain, impairment refers to the perception of pain; (c) a disability or restriction in normal activity; and (d) a handicap (in which the impairment or disability exerts an impact on normal social functioning). This chapter focuses on the measurement of pain as impairment.

CHARACTERISTICS OF A GOOD MEASURE OF PAIN

Pain measurement refers to the application of a specific metric to some dimension of pain. Pain is a multidimensional phenomenon (12). For example, pain has both a sensory dimension of intensity (how strong the pain sensation is) and affective (how upsetting the pain is). Consequently, a good measure should clearly identify and define which dimension is to be measured. It should accurately reflect the individual's subjective experience and be responsive to gradations in pain (an ordinal measure) and not just the presence or absence of pain (a nominal measure). Whether interval data (how much more or less pain) can be generated from a measure of pain depends on the perceived equality of the intervals, as interval scales are linear, based on repeatable units of equal value.[1] It should be noninvasive, developmentally appropriate, inexpensive, and potentially usable at the bedside. The psychometric properties that are required of a good pain measure are validity, reliability, sensitivity, and specificity (13).

Validity (from the Latin *validus* meaning strong) refers to the strength or robustness of the measure; this is generally defined as the extent to which a test measures what it is intended to measure. As there is no gold standard for pain measurement, evidence of validity may have to be assembled from a number of sources, both convergent (supported by other evidence of pain, e.g., behavioral) and divergent (supported by a zero or low score on some other measure such as the number of analgesics required). Reliability refers to the consistency of a measure; the greater the reliability is, the less discrepancy would appear on repeated measures if the construct being measured remained stable. In the case of pain, reliability refers to the degree to which variations in pain scores in individuals or groups reflect actual variation in pain levels.

The sensitivity of a measure of pain refers to the extent to which it can be relied on to pick up on the presence or degree of pain, whereas the specificity of a pain measure indicates the degree to which a score reflects only, for example, a selected aspect of pain, and is not influenced by other factors. Measures of pain-related affect, for example, are likely to be more sensitive than specific because they may identify aversive emotions, whereas these may not be purely pain related. The requirements for a pain measure in terms of reliability, sensitivity, and specificity will vary with the purpose of the measure.

---

[1]It has been proposed (B. M. Kiely, personal communication, 2001) that if increases in perceived pain intensity were plotted over time tolerable as a measure of pain, the relationship would not be linear, but a sigmoid curve, from which interval data cannot be generated. For example, the changes in perceived pain related to immersing one's hand in water that is being gradually heated are likely to be less steep at both very low and very high temperatures.

PEDIATRIC PAIN MEASURES

As noted in the introduction, pain is private and subjective and can only be accessed and measured by indirect methods. These methods include self-report, observation of behaviors that suggest pain, and physiologic and biologic measures. In the case of children, there may be additional barriers to obtaining information about their pain because of limited cognitive or linguistic skills or by the contingencies of pain reports or behaviors, for example, getting an injection or not being discharged from hospital. Nonetheless, several valid and reliable measures have been developed to measure children's pain. Several of these measures are discussed below.

Self-Report Measures

Self-report of pain essentially involves some intentional communication by the child

TABLE 8.1. *Recommended self-report measures in children*

Measure	Description	Indications for use	Advantages	Disadvantages
Self-report measures	Child is asked about intensity, rhythm, and variations in pain	Adequate cognitive and communicative abilities	Simple and efficient, can be administered easily	Subject to bias (e.g., demand characteristics, inaccurate or selective memory)
Poker chip tool (Hester et al., 1990)	Child chooses 1 to 4 chips ("pieces of pain")	4–8 yr old	Correlates with overt behaviors in injections, adequate convergent validity, partial support for discriminant validity	May be childish for older children
Faces scale (Bieri et al., 1990)	Faces indicating intensity were derived from children's drawings	6–8 yr old	Strong agreement among children about pain severity of faces and consistency of intervals, adequate test-retest reliability	
Visual analog scale (VAS)	Vertical or horizontal line with verbal, facial, or numerical anchors on a continuum of pain intensity	5 years and over	Reliable and valid (e.g., child report correlates with behavioral measures and with parent, nurse, physician ratings), versatile (can rate different dimensions on same scale)	Intervals on numerical scales may not be equal from a child's perspective
Oucher scale (Beyer and Wells, 1989)	6 photos of children's faces indicating intensity; 100-point corresponding vertical scale	3–12 yr	Reliable, adequate content validity, correlates with other VAS scales Presentation of both pictorial and numerical scales is applicable for broader age range	See VAS
Pain diary	Numerical ratings are repeated, along with recording of other relevant information (e.g., time, activity, medication)	Older child/ adolescent, measurement of chronic or recurrent pain (e.g., headache, limb pain, cancer pain)	Adequate interrater reliability between parent and child, useful in determining patterns of pain and in teaching self-management strategies (thereby providing a sense of mastery)	Requires commitment to record regularly and accurately, requires effort and prompting if moving from one situation to another (memory over time is rarely accurate)

about his or her experience of pain. Such communications could include verbal, gestural, numerical, pictorial, tactile, mechanical, or electronic modes of communication.

In Table 8.1, we summarize the best validated self-report measures that clinicians can use in everyday practice with the advantages and disadvantages of each. Simple training methods, usually requiring the child to rate past or hypothetical pains, have been used in the validation of most self-report measures (14). Young children and children with cognitive deficits or problems in communication may require more training (15). Flavell (16) noted that, at least in the context of mathematical tasks, training is not effective if the task is well beyond the child's cognitive capabilities.

Behavioral Measures of Pain

Specific types of distress behaviors (e.g., vocalization, facial expression, and body movement) have been associated with pain and are helpful in evaluating pain in children with limited communication skills. However, it may be difficult to discriminate between pain behaviors and behavior resulting from other sources of distress such as hunger or anxiety, so that the specificity of such measures may be less than their sensitivity. Reliability and validity are highest when measuring short, sharp pain (e.g., from injections or lumbar punctures). Measurement of longer lasting pain (such as postoperative pain) is more difficult because of the relatively rare occurrence of gross movements (17). However, Finke et al. report that the Children's and Infants Postoperative Pain Scale was both sensitive and specific in assessing postoperative analgesic needs in toddlers (18).

Two groups have investigated the use of facial responses to short, sharp pain in infants (19,20). Facial expressions offer one way to rate more subtle behaviors and, in infants, are relatively free of learning biases. Facial responses have not been investigated in older children, possibly because it is known that from around 4 years of age, children begin to manage their emotional expression and to mask their feelings. With preschool-age and older children, several behavioral rating scales are used to measure pain in response to medical procedures. These scales operationally define specific behaviors, such as gross motor movements and verbal behavior, as they occur during set intervals or phases of a procedure. Observers require specific training in their use, which makes these scales more time-consuming than self-report. Nonetheless, they are an important component to validating more subjective pain measures.

Table 8.2 describes four widely used behavioral rating scales: the Procedural Rating Scale (20), the Observational Scale of Behavioral Distress (21), the Children's Hospital of Eastern Ontario Pain Scale (22), and the Gauvain-Piquard rating scale (23). Because the Children's Hospital of Eastern Ontario Pain Scale is the most easily learned of the scales and has been well validated for short, sharp pain, it is presented in its entirety in Table 8.3. A variant of behavioral measures is to have adults observe a child and rate how much pain they think a child is experiencing on a visual analog scale. This approach is efficient and appears to be valid because these ratings correlate well with the child's own self-report (24). Chambers et al. (25) developed the Parent's Postoperative Pain Rating Scale, which is based on this principle. Parents are asked to rate their children's pain by noting changes in the frequency of a number of behaviors.

Biologic Measures

As with behavioral measures of pain, biologic measures cannot discriminate well between physical responses to pain and other forms of stress to the body. Furthermore, most studies of biologic measures have involved infants and have generally assessed short, sharp pain. Although there are sufficient data on the validity of heart rate, transcutaneous oxygen, sweating, and electroencephalography in certain circumstances, heart rate is probably the simplest and easiest to measure. However, heart rate as a measure of pain is still not fully understood, and caution must be used in its interpretation.

TABLE 8.2. *Pain as impairment: recommended behavioral measures in children*

Measure	Description	Indications for use	Advantages	Disadvantages
Behavioral measures	Direct observation of overt behaviors, usually measured repeatedly at regular intervals, according to time or phase of procedure	Very young children, used with self-report, best reliability and validity are for short, sharp pain	Useful when child is unable to rate pain, less subject to bias than self-report	Not as well-validated for longer lasting pain or for subtle behaviors (e.g., guarding wound), difficult to discriminate between pain and distress
Procedural rating scale (Katz et al., 1980) and observational scale of behavioral distress (OBSD) (Jay et al., 1983)	10 observed behaviors: crying, screaming, physical restraint, verbal resistance, requests for emotional support, muscular rigidity, verbal pain expression, flailing, nervous behavior, and information seeking	Originally used for bone marrow aspirations and lumbar punctures, but appropriate for any short, sharp pain	Satisfactory interrater reliability OBSD correlates with self-report of pain and anxiety	Requires training of observers
Children's Hospital of Eastern Ontario (CHEOPS) (McGrath et al., 1985)	6 observed behaviors: crying facial expression, verbal expression, torso position, and leg position	Originally used for postoperative pain and needle pain	Easy to learn and use, interrater reliability = 0.80; concurrent validity	Insensitive to long-term pain
Gauvain-Piquard rating scale (Gauvain-Piquard et al., 1987)	15 behaviors divided into 3 subscales: pain behaviors (e.g., guarding wound), anxiety behaviors (e.g., nervousness), psychomotor alterations (e.g., withdrawal)	Validated with 2- to 6-yr olds, used for long-term pain in pediatric oncology patients	Adequate interrater reliability and sensitivity to differences in children	

DEVELOPMENTAL ISSUES IN PAIN MEASUREMENT

In the following sections, we discuss the implications of developmental change with age in relation to children's ability to report on their pain, referring to Piaget's stages of cognitive development, the less well-known literature on children's understanding of measurement (26), and children's understanding of numbers (16,27–30).

Preschool-Age Children (Ages 1 to 5 Years)

Children in this age range present a particular challenge in terms of pain measurement, especially before 3 years of age. The cognitive, linguistic, and social competencies of toddlers limit the range of measurement options. Further, when toddlers are ill, it is more difficult to engage them in tasks that do not fall in the range of activities that would normally interest them.

Testability

Cooperation with self-report/formal measures of pain depends in part on the testability of the child, i.e., the child's ability to attend to and address a specific task without assimilating it into some egocentric play schema (16).

TABLE 8.3. *Behavioral definitions and scoring of Children's Hospital of Eastern Ontario Pain Scale*

Item	Behavior	Score	Definition
Cry	No cry	1	Child is not crying
	Moaning	2	Child is moaning or quietly vocalizing; silent cry
	Crying	2	Child is crying, but the cry is gentle or whimpering
	Scream	3	Child is in a full-lunged cry, sobbing, may be scored with complaint or without complaint
Facial	Composed	1	Neutral facial expression
	Grimace	2	Score only if definite negative facial expression
	Smiling	0	Score only if positive facial expression
Child Verbal	None	1	Child not talking
	Other complaints	1	Child complains, but not about pain, e.g., "I want to see Mommy" or "I am thirsty"
	Pain complaints	2	Child complains about pain
	Both complaints	2	Child complains about pain and about other things, e.g., "I hurt, I want Mommy"
	Positive	0	Child makes any positive statement or talks about other things without complaint
Torso	Neutral	1	Body (not limbs) is at rest, torso is inactive
	Shifting	2	Body is in motion in a shifting or serpentine fashion
	Tense	2	Body is arched or rigid
	Shivering	2	Body is shuddering or shaking involuntarily
	Upright	2	Child is in vertical or upright position
	Restrained	2	Body is restrained
Touch	Not touching	1	Child is not touching or grabbing at wound
	Reach	2	Child is reaching for but not touching wound
	Touch	2	Child is gently touching wound or wound area
	Grab	2	Child is grabbing vigorously at wound
	Restrained	2	Child's arms are restrained
Legs	Neutral	1	Legs may be in any position but are relaxed, includes gentle swimming or serpentine-like movements
	Squirming/kicking	2	Definitive uneasy or restless movements in the legs and/or striking out with foot or feet
	Drawn up/tensed	2	Legs tensed and/or pulled tightly to body and kept there
	Standing	2	Standing, crouching, or kneeling
	Restrained	2	Child's legs are being held down

From McGrath PJ, Johnson G, Goodman JT, et al. Advances in pain research and therapy. In: Fields HL, Dubner R, Cervero F, eds. *The CHEOPS: A behavioral scale to measure post-operative pain in children.* New York: Raven Press, 1985:395–402, with permission.

Children in general develop this ability around 4 years of age (16). Younger children's communication with relative strangers in hospital settings may also be confounded by mutual unintelligibility of speech and by stranger anxiety, suggesting that behavioral rating scales, including facial expression and the reports of parents/caregivers familiar with the child in health, offer the best methods of pain assessment and measurement in children aged 1 to 3 or 4 years. However, toddlers can show considerable concentration and perseverance in completing tasks in the context of play. The challenge of obtaining information from preschoolers through familiarity, play, and "ideal discourse" is discussed by Champion et al. (31).

Preoperational Thinking and Pain Measurement

Although 4- and 5-year-old children can comply with some self-report measures, their ability to do so is likely to be influenced by the cognitive characteristics of the preoperational stage (approximately 2 to 6 or 7 years) described by Piaget (16). The child's thinking, especially in the earlier years of this stage, tends to be egocentric, concrete, and perceptually dominated. The nature of these cognitive characteristics and their implications for pain measurement are discussed below.

Egocentric Thought

Egocentric thinking refers to young children's relative lack of awareness of the boundaries separating their thoughts from those of others. Preschool children may assume that others know how much they hurt, and therefore the task of communicating pain through pain measures may appear less salient to this age group than to older children (8). For example, McCaffery (32) described a 3-year-old girl who, when asked about her tummy pain, impatiently raised her skirt and exclaimed "There—can't you see it?" Furthermore, young children's heteronomous view of adults as all-powerful and all-seeing (33) may also predispose them to believe that adults know how much they hurt.

Concrete Thinking

Although preoperational thinking is representational in nature, it tends to operate very much in terms of concrete and static images of reality rather than abstract schematic signs (16). This concrete nature of young children's thinking may influence their understanding of pain measurement scales. These difficulties could arise because of a lack of comprehension of the instructions and/or the anchor words used. Simple, concrete anchor words, e.g., "no hurt" to "biggest hurt" (3) are obviously preferable to relatively long, complex, and hypothetical terms such as "least pain sensation possible . . . most intense pain sensation possible" (34). Even "worst pain possible/imaginable" may pose problems for younger children because these phrases require some implicit understanding of the abstract concept of possibility (16). Also, with regard to children's understanding of the word worst, Gaffney (8) found that 5- and 6-year-old children had difficulty in responding to the sentence completion item "The worst thing about pain is . . . " Although not certain, it is probable that it was the word worst, as the most complex of the words used in this phrase, made it difficult for the children to respond to and complete.

Concrete Thinking and Dimensions of Pain

Concrete thinking may also influence the dimensions of pain that can be measured in young children. As the sensory and affective dimensions of pain referred to earlier probably influence each other reciprocally, making it difficult for even adults to separate these dimensions, the potential therapeutic value of measures of pain-related affect has prompted attempts to measure this dimension of pain in children. However, it has proved difficult with children younger than approximately 8 years of age (31,34). It has been demonstrated previously that children's ability to quantify different dimensions of continuous quantities follows a developmental pattern (27). As might be expected, children can quantify concrete dimensions before more abstract, less perceptually obvious dimensions. For example, quantity/amount is quantified before weight, weight before volume, and volume before density. With regard to dimensions of pain, the physical sensory dimension is conceptualized by children earlier than the affective dimension and thus is presumably quantifiable earlier. Young children (5 to 7 years of age) define and describe pain in concrete, physical/sensory terms, whereas affective themes begin to be added around the age of 7 to 8 years of age, with girls preceding boys in this ability (7). Gaffney (8) found that in response to a sentence-completion item on the effects of pain ("A pain can make you . . . ") only one of 194 5- to 7-year-old children used an affective label (sad), whereas the majority responded with sick, cry, or sore. It is possible that young children use the word cry to express the emotional reaction to pain. The use of affective terms and their variety and complexity increased significantly with age in response to the item cited above but did not become well established until between 10 and 12 years of age in this sample of healthy schoolchildren. Although it might be expected that recent experience of pain would increase reports of pain-related affect, Champion et al. (31) and Goodenough et al. (34) reported a similar developmental pattern of difficulty in obtaining pain affect ratings after venipuncture from children younger than 8 years of age using a visual analog format. These results highlight the time lag that can occur between experiencing states and being able to think about, objectify, or quantify them because very young children do show emotional reactions to painful stimuli, as clearly illustrated by Craig (35) in a series of photographs of toddlers during and after inoculation. Also, from approximately 2 years of age, children are beginning to use emotional labels such as happy, sad, and mad (36). Nevertheless, a conscious awareness of emotional states as being evoked by or being connected to pain does not appear to develop until much later.

Although the task of rating pain on some affective dimension may be too abstract for children younger than approximately 8 years of age, strategies that examine how the child feels either during or after pain using either a faces scale such as the Facial Affective Scale (37) or a visual analog scale are likely to be more successful in obtaining information on pain-related affect in young children. Chambers and Craig (38) reported that 5- and 6-year-old children could rate on a Likert scale how good or bad they would feel in particular situations, although they used the extremes of the scale more than older children. A pertinent issue in tasks that ask a child to rate how he/she feels using some emotional label is that there may be a developmental pattern in the recognition or objectification of different kinds of emotions. Cartoon depictions of some affective states (happy and sad) are recognized more reliably by preschoolers and first graders than those depicting fear or anger (39), and there is a developmental pattern in children's use of emotional terms (36).

Perceptually Dominated Thinking

Perceptually dominated thinking refers to the young child's tendency to focus on the more perceptually obvious aspects of a situation (16) and neglect less obvious and possibly divergent features. This may also influence young children's use of pain measures because a problem encountered in both visual analog scales and faces scales is the frequency with which end points are selected (31). Because end points are perceptually stronger than mid portions, it is likely that the perceptually dominated nature of preoperational thinking influences this selection (26) so that strategies that would minimize this tendency are desirable. The design of an interactive faces scale (34), other electronic measures (40), and the removal of unnecessary corners at the end of visual analog lines may be helpful.

Preschool Children's Understanding of Measurement

Because the process of measurement is based on a number of assumptions that are not necessarily shared by children (26), studies of children's spontaneous approaches to tasks involving measurement may offer insights into measuring pain in children. These studies by Piaget and colleagues (26) describe the strategies used by children before the development of the logic underlying the measurement of most continuous quantities (that is, the addition of equal arbitrary subunits) at 8 to 9 years of age. When asked to reproduce a tower of bricks placed on a higher table and separated by a screen, 4- and 5-year-old children used global visual estimates of the relative heights. Piaget noted that, generally, children find perceptual comparisons easier than adults and are often more accurate. He suggested that children show a blind faith in their visual estimates, which tends to preclude "the wish to know of more exact ways of measuring" (26) because these children tended to ignore the measurement aids with which they were supplied.

Piaget and colleagues (26) also highlighted the important finding that children use body parts to help them perform measurements. For example, 5- to 7-year-old children used body level and arm, hand, and finger spans as ways of measuring, again in preference to supplied aids such as rulers and pieces of string because for younger children, "this technique carries greater conviction." This spontaneous use of body parts as measures indicates that this approach comes naturally to young children and is therefore an area that merits further investigation in the context of pain measurement.

Preschool Children's Understanding of Numbers

Children's ability to use numerical rating scales is obviously dependent on their understanding of numbers. Although 4- and 5-year-old children have a global, intuitive grasp of the quantitative meaning of small numbers (28) and can count small sets of numbers (29), counting and understanding the quantitative significance of numbers are two separate developments. To use Chi's (41) metaphor, these developing abilities are stored in different "files" that do not begin to "merge" until approximately 6 years of age, providing a new conceptual structure that underpins the quantitative understanding of number names. Furthermore, this conceptual understanding of number is not an all-or-nothing event: it develops first in relation to the smallest numbers and is only gradually extended to larger and larger number sets (16). As a result, smaller numbers are inherently more meaningful as larger numbers may progressively lose their quantitative significance and become merely counting tags. With young children, the use of numbers tends to be idiosyncratic and unreliable; Gelman and Baillargeon (30) stated that although very young children grasp many of the principles involved in counting, they tend to apply them in an idiosyncratic manner (e.g., two, six, nine, eleven to represent one, two, three, four), and a large number might be "forty-nine a hundred."

Measures Appropriate for Use with Preschool-Age Children

Although children younger than the age of 3 to 4 years cannot generally comply with self-report measures, measures of pain intensity used in older preschool children include visual analog scales, faces scales, the Poker Chip Tool, and the Finger Span Test. The basic task demand of these measures appears to require the child to estimate or indicate his or her pain as part of a whole or maximum value defined by anchors. When considering whether children can or cannot "do" these tasks, it may be worth recalling, as Kuhn (42) pointed out, that the development of skills and strategies during childhood proceeds along a continuum from implicit to explicit mastery rather than a sudden transition from failure to success on a given task. An explicit understanding of proportionality may therefore not be necessary for children to use these measures. The concrete and global nature of young children's thinking has, in fact, the advantage of predisposing them to a belief in wholes rather than infinities, as, for example, children believe in the existence of some "biggest number" (30); as noted previously, they use global perceptual estimates in measuring tasks that they may also use in pain measures. These "raw perceptual intuitions" (27) cannot, by definition, depend much on explicit seriation and classification. Perhaps the basic demands of pain measures, although they may appear abstract or difficult for young children, are not incongruent with "their spontaneous attitude of mind" (16), provided that the instructions and anchor words used are developmentally appropriate. In fact, it is possible that the idea of indicating one's pain on a line on a page may seem in some ways less strange to children than to adults.

Visual Analog Scales

Visual analog scales have been used to measure pain in preschool-age children (34). However, there have been concerns regarding the apparent abstractness of the visual analog scale format in relation to its use with young children (13,31). In some versions, efforts have been made to make them more concrete by the addition of subunits or numbers. Visual analog scales without subunits are, in fact, more congruent with young children's understanding of measurement as "intensive" (without subunits) as opposed to the "extensive" subunit-based approach of older children and adults (26) in allowing a global perceptual estimate to be made. Another issue in the use of visual analog scales is that they require the user to have some implicit grasp that the line separating the anchors represents a continuum. Research by Piaget and Inhelder (27) indicates that young children have an intuitive grasp of linear continua because when asked to estimate relative quantities of beads (less, more, or the same) that were beyond their ability to count, young children accomplished this task easily if asked which pile of beads would make the longest or shortest necklace, indicating some implicit understanding of linear wholes.

A disadvantage of visual analog scales is they require more cross-modal translation than faces scales, which, as discussed below, are more direct and involve less labeling of states. Also, in childhood, the upper end of the visual analog scale continuum or whole is likely to be less static than in adults, changing with pain experiences and the ability to objectify, label, and remember them. Perceptual dominance, the tendency to focus on perceptually strong aspects of a situation, as noted earlier, may influence the child to focus on visual analog scale end points.

Faces Scales

Faces scales as measures of pain have the advantages of being more direct and involving less cross-modal translation than visual analog scales. It appears that young children can discriminate degrees of pain intensity in facial expressions, but the development of this ability requires systematic investigation (31). Children's ability to discriminate pain-related affect may depend on the affect depicted because some emotions may be discriminated earlier than others (39).

The number of faces used in faces scales is an important issue. Champion et al. (31) noted that children younger than 5 years of age have difficulty with more than four or five choices. This difficulty parallels their ability to count meaningfully and is presumably related to the limited information-processing capacity of the early preoperational period (28). Illness and pain may further reduce this limited information-processing capacity, and too many options may augment children's tendency to focus on end points. Although Chambers and Craig (38) have shown that an increase from three to five options on a Likert scale did not have this effect, it could occur with larger numbers of options. Interactive computer-based scales (40) could reduce the tendency to select end points. Champion and colleagues (31) are working on developing an interactive faces scale that can be manipulated electronically to increase or decrease the depiction of pain. This format would be congruent with young children's understanding of "less, more, or the same" as perceptually (how it looks) rather than conceptually based (27).

The Poker Chip Tool

This tool, developed by Hester and colleagues (43), which requires children to rate their pain by selecting one to four "pieces of hurt" concretely represented by poker chips, has been widely and effectively used with young children. This tool has the advantage of having some resemblance to a game. Also, analysis of the instructions shows that the Poker Chip Tool is not number dependent and can be done on the basis of the global quantification model (a little, when I add more, gives a lot) proposed by Case (28) as typical of preschoolers' understanding of quantity.

The Finger Span Test

This test, developed by Franzen and Ahlquist (44), is the only formal body-based measure of which we are aware. The child is asked to estimate their pain by holding the thumb and forefinger together to indicate no pain and as far apart as possible to indicate maximum pain, and a pain measure is obtained by the distance between thumb and forefinger as a proportion of the maximum distance. As noted above, body-based measures are natural to children, and even though they are more difficult to quantify because the maximum value will vary between individuals, informal reports indicate that this format is being used clinically and therefore should be evaluated for validity and reliability.

School-Age Children (6 to 12 Years)

This age range spans three cognitive developmental stages, from the end of the preoperational through concrete operations and into early formal operations. The characteristics of preoperational thinking (described in the previous section) decline with the emergence of concrete operations at 7 to 8 years of age. Several skills become operationally based and thus explicit between approximately 7 and 10 years of age, including measurement, classification, and seriation. As was noted previously in relation to the quantification of different dimensions, seriation (the ability to accurately place in ascending or descending order) of different dimensions of a quantity also follows a developmental sequence from concrete to abstract, so that children should be able to seriate concrete, physical aspects of pain before the more abstract, affective dimensions.

With regard to measure of pain-related affect, Gaffney (8) found that children's objectification of pain starts to extend from the physical to include the affective aspects between the ages of 7 and 10 but is not well established until 10 or 11 years of age. Champion et al. (31) and Goodenough et al. (34) reported that girls are more advanced than boys in their ability to give separate ratings of pain-related affect. The unpublished Gaffney data previously mentioned also showed girls to be approximately 2 years ahead of boys in their use of various affective terms related to pain. This gap was found to remain until approximately age 14 when boys' abilities caught up. These findings are consistent with previous work that showed that girls tend to be more emotionally and socially oriented than boys (45,46).

Adolescents

During the period of early formal operations (ages 11 to 14 years), there is an increasing emphasis on the psychologic aspects of pain that are now extended to psychosocial effects (9). Because adolescence is a period of considerable introspection during which self-concepts change from concrete to abstract psychologic characteristics (47), most adolescents are able to report on pain-related affect and have developed a more complex pain vocabulary (9). Adolescent thought is less confined to the present than that of earlier cognitive stages. Being more future oriented, it is possible that worry about the significance of pain in terms of recurrence of illness, future disability or disfigurement may influence pain measurement.

Children and Adolescents with Cognitive and Communicative Difficulties

A long-neglected area that is now receiving attention is that of identifying and beginning to measure pain in children who have significant difficulties in communicating to others about their pain (48). These children include those with mental retardation, metabolic disorders, autism, severe brain injury, and communication difficulties because of neuromuscular disorders or loss of hearing or vision. Initial attempts to address this problem have consisted of asking parents or caregivers to identify the cues that indicate pain or discomfort in the child (48). However, because many indicators of pain or comfort are unique to the individual, individualized assessment and measurement will always be required.

Another approach to this important problem has been to collect data on common sources of pain in some of these populations (48). This approach acknowledges that, when caring for children with communication difficulties, the onus should be on clinicians/caregivers to have a high index of suspicion of common pain sources in particular groups of patients. This survey should provide valuable information from people experienced in the field on the sources and prevalence of painful conditions in some of these groups (for example, painful gastroesophageal reflux, spasm, or constipation in children with cerebral palsy). This could be a major contribution to increasing comfort in children with communication difficulties because in many situations pain may be alleviated by addressing the source (e.g., acid reflux or the need for repositioning) rather than the administration of analgesia.

FUTURE DIRECTIONS

Clinical Practice

Clinical pediatric practice is likely to see increasing utilization of pain measurement. Ideally, a pain flow chart to record measures over time should be standard in patients' charts. Measuring and recording pain in this way, apart from according pain some status as the fifth vital sign, will over time provide valuable information on patients' perceptions of various types and dimensions of pain across age, gender, and diagnosis. This in turn should lead to improved diagnosis and preemption and treatment of pain (including pain in children with communication problems), in accordance with the draft standards for pain assessment and management of the Child Friendly Healthcare Initiative supported by World Health Organization and United Nations International Children's Emergency Fund.

Research

As mentioned in the introduction to this chapter, we need to develop our understanding of measurement along with our understanding of pain and of children. We need to consider how the act of measurement might change what is being measured, i.e., the perception of pain. This limitation, described in physics as the Heisenberg uncertainty principle, is often observed in medical practice, as, for example, in measuring blood pressure. Historically, the ability to measure continuous quantities has proceeded in tandem with the understanding of what is being measured (30). Therefore, as our knowledge of pain improves, so will our ability to measure it.

The literature on the measurement of pain in children contains very little information on pain measurement as a process. This needs to be looked at from the perspective of children—what approaches or strategies they use at different ages, rather than what they "can" or "cannot" do. This is, in fact, what Piaget's approach to understanding how children think was based on—not whether children got the right or wrong answer to a problem, but how they arrived at their particular conclusion. He amassed his vast research, aimed at uncovering "the spontaneous attitude of mind" underlying children's apparently idiosyncratic logic, by developing his "clinical method," a kind of gentle, simple, but persistent querying of how the child was thinking. That this is relevant to pain measurement is illustrated by an anecdote shared by a participant at International Symposium on Paediatric Pain 2000, who recounted that an 8-year-old boy chose 10 of 10 on a scale to describe his pain, although he seemed comfortable. On questioning, it emerged that he perceived 10 of 10 to be a "good" score, whereas 0 of 10 was "bad," based on his school marking system. Piaget's clinical method could be studied and adapted to investigate how children actually decide on a face, a number, or a point on a scale, perhaps initially with healthy children after a short procedure such as vaccination.

Some specific issues as well as general approaches could be investigated. von Baeyer and colleagues (personal communication, 2001) are currently examining children's understanding of anchor words. How children scan faces in faces scales and whether photographs and cartoon depictions are scanned similarly could be analyzed. How children use anchors in visual analog scales, if the use of mechanical sliders changes how children use these scales, and whether vertical presentation of the visual analog scale to children is preferable are issues that could be investigated. Research is also needed into what items or terms should be used in pain scales, based on suggestions by children themselves. It is likely that much informal information on these and related issues exists among regular users of measures in both practice and research, but it needs to be shared and analyzed.

SUMMARY

In this chapter, we focused on the developmental factors that may influence children's ability to comply with pain measurement, emphasizing that children may be able to perform some tasks on the basis of implicit rather than explicit understanding of the concepts involved. We highlighted the need for investigation into the strategies that children of different ages actually use while using self-report measures. Such information would lead to a clearer understanding of children's perspective on pain measurement and thereby contribute to better pain measurement.

REFERENCES

1. McGrath PJ, Unruh A. *Pain in children and adolescents*. Amsterdam: Elsevier, 1987.
2. Ross DM, Ross SA. Assessment of pediatric pain. *Issues Comprehens Nurs* 1988;11:73–91.
3. Beyer JE, Wells N. The assessment of pain in children. *Pediatr Clin North Am* 1989;36:837–854.
4. Savedra MC, Tesler MD. Assessing children's and adolescent's pain. *Pediatrician* 1989;16:24–29.
5. McGrath PA. *Pain in children: nature, assessment, treatment*. New York: Guilford, 1990.
6. Finley GA, McGrath PJ. *Measurement of pain in infants and children*. Seattle: IASP Press, 1998.
7. Gaffney A, Dunne EA. Developmental aspects of children's definitions of pain. *Pain* 1986;26:105–117.
8. Gaffney A. Pain: perspectives in childhood [Dissertation]. Cork: University College, 1987.
9. Gaffney A. How children describe pain: s study of words and analogies used by 5 to 14 year-olds. In: Dubner R, Gebhart GF, Bond MR, eds. *Proceedings of the 5th World Congress on Pain*. Amsterdam: Elsevier, 1988:341–347.
10. World Health Organization. *International classification of impairments, disabilities, and handicaps*. Geneva: World Health Organization, 1980.
11. Matthews JR, McGrath PJ, Pigeon H. Assessment and measurement of pain in children. In: Schechter NL, Berde CB, Yaster M, eds. *Pain in infants, children, and adolescents*. Baltimore: Williams & Wilkins, 1993: 97–111.
12. International Association for the Study of Pain Task Force on Taxonomy. *Classification of chronic pain: descriptions of chronic pain syndromes and definitions of pain terms*, 2nd ed. Seattle: IASP Press, 1994.
13. Johnston CC. Psychometric issues in the measurement of pain. In: Finley GA, McGrath PJ, eds. *Measurement of pain in infants and children*. Seattle: IASP Press, 1998.
14. Bieri D, Reeve RA, Champion GD, et al. The Faces Pain Scale for the self-assessment of the severity of pain experienced by children: Development, initial validation, and preliminary investigation for ratio scale properties. *Pain* 1990;41:139–150.
15. Fanurik D, Koh JL, Schmitz ML, et al. Pain assessment and treatment in children with cognitive impairment: a survey of nurses' and physicians' beliefs. *Clin J Pain* 2000;15:304–312.
16. Flavell JH. *The developmental psychology of Jean Piaget*. New York: Von Nostrand Reinhold, 1963.
17. Johnston CC, Strada ME. Acute pain response in infants: a multidimensional description. *Pain* 1986;24: 373–382.
18. Finke W, Buttner W, Reckert S, et al. Respiratory and circulatory items as predictors of the postoperative analgesic demand in newborns and infants. *Anasthesiol Intensivmed Notfallmed Schmerzther* 1999;34:747–757.
19. Grunau RVE, Craig KD. Pain expression in neonates: facial action and cry. *Pain* 1987;28:395–410.
20. Katz ER, Kellerman J, Siegel SE. Distress behavior in children with cancer undergoing medical procedures: developmental considerations. *J Consult Clin Psychol* 1980;48:356–365.
21. Jay SM, Ozolina M, Elliott C, et al. Assessment of children's distress during painful medical procedures. *J Health Psychol* 1983;2:133–147.
22. McGrath PJ, Johnson G, Goodman JT, et al. The CHEOPS: a behavioral scale to measure postoperative pain in children. In: Fields HL, Dubner R, Cervero F, eds. *Advances in pain research and therapy*. New York: Raven Press, 1985:395–402.
23. Gauvain-Piquard A, Rodary C, Rezvani A, et al. Pain in children aged 2-6 years: a new observational rating scale elaborated in a pediatric oncology unit—preliminary report. *Pain* 1987;31:177–188.
24. O'Hara M, McGrath PJ, D'Astous J, et al. Oral morphine versus injected meperidine (Demerol) for pain relief in children after orthopedic surgery. *J Pediatr Orthop Surg* 1987;7:78–82.
25. Chambers CT, Reid GJ, McGrath PJ, et al. Development and preliminary validation of a postoperative pain measure for parents. *Pain* 1996;68:307–313.
26. Piaget J, Inhelder B, Smezinska A. *The child's conception of geometry*. London: Routledge and Kegan Paul, 1960.
27. Piaget J, Inhelder B. *The child's construction of quantities*. London: Routledge and Kegan Paul, 1977.
28. Case R. Preschool children's understanding of quantity. In: Damon W, ed. *Handbook of child psychology, volume 2*, 5th ed. New York: John Wiley & Sons, 1998.
29. Gelman R. Counting in the preschooler: what does and does not develop? In: Siegler R, ed. *Children's thinking: what develops?* Hillsdale, NJ: Lawrence Erlbaum, 1978:213–242.

30. Gelman R, Baillargeon R. A review of some Piagetian concepts. In: Mussen P, ed. *Handbook of child psychology*, 4th ed. New York: John Wiley & Sons, 1983.
31. Champion GD, Goodenough B, von Baeyer C, et al. Measurement of pain by self-report. In: Finley GA, McGrath PJ, eds. *Measurement of pain in infants and children*. Seattle: IASP Press, 1998.
32. McCaffery M. Pain relief for the child: problem areas and selected non-pharmacological methods. *Pediatr Nurs* 1977;3:11–16.
33. Piaget J. *The moral judgement of the child*. Harmondsworth, UK: Penguin Books, 1977.
34. Goodenough B, Thomas W, Champion GD, et al. Unravelling age effects and sex differences in needle pain: ratings of sensory intensity and unpleasantness of venipuncture pain by children and their parents. *Pain* 1999;80:179–190.
35. Craig KD. The facial display of pain. In: Finley GA, McGrath PJ, eds. *Measurement of pain in infants and children*. Seattle: IASP Press, 1998.
36. Bloom L. Language acquisition in its developmental context. In: W. Damon ed. *Handbook of child psychology*, 5th ed. New York: John Wiley & Sons, 1998.
37. McGrath PA, Seifert CE, Speechley KN, et al. A new analogue scale for assessing children's pain: an initial validation study. *Pain* 1996;64:435–443.
38. Chambers CT, Craig KD. Smiling face as anchor for pain intensity scales—reply. *Pain* 2001;89:297–300.
39. Borke H. Interpersonal perception of young children: egocentrism or empathy? *Dev Psychol* 1971;5:263–269.
40. Calam RM, Jimmieson P, Cox AD, et al. Can computer based assessment help us to understand children's pain? *Eur J Anaesthesiol* 2000;17:284–288.
41. Chi MTH. Conceptual change with and across ontological categories. In: Giere R, ed. *Cognitive models of science: Minnesota studies in the philosophy of science*. Minneapolis: University of Minnesota Press, 1994.
42. Kuhn D. Afterword. In: Kuhn D, Siegler R, eds. *Cognition, perception, and language*. New York: John Wiley & Sons, 1998.
43. Hester NO, Foster R, Kristensen K. Measurement of pain in children: generalizability and validity of the pain ladder and the poker-chip tool In: Tyler DC, Krane EJ, eds. *Advances in pain research and therapy, volume 15: pediatric pain*. New York: Raven Press, 1990:79–84.
44. Franzen OG, Ahlquist ML The intensive aspect of information processing in the intradental A-delta systems in man: a psychophysiological analysis of sharp dental pain. *Behav Brain Res* 1989;33:1–11.
45. Bull NJ. *Moral judgement from childhood to adolescence*. London: Routledge and Kegan Paul, 1969.
46. Kagan J. The psychology of sex differences. In: Kagan J, ed. *The growth of the child*. London: Methuen, 1979.
47. Harter S, Whitesell NR. Developmental changes in children's understanding of single, multiple, and blended emotion concepts. In: Saarni C, Harris PL, eds. *Children's understanding of emotion*. Cambridge: Cambridge University Press, 1989.
48. Breau LM, McGrath PJ, Camfield C, et al. Preliminary validation of an observational pain checklist for persons with cognitive impairments and inability to communicate verbally. *Dev Med Child Neurol* 2000;42:609–616.

9

Cultural Considerations in Children's Pain

Bruce A. Bernstein and Lee M. Pachter

Culture is the way of life of a people. It consists of conventional patterns of thought and behavior, including values, beliefs, rules of conduct, political organization, economic activity, and the like, which are passed on from one generation to the next by learning—and not by inheritance (1).

The observation that culture or ethnicity is important in assessing and managing children's pain is an axiom in the pediatric pain literature (2–4). In fact, several national health care societies have made an awareness of "culture" with regard to pain control an official policy matter. The American Nurses Association, for example, in their policy statement on cultural diversity in nursing practice, maintains that "culture is one of the organizing concepts upon which nursing is based and defined" and recommends a range of culturally sensitive practices (5). In its pediatric *Operative and Medical Procedures* assessment guidelines, the U.S. Agency for Health Care Policy and Research notes "children who may have difficulty communicating their pain require particular attention. This includes...children from families where the level of education or cultural background differs significantly from that of the health care team." It is further recommended that, as part of their assessments, providers "elicit from the family culturally determined beliefs about pain and medical care" (6).

The precise contribution or issues that specific cultures bring to pediatric pain experience and control, however, are more ambiguous than might be expected from these positions. Our objective in this chapter is to review current knowledge and thinking about this matter and to reflect on clinical and research implications of what we know.

THEORETIC BASIS

The theoretic principles underlying the idea that culture[1] is influential in pain experience include:

1. The knowledge of individual variation in the perception of and response to apparently similar painful stimuli and illness conditions (8,9);
2. The belief that pain experience is mediated by cognitive or psychologic factors, especially anxiety, attention, emotion, fear, depression, fatigue, and the underlying attitudes of the patient toward pain and illness (10–15);
3. The recognition of differing explanatory models or cultural constructions of illness experience between cultural groups (which may be substantially different from biomedical models) (16–18);
4. The assumption that concepts of the meaning of and behavioral norms in re-

[1]Culture is an ethereal concept with a multitude of definitions, usually including in some form a set of cognitive features (e.g., beliefs, values), public and private behaviors, habits, and traditions that are shared within distinct populations. Cultures typically include ideals, values, and strategies, often expressed in precepts and aphorisms, for dealing with pain and suffering. Ethnicity or ethnic group, often used synonymously with culture in the medical literature, has a subtly different meaning for social scientists, connoting a social group within a larger cultural and social system, which self-identifies and is identified as such by the larger society based on a matrix of cultural and/or physical traits (7). It makes sense, therefore, to speak of the culture of an ethnic group, but not the ethnicity of a culture.

sponse to pain and other aspects of illness are learned from parents, other people, and experiences in the social environment (2,19–21).

Acute or chronic pain and the experience of illness always occur within a cultural context. This includes the cultural or ethnic background of the individual and the social setting in which events unfold. Cultural factors, therefore, might reasonably be expected to influence all aspects of the typical sequence of a painful episode—perception of pain (threshold), tolerance, behavioral/emotional response, individual and outside strategies to address the pain (coping, treatments), and response to these strategies.

More specifically, culture is often hypothesized to be a determinant of an individual's subjective experience of pain and suffering, i.e., the private or internal perception of how and how much a particular occurrence or condition hurts. Culture also undoubtedly plays a significant role in shaping patterns of behavior in response to pain. Although research on the development of pain behavior is limited, there is little dispute that much of it is substantially learned via mechanisms such as modeling, direct explanations and instructions, and experience of what others do in response to signals of distress (19,22,23). In addition to strongly influencing the meaning of pain for the individual, culture provides models for appropriate forms of communication and coping strategies in response to pain. To the extent that subjective experience and response to pain can be separated, therefore, members of different cultures might be expected to respond differently to similar types or amounts of pain.

This is not to suggest that all members of a particular cultural or ethnic group can be stereotyped to have a discrete set of beliefs and behaviors. Substantial *intracultural variation* exists within any cultural group. Individuals and families form *personal health styles* that incorporate modal cultural health beliefs and behaviors with personal past experience, education, individual style, and current circumstances.

Acquisition of culture begins in infancy and continues throughout childhood and into adult life. Through both passive and active processes, the child learns which types of behavior are appropriate for different situations as well as the degree of allowable variation from the norm. Thus, culture would be expected to influence pain experience and behavior beginning in early childhood. In addition, patterns of parent and other adult interactions with children in pain would be expected to reflect culturally based attitudes toward child-rearing, pain, and illness. These attitudes might also affect health care seeking behavior, decisions, and interactions with providers.

Although the theoretic argument is substantial, empiric details concerning the influence of culture on children's pain are limited. Most studies addressing culture and pain reported in the literature have been conducted with adults. Even if the influence of culture on adult pain were well specified, the applicability of this knowledge to pediatric populations would need further specification. To make matters worse, the adult data, in aggregate, provide an ambiguous picture of the role of culture in pain experience and response.

METHODOLOGIC ISSUES

Several methodologic challenges impede the development of a reliable, generalized perspective on the role of culture in children's pain. Definition and measurement of pain are variable. Ethical considerations constrain generation of some types of comparative data. In addition, the "file drawer problem," in meta-analytic terminology, is a significant obstacle to forming firm conclusions from the literature. That is, in assessing the empiric information, we are likely to be missing results of studies in which comparisons between cultural groups were made but no significant differences were found.

Perhaps the most serious impediment to synthesizing available data has been the lack of standard and rigorously applied criteria for categorizing an individual's culture or ethnic group. Categorization criteria include appearance as assessed by researchers or clinical staff, notations (usually of anonymous origin) on clinical records, and self-description. Many reports do not specify the method for identifying cultural group. *Culture* and *ethnicity* are frequently confounded with *race*, a concept based primarily on physical appearance and presumed genotypic similarities of populations. The notion of race appears to be more concrete for some researchers. Racial groups (e.g., white, black, Hispanic, Oriental), however, may actually be heterogeneous with regard to cultural factors likely to be of interest in the study of pain. The construct of race has itself undergone considerable re-examination among human biologists in the past decade (24), and whether race is a meaningful concept remains a controversial matter. The American Association of Physical Anthropologists, for example, in their 1996 statement on biologic aspects of race, maintain "pure races, in the sense of genetically homogenous populations, do not exist in the human species today, nor is there any evidence that they have ever existed in the past.... There is no national, religious, linguistic or cultural group or economic class that constitutes a race" (25).

Because of the unscientific nature of the terms *culture*, *ethnicity*, and *race* as used in the medical literature, several public health researchers advocate de-emphasis of these categories, suggesting they do little more than advance stereotypes (26–28). Ethnic and racial categories, however, although ambiguous on close examination, are in fact conventionally recognized and the basis of substantial thought and research in medicine. Thus, with the methodologic caveats noted, it makes sense to briefly review the adult literature on pain and culture, emphasizing aspects that might be important in thinking about children.

ADULT DATA ON CULTURE AND PAIN

Systematic study of the role of culture in adult pain first appeared in the scientific literature in the early 1940s with the reports of Sherman (29) and Chapman and Jones (30). Available data can be categorized into essentially three types: descriptive ethnomedical material focused on health beliefs and practices, some addressing pain issues specifically; observations and comparative studies of clinical pain; and experimental pain studies conducted in laboratory settings.

Ethnomedicine

An extensive literature detailing the unique cultural constructions of illness of a large number of culturally distinct populations has accumulated over the past half century (16–18,31). Even the more general discussions of health beliefs and practices may provide useful insights into the suffering and pain behaviors of specific cultural group members. In a literature review introducing a study with facial pain patients, Lipton and Marbach (32) listed 29 cultural groups for which various aspects of the clinical pain experience have been addressed. Several ethnographic reports have appeared subsequently, adding to the cross-cultural database (33–39). These reports tend to rely on qualitative methodologies and examine traits such as concepts of illness, patterns of pain perception and expression (e.g., language, body awareness), cultural ideals, and characteristic patterns of response to pain and suffering.

A more extensive review of this literature is beyond the scope of this discussion. The nature and utility of this type of data, however, are illustrated by Sargent's (33) description of the Bariba, a major West African ethnic group of sedentary agriculturists inhabiting Northern Benin and Nigeria. Based on interviews with Bariba women, indigenous midwives, and other key informants and on observations of deliveries, Sargent described a cultural ideal of stoicism in the face of pain, apparent in the mythology and proverbs of this group as well as evident in public pain behavior.

The Bariba, in her analysis, conceptualized pain response in the context of shame and honor. "To display pain," one informant told her, "would indicate a lack of courage. Cowardice, in Bariba tradition, is the essence of shame and rather than live in shame, a true Bariba would kill himself." Proscriptions for displays of pain are described for women in childbirth, men wounded in war, and boys and girls undergoing circumcision. Typical expressions of pain in this culture included "(the sound) *wee*, clicking of the teeth and shaking one hand in the air." These behaviors were often met with mockery. Bariba expressed a fatalistic attitude toward pain, saying that either they would die or not, and, either way, crying out would have no effect.

The report, therefore, describes a cultural construction of pain including an ideology concerning its meaning, familiar patterns of pain behavior, and mechanisms for teaching and maintaining appropriate responses. The clinical implications that these types of observations suggest are exemplified by the comments of Honeyman and Jacobs (40) on their experience providing health care to a small aboriginal population living in the central Australia desert. While assessing the presence of low back pain, they were struck by their patients' high pain tolerance relative to Western or European standards. This behavior began in early childhood and featured a denial or unwillingness to talk about pain. Pain was not viewed as a health problem; thus, people were not motivated to consult physicians about its occurrence. One would expect, therefore, that serious painful disease would likely be presented later in its course or not to physicians unless special efforts to elicit symptoms were made.

Comparative Studies of Clinical Pain

The empiric evidence supporting the importance of culture in pain is based substantially on a number of studies comparing cultural groups in various dimensions of clinical pain experience. Zborowski's (41,42) research conducted in the early 1950s with male patients in a New York veterans' hospital is generally accorded seminal status in this tradition. Drawing on ethnographic data collected over a 3-year period, Zborowski articulated a framework for the study of culture and pain response. This included (a) a rationale for categorizing ethnic groups; (b) exploration of culturally specific attitudes directly related to the quality of pain and suffering, notably the meaning of the pain for the patient; (c) an accounting of attitudes or cultural traits indirectly related to pain experience, such as present versus future time orientation, and (d) eliciting self-assessments of response styles.

In his paper and subsequent monograph, Zborowski provided classic descriptions of typical ethnic styles in the experience of pain. Jewish and Italian patients described themselves and were observed to be emotional, expressive, and dramatic about their pain and generally uninhibited about communicating their distress to others. "Old Americans" (individuals of white Anglo-Saxon ancestry whose ancestors had for several generations been born in the United States) and Irish were less emotional and expressive than the former groups and more likely to want to hide or, in the case of the Irish, deny their pain. With Zborowski's reports, the pain response patterns of Old Americans became identified as representing the dominant culture and the expectation of the medical system, and this group became a reference group for future studies.

Several comparative studies have been conducted since Zborowski's research. Outcome measures have typically been patients' subjective assessments of pain qualities such as intensity, interference with normal functioning, attitudes toward pain being experienced, presenting symptoms, pain language, anxiety, health care seeking behavior, and coping. These have been supplemented in some cases by the observations and assessments of physicians and others, including quantification of analgesia consumption. In keeping with methodologic developments, pain outcome measures have become increasingly quantitative and have relied more on standardized assessment tools such as the McGill Pain Questionnaire. A range of two to six groups has been compared. However, the cultural groups included and associated clinical circumstances or pathologies have not been the same across studies. The majority includes Anglo Americans (43–46), Anglo Canadians (47), or whites (48–54). Other groups include Italian Americans or immigrants (32,55–58), Italian Australians (58), Italian and Irish Catholics (59), Irish Americans or immigrants (32,55, 56), Jewish Americans (32,56), blacks (32,48, 53,54,56,60–63), African Americans (49), Hispanics (48,49,61,64), Puerto Ricans in the United States (32,54,63), Australians (40,58), American Indians (61), East Indians, Ukrainians and Hutterites (47), Polish Americans and French Canadians (57), Chinese (45,65–67), Japanese (44,65), Koreans (68), Asians (60, 69), Jamaican immigrants (69), and Scandinavians (66,67). Painful conditions addressed have included arthritis, cancer, childbirth, chronic pain, facial pain, fibromyalgia, heart disease, long-bone fractures, low back pain, and postoperative pain. Several more extensive summaries of these data are available (32,70–73).

Most of these reports describe some significant variation in pain outcomes comparing some, but usually not all, cultural groups studied. Differences in pain response outcomes are more typically found than differences in pain perception and ratings of intensity. The data, however, are contradictory with regard to a consistent pattern comparing cultures. There is a tendency, particularly in the earlier data, for Anglo individuals to report less pain intensity and response than other groups, but this is not always the case. A model that equally fits the data is that subjects who are members of the majority cultural group or who more closely match the ethnicity of the care providers are more likely to report lower pain intensity and demonstrate less response than their minority counterparts. Minority and lower socioeconomic status groups tend to present with more advanced disease and carry higher pain burdens.

A handful of studies concerning analgesia consumption has added an important dimension to the exploration of culture and pain control. In 1981, Streltzer and Wade (65) reported findings of a study of narcotic administration during the first five postoperative days among 270 patients who underwent cholecystectomy representing five ethnic groups at two major Honolulu hospitals. White and Hawaiian patients received significantly more analgesia, expressed as meperidine milligram equivalents, than Filipino, Japanese, and Chinese patients. After controlling for age, gender, and a number of other demographic variables, ethnicity predicted a small but significant portion of the variance in analgesia use. "Whether this reflects ethnic differences in analgesic requirements," the authors observed "or...cultural bias in treatment remains to be determined."

A few subsequent studies have generated additional data on the question but not a definitive answer. Todd et al. (74) reviewed analgesia prescription for 139 patients presenting in a Los Angeles emergency department with long bone fractures. Hispanic patients were significantly less likely to be prescribed analgesia than non-Hispanic whites. Todd et al. and another group of researchers later published a similar study of 217 long bone fracture patients at an Atlanta emergency department (75). In this study, black patients were significantly less likely than whites to receive analgesia. In both studies, ethnicity remained significant when controlling for potential confounding variables such as time since the injury and need for fracture reduction. Choi et al. (76), in contrast, found no difference in analgesia administration for patients with long bone fractures in a London hospital according to ethnic group (white, Bangladeshi, and other). Ng et al. (77) studied postoperative analgesia among 250 white, black, and Hispanic patients hospitalized for open reduction and internal fixation of a limb fracture. White patients received significantly more daily morphine equivalents than Hispanics, with blacks intermediate but not statistically different from these two groups. In another study in San Diego, CA, Ng et al. (78) compared patient-controlled analgesia for post-operative pain (head, neck, torso, and extremities) among 454 Asian, black, Hispanic, and white subjects. No differences were found in the amount of narcotic self-administered, but significant differences, controlling for potential confounders, were found in the amount prescribed according to ethnic group.

Pain assessment factors, particularly language and cross-cultural communication issues, are logical objects of study for insights into these findings. Studies of cross-cultural issues in pain assessment are limited, however. Todd et al. (79) compared patient and emergency department physician assessments of pain severity for 69 Hispanic and 139 non-Hispanic white level I trauma center patients in Los Angeles. No significant differences in patient severity ratings, physician severity ratings, or disparities between physician and patient ratings in association with ethnic group were found. Calvillo and Flaskerud (43), in a study of 22 Mexican-American and 38 Anglo-American female cholecystectomy patients found that, although patient ratings were not significantly different between cultural groups, nurses rated the pain experienced as significantly greater among the Anglo-American women (43). Similarly, Sheiner et al. (80), in a study in Israel with 225 Jewish and 192 Bedouin parturients, found that labor pain intensity was no different between ethnic groups as rated by patients but was rated higher for Jewish than Bedouin women by the study observers—a Jewish physician and midwife. Harrison et al. (81) studied 50 Arabic-speaking patients hospitalized in a government general hospital in the United Arab Emirates. Patient pain ratings were compared with ratings by two nurses for each patient who had provided major care, one Arabic- and one non-Arabic speaker. Patient ratings were significantly correlated with ratings of nurses who spoke Arabic, but not with those of non-Arabic speakers.

Pharmacogenetics associated with ethnic or racial groups are also theoretically worth exploring with respect to analgesic requirements and consumption. A few studies are available; almost all compared Asian and white groups. Findings from pharmacokinetic studies include lower clearance rates of acetaminophen in Asians compared with whites (82), a higher excretion of unchanged drug after a single oral dose of codeine in Chinese compared with whites (83), and a lower response to morphine as reflected by respiratory and cardiovascular parameters but greater gastrointestinal symptoms in Chinese compared with whites (84). In addition to the study of Streltzer and Wade of patients who underwent cholecystectomy reviewed above (65), additional studies have found decreased opioid demand or requirement for Asians versus whites in various clinical circumstances, i.e., cesarean section (85), abdominal surgery (86,87), and appendectomy (88). In contrast, in addition to the Ng et al. (78) surgery study, two studies of postsurgical patients found no differences in analgesia requirements comparing these groups (89,90). Available data were reviewed by Wood et al. (91) and Lee et al. (92). Differences tend to be small and the populations represented are limited; thus, the clinical implications of these data are unclear.

Failure to adequately address intracultural variation is a generic shortcoming in these studies. More recently, quantification of dimensions that vary intraculturally, such as socioeconomic status, is being included in research designs. Acculturation (93) is of particular interest, following the hypothesis that a cultural or ethnic group, particularly an immigrant population, tends to acculturate to the dominant society. Thus, Lipton and Marbach (32) included sociodemographic variables, social assimilation, cultural assimilation, psychologic distress, and clinical variables along with ethnic group categorization as independent variables in a study of the pain perceptions of patients with face pain. The list of independent variables in a study of chronic pain in six ethnic groups by Bates et al. (57) included sociodemographic characteristics, "heritage consistency," locus of control, and clinical characteristics.

These data indicate that cultural differences in pain experience, in particular differences in response, can be demonstrated by comparing a number of ethnic groups in a wide variety of situations. The mix of ethnic groups, outcome measures, and clinical conditions, however, makes it inappropriate to generalize beyond this broad conclusion. Frequently, intracultural variation in the pain experience, however measured, is the same as or greater than intercultural differences.

Experimental Pain

Investigation of experimental pain has paralleled that of clinical pain since the 1940s. Typically, subjects are grouped according to cultural or ethnic group—actually often race—and exposed to a standardized unpleasant stimulus. These have included measured amounts of radiant heat, contact heat, pressure, electric shock, and exposure to cold water. Pain sensation variables (primarily threshold, unpleasantness, and tolerance) have been the outcomes studied.

Since 1943, at least 15 of these studies have been published, involving comparisons of two or more ethnic groups (29,30,44,94–105). Anglo Americans, whites, blacks, African Americans, Orientals, and groups based on religious affiliation account for most of the ethnic categories studied. Zatzick and Dimsdale (106) reviewed a majority of these studies in detail.

Although these studies provide ambiguous information about culture and pain, with little speculation about what may underlie their findings, several have had important impacts on the evolution of thinking on this matter. Two sets of studies comparing Christian and Jewish subjects revealed differences in pain response parameters (tolerance, autonomic variables). On retesting Jewish subjects, Lambert et al. (97) found a significant increase in pain tolerance among the subjects who were told that Protestants "could take more pain." Poser (98) added an additional significant variable: *the ethnicity of the examiner*. In his study, Jewish subjects tested twice for pressure pain demonstrated significantly larger pain sensitivity ranges (difference between pain threshold and tolerance) when the experimenter was Christian than when he or she was Jewish. A study by Woodrow et al. (102) of tolerance to pain induced by mechanical pressure on the Achilles tendon conducted with 41,119 subjects is frequently cited as evidence of ethnic differences in pain experience. Whites were found to be statistically significantly more tolerant than blacks, who were in turn significantly more tolerant than Orientals. Although the sample size is large, the groups in these studies are broadly categorized. Race was determined "by observation of the subject's skin color," and no data on ethnicity of the examiners were collected. Two additional studies in the southeastern United States comparing African-American and white subjects' sensitivity to thermal pain have recently been published (104,105). Similar findings of lower pain tolerance in African Americans were noted. The designs also featured similar classification problems, while one study included an analysis of the effect of examiner's race.

These experimental pain studies have consistently found that pain threshold does not vary across ethnic groups. However, all the studies found differences between ethnic groups in some pain parameter, usually some measure of pain tolerance. Because of differences in the type of experimental pain utilized, inconsistencies in how groups were constituted, and an inconsistent matrix of findings, further conclusions such as characterization of pain response profiles for specific ethnic groups are not supported. It is also well recognized that experimental pain may be a useless model for clinical pain.

DATA ON CHILDREN, CULTURE, AND PAIN

Only a few studies address culture and children's pain. Attention has been paid to the cross-cultural validity and reliability of assessment tools. Pain concepts and language among children have been explored within a few cultures. In a few cases, cultural differences in the pain experience of children with similar pathologies have been observed.

Cultural Differences in Children's Pain Description

Few empiric data are available concerning the effect of culture on children's perceptions and communication about painful episodes. Abu-Saad (107,108) studied a sample of Latin-American, Arab-American, and Chinese-American children aged 9 to 12 years attempting to see whether the children in these groups described their pain experiences in different terms. Through semistructured interviews, the children answered open-ended questions about causes, descriptions, colors, coping mechanisms, and a range of feelings about pain.

Minimal cross-cultural differences were found. In all cultural groups, most pain descriptors centered on sensory terms. The Chinese-American and Arab-American children listed more affective and evaluative terms than the Latin-American children did. In general, the Arab-American children provided more responses per child than children of the other ethnic groups. With regard to causes of pain, Latin-American children most often listed aches and pains (such as headaches, stomach aches, and earaches), Arab-American and Chinese-American children most often listed falls, and Chinese-American children often described psychologic causes such as "people making fun of me." No statistical analyses evaluating the strength or significance of these findings were included. The children studied were all first-generation Americans, and interviews were all conducted in English. Thus, these children were likely to have been highly acculturated to the American lifestyle.

Abu-Saad (109) reported similar data among samples of Dutch children. Pain descriptions of Arabic children are included in a study by Harrison et al. (110). The research of Gaffney (111) on Irish children and that of Savedra et al. (112) on American children also provide data about the development of children's pain language and concepts in a unicultural context.

Cultural patterns in parents' attitudes and instructions concerning children's pain are theoretically important with regard to the development of pain concepts and behaviors, but surprisingly little has been published in this area. A study by Fritz et al. (113) with Vietnamese refugees exploring parenting beliefs, discipline techniques, and parental expectations of children's reactions to pain suggests the potential value of this research direction. Data were collected via interpreter-assisted, semistructured interviews with 14 parents recently resettled in a northeastern U.S. city. Most respondents were unfamiliar with Western-style medicine and relied on traditional techniques—balms, cupping, and coin rubbing for first-line treatment of pain. Sickness, evil spirits, and imbalance in life's elements were identified as causes of pain. Although crying and complaints were acceptable for young children, older children (age 8 and older) were expected to respond stoically to pain and not to be comforted with physical affection.

Cross-Cultural Issues in the Validity of Pain Assessment

A few studies explored the validity and reliability of standard pediatric pain assessment strategies in non-Anglo populations. Pfefferbaum et al. (114) and Adams (115) studied the influence of cultural heritage and acculturation on the perception and expression of pain in a group of Anglo and Hispanic (predominantly Mexican-American) oncology patients between the ages of 3 and 15. Outcome measures included two self-reports: the Faces Scale (116) and the Children's Procedural Interview, a postprocedure, structured interview developed for the study, and two observational assessments: the Procedure Behavior Check List (PBCL) (117), and caregiver ratings. The study assessed the validity and reliability of these instruments in both the Anglo and Hispanic groups studied and examined differences between the two groups regarding perception and assessment of painful episodes.

For the PBCL, although construct validity (as measured by correlation between PBCL and scores on the Faces Scale) was determined to be high in both groups, concurrent validity (correlation between PBCL and caregiver assessments) was low in the Hispanic sample. Similarly, reliability (as measured by Cronbach α) was high (0.78) for the Anglo children but low (0.54) for the Hispanic sample. The reliability coefficients for the Children's Procedural Interview and Faces Scale were high in both groups. These findings suggest that observational scales (specifically the PBCL) and interviews may not be as reliable for pain assessment as self-report scales in Hispanic study groups. This appears to make intuitive sense, especially if the rater or observer is a non-Hispanic. The Faces Scale appears to be a reliable self-report instrument in this Hispanic population. The fact that this type of scale is less language bound may account for some of this success.

Aun et al. (118) provided another study evaluating the cultural appropriateness of a standard assessment method with their investigation of the optimal spatial orientation of visual analog scales in a Chinese patient population. Written Chinese characters are read vertically downward and from right to left. The authors hypothesized that this fact may make traditional Western visual analog scales (which are normally oriented horizontally and from left to right) less appropriate in their patient population. They found that the use of vertically oriented visual analog scales resulted in less error than horizontally oriented scales. This finding suggests that cultural background may influence in unexpected ways the reliability of pain assessment tools developed in a single cultural context.

The development and validation by Beyer and Knott (119) of the African-American and Hispanic versions of the Oucher Scale have been an important accomplishment in addressing this issue. The Oucher Scale, which is routinely employed in children's pain management and research, was originally developed in 1980 as self-report of pain intensity for white children 3 to 12 years old (120). Children are provided with a set of six photographs of children's faces representing apparently little to very substantial discomfort. The new versions feature culturally specific photographs, that is pictures of children who more closely match the physical characteristics of African-American and Hispanic children. These tools, therefore, address cultural issues in accuracy of pain assessment. They were also designed to promote cultural sensitivity and self-esteem for minority, nonwhite children within the majority health care system.

Cultural Differences in the Clinical Pain Experience of Children

Because theories of cultural influences on pain experience are based essentially on cognitive factors, little ethnically associated effects on infant pain would be expected. Therefore, findings of ethnic group differences in infants' responses to injections in two studies are surprising. Lewis et al. (121) compared behavioral and cortisol responses of Japanese and American white 4-month-old infants after routine inoculation. The white infants had a significantly more intense initial affective response and a longer latency to quiet than the Japanese infants. The Japanese infants, however, had a greater cortisol response. In a subsequent study, Rosmus et al. (122) compared behavioral response to injections as measured by the Neonatal Facial Coding System of 26 Canadian born-Chinese and 26 non-Chinese 2-month-old infants. A multivariate analysis of variance found one facial (brow bulge) and two cry (duration and cry bursts) parameters to be significantly greater for Chinese infants. Researchers hypothesized that contextual variables, such as mother–infant interaction factors and ability to sustain arousal, might be responsible for the differences. They also observed that the contrasting findings of these two studies underscore the dangers of collapsing individuals into broad categories such as "Asian."

A few other studies are available comparing the clinical pain experience of children in different ethnic groups. These are primarily associated with procedure and postoperative pain. Pfefferbaum et al. (114), for example, evaluated differences between Hispanic and Anglo oncology patients in pain perception after an invasive diagnostic procedure (either spinal tap or bone marrow aspiration). Scores on the Faces Scale were similar in both groups. The only ethnic differences found were in parental level of anxiety, as measured by the state-trait anxiety inventory (123), on which the Hispanic parents scored significantly higher.

van Aken et al. (21) studied 60 Dutch and 115 American children ranging in age from 8 months to 18 years undergoing cancer diagnostic procedures. Their study involved assessment of pain response with the Procedure Behavior Rating Scale during three phases of the procedure. Multivariate analyses of variance found no significant differences in overall distress between cultures, although several significant interactions with age and phase were noted. Americans demonstrated more anxiety and greater distress, particularly at younger ages. The researchers were unable to unravel the effects of culture or national location from differences in setting—the larger, impersonal American clinic versus the smaller, more personal health care setting of the Dutch sample.

Bohannon (124) compared the surgery-related pain experience of 25 African-American and 30 white 3- to 7-year-old children in a Miami hospital. Outcomes included physiologic variables (vital signs), a pain self-report (Wong Baker Faces), and a behavioral observation (Children's Hospital of Eastern Ontario Pains Scale). African-American children had significantly higher physiologic parameters and lower behavioral distress scores as assessed by observation. No significant difference was found in self-report of pain or amounts of pain medication administered.

Hu et al. reported lower levels of analgesia in a sample of Chinese pediatric burn (125) and surgical (herniorrhaphy and appendectomy) (126) patients compared with "levels common for children in Western countries with comparable injuries or procedures." Their hypothesis that "pain tolerance of Chinese children might be higher than that of Occidentals" clearly requires further exploration with studies in which pathology and availability of analgesia can be accurately compared across groups.

A study conducted in London by Thomas and Rose (69) on pain associated with ear piercing found ethnic differences in pain intensity ratings as self-reported on the pain-related index subscale of the McGill Pain Questionnaire. Subjects were 28 Afro West Indians, 28 Anglo Saxons and 28 Asians aged 15 to 25 years. Afro West Indians gave the ear piercing pain significantly lower pain ratings than Anglo Saxons and Asians, who were not different from one another. Subjects were also asked to rate their coping ability and their sense of their parents' reaction to minor injury when they were young, both on a five-point scale. Coping and parents' response ratings were significantly negatively correlated (i.e., greater ability to cope was associated with less parental concern). However, neither of these variables was significantly correlated with pain intensity ratings.

Virtually no studies have been reported concerning cross-cultural variation in children's pain experience associated with chronic illness. In a study with adolescent oncology patients in San Antonio, TX, Zeltzer and LeBaron (127) found no significant differences between Mexican-American and Anglo-American children in trait anxiety or impact of illness, measured with a standard battery of psychologic tests. The cultural context of chronic disease and pain has received substantial attention in the adult literature and would be a logical research focus with respect to children's pain.

RESEARCH AND CLINICAL IMPLICATIONS

It is well accepted that culture or ethnicity is an important consideration with respect to children's pain, manifesting its influence through attitudes such as the meaning of illness and pain and through learned behavior patterns and norms. However, empiric data on differences in pain experience and response patterns comparing children of various cultures are limited.

There is also limited information on how children's concepts of meaning and learned behavior with respect to pain develop. That researchers and summarists mean different things by "culture" and "ethnicity" further complicates the inquiry. Frequently, the groupings do not differentiate on the basis of the shared characteristics, such as explanatory models of illness, that would be expected to be associated with differences in pain experience; thus, the frequent finding that intracultural variation is as large or larger than that between cultures should not surprise us.

It is not clear exactly what it is about culture or ethnicity among *children* that we should be aware of or study with respect to pain. Consequently, there is no well-accepted model for grouping cultures or ethnic groups. No formula, therefore, factors the importance of culture into the assessment of pain and effectiveness of its management in children.

Despite the ambiguities, however, our recommendation is that clinical care and research concerned with children's pain should be undertaken with a culturally sensitive approach (128,129). An awareness of culture must be used with caution. Care must be taken to avoid reliance on stereotypes, with the misinterpretation and alienation that these may engender. It is our contention, however, that health care will be of higher quality when the culture of the patient and his or her family is not ignored. It may be helpful to take the view that a patient's identification with a cultural or ethnic group constitutes a probability that the patient will experience pain and respond to suffering in ways that can be better understood by awareness of the patient's culture.

Although the data do not support global or universal propositions about the influence of specific cultures, a substantial number of studies have demonstrated cultural differences in pain experience in specific settings. There are likely benefits, therefore, to reflection on culture and pain issues in local contexts.

In the clinical setting, important cultural considerations may include beliefs about causes of illness and implications of pain, use of folk healers and remedies, acceptability and efficacy of various pain management strategies (e.g., acupuncture, cognitive strategies), and expectations for and normative styles of interaction with health care providers. Clinicians should become familiar with the beliefs and practices common to the cultural groups that they serve, be willing to elicit information concerning these matters in a nonjudgmental manner, and accommodate cultural practices in keeping with acceptable medical practice. Assessing a child's or parent's level of acculturation may be helpful in determining the degree to which the patient adheres to culturally mediated beliefs, knowledge, and attitudes concerning pain.

A wide range of research on cultural influences in pain experience focused specifically on childhood would be welcome, given the paucity of information in this area. This includes more ethnographic information about culturally based attitudes and expectations regarding children's pain experience and behavior as well as cross-cultural comparisons of clinical pain in pediatric populations. In addition, the role of culture for children with chronically painful conditions has received little attention.

Special attention should be given to appropriately categorizing the culture or ethnicity of subjects included in pain studies. Studies employing broad, racially based groupings provide heterogeneous samples and are not likely to advance our understanding. Specific ethnic groups [e.g., Haitians, Jamaicans, and southern U.S. African Americans (rather than blacks); and Puerto Ricans and Mexicans (rather than Hispanics)] should be identified (130–133). Research is further strengthened by measurement of intracultural variation—

levels of acculturation and socioeconomic status, in particular.

A second axiom of the pediatric pain literature is that children's pain tends to be undertreated (134). It may be useful in this context to view the encounter between the child and health care provider as an interaction of two cultures, one being the culture of medicine (135,136). Adequate pain assessment and management may require some special effort in language, appreciation of expectation, and meaning of behaviors, but these issues should be overcome with the careful assessment, communication, and adjustment of therapies that have become the current standard of care in addressing children's pain.

REFERENCES

1. Hatch E. Culture. In: Kuper A, Kuper J, eds. *The social science encyclopedia.* London: Routledge & Kegan Paul, 1985:178–179.
2. McGrath P, Unruh A. *Pain in children and adolescents.* Amsterdam: Elsevier, 1987.
3. Ross D, Ross S. *Childhood pain: current issues, research and management.* Baltimore: Urban & Schwarzenberg, 1988.
4. Zeltzer L, Anderson C, Schechter N. Pediatric pain: current status and new directions. *Curr Probl Pediatr* 1990;20:411–486.
5. Anonymous. Position statement on cultural diversity in nursing practice. *Maryland Nurse* 1995;14:7.
6. Agency for Health Care Policy Research. *Quick reference guide for clinicians: acute pain management in infants, children, and adolescents: operative and medical procedures* (AHCPR Pub. No. 92-0019). Rockville, MD: U.S. Department of Health and Human Services, 1992.
7. Tumin M. Ethnic group. In: Gould J, Kilb W, eds. *A dictionary of the social sciences.* New York: Macmillan, 1964:243.
8. Clark J, Bindra D. Individual differences in pain thresholds. *Can J Psychol* 1956;10:69–76.
9. Gracely R. Methods of testing pain mechanisms in normal man. In: Wall P, Melzack R, eds. *Textbook of pain.* Edinburgh: Churchill-Livingstone, 1989: 257–268.
10. Beecher H. Relationship of significance of wound to pain experienced. *JAMA* 1956;161:1609–1613.
11. Melzack R, Wall P. Pain mechanisms: a new theory. *Science* 1965;150:971–979.
12. Melzack R. Neurophysiological foundation of pain. In: Sternback R, ed. *The psychology of pain.* New York: Raven Press, 1986:1–24.
13. LaVigne J, Schulein M, Hahn Y. Psychological aspects of painful medical conditions in children: I. Developmental aspects and assessment. *Pain* 1986;27: 133–147.
14. LaVigne J, Schulein M, Hahn Y. Psychological aspects of painful medical conditions in children: II. Personality factors, family characteristics, and treatment. *Pain* 1986;27:147–169.
15. McGrath P, Craig K. Developmental and psychological factors in children's pain. *Pediatr Clin North Am* 1989;36:823–836.
16. Kleinman A, Eisenberg L, Good B. Culture, illness and care. *Ann Intern Med* 1977;88:251–258.
17. Harwood A. *Ethnicity and medical care.* Cambridge, MA: Harvard University Press, 1981.
18. Rubel A, Hass M. Ethnomedicine. In: Johnson T, Sargent C, eds. *Medical anthropology: contemporary theory and method,* rev. ed. New York: Praeger, 1996: 113–130.
19. Craig K. Social modeling influences: pain in context. In: Sternback R, ed. *The psychology of pain.* New York: Raven Press, 1986:67–95.
20. Bates M. Ethnicity and pain: a biocultural model. *Soc Sci Med* 1987:24:47–50.
21. van Aken MA, van Lieshout CF, Katz ER, et al. Development of behavioral distress in reaction to acute pain in two cultures. *J Pediatr Psychol* 1989;14: 421–432.
22. Burdette B, Gale E. Pain as a learned response: a review of behavioral factors in chronic pain. *J Am Dent Assoc* 1988;116:881–885.
23. Mikail S, von Beyer C. Pain, somatic focus, and emotional adjustment in children of chronic headache sufferers and controls. *Soc Sci Med* 1990;31:51–59.
24. Cartmill M. The status of the race concept in physical anthropology. *Am Anthropol* 1988;100:651–660.
25. American Association of Physical Anthropologists. AAPA statement on biological aspects of race. *Am J Phys Anthropol* 1996;101:569–570.
26. Bhopal R, Donaldson L. White, European, western, Caucasian, or what? Inappropriate labeling in research on race, ethnicity, and health. *Am J Public Health* 1998;88:1303–1307.
27. Fullilove MT. Comment: abandoning "race" as a variable in public health research—an idea whose time has come. *Am J Public Health* 1998;88:1297–1298.
28. Rivara FP. Use of the terms *race* and *ethnicity*. *Arch Pediatr Adolesc Med* 2000;155:119.
29. Sherman E. Sensitivity to pain. *CMAJ* 1943;48: 437–441.
30. Chapman W, Jones C. Variations in cutaneous and visceral pain sensitivity in normal subjects. *J Clin Invest* 1944;23:81–91.
31. Landy D. *Culture, disease and healing.* New York: Macmillan, 1977.
32. Lipton J, Marbach J. Ethnicity and the pain experience. *Soc Sci Med* 1984;12:1279–1298.
33. Sargent C. Between death and shame: dimensions of pain in Bariba culture. *Soc Sci Med* 1984;19: 1299–1304.
34. Reizian A, Meleis A. Arab-Americans' perceptions of and responses to pain. *Crit Care Nurs* 1986;6:30–37.
35. Migliore S. Punctuality, pain, and time-orientation among Sicilian-Canadians. *Soc Sci Med* 1989;28: 851–859.
36. Morse J. Cultural variation in behavioral response to parturition: childbirth in Fiji. *Med Anthropol* 1989;12: 35–54.
37. Pugh J. The semantics of pain in Indian culture and medicine. *Cult Med Psychiatry* 1991;15:19–43.

38. Villarruel A. Mexican-American cultural meanings, expressions, self-care and dependent-care actions associated with experiences of pain. *Res Nurs Health* 1995;18:427–436.
39. Beck SL. An ethnographic study of factors influencing cancer pain management in South Africa. *Cancer Nurs* 2000;23:91–100.
40. Honeyman P, Jacobs E. Effects of culture on back pain in Australian aboriginals. *Spine* 1996;21:841–843.
41. Zborowski M. Cultural components in response to pain. *J Soc Issues* 1952;8:16–30.
42. Zborowski M. *People in pain*. San Francisco: Jossey-Bass, 1969.
43. Calvillo E, Flaskerud J. Evaluation of the pain response by Mexican American and Anglo American women and their nurses. *J Adv Nurs* 1993;18:451–459.
44. Chapman C, Toru S, Martin R, et al. Comparative effects of acupuncture in Japan and the United states on dental pain perception. *Pain* 1982;12:319–328.
45. Cleeland C, Nakamura Y, Mendoza T, et al. Dimensions of the impact of cancer pain in a four country sample: new information from multidimensional scaling. *Pain* 1996;67:267–273.
46. Lee M, Essoka G. Patient's perception of pain: comparison between Korean-American and Euro-American obstetric patients. *J Cult Diversity* 1998;5:29–37.
47. Morse J, Morse R. Cultural variation in the inference of pain. *J Cross Cult Psychol* 1988;19:232–242.
48. Andersen RE, Crespo CJ, Ling SM, et al. Prevalence of significant knee pain among older Americans: results from the Third National Health and Nutrition Examination Survey. *J Am Geriatr Soc* 1999;47: 1435–1438.
49. Anderson KO, Mendoza TR, Valero V, et al. Minority cancer patients and their providers: pain management attitudes and practice. *Cancer* 2000;88:1929–1938.
50. Bell M, Reeves K. Postoperative pain management in the non-Hispanic white and Mexican American older adult. *Semin Perioper Nurs* 1999;8:7–11.
51. Jordan MS, Lumley MA, Leisen JCC. The relationships of cognitive coping and pain control beliefs to pain and adjustment among African-American and Caucasian women with rheumatoid arthritis. *Arthritis Care Res* 1998;11:80–88.
52. Johnson-Umezulike JM. A comparison of pain perception of elderly African Americans and Caucasians. *Nurs Connect* 1999;12:5–12.
53. Summers RL, Cooper GJ, Carlton FB, et al. Prevalence of atypical chest pain descriptions in a population from the southern United States. *Am J Med Sci* 1999;318: 142–145.
54. Weisenberg M, Kreindler M, Schachat R, et al. Pain: anxiety and attitudes in black, white and Puerto Rican patients. *Psychosom Med* 1975;37:123–134.
55. Koopman C, Eisenthal S, Stoeckle J. Ethnicity in the reported pain, emotional distress, and requests of medical outpatients. *Soc Sci Med* 1985;18:487–490.
56. Flannery R, Sos J, McGovern P. Ethnicity as a factor in the expression of pain. *Psychosomatics* 1981;22: 39–50.
57. Bates M, Rankin-Hill L, Sanchez-Ayendez M. The effects of the cultural context of health care on treatment of and response to chronic pain and illness. *Soc Sci Med* 1997;45:1433–1447.
58. Pesce G. Measurement of reported pain of childbirth: a comparison between Australian and Italian subjects. *Pain* 1987;31:87–92.
59. Zola I. Culture and symptoms—an analysis of patients' presenting complaints. *Am Soc Rev* 1966;31: 615–630.
60. Faucett J, Gordon N, Levine J. Differences in postoperative pain severity among four ethnic groups. *J Pain Symptom Manage* 1994;9:383–389.
61. Gaston-Johansson F, Albert M, Fagan E, et al. Similarities in pain descriptions of four different ethnic groups. *J Pain Symptom Manage* 1990;5:94–100.
62. Haywood L, Ell K, deGuman M, et al. Chest pain admissions: characteristics of black, Latino, and white patients in low- and mid-socioeconomic strata. *J Natl Med Assoc* 1993;85:749–757.
63. Garron D, Leavitt F. Demographic and affective covariates of pain. *Psychosom Med* 1979;41:525–535.
64. Bates M, Edwards W. Ethnic variations in the chronic pain experience. *Ethnicity Dis* 1992;2:63–83.
65. Streltzer J, Wade T. The influence of cultural group on the undertreatment of postoperative pain. *Psychosom Med* 1981;43:397–403.
66. Moore R, Niller M, Weinstein P, et al. Cultural perceptions of pain and pain coping among patients and dentists. *Commun Dent Oral Epidemiol* 1986;14:327–333.
67. Moore R, Brodegaard I, Mao T, et al. Acute pain and use of local anesthesia: tooth drilling and childbirth labor pain beliefs among Anglo-Americans, Chinese, and Scandinavians. *Anesth Prog* 1998;45:29–37.
68. Ramer L, Richardson J, Cohen M, et al. Multimeasure pain assessment in an ethnically diverse group of patients with cancer. *J Transcult Nurs* 1999;10:94–101.
69. Thomas VJ, Rose FD. Ethnic differences in the experience of pain. *Soc Sci Med* 1991;39:1063–1066.
70. Wolff B, Langley S. Cultural factors and the response to pain: a review. *Am Anthropol* 1968;70:494–501.
71. Wolff B. Ethnocultural factors influencing pain and illness behavior. *Clin J Pain* 1985;1985:23–30.
72. Martinelli A. Pain and ethnicity: how people of different cultures experience pain. *AORN J* 1987;46: 273–281.
73. Dimsdale JE. Stalked by the past: the influence of ethnicity on health. *Psychosom Med* 2000;61:161–170.
74. Todd K, Samaroo N, Hoffman J. Ethnicity as a risk factor for inadequate emergency department analgesia. *JAMA* 1993;269:1537–1539.
75. Todd KH, Deaton C, D'Adamo AP, et al. Ethnicity and analgesic practice. *Ann Emerg Med* 2000;35:11–16.
76. Choi DMA, Yate P, Coats T, et al. Ethnicity and prescription of analgesia in an accident and emergency department: cross sectional study. *BMJ* 2000;320: 980–981.
77. Ng B, Dimsdale JE, Shrag GP, et al. Ethnic differences in analgesic consumption for postoperative pain. *Psychosom Med* 1996;58:125–129.
78. Ng B, JE D, Rollnik J, et al. The effect of ethnicity on prescriptions for patient-controlled analgesia for postoperative pain. *Pain* 1996;66:9–12.
79. Todd KH, Lee T, Hoffman JR. The effect of ethnicity on physician estimates of pain severity in patients with isolated extremity trauma. *JAMA* 1994;271:925–928.
80. Sheiner EK, Sheiner E, Shoham-Vardi I, et al. Ethnic differences influence care givers' estimates of pain during labor. *Pain* 1999;81:299–305.
81. Harrison A, Busabir A, al-Kaabi A, et al. Does sharing

a mother-tongue affect how closely patients and nurses agree when rating the patient's pain, worry and knowledge? *J Adv Nurs* 1996;24:229–235.
82. Mucklow J, Fraser H, Burpitt C, et al. Environmental factors affecting paracetamol metabolism in London factory and office workers. *Br J Clin Pharmacol* 1980; 10:67–74.
83. Yue Q, Svensson J, Alm C, et al. Interindividual and interethnic differences in the demethylation and glucuronidation of codeine. *Br J Clin Pharmacol* 1989; 28:629–637.
84. Zhou H, Sheller J, Wood AW. Caucasians are more sensitive than Chinese to the cardiovascular and respiratory effects of morphine but less to the gastrointestinal side effects. *Clin Res* 1990;38:7A.
85. Carnie J, Perks D. The pattern of postoperative analgesic administration in non-English speaking Asian women following caesarean section. *Ann R Coll Surg Engl* 1984;66:365–366.
86. Houghton IT, Chan K, Wong YC, et al. Pethidine pharmacokinetics after intramuscular dose: a comparison in Caucasian, Chinese and Nepalese patients. *Methods & Findings in Experimental & Clinical Pharmacology* 1992;14:451–458.
87. Houghton I, Aun C, Gin T, et al. Inter-ethnic differences in postoperative pethidine requirements. *Anaesth Intensive Care* 1992;20:52–55.
88. McDonald D. Gender and ethnic stereotyping and narcotic analgesic administration. *Res Nurs Health* 1994; 17:45–49.
89. Aun C, Houghton I, Chan K, et al. A comparison of alfentanil requirements in European and Asian Patients during general anaesthesia. *Anaesth Intensive Care* 1988;16:396–404.
90. Tsui S, Lo R, Tong W, et al. A clinical audit for postoperative pain control on 1443 surgical patients. *Acta Anaesthesiol Sin* 1995;33:137–148.
91. Wood AJJ, Zhou HH. Ethnic differences in drug disposition and responsiveness. *Clin Pharmacokinet* 1991;20:350–373.
92. Lee A, Gin T, Oh T. Opioid requirements and responses in Asians. *Anaesth Intensive Care* 1997;25: 665–670.
93. Richman J, Gavira M, Flaherty J, et al. The process of acculturation: theoretical perspectives and an empirical investigation in Peru. *Soc Sci Med* 1987;25: 839–847.
94. Clark W, Clark S. Pain response in Nepalese porters. *Science* 1980;209:410–411.
95. Walsh N, Schoenfield L, Ramamurthy S, et al. Normative model for cold pressor test. *Am J Phys Med Rehabil* 1989;68:6–11.
96. Meehan J, Stoll A, Hardy J. Cutaneous pain threshold in native Alaskan-Indian and Eskimo. *J Appl Physiol* 1954;6:397–400.
97. Lambert W, Libman E, Poser E. The effect of increased salience of a membership group on pain tolerance. *J Pers* 1960;38:350–357.
98. Poser E. Some psychosocial determinants of pain tolerance. Paper presented at the XVIth International Congress of Psychology, Washington, DC, 1963.
99. Mersky H, Spear F. The reliability of the pressure algometer. *Br J Soc Clin Psychol* 1964;3:130–136.
100. Sternbach R, Tursky B. Ethnic differences among housewives in psychological and skin potential responses to electric shock. *Psychophysiology* 1967;1: 241–246.
101. Tursky B, Sternbach R. Further physiological correlates of ethnic differences in responses to shock. *Psychophysiology* 1967;4:67–74.
102. Woodrow K, Friedman G, Siegelaub A, et al. Pain tolerance: differences according to age, sex, and race. *Psychosom Med* 1972;34:548–556.
103. Knox V, Shum K, McLaughlin D. Response to cold pressor pain and to acupuncture analgesia in oriental and occidental subjects. *Pain* 1977;4:49–57.
104. Edwards R, Fillingim R. Ethnic differences in thermal pain responses. *Psychosom Med* 1999;61:346–354.
105. Sheffield D, Biles PL, Oram H, et al. Race and sex differences in cutaneous pain perception. *Psychosom Med* 2000;62:517–523.
106. Zatzick D, Dimsdale J. Cultural variations in response to painful stimuli. *Psychosom Med* 1990;52:544–557.
107. Abu-Saad H. Cultural components of pain: the Asian American child. *Child Health Care* 1984;13:11–14.
108. Abu-Saad H. Cultural group indicators of pain in children. *Matern Child Nurs J* 1984;13:187–193.
109. Abu-Saad H. Toward the development of an instrument to assess pain in children: Dutch study. In: Tyler D, Krane E, eds. *Advances in pain therapy research*. New York: Raven Press, 1990:101–106.
110. Harrison A. Arabic children's pain descriptions. *Pediatr Emerg Care* 1991;7:199–203.
111. Gaffney A. How children describe pain: a study of words and analogies used by 5- to 14-year-olds. In: Dubner R, Gebhart C, Bond M, eds. *Proceedings of the Vth World Congress on Pain, volume 3: pain research and clinical management*. Amsterdam: Elsevier, 1988.
112. Savedra M, Givvons P, Tesler M, et al. How do children describe pain: a tentative assessment. *Pain* 1982; 14:95–104.
113. Fritz K, Schechter N, Bernstein B. Cultural components of pain behavior in Vietnamese refugee children. *J Pain Symptom Manage* 1991;6:205(abst).
114. Pfefferbaum B, Adams J, Aceves J. The influence of culture on pain in Anglo and Hispanic children with cancer. *J Am Acad Child Adolesc Psychiatry* 1990;29: 642–647.
115. Adams J. A methodological study of pain assessment in Anglo and Hispanic children with cancer. In: Tyler D, Krane E, eds. *Advances in pain therapy research*. New York: Raven Press, 1990:43–51.
116. Kuttner L, LePage T. Face scales for the assessment of pediatric pain: a critical review. Canadian *J Behav Sci* 1989;21:198–209.
117. LaBaron S, Zeltzer L. Assessment of acute pain and anxiety in children and adolescents by self-reports, observer reports, and a behavior checklist. *J Consult Psychol*1984;52:729–738.
118. Aun C, Lam Y, Collett B. Evaluation of the use of visual analogue scale in Chinese patients. *Pain* 1986; 27: 215–221.
119. Beyer J, Knott C. Construct validity estimation for the African-American and Hispanic versions of the Oucher Scale. *J Pediatr Nurs* 1998;13:20–31.
120. Beyer J. *The Oucher: a user's manual and technical report*. Denver: University of Colorado Health Sciences Center, 1988.
121. Lewis M, Ramsay D, Kawakami K. Differences be-

tween Japanese infants and Caucasian American infants in behavioral and cortisone response to inoculation. *Child Dev* 1993;64:1722–1731.
122. Rosmus C, Johnson CC, Chan-Yip A, et al. Pain response in Chinese and non-Chinese Canadian infants: is there a difference? *Soc Sci Med* 2000;51:175–184.
123. Spielberger C. *Manual for the state-trait inventory*. Palo Alto, CA: Consulting Psychologists Press, 1983.
124. Bohannon AS. Physiological, self report and behavioral ratings of pain in three to seven year old African-American and Anglo-American children. [Ph.D. Dissertation]. Miami: University of Miami, 1995.
125. Hu Y, Zhang G, Chen Z. Pain after burn injuries among Chinese children: a further study on transcultural and ethnic differences of pain. *J Pain Symptom Manage* 1991;6:155(abst).
126. Hu Y, Zhang G, Chen Z. Evaluation of pain tolerance of children in Xinjiang, China, from analgesic measures for surgery . *J Pain Symptom Manage* 1991;6: 205(abst).
127. Zeltzer L, LeBaron S. Does ethnicity constitute a risk factor in the psychological distress of adolescents with cancer? *J Adolesc Health Care* 1985;6:8–11.
128. Pachter L. Cultural issues in pediatric care. In: Nelson WE, Behrman RE, Kliegman RM, Arvin AM, eds. *Nelson textbook of pediatrics*, 15th ed. Philadelphia: WB Saunders, 1996:16–18.
129. Banoub-Baddour S, Laryea M. A culturally sensitive perspective on pain in young children diagnosed with cancer. *J Pain Symptom Manage* 1991;6:204(abst).
130. Hayes-Bautista D. Latino terminology: conceptual basis for standardized terminology. *Am J Public Health* 1987;77:61–68.
131. Friedman D, Cohen B, Dunn V, et al. Ethnic variation, maternal risk characteristics among blacks—Massachusetts, 1987–1988. *JAMA* 1991;266:327–328.
132. Yu E. The health risks of Asian-Americans. *Am J Public Health* 1991;81:1391–1393.
133. Hahn R. The state of federal health statistics on racial and ethnic groups. *JAMA* 1992;267:268–271.
134. Schechter N. The undertreatment of pain in children: an overview. *Pediatr Clin North Am* 1989;36:781–794.
135. Stein H. *American medicine as culture*. Boulder, CO: Westview Press, 1990.
136. Rhodes L. Studying biomedicine as a cultural system. In: Sargent C, Johnson T, eds. *Medical anthropology: contemporary theory and methods*, rev. ed. Westport, CT: Praeger, 1996:165–182.

10

The Ethics of Pain Control in Infants and Children

Gary A. Walco, Jeffrey P. Burns, and Robert C. Cassidy

As has been discussed throughout this text, infants and young children often receive little attention to their pain and are forced to endure a great deal of untreated suffering. Despite major advances in understanding pain mechanisms in developing organisms, assessing pain in the young, and generating innovative treatment approaches to pain, there remains a consistent disparity between what is available technologically and what is practiced clinically (1,2). This gap raises an urgent ethical question: Is the apparent undertreatment of pain in infants and children ethically justifiable? The intent of this chapter is to discuss the possible justifications for this undertreatment. In addition, the basic paradigm used to explore those clinical issues is applied to ethical concerns pertaining to end-of-life care, placebo controls, and the use of experimental pain paradigms in children.

THE UNDERTREATMENT OF PAIN IN CHILDREN

At first glance, it might seem ridiculous to try to justify not treating pain. In numerous papers, it is asserted that alleviating pain and suffering are ethical imperatives in the practice of medicine or nursing (3,4). Some have gone one step further by raising arguments about whether pain relief or anesthesia is the *right* of all patients (5,6). If we speak of inalienable rights, by definition these are deemed to be inherent and absolute. Thus, if we assert that pain relief is a right in medical settings, we imply that all individuals in all situations are entitled to experience no pain. In other words, pain relief would be deemed an absolute, regardless of cost, and there would be no justification for unrelieved pain.

However, the issue is not so straightforward because pain is not always an unqualified evil and pain relief interventions are not always of unqualified benefit. The determinative principle of responsible medical care is not "Do no *hurt*." It is, "Do no *harm*." The difference is that the most appropriate medical treatment may entail hurting a patient. It only becomes harmful when the amount of hurt or suffering is greater than necessary to achieve the intended benefit.

Here lies the basic ethical challenge to caregivers: Because pain seems harmful to patients, and caregivers are categorically committed to preventing harm to their patients, not using all the available means of relieving pain must be justified. Three types of possible justifications for undertreating pain have been described (7): (a) a *revisionist* justification—the pain is not that bad, (b) a *comparative* justification—the burdens of relieving the pain are greater than the burdens of unrelieved pain, and (c) a *pragmatic* justification—unrelieved pain is necessary to gain something better.

The Revisionist Justification

Pain, by definition, is a subjective experience and therefore the usual objective data on which medical decisions are based are not as readily available. As a result, physicians rely on their knowledge of the pathophysiologic condition and their observations of pain behavior as well as patients' self-reports to make judgments about individuals' experiences of pain. Thus, patients' reports of pain are not taken at simple face value but revised in the context of other factors. The fact that pain is undertreated suggests that the relationships among pain, the severity of the pathophysiology, and pain behavior are not direct and/or that caregivers are not objective behavioral observers (8).

The revision of patients' pain expressions persists, despite the fact that adults and older children have the language and cognitive skills needed to make their discomfort known to others in relatively precise terms. It is commonly accepted that children as young as 3 to 4 years of age are able to report on various aspects of pain including site, relative intensity, and some sensory components (9). In addition, with development comes increased differentiation of affect and behavioral responses, such that elements of specific pain-related behaviors may be documented more reliably (10).

Without language skills or intentional means of making specific needs known, as with neonates, the potential for the revision or denial of pain indicators is even greater. As discussed by Anand and Craig (11), our working definitions of pain should be revised to include those who are incapable of self-report. Clearly, efferent responses to pain (including self-report) are linked to antecedent afferent elements, but the precise relationship between these two is context specific and must include developmental components (12). Without such broader concepts, it would be very easy to ignore or dismiss pain indicators displayed by infants because they do not conform to our usual expectations of pain responses.

For a given pathophysiologic condition, there is often the mistaken assumption that there is a "correct" amount of pain. In other words, some clinicians believe that there is (or should be) a uniform pain response based on the amount and nature of, for example, tissue damage. Data from studies with older children, however, have shown significant individual variability in clinical pain experiences (13,14) as well as among more basic factors such as pain threshold (15). Therefore, the nociceptive stimulation associated with a specific pathophysiologic condition accounts for only a small percentage of the variance associated with individuals' pain experiences, and more accurate assessment must include developmental and contextual factors.

Although our sophistication in assessing pain-related behaviors in the young has expanded dramatically (see Chapters 7 and 8), far too often this knowledge is not applied clinically and caregivers are not entirely objective observers. Rather, judgments regarding pain assessment and intervention become subject to observers' deep-seated values. Thus, indicators of pain and distress are attributed to other, more benign factors. Our needs may also lead us to downplay a child's suffering to alleviate our own feelings of inadequacy from not relieving enough of the child's distress. The result is that pain behavior is reinterpreted, minimized, or ignored.

The feelings of caregivers (both professional and familial) and their resulting judgments also may be insulated by ignorance about children's pain. For example, until relatively recently, many believed that very young infants did not have the neurologic capacity to experience pain, and, even if they did, it would not be remembered or have any lasting deleterious effects. We now have evidence indicating that these views are wrong. The peripheral and central nervous system structures involved in nociception develop during the second and third trimesters of gestation (14,16), and evidence indicates that nociceptive pathways, although still developing, are in place and functional in even premature infants (17,18) (see Chapter 3 for more details).

Although these studies make it clear that neonates *can* feel pain, data from studies focused on physiologic and behavioral parameters demonstrate that infants *do* experience pain. As discussed in Chapter 7, a number of physiologic response parameters have been associated with pain in newborns. These include sympathetic nervous system responses to painful stimuli, such as circumcision (19), as well as documented changes in hormonal and metabolic status resulting from poorly treated postoperative pain (20,21).

Another discredited notion is that young children's pain is not displayed reliably and therefore cannot be measured accurately. Realistically, crying is a primary means for infants to communicate needs, but crying may also represent pain and distress. As a result, the distinctions between "pain behavior" and "nonpain behavior" are not nearly as clearly defined as it might be in older individuals. However, some significant distinctions may certainly be made, as exemplified by the work of Grunau and Craig (22). They provided a series of studies focusing on characteristic facial components of a pain response that are relatively distinctive and measurable. Similar data have been generated on infants' cries as interpreted with spectrographic analyses (23). The reader is referred to Chapter 7 for a more in-depth discussion of these issues, but suffice it to say that, based on physiologic and behavioral indices, it is clear that even the very youngest children feel pain, they respond to pain, and those responses are measurable.

Especially because children are incapable of advocating for themselves, it is up to caregivers to use available strategies to observe them sensitively, assess their conditions objectively, and treat them effectively. The technology to assess pain in children reliably and validly is available and should be applied clinically. Denial of relief from pain that is proportionate to the child's expressed need for such relief must be judged an unjustified harm, unless such deprivation serves a substantially greater good.

The Comparative Justification

Even if we accept newborns' and children's pain as a reality, we still need to weigh the benefits and risks of unrelieved pain against those of pain relief. In some circumstances, a responsible conclusion might be that the harm of unrelieved pain is less severe than the harm of pain relief. The comparative justification may lead one to choose pain as the lesser evil over the potentially deleterious effects of analgesic medication. Concerns have focused on (a) the method of analgesic administration, (b) the danger of side effects, and (c) the long-term consequences of use, such as addiction. Especially because we view young children as vulnerable, fragile, and in need of our protection, concerns for such negative effects may be even greater than in the rest of the population.

In the past, management of moderate to severe acute pain in children involved the parenteral administration of opioids, often intramuscularly. Thus, the child had to endure the discomfort of a needle puncture to gain the relatively distant and temporary benefit of pain relief. Although this practice has diminished as other routes of administration continue to be tested and shown to be effective (see Chapter 38), it has not been eliminated.

In instances in which injections are necessary for analgesia or anesthesia, innovative problem solving may also come into play. Penile nerve blocks have been shown to be an effective means of reducing circumcision pain (24). Practitioners often decline their use, however, claiming that the pain of injections is as bad as the pain of circumcision. As suggested by Yaster et al. (25), however, using a smaller needle (25 gauge) virtually eliminates this problem, and the infant may get "economic" relief. In addition, use of topical anesthetics before injections eliminates discomfort. This was clearly shown among children with cancer undergoing lumbar punctures who used cognitive-behavioral strategies and an application of lidocaine-prilocaine cream (EMLA) before injections of buffered lidocaine. Pain scores were absolutely minimal, whereas expressions of self-control and effectiveness were extremely high (26).

A second major concern in using analgesic medications is side effects, most notably respiratory depression. Although the potential for these difficulties is not disputed, in deciding whether the risk outweighs the potential benefit to the child, one must consider two key issues: (a) Is the risk of respiratory problems greater in children than adults? (b) Do side effects associated with narcotics, including respiratory depression, pose a serious and irreversible threat?

Opioid agonists, such as morphine, reduce the sensitivity of brainstem respiratory centers to hypercarbia and hypoxia, interfering with pontine and medullary ventilatory centers that regulate the rhythm of breathing. The results are prolonged pauses between breaths and periodic breathing patterns (27). In the past, studies of the incidence of respiratory depression were generally anecdotal in nature (28–31), and thus conclusive statements about the frequency of such difficulties were not available. Recent clinical series indicate relatively low rates of respiratory depression among patients receiving opioids. For example, Bozkurt et al. (32) found only that among 175 children receiving single-injection lumbar epidural morphine for postoperative pain, only two (1.1%) showed signs of respiratory depression. Gibbons et al. (33) described a higher rate of respiratory depression among young burn patients (8% to 11%), but this appeared attributable to relatively high doses of opioids and/or pairing them with other sedating agents.

The risk of respiratory depression in neonates has been a topic of some debate, although recent data are more definitive. Based principally on studies with rat pups, Yaster and Maxwell (27) concluded that newborns appear to be more sensitive to the respiratory depressant effects of opioids than older individuals. Marsh et al. (34) comprehensively reviewed aspects of the opiate system in newborns and concluded the opposite. They stated, "We now have much more knowledge of morphine pharmacokinetics and the activity of its metabolites, and it is possible that if equi-analgesic rather than 'scaled down' adult doses are given, the risk of serious respiratory depression would be no greater." Similar conclusions were drawn by Kart et al. (35) in their review of the literature. Finally, a recent statement on pain and stress in the neonate issued by the American Academy of Pediatrics and the Canadian Paediatric Society (36) acknowledges the risk of respiratory depression in the young but encourages responsible use of medications, not their avoidance.

These data should not be interpreted to mean that opioids present no risks. Gill et al. (30) concluded that although respiratory depression in pediatric patients, including neonates, occurs infrequently, it may still have serious consequences. By carefully considering dose, route, and method of administration, identifying predisposing factors, and providing adequate monitoring, risks can be reduced greatly. There are a number of clinical warning signs that indicate impending respiratory depression, and most difficulties may be averted with simple dose reductions. Finally, because agents are available to reverse the effects of opioids, the condition can be treated effectively if it occurs.

A third major concern among both parents and physicians in utilizing opioids is the potential for drug addiction (37,38). To assess this risk, one must distinguish between physical dependence (a physiologically determined state in which symptoms of withdrawal would occur if the medication were not administered) and addiction (a psychologic obsession with the drug). Physical dependence is an expected phenomenon that is easily managed by tapering drug doses over time to avoid withdrawal syndromes. Addiction to narcotics is rare among adults treated for disease-related pain and appears to depend more on psychosocial factors than on the disease or the pharmacokinetics of medically prescribed narcotics themselves (39). Studies of children treated for pain associated with sickle cell disease (40,41) or postoperative recovery (31) have found virtually no risk of addiction associated with the administration of narcotics. Based on the available incidence data, as well as what is known about the psychology of drug addiction, there are no known physiologic or psychologic characteristics of children that make them vulnerable to drug addiction.

In addition to evaluating the "costs" of using analgesics, among very young children there are also potential long-term "costs" of untreated pain. The studies by Fitzgerald and colleagues with rats and human neonates have shed light on this issue. In rat pups, it was shown that tissue damage in the early postnatal period causes a profound and lasting sprouting response of local sensory nerve terminals (42). This in turn results in hyperinnervation, which remains evident in adult rats well after the wound has healed. An implication is that in the neonatal period, peripheral nerve networks are going through a process of increasing differentiation. When repeatedly insulted with painful stimuli, this process is altered such that lower levels of stimulation potentiate relatively significant nociceptive responses. Indeed, human neonates undergoing repeated heal lancing demonstrated a similar hyperalgesic response (43).

Other clinical research findings support these concerns. Taddio et al. (44) focused on reactions to routine vaccination at 4 and 6 months of age among three groups of male infants: those who were uncircumcised, those who were circumcised within 5 days of birth using a topical anesthetic (lidocaine-prilocaine cream) for pain management, and those who were circumcised with a placebo topical cream. When these children came in for their routine vaccinations, they were videotaped so that a number of pain behaviors could be evaluated, including facial action (brow bulge, nasolabial furrow, eyes squeezed shut) and cry duration and a visual analog scale score for pain was assigned. Analyses showed greater pain responses across the board in boys who were circumcised without local anesthesia in contrast to those who were uncircumcised. In addition, visual analog scores were significantly different between boys circumcised with lidocaine-prilocaine cream versus those with the placebo cream. Relevant variables, such as temperament, age, weight, time since last feeding, time of last sleep before vaccination, and ingestion of acetaminophen, did not correlate with pain indices. Thus, early, untreated pain experiences appear to sensitize the child to subsequent painful experiences.

In conclusion, the administration of analgesic medication depends on an analysis of relative benefits and risks. An overestimation of the risk of analgesic use leads to an underestimation of the harm of untreated pain. When analgesics are administered properly, the risks of respiratory depression or addiction are actually very low. Available data also indicate the risks of long-term sequelae of untreated pain may be rather high. Any comparative justification for withholding pain relief must be rigorously controlled by a careful analysis of all the risks and benefits and the disciplined use of empiric data, not speculation or undocumented lore.

The Pragmatic Justification

The pragmatic justification authorizes using some means that in and of themselves are bad, if the end they serve is good. Its classic formulation is "the end justifies the means." For caregivers, pain is often viewed as a means to an end. Pain is not judged to be good or bad in and of itself, but rather by how it affects the goals of therapy (e.g., cure of disease, prevention of death, improvement of function). For clinicians, suffering may be ethically acceptable if it is therapeutically beneficial. For example, pain evoked during physical examination may help diagnose occult conditions.

However, an end does not justify any means. An acceptable justification must meet the test of proportionality. There must be a positive proportionality between the value of the end and the burdens of the means. Treatment is a package deal, and our ethical duty is to design the package with the greatest possible benefit and the least possible suffering. Therefore, the claim of pragmatic justification is defensible only after we have carefully tested both the means and ends involved in each individual case.

For the end to justify the means, the end must be a substantial and realizable good, and the means used to achieve that good must be reasonably expected to prove effective. Thus, to use pain as a therapeutic instrument, a pragmatic "morality of means" test must be passed. This test has three component challenges: First, *is the pain useful?* We must be able to affirm that there is a reasonable probability that using the pain will really achieve the end that is sought. Second, *is the pain necessary?* Using pain is justified only when there is no other less noxious means available. Pain must be the instrument of last resort. Third, *is the pain the least possible?* We must do all we can to assure that only the minimal amount of pain remains. Because the suffering of a child pays for the price of therapeutic gain, we must be exquisitely economical.

In addition to passing the morality of means test, pragmatic justification requires a "morality of ends" test. Those who justify pain on pragmatic grounds usually invoke two major ends: therapeutic guidance and character development. For the therapeutic guidance purpose, pain may be viewed as useful to determine the nature and extent of an illness. For example, pain responses observed while palpating an abdomen may serve as an important means of diagnosing an ailment. Completely relieving pain might cloud the physician's judgment and thereby actually harm the patient. One must weigh the benefits of immediate relief against the benefits of long-term cure or better recovery. In such circumstances, however, pain not kept to a minimum, both in terms of intensity and duration, would be unjustified and therefore unethical.

The second end used to justify the means, character development, is much more ethically dubious. This moralistic theory champions particular character traits such as courage, self-discipline, independence, and self-sacrifice. Although in some settings, promoting such heroic virtues may be ethically defensible, in a medical context, they become extremely questionable. Imposing the additional burden of character development on infants and children already encumbered by sickness reflects a lack of compassion and denies them respect for the significance of their current suffering.

DECISION MAKING AND PALLIATIVE CARE

Pain management and palliative care in children is a unique endeavor, but many of the principles devised for adult patients apply. A large multicenter study, the Study to Understand Prognoses and Preferences for Outcomes and Risks of Treatments (SUPPORT), was a controlled clinical trial at five teaching hospitals in the United States sponsored by the Robert Wood Johnson Foundation to improve care for seriously ill adult patients (45). Physicians in the intervention group received estimates of the likelihood of 6-month survival, patient preferences for cardiopulmonary resuscitation, and the likelihood of functional disability at 2 months. A specifically trained nurse had multiple contacts with the patient and family and provided direct feedback to the medical rounding team on patient preferences for life-sustaining treatment and encouraged attention to pain control.

Despite the provision of direct feedback to the care team, the intervention failed to improve care or patient outcomes. In particular, surrogates reported that 50% of patients who could communicate reported moderate or severe pain at least half of the time during their last 3 days of life. Nearly 15% reported extremely severe pain or moderately severe pain occurring at least half of the time, and nearly 15% of those patients with pain were dissatisfied with its control. After adjustment for confounding variables, dissatisfaction with pain control was more likely among patients with more severe pain, greater anxiety, depression, alteration of mental status, and lower reported income; dissatisfaction with pain control also varied among study hospitals and by physician specialty.

Studies of satisfaction with pain control in pediatric patients also raise concerns about the care provided to critically ill children. Sirkia (46) examined satisfaction with pain control in 100 pediatric patients with cancer treated at the Children's Hospital, University of Helsinki, Finland, who died between 1987 and 1992. Parenteral morphine was administered to 40 children, principally as a continuous infusion through a central venous line. The dose of morphine was 0.8 mg/kg per day at the start and was increased to an average of 4.9 mg/kg per day (range, 0.2 to 55). Of the 62 children who received regular pain medication, 81% of families reported that the analgesia appeared adequate, whereas nearly one of every five family respondents felt that the analgesia did not sufficiently relieve their child's suffering.

More recently, Wolfe and colleagues (47) found that 89% of 103 parents whose children died of cancer in a hospital setting reported that their child experienced suffering "a lot" or "a great deal" from at least one symptom in their last month of life. Of the children who were treated for specific symptoms, interventions were successful, by the parents' assessments, in only 27% of those with pain and in only 16% of those with dyspnea. These data suggest the need for more effective management of patient suffering and clearer communication with parents in the care of children who are dying of cancer.

Investigators have also described the attitudes and practice of clinicians in providing sedation and analgesia to dying children as life-sustaining treatment is withdrawn. A prospective case series of 53 consecutive patients who died after the withdrawal of life-sustaining treatment in the pediatric intensive care unit at three teaching hospitals in Boston found that clinicians frequently escalate the dose of sedatives or analgesics to dying patients as life-sustaining treatment is withdrawn (48). Pediatric critical care physicians and nurses cited patient-centered reasons as their principal justification for this practice. The study found that sedatives and/or analgesics were administered to 47 (89%) of these patients. Those who were comatose were less likely to receive these medications. Physicians and nurses cited treatment of pain, anxiety, and air hunger as the most common reasons and hastening death as the least common reason for administration of these medications. Hastening death was viewed as an "acceptable, unintended side effect" of terminal care by 91% of physician-nurse matched pairs. The mean dose of sedatives and analgesics nearly doubled as life support was withdrawn, and the degree of escalation in dose did not correlate with clinicians' views on hastening death.

This raises the dilemma regarding the appropriate dose of sedatives or analgesics to administer to a dying patient. An ethical rule that is frequently cited as an answer to this question is the doctrine of double effect, which distinguishes between prohibited "death causing" and permitted "death-hastening" analgesic administration to terminally ill patients (49). The doctrine states that when an action has two effects, one of which is inherently good and the other is inherently bad, that action can be justified if certain conditions are met.

The four requirements for the doctrine of double effect are as follows. (a) The action in itself must be good or at least morally indifferent. (b) The agent must intend only the good effect and not the evil effect. The evil effect is foreseen, but not intended—it is allowed but not sought. In the case of administering morphine to a terminally ill patient, the physician must intend only the relief of the patient's pain and suffering. Respiratory depression and the potential for an earlier death are foreseen complications but are not sought. (c) The evil effect cannot be a means to the good effect. For example, by administering potassium chloride or neuromuscular blockade as interventions for palliative care, the evil effect (death) becomes the means to the good effect (relief from suffering). By contrast, morphine does not depend on the patient's death to achieve effective pain relief. (d) The good intended must outweigh the evil permitted. In the case of an imminently dying patient, the benefit of pain relief outweighs the risk of hastening death. This would not be true if the patient were not terminally ill. For example, if otherwise healthy patients required so much morphine for pain control that they developed serious respiratory depression, they should be placed on a ventilator, not allowed to die.

Whether double effect reasoning is a necessary or sufficient guide for morally permissible administration of sedation and analgesia in terminal care is controversial (50–53). Critics of the doctrine of double effect argue that it is dependent on an overly simplistic notion of intent that is impossible to verify externally. These critics believe that the only morally relevant consideration is the informed consent of the patient, not the intentions of the clinicians. Still other critics claim that a strict interpretation of the doctrine of double effect prohibits any action that could be interpreted as intentionally causing death. Therefore, according to this critique, the doctrine of double effect may actually result in unnecessary patient suffering because clinicians will be reluctant to treat pain at the end-of-life to avoid any appearance of intentionally causing death.

In the pediatric end of life care, however, there are no viable alternatives to double effect reasoning in guiding permissible clinical conduct. Most terminally ill children cannot express their wishes for terminal care, and, especially in intensive care, most will experience a rapid decline in comfort as life support (such as mechanical ventilation) is withdrawn. Double effect reasoning provides a defensible rationale for adequate palliation for practitioners who support neither euthanasia at one extreme nor the practice of allowing patients to die with untreated suffering on the other.

What is the difference between practice by the doctrine of double effect and the performance of euthanasia? The key difference lies in the intention of the physician. Although the full intentions and motives of another cannot be validated with certainty, if the physician's intention is treatment of the patient's pain and suffering and the only effective means is increased medication, the administration of analgesics and sedatives is ethically permitted under the doctrine of double effect. When the physician's intention is to kill the patient, then the line between accepted practice and euthanasia has been crossed.

How much is too much analgesia or sedation for a terminally ill child? There is no arbitrary amount of narcotic that is necessarily too much, or too little, in any given case. Brody and colleagues (54) expressed the views of many experts on pain and symptom management: "The optimal dose of morphine for relief of pain or dyspnea is determined by increasing the dose until the patient responds. Patients who have not previously received opioids should be given low doses initially, which should be rapidly increased until symptoms are relieved. For patients with particularly severe or acute symptoms, rapid titration requires that an experienced clinician be at the bedside." Regardless of the dosing scheme that is required to treat pain and suffering effectively, it should be standard medical practice to thoroughly document the signs and symptoms of suffering that the clinicians observe, the rationale behind the regimen chosen to treat these symptoms, the careful monitoring of the efficacy of the regimens, and the responsive and responsible adjustment of the regimen to provide optimal palliative care.

PLACEBO-CONTROLLED CLINICAL TRIALS

Recent guidelines from the U.S. Food and Drug Administration are aimed at increasing the inclusion of children in clinical trials of new medications, including analgesics (55). A traditional approach, still invoked in pediatric trials today, includes the use of a placebo control group (56). In other words, to demonstrate the efficacy of a given medication, it is tested against a control group that receives an inert substance believed to have no clinical benefit whatsoever. In the case of pain research, this implies that a group of children must endure pain so that a drug may be shown to be efficacious and thus gain Food and Drug Administration approval. The serious ethical question in this instance, and in human experimentation in general, focuses on how much some persons may be burdened for the benefit of others.

In principle, the welfare of the individual patient is of chief concern (57). However, the advancement of scientific knowledge and its substantial and indisputable benefits for many other persons is also of appropriate concern and should be weighted along with the concerns for the individual. Thus, some risk to the subject is balanced against potential benefit to the subject and others. The challenge that is difficult for any placebo-controlled trial to meet arises from the fact that by substituting a placebo for an active clinical control imposes additional risk with no chance of compensatory benefit for the subject in the control arm of the study. Therefore, placebo-controlled trials must address two major ethical concerns: (a) a heightened standard of informed consent and (b) a decreased level of acceptable risk.

A Heightened Standard of Consent

Informed consent has become one of the established pillars of ethical research. The first principle of the Nuremberg Code (58) is: "The voluntary consent of the human subjects is absolutely essential." For placebo trials, researchers must demonstrate (at a minimum to their institutional review boards) that they have met a heightened standard of informed consent. Specifically, subjects must show that they fully comprehend the nature and significance of a placebo-controlled trial and, most important, the additional risks that may occur for those assigned to the placebo group. Subjects must show that they fully grasp that the placebo is honestly expected to have no therapeutic benefit. Obviously, these are major issues when the intent of the study is to reduce or alleviate pain.

The situation is further complicated by the fact that in studies with minors, informed consent is given by a parent or guardian. Thus, the researcher must also gain assent from minor children, disclosing to them all the risks and benefits of the study, including a chance that they will receive a medication that is thought to be inert.

Decreased Level of Acceptable Risk

A subject's fully educated choice is not sufficient by itself to justify the degree of risk posed by some placebo-controlled trials. The researchers (and Institutional Review Board reviewers) are still ethically obligated to make extraordinary efforts to produce a study design in which the risks are reduced to an acceptable level by meeting three tests (similar to the pragmatic justification discussed above): (a) *Have the risks been fully minimized?* Has everything possible been done to reduce the amount of potential risk to the placebo subjects to the absolute minimum possible? This is the first requirement set by the Federal Regulations for Institutional Review Board approval of human subjects research. (b) *Are the remaining risks minimal?* Does being put on placebo create more than "minimal risk" for those human subjects? Even after all possible efforts have been made to minimize the risks to the placebo subjects, the remaining risk may still be unacceptably high. (c) *Are those minimal risks truly necessary?* Are there other means of maintaining the validity of the study without subjecting participants to even minimal levels of risk?

In a footnote to a chapter on pediatric analgesic trials (59), Rogers specifically states that the use of placebo controls in children should be avoided. She feels that the impact of including such a group would lead to decreased enrollment in studies because of untreated pain. Experimental designs using lower and upper dosages of test and standard medication may be used and crossover models may be employed so that subjects are their own controls, rather than involving a group untreated for pain. Thus, it is clearly in the best interest of both patients and researchers who wish to accrue subjects for pediatric analgesic trials to minimize or avoid the use of placebos in demonstrating the effectiveness of new agents.

EXPERIMENTALLY INDUCED PAIN STUDIES WITH CHILDREN

To assess systematically the relationship between pain and other related factors, it is important to experimentally control elements of the pain experience. This may be done through laboratory studies in which pain is stimulated through various channels, tapping into pain threshold (the lowest level of stimulation labeled as pain), pain tolerance (the highest level of stimulation that a subject might endure), and pain responsiveness (nature of pain experience in response to controlled stimuli). For example, studies have been conducted to assess the effects of age, site of stimulation, and gender on mechanical pain thresholds with healthy children between the ages of 6 and 17 years (60). Others have examined the relationship between pain threshold and diseases such as juvenile arthritis (61–63), sickle cell disease (61,64), and recurrent abdominal pain (65). Finally, others have used experimental pain paradigms to study or facilitate coping with clinical pain (66–68). A comprehensive review of these studies is beyond the scope of this chapter.

In an editorial on the ethics of laboratory-induced pain in children, McGrath (69) presented a balanced perspective. First, she pointed out the benefits of such research, including further elucidating complex nociceptive mechanisms, especially as related to developmental factors, and further alleviating pain through demonstrating the effectiveness of analgesics and other interventions for pain and coping. After recognizing ethical concerns, McGrath goes on to say that experimental pain paradigms should be judged by the same criteria that one would use to judge any study in which subjects are at risk. First, the validity of the study should be assessed and possible benefits appreciated. Once the methodology is clear, the specific type of experimental pain should be considered and appropriate stimulus levels assigned. She recommends the least stimulation necessary to accomplish the study objectives. This should then be balanced against the potential risk and if there is great benefit to either the child or society at large, the research would be deemed ethical.

Such reasoning is precisely consistent with the pragmatic justification described above. It would be ethical to use research paradigms involving nonclinical pain if (a) it would be a valid means of gaining the needed information, (b) it was the only means by which the information could be obtained, and (c) a minimum amount of stimulation was used. In other words, the demands of a morality of means tests as well as a morality of ends test would be satisfied. In addition, elements of informed consent and assent from the minor would be imperative. It is important to note that when experimenters are sensitive to the issues and these safeguards are in place, experimental pain paradigms actually pose little threat to the subjects and many find the experience informative (61,70).

CONCLUSION

It would be fairly easy to ignore the demands of pain management posed by infants and young children. Often they are incapable of rationally communicating their own needs or desires and one might feel little or no obligation to explain or justify their treatment to them. As evidenced by the material in this book, however, in recent years there has been increasing scientific knowledge related to the mechanisms, behavior, assessment, and treatment of pain in the young as well as the deleterious physiologic and psychologic effects of untreated pain.

The assessment and treatment of pain in infants and children are important parts of pediatric practice. This issue is of little debate as the standards of care, as mandated by significant regulatory agencies such as the Joint Commission for the Accreditation of Health Organizations (71), insist on the regular assessment and appropriate treatment of pain in all patients across settings. Thus, it is expected that health professionals will provide care that reflects the technologic growth of the field, thereby minimizing unnecessary pain and distress in the young, both throughout their lives and at the end of life.

Additional ethical concerns have been raised regarding scientific studies involving children, both in the development and validation of analgesic interventions and with regard to experimentally induced pain. Many of the same standards invoked in evaluating the clinical treatment of pain apply to this arena as well. A careful cost–benefit analysis of the study must be conducted, recognizing that pain in a child is a potential cost and that, therefore, the possible benefits derived from the study must be very great.

ACKNOWLEDGMENT

The authors thank Neil Schechter, M.D., for his contributions to previous manuscripts.

REFERENCES

1. McLaughlin CR, Hull JG, Edward WH, et al. Neonatal pain: a comprehensive survey of attitudes and practices. *J Pain Symptom Manage* 1993;8:7–16.
2. Porter FL, Wolf CM, Gold J, et al. Pain and pain management in newborn infants: a survey of physicians and nurses. *Pediatrics* 1997;100:626–632.
3. Emanuel EJ. Pain and symptom control. Patient rights and physician responsibilities. *Hematol Oncol Clin North Am* 1996;10:41–56.
4. Kachoyeanos MK, Zollo MB. Ethics in pain management of infants and children. *Am J Mater Child Nurs* 1995;20:142–147.
5. Von Gunten CF, von Roenn JH. Barriers to pain control: ethics & knowledge. *J Palliative Care* 1994;10:52–54.
6. Pellegrino ED. Emerging ethical issues in palliative care. *JAMA* 1998;279:1521–1522.
7. Walco GA, Cassidy RC, Schechter NL. Pain, hurt, and harm: the ethics of pain control in infants and children. *N Engl J Med* 1994;331:541–544.
8. Nolan K. Ethical issues in pediatric pain management. In: Schechter NL, Berde CB, Yaster M, eds. *Pain in infants, children, and adolescents*. Baltimore: Williams & Wilkins, 1993:123–132.
9. McGrath PA. *Pain in children: nature, assessment, and treatment*. New York: Guilford Press, 1990.
10. Walco GA, Harkins SW. Lifespan developmental approaches to pain. In: Gatchel RJ, Turk DC, eds. *Psychosocial factors in pain: evolution and revolutions*. New York: Guilford Publications, 1999:107–117.
11. Anand KJS, Craig KD. New perspectives on the definition of pain. *Pain* 1996;67:3–6.
12. McGrath PJ, Frager G. Psychological barriers to optimal pain management in infants and children. *Clin J Pain* 1996;12:135–141.
13. Ilowite NT, Walco GA, Pochaczevsky R. Assessment of pain in patients with juvenile rheumatoid arthritis: relation between pain intensity and degree of joint inflammation. *Ann Rheum Dis* 1992;51:343–346.
14. Petrie A. *Individuality in pain and suffering*. Chicago: University of Chicago Press, 1967.
15. Walco GA, Dampier CD, Hartstein G, et al. The relationship between recurrent clinical pain and pain threshold in children. In: Tyler DC, Krane EJ, eds. *Advances in pain research and therapy.volume 15: pediatric pain*. New York: Raven Press, 1990:333–340.
16. Anand KJS, Carr DB. The neuroanatomy, neurophysiology and neurochemistry of pain, stress, and analgesia in newborns, infants, and children. *Pediatr Clin North Am* 1989;36:795–822.
17. Anand KJS, Hickey PR. Pain and its effects in the human neonate and fetus. *N Engl J Med* 1987;317: 1321–1329.
18. Fitzgerald M, Anand KJS. Developmental neuroanatomy and neurophysiology of pain. In: Schechter NL, Berde CB, Yaster M, eds. *Pain in infants, children, and adolescents*. Baltimore: Williams & Wilkins, 1993: 11–31.
19. Williamson PS, Williamson ML. Physiological stress reduction by local anesthetic during newborn circumcision. *Pediatrics* 1983;71:36–40.
20. Anand KJS, Sippell WG, Aynsley-Green A. Randomized trial of fentanyl anaesthesia in preterm babies undergoing surgery: effects on stress response [erratum published in *Lancet* 1987;1:234]. *Lancet* 1987;1: 62–66.
21. Anand KJS, Hickey PR. Randomised trial of high-dose sufentanil anesthesia in neonates undergoing cardiac surgery: effects on metabolic stress response. *Anesthesiology* 1987;67:A502.
22. Craig KD. The facial display of pain. In: Finley GA, McGrath PJ, eds. *Progress in pain research and management: volume 10: measurement of pain in infants and children*. Seattle: IASP Press, 1998:103–121.
23. Levine JD, Gordon NC. Pain in prelingual children and its evaluation by pain-induced vocalization. *Pain* 1982; 14:85–93.
24. Dalens B. Peripheral nerve blockade in the management of postoperative pain in children. In: Schechter NL, Berde CB, Yaster M, eds. *Pain in infants, children, and adolescents*. Baltimore: Williams & Wilkins, 1993: 261–280.
25. Yaster M, Krane EJ, Kaplan RF, et al. *Pediatric pain management and sedation handbook*. St. Louis: Mosby, 1997.
26. Walco GA, Conte PM, Labay LE, et al. Procedural distress in pediatric oncology. Paper presented at the 5th International Symposium on Paediatric Pain, June 2000, London.
27. Yaster M, Maxwell LG. Opioid agonists and antagonists. In: Schechter NL, Berde CB, Yaster M, eds. *Pain in infants, children, and adolescents*. Baltimore: Williams & Wilkins, 1993:145–171.
28. Beasley SW, Tibballs J. Efficacy and safety of continuous morphine infusion for postoperative analgesia in the pediatric surgical ward. *Aust N Z J Surg* 1987;57:233–237.
29. Dilworth NM, MacKellar A. Pain relief for the pediatric surgical patient. *J Pediatr Surg* 1987;22:264–266.
30. Gill AM, Cousins A, Nunn AJ, et al. Opiate-induced respiratory depression in pediatric patients. *Ann Pharmacother* 1996;30:125–129.
31. McCaffery M, Wong DL. Nursing interventions for pain control in children. In: Schechter NL, Berde CB, Yaster M, eds. *Pain in infants, children, and adolescents*. Baltimore: Williams & Wilkins, 1993:295–316.
32. Bozkurt P, Kaya G, Yeker Y. Single-injection lumbar epidural morphine for postoperative analgesia in children: a report of 175 cases. *Reg Anesth* 1997;22:212–217.
33. Gibbons J, Honari SR, Sharar SR, et al. Opiate-induced respiratory depression in young pediatric burn patients. *J Burn Care Rehabil* 1998;19:225–229.

34. Marsh DF, Hatch DJ, Fitzgerald M. Opioid systems and the newborn. *Br J Anaesth* 1997;79:787–795.
35. Kart T, Christup LL, Rasmussen M. Recommended use of morphine in neonates, infants and children based on a literature review: part 2—clinical use. *Paediatr Anaesth* 1997;7:93–101.
36. American Academy of Pediatrics, Canadian Paediatric Society. Policy statement: prevention and management of pain and stress in the neonate. *Pediatrics* 2000;105: 454–461.
37. Craig KD, Lilley CM, Gilbert CA. Social barriers to optimal pain management in infants and children. *Clin J Pain* 1996;12:232–242.
38. McGrath PJ. Attitudes and beliefs about medication and pain management in children. *J Palliat Care* 1996;12: 46–50.
39. Chapman CR, Hill HF. Prolonged morphine self-administration and addiction liability: evaluation of two theories in a bone marrow transplant unit. *Cancer* 1989; 63:1636–1644.
40. Morrison RA. Update on sickle cell disease: incidence of addiction and choice of opioid in pain management. *Pediatr Nurs* 1991;17:503.
41. Pegelow CH. Survey of pain management therapy provided for children with sickle cell disease. *Clin Pediatr* 1992;31:211–214.
42. Reynolds ML, Fitzgerald M. Long-term sensory hyperinnervation following neonatal skin wounds. *J Comp Neurol* 1995;358:487–498.
43. Fitzgerald M, Millard C, McIntosh N. Cutaneous hypersensitivity following peripheral tissue damage in newborn infants and its reversal with topical anaesthesia. *Pain* 1989;39:31–36.
44. Taddio A, Katz J, Ilersich AL, et al. Effect of neonatal circumcision on pain response during subsequent routine vaccination. *Lancet* 1997;349:599–603.
45. The SUPPORT Principal Investigators. A controlled trial to improve care for seriously ill hospitalized patients. The study to understand prognoses and preferences for outcomes and risks of treatments (SUPPORT) [published erratum appears in *JAMA* 1996 24;275: 1232]. *JAMA* 1995;274:1591–1598.
46. Sirkia K. Pain medication during terminal care of children with cancer. *J Pain Symptom Manage* 1998;15:220–226.
47. Wolfe J, Grier HE, Klar N, et al. Symptoms and suffering at the end of life in children with cancer. *N Engl J Med* 2000;342:326–333.
48. Burns JP, Mitchell C, Outwater KM, et al. End-of-life care in the pediatric intensive care unit after the forgoing of life-sustaining treatment. *Crit Care Med* 2000; 28:3060–3066.
49. Garcia J. Double effect. In: Reich WT, ed. *Encyclopedia of bioethics. Volume 2*. New York: Simon and Schuster, 1995:515–544.
50. Quill TE, Dresser R, Brock DW. The rule of double effect: a critique of its role in end-of-life decision making. *N Engl J Med* 1997;337:1768–1771.
51. Fohr SA. The double effect of pain medication: separating myth from reality. *J Palliat Med* 1998;1:315–328.
52. Brody H. Physician-assisted suicide in the courts: moral equivalence, double effect, and clinical practice. *Minn Law Rev* 1998;82:939–963.
53. Kamm FM. The doctrine of double effect: reflections on theoretical and practical issues. *J Med Philos* 1991;16: 571–585.
54. Brody H, Campbell ML, Faber-Langendoen K, et al. Withdrawing intensive life-sustaining treatment: recommendations for compassionate clinical management. *N Engl J Med* 1997;336:652–657.
55. Buck ML. The FDA Modernization Act of 1997: impact on pediatric medicine. *Pediatr Pharmacother* 2000;6: 612–614.
56. Wright IV C. Pediatric pain studies: the impact of regulations on research and development. Paper presented at the 20th Annual Scientific Meeting of the American Pain Society, April 2001, Phoenix, AZ.
57. AMA Council on Ethical and Judicial Affairs. *Code of medical ethics, current opinions with annotations*. Chicago: American Medical Association, 1994:12.
58. The Nuremberg Code, 1949. Reprinted in: Levin R. *Ethics and regulation of clinical research.* Baltimore: Urban and Schwarzenberg, 1986: 425–426.
59. Berde CB. Pediatric analgesic trials. In: Max M, Portenoy R, Laska E, eds. *Advances in pain research and therapy: volume 18: the design of analgesic clinical trials*. New York: Raven Press, 1991:445–455.
60. Hogeweg JA, Kuis W, Oostendorp RA, et al. The influence of site of stimulation, age, and gender on pain threshold in healthy children. *Phys Ther* 1996;76: 1331–1339.
61. Walco GA, Dampier CD, Hartstein G, et al. The relationship between recurrent clinical pain and pain threshold in children. In: Tyler DC, Krane EJ, eds. *Advances in pain research and therapy: volume 15: pediatric pain*. New York: Raven Press, 1990:333–340.
62. Hogeweg JA, Kuis W, Oostendorp RA, et al. General and segmental reduced pain thresholds in juvenile chronic arthritis. *Pain* 1995;62:11–17.
63. Hogeweg JA, Kuis W, Huygen AC, et al. The pain threshold in juvenile chronic arthritis. *Br J Rheumatol* 1995;34:61–67.
64. Gil KM, Edens JL, Wilson JJ, et al. Coping strategies and laboratory pain in children with sickle cell disease. *Ann Behav Med* 1997;19:22–29.
65. Alfven G. The pressure pain threshold (PPT) of certain muscles in children suffering from recurrent abdominal pain of non-organic origin. An algometric study. *Acta Paediatr* 1993;82:481–483.
66. Zeltzer LK, Fanurik D, LeBaron S. The cold pressor paradigm in children: feasibility of an intervention model (part II). *Pain* 1989;37:305–313.
67. Fanurik D, Zeltzer LK, Roberts MC, et al. The relationship between children's coping styles and psychological interventions for cold pressor pain. *Pain* 1993;53: 213–222.
68. Siegel LJ. Increasing pain tolerance through self-efficacy training. *J Pain Symptom Manage* 1991;6:144.
69. McGrath PA. Inducing pain in children—a controversial issue. *Pain* 1993;52:255–257.
70. LeBaron S, Zeltzer L, Fanurik D. An investigation of cold pressor pain in children (part I). *Pain* 1989;37:161–171.
71. Joint Commission on Accreditation of Healthcare Organizations. *Comprehensive accreditation manual for hospitals: the official handbook.* Oakbrook Terrace, IL: Joint Commission on Accreditation of Healthcare Organizations, 2000.

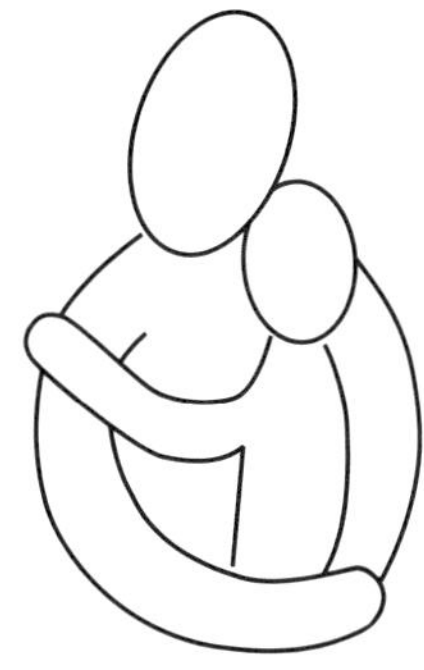

PART II

Therapeutic Interventions

11

Nonsteroidal Anti-inflammatory Drugs in Pediatric Pain Management

Eeva-Liisa Maunuksela and Klaus T. Olkkola

The nonsteroidal anti-inflammatory drugs (NSAIDs), also referred to as antipyretic analgesics and peripherally active nonopioid analgesics, are a large group of various drugs having a similar mode of action. These agents reduce the metabolism of arachidonic acid to prostaglandins. The reference substance is acetylsalicylic acid (aspirin), which has been in clinical use since the latter part of the nineteenth century. Interestingly, its exact mechanism of action remained unknown until the early 1970s.

The NSAIDs are one of the most frequently used group of drugs and, in relation to their wide consumption, are very safe. Several preparations of this group of drugs have been used in large doses for more than 10 years, revealing no or rare side effects. Unlike opioids, NSAIDs neither affect ventilation nor produce physical dependence. They are suitable for use as primary analgesics for all types of pain.

In the 1990s, awareness of undertreatment of surgical pain (1) led to a great number of clinical trials to study whether part of the need for analgesics could be covered by regular administration of NSAIDs. These drugs have opioid-sparing effects if administered intravenously, orally, or rectally (2–5).

MECHANISM OF ACTION

Arachidonic acid, normally stored in cell membranes, is released when membranes are perturbed, e.g., with inflammation or trauma. The metabolism of arachidonic acid through the cyclooxygenase (COX) pathway leads to the production of various prostaglandins and thromboxanes and through the lipoxygenase pathway results in the production of leukotrienes (Fig. 11.1). When the COX pathway is blocked by NSAIDs, the arachidonic acid metabolism is shunted, creating excessive levels of leukotrienes. This mechanism is probably responsible for aspirin-induced asthma. The COX products are potent vasodilators and hyperalgesic agents and contribute significantly to the erythema, swelling, and pain associated with inflammation. All cells, except red blood cells, are capable of producing prostaglandins and thromboxanes. In various organs, prostaglandins and thromboxanes mediate various physiologic functions that are interfered with by the inhibition of the COX enzyme.

Two different COX isoenzymes have been identified, a constitutive COX (COX-1) and an inducible COX (COX-2) (6). Most anti-inflammatory analgesics block the function of both isoenzymes and produce the useful effects and side effects. The prostanoids produced by the COX-1 isoenzyme protect the gastric mucosa, regulate renal blood flow, and induce platelet aggregation. In other words, COX-1 blockade is mainly responsible for the unwanted effects of anti-inflammatory analgesics. Following trauma and inflammation, the amount of COX-2 is increased. By blocking the function of COX-2 isoenzyme, it is possible to produce the beneficial effects of anti-inflammatory analgesics. The ability of NSAIDs to inhibit COX activity varies, and the ratio of COX-2/COX-1 inhibition varies in different NSAIDs (6). None of the modern COX-2-inhibiting NSAIDs has been studied in children.

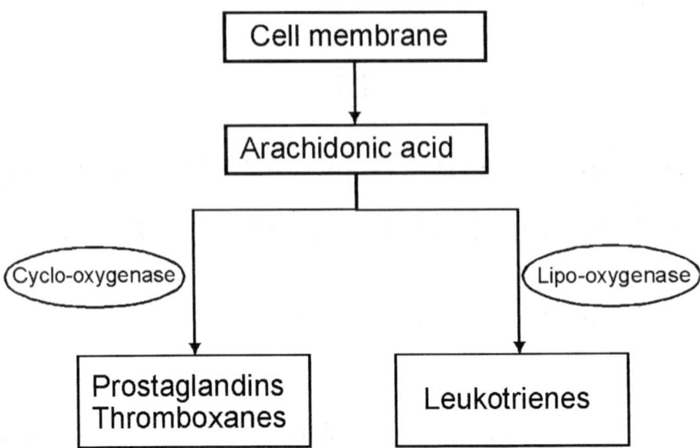

FIG. 11.1. Metabolism of arachidonic acid.

Alone, prostaglandins do not cause pain but do sensitize the nerve endings to perceive an ordinary nonpainful stimulus as pain. They are synergistic with other inflammatory mediators such as bradykinin and histamine. NSAIDs appear to act primarily through the inhibition of COX, thereby blocking the synthesis of prostaglandin and thromboxane. Much effort has been made to evaluate the anti-inflammatory effect of NSAIDs compared with their analgesic properties. The specific mechanism through which these drugs produce analgesia is not known. Although the degree of the anti-inflammatory effect of the various NSAIDs varies, the analgesic efficacy of all preparations is essentially the same. Typical for this whole group of drugs is the so-called analgesic "ceiling effect," i.e., after a certain level, increasing the dose does not increase analgesia. Conversely, in therapeutic doses NSAIDs do not have central depressing effects. This differentiates NSAIDs from the opioid analgesics. Clinically, the various compounds differ in spectrum and degree of side effects.

INDICATIONS

As analgesics, NSAIDs are effective in rheumatoid arthritis; various joint, bone, and muscle pains; back pain; headache; dental pain; and menstrual pains. An important indication for their use is bone and joint trauma, including fractures where swelling is a major component producing pain. Parenteral preparations of NSAIDs are successfully used for ureteral and biliary colic in adults. Since the late 1970s, the use of intravenous NSAIDs as a continuous infusion for postoperative pain has been increasing, although intravenous (i.v.) bolus doses combined with opioids were already in use for postoperative pain in the 1960s (unpublished personal observation).

In pediatrics, NSAIDs are used most commonly to treat juvenile rheumatoid arthritis (JRA). The effects of long-term use, including unwanted effects, have primarily been observed in these patients (7). NSAIDs are also used as antipyretics (8,9) for fever and infection as in the common cold and otitis media. Indomethacin promotes the closure of a patent ductus arteriosus in newborn and preterm infants (10). In small doses, aspirin inhibits platelet aggregation, and in some conditions, indomethacin and diclofenac have been successful in treating nocturnal enuresis (11,12). Pediatric postoperative analgesia has been studied with several old and new preparations administered in various ways. The prerequisites of day-case surgery have aroused special interest in the use of NSAIDs in children.

NSAIDs are the second step (mild to moderate pain) in the World Health Organization's step-wise ladder of pain therapy. When combined with opioids in a multimodal therapeutic treatment plan, NSAIDs are also used in the treatment of severe, long-lasting pain such as cancer pain. They are also useful in the treatment of recurrent pain problems such as sickle-cell vaso-occlusive crisis pain.

PHARMACOKINETICS AND PHARMACODYNAMICS

Although NSAIDs have been used, at least to some extent, for managing chronic rheumatoid pain in children, their use for treating children's acute pain has been studied in large scale only since the 1990s. The pharmacokinetics of various NSAIDs in infants and children has been studied, but there appears to be little information about the concentration–effect relationship (13). A summary comparing the elimination half-lives of NSAIDs in children of various ages with those of adults is presented in Table 11.1.

Acetaminophen is perhaps the most popular analgesic in pediatric practice. It is thought to be effective through inhibition of COX in the central nervous system, producing analgesia comparable with the other NSAIDs. It does not inhibit prostaglandin synthesis in other tissues nor exhibit any significant anti-inflammatory or NSAID side effects in doses used traditionally.

Analgesic plasma concentrations of acetaminophen are not known but concentrations of 10 to 20 μg/mL are thought to be effective as antipyretics (8,9). After oral doses of 10 to 15 mg/kg, these concentrations may be reached in 30 minutes. After rectal administration, the absorption is variable; maximal concentrations usually occur at 2 to 3 hours and reach these levels with doses of more than 40 mg/kg (13–17).

The elimination of acetaminophen is mainly through glucuronidation and sulfation. A small amount is eliminated by oxidation through cytochrome P-450. With an overdose, the oxidation increases and the metabolite *N*-acetyl-*p*-benzocinon-imine causes death of liver cells. The risk for liver toxicity is significant if the single dose exceeds 150 mg/kg orally. There are recent reports of fulminant hepatic failure after accidental overdosing in young children (18–20). Plasma concentration 150 to 200 μg/mL is considered indication for starting therapeutic measures (21). Active therapy with oral or preferably i.v. *N*-acetylcysteine has been shown effective (22).

Acetaminophen is a safe analgesic when used in therapeutic doses. Even the newborn is able to metabolize it; the elimination rate is similar in neonates, children, and adults (17,23).

Acetylsalicylic acid (aspirin), the oldest NSAID, still enjoys wide use, especially in chronic conditions like JRA. Because its use in small children increases the risk of Reye syndrome, including liver damage and central nervous system symptoms, aspirin must be administered cautiously (24). The elimination of aspirin is slowed at higher salicylate concentrations. In neonates, elimination of aspirin is significantly slower than in adults but appears to reach adult values within the first year of life (25).

Indomethacin is an effective anti-inflammatory agent. In neonates, it is used primarily for the closure of patent ductus arteriosus. Its elimination is markedly delayed in premature infants compared with adults (26). However, children metabolize and eliminate indomethacin the same as adults do by 1 year of age (27). Used as an analgesic, indomethacin has fewer side effects in small children than in

TABLE 11.1. *Terminal elimination half-lives of different nonsteroidal anti-inflammatory drug used in infants, children, adolescents, and adults*

Drug	Premature infants	<10 d	1–7 yr	7–15 yr	Adults
Acetaminophen		4.9	4.5	4.4	3.6
Diclofenac			1.3		1.1
Indomethacin	20.7	14.7	8.5		7.1
(S)-Ketorolac				6.8	6.2
Naproxen				12	12
Piroxicam				35	55
Propacetamol		3.5	2.1	1.6	3.6

adults. Although indomethacin is reported to decrease urinary output and cause weight gain and hyponatremia in premature infants, this has not been clinically observed by the age of 1 year (2,28).

Ibuprofen is known as an effective analgesic with only few side effects. Recently, it was introduced as a nonprescription analgesic/antipyretic for use in children. It has several useful formulations that vary in different countries. An oral solution of 5 to 10 mg/kg has been shown to be effective as an antipyretic. For analgesia, single doses of 10 to 15 mg/kg are thought to be effective (3,29), and in long-term use, 40 mg/kg per day has been safe (30). The peak serum concentration appears in an hour, but, as with acetaminophen, the peak antipyretic effect is delayed until 2.5 to 3 hours after administration (8,9). The antipyretic effect is greater and longer lasting than that of 12.5 mg/kg acetaminophen.

The plasma concentration range for ibuprofen in children (5 to 10 mg/kg oral solution) appears to be similar to that in adults after a 400-mg dose. The ibuprofen elimination in children with JRA is the same as that in adults, $t_{1/2}$ of 1 to 3 hours (30). In young febrile children, the terminal elimination rate is reported to be somewhat faster, 0.8 to 1.2 hours. The volume of distribution and clearance seemed to be less in children older than 2.5 years compared with younger children. These developmental changes might be owing to age-dependent protein binding (9).

Diclofenac, ketoprofen, ketorolac, naproxen, and piroxicam are anti-inflammatory analgesics claimed to exhibit fewer side effects than the older agents aspirin and indomethacin, at least in adults. Diclofenac is eliminated mainly through metabolism. Because its plasma clearance is approximately two times higher in children than in adults, its maintenance dose, calculated on a milligram per body weight basis, must be higher in children to achieve equal steady-state concentrations (31). The elimination half-life of diclofenac is at the same level in children as it is in adults; the elimination of ketoprofen occurs at similar rates as well (32).

In children, ketorolac is eliminated as rapidly as in adults. The plasma clearance of ketorolac is higher in children, indicating a higher dose requirement (33,34). The elimination half-life of naproxen varied between 10 and 14 hours, similar to that observed in adults (35). Piroxicam is an anti-inflammatory agent with a long duration of action that allows dosing only once daily. In children, its elimination half-life is 30 to 35 hours, approximately 20 hours shorter than in adults. This seems to be caused by the higher clearance of piroxicam in children because the volume of distribution is similar to that in adults (36).

EFFICACY AND CLINICAL USE

JRA is a heterogeneous disease, a group of different chronic joint inflammations of unknown cause. A child with JRA does not appear to be in pain and moves seemingly without difficulty, although in a manner different from that of a healthy child. Aches in the joints are rarely a dominant symptom in a child but may appear after exercise in a long-lasting disease. Some difficulties in the efficacy studies of NSAIDs result from the heterogeneity of the disease as well as in the assessment (7,37).

NSAIDs are considered first choice for treatment of all forms of JRA (38). Aspirin is the least expensive, physicians have a lot of experience with it, and no other NSAID has proved more effective. However, in the 1990s, the efficacy and tolerance of tolmetin, naproxen, and diclofenac were found equal, and they and flurbiprofen, ibuprofen, and ketoprofen have been found useful and well tolerated in children with JRA. All experience in the long-term use of NSAIDs in children comes from the patients with JRA (7,39–42).

ACUTE PAIN AND FEVER

Acetaminophen is the most commonly used analgesic and antipyretic in children. With commonly used doses, 10 to 15 mg/kg every 6 to 8 hours or as single boluses known to be effective in the treatment of fever, acetaminophen has not proved to be effective as an analgesic (43–47).

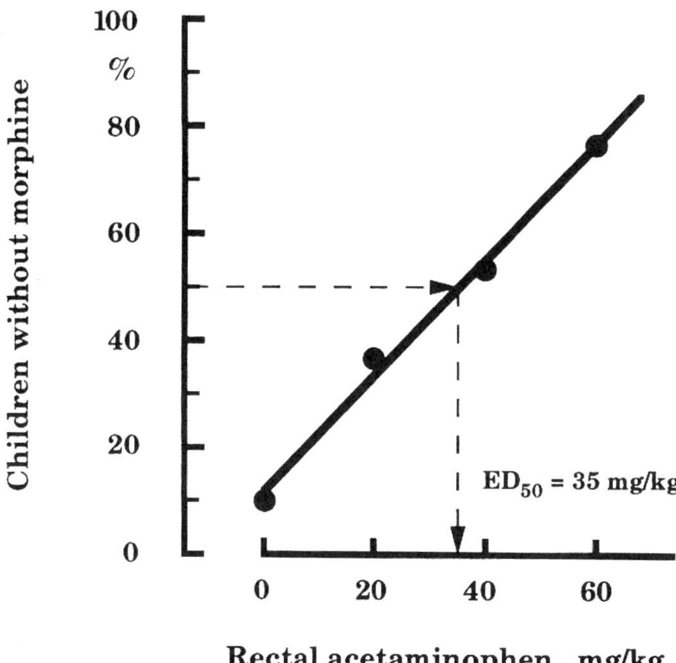

FIG. 11.2. Correlation between the dose of rectal acetaminophen in a pediatric day-case surgery and the percentage of children who did not need postoperative rescue morphine. (From Korpela R, Korvenoja P, Meretoja OA. Morphine sparing effect of acetaminophen in pediatric day-case surgery. *Anesthesiology* 1999;91:442–447, with permission.)

An oral dose of 20 mg/kg was effective, but a rectal dose of as much as 20 to 35 mg/kg was ineffective for tonsillectomy/appendectomy pain (14,16,48,49). It was recently shown that acetaminophen has a clear dose-related potency for postoperative pain in children, with significance reached with a 40- or 60-mg/kg dose (5) (Fig. 11.2). The median effective dose of rectal acetaminophen was 35 mg/kg; 20 mg/kg did not significantly reduce pain compared with placebo (Fig. 11.3). Propacetamol is an injectable prodrug of paracetamol (acetaminophen). Although unavailable in North America, it has been used extensively as a parenteral analgesic in France. Propacetamol is completely hydrolyzed within 6 minutes of administration; 1 g of the prodrug yields 0.5 g of paracetamol. It is a safe and pratical analgesic in children with established i.v. access (50).

The analgesic efficacy of 1 mg/kg diclofenac administered rectally (49), 10 mg ibuprofen administered orally (29), 40 mg/kg ibuprofen daily administered rectally (3,51), 5 mg/kg ketoprofen i.v. daily (52,53), 1 mg/kg ketorolac i.v. (46,54) has been shown in pediatric postoperative pain (55). In the 1990s, the use of preemptive and regular anti-inflammatory medication for pediatric day-case surgery was extensively studied (3,29,46,49,51–55). At equipotent doses, the analgesic effects, safety, and major side effect profiles of the antipyretic analgesics are similar (Table 11.2). Generally, 1 mg/kg rectal diclofenic = 10 mg/kg oral ibuprofen = 40 mg/kg rectal acetaminophen = 5 mg/kg i.v. ketoprophen = 0.5 mg/kg i.v. ketorolac.

CONTRAINDICATIONS AND UNWANTED EFFECTS

Based on their mechanism of action, the NSAIDs inhibiting COX-1 and COX-2 enzymes are able to cause gastrointestinal (GI)

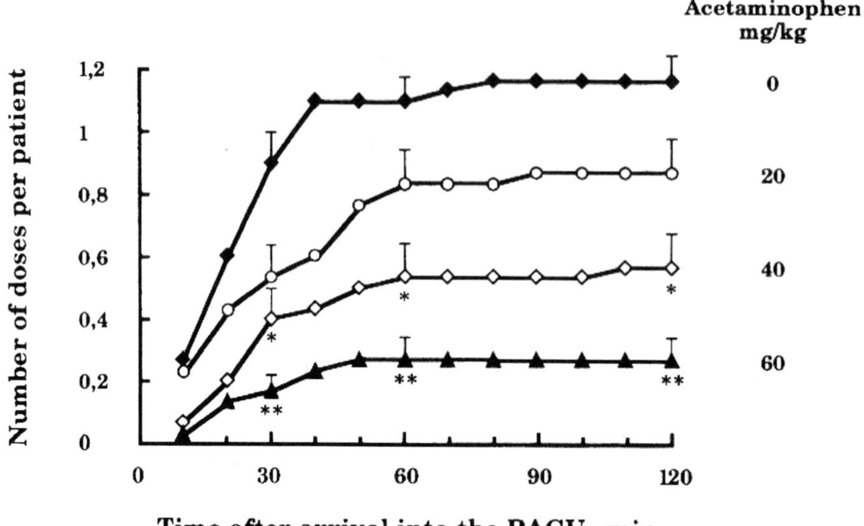

FIG. 11.3. Average number of morphine doses required in children who received 0, 20, 40, or 60 mg/kg acetaminophen rectally. Acetaminophen had a clear morphine-sparing effect: the number of morphine doses was smaller with the greater acetaminophen doses. *Single asterisk* denotes difference from the 0 mg/kg group, and *double asterisk* denotes significant difference from 0 and 20 mg/kg groups. Bars indicate standard error of the mean. (From Korpela R, Korvenoja P, Meretoja OA. Morphine sparing effect of acetaminophen in pediatric day-case surgery. *Anesthesiology* 1999;91: 442–447, with permission.)

irritation, disturbances in blood clotting, and renal function as well as bronchoconstriction.

In adult patients, the GI complaints are the most common side effects of NSAIDs. Arthrosis in elderly patients necessitates regular long-term pharmacotherapy. The risk of activation of a peptic ulcer or bleeding is significant. For these patients, the introduction of the selective COX-2 enzyme–blocking NSAIDs are advantageous. When treating acute pain and fever in children, the GI symptoms are not as common as in adult patients. When serious clinical adverse events were compared in more than 27,000 children younger than 2 years receiving short-term treatment of either acetaminophen or ibuprofen suspension, the risk was small and

TABLE 11.2. *Pediatric dosage of nonsteroidal anti-inflammatory drugs used as analgesics for nonchronic pain*

Drug	Single dose (mg/kg)	No. of daily doses	Maximum dose (mg/kg/d)
Acetaminophen	40–60 p.r. 20–30 p.o.	4	100
Aspirin	10–15	4–6	60
Diclofenac	1.0–2.0	3–4	?
Ibuprofen	10–15	3–4	40
Indomethacin	1	3	3
Ketoprofen	1.5	2–3	5
Ketorolac	0.5	3–4	?
Naproxen	10	2	20
Piroxicam	0.4	1	?
Propacetamol	20–40	4–6	200

?, lack of available data; p.r., per rectum; p.o., per os (orally).

did not vary by choice of medication (56). In two large studies on NSAIDs effects on the GI tract in patients with JRA, the authors concluded that although mild GI disturbances are frequent side effects associated with NSAID therapy, probably comparable with the rates found in adults taking NSAIDs, the number of children with JRA who experience clinically significant gastropathy appears to be low (57,58). The GI complaints are rare when treating postoperative pain in children with regular/continuous NSAIDs (3,53,54).

There has been special concern about the increased tendency of bleeding when NSAIDs are given perioperatively (59). They all inhibit platelet aggregation and prolong bleeding time. Acetaminophen is a weak COX-1 and COX-2 inhibitor (6) and therefore has been preferred as a nonopioid analgesic in patients at risk of bleeding disorders. However, *in vitro*, acetaminophen is also able to disturb platelet aggregation and, depending on the concentration, decreases platelet thromboxane B_2 synthesis (60). Although the bleeding time is increased after administration of most NSAIDs, it usually remains within normal values if the patient has a healthy clotting system (60,61). It is advisable to avoid pre- or intraoperative NSAID administration if the surgery involves large bleeding surfaces or the possibility of uncontrollable bleeding.

Studies on oral and i.v. ketoprofen and bleeding during and after adenoidectomy did not reveal any increased bleeding (52). There are controversial results on diclofenac and ketorolac in children during and after tonsillectomy (62–65). Rectal diclofenac, 3 mg/kg daily, was a poor analgesic as was 90 mg/kg acetaminophen daily, but there were no episodes of bleeding (66). After 1 mg/kg preoperative ketorolac, extra measures were required to obtain hemostasis and there was greater blood loss compared with 35 mg/kg acetaminophen administered rectally. Both were poor analgesics (67). The different results might be owing to different doses and timing. For the analgesic effect, it is better to give the NSAID early, but to avoid bleeding, it is wise to give it after the primary hemostasis has taken place. Tonsillectomy pain lasts for several days and requires opioids to control the pain. We would rely on intraoperative short-acting opioids and start the NSAID at the end of surgery, when bleeding is under control.

The effects of NSAIDs on healthy kidneys are negligible (68). If the renal circulation is affected by hypotension, hypovolemia, or cardiac insufficiency or there is a preexisting renal disease, blocking COX may result in oliguria or anuria. Therefore, it is important to inform parents of febrile children or children with day-case surgery to ensure adequate intake of fluids. After tonsillectomy/adenoidectomy, painless swallowing is an important factor that promotes drinking.

Aspirin-induced asthma, bronchospasm after ingestion of aspirin or other NSAIDs, is experienced by 8% to 20% of adults with asthma. The reaction is potentially fatal. It is reported to rarely occur in children (56). NSAIDs should be used with caution in children with asthma. Conventional doses of acetaminophen are thought to be safe in children with asthma.

There are experimental laboratory reports of the effects of NSAIDs on healing of bowel anastomoses and bone fractures. There are no clinical data to support this. In Europe, various NSAIDs in large doses have been administered (ordered by orthopedic/GI surgeons) to these patients, adults as well as children, with good surgical and analgesic results.

PEDIATRIC ANALGESIC ADMINISTRATION

The same analgesics known to be effective in adults can be safely administered to children after the newborn period. The margin of safety for children is at least equal to that of adults. For successful analgesic treatment of pediatric patients, one must pay special attention to drug administration—the route of administration, correct dose and timing, and choice of analgesic drug (Table 11.2).

Although the management of mild to moderate pain rarely requires parenteral analgesic therapy, children who have a previously established i.v. catheter can be treated wth i.v.

NSAIDs. The i.v. preparations of NSAIDs can be added to the ordinary infusion without an expensive pump because NSAIDs do not produce any acute side effects. As long as the child needs an i.v. line, this route provides convenient, continuous analgesic administration with little additional cost.

The oral route is preferable whenever possible. In addition to use for long-term analgesic treatment at home, oral medication can often be administered for postoperative pain preemptively. When given preoperatively, NSAIDs can be mixed with other premedications. Rectal administration of medication postoperatively is widely used for young children. Acceptability and, accordingly, the availability of rectal preparations vary greatly in different cultures. Children consider it a better choice than injection. Suppositories might be useful in terminal care at home when oral administration is not possible. There are often difficulties in administering any medication to a child, making the use of preparations with a long-lasting effect advantageous.

It is common in enteral administration for the effect to occur relatively slowly. Oral or rectal medication used for acute pain must be administered well in advance, usually at least an hour before the effect is expected. Because of the mechanism of action, the analgesic effect of the NSAID is reached slowly when the drug is administered intravenously. There is no advantage in using the intramuscular route, particularly regarding bioavailability; the NSAIDs are almost completely absorbed when taken enterally. Furthermore, intramuscular injection does not provide a better or faster analgesic effect. The parenteral formulations cause considerable pain on injection.

The choice of analgesic should be based on the assumed severity, type, and duration of pain. The analgesic efficacy of the NSAIDs has been underestimated. When used properly, i.e., prescribing an adequate dose, allowing time for their full effect, and continuing the administration to keep the prostaglandin levels low, NSAIDs are able to control moderate and even some severe pain. Their margin of safety is wide, and no such individual variation occurs as with opioid analgesics. Because NSAIDs do not cause respiratory depression or other acute serious adverse effects, their preemptive administration is safe. The experience of postoperative pain is the most important single cause of long-lasting temper tantrums and untoward behavioral changes in children (69). Postoperative pain also seems to be a clear predictor of postoperative nausea and vomiting in children (5,45,48,70).

In the treatment of pediatric pain, prevention has special advantages because assessing pain is difficult and children cannot or do not understand how to ask for analgesic relief. For the same reasons, children benefit from regular or continuous analgesic administration in all types of pain management. Basic analgesia with regular oral/rectal administration or with a continuous i.v. infusion dramatically improves the general well-being of the child, compared with the ups and downs of as-needed medication. Today, the safety and lack of side effects of NSAIDs medication, together with the benefit of the child being free from pain, are appreciated.

The advantages of combining analgesics that have different modes of action have become familiar through cancer pain therapy. In the same light, better analgesic effect with fewer side effects should be available for treating other types of pain as well. The opioid-sparing effect of various NSAIDs in adults and children has been demonstrated. Although opioid analgesics are needed for visceral and other types of severe pain, the dose and side effects can be diminished with the simultaneous use of NSAIDs.

Many prejudices exist concerning use of analgesics in general—their potential to cause dependence and their seemingly harmful effects on children. As with any drug therapy, if patient and/or family compliance fails, treatment will not succeed. Information about analgesics and the principles of analgesic therapy should be explained not only for terminal cancer pain treatment but for postoperative pain treatment as well. Analgesic treatment should always be discussed with the child when possible and with the parents, enabling the medical staff to ascertain patient acceptance and parental understanding of the importance of regular administration and recognition of possible side effects.

REFERENCES

1. Schechter NL. The undertreatment of pain in children: an overview. *Pediatr Clin North Am* 1989;36:781–794.
2. Maunuksela E-L, Olkkola KT, Korpela R. Does prophylactic intravenous infusion of indomethacin improve the management of postoperative pain in children? *Can J Anaesth* 1988;35:123–127.
3. Maunuksela E-L, Ryhänen P, Janhunen L. Efficacy of rectal ibuprofen in controlling postoperative pain in children. *Can J Anaesth* 1992;39:226–230.
4. Teiriä H, Meretoja OA. PCA in pediatric orthopaedic patients: influence of a NSAID on morphine requirement. *Paediatric Anaesth* 1994;4:87–91.
5. Korpela R, Korvenoja P, Meretoja OA. Morphine sparing effect of acetaminophen in pediatric day-case surgery. *Anesthesiology* 1999;91:442–447.
6. Mitchell JA, Akarasereenont P, Thiemermann C, et al. Selectivity of nonsteroidal anti-inflammatory drugs as inhibitors of constitutive and inducible cyclo-oxygenase. *Proc Natl Acad Sci U S A* 1993;90:11693–11697.
7. Williams PL, Ansell BM, Bell A, et al. Multicenter study of piroxicam versus naproxen in juvenile chronic arthritis, with special reference to problem areas in clinical trials of nonsteroidal anti-inflammatory drugs in childhood. *Br J Rheumatol* 1986;25:67–71.
8. Brown RD, Wilson JT, Kearns GL, et al. Single-dose pharmacokinetics of ibuprofen and acetaminophen in febrile children. *J Clin Pharmacol* 1992;32:231–241.
9. Kelley MT, Walson PD, Edge JH, et al. Pharmacokinetics and pharmacodynamics of ibuprofen isomers and acetaminophen in febrile children. *Clin Pharmacol Ther* 1992;52:181–189.
10. Yeh TF, Goldbarg HR, Henek T, et al. Intravenous indomethacin therapy in premature infants with patent ductus arteriosus: causes of death and one-year follow-up. *Am J Dis Child* 1982;136:803–807.
11. Waili NS. Diclofenac sodium in the treatment of primary nocturnal enuresis: double blind cross-over study. *Clin Exp Pharmacol Physiol* 1986;13:139–142.
12. Waili NS. Indomethacin suppository to treat primary nocturnal enuresis: double-blind study. *J Urol* 1989; 142:1290–1292.
13. Andersson BJ, Holford NH, Wollard GA, et al. Perioperative pharmacodynamics of acetaminophen analgesia in children. *Anesthesiology* 1999;90:411–421.
14. Andersson B, Kanagasundarum S, Woolard G. Analgesic efficacy of paracetamol in children using tonsillectomy as a pain model. *Anaesth Intensive Care* 1996;24:669–673.
15. Montgomery CJ, McGormac JP, Reichert CC, et al. Plasma concentrations after high dose (45 mg/kg) rectal acetaminophen in children. *Can J Anaesth* 1995;42: 982–986.
16. Birmingham PK, Tobin MJ, Henthorn TK, et al. Twenty-four-hour pharmacokinetics of rectal acetaminophen in children. An old drug with new recommendation. *Anesthesiology* 1997;87:244–252.
17. Hansen TG, O'Brien K, Morton NS, et al. Plasma paracetamol concentrations and pharmacokinetics following rectal administration in neonates and young infants. *Acta Anaesth Scand* 1999;43:855–859.
18. Miles FK, Kamath R, Dorney SF, et al. Accidental paracetamol overdosing and fulminant hepatic failure in children. *Med J Aust* 1999;171:472–475.
19. Morton NS, Arana A. Paracetamol-induced fulminant hepatic failure in a child after 5 days of therapeutic doses. *Paediatr Anaesth* 1999;9:463–465.
20. Bauer M, Babel B, Giesen H, et al. Fulminant liver failure in a young child following repeated acetaminophen overdosing. *J Forensic Sci* 1999;44:1299–1303.
21. Rivera-Penera T, Gugig R, Davis J, et al. Outcome of acetaminophen overdose in pediatric patients and factors contributing to hepatotoxicity. *J Pediatr* 1997;130, 300–304.
22. Buckley NA, Whyte IM, O'Connell DL, et al. Oral or intravenous n-acetylcysteine: which is the treatment of choice for acetaminophen (paracetamol) poisoning? *J Toxicol Clin Toxicol* 1999;37:759–767.
23. Miller RP, Roberts RJ, Fisher LJ. Acetaminophen elimination kinetics in neonates, children and adults. *Clin Pharmacol Ther* 1976;19:284–294.
24. Khan AS, Kent J, Schonberger LB. Aspirin and Reye's syndrome. *Lancet* 1993;341:968.
25. Levy G, Garretson LK. Kinetics of salicylate elimination by newborn infants of mothers who ingested aspirin before delivery. *Pediatrics* 1974;53:201–210.
26. Barsh AR, Hickey DE, Graham TP, et al. Pharmacokinetics of indomethacin in the neonate: relation of plasma indomethacin levels to response to ductus arteriosus. *N Engl J Med* 1981;305:67–72.
27. Olkkola KT, Maunuksela E-L, Korpela R. Pharmacokinetics of postoperative intravenous indomethacin in children. *Pharmacol Toxicol* 1989;64:157–160.
28. Maunuksela E-L, Olkkola KT, Korpela R. Intravenous indomethacin as postoperative analgesic in children: acute effects on blood pressure, heart rate, body temperature and bleeding. *Ann Clin Res* 1987;19: 359–363.
29. Schatel BP, King SA, Thoden WR. Pain relief in children: a placebo-controlled study. *Clin Pharmacol Ther* 1991;49:154.
30. Mäkelä A-L, Lempiäinen M, Yrjänä T. Ibuprofen levels in serum and synovial fluid. *Scand J Rheumatol* 1981; 39:15–17.
31. Korpela R, Olkkola KT. Pharmacokinetics of intravenous diclofenac sodium in children. *Eur J Clin Pharmacol* 1990;38:293–295.
32. Lempiäinen M, Mäkelä AL. Determination of ketoprofen by high performance liquid chromatography from serum and urine: clinical application in children with juvenile rheumatoid arthritis. *Int J Clin Pharmacol Res* 1987;7:265–271.
33. Olkkola KT, Maunuksela E-L. The pharmacokinetics of postoperative intravenous ketorolac tromethamine in children. *Br J Clin Pharmacol* 1991;31:182–184.
34. Hamunen K, Maunuksela E-L, Sarvela J, et al. Stereoselective pharmacokinetics of ketorolac in children, adolescents and adults. *Acta Anaesth Scand* 1999;43:1041–1046.
35. Kauffmann RE, Bollinger RO, Wan SH, et al. Pharmacokinetics of naproxen in children. *Dev Pharmacol Ther* 1982;5:143–150.
36. Mäkelä AL, Olkkola KT, Mattila MJ. Steady state pharmacokinetics of piroxicam in children with rheumatic diseases. *Eur J Clin Pharmacol* 1991;41:79–81.
37. Lovell DJ, Walco JA. Pain associated with juvenile rheumatoid arthritis. *Pediatr Clin North Am* 1989;36: 1015–1027.

38. Cron RQ, Sharma S, Sherry DD. Current treatment by United States and Canadian pediatric rheumatologists. *J Rheumatol* 1999;26:2036–2038.
39. Leak AM, Richter MR, Klemens LE, et al. A crossover study of naproxen, diclofenac, and tolmetin in seronegative juvenile chronic arthritis. *Clin Exp Rheumatol* 1988;6:157–160.
40. Haapasaari J Wuolijoki E, Ylijoki H. Treatment of juvenile rheumatoid arthritis with diclofenac sodium. *Scand J Rheumatol* 1983;12:325–330.
41. Leak AM, Richter MR, St Cyr CH, et al. Flurbiprofen is as effective as naproxen in juvenile spondylitis. *J Rheumatol* 1986;13:664–665.
42. Brever EJ, Gianni E, Baum J, et al. Ketoprofen (Orudis) in the treatment of juvenile rheumatoid arthritis. A segment I study. *J Rheumatol* 1982;9:144–148.
43. Baer GA, Rorarius MGF, Kolehmainen S, et al. The effect of paracetamol or diclofenac administered before operation on postoperative pain and behavior after adenoidectomy in small children. *Anaesthesia* 1992;47:1078–1080.
44. Bertin L, Pons G, d'Athis P, et al. Randomized double-blind, multicenter controlled trial of ibuprofen versus acetaminophen (paracetamol) and placebo for treatment of symptoms of tonsillitis and pharyngitis in children. *J Pediatr* 1991;119:811–814.
45. Tobias DJ, Love S, Hersey S, et al. Analgesia after bilateral myringotomy and placement of pressure equalization tubes in children: acetaminophen versus acetaminophen with codeine. *Anesth Analg* 1995;81:496–500.
46. Watcha MF, Ramirez-Ruiz M, White PF, et al. Perioperative effects if ketorolac and acetaminophen in children undergoing bilateral myringotomy. *Can J Anaesth* 1992; 39:649–654.
47. Bennie RE, Boehringer LA, McMahon S, et al. Postoperative analgesia with preoperative oral ibuprofen or acetaminophen in children undergoing myringotomy. *Pediatr Anaesth* 1997;7:399–403.
48. Rusy LM, Houck CS, Sullivan LJ, et al. A double-blind evaluation of ketorolac tromethamine versus acetaminophen in pediatric tonsillectomy: analgesia and bleeding. *Anesth Analg* 1995;80:226–229.
49. Morton NS, O'Brien K. Analgesic efficacy of paracetamol and diclofenac in children receiving PCA morphine. *Br J Anaesth* 1999;82:715–717.
50. Grandy JC, Rod B, Boccard E, et al. Pharmacokinetics and antipyretic effects of an injectable pro-drug of paracetamol (proparacetamol) in children. *Pediatr Anaesth* 1992;2:291–295.
51. Kokki H, Hendolin H, Maunukseal E-L, et al. Ibuprofen in the treatment of postoperative pain in small children. A randomized double-blind placebo controlled parallel group. *Acta Anaesth Scand* 1994;38:467–472.
52. Kokki H, Nikanne E, Tuovinen K. I.v. intraoperative ketoprofen in small children during adenoidectomy: a dose-finding study. *Br J Anaesth* 1998;81:870–874.
53. Kokki H, Tuovinen K, Hendolin H. The effect of intravenous ketoprofen on postoperative epidural sufentanil analgesia in children. *Anesth Analg* 1999;88:1036–1041.
54. Maunuksela E-L, Kokki H, Bullingham RES. Comparison of iv ketorolac with morphine for postoperative pain in children. *Clin Pharmacol Ther* 1992;52:436–443.
55. Romsing J, Walther-Larsen S. Peri-operative use of nonsteroidal anti-inflammatory drugs in children. *Anaesthesia* 1997;52:73–83.
56. Lesko SM, Mitchell AA. The safety of acetaminophen and ibuprofen among children younger than two years old. *Pediatrics* 1999;104:e39.
57. Dowed JE, Cimaz R, Fink CW. Nonsteroidal anti-inflammatory drug-induced gastroduodenal injury in children. *Arthritis Rheum* 1995;38:1225–1231.
58. Keenan GF, Gianni EH, Athreya BH. Clinically significant gastropathy associated with nonsteroidal anti-inflammatory drug use in children with juvenile rheumatoid arthritis. *J Rheumatol* 1995;22:1149–1151.
59. Souter JA, Fredman B, White PF. Controversies in the perioperative use of nonsteroidal anti-inflammatory drugs. *Anesth Analg* 1994;79:1178–1190.
60. Niemi TT, Backman JT, Syrjälä MT, et al. Platelet dysfunction after intravenous ketorolac or proparacetamol. *Acta Anaesth Scand* 2000;44:69–74.
61. Niemi TT, Taxell C, Rosenberg PH. Comparison of the effects of intravenous ketoprofen, ketorolac and diclofenac on platelet function in volunteers. *Acta Anaesth Scand* 1997;41:1353–1358.
62. Gunter JB, Varughese AM, Harrington JF, et al. Recovery and complications after tonsillectomy in children: a comparison of ketorolac and morphine. *Anesth Analg* 1995;81:1136–1141.
63. Splinter WM, Rhine EJ, Roberts DW, et al. Preoperative ketorolac increases bleeding after tonsillectomy in children. *Can J Anaesth* 1996;43:560–563.
64. Römsing J, Östergaard D, Welther-Larssen S, et al. Analgesic efficacy and safety of preoperative versus postoperative ketorolac in pediatric tonsillectomy. *Acta Anaesth Scand* 1998;42:770–775.
65. Robinson PM, Ahmed I. Diclofenac and post-tonsillectomy haemorrhage. *Clin Otolaryngol* 1994;19:344–345.
66. Römsing J, Ostergaard D, Drozdziewicz D, et al. Diclofenac or acetaminophen for analgesia in pediatric tonsillectomy outpatients. *Acta Anaesth Scand* 2000;44: 291–295.
67. Rusy LM, Houck CS, Sullivan LJ, et al. A double-blind evaluation of ketorolac tromethamine versus acetaminophen in pediatric tonsillectomy: analgesia and bleeding. *Anesth Analg* 1995;80:226–229.
68. Kenny GNC. Potential renal, haematological and allergic adverse effects associated with nonsteroidal anti-inflammatory drugs. *Drugs* 1992;44[Suppl 5]:31–37.
69. Kotiniemi LH, Ryhänen PT, Moilanen IK. Behavioral changes in children following day-case surgery: a 4-week follow-up of 551 children. *Anaesthesia* 1998;52: 570–576.
70. Kotiniemi LH, Ryhänen PT, Valanne J, et al. Postoperative symptoms at home following day-case surgery in children: a multicenter survey of 551 children. *Anaesthesia* 1998;52:563–569.

12

Opioid Agonists and Antagonists

Myron Yaster, Sabine Kost-Byerly, and Lynne G. Maxwell

Historically, opium and its derivatives (e.g., paregoric, morphine) were used for the treatment of diarrhea (dysentery) and pain. The beneficial psychologic and physiologic effects of opium, as well as its toxicity and potential for abuse, have been well known to physicians and the public for centuries (1,2). In 1680, Sydenham wrote, "Among the remedies which it has pleased Almighty God to give man to relieve his sufferings, none is so universal and so efficacious as opium." Conversely, many physicians throughout the ages have underused opium when treating patients in pain because of their fear that their patients would be harmed by its use. In the current era, addiction is particularly feared. Opium's easy availability, despite every effort by the government to control it, has resulted in a scourge of addiction that has devastated large segments of our population. Until and unless we can separate opium's dark consequences (yin) from its benefits (yang), innumerable numbers of patients will suffer unnecessarily. The purpose of this chapter is to delineate the role of opioid receptors in the mechanism of opioid analgesia, to highlight recent advances in opioid pharmacology and therapeutic interventions, and to provide a pharmacokinetic and pharmacodynamic framework regarding the use of opioids in the treatment of childhood pain.

TERMINOLOGY

The terminology used to describe potent analgesic drugs is constantly changing (2–4). They are commonly referred to as narcotics (from the Greek *narco*, to deaden), opiates (from the Greek *opion*, poppy juice, for drugs derived from the poppy plant), opioids (for all drugs with morphine-like effects, whether synthetic or naturally occurring), or euphemistically as strong analgesics (when the physician is reluctant to tell the patient or the patient's family that narcotics are being used) (2,5,6). Furthermore, the discovery of endogenous endorphins and opioid receptors has necessitated the reclassification of these drugs into agonists, antagonists, and mixed agonist–antagonists based on their receptor binding properties (2,6–11).

OPIOID RECEPTORS

Over the past 20 years, multiple opioid receptors and subtypes have been identified and classified (Table 12.1) (2,6–11). An understanding of the complex nature and organization of these multiple opioid receptors is essential for an adequate understanding of the response to and control of pain (12). In the central nervous system, there are four primary opioid receptor types, designated μ (for morphine), κ, δ, and σ. Recently, the μ, κ, and δ receptors have been cloned and have yielded invaluable information of receptor structure and function (13–16).

The μ receptor is further subdivided into μ_1 (supraspinal analgesia) and μ_2 (respiratory depression, inhibition of gastrointestinal motility, and spinal analgesia) subtypes (7,17,18). When morphine and other μ agonists are given systemically, they act predominantly through supraspinal μ_1 receptors. The κ and δ receptors have been subtyped as well, and other receptors and subtypes will surely

TABLE 12.1. *Classification of opioid receptors*

Receptor	Prototype agonist	CNS location	Effects
μ	Morphine, fentanyl, meperidine, codeine, methadone, hydromorphone,	Brain (laminae III and IV of the cortex, thalamus, periaqueductal gray), spinal cord (substantia gelatinosa)	μ_1, supraspinal analgesia, dependence; μ_2, respiratory depression, inhibition of gastrointestinal motility, bradycardia ++ sedation
κ	Ketocyclazocine, dynorphin, ? butorphanol	Brain (hypothalamus, periaqueductal gray, claustrum), spinal cord (substantia gelatinosa)	Spinal analgesia, ++++ sedation, miosis, inhibition of antidiuretic hormone release
δ	Enkephalins, DADL	Brain (pontine nucleus, amygdala, olfactory bulbs, deep cortex)	Analgesia, euphoria
σ	*N*-allylnormetazocine, phencyclidine, ? ketamine		Dysphoria, hallucinations, psychomotor stimulations

be discovered as research in this area continues (19).

The differentiation of agonists and antagonists is fundamental to pharmacology. A neurotransmitter is defined as having agonist activity, whereas a drug that blocks the action of a neurotransmitter is an antagonist (20–24). By definition, receptor recognition of an agonist is "translated" into other cellular alterations (i.e., the agonist initiates a pharmacologic effect), whereas an antagonist occupies the receptor without initiating the transduction step (i.e., it has no intrinsic activity or efficacy) (25). The intrinsic activity of a drug defines the ability of the drug–receptor complex to initiate a pharmacologic effect. Drugs that produce less than a maximal response have a lower intrinsic activity and are called partial agonists. Partial agonists also have antagonistic properties because by binding the receptor site, they block access of full agonists to the receptor site. Morphine and related opiates are μ agonists, and drugs that block the effects of opiates at the μ receptor, such as naloxone, are designated antagonists. The opioids most commonly used in the management of pain are μ agonists (Tables 12.2–12.4). These include morphine, meperidine, methadone, codeine, oxycodone, and the fentanyls. Mixed agonist–antagonist drugs act as agonists or partial agonists at one receptor and antagonists at another receptor. Mixed (opioid) agonist–antagonist drugs include pentazocine (Talwin), butorphanol (Stadol), nalorphine, dezocine (Dalgan), and nalbuphine (Nubain). Most of these drugs are agonists or partial agonists at the κ and σ receptors and antagonists or partial agonists at the μ receptor (Table 12.3). Thus, these drugs produce antinociception alone and dose dependently antagonize the effects of morphine. Buprenorphine (Buprenex) is considered a partial agonist at the μ and κ receptors.

Over the past 20 years, three distinct families of endogenous neuropeptides with opioid activity have been identified: the enkephalins, the endorphins (from endogenous morphine), and the dynorphins. Each family is derived from a distinct precursor polypeptide: proenkephalin, pro-opiomelanocortin, and prodynorphin, respectively. These precursor polypeptides are distributed in a specific anatomic fashion and are not necessarily confined to the central nervous system. Proenkephalin contains the amino acid sequence for met- and leuenkephalin and is located primarily in the spinal cord, periaqueductal gray, amygdala, hippocampus, cerebral cortex, and in areas that regulate autonomic and neuroendocrinologic function, primarily the anterior pituitary gland. It is also found in the adrenal medulla and the nerve plexii of the stomach and small intestine. Pro-opiomelanocortin contains the amino acid sequence

TABLE 12.2. *Commonly used μ agonist drugs*

Agonist	Equipotent i.v. dose (mg/kg)	Duration (hr)	Bioavailability (%)	Comments
Morphine	0.1	3–4	20–40	Seizures in newborns, also in all patients at high doses; histamine release, vasodilation—avoid in asthmatics and in circulatory compromise; MS Contin 8–12-hr duration
Meperidine	1.0	3–4	40–60	Catastrophic interactions with monoamine oxidase inhibitors; tachycardia, negative inotrope; metabolite produces seizures, not recommended for long-term use
Methadone	0.1	6–24	70–100	Can be given i.v. even though the package insert says subcutaneously or intramuscularly
Fentanyl	0.001	0.5–1		Bradycardia, minimal hemodynamic alterations; chest wall rigidity (>5 μg/kg rapid i.v. bolus), prescribe naloxone or paralyze with succinylcholine or pancuronium; transdermal patch available for chronic pain, contraindicated in acute pain
Codeine	1.2	3–4	40–70	Oral route only, prescribe with acetaminophen
Hydromorphone (Dialaudid)	0.015–0.02	3–4	40–60	Causes less central nervous system depression than morphine, less itching and nausea than morphine, can be used in intravenously and epidural patient-controlled analgesia
Oxycodone (component opioid in Tylox)	0.15	3–4	50	A third less than morphine but with better oral bioavailability, often used when weaning from intravenous to oral medication; available as a continuous-release preparation

TABLE 12.3. *Action of opioids at receptor subtypes*

Agent	Receptor subtype		
	μ	κ	σ
Morphine	Agonist	Agonist	Minimal effect
Meperidine	Agonist		
Fentanyl	Agonist		
Codeine	Agonist		
Naloxone (Narcan)	Antagonist	Antagonist	Antagonist
Naltrexone (Trexal)	Antagonist		
Pentazocine (Talwin)	Antagonist	Agonist	
Butorphanol (Stadol)	Minimal effect	Agonist	Agonist
Nalbuphine (Nubain)	Antagonist	Partial agonist	Agonist
Buprenorphine	Partial agonist	Agonist	Agonist

TABLE 12.4. *Physiologic effects of opioids by organ system*

- I. Central nervous system
  - A. Analgesia
  - B. Sedation
  - C. Dysphoria and euphoria
  - D. Nausea and vomiting
  - E. Miosis
  - F. Seizures
  - G. Psychotomimetic behaviors, excitation
- II. Respiratory system
  - A. Antitussive
  - B. Respiratory depression (decreased minute ventilation)
    - 1. Decreased respiratory rate
    - 2. Decreased tidal volume
    - 3. Decreased ventilatory response to carbon dioxide
  - C. Bronchospasm
    - 1. Morphine releases histamine
- III. Cardiovascular system
  - A. Heart rate
    - 1. Bradycardia (fentanyl, morphine)
    - 2. Tachycardia (meperidine)
  - B. Minimal effects on cardiac output
  - C. Vasodilation, venodilation
    - 1. Morphine >>> other opioids, ? histamine effect
- IV. Gastrointestinal system
  - A. Decreased intestinal motility and peristalsis
    - 1. Therapy for diarrhea
    - 2. Side effect + constipation
  - B. Increased sphincter tone
    - 1. Sphincter of Oddi
    - 2. Ileocolic
- V. Urinary system
  - A. Increased tone
    - 1. Ureters
    - 2. Bladder
    - 3. Detrusor muscles of the bladder

for melanocyte-stimulating hormone, adrenocorticotropic hormone, and β endorphin. It is found primarily in the cortex and the arcuate nucleus. Finally, prodynorphin contains the amino acid sequence for dynorphin and endorphin and is often distributed together with proenkephalin.

The μ receptor and its subspecies and the δ receptor produce analgesia, respiratory depression, euphoria, and physical dependence. Morphine is 50 to 100 times weaker at the δ than the μ receptor. By contrast, the endogenous opiate-like neurotransmitter peptides known as the enkephalins tend to be more potent at the δ and κ than the μ receptors. The κ receptor, located primarily in the spinal cord, produces spinal analgesia, miosis, and sedation with minimal associated respiratory depression. Indeed, this may have important clinical significance. As tolerance develops, increasing doses of morphine are required to produce effective analgesia. It is intriguing to speculate that at higher doses, the analgesia produced by morphine occurs by its δ and κ effects rather than by its μ agonist activity. Alternatively, when administered spinally, morphine and other μ agonists achieve cerebrospinal fluid levels that are log concentrations higher than can be achieved by more conventional routes of drug administration. Indeed, when administered by this route, the concentration of μ agonists may be high enough to produce analgesia via the κ receptor. Finally, the σ receptor is responsible for the psychotomimetic effects observed with some opiate drugs, particularly the mixed agonist–antagonist drugs. These effects include dysphoria and hallucinations.

Several studies suggest that the respiratory depression and analgesia produced by μ agonists involve different receptor subtypes (26–28). Other studies have disputed these findings (19,29). These receptors change in number in an age-related fashion and can be blocked by naloxone. Pasternak and colleagues (26,27), working with newborn rats, showed that 14-day-old rats are 40 times more sensitive to morphine analgesia than 2-day-old rats. Nevertheless, morphine depresses the respiratory rate in 2-day-old rats to a greater degree than in 14-day-old rats. Thus, the newborn may be particularly sensitive to the respiratory depressant effects of the commonly administered opioids in what may be an age-related receptor phenomenon (30). Obviously, this has important clinical implications for the use of narcotics in the newborn.

The μ, δ, and κ are distinct receptors but produce analgesia primarily by inhibiting synaptic transmission in the central nervous system and the myenteric plexus. They are usually found on the presynaptic nerve terminal and decrease the release of excitatory neurotransmitters from terminals carrying nociceptive stimuli. As a result, neurons are hyperpolarized, which suppresses spontaneous discharge and evoked responses. These receptors are coupled to guanosine 5′-triphosphate (GTP)–binding regulatory proteins (G proteins) and regulate transmembrane signaling by regulating adenosine 3′,5′-cyclic monophosphate (cyclic AMP), various ion (K, Ca, Na) channels and transport proteins, and phospholipases C and A_2 (diacylglycerol and inositol triphosphate activation of protein kinase C) (8,31,32).

G proteins are made of three subunits designated α, β, and γ (Fig. 12.1). The recognition site of the G protein faces the exterior of the lipid cell membrane to facilitate access of water-soluble endogenous ligands and drugs, whereas the catalytic site faces the interior of the cell. After binding of an agonist to an opioid receptor, GTP binds to the α unit of the G protein, which then dissociates from the β and γ subunits. The GTP-bound α unit interacts with the membrane-bound effector, for example, adenylate cyclase to produce or inhibit the secondary messenger cyclic AMP. When GTP is hydrolyzed to guanosine 5′-diphosphate by a GTPase on the α unit, the 5′-diphosphate α unit rejoins the β and γ subunits on the G protein and turns off the transmembrane signal. Several receptors may activate a single G protein. One receptor can also regulate many G proteins. One G protein can regulate several effectors, such as activation of a calcium channel or a phospholipase or release of intracellular calcium stores, and one effector can be activated by several G proteins.

Signal transduction from opioid receptors occurs via bonding to inhibitory G proteins (G_i and G_o). Analgesic effects are mediated by decreased neuronal excitability from an inwardly rectifying K^+ current, decreased cyclic AMP production, increased nitric oxide synthesis, and the production of 12-lipoxygenase metabolites. Synergism between opioids and nonsteroidal anti-inflammatory drugs occurs from the availability of greater amounts of arachidonic acid for metabolism by 12-lipoxygenase pathway, after blockade of prostaglandin production in the cyclooxygenase pathway by nonsteroidal anti-inflammatory drugs (33).

Ligand-induced conformational changes may also play a role in receptor-induced biologic responses. Evidence of this may lie in the puzzling findings that agonists with similar affinities can have different potencies (34,35). Opioids exert their analgesic effects supraspinally, at the level of the brainstem, spinally by inhibiting nociceptive input, and peripherally when pain is produced by inflammation or a sympathetic pain syndrome (36,37). Supraspinal injections of μ, κ, and δ agonists produce naloxone-sensitive analgesia. That opioids cause analgesia at a spinal site has led to increasing use of extradural or spinal administration of opioids for pain relief. Some drugs, such as meperidine and fentanyl, possess additional local anesthetic activity, and this may increase their ability to produce pain relief via the spinal or extradural route (38). It is most likely that the spinal analgesic activity of opioids is mediated via μ receptors because these make up the largest proportion of receptors in the spinal cord. These receptors are found close to the C-fiber terminals in lamina I and in the substantia gelatinosa. Very small doses of μ agonists actually enhance C-fiber activity: this effect is not shared by δ agonists and may account for the itching seen after spinal opioid injections. Powerful analgesic effects in inflammatory pain may be obtained with opioids acting at peripheral receptors. Indeed, morphine injected intra-articularly has been shown to provide pain relief after arthroscopic knee surgery (36,39,40).

Pain pathways and their modulation involve many neurotransmitters in addition to the endogenous opioids. Recently, much research has involved the roles that the excitatory amino acids glutamate and aspartate, the catecholamine norepinephrine, and the cholecystokinin peptides have in pain pathways and in modulation of opioid analgesic activity. The excitatory amino acids glutamate and aspartate combine with at least five subtypes of receptor, known as *N*-methyl-D-aspartate (NMDA), α-amino-3-hydroxy-5-methyl-4 isoxazole propi-

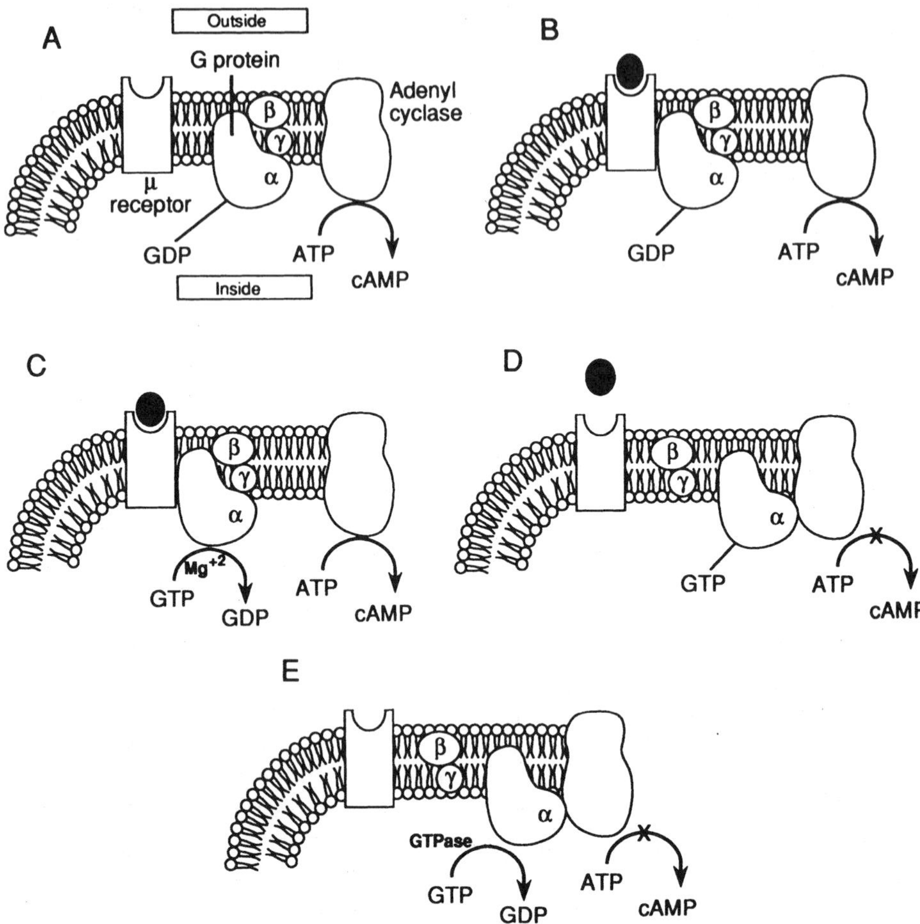

FIG. 12.1. G-protein cycling. **A:** In the inactive state, the binding of the opioid receptor is unoccupied. The heterotrimeric G protein is coupled to neither the receptor nor the effector and the α subunit is bound by guanosine 5′-diphosphate (*GDP*). **B:** An opioid agonist binds to the receptor. This results in a conformational change in its structure, facilitating contact with the G protein. **C:** The affinity of GDP for the α subunit of the G protein is decreased, and in the presence of magnesium ions (Mg^{2+}) is replaced by guanosine 5′-triphosphate (*GTP*). **D:** The GTP-bound α subunit of the G protein dissociates from its q dimer and couples to the effector. The affinity of the receptor for its agonist decreases and the agonist leaves its receptor binding site. **E:** The intrinsic GTPase in the dissociated α subunit is now activated and hydrolyzes the bound GTP into guanosine 5′-diphosphate, releasing inorganic phosphate (P_i). *ADP*, adenosine diphosphate; *ATP*, adenosine triphosphate; *cAMP*, adenosine 3′,5′-cyclic monophosphate. (Modified from Maze M, Tranquilli W. Alpha-2 adrenoceptor agonists: defining the role in clinical anesthesia. *Anesthesiology* 1991;74:581–605, with permission.)

onic acid (AMPA) (previously quisqualate), kainate, L-2-amino-4-phosphonobutyrate, and metabotropic, and modulate opioid analgesia. The NMDA receptor has been characterized the best and is known to be part of a ligand-gated ion channel (41). Low-frequency stimulation of C fibers leads to a gradual increase in wide dynamic range neuronal discharge, which is termed central facilitation or windup. Windup amplifies pain afferent transmission. The NMDA receptor is responsible for windup (42). Unlike the AMPA receptor that is activated by excitatory amino acids and results in short-lasting neuronal activation, NMDA receptor activation is complicated, requiring occupation by the endogenous agonist glutamate, the presence of glycine, and the removal of a Mg^{2+}-dependent channel block ("plug"). The removal of the Mg^{2+} plug results in slow, summating, and prolonged depolarization of second-order neurons. Drugs that block the NMDA receptor such as ketamine, dextromethorphan, and perhaps very low dose naloxone and methadone may have an important role in pain management (43–45). We now know that even a single opioid dose may elicit adaptive changes in the nervous system, leading to the attenuation of the effect of the opioid. Activation of the NMDA receptor constitutes an important step in these adaptive changes. Stimulation of NMDA receptors after opioid treatment may reduce the magnitude and duration of opioid-induced antinociception. Thus, blockade of NMDA receptors may be expected to acutely enhance opioid-induced antinociception (46).

Agonists at α_2 receptors, such as dexmedetomidine, have both sedative and analgesic activity and reduce the dose requirements for intravenous and inhalation anesthetics and opioid drugs. Spinally and intravenously administered α_2 agonists can potentiate the analgesic properties of opioids and local anesthetics. Whether they can produce analgesia on their own is controversial (47–52).

STRUCTURE–ACTIVITY RELATIONSHIPS OF OPIOID AGONISTS

The alkaloids of opium can be divided into two distinct chemical classes: the phenanthrenes and the benzylisoquinolines (Fig. 12.2). Both are alkaloids, but only the phenanthrenes (morphine, codeine, and thebaine, a precursor for etorphine) are active. The phenanthrenes are composed of three 14-

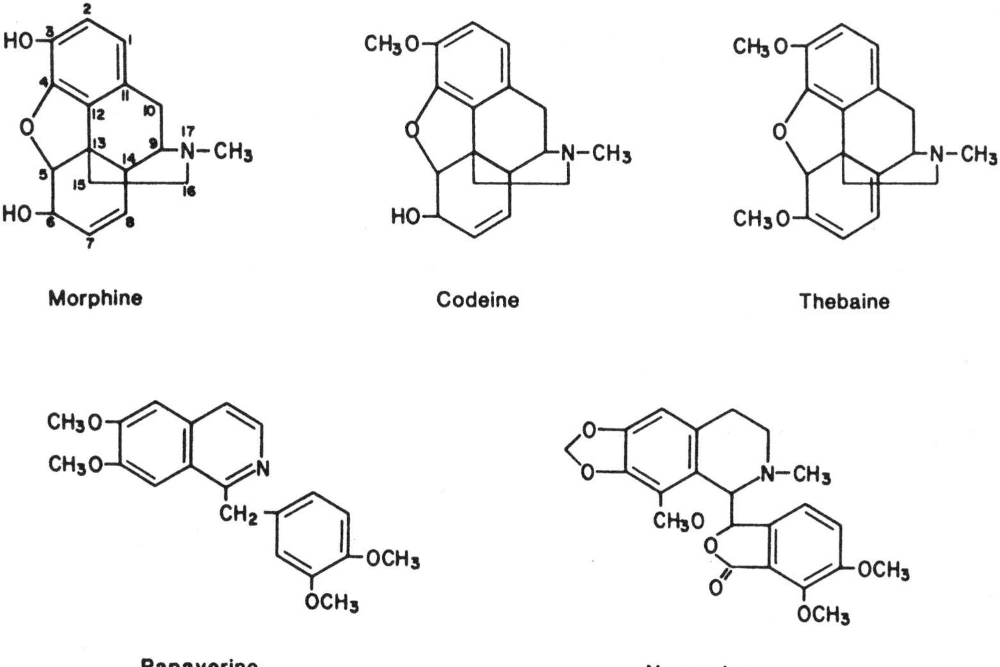

FIG. 12.2. The alkaloids of opium can be divided into two distinct chemical classes, namely, the phenanthrenes and the benzylisoquinolines, and are depicted.

carbon rings and a fourth piperidine ring that includes a tertiary nitrogenous amine. The tertiary amine nitrogen is highly ionized and makes the molecule water soluble. Semisynthetic opioids are made by simple modifications of the morphine molecule. Examples include codeine and heroin. Synthetic opioids, conversely, contain the phenanthrene nucleus of morphine but are manufactured by synthesis rather than by chemical modification of morphine. These synthetic opioids include methadone derivatives, benzomorphan derivatives (pentazocine), and phenylpiperidine derivatives (meperidine, fentanyl).

OPIOID DRUG SELECTION

Many factors are considered when deciding which is the appropriate opioid analgesic to administer to a patient in pain. These include pain intensity, patient age, coexisting disease, potential drug interactions, treatment history, physician preference, patient preference, and route of administration. The idea that some opioids are weak (e.g., codeine) and others strong (e.g., morphine) is outdated. All are capable of treating pain regardless of its intensity if the dose is adjusted appropriately. At equipotent doses, most opioids have similar effects and side effects (Table 12.2) Characteristics of selected μ opioid agonist drugs are listed for quick reference in Tables 12.2 through 12.4.

Morphine

Morphine (from Morpheus, the Greek god of sleep) is the gold standard for analgesia with which all other opioids are compared. When low doses [0.1 $mg \cdot kg^{-1}$ (intravenous or intramuscular)] are administered to otherwise unmedicated patients in pain, analgesia usually occurs without loss of consciousness. The relief of tension, anxiety, and pain usually results in drowsiness and sleep as well. Older patients with discomfort and pain usually develop a sense of well-being and/or euphoria after morphine administration. Interestingly, when morphine is given to pain-free adults, they may show the opposite effect, i.e., dysphoria and increased fear and anxiety. Mental clouding, drowsiness, lethargy, an inability to concentrate, and sleep may occur after morphine administration even in the absence of pain. Less advantageous central nervous system effects of morphine include nausea and vomiting, pruritus (especially around the nose), miosis, and, at high doses, seizures (53). Seizures are a particular problem in the newborn because they may occur at commonly prescribed doses (0.1 mg/kg) (Table 12.2) (54–57).

Although morphine produces peripheral vasodilation and venous pooling, it has minimal hemodynamic effects (e.g., cardiac output, left ventricular stroke work index, pulmonary artery pressure) in normal, euvolemic, supine patients. The vasodilation associated with morphine is primarily owing to its histamine-releasing effects. The magnitude of morphine-induced histamine release can be minimized by limiting the rate of morphine infusion to 0.025 to 0.05 mg/kg per minute, by keeping the patient in a supine to a slightly head down (Trendelenburg) position, and by optimizing intravascular volume. Significant hypotension may occur if sedatives such as diazepam are concurrently administered with morphine or if a patient suddenly changes from a supine to a standing position. Otherwise, it produces virtually no cardiovascular effects when used alone. It causes significant hypotension in hypovolemic patients and its use in trauma patients is therefore limited.

Morphine (and all other narcotics at equipotent doses) produces a dose-dependent depression of ventilation primarily by reducing the sensitivity of the brainstem respiratory centers to hypercarbia and hypoxia. Opioid agonists also interfere with pontine and medullary ventilatory centers that regulate the rhythm of breathing. This results in prolonged pauses between breaths and periodic breathing patterns. This explains the classic clinical picture of opioid-induced respiratory depression. Initially, respiratory rate is affected more than tidal volume, but as the dose of morphine is increased, tidal volume becomes affected as well. Increasing the dose further results in apnea.

The most sensitive means of measuring the respiratory depression produced by any drug is measuring the reduction in the slope of the carbon dioxide response curve and by the depression of minute ventilation (milliliters per kilogram) that occurs at P_{CO_2} = 60 mm Hg. Morphine shifts the carbon dioxide response curve to the right and also reduces its slope. This is demonstrated in Figure 12.3. The combination of any opioid agonist with any sedative produces more respiratory depression than when either drug is administered alone (Fig. 12.3) (58,59). Clinical signs that predict impending respiratory depression include somnolence, small pupils, and small tidal volumes. Aside from newborns, patients who are at particular risk of opioid-induced respiratory depression include those with an altered mental status, those who are hemodynamically unstable, those who have a history of apnea or disordered control of ventilation, or those who have a known airway problem. Morphine also depresses the cough reflex by a direct effect on the cough center in the medulla and is not related to its effects on ventilation. It also depresses the sense of air hunger that occurs when arterial carbon dioxide levels rise. This explains morphine's use as a sedative in terminally ill patients and critically ill patients who are "fighting the ventilator."

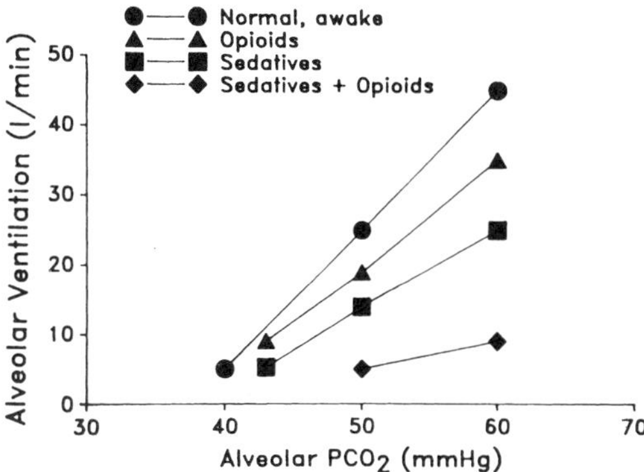

FIG. 12.3. The relationship between ventilation and carbon dioxide is represented by a family of curves. Each curve has two parameters: an intercept and slope. Sedatives and opioids shift the position and slope to the right. The combination of drugs produces the most profound effects. (From Yaster M, Nichols DG, Deshpande JK, et al. Midazolam-fentanyl intravenous sedation in children: case report of respiratory arrest. *Pediatrics* 1990;86:463–467, with permission.)

Morphine (and all other narcotics at equipotent doses) inhibits intestinal smooth muscle motility. This decrease in peristalsis of the small and large intestine and increase in tone of the pyloric sphincter, ileocecal valve, and anal sphincter explains the historic use of opioids in the treatment of diarrhea as well as its side effect of constipation when treating chronic pain. Indeed, the use of opium to treat dysentery (diarrhea) preceded its use in Western medicine for analgesia. The gastrointestinal tract is very sensitive to opioids even at low doses. In the rat, four times more morphine is needed to produce analgesia than is needed to slow gastrointestinal motility (60). Opioids affect the bowel centrally and, by direct action on the gut, μ and δ opioid receptor sites. In fact, loperamide, an opioid receptor agonist with limited ability to cross the blood–brain barrier is used clinically to treat diarrhea, suggesting that direct, local gut action is present in the opioid-constipating effect in diarrhea. Tolerance to the constipating effects of morphine is minimal. Because of this, we routinely prescribe laxatives or stool softeners for patients expected to be treated with morphine (and all other opioids) for more than 2 or 3 days. Alternatively, naloxone, a nonselective opioid antagonist, can prevent or treat opioid-induced constipation. Unfortunately, it also antagonizes opioid-induced analgesia. Yuan et al. (61), in a series of experiments, demonstrated that methylnaltrexone, a quaternary derivative of naltrexone, can selectively block the peripheral effects of opioids (constipation) without affecting analgesia (61). This drug may be useful for other opioid-induced side effects such as pruritus (62).

Morphine potentiates biliary colic by causing spasm of the sphincter of Oddi and should be used with caution in patients with, or at risk of, cholelithiasis (e.g., sickle cell disease). This effect is antagonized by naloxone and glucagon (2 mg intravenously in adult patients). Biliary colic can be avoided by using mixed agonist–antagonist opioids such as pentazocine. Whether other pure μ agonists such as meperidine or fentanyl produce less biliary spasm than morphine is disputed in the literature. Some studies show that meperidine produces less biliary spasm than morphine and others show that at equianalgesic doses they produce virtually identical increases in common bile duct pressure.

The nausea and vomiting that are seen with morphine administration are caused by stimulation of the chemoreceptor trigger zone in the brainstem (63). This may reflect the role of opioids as partial dopamine agonists at dopamine receptors in the chemoreceptor trigger zone and the use of dopamine antagonists such droperidol (a butyrophenone) or chlorpromazine (a phenothiazine) in the treatment of opioid-induced nausea and vomiting. Morphine increases tone and contractions in the ureters, bladder, and detrusor muscles of the bladder, which may make urination difficult. This may also explain the increased occurrence of bladder spasm and pain that occur when morphine is used to treat patients who have undergone bladder surgery.

Regardless of its route of administration, morphine (and fentanyl) commonly produces pruritus that can at times be maddening and impossible to treat. Indeed, some patients refuse opioid analgesics because they would rather hurt than itch. Opioid-induced itching is caused either by the release of histamine and histamine's effects on the peripheral nociceptors or by central μ receptor activity (64,65). Traditional antihistamines such as diphenhydramine and hydroxyzine are commonly used to treat this side effect. Additionally, there is increasing use of low-dose μ antagonists (naloxone and nalmefene) and mixed agonist–antagonists (butorphanol) in the treatment of opioid-induced pruritus (66–68). Interestingly, these latter agents may also be effective for nonopioid-induced pruritus such as the itching that accompanies end-stage liver and kidney disease (69).

There is now a considerable body of literature that demonstrates a modulatory function of the immune system by opioids. This modulation takes the form of an alteration in the biochemical and proliferative properties of the various cellular components of the immune system (70). Vertebrates and invertebrates have been shown to possess a peptide that is a proenkephalin and has a strong antibacterial action. This peptide is called enkelytin (proenkephalin A), and there is a strong sequence homology between invertebrate and mammalian enkelytin system (71,72). It has been suggested that immune or neural signaling leads to enhanced proenkephalin proteolytic cleaving, thereby causing the release of both opioid peptides and enkelytin simultaneously. This scenario would allow a two-pronged attack. Opioid peptides would modulate neutrophil chemotaxis, phagocytic activity, and the secretion of cytokines, while the simultaneously liberated enkelytin would exert an antibacterial action.

Moreover, inflammatory mediators have been shown to modify the release of opioid peptides from immune system cells and from cells of the peripheral and central nervous systems. The potential effects of exogenously administered opioids on the immune system cannot be ignored. Opioids released from cells of the immune system may modulate the release of cytokines from the same and other cells of the immune system (73). Additionally, it has been suggested that T lymphocytes may act as a vector to deliver β endorphin to inflamed tissues. The significance of this hypothesis is that it would allow the potential for highly specific opioid control of peripheral analgesia by targeted delivery of β endorphin directly to sites of inflammation. This would maximize the potential analgesic and anti-inflammatory effects of endogenous opioids acting at peripheral receptors and by inhibiting the release of the inflammatory peptide substance P from primary afferent neurons (74,75). Conversely, chronic morphine treatment is a mechanism used in laboratory experiments to render mice immunocompromised, and parenteral drug abuse is a significant risk factor for contracting human immunodeficiency virus-1 (76,77). Furthermore, interferon γ–stimulated natural killer cell cytotoxicity is significantly suppressed after short-term exposure to morphine in humans (78).

Finally, *tolerance* and *physical dependence* with repeated opioid administration is a characteristic common to all opioid agonists. *Tolerance* is the development of a need to increase the dose of opioid agonist to achieve the same analgesic effect previously achieved with a lower dose. Tolerance usually develops after 10 to 21 days of morphine administration, although the constipating and miotic actions of morphine may persist. Additionally, cross-tolerance develops between all the μ opioid agonists. *Physical dependence*, sometimes referred to as neuroadaptation, is caused by repeated administration of an opioid that necessitates the continued administration of the drug to prevent the appearance of a withdrawal or abstinence syndrome that is characteristic of that particular drug. It usually occurs after 2 to 3 weeks of morphine administration but may occur after only just a few days of therapy. Very young infants treated with very high dose fentanyl infusions after surgical repair of congenital heart disease and/or those who required extracorporeal membrane oxygenation have been identified to be at particular risk (79–82). Several studies have suggested that the intrinsic efficacy of an opioid analgesic can determine, in part, the degree of tolerance to that agent. Specifically, animal and human studies have demonstrated that the tolerance that develops to equieffective doses of opioid analgesics with high intrinsic efficacy is less than the tolerance that develops to lower intrinsic efficacy compounds (83,84). Additionally, these effects occur more rapidly after continuous infusion compared with intermittent dosing (85).

Tolerance develops to some drug effects much more rapidly than to other effects of the same drug. For example, tolerance develops rapidly to opioid-induced euphoria and respiratory depression but much more slowly to the gastrointestinal effects. Opioids given acutely or long term induce the downregulation, internalization, and desensitization of opioid receptors (86). These changes in receptor number and affinity do not explain the entire phenomenon of tolerance (87,88). Rather, subreceptor and intracellular mechanisms, including changes in the regulation of second- and third-degree messenger systems (upregulation of cyclic AMP, phosphorylation of protein kinases), cross-talk with other receptor systems (NMDA), and changes in G proteins and other effector proteins, also play an important role (87,88). *In vitro* and *in vivo* evidence indicates that the desensitization of G protein–coupled receptors involves the phosphorylation of G protein–coupled receptors and subsequent binding of regulatory proteins called β arrestins (89–91). Using a knockout mouse lacking β arrestin, Bohn et al. (89) reported that desensitization of the μ opioid receptor did not occur in these animals after chronic morphine exposure and that these animals fail to develop nociceptive tolerance. Interestingly, the absence of β arrestin in the knockout mice did not prevent the development of dependence and withdrawal, suggesting that the two phenomena are not linked (89). Thus, in the future, tolerance may be prevented by using NMDA receptor (or low-dose opioid receptor) blockade (92,93).

When physical dependence has been established, discontinuation of an opioid agonist produces a *withdrawal* syndrome within 24 hours of drug cessation. Opioids cause an initial inhibition of neuronal adenylyl cyclase. Continued treatment (or abuse) results in gradual upregulation of cyclic AMP to pretreatment levels and thus tolerance. Cessation of therapy releases the tolerant neurons from opioid inhibition of adenylyl cyclase leading to a rebound increase in cyclic AMP production and symptoms of withdrawal (94). Symptoms reach their peak within 72 hours and include abdominal cramps, vomiting, diarrhea, tachycardia, hypertension, diaphoresis, restlessness, and insomnia. The symptoms can be terminated with very low doses of opioid agonist and can be ameliorated with α_2 agonists such as clonidine in doses of 3 to 5 μg/kg.

Physical dependence must be differentiated from addiction. *Addiction* is a term used to connote a severe degree of drug abuse and dependence that is an extreme of behavior, in which drug use pervades the total life activity of the user, and of the range of circumstances in which drug use controls the user's behavior. Patients who are addicted to opioids often spend large amounts of time acquiring or using the drug, abandon social or occupational activities because of drug use, and continue to use the drug despite adverse psychologic or physical effects. In a sense, addiction is a subset of physical dependence. Anyone who is addicted to an opioid is physically dependent; however, not everyone who is physically dependent is addicted. Patients appropriately treated with morphine and other opioid agonists for pain can become tolerant and physically dependent. They rarely, if ever, become addicted.

Pharmacokinetics

To relieve or prevent pain, the agonist must get to the receptor in the central nervous system (Fig. 12.4). There are essentially two ways that this occurs: either by the bloodstream (after intravenous, intramuscular, oral, nasal, transdermal, or mucosal administration) or by direct application (intrathecal or epidural) into the cerebrospinal fluid (CSF) (12,95,96). Agonists administered via the bloodstream must

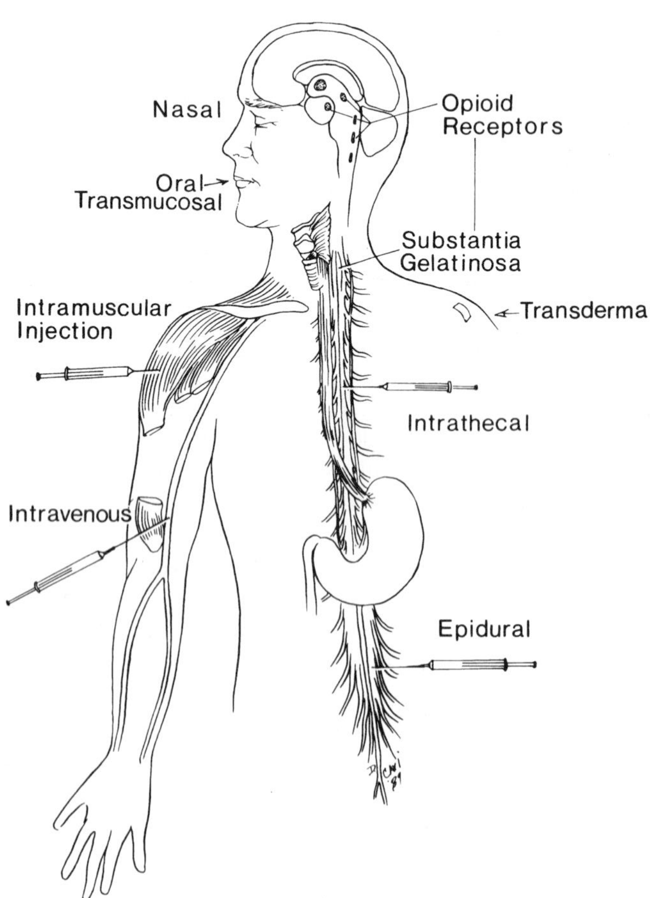

FIG. 12.4. Location of opioid receptors within the central nervous system. Opioids reach the receptor after parenteral (intravenous, intramuscular), spinal (intrathecal, epidural), enteral (mouth, nose), or transdermal administration.

cross the blood–brain barrier, a lipid membrane interface between the endothelial cells of the brain vasculature and the extracellular fluid of the brain, to reach the receptor. Normally, highly lipid-soluble agonists, such as fentanyl, rapidly diffuse across the blood–brain barrier, whereas agonists with limited lipid solubility, such as morphine, have limited brain uptake (97–101). The blood–brain barrier may be immature at birth and is known to be more permeable to morphine. Way et al. (102) demonstrated that morphine concentrations were two to four times greater in the brains of younger rats than older rats despite equal blood concentrations. Obviously, the immaturity of the blood–brain barrier has less of an effect on highly lipid-soluble agents like fentanyl (103).

Spinal administration, either intrathecally or epidurally, bypasses the blood and directly places an agonist into the CSF, which bathes the receptor sites in the spinal cord (substantia gelatinosa) and brain. This "backdoor" to the receptor significantly reduces the amount of agonist needed to relieve pain (104). After spinal administration, opioids are absorbed by the epidural veins and redistributed to the systemic circulation where they are metabolized and excreted. Hydrophilic agents, such as morphine, cross the dura more slowly than more lipid-soluble agents such as fentanyl or meperidine (105). This physicochemical property is responsible for the more prolonged duration of action of spinal morphine and its very slow onset of action after epidural administration (12,106,107).

Although it would be desirable to adjust opioid dosage based on the concentration of drug achieved at the receptor site, this is rarely feasible. The alternative is to measure blood or plasma concentrations and model how the body handles a drug. Pharmacokinetic studies thereby help the clinician select suitable routes, timing, and dosing of drugs to maximize a drug's dynamic effects (see Chapter 5).

After administration, the disposition of a drug is dependent on distribution ($t_{1/2}\alpha$) and elimination. The terminal half-life of elimination ($t_{1/2}\beta$) is directly proportional to the volume of distribution (Vd) and inversely proportional to the total body clearance (Cl) by the following formula:

$$t_{1/2}\beta = 0.693 \times (Vd/Cl).$$

Thus, a prolongation of the $t_{1/2}\beta$ may be owing to either an increase in a drug's volume of distribution or a decrease in its clearance.

The liver is the major site of biotransformation for most opioids. The major metabolic pathway for most opioids is oxidation. The exceptions are morphine and buprenorphine, which primarily undergo glucuronidation, and remifentanil, which is cleared by ester hydrolysis (108–110). Many of these reactions are catalyzed in the liver by microsomal mixed-function oxidases that require the cytochrome P_{450} system, nicotinamide adenine dinucleotide phosphate, and oxygen. The cytochrome P_{450} system is very immature at birth and does not reach adult levels until the first month or two of life (111,112). This immaturity of this hepatic enzyme system may explain the prolonged clearance or elimination of some opioids in the first few days to weeks of life. In contrast, the P_{450} system can be induced by various drugs (phenobarbital) and substrates and matures regardless of gestational age. Thus, it may be the age from birth and not the duration of gestation that determines how premature and full-term infants metabolize drugs. Greeley et al. (113) demonstrated that sufentanil is more rapidly metabolized and eliminated in 2- to 3-week-old infants than newborns younger than 1 week of age.

Morphine is primarily glucuronidated into two forms: an inactive form (morphine-3-glucuronide) and an active form (morphine-6-glucuronide). Both glucuronides are excreted by the kidney. In patients with renal failure or with reduced glomerular filtration rates (e.g., neonates), the morphine 6-glucuronide can accumulate and cause toxic side effects including respiratory depression. This is important to consider not only when prescribing morphine but when administering other opioids that are metabolized into morphine such as methadone and codeine.

The pharmacokinetics of opioids in patients with liver disease requires special attention. Oxidation of opioids is reduced in patients with hepatic cirrhosis, resulting in decreased drug clearance (meperidine, dextropropoxyphene, pentazocine, tramadol, and alfentanil) or increased oral bioavailability caused by a reduced first-pass metabolism (meperidine, pentazocine, and dihydrocodeine). Although glucuronidation is thought to be less affected in liver cirrhosis, the clearance of morphine is decreased and oral bioavailability increased. The consequence of reduced drug metabolism is the risk of accumulation in the body, especially with repeated administration. Lower doses or longer administration intervals should be used to minimize this risk. Meperidine poses a special concern because it is metabolized into normeperidine, a toxic metabolite that causes seizures and accumulates in liver disease (114,115). Conversely, drugs that are inactive but are metabolized in the liver into active forms such as codeine may be ineffective in patients with liver disease. Finally, the disposition of a few opioids, such as fentanyl, sufentanil, and remifentanil, appears to be unaffected in liver disease, and these are the drugs that we use preferentially in managing pain in patients with liver disease (116).

The pharmacokinetics of morphine has been extensively studied in adults, older children, and premature and full-term newborns (55–57,117–120). After an intravenous bolus, 30% of morphine is protein bound in the adult compared with only 20% in the newborn. This increase in unbound (free) morphine allows a greater proportion of active drug to penetrate the brain. This may explain, in part, the observation of Way et al. (102,121) of increased brain levels of morphine in the newborn and its more profound respiratory depressant effects. The elimination half-life of morphine in adults and older children is 3 to 4 hours and is consistent with its duration of analgesic action (Table 12.5). The $t_{1/2}\beta$ is more than twice as long as in newborns younger than 1 week of age than in older children and adults and is even longer in premature infants and children requiring pressor support (55,82,122,123). Clearance is similarly decreased in the newborn compared with the older child and adult (Table 12.5). Thus, infants younger than 1 month of age attain higher serum levels that decline more slowly than older children and adults. This may also account for the increased respiratory depression associated with morphine in this age group (30).

Interestingly, the half-life of elimination and clearance of morphine in children older than 1 to 2 months of age is similar to that in adults. Thus, the hesitancy in prescribing and administering morphine in children younger than 1 year of age may not be warranted. Conversely, the use of any opioid in children younger than 2 months of age, particularly those born prematurely, must be limited to a monitored, intensive care unit setting not only because of pharmacokinetic and dynamic reasons but because of immature ventilatory responses to hypoxemia, hypercarbia, and airway obstruction in the neonate (124–127).

Suggested Dosage

The "unit" dose of intravenously administered morphine is 0.1 mg/kg and is modified based on patient age and disease state (Table 12.2). To minimize the complications associated with intravenous morphine (or any opioid) administration, we always recommend *titration of the dose at the bedside* until the

TABLE 12.5. *Morphine pharmacokinetics*[a]

	Premature	Full-term	Adult
Elimination half life (T 1/2 β)	7.4±1.7	6.7±4.6	3.0±1.5
Clearance (mL/kg/min)	9.6±4.0	15.5±10.0	20±2.0
Volume of distribution (Vd) (L/kg)	5.18±1.6	2.9±2.1	5.2±2.2

[a]Because of individual variability, the dose of morphine should be titrated individually.

desired level of analgesia is achieved. Based on its relatively short half-life (3 to 4 hours), one would expect older children and adults to require morphine supplementation every 2 to 3 hours when being treated for pain, particularly if the morphine is administered intravenously (Fig. 12.5) (3,128). This has led to the recent use of continuous infusion regimens of morphine (0.02 to 0.03 mg/kg per hour) and patient-controlled analgesia (PCA) (see below), which maximize pain-free periods (129–134). Alternatively, longer acting agonists such as methadone (see below) maybe used (135–139). Finally, only approximately 20% to 30% of an orally administered dose of morphine reaches the systemic circulation (140,141). When converting a patient's intravenous morphine requirements to oral maintenance, one needs to multiply the intravenous dose by three to five times (Table 12.2). Oral morphine is available as a liquid, tablet, and sustained-release preparations

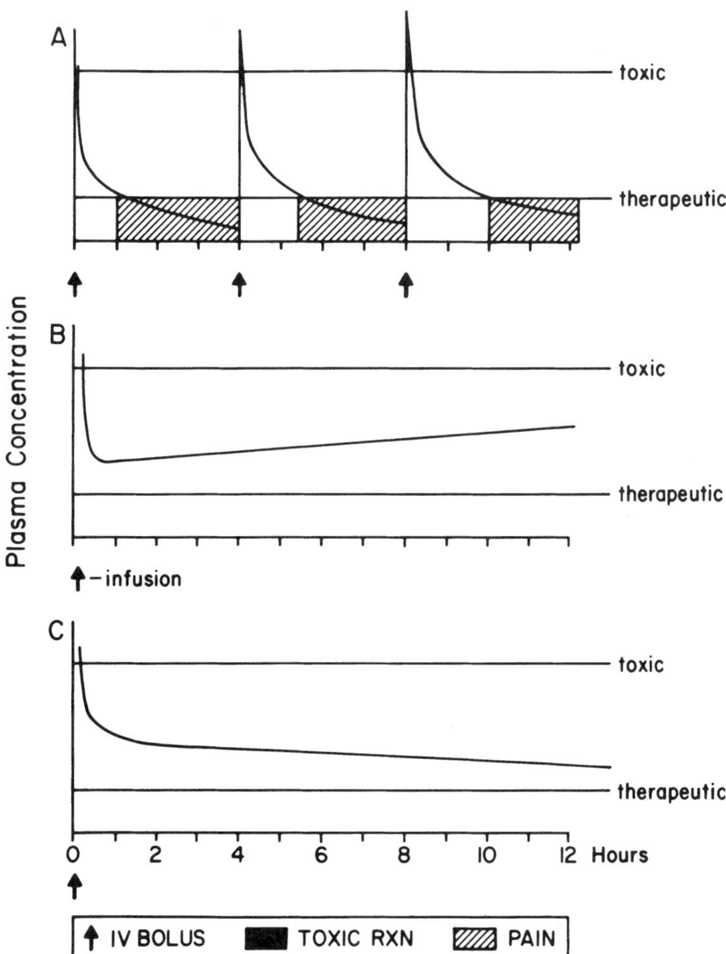

FIG. 12.5. Simulated blood concentration–dose relationships for opioids by different administration regimens. **A:** Intravenous bolus administration of morphine sulfate (elimination half-life is 4 hours) every 4 hours. **B:** Intravenous bolus administration of morphine sulfate followed by a continuous infusion. **C:** Intravenous bolus administration of methadone (elimination half-life is 19 hours). Note the absence of pain periods in **B** and **C**. (From Yaster M, Deshpande JK, Maxwell LG. The pharmacologic management of pain in children. *Compr Ther* 1989;15:14–26, with permission.)

[morphine sulfate (MS Contin)]. Unfortunately, not all sustained-release products are the same. There are several modified release formulations of morphine with recommended dose intervals of either 12 or 24 hours, including tablets (MS Contin, Oramorph SR), capsules (Kapanol, Skenan), suspension, and suppositories. Orally administered solid dose forms are most popular, but significant differences exist in the resultant pharmacokinetics and bioequivalence status of morphine after single doses and at steady state (142). Rectal administration is not recommended because of extremely irregular absorption (6% to 93% bioavailability) (143).

Fentanyl(s)

Because of its rapid onset (usually less than 1 minute) and brief duration of action (30 to 45 minutes), fentanyl has become a favored analgesic for short procedures, such as bone marrow aspirations, fracture reductions, suturing lacerations, endoscopy, and dental procedures. Fentanyl is approximately 100 (50 to 100) times more potent than morphine [the equianalgesic dose is 0.001 mg·kg^{-1} (Table 12.2)] and is largely devoid of hypnotic or sedative activity. Sufentanil is a potent fentanyl derivative and is approximately ten times more potent than fentanyl. It is most commonly used as the principle component of cardiac anesthesia and is administered in doses of 15 to 30 μg/kg. Alfentanil is approximately five to ten times less potent than fentanyl and has an extremely short duration of action, usually less than 15 to 20 minutes. Remifentanil (Ultiva) is a new μ opioid receptor agonist with unique pharmacokinetic properties. It is approximately ten times more potent than fentanyl and must be given by continuous intravenous infusion because it has an extremely short half-life (144,145).

Fentanyl's ability to block nociceptive stimuli with concomitant hemodynamic stability is excellent and makes it the drug of choice for trauma, cardiac, or intensive care unit patients. Furthermore, in addition to its ability to block the systemic and pulmonary hemodynamic responses to pain, fentanyl also prevents the biochemical and endocrine stress (catabolic) response to painful stimuli that may be so detrimental in the seriously ill patient. Fentanyl does have some serious side effects, namely, the development of glottic and chest wall rigidity after rapid infusions of 0.005 mg·kg^{-1} or greater and the development of bradycardia. The cause of the glottic and chest wall rigidity is unclear, but its implications are not, i.e., it may make ventilation difficult or impossible. Chest wall rigidity can be treated with either muscle relaxants, such as succinylcholine or pancuronium, or with naloxone.

Pharmacokinetics

Fentanyl, like morphine, is primarily glucuronidated into inactive forms that are excreted by the kidney. It is highly lipid soluble and is rapidly distributed to tissues that are well perfused, such as the brain and heart. Normally, the effect of a single dose of fentanyl is terminated by rapid redistribution to inactive tissue sites such as fat, skeletal muscles, and lung rather than by elimination. This rapid redistribution produces a dramatic decline in the plasma concentration of the drug. In this manner, its very short duration of action is very much akin to other drugs whose action is terminated by redistribution such as thiopental. However, after multiple or large doses of fentanyl (e.g., when it is used as a primary anesthetic agent or when used in high-dose or lengthy continuous infusions), prolongation of effect occurs because elimination and not distribution determines the duration of effect. Indeed, it is now clear that the duration of drug action for many drugs is not solely the function of clearance or terminal elimination half-life but rather reflects the complex interaction of drug elimination, drug absorption, and rate constants for drug transfer to and from sites of action ("effect sites"). The term *context-sensitive half-time* refers to the time for drug concentration at idealized effect sites to decrease by half (143). The context-sensitive half-time for fentanyl increases dramatically when it is administered by continuous infusion (146,147). In newborns receiving fentanyl infusions for more than 36 hours, the context-sensitive half-life was longer than 9 hours after cessation of the infusion (148). Even single doses of fentanyl may have prolonged effects in the newborn, particularly those neonates with abnormal or decreased liver blood flow after acute illness or abdominal surgery (149–152). Additionally, some conditions that may raise intra-abdominal pressure may further decrease liver blood flow by shunting blood away from the liver via the still patent ductus venosus (152–155).

Fentanyl and its structurally related relatives sufentanil, alfentanil, and remifentanil are highly lipophilic drugs that rapidly penetrate all membranes including the blood–brain barrier. After an intravenous bolus, fentanyl is rapidly eliminated from plasma as the result of its extensive uptake by body tissues. The fentanyls are highly bound to α_1-acid glycoproteins in the plasma, which are reduced in the newborn (156,157). The fraction of free unbound sufentanil is significantly increased in neonates and children younger than 1 year of age (19.5 ± 2.7% and 11.5 ± 3.2%, respectively) compared with older children and adults (8.1 ± 1.4% and 7.8 ±1.5%, respectively), and this correlates with levels of α_1-acid glycoproteins in the blood.

Fentanyl pharmacokinetics differ among newborn infants, children, and adults. The total body clearance of fentanyl is greater in infants 3 to 12 months of age than in children older than 1 year of age or adults (18.1 ± 1.4, 11.5 ± 4.2, and 10.0 ± 1.7 $mL{\cdot}kg^{-1}{\cdot}min^{-1}$, respectively) and the half-life of elimination is longer (233 ± 137, 244 ± 79, and 129 ± 42 minutes, respectively) (158). The prolonged elimination half-life of fentanyl from plasma has important clinical implications. Repeated doses of fentanyl for maintenance of analgesic effects lead to accumulation of fentanyl and its ventilatory depressant effects (158–161). Very large doses (0.05 to 0.10 $mg{\cdot}kg^{-1}$ as used in anesthesia) may be expected to induce long-lasting effects because plasma fentanyl levels will not fall below the threshold level at which spontaneous ventilation occurs during the distribution phases. Conversely, the greater clearance of fentanyl in infants older than 3 months of age produces lower plasma concentrations of the drug and may allow these children to tolerate more drug without respiratory depression (150,158). In adult studies, the mean plasma concentration of fentanyl needed to produce analgesia varies between 0.5 and 1.5 ng/mL (162,163).

Alfentanil has a shorter half-life of elimination and redistribution than fentanyl, may cause less postoperative respiratory depression than either morphine or fentanyl, and is often given by infusion. Following a bolus and continuous infusion, Gronert et al. (164) found very little respiratory depression when alfentanil was used intraoperatively even in very young infants. The pharmacokinetics of alfentanil differs in the neonate compared with older children. Compared with older children, premature infants demonstrated a significantly larger apparent volume of distribution (1.0 ± 0.39 versus 0.48 ± 0.19 L/kg), a smaller clearance (2.2 ± 2.4 versus 5.6 ± 2.4 mL/kg/min), and a markedly prolonged elimination half-life (525 ± 305 versus 60 ± 11 minutes) (165).

The pharmacokinetics of remifentanil are characterized by small volumes, rapid clearances, and low variability compared with other intravenous anesthetic drugs (108–110, 144,145,166). The drug has a rapid onset of action (half-time for equilibration between blood and the effect compartment is 1.3 minutes) and a short context-sensitive half-life (3 to 5 minutes). The latter property is attributable to hydrolytic metabolism of the compound by nonspecific tissue and plasma esterases. Virtually all (99.8%) of an administered remifentanil dose is eliminated during the α half-life (0.9 minutes) and β half-life (6.3 minutes). The pharmacokinetics of remifentanil suggests that within 10 minutes of starting an infusion, remifentanil nearly reaches steady state. Thus, changing the infusion rate of remifentanil produces rapid changes in drug effect. The rapid metabolism of remifentanil and its small volume of distribution mean that remifentanil does not accumulate. Discontinuing the drug rapidly stops its effects regardless of how long it was being administered (146,147). Finally, the primary metabolite has little biologic activity, making it safe even in patients with renal disease.

Suggested Dosage

When used to provide analgesia for short procedures, fentanyl is often administered intravenously in doses of 1 to 3 μg/kg. However, if any sedative (e.g., midazolam or chloral hydrate) is administered concomitantly, respiratory depression is potentiated and the dose of both drugs must be reduced (Fig. 12.3) (58). Fentanyl can also be used in the intensive care unit or the operating room to provide virtually complete anesthesia in doses of 10 to 50 μg/kg (167,168). The lower dose is often used to provide anesthesia for intubation, particularly in the newborn and in head trauma, cardiac, and hemodynamically unstable patients. Continuous infusions of fentanyl are often used to provide analgesia and sedation in intubated and mechanically ventilated patients, particularly those on extracorporeal membrane oxygenation. After a loading dose of 10 μg/kg, an infusion is begun of 2 to 5 μg/kg per hour. Rapid tolerance develops, and an increasing dose of fentanyl is required to provide satisfactory analgesia and sedation (see above). It can also be administered via PCA pumps usually in doses of 0.5 μg/kg per bolus dose (see below). Remifentanil is increasingly being used as an intraoperative analgesic and may have a role in postoperative pain and sedation management. In the operating room, it is administered via a bolus (0.5 to 1 μg/kg) followed by an infusion that ranges between 0.1 and 1 μg/kg per minute.

Sufentanil, which is five to ten times more potent than fentanyl, can be administered intranasally in doses of 1.5 to 3.0 μg/kg and produces effective analgesia and sedation within 10 minutes of administration (169). Higher doses (4.5 μg/kg) produce untoward side effects including chest wall rigidity, convulsions, respiratory depression, and increased postoperative vomiting (169). Another exciting alternative to intravenous or intramuscular injection is the fentanyl lollipop or oral transmucosal fentanyl citrate (170–173). In doses of 15 to 20 μg/kg, this is an effective, nontraumatic method of premedication that is self-administered and extremely well accepted by children (173). Side effects include facial pruritus (90%), slow onset time (25 to 45 minutes to peak effect), and an increase in gastric volume compared with unpremedicated patients [15.9 ± 10.8 mL compared with 9.0 ± 6.2 mL (mean ± standard deviation)]. Finally, transdermal fentanyl preparations are now available to provide sustained plasma fentanyl concentrations. This has great potential use in the treatment of cancer and other chronic pain.

Meperidine

Meperidine (Demerol), also known as pethidine, is a synthetic narcotic derived from phenylpiperidine. It is most commonly used in children either as a premedicant for anesthesia (or sedation) or as a treatment for postoperative pain. Although it is ten times less potent than morphine, it has pharmacokinetic properties that are otherwise quite similar to it. Meperidine is a μ agonist that binds to opioid receptors in the central nervous system and can produce analgesia, sedation, euphoria, dysphoria, miosis, and respiratory depression. At equianalgesic doses (Table 12.2), there is little quantitative or qualitative difference between meperidine and morphine in producing these effects. Meperidine stimulates the chemoreceptor trigger zone in the brainstem to the same degree that morphine does and may thereby produce either nausea or vomiting or both (Table 12.4).

Meperidine differs from morphine in that large doses (toxic levels) may produce slow waves on the electroencephalogram. Additionally, high levels of meperidine's principal metabolite, normeperidine, may produce tremors, muscle twitches, hyperactive reflexes, and convulsions (114,115). Because of the accumulation of this metabolite, the prolonged use of meperidine should be discouraged, if not avoided completely.

It is unique among all the opioids in that in prevents or stops shivering (174). It is frequently used for this purpose in patients who shiver after amphotericin administration, blood product (particularly platelet) transfusions, or general anesthesia or who are hypothermic. Similarly, severe, catastrophic reactions may follow the administration of meperidine to patients who are being treated with monoamine oxidase inhibitors and in patients with untreated hyperthyroidism. Specifically, excitation, hyperpyrexia, delirium, and seizures may occur when meperidine is given to patients on monoamine oxidase inhibitors. These symptoms are often misdiagnosed and attributed to other processes and not to the drug–drug interaction. Unfortunately, any and all of these symptoms may lead to death. Like meperidine's effects on shivering, this property is unique to meperidine and does not occur with other μ agonists.

At equipotent doses (1.0 mg/kg) (Table 12.2), meperidine's effects on respiration and gastrointestinal motility are similar to those of the other opioid analgesics. Meperidine is a potent respiratory depressant and antitussive. Unlike morphine, meperidine depresses minute ventilation through a primary reduction in tidal volume rather than a reduction in respiratory rate. It depresses intestinal smooth muscle motility and exerts a spasmogenic effect on intestinal smooth muscle. Thus, gastric motility is decreased, and the gastric emptying time of the stomach is increased. Some studies suggest that meperidine exerts less of an effect on the biliary tract, including the common bile duct, than morphine. Specifically, at equianalgesic doses, biliary tract pressure rises to a lesser extent after meperidine than morphine administration, making it a preferred agent for biliary colic. This point is often disputed in the literature (see above). Finally, meperidine, unlike the other opioids, depresses cardiac output by approximately 20% and produces a tachycardia when it is administered intravenously.

Pharmacokinetics

Meperidine, like morphine and fentanyl, is nearly completely metabolized in the liver with a plasma half-life of elimination of approximately 3 hours. Unlike morphine and fentanyl, the principal metabolic pathways involved in meperidine metabolism are hydrolysis and *N*-demethylation. The latter process produces normeperidine, which is principally responsible for the sedative and convulsive effects of meperidine. Normeperidine is approximately one-half as active as meperidine as an analgesic but twice as active a convulsant. The levels of normeperidine may be increased by ingestion of large doses or because of enzyme induction. Urinary excretion of the metabolites is responsible for final elimination of the drug, whereas approximately one-third of meperidine is demethylated into normeperidine, a metabolite that is one-half as active as meperidine as an analgesic but twice as active as a convulsant. Because of the propensity of normeperidine to produce seizures and hallucinations, we believe that meperidine should not be routinely prescribed for chronic pain management or in patients with known seizure disorders.

Suggested Dosage

Meperidine is effective whether administered orally or parenterally. The drug is extremely well absorbed from the gastrointestinal tract and has a bioavailability of approximately 50%, making it among the most prescribed oral narcotics. It is available in both liquid (syrup) and tablet form. Typically, meperidine, 1 to 3 mg/kg, can exert analgesic effects within 15 to 30 minutes of oral administration and achieves peak plasma concentrations within 1 to 2 hours of ingestion. Intramuscular injection, 1 mg/kg, which we believe is an unacceptable route of routine drug administration, provides a more rapid onset of analgesia (approximately 10 minutes) and reaches a peak effect within 60 minutes of administration. Obviously, plasma concentrations may show marked variability after intramuscular injection based on an individual patient's state of peripheral perfusion and results in inadequate, fluctuating, and unpredictable blood concentrations.

Meperidine is commonly administered intramuscularly for moderate to severe pain or as part of a lytic (sedative) cocktail [comprising meperidine, promethazine, and chlorpromazine and known as MPC (or as DPT for the brand names Demerol, Phenergan, and Thorazine)] in a dose of 1 to 2 $mg{\cdot}kg^{-1}$. We do not recommend intramuscular administration of analgesics (or any drug) in children nor do we advocate the use of the lytic cocktail. In fact, we consider the lytic cocktail to be an archaic and frankly dangerous sedative combination. We mention this Darwinian approach to sedation only to condemn its continued use. Although an intramuscular injection results in higher sustained plasma levels of meperidine and longer pain-free intervals, it is clear that children will often suffer in silence to avoid yet another pain, namely, the "shot." When administered intravenously (1 $mg{\cdot}kg^{-1}$) for pain control, meperidine offers few advantages over morphine and must be given cautiously and *by titration at the bedside*. A much smaller intravenous dose (0.25 to 0.5 mg/kg) effectively prevents or stops shivering. Based on meperidine's plasma half-life of elimination, the frequency of administration ranges between 3 and 4 hours.

Methadone

Primarily thought of as a drug to treat or wean opioid-addicted or -dependent patients, methadone is increasingly being used for postoperative pain relief and for the treatment of intractable pain (4,136–138,175). It is noted for its slow elimination, very long duration of effective analgesia, and high oral bioavailability (Table 12.2). Methadone is metabolized extremely slowly and has a very prolonged duration of action based in part on the fact that its principle metabolite is morphine. The $t_{1/2}\beta$ of methadone averages 19 hours and clearance averages 5.4 $mL{\cdot}min^{-1}{\cdot}kg^{-1}$ in children 1 to 18 years of age (139).

Methadone has the longest $t_{1/2}\beta$ of any of the commonly available opiates and may provide 12 to 36 hours of analgesia after a single intravenous or oral dose (4,136–138,175). Pharmacokinetically, children are indistinguishable from young adults. Because a single dose of methadone can achieve and sustain a high drug plasma level, it is a convenient way to provide prolonged analgesia without requiring an intramuscular injection (Fig. 12.5). Indeed, when administered either orally or intravenously, it may be viewed as an alternative to the use of continuous intravenous opioid infusions. Berde et al. (4,175) recommend loading patients with an initial dose of intravenous methadone, 0.1 to 0.2 $mg{\cdot}kg^{-1}$, and then titrating in 0.05-$mg{\cdot}kg^{-1}$ increments every 10 to 15 minutes until analgesia is achieved. Supplemental methadone can be administered in 0.05- to 0.1-$mg{\cdot}kg^{-1}$ increments by slow intravenous infusion every 4 to 12 hours as needed. Berde et al. (4,175) also reported the use of small incremental doses administered by "sliding scale." "Small increments of methadone are administered intravenously over 20 minutes every 4 hours via a 'sliding' scale on a 'reverse prn' (the nurse asks the patient) basis: 0.07 to 0.08 mg/kg for severe pain, 0.05 to 0.06 mg/kg for moderate pain, 0.03 mg/kg for little or no pain, if the patient is alert, and no drug if the patient has little pain and is somnolent" (4,175). The influence of pathophysiology on the pharmacokinetics and pharmacodynamics of methadone is unknown primarily because its use as an analgesic is a relatively recent phenomenon. Dosing decisions in the very young and in patients with various end-organ diseases must be made conservatively.

Additionally, we and others are using methadone and sustained-relief morphine to wean patients who have become physically dependent on opioids after prolonged analgesic therapy (86,176,177). When used to treat dependence and withdrawal symptoms, clonidine, an α_2 agonist, can be concomitantly administered in doses of 5 μg/kg to significantly reduce withdrawal symptomatology. Finally, because methadone is extremely well absorbed from the gastrointestinal tract and has a bioavailability of 80% to 90%, it is extremely easy to convert intravenous dosing regimens to oral ones. Recently, the conversion dose of morphine to methadone has been challenged. Traditionally, it has been thought that the ratio of morphine to methadone was approximately 1:1; it now appears that it is closer to 1:0.25 or even 1:0.1 (43,178–180). Underestimating methadone's potency substantially increases the risk of potential life-threatening toxicity. The unexpected finding that methadone is more potent as a respiratory depressant and sedative than was predicted by published conversion ratios is sometimes referred to as *incomplete cross-tolerance*. Incomplete cross-tolerance for methadone may be owing to its antagonist actions at the NMDA receptor (44,45,93).

Hydromorphone

Hydromorphone, a derivative of morphine, is an opioid with appreciable selectivity for μ opioid receptors. It is noted for its rapid onset and 4- to 6-hour duration of action. It differs from its parent compound morphine in that it is five times more potent and ten times more lipid soluble and does not have an active metabolite (130,181). Its elimination half-life is 3 to 4 hours and, like morphine and meperidine, shows very wide intrasubject pharmacokinetic variability. Hydromorphone is far less sedating than morphine and is thought by many to be associated with fewer systemic side effects. Indeed, it is often used as an alternative to morphine in intravenous PCA or when morphine produces too much sedation or nausea. Additionally, hydromorphone is receiving renewed attention as an alternative morphine for treatment of prolonged cancer-related pain because it can be prepared in more concentrated aqueous solutions than morphine.

Hydromorphone is effective when administered intravenously, subcutaneously, epidurally, and orally (130,182). The intravenous route of administration is the most commonly used technique in the intensive care unit. After a loading dose of 0.005 to 0.015 mg/kg, a continuous infusion ranging from 0.003 to 0.005 mg/kg per hour is started. Supplemental boluses of 0.003 to 0.005 mg/kg are administered by either the nurse or patient as needed. When administered epidurally, one can use either continuous infusions [0.001 to 0.003 mg/kg per hour (the adult dose is 0.15 to 0.3 mg per hour)] or continuous infusions with patient-controlled boluses [0.001 to 0.003 mg/kg per bolus (the adult dose is 0.15 to 0.3 mg per bolus)].

Codeine

Codeine is a μ opioid agonist that is most frequently used as an antitussive and an agent to treat pain in children and adults. It is a phenanthrene alkaloid and derived from morphine. Although effective when administered either orally or parenterally, it is most commonly administered in the oral form, usually in combination with acetaminophen (or aspirin). In equipotent doses (Tables 12.2 and 12.3), codeine's efficacy as an analgesic and respiratory depressant approaches that of morphine. In addition, codeine shares with morphine and the other opioid agonists common effects on the central nervous system including sedation, respiratory depression, and stimulation of the chemoreceptor trigger zone in the brainstem. It also delays gastric emptying and can increase biliary tract pressure. Codeine is very nauseating; many patients claim that they are allergic to it because it so commonly induces vomiting. There are much fewer nausea and vomiting problems with oxycodone. Because of this, oxycodone and hydrocodone are now preferred oral opioids. Finally, codeine has potent antitussive properties that are similar to those of most other opioids and is most commonly prescribed for this effect.

Codeine has a bioavailability of approximately 60% after oral ingestion. The analgesic effects occur as early as 20 minutes after ingestion and reach a maximum at 60 to 120 minutes. The plasma half-life of elimination is 2.5 to 3 hours. Codeine undergoes nearly complete metabolism in the liver before its final excretion in urine. Interestingly, the analgesic effects of codeine are not owing to codeine itself; rather, it must be first metabolized via O-demethylation into morphine through a pathway dependent on the P-450 subtype 2D6 (CYP2D6). Only approximately 5% to 10% of an administered codeine dose is demethylated in the liver into morphine (183,184). A significant portion of the population (ranging between 4% and 10%), depending on ethnic group (e.g., Chinese), lacks CYP2D6, and these patients achieve very little analgesia (or respiratory depression) when they receive codeine (183,184).

Oral codeine is usually prescribed in combination with either acetaminophen or aspirin. It is available as a liquid or tablet (185). If prescribing codeine, we recommend the premixed combination compound for most children because when prescribed as a single agent, codeine is not readily available in liquid form at most pharmacies and is almost twice as expensive as the combined form. Furthermore, acetaminophen potentiates the analgesia produced by codeine and allows the practitioner to use less opioid and yet achieve satisfactory analgesia. Nevertheless, it is important to understand that all combination preparations of acetaminophen may result in inadvertently administering a hepatotoxic acetaminophen dose when increasing doses are given for uncontrolled pain (185–188). Acetaminophen toxicity may result from a single toxic dose, repeated ingestion of large doses of acetaminophen (e.g., in adults, 7.5 to 10 g daily for 1 to 2 days; in children, 60 to 420 mg/kg daily for 1 to 42 days), or long-term ingestion (186–188).

Codeine and acetaminophen are available as an elixir (120 mg acetaminophen and 12 mg codeine) and as "numbered" tablets, e.g., Tylenol Nos. 1, 2, 3, or 4. The number refers to how much codeine is in each tablet. Tylenol No. 4 has 60 mg codeine, No. 3 has 30 mg, No. 2 has 15 mg, and No. 1 has 7.5 mg. Progressive increases in dose are associated with a similar degree of respiratory depression, delayed gastric emptying, nausea, and constipation as with other opioid drugs. Although it is an effective analgesic when administered parenterally, intramuscular codeine has no advantage over morphine or meperidine (despite 100 years as the standard for neurosurgery). Intravenous administration of codeine is associated with serious complications including apnea and severe hypotension, probably secondary to histamine release. Therefore, we do not recommend the intravenous administration of this drug in children. Codeine is used for the treatment of mild to moderate pain (or cough), usually in an outpatient setting. Typically, it is prescribed in a dose of 0.5 to 1 $mg{\cdot}kg^{-1}$ with a concurrently administered dose of acetaminophen (10 $mg{\cdot}kg^{-1}$). Only approximately one-half of the analgesic dose is needed to treat a cough.

Oxycodone and Hydrocodone

Oxycodone (the opioid in Tylox and Percocet) and hydrocodone (the opioid in Vicodin and Lortab) are opiates that are frequently used to treat pain in children and adults, particularly for less severe pain or when patients are being converted from parenteral narcotics to enteral ones (Table 12.2) (133). Like codeine, oxycodone and hydrocodone are administered in the oral form, usually in combination with acetaminophen (Tylox, Percocet, Vicodin, Lortab, codeine 1, 2, 3, and 4) or aspirin (185).

In equipotent doses, oxycodone, hydrocodone, and morphine are equal as both analgesics and respiratory depressants. In addition, these drugs share with other narcotics common effects on the central nervous system including sedation, respiratory depression, and stimulation of the chemoreceptor trigger zone in the brainstem. Hydrocodone and oxycodone have a bioavailability of approximately 60% after oral ingestion. Oxycodone is metabolized in the liver into oxymorphone, an active metabolite, both of which may accumulate in patients with renal failure (189). The analgesic effects occur as early as 20 minutes after ingestion and reach a maximum at 60 to 120 minutes. The plasma half-life of elimination is 2.5 to 4 hours. Like oral codeine, hydrocodone and oxycodone are usually prescribed in combination with either acetaminophen or aspirin (Tylenol and codeine elixir, Percocet, Tylox, Vicodin, Lortab), and the same risk of acetaminophen-induced hepatotoxicity exists.

Hydrocodone is prescribed in a dose of 0.05 to 0.1 mg/kg. The elixir is available as 2.5 mg/5 mL combined with acetaminophen 167 mg/ 5 mL. As a tablet, it is available in hydrocodone doses between 2.5 to 10 mg, combined with 500 to 650 mg acetaminophen. Oxycodone is prescribed in a dose of 0.05 to 0.1 mg/kg. Unfortunately, the elixir is not available in most pharmacies. When it is, it comes in two forms: 1 and 20 mg/mL. Obviously, this has enormous implications and can easily lead to a catastrophic overdose. In tablet form, oxycodone is commonly available as Tylox (500 mg acetaminophen and 5 mg oxycodone) and as Percocet (325 mg acetaminophen and 5 mg oxycodone). Oxycodone is also available without acetaminophen in a sustained-release tablet for use in chronic pain. Like all time-release tablets, it must *not* be ground up and therefore cannot be administered through a gastric tube. Like sustained-release morphine, sustained-release oxycodone is for use only in opioid-tolerant patients with chronic pain, *not* for acute pain management. Also note that in patients with rapid gastrointestinal transit, sustained-release preparations may not be absorbed at all (liquid methadone may be an alternative) (185). Finally, oxycodone is very well absorbed rectally (190). Unfortunately, a rectal suppository is not commercially available, but the oral form can be given rectally to good effect.

OPIOID AGONIST–ANTAGONIST DRUGS

Mixed agonist–antagonist drugs act as agonists or partial agonists at one receptor and antagonists at another receptor. Mixed (opioid) agonist–antagonist drugs include, but are not limited to, buprenorphine, pentazocine, butorphanol, nalorphine, dezocine, and nalbuphine. Most of these drugs are agonists or partial agonists at the κ and σ receptors and antagonists at the μ receptor (Table 12.3). The primary advantage of these drugs is their ability to produce analgesia with limited respiratory depression. Additionally, they have a very low potential to produce opioid addiction. Their primary disadvantage is that an analgesic "ceiling effect" may be reached, such that increasing the dose of these drugs or adding a pure agonist does not produce additional analgesia. Furthermore, in physically dependent patients, these drugs can and do induce withdrawal symptoms. Based on animal and human studies, a rank order of intrinsic efficacy for these drugs is morphine ≥ dezocine = buprenorphine > butorphanol > nalbuphine (191).

Pentazocine

Pentazocine (Talwin) is a mixed agonist–antagonist that is derived from benzomorphan and is presumed to exert its agonist effects at the δ and κ receptors and its antagonist effects at the μ receptor. It is two to three times less potent than morphine and can be administered orally, parenterally, and epidurally. Epidural administration produces a rapid onset of analgesia that is shorter in duration than that produced by morphine (192). The most common side effects associated with pentazocine administration are sedation, diaphoresis, and dizziness. Sedation is prominent after epidural placement of pentazocine, presumably reflecting activation of κ receptors. However, nausea and vomiting are less common than with morphine. Dysphoria, including an intense fear of impending death, is associated with high doses of pentazocine, which has tended to limit its use. As mentioned previously, at equianalgesic doses, biliary tract pressure rises to a lesser extent after pentazocine than after administration of morphine, meperidine, or fentanyl (193). Finally, pentazocine produces an increase in plasma concentrations of catecholamines, which may account for increases in heart rate, systemic blood pressure, pulmonary artery blood pressure, and left ventricular end-diastolic pressure that accompany administration of this drug.

Pentazocine has an elimination half-life in adults of 2 to 3 hours. It is primarily biotransformed in the liver and excreted by the kidney. In adults, 20 to 30 mg pentazocine administered parenterally produces analgesia, sedation, and depression of ventilation similar to 10 mg morphine. Increasing the intramuscular dose to more than 30 mg does not produce proportionate increases in these responses. When administered orally, 50 mg is roughly equivalent in analgesic potency to 60 mg codeine.

Butorphanol

Butorphanol (Stadol) is an agonist–antagonist opioid that resembles pentazocine. Butorphanol has a greater affinity for κ receptors to produce analgesia than pentazocine and minimal affinity for σ receptors. Thus, compared with pentazocine, the analgesic effects of butorphanol are approximately 20 times greater and the incidence of associated dysphoria is very low. Common side effects of butorphanol, like all other agonist–antagonists, include sedation, nausea, and diaphoresis. Dysphoria, reported frequently with other opioid agonist–antagonists, is very infrequent after administration of butorphanol. Like pentazocine, analgesic doses of butorphanol increase systemic blood pressure, pulmonary artery blood pressure, and cardiac output and should be avoided in patients with heart disease. Also, just like pentazocine, the effects of butorphanol on the biliary and gastrointestinal tracts seem to be milder than those produced by morphine, meperidine, and fentanyl.

Butorphanol is available parenterally and intranasally. It is rapidly and almost completely absorbed after administration of an intramuscular injection or an intranasal spray. In adult postoperative patients, 1 mg intravenously or 2 mg administered intramuscularly produces analgesia and depression of ventilation similar to 10 mg morphine. For moderate to severe pain in adults, one spray (1 mg) in each nostril provides 2 hours of pain relief (194). The pediatric dose of butorphanol is 0.25 to 0.5 mg/kg intravenously or intranasally (195). Transnasal butorphanol has also been used (and abused) in patients with migraine headaches (196,197). The elimination half-life of butorphanol in adults is 2.5 to 3.5 hours. Finally, butorphanol is also quite effective when given epidurally and, unlike fentanyl and morphine, does not result in pruritus (66,198).

Nalbuphine

Nalbuphine (Nubain) is an agonist–antagonist opioid that is related chemically to oxymorphone and naloxone and is roughly equivalent on a milligram per kilogram basis to morphine. Just like the other agonist–antagonist drugs, sedation is its most common side effect. Conversely, the incidence of dysphoria is less than that produced by pentazocine and butorphanol. In contrast to these latter two drugs, nalbuphine does not increase systemic blood pressure, pulmonary artery blood pressure, heart rate, or atrial filling pressures and may therefore be a better drug to use in patients with heart disease (199). Its effects on biliary duct pressure are similar to those produced by pentazocine.

The antagonist effects of nalbuphine are speculated to occur at μ receptors. Consequently, if a ceiling effect is reached, the addition of pure μ agonist drugs may not be able to provide adequate analgesia. Conversely, the antagonist effects of nalbuphine at μ receptors can be used to a therapeutic advantage because of nalbuphine's ability to antagonize the lingering ventilatory depressant effects of opioid agonists while still maintaining analgesia. Intravenously administered nalbuphine, 10 to 20 mg, reverses postoperative depression of ventilation caused by fentanyl but maintains analgesia (200,201). It can also be used to treat opioid-induced pruritus (202). Nalbuphine can be administered orally, parenterally, or epidurally. Only approximately 20% to 25% of an orally administered dose of nalbuphine reaches the systemic circulation. When converting a patient's intravenous nalbuphine requirements to oral maintenance, one needs to multiply the intravenous dose by three to five times.

Buprenorphine

Buprenorphine (Buprenex) is the only partial agonist opioid drug. It is widely used in Europe both intravenously and sublingually in the treatment of moderate to severe pain (2). Because it undergoes significant first-pass metabolism when taken orally, it is not available in an enteral form.

Dextromethorphan

Dextromethorphan, a noncompetitive antagonist of the NMDA receptor, is the D isomer of the codeine analog of levorphanol. Unlike the L isomer, it has no addictive properties and fewer subjective side effects than codeine. Historically, dextromethorphan has been used as an antitussive but has recently been used, albeit with mixed results, in the treatment of acute and chronic pain primarily by blocking central sensitization (windup) (46,203). As discussed previously, central sensitization mainly results from the activation of NMDA receptors in the central nervous system triggered by long-lasting nociceptive afferent input. NMDA receptor antagonists such as dextromethorphan prevent the induction of central sensitization in experimental conditions. Although its duration of action as an NMDA receptor antagonist is unknown, the elimination half-life of orally administered dextromethorphan is approximately 8 hours, and its antitussive effect persists for 5 to 6 hours (2).

Although it has little or no analgesic effect, dextromethorphan potentiates morphine analgesia and may have a role in acute pain management (204). Indeed, combination drugs such as MorphiDex (morphine sulphate plus dextromethorphan hydrobromide) are now available (205). The mode of possible interaction between NMDA and opioid receptors that may underlie the observed potentiation between morphine and NMDA antagonists has been reviewed and discussed previously (206). Briefly, even a single opioid administration seems to elicit adaptive changes in the nervous system, leading to the attenuation of the effect of the opioid. Activation of the NMDA receptor constitutes an important step in these adaptive changes. Stimulation of NMDA receptors after opioid treatment may reduce the magnitude and duration of opioid-induced antinociception. Thus, blockade of NMDA receptors may be expected to acutely enhance opioid-induced antinociception.

Theoretically, dextromethorphan should be most effective in the treatment of chronic and neuropathic pain. Unfortunately, most studies have found it ineffective (207,208). Curiously, it may be more beneficial in the preemptive treatment of acute pain, for example, if given preoperatively. (209). Kawamata et al. (210) found that preemptive administration of 30 to 60 mg dextromethorphan reduced acute postoperative tonsillectomy pain in adults. Rose et al. (211) administered 0.5 to 1 mg/kg dextromethorphan to children for the same surgery and found no discernible effect.

PATIENT (PARENT AND NURSE) - CONTROLLED ANALGESIA

Because of the enormous individual variations in pain perception and opioid metabolism, fixed doses and time intervals make little sense. Based on the pharmacokinetics of the opioids, it should be clear that intravenous boluses of morphine may need to be given at intervals of 1 to 2 hours to avoid marked fluctuations in plasma drug levels. Continuous intravenous infusions can provide steady analgesic levels and are preferable to intramuscular injections and have been used with great safety and effectiveness in children (56,123,212). However, they are not a panacea because the perception and intensity of pain is not constant. For example, a postoperative patient may be very comfortable resting in bed and may require little adjustment in pain management. This same patient may experience excruciating pain when coughing, voiding, or getting out of bed. Thus, rational pain management requires some form of titration to effect whenever any opioid is administered. To give patients, and in some cases parents and nurses, some measure of control over their, or their children's, pain therapy, demand analgesia or PCA devices have been developed (129,133,213,214). These are microprocessor-driven pumps with a button that the patient presses to self-administer a small dose of opioid.

PCA devices allow patients to administer small amounts of an analgesic whenever they feel a need for more pain relief. The opioid, usually morphine, is administered either intravenously or subcutaneously (129,133,213). The dose of opioid, number of boluses per hour, and the time interval between boluses (the "lock-out period") are programmed into the equipment by the pain service physician to allow maximal patient flexibility and sense of control with minimal risk of overdose. Generally, because older patients know that if they have severe pain, they can obtain relief immediately, many prefer dosing regimens that result in mild to moderate pain in exchange for fewer side effects such as nausea or pruritus. The most commonly prescribed opioids for intravenous PCA are morphine, hydromorphone, and fentanyl. Typically, we initially prescribe morphine, 20 μg/kg per bolus, at a rate of five boluses per hour, with a 6- to 8-minute lock-out interval between each bolus (129,133,213). Variations include larger boluses (30 to 50 μg/kg), shorter time intervals (5 minutes), and so on. Hydromorphone may have fewer side effects than morphine and is often used when pruritus and nausea complicate morphine PCA therapy. Because it is five to seven times more potent than morphine, the size of the bolus dose is reduced to 3 to 4 μg/kg (130). The fentanyl equivalent is less clear. Although fentanyl is considered 50 to 100 times more potent than morphine when given as a single bolus, Monitto et al. (134) used a conversion of 40:1 in a study in which parents and nurses controlled the PCA pump. In this study, 0.5 μg/kg fentanyl was administered by continuous infusion, and bolus doses were 0.5 μg/kg.

The PCA pump computer stores within its memory how many boluses that the patient has received and how many attempts the patient has made to receive a bolus. This enables the physician to evaluate how well the patient understands the use of the pump and provides information to program the pump more efficiently. Many PCA units allow low background continuous infusions (morphine at 20 to 30 μg/kg per hour, hydromorphone at 3 to 4 μg/kg per hour, fentanyl 0.5 μg/kg per hour) in addition to self-administered boluses. This is sometimes called "PCA-Plus." A continuous background infusion is particularly useful at night and often provides more restful sleep by preventing the patient from awakening in pain. It also increases the potential for overdose (129,134,215). Although the adult literature on pain does not support the use of continuous background infusions, it has been our experience that continuous infusions are essential for both the patient and physician (i.e., fewer telephone calls, problems) (216). Indeed, in our practice, we usually use continuous background infusions when we prescribe intravenous (or epidural) PCA.

PCA requires a patient with enough intelligence and manual dexterity and strength to operate the pump. Thus, it was initially limited to adolescents and teenagers, but the lower age limit in whom this treatment modality can be used continues to fall. In fact, it has been our experience that any child able to play a video game can operate a PCA pump (5 to 6 years of age). Allowing parents or nurses to initiate a PCA bolus is controversial. In our practice, we empower nurses and parents to initiate PCA boluses and use this technology in children even younger than 1 year of age. In our experience, the incidence of common opioid-induced side effects is similar to that observed in older patients (134). Interestingly, respiratory depression is very rare but does occur, reinforcing the need for close monitoring and established nursing protocols. Difficulties with PCA include its increased costs, patient age limitations, and the bureaucratic (physician, nursing, and pharmacy) obstacles (protocols, education, storage arrangements) that must be overcome before its implementation. Contraindications include the patient's inability to push the bolus button (weakness, arm restraints), inability to understand how to use the machine, and desire not to assume responsibility for his/her own care.

INTRATHECAL/EPIDURAL OPIOID ANALGESIA

The presence of high concentrations of opioid receptors in the spinal cord makes it possible to achieve analgesia, in both acute and chronic pain, with small doses of opioids administered in either the subarachnoid or epidural spaces (Fig. 12.6) (12,106,217–219). By bypassing the blood and the blood–brain barrier, small doses of agonist are effective because they can reach the receptor by the backdoor (104). CSF opioid levels, particularly for morphine, are several thousand times greater than those achieved by the parenteral route (see below) (58,97). It is these high levels that produce the profound and prolonged analgesia that accompanies intrathecal/epidural opioid administration.

Yaksh (104) demonstrated in unanesthetized rats that intrathecal narcotics produced profound segmental analgesia that is dose dependent and reversible with naloxone. However, after 1 hour, rostral spread was evident, especially at higher doses (220,221). The passage of epidurally administered agonists across the dura into the CSF is dependent on the lipid solubility of the drug. Additionally, once in the CSF, opioids must pass from the water phase of the CSF into the lipid phase of the underlying neuraxis to reach the receptor. This too is dependent on lipid solubility. Hydrophilic agents such as morphine have a greater latency and duration of action than more lipid-soluble agents such as fentanyl (99,100). In contrast, the lipid-soluble agonists produce more segmental analgesia

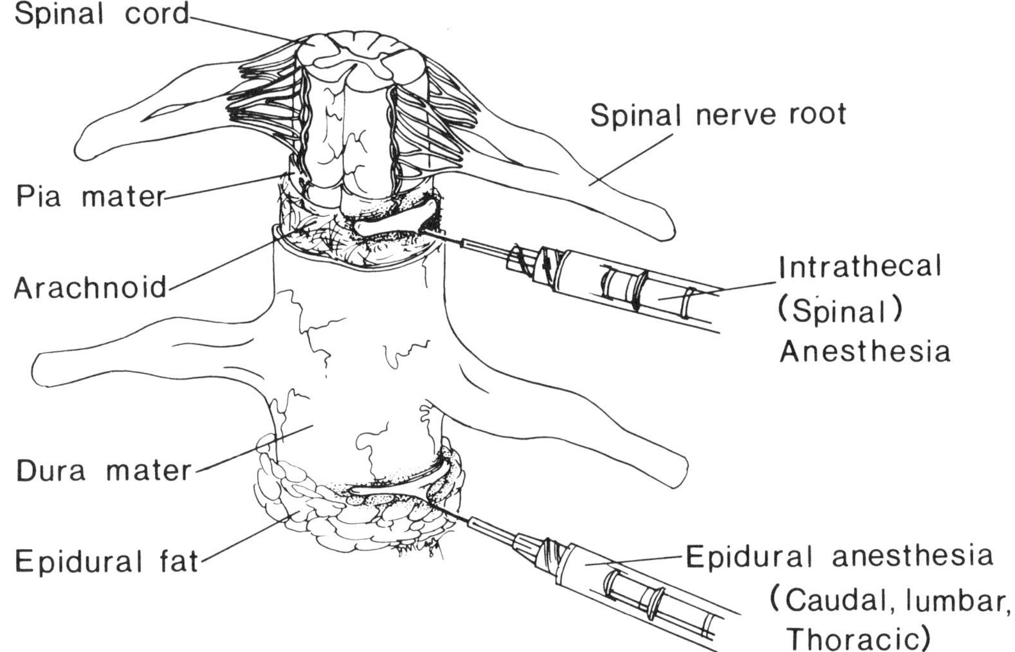

FIG. 12.6. The relationship between the spinal cord and its coverings, i.e., the pia matter, arachnoid, and dura are shown. In an intrathecal or "spinal" injection, the needle passes through the dura and arachnoid into the subarachnoid space, which contains cerebrospinal fluid. In an epidural injection, the needle passes through the ligamentum flavum but remains above the dura mater.

with less rostral spread than the less lipid soluble agonists (98,222).

Epidural morphine has been shown to provide effective postoperative analgesia after abdominal, thoracic, and cardiac surgery, even when administered via the caudal route (223—228). Krane et al. (224) reported that 0.03 mg/kg of caudal-epidural morphine is equally effective as 0.1 mg/kg in providing postoperative analgesia, although the higher dose provides a significantly longer duration of analgesia (13.3 ± 4.7 versus 10.0 ± 3.3 hours, respectively). The incidence of side effects was the same in both groups, although one patient receiving 0.1 mg/kg developed late respiratory depression. Therefore, these investigators suggest starting with the lower dose when using this technique. Whether even lower doses would be effective is unknown.

Spinal opiates produce analgesia without altering autonomic, sensory, or neuromuscular function. Additionally both light touch and proprioception are preserved. Paralysis and hypotension, therefore, are absent. Another critical advantage over local anesthetics is the availability of a specific opioid receptor antagonist, naloxone. Thus, unlike local anesthetics, spinal opioids allow patients to ambulate without orthostatic hypotension. Common side effects of intrathecal/epidural narcotics include facial or segmental pruritus, urinary retention, nausea and vomiting, and respiratory depression (105,229–232). These side effects occur with greater frequency when opioids are administered intrathecally instead of epidurally. Except for urinary retention, reversal of adverse side effects, with maintenance of adequate analgesia, can be achieved by using a low-dose (0.001 to 0.002 mg·kg^{-1}) naloxone infusion. Pruritus and nausea can also be treated with intravenous or oral diphenhydramine (Benadryl), 0.5 to 1.0 mg/kg or hydroxyzine (Vistaril, Atarax). Urinary retention is common after spinally administered opiates. The lower one's threshold (e.g., 4, 6, 8 hours) without voiding, the more common it is. Bladder catheterization relieves this problem.

Although rare, respiratory depression is a major risk when using intrathecal/epidural opioids. Attia et al. (232) demonstrated that the ventilatory response to carbon dioxide is depressed for as long as 22 hours after the administration of 0.05 mg·kg^{-1} of morphine epidurally. After intrathecal morphine administration (0.02 mg/kg), Nichols et al. (58) demonstrated in children varying in age from 3 months to 15 years significant depression of the ventilatory response to carbon dioxide for as long as 18 hours. The greatest respiratory depression correlated with the highest CSF morphine levels (2,863 ± 542 ng/mL), which occurred 6 hours after administration. This depression persisted despite a fall in CSF morphine levels 12 (641 ± 219 ng/mL) to 18 (223 ± 152 ng/mL) hours later. This confirms the clinical impression that respiratory depression usually occurs within the first 6 hours after the administration of epidural or intrathecal morphine but may occur as long as 18 hours afterward. Respiratory depression, hypoxemia, and obstructive apnea are more common in infants than in older children, even when morphine is administered in doses as low as 0.025 mg/kg (118).

In older children and adults, respiratory depression most commonly occurs when intravenous or intramuscular narcotics have been administered to supplement the intrathecal opioid. The risk of respiratory depression can be minimized if smaller doses of supplemental narcotics are used or through the epidural use of shorter acting, more lipid-soluble agents (fentanyl, sufentanil), which produce more segmental analgesia with little rostral spread. In contrast, because of their shorter duration of action, fentanyl and sufentanil are increasingly being administered by continuous epidural infusion, either alone or in combination with very dilute [1/16% (0.0625 mg/mL) or 0.1% (1.0 mg/mL)] bupivacaine concentrations. Typically, the epidural solution contains 1 to 2 μg/mL of fentanyl, with or without bupivacaine, and is administered at rates ranging between 0.2 and 1.0 ml/kg per hour. This provides effective analgesia for both postoperative and chronic cancer pain. Sufentanil (0.1 to 0.2 μg/kg), the only drug approved for epidural use by the U.S. Food and Drug Administration (FDA), has been shown to provide effective analgesia in children ranging in age from 4 to 12 years for approximately 2 hours.

Regardless of the opioid prescribed and its route of administration, a regular system of monitoring for respiratory depression is mandatory for safe use (233,234). Clinical signs that predict impending respiratory depression include somnolence, small pupils, and small tidal volumes. In addition, we insist on the use of oxyhemoglobin saturation monitoring (pulse oximetry) when instituting this therapy.

NOVEL ROUTES OF OPIOID ADMINISTRATION

Although opioids are traditionally administered parenterally (intravenous, intramuscular), spinally (intrathecal, epidural), and enterally (oral, rectal), the need for alternatives, particularly when treating children with either acute or chronic pain, has resulted in the development of novel routes of opioid administration. Some, such as transdermal and transmucosal administration, have achieved widespread use. Others such as intranasal, inhalational, and iontophoretic administration have not. All these modes of delivery can now be considered conventional, although few have been specifically tested or approved for use in children.

Transdermal and Transmucosal Fentanyl

Because fentanyl is extremely lipophilic, it can be readily absorbed across any biologic membrane including the skin. Thus, it can be given painlessly by new, nonintravenous routes of drug administration including the transmucosal (nose and mouth) and transdermal routes. The transdermal route is frequently used for the long-term administration of many drugs including scopolamine, clonidine, and nitroglycerin. A selective semipermeable membrane patch with a reservoir of drug allows the slow, steady-state absorption of drug across the skin. The patch is attached to the skin by a contact adhesive, which often causes skin irritation. Many factors, including body site, skin temperature, skin damage, ethnic group, and age, will affect the absorption of fentanyl across the skin.

Because fentanyl is painlessly absorbed across the skin, a substantial amount is stored in the upper skin layers, which then act as a secondary reservoir. The presence of a skin depot has several implications: It dampens the fluctuations of fentanyl effect, needs to be reasonably filled before significant vascular absorption occurs, and contributes to a prolonged residual fentanyl CP (plasma concentration) after patch removal. The amount of fentanyl remaining within the system and skin depot after removal of the patch is substantial. At the end of a 24-hour period, a fentanyl patch releasing drug at the rate of 100 mg per hour, 1.07 to 0.43 mg fentanyl (approximately 30% of the total delivered dose from the patch) remains in the skin depot. Thus, removing the patch does not stop the continued absorption of fentanyl into the body (235).

Because of its long onset time, inability to rapidly adjust drug delivery, and long elimination half-life, transdermal fentanyl is *contraindicated* for *acute* pain management. As stated above, the safety of this drug delivery system is compromised even further because fentanyl continues to be absorbed from the subcutaneous fat for almost 24 hours after the patch is removed. In fact, the use of this drug delivery system for acute pain has resulted in the death of an otherwise healthy patient. Transdermal fentanyl is applicable only for patients with chronic pain (e.g., cancer) or in opioid-tolerant patients. Even when transdermal fentanyl is appropriate, the vehicle imposes its own constraints: the smallest "denomination" of fentanyl patch delivers 25 μg of fentanyl per hour; the others deliver 50, 75, and 100 μg fentanyl per hour. Patches *cannot* be physically cut in smaller pieces to deliver less fentanyl. This often limits usefulness in smaller patients.

Conversely, the transmucosal route of fentanyl administration is extremely effective for acute pain relief and heralds a new era in the management of acute pain management in children. In this novel delivery technique, fentanyl is manufactured in a candy matrix (Fentanyl Oralet) attached to a plastic applicator (it looks like a lollipop); as the child sucks on the candy, fentanyl is absorbed across the buccal mucosa and is rapidly (10 to 20 minutes) absorbed into the systemic circulation (171,236–240). If excessive sedation occurs, the fentanyl is removed from the child's mouth by the applicator. It is more efficient than ordinary oral/gastric intestinal administration because transmucosal absorption bypasses the efficient first-pass hepatic metabolism of fentanyl that occurs after enteral absorption into the portal circulation. The Fentanyl Oralet has been approved by the FDA for use in children for premedication before surgery and for procedure-related pain (e.g., lumbar puncture, bone marrow aspiration) (241). It is also useful in the treatment of cancer pain and as a supplement to transdermal fentanyl (242). When administered transmucosally, fentanyl is given in doses of 10 to 15 μg/kg, is effective within 20 minutes, and lasts approximately 2 hours. Approximately 25% to 33% of the given dose is absorbed. Thus, when administered in doses of 10 to 15 μg/kg, blood levels equivalent to 3 to 5 μg/kg intravenous fentanyl are achieved. The major side effect, nausea and vomiting, occurs in approximately 20% to 33% of patients who receive it (243). This product is only available in hospital (and Surgicenter) pharmacies and, as with all sedative/analgesics, will require vigilant patient monitoring.

Intranasal Route

The intranasal route of opioid administration has long been favored by drug abusers and has only recently been used therapeutically. Rapid, painless, and safe, it is a reliable method of giving opioids to patients in whom there is no intravenous access or who cannot tolerate the parenteral route of drug administration. Fentanyl, sufentanil, and butorphanol are the most commonly administered intranasal opioids, although there are also reports of using oxycodone and meperidine by this route. Absorption of drug across the nasal mucosa depends on lipid solubility and has the advantage of avoiding first-pass metabolism. Unfortunately, there have been few pharmacokinetic studies involving intranasal opioids in children. In practice, fentanyl, sufentanil, and butorphanol produce analgesia within 10 to 30 minutes of intranasal administration.

Intranasal opioids can be administered either as a dry powder or dissolved in water or saline. Sufentanil has been given with a 1- or 3-mL syringe, nasal spray, or nasal dropper, and butorphanol has been formulated in an intranasal metered-dose spray (0.25 mg). Butorphanol has been used in the treatment of acute migraine headache, for postoperative pain relief after myringotomy and tube surgery, and for musculoskeletal pain (169,194,195,197). There are few reported side effects related specifically to the intranasal route of administration, presumably because, unlike midazolam, none of the opioids is particularly irritating. For example, 85% of children cried after intranasal midazolam compared with 28% of those receiving sufentanil as premedication for same-day outpatient anesthesia (244,245).

Inhalation

Nebulized or inhaled opioids are most commonly used in the palliative care of terminally ill patients with dyspnea (246). Although it is unclear whether inhaled opioids provide superior relief to patients with air hunger, anecdotal evidence and some adult literature have suggested that inhalation administration of opioids is not just another method of systemic administration of opioids but a way to specifically target opioid receptors in the lungs. Using immunoreactive techniques, opioid peptides have been detected in bronchial mucosal cells, and doses as low as 5 mg nebulized morphine have been reported to reduce significantly the sensation of breathlessness in patients with chronic lung disease (247).

Wide dosing ranges, concentrations, and volumes to be administered have been used.

Chandler (246) suggests starting opioid-naïve adults with 5 to 10 mg morphine every 4 hours and opioid-tolerant adults with 10 to 20 mg. Theoretically, there should be nearly total transmucosal absorption, but much of the dose is deposited in the nebulizer apparatus, with a bioavailability of only 5% to 30% (246). There are almost no studies using this technique in children. Based on extrapolation from adult literature, in our practice, we start with 4 hours of the child's usual intravenous opioid dose. This can be administered as the parenteral solution mixed with a few milliliters of saline, delivered via a portable oxygen tank and simple "neb mask" (such as that used to deliver albuterol). Opioid-naïve caregivers must not inhale the opioid aerosol. Nebulized morphine has been reported to cause bronchospasm in persons with underlying reactive airway disease. Nebulized fentanyl may cause fewer problems because it releases less histamine. Independent of special relief of dyspnea, using the nebulized route may satisfy the family and nurses that we are "doing something different" at a time when little can be done. Other studies suggest that simple nebulized saline may be as helpful as nebulized opioids. Finally, some work suggests that blow-by air can be as effective as blow-by oxygen (248).

Iontophoresis

Iontophoresis is a method of transdermal administration of ionizable drugs in which the electrically charged components are propelled through the skin by an external electric field. Several drugs, such as lidocaine, corticosteroids, morphine, and fentanyl, can be delivered iontophoretically (249–252). This technique is not completely painless, and some younger children object to its use.

OPIOID ANTAGONISTS

Naloxone

A discussion of opioid analgesics would be incomplete without mentioning the opioid antagonists. Naloxone is a pure opioid antagonist at the μ, δ, and κ receptors. It has virtually no agonist activity. It antagonizes the effects of pure agonist drugs, such as morphine, as well as the effects of mixed agonist–antagonist drugs, such as butorphanol. It is the most commonly used opioid antagonist in clinical practice today.

Naloxone is extremely potent and nonselective in its opioid reversal effects (Table 12.3). It not only antagonizes the sedation, respiratory depression, and gastrointestinal effects of the opioid agonists, but it reverses the analgesia as well. Indeed, the reversal of opioid agonists and their effects by antagonists must be accomplished with great caution, particularly in patients who have been receiving prolonged opioid therapy, exhibit opioid dependence, or are in extreme pain, because it may be accompanied by overt withdrawal symptoms. Occasionally, a life-threatening "overshoot" phenomenon may occur in these patients, with the development of tachypnea, tachycardia, hypertension, nausea and vomiting, and sudden death from ventricular fibrillation. Obviously, the magnitude of the withdrawal syndrome depends on the dose of naloxone administered and on the degree of the patient's physical dependence. It is our practice to employ mechanical ventilation as a safer alternative to using naloxone for treating narcotic-induced respiratory depression in dependent patients or in patients with severe pain.

Naloxone is a pure μ receptor antagonist and is effective in reducing and reversing (antagonizing) all opioid-related side effects in a dose-dependent manner (3,253). Thus, higher intravenous doses reverse opioid-induced analgesia and lower doses (naloxone infusion <1 μg/kg per hour) maintain analgesia and may prevent many of the nuisance side effects, such as pruritus and nausea and vomiting. In our clinical practice, we routinely treat patients who develop opioid-induced pruritus with low-dose intravenous naloxone infusions.

Over the past 5 years, several studies have been published suggesting that low-dose naloxone infusions may have an opioid-sparing effect and may prevent the development of tolerance (31,254–257). How low-dose naloxone improves analgesia is unclear, although it is believed to be related to inhibition of presynaptic (negative feed back) receptor blockade. Recently, Gan et al. (68) demonstrated the opioid-sparing effects and the reduction of side effects of low-dose naloxone infusions in adult patients receiving intravenous morphine PCA. Comparable studies have never been performed in children. This is done by administering 0.001 mg/kg naloxone as an intravenous bolus and then starting an infusion of 0.001 mg/kg per hour. When naloxone is administered to patients who have not received opioids, it produces minimal to no effects (except in patients in shock) and has no inherent properties that induce physical dependence or tolerance.

Naloxone is rapidly metabolized (by conjugation with glucuronic acid) in the liver and is best given parenterally because of its rapid first-pass extraction through the liver after oral administration. After intravenous administration, it reverses the effects of opioids virtually instantaneously. Unfortunately, it has a plasma elimination half-life of only 60 minutes and a duration of action that is much shorter than the agonists that it is used to reverse. Therefore, when naloxone is used to reverse narcotic-induced respiratory depression, patients must be monitored for the return of the depression, based on the half-life of the opiate agonist. This may require repeat intravenous doses, intramuscular (depot) injection, or a continuous intravenous infusion.

Naloxone is supplied as a parenteral solution (0.4 or 0.02 mg/mL). The standard initial dose for children and adults is 0.01 mg/kg given intravenously. If this dose does not result in the desired degree of clinical improvement, subsequent doses of 0.02, 0.04, 0.08, and 0.1 mg/kg may be administered in a stepwise manner. However, one must remember that this dose of naloxone also antagonizes the analgesic effects of most opioids. When used to reverse neonatal respiratory depression (caused by narcotics administered to the mother during labor), the usual initial resuscitation dose is the same as used for older children (0.01 mg/kg of the 0.02 mg/mL solution). If an intravenous route is not available, naloxone may be administered intramuscularly or subcutaneously.

Naltrexone

Naltrexone, like naloxone, is a relatively pure μ receptor antagonist. Unlike naloxone, it is highly effective when administered orally. Occasionally, it is used to detect or monitor for opioid addiction, particularly when drugs that are not easily detectable in urine screening (e.g., fentanyl) are suspected. Yuan et al. (61), in a series of experiments, demonstrated that methylnaltrexone, a quaternary derivative of naltrexone, does not cross the blood–brain barrier and can selectively block the peripheral effects of opioids (constipation) without affecting the central effects such as analgesia. This drug may also be useful for other opioid-induced peripheral side effects such as pruritus (62).

Ketamine

Ketamine is a phencyclidine derivative that was introduced with great fanfare as a "foolproof" method of providing anesthesia and analgesia to adults and children in the early 1970s (258,259). Initially, it was hoped that ketamine would become the "Swiss army knife" of analgesia and anesthesia and that it could be administered by nonanesthesiologists (258). Unfortunately, this, like many other claims about new drugs, turned out to be more wishful thinking than any resemblance to truth. Nevertheless, ketamine is an outstanding sedative, amnestic, and analgesic that is particularly useful in the treatment of procedure-related pain (e.g., catheterization, tracheal intubation, chest tube insertion, lumbar puncture, fracture reduction, dental work) and as an agent to induce anesthesia in patients with congenital heart disease, particularly those with right-to-left shunts (259–262). It is a potent analgesic even at subanesthetic plasma concentrations, and its analgesic and anesthetic effects may be mediated by different mechanisms. It is also an outstanding anesthetic agent in critically ill patients because it produces its effects with minimal perturbations of the cardiovascular and respiratory systems. It increasingly is being used in emergency departments, intensive care units, and procedure facilities for painful procedures (259,262).

When administered intravenously, 1 to 2 mg/kg ketamine rapidly (30 seconds) produces a state of general anesthesia, with a loss of consciousness and transient period of apnea that may last as long as 1 to 2 minutes. It maintains a period of unconsciousness, amnesia, and analgesia that may last for as long as 2 hours. The resulting anesthetic state is distinctly unusual in that patients appear awake, although they are unconscious. Loss of consciousness is heralded by the appearance of vertical or horizontal nystagmus. Patients become cataleptic with their eyes open in a fixed gaze and with their corneal and papillary reactions intact. Furthermore, depending on dose and route of administration, patients may continue to verbalize and respond to external stimuli. However, they often cannot connect or associate the stimulus actually being applied to their internal perceptions of what is happening. For example, a patient who has received ketamine for a kidney biopsy may complain during the insertion of the biopsy needle that his leg hurts or that he is hungry. Because of this, the anesthesia produced by ketamine is often called *dissociative anesthesia*. The mechanism by which ketamine anesthesia occurs is unknown, although recent investigations suggest that the mechanism of action is antagonism of NMDA, an excitatory amine at its receptor (263). The NMDA receptor may also represent a subgroup of the σ opiate receptor that blocks spinal nociceptive reflexes. Ketamine's affinity for opioid receptors is controversial but provides an attractive theory for its analgesic properties at central and spinal sites. Several animal studies have demonstrated cross-tolerance between the opiates and ketamine. This would be expected if there is a common receptor. Conversely, naloxone, an opioid receptor antagonist, does not reverse ketamine's analgesic properties. Ketamine also interacts with muscarinic cholinergic receptors within the central nervous system by decreasing the average lifetime of single channel currents activated by acetylcholine. Thus, centrally acting anticholinesterase agents, such as physostigmine, may antagonize some of ketamine's anesthetic effects.

Ketamine anesthesia has a hallucinatory quality; in fact, patients often describe vivid dreams, auditory and visual illusions, and extracorporeal experiences (a sense of floating outside one's body). These hallucinations may persist for hours or may recur ("flashback"), particularly on the nights (nightmares or night terrors) after ketamine administration. Nightmares are much more common in adults than in children. They have been reported in as many as 10% of adult patients, but in less than 5% of children. Indeed, nightmares and flashbacks are one of the most important reasons that ketamine's clinical use has been limited. Fortunately, the incidence of night terrors can be reduced or eliminated by the concomitant administration of virtually any benzodiazepine.

Ketamine is contraindicated in patients with increased intracranial pressure because it significantly increases cerebral blood flow and blood volume (264,265). Most anesthetic agents, such as the barbiturates, produce unconsciousness and thereby decrease the cerebral metabolic rate. This has the effect of reducing cerebral oxygen consumption, cerebral blood flow, and cerebral blood volume. This decrease in cerebral blood flow and volume decreases intracranial pressure, particularly in injured brains in which intracranial compliance is reduced. Ketamine, in contrast, is an excitatory hallucinogen that produces a coupled increase in both cerebral metabolism and blood flow. This has the effect of increasing intracranial pressure. Obviously, this may be catastrophic in patients with poor intracranial compliance. Additionally, ketamine depresses ventilation and may thereby cause an increase in arterial carbon dioxide concentrations (266,267). This further exacerbates ketamine's effects on intracranial pressure because hypercarbia is one of the most potent stimuli to raise cerebral blood flow and intracranial pressure.

Regardless of its route of administration, ketamine significantly increases mean arterial blood pressure, heart rate, and cardiac output and is therefore commonly used in patients who are in shock or who are cardiovascularly unstable. At first glance, this is surprising, because ketamine is a negative inotrope. However, its negative inotropy is more than counterbalanced by the fact that ketamine administration is associated with dramatic increases in sympathetic outflow and plasma catecholamine levels. The increase in plasma catecholamines that accompanies its administration accounts for ketamine's ability to raise blood pressure and cardiac output. This also means that if a patient is catecholamine depleted or blocked, ketamine administration may result in profound hypotension and even death.

Ketamine's effects on pulmonary vascular resistance are controversial (268,269). Morray et al. (260) demonstrated in spontaneously breathing children undergoing cardiac catheterization a significant rise in pulmonary vascular resistance after ketamine administration. Conversely, Hickey et al. (268) found no change in pulmonary vascular resistance after intravenous administration of 2 mg/kg ketamine in 14 children who had undergone cardiac surgery. These latter investigators concluded that cardiovascular hemodynamics, especially the pulmonary vascular resistance index, are minimally affected by ketamine in mildly sedated infants with congenital heart disease (268). This was true regardless of baseline pulmonary vascular resistance index, as long as the airway was patent and ventilation was normal. Furthermore, these investigators believed that partial airway obstruction, hypoventilation, or possible catecholamine depletion was responsible for the rise in pulmonary vascular resistance that was previously reported with ketamine use. This is further supported by the work of Greeley et al. (270), who demonstrated reversal of a right-to-left shunt during a tetralogy of Fallot episode and an increase in arterial oxygen saturation after ketamine administration.

Ketamine is a ventilatory depressant (266). It reduces the ventilatory response to carbon dioxide administration, although resting respiratory rate, tidal volume, end-tidal carbon dioxide concentration, and minute ventilation are unchanged. In fact, a continuous ketamine infusion of 40 μg/kg/minute has been shown to shift the carbon dioxide response curve to the right, without altering its slope. This perturbation of ventilatory control is most marked in former preterm neonates (271). Welborn et al. (267), studying spinal anesthesia in premature neonates who were younger than 51 weeks postconceptional age, found that a sedating dose of 1 to 2 mg/kg ketamine given intramuscularly led to prolonged apnea and bradycardia in eight of nine of infants studied (89%). None of the 11 infants receiving spinal anesthesia without sedation experienced similar problems (267).

Laryngeal reflexes remain relatively intact during ketamine anesthesia, but airway protection should not be presumed unless the airway is secured with an endotracheal tube. There are many reports in the literature of patients aspirating after ketamine administration, which should not be at all surprising. Any anesthetic agent that induces unconsciousness should be presumed to result in pulmonary aspiration of stomach contents when consciousness is lost. Patients should have no solid foods by mouth for at least 8 hours before ketamine administration and if this is not possible, "full-stomach" precautions (i.e., cricoid pressure, rapid-acting paralytics, tracheal intubation) should always be taken.

Ketamine is a potent bronchial smooth muscle relaxant, making it the ideal anesthetic and analgesic agent in patients with asthma. It increases pulmonary compliance both by direct action on the bronchial smooth muscles and by its ability to increase plasma catecholamine levels. In the rare event that asthmatics require intubation, ketamine is the best agent to use to induce anesthesia and to maintain sedation while the patient is being ventilated. Additionally, low doses may be used when invasive, painful procedures, such as arterial catheterization, must be performed in asthmatics in whom reason and distraction techniques fail.

Finally, ketamine increases salivary and bronchial mucous gland secretions, possibly through central cholinergic receptor stimulation. We have seen patients literally drown in their secretions and obstruct their airways after ketamine administration. We therefore recommend that whenever ketamine is given, a potent antisialogogue, such as 0.02 mg/kg atropine or 0.01 mg/kg glycopyrrolate be given concomitantly.

Pharmacokinetics

Ketamine is highly lipid soluble and, after a single intravenous bolus, swiftly crosses the blood–brain barrier to rapidly produce a loss of consciousness. Its uptake, distribution, and elimination from the body are remarkably similar to those of thiopental (272–274). Redistribution, rather than biotransformation and elimination, is responsible for ketamine's short duration of action. Its $t_{1/2}\alpha$ is only 11 to 16 minutes and its elimination half-life is 2.5 to 3 hours. Its 2- to 3-hour elimination half-life may explain why protracted emergence from ketamine anesthesia may occur.

Ketamine is *N*-demethylated by the liver's microsomal enzyme system (cytochrome P-450) to norketamine. This is followed by hydroxylation and conjugation to a glucuronide, which is a nonactive, water-soluble metabolite. Clearance is high at 20 mL/kg per minute and closely approximates total liver blood flow, giving ketamine a short elimination half-life of approximately 2 to 3 hours (Table 12.6). Reduction in liver blood flow by drugs such as cimetidine or by immaturity or intra-abdominal pathology may significantly prolong ketamine's terminal half-life of elimination ($t_{1/2}\beta$) and therefore its effects.

Dosage and Route of Administration

Ketamine is effective whether administered intravenously or intramuscularly (275–277). Enteral absorption after oral, rectal, or transmucosal administration has been both safe and effective (278,279). When administered in small doses (0.25 to 1.0 mg/kg intravenously or 3 to 5 mg/kg intramuscularly), ketamine provides very adequate sedation and analgesia for short painful procedures such as dressing changes in burn patients, fracture reductions, central line placement. This dose does not completely ablate unconsciousness and can be considered a "stun" dose. When administered intravenously in higher doses (2 to 4 mg/kg), it will induce general anesthesia and a complete loss of consciousness within 60 seconds of administration. Thus, ketamine is particularly useful when intubating asthmatics, children with congenital heart disease, and after trauma. Obviously, the dose of ketamine should be reduced in the presence of hypovolemia or catecholamine exhaustion.

Regardless of how it is administered or for what purpose, we strongly recommend that a benzodiazepine (0.05 mg/kg midazolam intravenously or 0.01 mg/kg intramuscularly) and an antisialagogue (0.02 mg/kg atropine intravenously or intramuscularly) be administered concomitantly. This is necessary to reduce the incidence of emergence delirium, nightmares, and increased salivation that are associated with ketamine use.

Ketamine may also be administered by continuous infusion in subanesthetic doses to provide continuous analgesia and sedation (280–282). In one study, five children were given ketamine via a bolus dose of 0.5 to 1.0 mg/kg followed by a continuous infusion of 10 to 15 μg/kg per minute for as long as 4 days (282). This provided very effective sedation and analgesia and suggests its possible use in asthmatics and children with complex congenital heart disease. The common adverse effects of hypersalivation and emergence delirium and night terrors can be prevented by the concomitant use of antisialogogues and benzodiazepines.

Tramadol

Tramadol, a synthetic 4-phenyl-piperidine analog of codeine, is a centrally acting synthetic analgesic that has been used for years in Europe and was approved by the FDA for adult use in the United States in 1995 (46,283). It is a racemic mixture of two enantiomers, (+)-tramadol and (−)-tramadol (46,284). The (+)-enantiomer has a moderate affinity for the μ opioid receptor, greater than that of the (−)-enantiomer. In addition, the (+)-enantiomer inhibits serotonin uptake, and the (−)-enantiomer blocks the reuptake of norepinephrine, complementary properties that result in a synergistic antinociceptive interaction between the two enantiomers. Tramadol may also produce analgesia as an α_2 agonist (285). A metabolite (O-desmethyltramadol) binds to opioid receptors with a greater affinity than the parent compound and could contribute to tramadol's analgesic effects as well. However, in most animal tests and human clinical trials, the analgesic effect of tramadol is only partially blocked by the opioid antagonist naloxone, suggesting an important nonopioid mechanism. Thus, tramadol provides analgesia synergistically by opioid (direct binding to the μ opioid receptor by the parent compound and its metabolite) and nonopioid mechanisms (an increase in central neuronal synaptic levels of two neurotransmitters, serotonin and norepinephrine). Finally, animal and human studies have suggested that tramadol may have a selective spinal action. Tramadol has been shown to provide effective, long-lasting analgesia after extradural administration in both adults and children and prolongs the duration of action of local anesthetics when used for brachial plexus and epidural blockade (286,287).

Tramadol's intravenous analgesic effect has been reported to be ten to 15 times less than that of morphine, with a more favorable side-effect profile (46,288). Unlike nonsteroidal anti-inflammatory drugs and opioid mixed agonist–antagonists (e.g., butorphanol, nalbuphine), the therapeutic use of tramadol has not been associated with clinically important side effects such as respiratory depression, constipation, and sedation. In addition, analgesic tolerance has not been a serious problem during repeated administration, and neither psychologic dependence nor euphoric effects are observed in long-term clinical trials. Thus, tramadol may offer significant advantages in the management of pain in children by virtue of its dual mechanism of action, its lack of a ceiling effect, and its minimal respiratory depression.

REFERENCES

1. Hamilton GR, Baskett TF. In the arms of Morpheus: the development of morphine for postoperative pain relief. *Can J Anaesth* 2000;47:367–374.
2. Reisine T, Pasternak G. Opioid analgesics and antagonists. In: Hardman JG, Limbird LE, eds. Goodman and Gilman's the pharmacologic basis of therapeutics. New York: McGraw-Hill, 1996:521–555.
3. Yaster M, Deshpande JK. Management of pediatric pain with opioid analgesics. *J Pediatr* 1988;113: 421–429.
4. Berde CB. Pediatric postoperative pain management. *Pediatr Clin North Am* 1989;36:921–940.
5. Mather LE, Cousins MJ. Pharmacology of opioids. Part 2. Clinical aspects. *Med J Aust* 1986;144: 475–481.
6. Stoelting RK. Opioid agonists and antagonists. In: Stoelting RK, ed. *Pharmacology and physiology in anesthetic practice*. Philadelphia: Lippincott–Raven, 1999:77–112.
7. Pasternak GW. Pharmacological mechanisms of opioid analgesics. *Clin Neuropharmacol* 1993;16:1–18.
8. Standifer KM, Pasternak GW. G proteins and opioid receptor-mediated signalling. *Cell Signal* 1997;9: 237–248.
9. Nagasaka H, Awad H, Yaksh TL. Peripheral and spinal actions of opioids in the blockade of the autonomic response evoked by compression of the inflamed knee joint. *Anesthesiology* 1996;85:808–816.
10. Satoh M, Minami M. Molecular pharmacology of the opioid receptors. *Pharmacol Ther* 1995;68:343–364.
11. Harrison LM, Kastin AJ, Zadina JE. Opiate tolerance and dependence: receptors, G-proteins, and antiopiates. *Peptides* 1998;19:1603–1630.
12. Sabbe MB, Yaksh TL. Pharmacology of spinal opioids. *J Pain Symptom Manage* 1990;5:191–203.
13. Mestek A, Chen Y, Yu L. Mu opioid receptors: cellular action and tolerance development. *NIDA Res Monogr* 1996;161:104–126.
14. Chen Y, Mestek A, Liu J, et al. Molecular cloning and functional expression of a mu-opioid receptor from rat brain. *Mol Pharmacol* 1993;44:8–12.
15. Raynor K, Kong H, Chen Y, et al. Pharmacological characterization of the cloned kappa-, delta-, and mu-opioid receptors. *Mol Pharmacol* 1994;45:330–334.
16. Yasuda K, Raynor K, Kong H, et al. Cloning and functional comparison of kappa and delta opioid receptors from mouse brain. *Proc Natl Acad Sci U S A* 1993; 90:6736–6740.
17. Callahan P, Pasternak GW. Opiate receptor multiplicity: evidence for multiple mu receptors. *Monogr Neural Sci* 1987;13:121–131.
18. Traynor JR, Elliott J. Delta-opioid receptor subtypes

and cross-talk with mu-receptors. *Trends Pharmacol Sci* 1993;14:84–86.
19. Knapp RJ, Malatynska E, Collins N, et al. Molecular biology and pharmacology of cloned opioid receptors. *FASEB J* 1995;9:516–525.
20. Pasternak GW. Multiple morphine and enkephalin receptors and the relief of pain. *JAMA* 1988;259: 1362–1367.
21. Millan MJ. Multiple opioid systems and pain. *Pain* 1986;27:303–347.
22. Lord JA, Waterfield AA, Hughes J, et al. Endogenous opioid peptides: multiple agonists and receptors. *Nature* 1977;267:495–499.
23. Wood PL. The significance of multiple CNS opioid receptor types: a review of critical considerations relating to technical details and anatomy in the study of central opioid actions. *Peptides* 1988;9[Suppl 1]:49–55.
24. Wood PL. Multiple opiate receptors: support for unique mu, delta and kappa sites. *Neuropharmacology* 1982;21:487–497.
25. Snyder SH. Drug and neurotransmitter receptors in the brain. *Science* 1984;224:22–31.
26. Zhang AZ, Pasternak GW. Ontogeny of opioid pharmacology and receptors: high and low affinity site differences. *Eur J Pharmacol* 1981;73:29–40.
27. Pasternak GW, Zhang A, Tecott L. Developmental differences between high and low affinity opiate binding sites: their relationship to analgesia and respiratory depression. *Life Sci*1980;27:1185–1190.
28. Pasternak GW, Wood PJ. Multiple mu opiate receptors. *Life Sci* 1986;38:1889–1898.
29. Fowler CJ, Fraser GL. Mu-, delta-, kappa-opioid receptors and their subtypes. A critical review with emphasis on radioligand binding experiments. *Neurochem Int* 1994;24:401–426.
30. Thornton SR, Compton DR, Smith FL. Ontogeny of mu opioid agonist anti-nociception in postnatal rats. *Brain Res Dev Brain Res* 1998;105:269–276.
31. Crain SM, Shen KF. Modulation of opioid analgesia, tolerance and dependence by Gs-coupled, GM1 ganglioside-regulated opioid receptor functions. *Trends Pharmacol Sci* 1998;19:358–365.
32. Crain SM, Shen KF. Modulatory effects of Gs-coupled excitatory opioid receptor functions on opioid analgesia, tolerance, and dependence. *Neurochem Res* 1996; 21:1347–1351.
33. Vaughan CW, Ingram SL, Connor MA, et al. How opioids inhibit GABA-mediated neurotransmission. *Nature* 1997;390:611–614.
34. Zaki PA, Keith DE Jr, Brine GA, et al. Ligand-induced changes in surface mu-opioid receptor number: relationship to G protein activation? *J Pharmacol Exp Ther* 2000;292:1127–1134.
35. Keith DE, Murray SR, Zaki PA, et al. Morphine activates opioid receptors without causing their rapid internalization. *J Biol Chem* 1996;271:19021–19024.
36. Stein C. Peripheral analgesic actions of opioids. *J Pain Symptom Manage* 1991;6:119–124.
37. Stein C. *Opioids in pain control: basic and clinical aspects*. Cambridge: Cambridge University Press, 1999.
38. Power I, Brown DT, Wildsmith JA. The effect of fentanyl, meperidine and diamorphine on nerve conduction in vitro. *Reg Anesth* 1991;16:204–208.
39. Stein C. The control of pain in peripheral tissue by opioids. *N Engl J Med* 1995;332:1685–1690.
40. Stein C. Peripheral mechanisms of opioid analgesia. Anesth Analg 1993;76:182–191.
41. Fisher K, Coderre TJ, Hagen NA. Targeting the N-methyl-D-aspartate receptor for chronic pain management. Preclinical animal studies, recent clinical experience and future research directions. *J Pain Symptom Manage* 2000;20:358–373.
42. Coderre TJ, Katz J, Vaccarino AL, et al. Contribution of central neuroplasticity to pathological pain: review of clinical and experimental evidence. *Pain* 1993;52: 259–285.
43. Gagnon B, Bruera E. Differences in the ratios of morphine to methadone in patients with neuropathic pain versus non-neuropathic pain. *J Pain Symptom Manage* 1999;18:120–125.
44. Gorman AL, Elliott KJ, Inturrisi CE. The d- and l-isomers of methadone bind to the non-competitive site on the N-methyl-D-aspartate (NMDA) receptor in rat forebrain and spinal cord. *Neurosci Lett* 1997;223:5–8.
45. Ebert B, Thorkildsen C, Andersen S, et al. Opioid analgesics as noncompetitive N-methyl-D-aspartate (NMDA) antagonists. *Biochem Pharmacol* 1998;56: 553–559.
46. Raffa RB. A novel approach to the pharmacology of analgesics. *Am J Med* 1996;101:40S–46S.
47. Meert TF, De Kock M. Potentiation of the analgesic properties of fentanyl-like opioids with alpha 2-adrenoceptor agonists in rats. *Anesthesiology* 1994;81: 677–688.
48. Ossipov MH, Harris S, Lloyd P, et al. An isobolographic analysis of the antinociceptive effect of systemically and intrathecally administered combinations of clonidine and opiates. *J Pharmacol Exp Ther* 1990; 255:1107–1116.
49. Ossipov MH, Lopez Y, Bian D, et al. Synergistic antinociceptive interactions of morphine and clonidine in rats with nerve-ligation injury. *Anesthesiology* 1997; 86:196–204.
50. Yaksh TL, Reddy SV. Studies in the primate on the analgetic effects associated with intrathecal actions of opiates, alpha-adrenergic agonists and baclofen. *Anesthesiology* 1981;54:451–467.
51. Monasky MS, Zinsmeister AR, Stevens CW, et al. Interaction of intrathecal morphine and ST-91 on antinociception in the rat: dose-response analysis, antagonism and clearance. *J Pharmacol Exp Ther* 1990;254: 383–392.
52. Loomis CW, Milne B, Cervenko FW. A study of the interaction between clonidine and morphine on analgesia and blood pressure during continuous intrathecal infusion in the rat. *Neuropharmacology* 1988;27:191–199.
53. Esmail Z, Montgomery C, Courtrn C, et al. Efficacy and complications of morphine infusions in postoperative paediatric patients. *Paediatr Anaesth* 1999;9: 321–327.
54. Lynn AM, Nespeca MK, Opheim KE, et al. Respiratory effects of intravenous morphine infusions in neonates, infants, and children after cardiac surgery. *Anesth Analg* 1993;77:695–701.
55. Lynn AM, Slattery JT. Morphine pharmacokinetics in early infancy. *Anesthesiology* 1987;66:136–139.
56. Koren G, Butt W, Chinyanga H, et al. Postoperative morphine infusion in newborn infants: assessment of disposition characteristics and safety. *J Pediatr* 1985; 107:963–967.

57. Koren G, Butt W, Pape K, et al. Morphine-induced seizures in newborn infants. *Vet Hum Toxicol* 1985; 27:519–520.
58. Nichols DG, Yaster M, Lynn AM, et al. Disposition and respiratory effects of intrathecal morphine in children. *Anesthesiology* 1993;79:733–738; discussion 25A.
59. Yaster M, Nichols DG, Deshpande JK, et al. Midazolam-fentanyl intravenous sedation in children: case report of respiratory arrest. *Pediatrics* 1990;86:463–467.
60. Yuan CS, Foss JF. Antagonism of gastrointestinal opioid effects. *Reg Anesth Pain Med* 2000;25:639–642.
61. Yuan CS, Foss JF, O'Connor M, et al. Methylnaltrexone for reversal of constipation due to chronic methadone use: a randomized controlled trial. *JAMA* 2000;283:367–372.
62. Yuan CS, Foss JF, O'Connor M, et al. Efficacy of orally administered methylnaltrexone in decreasing subjective effects after intravenous morphine. *Drug Alcohol Depend* 1998;52:161–165.
63. Watcha MF, White PF. Postoperative nausea and vomiting. Its etiology, treatment, and prevention. *Anesthesiology* 1992;77:162–184.
64. Jinks SL, Carstens E. Superficial dorsal horn neurons identified by intracutaneous histamine: chemonociceptive responses and modulation by morphine. *J Neurophysiol* 2000;84:616–627.
65. Kuraishi Y, Yamaguchi T, Miyamoto T. Itch-scratch responses induced by opioids through central mu opioid receptors in mice. *J Biomed Sci* 2000;7:248–252.
66. Gunter JB, McAuliffe J, Gregg T, et al. Continuous epidural butorphanol relieves pruritus associated with epidural morphine infusions in children. *Paediatr Anaesth* 2000;10:167–172.
67. Joshi GP, Duffy L, Chehade J, et al. Effects of prophylactic nalmefene on the incidence of morphine-related side effects in patients receiving intravenous patient-controlled analgesia. *Anesthesiology* 1999;90: 1007–1011.
68. Gan TJ, Ginsberg B, Glass PS, et al. Opioid-sparing effects of a low-dose infusion of naloxone in patient-administered morphine sulfate. *Anesthesiology* 1997;87: 1075–1081.
69. Bergasa NV, Alling DW, Talbot TL, et al. Effects of naloxone infusions in patients with the pruritus of cholestasis. A double-blind, randomized, controlled trial. *Ann Intern Med* 1995;123:161–167.
70. Stefano GB, Salzet B, Fricchione GL. Enkelytin and opioid peptide association in invertebrates and vertebrates: immune activation and pain. *Immunol Today* 1998;19:265–268.
71. Metz-Boutigue MH, Goumon Y, Lugardon K, et al. Antibacterial peptides are present in chromaffin cell secretory granules. *Cell Mol Neurobiol* 1998;18: 249–266.
72. Strub JM, Goumon Y, Lugardon K, et al. Antibacterial activity of glycosylated and phosphorylated chromogranin A-derived peptide 173-194 from bovine adrenal medullary chromaffin granules. *J Biol Chem* 1996; 271:28533–28540.
73. Carr DJ, Rogers TJ, Weber RJ. The relevance of opioids and opioid receptors on immunocompetence and immune homeostasis. *Proc Soc Exp Biol Med* 1996; 213:248–257.
74. Cabot PJ, Carter L, Gaiddon C, et al. Immune cell-derived beta-endorphin. Production, release, and control of inflammatory pain in rats. *J Clin Invest* 1997;100: 142–148.
75. Jessop DS. Neuropeptides: modulators of the immune system. *Curr Opin Endocrinol Diabetes* 1998;5:52–58.
76. Di Francesco P, Tavazzi B, Gaziano R, et al. Differential effects of acute morphine administrations on polymorphonuclear cell metabolism in various mouse strains. *Life Sci* 1998;63:2167–2174.
77. Di Francesco P, Gaziano R, Casalinuovo IA, et al. Antifungal and immunoadjuvant properties of fluconazole in mice immunosuppressed with morphine. *Chemotherapy* 1997;43:198–203.
78. Yeager MP, Colacchio TA, Yu CT, et al. Morphine inhibits spontaneous and cytokine-enhanced natural killer cell cytotoxicity in volunteers. *Anesthesiology* 1995;83:500–508.
79. Arnold JH, Truog RD, Scavone JM, et al. Changes in the pharmacodynamic response to fentanyl in neonates during continuous infusion. *J Pediatr* 1991;119:639–643.
80. Dagan O, Klein J, Bohn D, et al. Effects of extracorporeal membrane oxygenation on morphine pharmacokinetics in infants. *Crit Care Med* 1994;22: 1099–1101.
81. Franck LS, Vilardi J, Durand D, et al. Opioid withdrawal in neonates after continuous infusions of morphine or fentanyl during extracorporeal membrane oxygenation. *Am J Crit Care* 1998;7:364–369.
82. Geiduschek JM, Lynn AM, Bratton SL, et al. Morphine pharmacokinetics during continuous infusion of morphine sulfate for infants receiving extracorporeal membrane oxygenation. *Crit Care Med* 1997;25: 360–364.
83. Paronis CA, Holtzman SG. Development of tolerance to the analgesic activity of mu agonists after continuous infusion of morphine, meperidine or fentanyl in rats. *J Pharmacol Exp Ther* 1992;262:1–9.
84. Sosnowski M, Yaksh TL. Differential cross-tolerance between intrathecal morphine and sufentanil in the rat. *Anesthesiology* 1990;73:1141–1147.
85. Duttaroy A, Yoburn BC. The effect of intrinsic efficacy on opioid tolerance. *Anesthesiology* 1995;82: 1226–1236.
86. Suresh S, Anand KJ. Opioid tolerance in neonates: mechanisms, diagnosis, assessment, and management. *Semin Perinatol* 1998;22:425–433.
87. Nestler EJ, Aghajanian GK. Molecular and cellular basis of addiction. *Science* 1997;278:58–63.
88. Nestler EJ. Under siege: the brain on opiates. *Neuron* 1996;16:897–900.
89. Bohn LM, Gainetdinov RR, Lin FT, et al. Mu-opioid receptor desensitization by beta-arrestin-2 determines morphine tolerance but not dependence. *Nature* 2000; 408:720–723.
90. Ferguson SS, Barak LS, Zhang J, et al. G-protein-coupled receptor regulation: role of G-protein-coupled receptor kinases and arrestins. *Can J Physiol Pharmacol* 1996;74:1095–1110.
91. Pitcher JA, Freedman NJ, Lefkowitz RJ. G protein-coupled receptor kinases. *Annu Rev Biochem* 1998;67: 653–692.
92. Trujillo KA. Effects of noncompetitive N-methyl-D-aspartate receptor antagonists on opiate tolerance and physical dependence. *Neuropsychopharmacology* 1995; 13:301–307.
93. Trujillo KA, Akil H. Inhibition of morphine tolerance

and dependence by the NMDA receptor antagonist MK-801. *Science* 1991;251:85–87.
94. Suresh S, Anand KJ. Opioid tolerance in neonates: mechanisms, diagnosis, assessment, and management. *Semin Perinatol* 1998;22:425–433.
95. Yaksh TL, Al Rodhan NR, Jensen TS. Sites of action of opiates in production of analgesia. *Prog Brain Res* 1988;77:371–394.
96. Yaksh TL. New horizons in our understanding of the spinal physiology and pharmacology of pain processing. *Semin Oncol* 1993;20[Suppl 1]:6–18.
97. Greene RF, Miser AW, Lester CM, et al. Cerebrospinal fluid and plasma pharmacokinetics of morphine infusions in pediatric cancer patients and rhesus monkeys. *Pain* 1987;30:339–348.
98. Plummer JL, Cmielewski PL, Reynolds GD, et al. Influence of polarity on dose-response relationships of intrathecal opioids in rats. *Pain* 1990;40:339–347.
99. Gourlay GK, Cherry DA, Plummer JL, et al. The influence of drug polarity on the absorption of opioid drugs into CSF and subsequent cephalad migration following lumbar epidural administration: application to morphine and pethidine. *Pain* 1987;31:297–305.
100. Gourlay GK, Cherry DA, Cousins MJ. Cephalad migration of morphine in CSF following lumbar epidural administration in patients with cancer pain. *Pain* 1985; 23:317–326.
101. Gourlay GK, Murphy TM, Plummer JL, et al. Pharmacokinetics of fentanyl in lumbar and cervical CSF following lumbar epidural and intravenous administration. *Pain* 1989;38:253–259.
102. Way WL, Costley EC, Way EL. Respiratory sensitivity of the newborn infant to meperidine and morphine. *Clin Pharmacol Ther* 1965;6:454–461.
103. Bragg P, Zwass MS, Lau M, et al. Opioid pharmacodynamics in neonatal dogs: differences between morphine and fentanyl. *J Appl Physiol* 1995;79:1519–1524.
104. Yaksh TL. Pharmacology and mechanisms of opioid analgesic activity. *Acta Anaesthesiol Scand* 1997;41: 94–111.
105. Etches RC, Sandler AN, Daley MD. Respiratory depression and spinal opioids. *Can J Anaesth* 1989;36: 165–185.
106. Cousins MJ, Mather LE. Intrathecal and epidural administration of opioids. *Anesthesiology* 1984;61: 276–310.
107. Yaksh TL. The spinal pharmacology of acutely and chronically administered opioids. *J Pain Symptom Manage* 1992;7:356–361.
108. Minto CF, Schnider TW, Shafer SL. Pharmacokinetics and pharmacodynamics of remifentanil. II. Model application. *Anesthesiology* 1997;86:24–33.
109. Minto CF, Schnider TW, Egan TD, et al. Influence of age and gender on the pharmacokinetics and pharmacodynamics of remifentanil. I. Model development. *Anesthesiology* 1997;86:10–23.
110. Burkle H, Dunbar S, Van Aken H. Remifentanil: a novel, short-acting, mu-opioid. *Anesth Analg* 1996;83: 646–651.
111. Tateishi T, Nakura H, Asoh M, et al. A comparison of hepatic cytochrome P450 protein expression between infancy and postinfancy. *Life Sci* 1997;61:2567–2574.
112. Hakkola J, Tanaka E, Pelkonen O. Developmental expression of cytochrome P450 enzymes in human liver. *Pharmacol Toxicol* 1998;82:209–217.
113. Greeley WJ, de Bruijn NP. Changes in sufentanil pharmacokinetics within the neonatal period. *Anesth Analg* 1988;67:86–90.
114. Plummer JL, Gourlay GK, Cmielewski PL, et al. Behavioural effects of norpethidine, a metabolite of pethidine, in rats. *Toxicology* 1995;95:37–44.
115. Szeto HH, Inturrisi CE, Houde R, et al. Accumulation of normeperidine, an active metabolite of meperidine, in patients with renal failure of cancer. *Ann Intern Med* 1977;86:738–741.
116. Tegeder I, Lotsch J, Geisslinger G. Pharmacokinetics of opioids in liver disease. *Clin Pharmacokinet* 1999; 37:17–40.
117. McRorie TI, Lynn AM, Nespeca MK, et al. The maturation of morphine clearance and metabolism. *Am J Dis Child* 1992;146:972–976.
118. Haberkern CM, Lynn AM, Geiduschek JM, et al. Epidural and intravenous bolus morphine for postoperative analgesia in infants. *Can J Anaesth* 1996;43: 1203–1210.
119. Dahlstrom B, Tamsen A, Paalzow L, et al. Patient-controlled analgesic therapy, Part IV: pharmacokinetics and analgesic plasma concentrations of morphine. *Clin Pharmacokinet* 1982;7:266–279.
120. Bhat R, Chari G, Gulati A, et al. Pharmacokinetics of a single dose of morphine in preterm infants during the first week of life. *J Pediatr* 1990;117:477–481.
121. Kupferberg HJ, Way EL. Pharmacologic basis for the increased sensitivity of the newborn rat to morphine. *J Pharmacol Exp Ther* 1963;141:105–109.
122. Dagan O, Klein J, Bohn D, et al. Morphine pharmacokinetics in children following cardiac surgery: effects of disease and inotropic support. *J Cardiothorac Vasc Anesth* 1993;7:396–398.
123. Lynn AM, Opheim KE, Tyler DC. Morphine infusion after pediatric cardiac surgery. *Crit Care Med* 1984; 12:863–866.
124. Martin RJ, DiFiore JM, Jana L, et al. Persistence of the biphasic ventilatory response to hypoxia in preterm infants. *J Pediatr* 1998;132:960–964.
125. Martin RJ, DiFiore JM, Korenke CB, et al. Vulnerability of respiratory control in healthy preterm infants placed supine. *J Pediatr* 1995;127:609–614.
126. Cohen G, Malcolm G, Henderson-Smart D. Ventilatory response of the newborn infant to mild hypoxia. *Pediatr Pulmonol* 1997;24:163–172.
127. Moss TJ, Jakubowska AE, McCrabb GJ, et al. Ventilatory responses to progressive hypoxia and hypercapnia in developing sheep. *Respir Physiol* 1995;100:33–44.
128. Golianu B, Krane EJ, Galloway KS, et al. Pediatric acute pain management. *Pediatr Clin North Am* 2000; 47:559–587.
129. Berde CB, Lehn BM, Yee JD, et al. Patient-controlled analgesia in children and adolescents: a randomized, prospective comparison with intramuscular administration of morphine for postoperative analgesia. *J Pediatr* 1991;118:460–466.
130. Collins JJ, Geake J, Grier HE, et al. Patient-controlled analgesia for mucositis pain in children: a three- period crossover study comparing morphine and hydromorphone. *J Pediatr* 1996;129:722–728.
131. Mackie AM, Coda BC, Hill HF. Adolescents use patient-controlled analgesia effectively for relief from prolonged oropharyngeal mucositis pain. *Pain* 1991; 46:265–269.

132. McNeely JK, Trentadue NC. Comparison of patient-controlled analgesia with and without nighttime morphine infusion following lower extremity surgery in children. *J Pain Symptom Manage* 1997;13:268–273.
133. Yaster M, Billett C, Monitto C. Intravenous patient controlled analgesia. In: Yaster M, Krane EJ, Kaplan RF, et al., eds. *Pediatric pain management and sedation handbook*. St. Louis: Mosby Year Book, 1997:89–112.
134. Monitto CL, Greenberg RS, Kost-Byerly S, et al. The safety and efficacy of parent-/nurse-controlled analgesia in patients less than six years of age. *Anesth Analg* 2000;91:573–579.
135. Gourlay GK, Wilson PR, Glynn CJ. Methadone produces prolonged postoperative analgesia. *BMJ* 1982;284:630–631.
136. Gourlay GK, Wilson PR, Glynn CJ. Pharmacodynamics and pharmacokinetics of methadone during the perioperative period. *Anesthesiology* 1982;57:458–467.
137. Gourlay GK, Willis RJ, Wilson PR. Postoperative pain control with methadone: influence of supplementary methadone doses and blood concentration–response relationships. *Anesthesiology* 1984;61:19–26.
138. Gourlay GK, Willis RJ, Lamberty J. A double-blind comparison of the efficacy of methadone and morphine in postoperative pain control. *Anesthesiology* 1986;64:322–327.
139. Berde CB, Beyer JE, Bournaki MC, et al. Comparison of morphine and methadone for prevention of postoperative pain in 3- to 7-year-old children. *J Pediatr* 1991;119:136–141.
140. Gourlay GK, Cherry DA, Cousins MJ. A comparative study of the efficacy and pharmacokinetics of oral methadone and morphine in the treatment of severe pain in patients with cancer. *Pain* 1986;25:297–312.
141. Gourlay GK, Plummer JL, Cherry DA, et al. Influence of a high-fat meal on the absorption of morphine from oral solutions. *Clin Pharmacol Ther* 1989;46:463–468.
142. Gourlay GK. Sustained relief of chronic pain. Pharmacokinetics of sustained release morphine. *Clin Pharmacokinet* 1998;35:173–190.
143. Lundeberg S, Beck O, Olsson GL, et al. Rectal administration of morphine in children. Pharmacokinetic evaluation after a single-dose. *Acta Anaesthesiol Scand* 1996;40:445–451.
144. Glass PS. Remifentanil: a new opioid. *J Clin Anesth* 1995;7:558–563.
145. Glass PS, Gan TJ, Howell S. A review of the pharmacokinetics and pharmacodynamics of remifentanil. *Anesth Analg* 1999;89[Suppl 4]:S7–S14.
146. Hughes MA, Glass PS, Jacobs JR. Context-sensitive half-time in multicompartment pharmacokinetic models for intravenous anesthetic drugs. *Anesthesiology* 1992;76:334–341.
147. Scholz J, Steinfath M, Schulz M. Clinical pharmacokinetics of alfentanil, fentanyl and sufentanil. An update. *Clin Pharmacokinet* 1996;31:275–292.
148. Santeiro ML, Christie J, Stromquist C, et al. Pharmacokinetics of continuous infusion fentanyl in newborns. *J Perinatol* 1997;17:135–139.
149. Koehntop DE, Rodman JH, Brundage DM, et al. Pharmacokinetics of fentanyl in neonates. *Anesth Analg* 1986;65:227–232.
150. Hertzka RE, Gauntlett IS, Fisher DM, et al. Fentanyl-induced ventilatory depression: effects of age. *Anesthesiology* 1989;70:213–218.
151. Gauntlett IS, Fisher DM, Hertzka RE, et al. Pharmacokinetics of fentanyl in neonatal humans and lambs: effects of age. *Anesthesiology* 1988;69:683–687.
152. Kuhls E, Gauntlett IS, Lau M, et al. Effect of increased intra-abdominal pressure on hepatic extraction and clearance of fentanyl in neonatal lambs. *J Pharmacol Exp Ther* 1995;274:115–119.
153. Yaster M, Scherer TL, Stone MM, et al. Prediction of successful primary closure of congenital abdominal wall defects using intraoperative measurements. *J Pediatr Surg* 1989;24:1217–1220.
154. Masey SA, Koehler RC, Buck JR, et al. Effect of abdominal distension on central and regional hemodynamics in neonatal lambs. *Pediatr Res* 1985;19:1244–1249.
155. Yaster M, Buck JR, Dudgeon DL, et al. Hemodynamic effects of primary closure of omphalocele/gastroschisis in human newborns. *Anesthesiology* 1988;69:84–88.
156. Wilson AS, Stiller RL, Davis PJ, et al. Fentanyl and alfentanil plasma protein binding in preterm and term neonates. *Anesth Analg* 1997;84:315–318.
157. Wood M. Plasma drug binding: implications for anesthesiologists. *Anesth Analg* 1986;65:786–804.
158. Singleton MA, Rosen JI, Fisher DM. Plasma concentrations of fentanyl in infants, children and adults. *Can J Anaesth* 1987;34:152–155.
159. Koehntop DE, Rodman JH, Brundage DM, et al. Pharmacokinetics of fentanyl in neonates. *Anesth Analg* 1986;65:227–232.
160. Murphy MR, Hug CC Jr, McClain DA. Dose-independent pharmacokinetics of fentanyl. *Anesthesiology* 1983;59:537–540.
161. McClain DA, Hug CC Jr. Intravenous fentanyl kinetics. *Clin Pharmacol Ther* 1980;28:106–114.
162. Gourlay GK, Kowalski SR, Plummer JL, et al. Fentanyl blood concentration-analgesic response relationship in the treatment of postoperative pain. *Anesth Analg* 1988;67:329–337.
163. Glass PS, Estok P, Ginsberg B, et al. Use of patient-controlled analgesia to compare the efficacy of epidural to intravenous fentanyl administration. *Anesth Analg* 1992;74:345–351.
164. Gronert BJ, Davis PJ, Cook DR. Continuous infusions of alfentanil in infants undergoing inguinal herniorrhaphy. *Paediatr Anaesth* 1992;2:105–109.
165. Davis PJ, Killian A, Stiller RL, et al. Pharmacokinetics of alfentanil in newborn premature infants and older children. *Dev Pharmacol Ther* 1989;13:21–27.
166. Kapila A, Glass PS, Jacobs JR, et al. Measured context-sensitive half-times of remifentanil and alfentanil. *Anesthesiology* 1995;83:968–975.
167. Robinson S, Gregory GA. Fentanyl-air-oxygen anesthesia for ligation of patent ductus arteriosus in preterm infants. *Anesth Analg* 1981;60:331–334.
168. Yaster M. The dose response of fentanyl in neonatal anesthesia. *Anesthesiology* 1987;66:433–435.
169. Henderson JM, Brodsky DA, Fisher DM, et al. Preinduction of anesthesia in pediatric patients with nasally administered sufentanil. *Anesthesiology* 1988;68:671–675.
170. Stanley TH, Leiman BC, Rawal N, et al. The effects of oral transmucosal fentanyl citrate premedication on preoperative behavioral responses and gastric volume and acidity in children. *Anesth Analg* 1989;69:328–335.
171. Streisand JB, Stanley TH, Hague B, et al. Oral trans-

mucosal fentanyl citrate premedication in children. *Anesth Analg* 1989;69:28–34.
172. Feld LH, Champeau MW, van Steennis CA, et al. Preanesthetic medication in children: a comparison of oral transmucosal fentanyl citrate versus placebo. *Anesthesiology* 1989;71:374–377.
173. Nelson PS, Streisand JB, Mulder SM, et al. Comparison of oral transmucosal fentanyl citrate and an oral solution of meperidine, diazepam, and atropine for premedication in children. *Anesthesiology* 1989;70:616–621.
174. Kurz M, Belani KG, Sessler DI, et al. Naloxone, meperidine, and shivering. *Anesthesiology* 1993;79: 1193–1201.
175. Shannon M, Berde CB. Pharmacologic management of pain in children and adolescents. *Pediatr Clin North Am* 1989;36:855–871.
176. Yaster M, Kost-Byerly S, Berde C, et al. The management of opioid and benzodiazepine dependence in infants, children, and adolescents. *Pediatrics* 1996;98: 135–140.
177. Tobias JD. Tolerance, withdrawal, and physical dependency after long-term sedation and analgesia of children in the pediatric intensive care unit. *Crit Care Med* 2000;28:2122–2132.
178. Ripamonti C, De Conno F, Groff L, et al. Equianalgesic dose/ratio between methadone and other opioid agonists in cancer pain: comparison of two clinical experiences. *Ann Oncol* 1998;9:79–83.
179. Lawlor PG, Turner KS, Hanson J, et al. Dose ratio between morphine and methadone in patients with cancer pain: a retrospective study. *Cancer* 1998;82:1167–1173.
180. Ripamonti C, Groff L, Brunelli C, et al. Switching from morphine to oral methadone in treating cancer pain: what is the equianalgesic dose ratio? *J Clin Oncol* 1998;16:3216–3221.
181. Bruera E, Pereira J, Watanabe S, et al. Opioid rotation in patients with cancer pain. A retrospective comparison of dose ratios between methadone, hydromorphone, and morphine. *Cancer* 1996;78:852–857.
182. Goodarzi M. Comparison of epidural morphine, hydromorphone and fentanyl for postoperative pain control in children undergoing orthopaedic surgery. *Paediatr Anaesth* 1999;9:419–422.
183. Caraco Y, Sheller J, Wood AJ. Impact of ethnic origin and quinidine coadministration on codeine's disposition and pharmacodynamic effects. *J Pharmacol Exp Ther* 1999;290:413–422.
184. Caraco Y, Sheller J, Wood AJ. Pharmacogenetic determination of the effects of codeine and prediction of drug interactions. *J Pharmacol Exp Ther* 1996;278: 1165–1174.
185. Krane EJ, Yaster M. Transition to less invasive therapy. In: Yaster M, Krane EJ, Kaplan RF, et al., eds. *Pediatric pain management and sedation handbook*. St. Louis: Mosby Year Book, 1997:147–162.
186. Heubi JE, Barbacci MB, Zimmerman HJ. Therapeutic misadventures with acetaminophen: hepatotoxicity after multiple doses in children. *J Pediatr* 1998;132:22–27.
187. Kearns GL, Leeder JS, Wasserman GS. Acetaminophen overdose with therapeutic intent. *J Pediatr* 1998;132:5–8.
188. Rivera-Penera T, Gugig R, Davis J, et al. Outcome of acetaminophen overdose in pediatric patients and factors contributing to hepatotoxicity. *J Pediatr* 1997;130: 300–304.
189. Kirvela M, Lindgren L, Seppala T, et al. The pharmacokinetics of oxycodone in uremic patients undergoing renal transplantation. *J Clin Anesth* 1996;8:13–18.
190. Leow KP, Cramond T, Smith MT. Pharmacokinetics and pharmacodynamics of oxycodone when given intravenously and rectally to adult patients with cancer pain. *Anesth Analg* 1995;80:296–302.
191. Morgan D, Cook CD, Smith MA, et al. An examination of the interactions between the antinociceptive effects of morphine and various mu-opioids: the role of intrinsic efficacy and stimulus intensity. *Anesth Analg* 1999;88:407–413.
192. Kalia PK, Madan R, Saksena R, et al. Epidural pentazocine for postoperative pain relief. *Anesth Analg* 1983;62:949–950.
193. Radnay PA, Duncalf D, Novakovic M, et al. Common bile duct pressure changes after fentanyl, morphine, meperidine, butorphanol, and naloxone. *Anesth Analg* 1984;63:441–444.
194. Scott JL, Smith MS, Sanford SM, et al. Effectiveness of transnasal butorphanol for the treatment of musculoskeletal pain. *Am J Emerg Med* 1994;12:469–471.
195. Bennie RE, Boehringer LA, Dierdorf SF, et al. Transnasal butorphanol is effective for postoperative pain relief in children undergoing myringotomy. *Anesthesiology* 1998;89:385–390.
196. Melanson SW, Morse JW, Pronchik DJ, et al. Transnasal butorphanol in the emergency department management of migraine headache. *Am J Emerg Med* 1997;15:57–61.
197. Elenbaas RM, Iacono CU, Koellner KJ, et al. Dose effectiveness and safety of butorphanol in acute migraine headache. *Pharmacotherapy* 1991;11:56–63.
198. Ackerman WE, Juneja MM, Kaczorowski DM, et al. A comparison of the incidence of pruritus following epidural opioid administration in the parturient. *Can J Anaesth* 1989;36:388–391.
199. Roth A, Keren G, Gluck A, et al. Comparison of nalbuphine hydrochloride versus morphine sulfate for acute myocardial infarction with elevated pulmonary artery wedge pressure. *Am J Cardiol* 1988;62: 551–555.
200. Bailey PL, Clark NJ, Pace NL, et al. Antagonism of postoperative opioid-induced respiratory depression: nalbuphine versus naloxone. *Anesth Analg* 1987;66: 1109–1114.
201. Moldenhauer CC, Roach GW, Finlayson DC, et al. Nalbuphine antagonism of ventilatory depression following high-dose fentanyl anesthesia. *Anesthesiology* 1985;62:647–650.
202. Kendrick WD, Woods AM, Daly MY, et al. Naloxone versus nalbuphine infusion for prophylaxis of epidural morphine-induced pruritus. *Anesth Analg* 1996;82: 641–647.
203. Weinbroum AA, Rudick V, Paret G, et al. The role of dextromethorphan in pain control. *Can J Anaesth* 2000;47:585–596.
204. Plesan A, Hoffmann O, Xu XJ, et al. Genetic differences in the antinociceptive effect of morphine and its potentiation by dextromethorphan in rats. *Neurosci Lett* 1999;263:53–56.
205. Katz NP. MorphiDex (MS:DM) double-blind, multiple-dose studies in chronic pain patients. *J Pain Symptom Manage* 2000;19[Suppl 1]:S37–S41.
206. Wiesenfeld-Hallin Z. Combined opioid-NMDA antag-

onist therapies. What advantages do they offer for the control of pain syndromes? *Drugs* 1998;55:1–4.

207. Sang CN. NMDA-receptor antagonists in neuropathic pain: experimental methods to clinical trials. *J Pain Symptom Manage* 2000;19[Suppl 1]:S21–S25.
208. McQuay HJ, Carroll D, Jadad AR, et al. Dextromethorphan for the treatment of neuropathic pain: a double-blind randomised controlled crossover trial with integral n-of-1 design.. *Pain* 1994;59:127–133.
209. Chia YY, Liu K, Chow LH, et al. The preoperative administration of intravenous dextromethorphan reduces postoperative morphine consumption. *Anesth Analg* 1999;89:748–752.
210. Kawamata T, Omote K, Kawamata M, et al. Premedication with oral dextromethorphan reduces postoperative pain after tonsillectomy. *Anesth Analg* 1998;86: 594–597.
211. Rose JB, Cuy R, Cohen DE, et al. Preoperative oral dextromethorphan does not reduce pain or analgesic consumption in children after adenotonsillectomy. *Anesth Analg* 1999;88:749–753.
212. Olkkola KT, Maunuksela EL, Korpela R, et al. Kinetics and dynamics of postoperative intravenous morphine in children. *Clin Pharmacol Ther* 1988;44:128–136.
213. Schechter NL, Berrien FB, Katz SM. The use of patient-controlled analgesia in adolescents with sickle cell pain crisis: a preliminary report. *J Pain Symptom Manage* 1988;3:109–113.
214. Lehmann KA. New developments in patient-controlled postoperative analgesia. *Ann Med* 1995;27:271–282.
215. Doyle E, Robinson D, Morton NS. Comparison of patient-controlled analgesia with and without a background infusion after lower abdominal surgery in children. *Br J Anaesth* 1993;71:670–673.
216. Parker RK, Holtmann B, White PF. Patient-controlled analgesia. Does a concurrent opioid infusion improve pain management after surgery? *JAMA* 1991;266: 1947–1952.
217. Yaksh TL. Opioid receptor systems and the endorphins: a review of their spinal organization. *J Neurosurg* 1987;67:157–176.
218. Yaksh TL. Multiple opioid receptor systems in brain and spinal cord: part 2. *Eur J Anaesthesiol* 1984;1: 201–243.
219. Yaksh TL. Spinal opiate analgesia: characteristics and principles of action. *Pain* 1981;11:293–346.
220. Yaksh TL, Rudy TA. Studies on the direct spinal action of narcotics in the production of analgesia in the rat. *J Pharmacol Exp Ther* 1977;202:411–428.
221. Yaksh TL, Rudy TA. Analgesia mediated by a direct spinal action of narcotics. *Science* 1976;192: 1357–1358.
222. Gourlay GK, Murphy TM, Plummer JL, et al. Pharmacokinetics of fentanyl in lumbar and cervical CSF following lumbar epidural and intravenous administration. *Pain* 1989;38:253–259.
223. Krane EJ, Jacobson LE, Lynn AM, et al. Caudal morphine for postoperative analgesia in children: a comparison with caudal bupivacaine and intravenous morphine. *Anesth Analg* 1987;66:647–653.
224. Krane EJ, Tyler DC, Jacobson LE. The dose response of caudal morphine in children. *Anesthesiology* 1989; 71:48–52.
225. Rasch DK, Webster DE, Pollard TG, et al. Lumbar and thoracic epidural analgesia via the caudal approach for postoperative pain relief in infants and children. *Can J Anaesth* 1990;37:359–362.
226. Dalens B, Tanguy A, Haberer JP. Lumbar epidural anesthesia for operative and postoperative pain relief in infants and young children. *Anesth Analg* 1986;65: 1069–1073.
227. Dalens B, Tanguy A. Intrathecal morphine for spinal fusion in children. *Spine* 1988; 13(5):494–498.
228. Serlin S. Single-dose caudal epidural morphine in children: safe, effective, and easy. *J Clin Anesth* 1991; 3:386–390.
229. Penon C, Negre I, Ecoffey C, et al. Analgesia and ventilatory response to carbon dioxide after intramuscular and epidural alfentanil. *Anesth Analg* 1988;67:313–317.
230. Negre I, Gueneron JP, Jamali SJ, et al. Preoperative analgesia with epidural morphine. *Anesth Analg* 1994; 79:298–302.
231. Benlabed M, Ecoffey C, Levron JC, et al. Analgesia and ventilatory response to C02 following epidural sufentanil in children. *Anesthesiology* 1987;67:948–951.
232. Attia J, Ecoffey C, Sandouk P, et al. Epidural morphine in children: pharmacokinetics and CO2 sensitivity. *Anesthesiology* 1986;65:590–594.
233. Tyler DC, Krane EJ. Epidural opioids in children. *J Pediatr Surg* 1989;24:469–473.
234. Krane EJ. Delayed respiratory depression in a child after caudal epidural morphine. *Anesth Analg* 1988;67: 79–82.
235. Grond S, Radbruch L, Lehmann KA. Clinical pharmacokinetics of transdermal opioids: focus on transdermal fentanyl. *Clin Pharmacokinet* 2000;38:59–89.
236. Schechter NL, Weisman SJ, Rosenblum M, et al. The use of oral transmucosal fentanyl citrate for painful procedures in children. *Pediatrics* 1995;95:335–339.
237. Goldstein-Dresner MC, Davis PJ, Kretchman E, et al. Double-blind comparison of oral transmucosal fentanyl citrate with oral meperidine, diazepam, and atropine as preanesthetic medication in children with congenital heart disease. *Anesthesiology* 1991;74:28–33.
238. Stanley TH, Hague B, Mock DL, et al. Oral transmucosal fentanyl citrate (lollipop) premedication in human volunteers. *Anesth Analg* 1989;69:21–27.
239. Ashburn MA, Lind GH, Gillie MH, et al. Oral transmucosal fentanyl citrate (OTFC) for the treatment of postoperative pain. *Anesth Analg* 1993;76:377–381.
240. Streisand JB, Varvel JR, Stanski DR, et al. Absorption and bioavailability of oral transmucosal fentanyl citrate. *Anesthesiology* 1991;75:223–229.
241. Dsida RM, Wheeler M, Birmingham PK, et al. Premedication of pediatric tonsillectomy patients with oral transmucosal fentanyl citrate. *Anesth Analg* 1998;86:66–70.
242. Portenoy RK, Payne R, Coluzzi P, et al. Oral transmucosal fentanyl citrate (OTFC) for the treatment of breakthrough pain in cancer patients: a controlled dose titration study. *Pain* 1999;79:303–312.
243. Epstein RH, Mendel HG, Witkowski TA, et al. The safety and efficacy of oral transmucosal fentanyl citrate for preoperative sedation in young children. *Anesth Analg* 1996;83:1200–1205.
244. Zedie N, Amory DW, Wagner BK, et al. Comparison of intranasal midazolam and sufentanil premedication in pediatric outpatients. *Clin Pharmacol Ther* 1996;59: 341–348.
245. Karl HW, Keifer AT, Rosenberger JL, et al. Compari-

son of the safety and efficacy of intranasal midazolam or sufentanil for preinduction of anesthesia in pediatric patients. *Anesthesiology* 1992;76:209–215.
246. Chandler S. Nebulized opioids to treat dyspnea. *Am J Hosp Palliat Care* 1999;16:418–422.
247. Bostwick DG, Null WE, Holmes D, et al. Expression of opioid peptides in tumors. *N Engl J Med* 1987;317: 1439–1443.
248. Booth S, Kelly MJ, Cox NP, et al. Does oxygen help dyspnea in patients with cancer? *Am J Respir Crit Care Med* 1996;153:1515–1518.
249. Zempsky WT, Ashburn MA. Iontophoresis: noninvasive drug delivery. *Am J Anesthesiol* 1998;25:158–162.
250. Ashburn MA, Gauthier M, Love G, et al. Iontophoretic administration of 2% lidocaine HC1 and 1:100,000 epinephrine in humans. *Clin J Pain* 1997;13:22–26.
251. Ashburn MA, Streisand J, Zhang J, et al. The iontophoresis of fentanyl citrate in humans. *Anesthesiology* 1995;82:1146–1153.
252. Ashburn MA, Stephen RL, Ackerman E, et al. Iontophoretic delivery of morphine for postoperative analgesia. *J Pain Symptom Manage* 1992;7:27–33.
255. Yaster M, Krane EJ, Kaplan RF, et al. *Pediatric pain management and sedation handbook*. St. Louis: Mosby Year Book, 1997.
254. Taiwo YO, Basbaum AI, Perry F, et al. Paradoxical analgesia produced by low doses of the opiate-antagonist naloxone is mediated by interaction at a site with characteristics of the delta opioid receptor. *J Pharmacol Exp Ther* 1989;249:97–100.
255. Ueda H, Fukushima N, Kitao T, et al. Low doses of naloxone produce analgesia in the mouse brain by blocking presynaptic autoinhibition of enkephalin release. *Neurosci Lett* 1986;65:247–252.
256. Levine JD, Gordon NC. Method of administration determines the effect of naloxone on pain. *Brain Res* 1986;365:377–378.
257. Yoburn BC, Duttaroy A, Shah S, et al. Opioid antagonist-induced receptor upregulation: effects of concurrent agonist administration. *Brain Res Bull* 1994;33: 237–240.
258. White PF, Way WL, Trevor AJ. Ketamine—its pharmacology and therapeutic uses. *Anesthesiology* 1982; 56:119–136.
259. Green SM, Johnson NE. Ketamine sedation for pediatric procedures: part 2, review and implications. *Ann Emerg Med* 1990;19:1033–1046.
260. Morray JP, Lynn AM, Stamm SJ, et al. Hemodynamic effects of ketamine in children with congenital heart disease. *Anesth Analg* 1984;63:895–899.
261. Reich DL, Silvay G. Ketamine: an update on the first twenty-five years of clinical experience. *Can J Anaesth* 1989;36:186–197.
262. Green SM, Nakamura R, Johnson NE. Ketamine sedation for pediatric procedures: part 1, a prospective series. *Ann Emerg Med* 1990;19:1024–1032.
263. Yamamura T, Harada K, Okamura A, et al. Is the site of action of ketamine anesthesia the N-methyl-D-aspartate receptor? *Anesthesiology* 1990;72:704–710.
264. Sari A, Okuda Y, Takeshita H. The effect of ketamine on cerebrospinal fluid pressure. *Anesth Analg* 1972;51: 560–565.
265. Takeshita H, Okuda Y, Sari A. The effects of ketamine on cerebral circulation and metabolism in man. *Anesthesiology* 1972;36:69–75.
266. Hamza J, Ecoffey C, Gross JB. Ventilatory response to CO2 following intravenous ketamine in children. *Anesthesiology* 1989;70:422–425.
267. Welborn LG, Rice LJ, Hannallah RS, et al. Postoperative apnea in former preterm infants: prospective comparison of spinal and general anesthesia. *Anesthesiology* 1990;72:838–842.
268. Hickey PR, Hansen DD, Cramolini GM, et al. Pulmonary and systemic hemodynamic responses to ketamine in infants with normal and elevated pulmonary vascular resistance. *Anesthesiology* 1985;62:287–293.
269. Wolfe RR, Loehr JP, Schaffer MS, et al. Hemodynamic effects of ketamine, hypoxia and hyperoxia in children with surgically treated congenital heart disease residing greater than or equal to 1,200 meters above sea level. *Am J Cardiol* 1991;67:84–87.
270. Greeley WJ, Stanley TE 3, Ungerleider RM, et al. Intraoperative hypoxemic spells in tetralogy of Fallot. An echocardiographic analysis of diagnosis and treatment. *Anesth Analg* 1989;68:815–819.
271. Tashiro C, Matsui Y, Nakano S, et al. Respiratory outcome in extremely premature infants following ketamine anaesthesia. *Can J Anaesth* 1991;38:287–291.
272. Grant IS, Nimmo WS, McNicol LR, et al. Ketamine disposition in children and adults. *Br J Anaesth* 1983; 55:1107–1111.
273. Malinovsky JM, Servin F, Cozian A, et al. Ketamine and norketamine plasma concentrations after i.v., nasal and rectal administration in children. *Br J Anaesth* 1996;77:203–207.
274. Grant IS, Nimmo WS, Clements JA. Pharmacokinetics and analgesic effects of i.m. and oral ketamine. *Br J Anaesth* 1981;53:805–810.
275. Hannallah RS, Patel RI. Low-dose intramuscular ketamine for anesthesia pre-induction in young children undergoing brief outpatient procedures. *Anesthesiology* 1989;70:598–600.
276. Schmid RL, Sandler AN, Katz J. Use and efficacy of low-dose ketamine in the management of acute postoperative pain: a review of current techniques and outcomes. *Pain* 1999;82:111–125.
277. Parker RI, Mahan RA, Giugliano D, et al. Efficacy and safety of intravenous midazolam and ketamine as sedation for therapeutic and diagnostic procedures in children. *Pediatrics* 1997;99:427–431.
278. Tanaka M, Sato M, Saito A, et al. Reevaluation of rectal ketamine premedication in children: comparison with rectal midazolam. *Anesthesiology* 2000;93: 1217–1224.
279. Sekerci C, Donmez A, Ates Y, et al. Oral ketamine premedication in children (placebo controlled double-blind study). *Eur J Anaesthesiol* 1996;13:606–611.
280. Cederholm I, Bengtsson M, Bjorkman S, et al. Long term high dose morphine, ketamine and midazolam infusion in a child with burns. *Br J Clin Pharmacol* 1990;30:901–905.
281. Hartvig P, Larsson E, Joachimsson PO. Postoperative analgesia and sedation following pediatric cardiac surgery using a constant infusion of ketamine. *J Cardiothorac Vasc Anesth* 1993;7:148–153.
282. Tobias JD, Martin LD, Wetzel RC. Ketamine by continuous infusion for sedation in the pediatric intensive care unit. *Crit Care Med* 1990;18:819–821.
283. Minto CF, Power I. New opioid analgesics: an update. *Int Anesthesiol Clin* 1997;35:49–65.

284. Raffa RB, Friderichs E, Reimann W, et al. Complementary and synergistic antinociceptive interaction between the enantiomers of tramadol. *J Pharmacol Exp Ther* 1993;267:331–340.
285. Desmeules JA, Piguet V, Collart L, et al. Contribution of monoaminergic modulation to the analgesic effect of tramadol. *Br J Clin Pharmacol* 1996;41:7–12.
286. Kapral S, Gollmann G, Wald B, et al. Tramadol added to mepivacaine prolongs the duration of an axillary brachial plexus blockade. *Anesth Analg* 1999;88: 853–856.
287. Prosser DP, Davis A, Booker PD, et al. Caudal tramadol for postoperative analgesia in pediatric hypospadias surgery. *Br J Anaesth* 1997;79:293–296.
288. Naguib M, Seraj M, Attia M, et al. Perioperative antinociceptive effects of tramadol. A prospective, randomized, double-blind comparison with morphine. *Can J Anaesth* 1998;45:1168–1175.

13

Treatment of Pediatric Pain with Nonconventional Analgesics

Elliot J. Krane, Michael S. Leong, Brenda Golianu, and Yvonne Y. Leong

Acute traumatic and surgical injuries produce a type of pain known as *nociceptive pain* and are managed with conventional analgesic medications (e.g., nonsteroidal anti-inflammatory drugs, weak or strong opioids) or by physical means (e.g., ice or heat). However, less common diseases such as peripheral neuropathies, central pain syndromes, and the diseases that are categorized under the rubric complex regional pain syndromes (CRPS) types 1 and 2 are associated with *neuropathic pain*. Neuropathic pain is more challenging to treat and generally requires therapy with both conventional and nonconventional analgesics, i.e., medications not traditionally thought of as possessing analgesic properties.

NEUROPATHIC PAIN SYNDROMES

Neuropathic pain is caused by injury or degeneration of peripheral nerves or the pain pathway in the central nervous system (CNS). Because of the loss of normal nociceptive pathways, normal inhibitors of pain and descending modulators of nociception are no longer fully operant. Consequently, conventional analgesic medications are often only partially effective or are completely ineffective in alleviating associated pain.

The clinical signs of neuropathic pain cover a broad range of symptoms but are most often stereotypic: pain is typically perceived as severe and lancinating or continuously burning. Most often, light mechanical stimulation of the affected body part is associated with severe pain (allodynia). What is ordinarily a mildly noxious stimulus is felt as unusually painful (hyperalgesia) and is perceived over a spatially extended area of the body (hyperpathia).

Nociceptive, or conventional, pain is caused by injury to, stimulation of, or inflammation of nearby peripheral nociceptors, such as high-threshold mechanoreceptors. Neuropathic pain does *not* involve stimulation or activity of the peripheral nociceptors but rather the nociceptive pathways proximal to the nociceptors. As such, this leaves the "target tissues" of those pathways in a state of abnormal sensory potential. Multiple mechanisms are responsible for the changes within the CNS that lead to the neuropathic state; the plasticity of the CNS in this regard closely resembles the changes in the pain system leading to activation-dependent autosensitization, collectively known as "windup."

The processes of central sensitization are receiving increased attention in basic and clinical research and deserve a note of attention here. Although it involves modulation of the primary afferent terminal and interneurons in the dorsal horn as well, the most important elements of central sensitization are found at the level of the wide dynamic range neurons concentrated in lamina V of the dorsal horn (Fig. 13.1). Nerve transmission in the dorsal horn begins with the afferent stimulus causing release of glutamate, substance P, and other neurotransmitters from the primary afferent. Glutamate then activates the α-amino-3-hydroxy-5-methyl-4-isoxazole proprionic acid (AMPA) receptor, a rapid and complete depolarization. These changes then elicit membrane depolar-

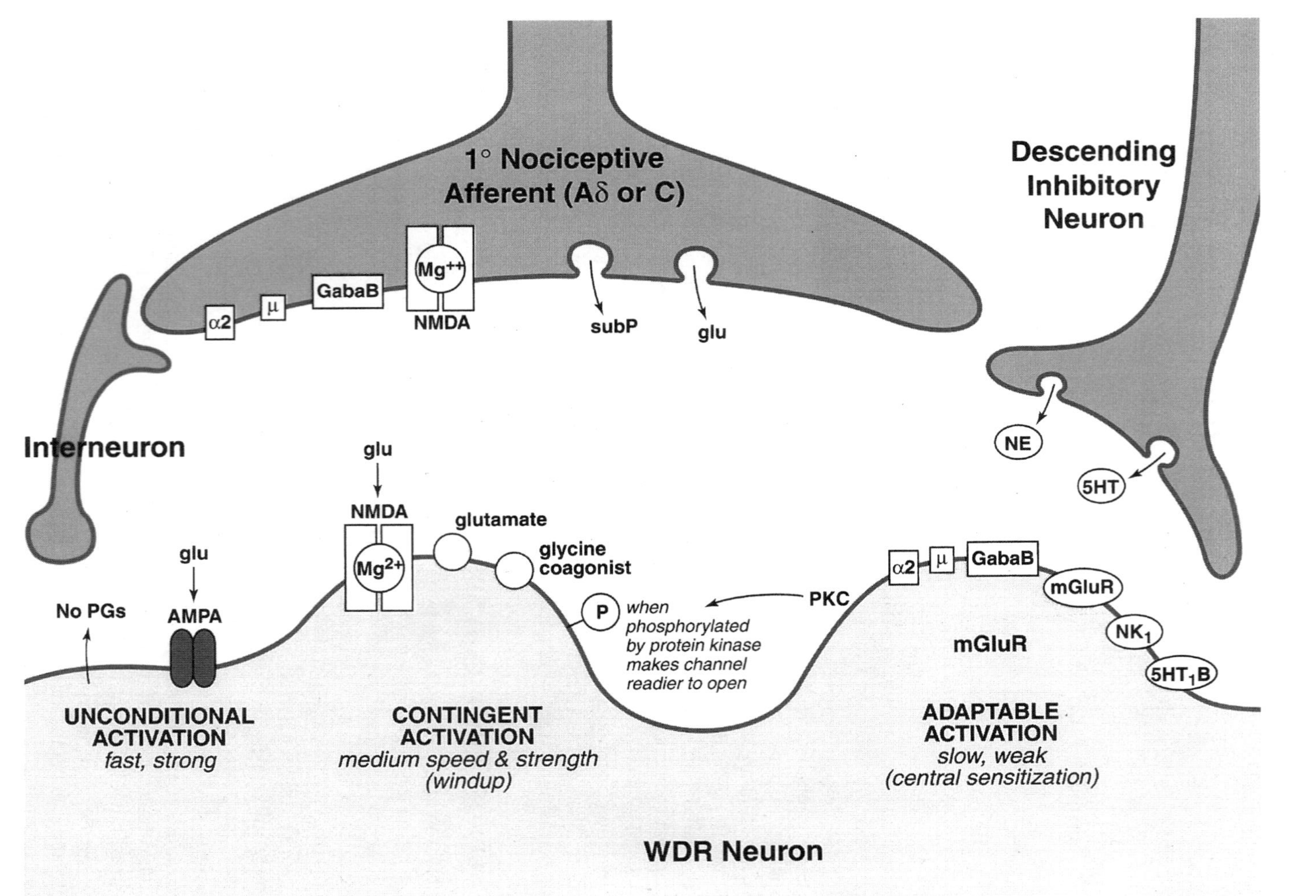
1° Nociceptive Afferent (Aδ or C)
Descending Inhibitory Neuron
Interneuron
α2
μ
GabaB
Mg++
NMDA
subP
glu
NE
5HT
glu
NMDA
Mg2+
glutamate
glycine coagonist
glu
AMPA
No PGs
P
when phosphorylated by protein kinase makes channel readier to open
PKC
α2
μ
GabaB
mGluR
NK1
5HT1B
mGluR
UNCONDITIONAL ACTIVATION
fast, strong
CONTINGENT ACTIVATION
medium speed & strength (windup)
ADAPTABLE ACTIVATION
slow, weak (central sensitization)
WDR Neuron

ization in the wide dynamic range neuron. *N*-methyl-D-aspartate (NMDA) receptors, also found in the wide dynamic range neuron, are activated more slowly (within seconds) and allow facilitated conduction and summation of action potentials.

Windup is an early and important component of central sensitization. With continued nociceptive input, the process then continues with the activation of other receptors, together referred to as the metabotropic glutamate receptors. These receptors require minutes to hours to become activated and begin a chain of translational events mediated by second messengers.

One of the key events is the phosphorylation of the NMDA receptor itself via protein kinase C. This phosphorylation then increases the activity of the NMDA receptor further and propagates the cycle of central sensitization. These events, however, can be intensely modulated by opioids, α_2 agonists, NMDA antagonists, norepinephrine, GABA (γ-aminobutyric acid)-minergic, serotonergic, and other agents. The clinical applications of these findings are still being developed, but the effects will likely be far reaching.

For example, in one study, patients who received dextromethorphan, an NMDA antagonist, required less analgesia after hysterectomy than patients who did not receive it (1). McQuay et al. (2) showed that in patients undergoing surgery, regional anesthesia resulted in increased time to postoperative analgesic request, as well as reduced overall need for analgesics. Finally, patients who had received 72 hours of epidural blockade before lower limb amputation had both less pain postoperatively and less phantom limb pain at 1-year follow-up (3).

Injured peripheral nerves respond to trauma by sending out sprouts of growth processes both in the periphery and in the CNS. A fibers in particular show central reorganization, sprouting from their deep dorsal horn laminar location up into that part of the spinal cord where C fibers normally terminate and make functional synapses (4,5). This proliferation in turn leads to the formation of abnormal synaptic connections in the CNS that persist over time.

For example, the injury of a peripheral nerve that ordinarily conducts touch sensation may result in the affected neurons sending out sprouts to lamina II of the dorsal horn of the spinal cord, an area in which only small unmyelinated pain fibers from the periphery normally synapse. Not only does this process lead to the perception of pain to light touch, but the new synapses are formed without the normal receptors and connections that modulate pain, that is, without the analgesic effect of endogenous opioids, α agonists, and so forth. This results in the perception of pain, allodynia, and hyperpathia refractory to ordinary analgesics.

Furthermore, injured and regenerating nerves are prone to spontaneous, unstimulated electrical activity. Spontaneous action potentials lead to the perception of continuous pain unrelated to stimulation of distal tissue injury or healing and to cell death in the superficial laminae of the dorsal horn where inhibitory interneurons are concentrated (4).

A more extensive discussion of neuropathic pain is found in Chapter 34.

FIG. 13.1. The most important elements of central sensitization are found at the level of the wide dynamic range (*WDR*) neurons concentrated in lamina V of the dorsal horn. Nerve transmission in the dorsal horn begins with the afferent stimulus causing release of glutamate, substance P, and other neurotransmitters from the primary afferent. Glutamate then activates the α-amino-3-hydroxy-5-methyl-4-isoxazole proprionic acid (*AMPA*) receptor, a rapid and complete depolarization. These changes then elicit membrane depolarization in the WDR neuron. Then *N*-methyl-D-aspartate (*NMDA*) receptors, also found in the WDR neuron, are activated more slowly (within seconds) and allow facilitated conduction and summation of action potentials. This initial activation of the NMDA receptor is referred to as windup. *PKC*, protein kinase C.

Clearly, the creation of these aberrant nociceptive pathways and the spontaneous activity of injured and regenerating neurons require a therapeutic approach to pain that differs from the management of more conventional nociceptive pain (6). Experience has shown that the use of membrane-stabilizing drugs (7), tricyclic antidepressants (TCAs) (8–10), and anticonvulsants (11) is effective for these pain syndromes.

The management of pediatric neuropathic pain is made difficult by the absence of any evidence-based research with children. Our practices are largely based on the perceptions and beliefs of individual clinicians or are extrapolated from accepted strategies in adults that are often derived more from anecdotal experience and perceptions than evidence-based medicine. Note that there are few codified "per kilogram" pediatric guidelines for many of the treatments that are described below and that there are few published evidence-based studies to validate their use. Many of the recommendations described below are based on our or other anecdotal experience and/or extrapolation from evidence-based studies concerning adult patients. Recommended dosages are generally extrapolated from dosages that are well accepted for other pediatric indications.

MEMBRANE STABILIZERS

Intravenous Lidocaine

Lidocaine is beneficial in the treatment of neuropathic pain states by blocking conduction of sodium channels in peripheral and central neurons and therefore reducing spontaneous impulse firing (12,13). Furthermore, the effectiveness of intravenous lidocaine in producing analgesia is a predictor of the subsequent efficacy of oral mexiletine both in the treatment of cardiac arrhythmia (14) and neuropathic pain (15). Although animal studies have shown that intravenous lidocaine alleviates tactile allodynia in rats (16), human studies have found no association between reduction in allodynia and pain relief (4). Typically, intravenous lidocaine is administered to a target plasma lidocaine level of 2 to 5 μg/mL (17–19).

There are few reports of the use of lidocaine for the treatment of neuropathic pain states in children. Wallace et al. (20) used intravenous lidocaine to control pain after anti-GD2 antibody therapy in children with neuroblastoma using intravenous lidocaine at 2 mg/kg over 30 minutes followed by 1 mg/kg per hour. Compared with a morphine infusion (0.05 to 0.1 mg/kg per hour), lidocaine was associated with improved mobility and decreased supplemental analgesic requirements. Of note, extended use of lidocaine infusions over 4 days was associated with an increased incidence of nausea.

Our clinical experience confirms that lidocaine is useful for treatment of pediatric neuropathic conditions. We routinely employ lidocaine as an adjunct medication for pain syndromes refractory to conventional therapy, such as the pain of mucositis after bone marrow transplantation and refractory cancer pain (20,21), and in neuropathic pain states such as CRPS-1, CRPS-2, erythromelalgia, and painful neuropathies to predict the efficacy of mexiletine (see below).

Because lidocaine pharmacokinetics are similar in children and adults, dosing schedules for children should correlate reasonably with published experience in adults. Lidocaine plasma levels are readily available in most clinical laboratories to assure that infusions are delivering an effective dose without producing toxicity. The most accurate way to deliver intravenous lidocaine is by a computerized infusion, a technique utilized in our adult pain clinic in which our protocol calls for an initiating bolus of lidocaine equal to 1 mg/kg over 5 minutes, with a subsequent infusion of lidocaine at a rate of 1 mg/kg per hour. Blood levels are checked every 8 hours, and the lidocaine infusion is adjusted to target a blood level between 2 and 5 μg/mL. Patients with hepatic or renal insufficiency need dose adjustments (halving the dose of bolus or infusion) to prevent toxicity.

Mexiletine (Mexitil)

Originally used as an oral cardiac antiarrhythmic analog of lidocaine, mexiletine is

TABLE 13.1. *Mexiletine dosing schedule for children*

Day	Morning (no. of tablets)	Mid-day (no. of tablets)	Bedtime (no. of tablets)
1			1
2			1
3			1
4	1		1
5	1		1
6	1		1
7	1	1	1
8	1	1	1
9	1	1	1
10	1	1	2
11	1	1	2
12	1	1	2
13	1	1	2
14	2	1	2
15	2	1	2
16	2	1	2
17	2	1	2
18+	2	2	2

Mexiletine is available as 150-, 200-, 250-, and 300-mg tablets. The target dose is 10 to 15 mg/kg. (From Krane EJ. Mexiletine dosing schedule. http://pedsanesthesia.stanford.edu/guide/guideline-mexiletine.html, 1999, with permission.)

used by most pain treatment centers as an oral analog to lidocaine to treat neuropathic pain. The original antiarrhythmic studies for lidocaine showed that it was a useful predictor for the antiarrhythmic efficacy of mexiletine and tocainide. Tocainide, unfortunately, produces significant toxicity such as blood dyscrasias and interstitial pneumonitis. Mexiletine, conversely, is without such toxicity and is much better tolerated. Dejgard et al. (22) reported a dose of mexiletine as high as 10 mg/kg daily to treat diabetic neuropathy. Mexiletine was used with at similar doses by Chabal et al. (23) in adults to treat peripheral nerve injuries. Chabal et al. commented that most subjects required a daily dose of mexiletine of 10 mg/kg for pain, whereas the usual range for treatment of cardiac arrhythmias is between 10 and 15 mg/kg.

A review of the pediatric literature shows no pharmacologic or pharmacokinetic difference in the absorption or metabolism of mexiletine between children and adults. Mexiletine is frequently associated with untoward gastrointestinal side effects, most commonly nausea and vomiting, as well as sedation, confusion, difficulty concentrating, diplopia, blurred vision, and ataxia, although gradual introduction of the drug and progressive escalation of the dose is ordinarily successful in reducing this side effect, as illustrated in Table 13.1.

ANTICONVULSANTS

Carbamazepine (Tegretol)

Carbamazepine is an older antiepileptic used to treat neuropathic pain via sodium channel blockade. Carbamazepine can be administered in oral (100 to 200 mg) and suspension formulations (100 mg/5 mL). Recommended dosing schedules for children older than 6 years of age start at 10 mg/kg daily in two divided doses to a usual maintenance dose of 15 to 30 mg/kg daily in two to four divided doses per day. Blood levels (therapeutic 4 to 12 μg/mL) can be obtained but do not necessarily correlate with analgesia for neuropathic pain.

Metabolism and adverse effects are significant with carbamazepine. Carbamazepine is hepatically metabolized, limiting its usefulness patients with hepatic insufficiency. Moreover, adverse effects are common including hematologic (aplastic anemia, agranulocytosis), cardiovascular (congestive heart failure, syncope, arrhythmia), CNS (sedation, dizziness, fatigue, slurred speech, ataxia), and even hepatitis (24). A complete blood count should be obtained before initiating this antiepileptic drug and should be repeated every 3 to 6 months. Although a classic agent for the management of neuropathic pain, carbamazepine is no longer a first-line drug, particularly for a child or adult who may have hematologic alterations or hepatic dysfunction.

Sodium Valproate (Depakote)

Valproic acid is an antiepileptic drug that has been used to treat neuropathic pain states and associated mood disturbances. The mood-stabilizing effect of valproic acid is especially useful for the management of agitation or mania associated with pain. The drug also is effective and approved by the U.S. Food and Drug Administration for the management of migraine headaches, but because of significant side effects, valproate is not usually a first-line agent unless mood stabilization is a desired co-end point of treatment.

The mechanism of action for valproate is unclear. The drug has a wide spectrum of anticonvulsant applications; therefore, multiple mechanisms of action are proposed. Loscher (25) describes at least three mechanisms. Valproate increases GABA synthesis and release, which may partially explain its efficacy in treating central pain. Valproate also attenuates neuronal excitation induced by NMDA-type glutamate receptors. NMDA receptors have some correlation with centralization of neuropathic pain states or the windup phenomenon. Moreover, valproate has direct effects on excitable membranes and acts as a membrane stabilizer, similar to intravenous lidocaine and mexiletine.

Valproate is available as an oral tablet, syrup, and rectal suppository. Dosing starts at 10 to 15 mg/kg per day to a maximum of 30 to 60 mg/kg per day. The drug has a half-life in children of 6 to 18 hours, with a peak effect 4 hours after administration. Plasma concentration does not correlate with toxicity, seizure control, or analgesia. Valproate is protein bound (80% to 95%) and metabolized by glucuronidation and other oxidative pathways.

Adverse effects can be significant. Typical toxic effects within the first several months include anorexia, nausea/vomiting, sedation, and weight gain or loss. Valproate may cause hepatotoxicity and hepatic dysfunction in 5% to 30% of patients. Other less common adverse effects include hyperammonemia, pancreatitis, and platelet dysfunction. For these reasons, valproate is not a first-line agent. Liver function tests should be performed before initiation of valproate treatment and then every month for the next 6 months. Symptoms such as malaise, lethargy, gastrointestinal symptoms, and easy bruising may indicate liver dysfunction and lead to immediate laboratory evaluation and discontinuation of the drug (26).

Gabapentin (Neurontin)

Gabapentin is a compound that was originally synthesized as a GABA-ergic drug to treat spasticity. It was later found to be more effective as a potent anticonvulsant for treating partial seizures and generalized tonic-clonic seizures (27,28). At this time, the mechanism of action of this agent is unclear. Gabapentin may enhance extracellular GABA levels by reversing GABA transport in a unique way. The compound does not reduce voltage-sensitive sodium channels or affect NMDA receptors. On a biochemical level, gabapentin may inhibit a branched chain amino acid transferase, ultimately producing a decreased level of glutamate, an excitatory amino acid that may be important in nerve transmission. Increased activity of glutamate dehydrogenase and glutamic acid decarboxylase has also been noted in gabapentin-treated animals, further decreasing levels of glutamate.

The most remarkable clinical feature of gabapentin is its few and infrequent side effects or dose-limiting factors. In fact, it is safe to say that of the many agents described in this chapter for the management of pain, none has a more benign side effect or toxicity profile.

Gabapentin is not protein bound; therefore, distribution is not affected by alterations in hepatic function. Gabapentin is not metabolized and therefore does not induce hepatic enzymes. Gabapentin elimination is entirely by renal excretion. Dosage must therefore be adjusted proportionally to the reduction in creatinine clearance.

Side effects are predominantly limited to the CNS: somnolence, dizziness, ataxia, nystagmus, and tremor. These effects are dose related and usually minor.

The dose for adults ranges from 300 to 5,600 mg daily. Gabapentin has a biologic half-life of 5 to 9 hours and therefore is typically prescribed on a three times daily schedule. Higher doses (e.g., >20 mg/kg daily) require more frequent administration because gastrointestinal absorption depends on an L-amino acid transporter in the gastrointestinal tract that may become saturated at higher gabapentin doses, producing diarrhea.

The use of gabapentin has been well described in the pediatric literature, using doses from 5 to 30 mg/kg for the management of seizure disorders (29,30). Behavioral side effects of gabapentin in children have been described as intensification of baseline behaviors including tantrums, hyperactivity, oppositional behavior, fighting, and increased anger (31). A disinhibition theory similar to one seen with benzodiazepine therapy has been postulated as the cause.

Gabapentin has been unambiguously found to be beneficial in treating chronic neuropathic pain syndromes in adults. Mellick and Mellick (32) described the use of gabapentin in complex regional pain syndrome type I, in which significant pain relief and possible reversal of the disease process was found. Controlled studies by Robotham et al. (33) for postherpetic neuralgia and Backonja et al. (34) for neuropathy secondary to diabetes mellitus also suggest efficacy of treatment in these neuropathic pain conditions. Backonja et al. additionally found that gabapentin therapy had a positive effect on mood.

In the treatment of pain in the pediatric population, reports are few, limited mostly to case reports and small series (35). Since the initiation of use of gabapentin, however, its clinical utility has far outpaced the published data. In part, this may be owing to the relative paucity of agents useful in neuropathic pain and the significant side effects of these agents. In our clinic, gabapentin is frequently used as a first- or second-line agent for the treatment of neuropathic pain, initially at 10 mg/kg and gradually escalating over several weeks to a maximum of 50 mg/kg. The daily dose may be titrated to as much as 70 mg/kg daily depending on clinical response and side effects (36).

TRICYCLIC ANTIDEPRESSANTS

Depression and other psychologic symptoms such as anxiety and anger accompany many chronic pain conditions. Originally, patients with chronic pain were treated for depression and coincidentally found significant pain relief independent of the mood-altering affect of antidepressant medication. Subsequent studies by Max et al. (37) and others (38,39) showed statistically significant relief in treating neuropathic pain syndromes.

TCAs have consistently been shown to be the single most efficacious class of alternative analgesic drugs for neuropathic pain of a variety of origins, including postherpetic neuralgia, painful neuropathies, traumatic nerve injury, and trigeminal neuralgia. For this reason and because of the beneficial antidepressant and sedative properties of these drugs, they are usually the first-line alternative analgesic drugs chosen to manage neuropathic pain and other opioid-resistant pain states (7–9,40–42).

All TCAs that have been tested have equal efficacy at therapeutic doses. Although most antidepressants take 4 to 6 weeks to reach their full antidepressant effect, the onset of analgesic effect is less clear but is almost certainly much shorter than that for the antidepressant effect (Fig. 13.1).

The pharmacology of TCAs is well defined. The antidepressant mechanism of action of TCAs is the reuptake inhibition of serotonin and norepinephrine from synaptic junctions in the CNS. Each TCA has varying degrees of effect on serotonin and norepinephrine levels, depending on whether the drug is a primary or tertiary amine (43). The analgesic mechanism is less well defined. TCAs have been demonstrated to block both Na^+ and Ca^{2+} gated channels and inhibit the NMDA receptor (44–46).

TCAs have a high first-pass metabolism by the liver after absorption from the gastrointestinal tract. They are highly protein bound in plasma to α_1-acid glycoprotein. TCAs are lipophilic molecules and therefore accumulate in the body's fat stores; biologic half-lives are quite long (1 to 4 days).

In patients, there is wide plasma TCA level variability owing to genetic cytochrome P-450 polymorphism. TCAs are metabolized by the drug-metabolizing isozyme cytochrome P-450 2D6 (debrisoquin hydroxylase). The biochemical activity of the cytochrome P-450 2D6 is reduced in a subset of the white population (approximately 7% to 10% of whites are so-called "poor metabolizers"); reliable estimates of the prevalence of reduced P-450 2D6 isozyme activity among Asian, African, and other populations are not yet available. Poor metabolizers have higher than expected plasma concentrations of TCAs when given usual doses. Depending on the fraction of drug metabolized by P-450 2D6, the increase in plasma concentration may be small or quite large (eightfold increase in plasma level of the TCA). This is also seen in the metabolism of codeine into morphine.

In addition, some drugs inhibit the activity of this isozyme and make normal metabolizers resemble poor metabolizers. An individual who is stable on a given dose of TCA may become abruptly toxic when given one of these inhibiting drugs as concomitant therapy. The drugs that inhibit cytochrome P-450 2D6 include some that are not metabolized by the enzyme (e.g., quinidine, cimetidine) and many that are substrates for P-450 2D6 (e.g., many other antidepressants, phenothiazines, and the type 1C antiarrhythmics propafenone and flecainide). Although all the selective serotonin reuptake inhibitors (SSRIs), e.g., fluoxetine, sertraline, and paroxetine, inhibit P-450 2D6, they may vary in the extent of inhibition. The extent to which SSRI–TCA interactions may pose clinical problems depends on the degree of inhibition and the pharmacokinetics of the SSRI involved. Nevertheless, caution is indicated in the coadministration of TCAs with any of the SSRIs and in switching from one class to the other. Of particular importance, sufficient time must elapse before initiating TCA treatment in a patient being withdrawn from fluoxetine, given the long half-life of the parent and active metabolite (at least 5 weeks may be necessary).

All TCAs cause the same side effects but differ in their side effect profile. Typical side effects of TCAs are dose related and include antihistaminic (H1 and H2) effects, causing sedation and increased gastric pH; antimuscarinic effects, producing dry mouth (xerostomia), impaired visual accommodation, urinary retention, and constipation; α-adrenergic blockade, causing orthostatic hypotension; weight gain; and, most significantly, a quinidine-like effect. The last can cause QRS widening on the electrocardiogram, causing a prolonged QTc-like syndrome. As early as 1990 in *The Medical Letter* and as recently as 1997, reports of the sudden death of children have raised concerns of life-threatening arrhythmias (47,48). Sudden deaths in children treated with TCA may be idiosyncratic. Desipramine (Norpramin) and imipramine (Tofranil) in particular seem to produce greater changes in baseline electrocardiography, specifically increased QRS duration.

Antidepressants therefore have many uses in pain medicine. These agents, shown in Figure 13.2, are used to treat depression, anxiety, sleep disturbance, and, of course, pain.

Amitriptyline (Elavil)

Collins et al. (49) retrospectively described eight children, ages 5 to 17 years, in whom intravenous amitriptyline was effective in treat-

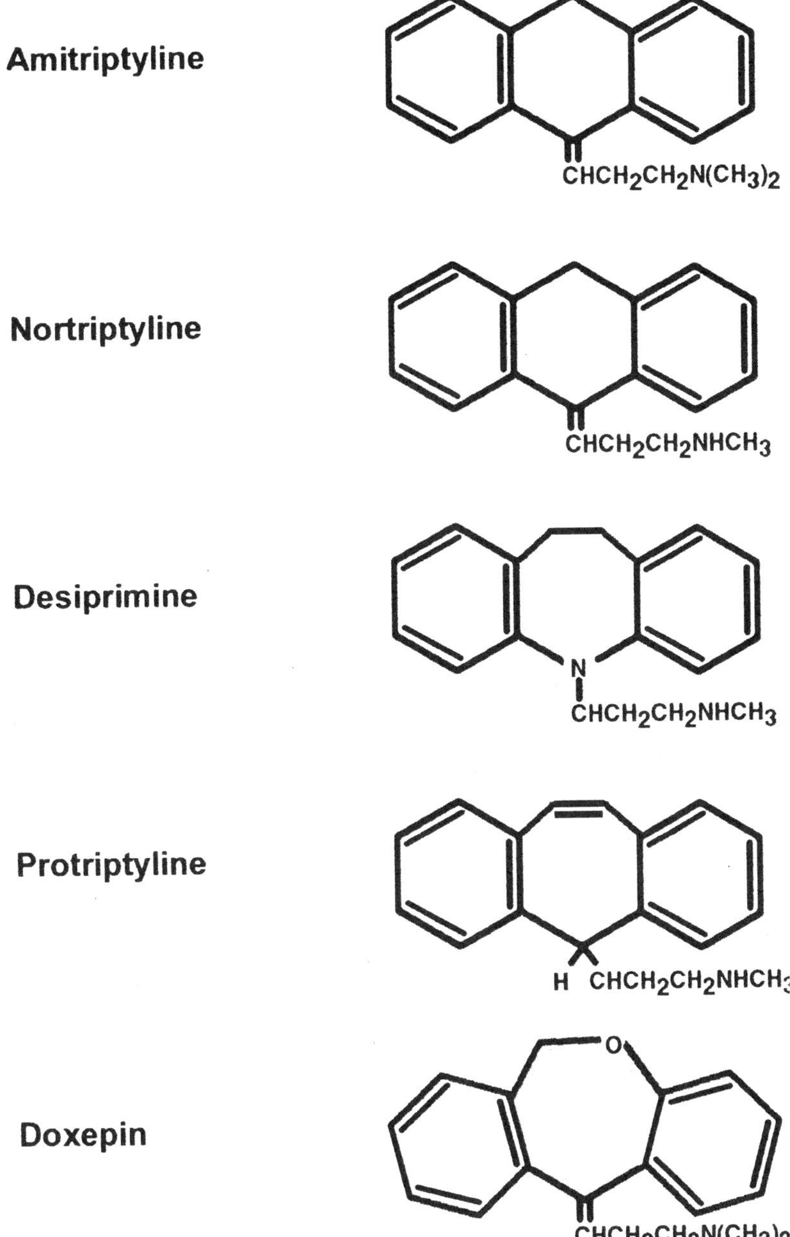

FIG. 13.2. The chemical structures of tricyclic antidepressants commonly used for the management of pain syndromes.

ing neuropathic pain, depression, and sleep disturbance and as an adjuvant for opioid analgesia. The calculation of initial intravenous dose for amitriptyline naïve children was 0.2 mg/kg daily, with ultimate doses of 0.05 to 2.4 mg/kg daily given intravenously. Side effects in addition to those listed above included dysphoria, which might have been secondary to concurrent opioids, and extrapyramidal effects that resolved with diphenhydramine.

Although children may be rapid metabolizers of amitriptyline and therefore require a twice-daily dosing schedule, a single daily dose is usually first used until a side effect profile is established for individual patients. The most prominent and consistent side effect is somnolence; therefore, the daily dose is generally given before bedtime. A recommended initial dose is 0.05 mg/kg daily escalating over a period of 3 to 4 weeks to approximately 0.5 to 1 mg/kg daily is generally sufficient for pain management, although higher doses have been used in the past for mood elevation. Amitriptyline may also be parenterally administered as an intramuscular injection using approximately one-third to one-half of the oral dose. The intramuscular preparation currently marketed may also be administered intravenously over a period of 2 hours, to mimic the absorption of an intramuscular injection.

The utility of routine measurement of plasma drug levels in pain management is dubious because no correlation has been shown between plasma drug levels and analgesia. However, plasma levels may identify a rapid or slow metabolizer, confirm patient/parent compliance with prescription, and optimization of dose before discontinuation of trial (50).

Nortriptyline (Pamelor)

Nortriptyline is a compound with a pharmacology that is virtually identical to that of amitriptyline, but because of the demethylation of the terminal amide group, the side effect profile is superior to that of amitriptyline, particularly in regard to its sedative and antimuscarinic effects.

Although published experience with nortriptyline is lacking in pediatrics, experience shows that it is equally effective and preferable when daytime somnolence limits the use of amitriptyline.

Desiprimine (Norpramin)

Desipramine has been reported to be associated with sudden death in several pediatric cases; therefore, its use has been abandoned for the management of pain in children.

Selective Serotonin Reuptake Inhibitors

Although most useful to treat clinical signs of depression complicating the management of chronic pain, most SSRIs are less effective than TCAs as specific analgesics, although Sindrup et al. (51) found some benefit in using paroxetine (Paxil) to treat diabetic neuropathies, especially when patients could not tolerate the side effects of TCAs. The notable exception to the absence of analgesic properties with this newest class of antidepressants is venlafaxine.

Venlafaxine (Effexor)

Venlafaxine is a novel SSRI chemically unrelated to other SSRIs but chemically similar to the opioid tramadol (Ultram) (Fig. 13.3) (52).

The mechanism of the antidepressant action of venlafaxine in humans is believed to be the same as with other SSRIs, associated with its potentiation of neurotransmitter activity in the CNS as with other SSRIs: preclinical studies have shown that venlafaxine and its active metabolite, O-desmethylvenlafaxine, are potent inhibitors of neuronal serotonin and norepinephrine reuptake and weak inhibitors of dopamine reuptake.

That venlafaxine is analgesic is seen in studies in animals that show that venlafaxine is effective in reversing chronic neuropathic pain secondary to thermal hyperalgesia and in addition is effective in treating the hyperalge-

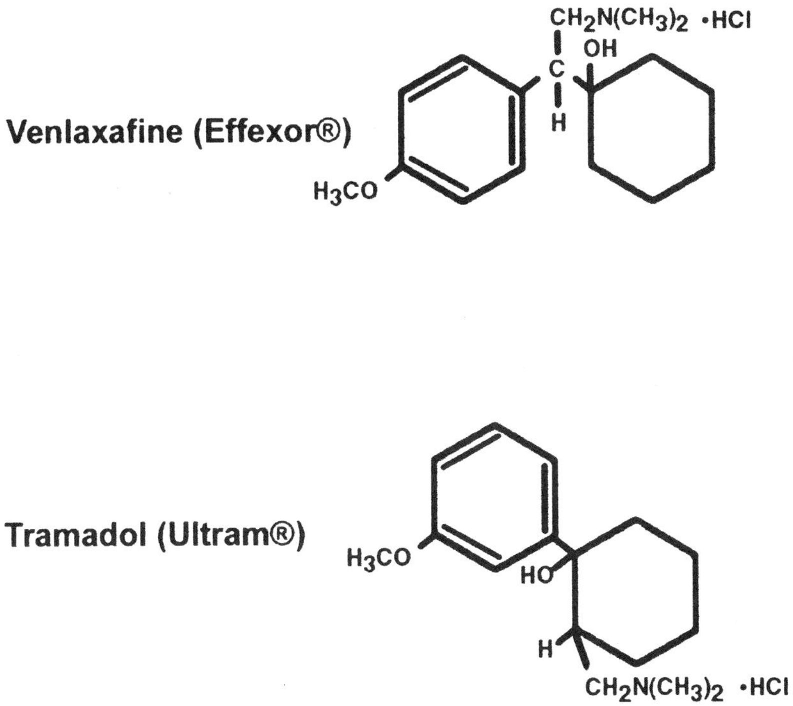

Venlaxafine (Effexor®)

Tramadol (Ultram®)

FIG. 13.3. The chemical structures of venlafaxine (Effexor) **(top)** and tramadol (Ultram) **(bottom)** demonstrate the chemical similarity between these two antidepressant and analgesic substances, respectively.

sia of neuropathic pain owing to chronic sciatic nerve constriction injury in rats (53).

Venlafaxine-induced antinociception is significantly inhibited by naloxone, nor-BNI, and naltrindole, but not by β FNA or naloxonazine, implying involvement of κ_1 and δ opioid mechanisms. When adrenergic and serotonergic antagonists are used, yohimbine, but not phentolamine or metergoline, decreased antinociception elicited by venlafaxine, implying a clear α_2- and a minor α_1-adrenergic mechanism of antinociception. Therefore, the antinociceptive effect of venlafaxine is mainly influenced by the κ and δ opioid receptor subtypes combined with the α_2-adrenergic receptor. These results suggest a potential use of venlafaxine in the management of some pain syndromes. However, further research is needed to establish both the exact clinical indications and the effective doses of venlafaxine when prescribed for neuropathic pain (54).

α-AGONISTS

Clonidine (Catapres, Duraclon Injection)

α_2 Receptors are located on primary afferent terminals (both peripheral and spinal endings) in the superficial laminae of the dorsal horn of the spinal cord and within several brainstem nuclei. The analgesic effect of clonidine may be at all three sites, with each site's relative contribution to its analgesic effect being unclear. Most studies support a direct and primary spinal analgesic action of clonidine. Supportive data for this conclusion are the facts that the relative potency of epidural clonidine to intravenous clonidine is 2:1, clonidine has a lipophilicity similar to fentanyl, the duration of analgesia of epidural clonidine is 3 to 5 hours, and spinal administration of clonidine results in a peak analgesic effect within 30 to 60 minutes with a duration of as long as 6 hours (55,56).

Clonidine increases the release of acetylcholine at the dorsal horn, activating spinal cord acetylcholine receptors (Fig. 13.1). This enhances sensory and motor block of C and Aδ fibers by local anesthetics by increasing potassium conductance. Clonidine is therefore thought to have applications in the treatment of chronic pain, particularly neuropathic pain.

Clonidine has not been unequivocally demonstrated to provide analgesia in peripheral neuropathic pain states. Transdermal clonidine patches in painful diabetic neuropathy have been effective only in a subset of adult patients (57,58). Adults with postherpetic neuralgia responded to oral clonidine (0.2 mg) in one placebo-controlled clinical trial (59).

Recent studies using clonidine in central and peripheral blockade show that it is coanalgesic when used with either local anesthetics or opioids in epidural, intrathecal, or peripheral blocks (60,61). Finally, intrathecal administration of clonidine has been shown to reduce intractable muscle spasms in patients with spinal cord injuries.

With regard to the pediatric literature, most studies have been performed using clonidine in combination with a bupivacaine epidural analgesia in the *acute* surgical pain setting. Motsch et al. (62) studied a group of 40 children undergoing minor surgical procedures. They found that combined caudal analgesia with bupivacaine and clonidine (5 μg/kg) was superior to local anesthetic alone, as determined by both duration and intensity of analgesia. However, children had decreased blood pressure and sedation for the first 3 postoperative hours. This observed effect is consistent with the known duration of epidural clonidine in adults. Other authors have studied caudal analgesia using bupivacaine and clonidine (1 to 2 μg/kg) with bupivacaine. This dose of clonidine was seen to decrease mean arterial pressure but not to cause bradycardia or respiratory depression (63–65). There are at present no clinical trials that describe the use of clonidine in chronic or neuropathic pain states.

Adverse effects of clonidine include a dose-dependent decrease in blood pressure. Action at the nucleus tractus solitarius and locus ceruleus decrease peripheral sympathetic tone. Further action at the lateral reticular nucleus causes hypotension and an antiarrhythmogenic action. Neuraxial administration inhibits sympathetic preganglionic neurons in the spinal cord, and heart rate may decrease secondary to a depression in atrioventricular nodal conduction, especially when clonidine is administered in the thoracic epidural or intrathecal spaces.

Clonidine produces sedation, which may be a desirable side effect in many circumstances. This side effect is localized to the activity in the locus ceruleus. The sedation of clonidine is dose dependent between 50 and 900 μg, or between approximately 1 and 10 μg/kg, regardless of route of administration. Epidural clonidine has a rapid onset of sedation within 20 minutes. Clonidine alone does not induce respiratory depression nor potentiate respiratory depression from opioids.

Sudden cessation of clonidine treatment, regardless of the route of administration and including after prolonged epidural administration, has in some cases resulted in symptoms similar to those of opioid abstinence syndrome, such as nervousness, agitation, headache, and tremor, accompanied or followed by a rapid rise in blood pressure.

The experience in adult patients with cancer with intractable pain suggests an initial epidural dose of 30 to 150 μg followed by a continuous infusion of 8 to 400 μg daily is effective for somatic pain management.

Extrapolation from experience in adults and our unpublished clinical experience suggests an initial dose of epidural clonidine of 1 to 2 μg/kg should also be appropriate either in the subarachnoid or epidural spaces, followed by an infusion of local anesthetic and clonidine at 0.02 to 0.1 μg/kg per hour, titrating as needed to a maximum of 0.2 μg/kg per hour, while observing for undesired hemodynamic effects or sedation (Table 13.2).

Capsaicin

Capsaicin is the chemical substance in chili peppers that creates their spiciness and heat. In 1997, a gene that encoded for a receptor

TABLE 13.2. *Summary of unconventional analgesics useful in the management of pain in children*

Drug	Indications and uses	Pediatric dosing	Toxicity and notes
Lidocaine	Neuropathic pain, refractory visceral pain	150 μg/kg per hr	Measure plasma level every 8–12 hr and maintain 2–5 μg/mL
Mexiletine	See lidocaine	See Table 13.1	Sedation, fatigue, confusion, nausea, hypotension
Carbamazepine	Trigeminal neuralgia, neuropathic pain, migraine prophylaxis	15–30 mg/kg	Blood dyscrasias, monitor plasma level and periodic CBC
Valproate	Neuropathic pain, migraine prophylaxis, mood lability	10–60 mg/kg	Blood dyscrasias, hepatotoxicity, dose divided t.i.d., monitor plasma level, periodic CBC and LFTs
Gabapentin	Neuropathic pain, migraine prophylaxis	5–30 mg/kg	Dose divided t.i.d. or q.i.d., escalate dose over several weeks to target dose
Amitriptyline, nortriptyline	Neuropathic pain, migraine prophylaxis	0.05–2 mg/kg	Escalate dose over several weeks to target dose, dose given h.s., obtain screening ECG before use, contraindicated in prolonged QTc
Venlafaxine	Chronic pain with depression, neuropathic pain	1–2 mg/kg	Dose divided b.i.d. or t.i.d., caution when used with TCAs or other SSRIs because of reported arrhythmias
Clonidine	Neuropathic pain, visceral pain, postoperative pain	0.05–0.2 μg/kg per hr	By oral, transdermal, or continuous epidural infusion; may produce hypotension, bradycardia, somnolence

CBC, complete blood count; t.i.d., three times a day; LFTs, liver function tests; q.i.d., four times daily; h.s., at bedtime; ECG, electrocardiogram; b.i.d., twice a day; TCAs, tricyclic antidepressants; SSRIs, selective serotonin reuptake inhibitors.

specific for capsaicinoids was identified. The capsaicin-gated vanilloid receptor 1 is a fatty acid receptor present only on C fibers, that, when activated, produces desensitization or degeneration of the sensory afferent (66). This phenomenon has led to the use of capsaicin for the management of chronic pain states, particularly those associated with burning cutaneous dysesthesias and mechanical allodynia (67). However, there are some conditions for which capsaicin is ineffective, such as peripheral neuropathy associated with acquired immune deficiency syndrome (68) and neuropathic pain associated with nerve injury (69). Overall, outcome studies show that the number needed to treat with capsaicin varies from 2.5 in painful diabetic neuropathy to 5.9 in other disorders (10). This is not an impressively effective treatment modality, and the inconvenience of the necessity to spread a cream over a large affected body surface further mitigates against its use.

Chronic application of capsaicin leads to depletion of substance P from cutaneous C fibers and ultimately degeneration of C fibers, thus some degree of analgesia. However, acute cutaneous application of capsaicin produces a complex sensation that changes in intensity and quality as a function of time and is characterized by sting, prick, burn, and pain sensations (70). The painful sensations and inconvenience associated with acute application of capsaicin to affected skin clearly limit its usefulness in pediatric pain medicine. Furthermore, there are no published reports of the use of capsaicin in children.

CONCLUSIONS

Nociceptive pain may be adequately treated with conventional opioid and nonopioid analgesic drugs; however, many neuropathic pain states are refractory to conventional analgesic drugs. For these conditions, use of a number of drugs not traditionally considered analgesic and not developed by the pharmaceutical industry for their analgesic properties is effective (Fig. 13.4). These drugs are effective

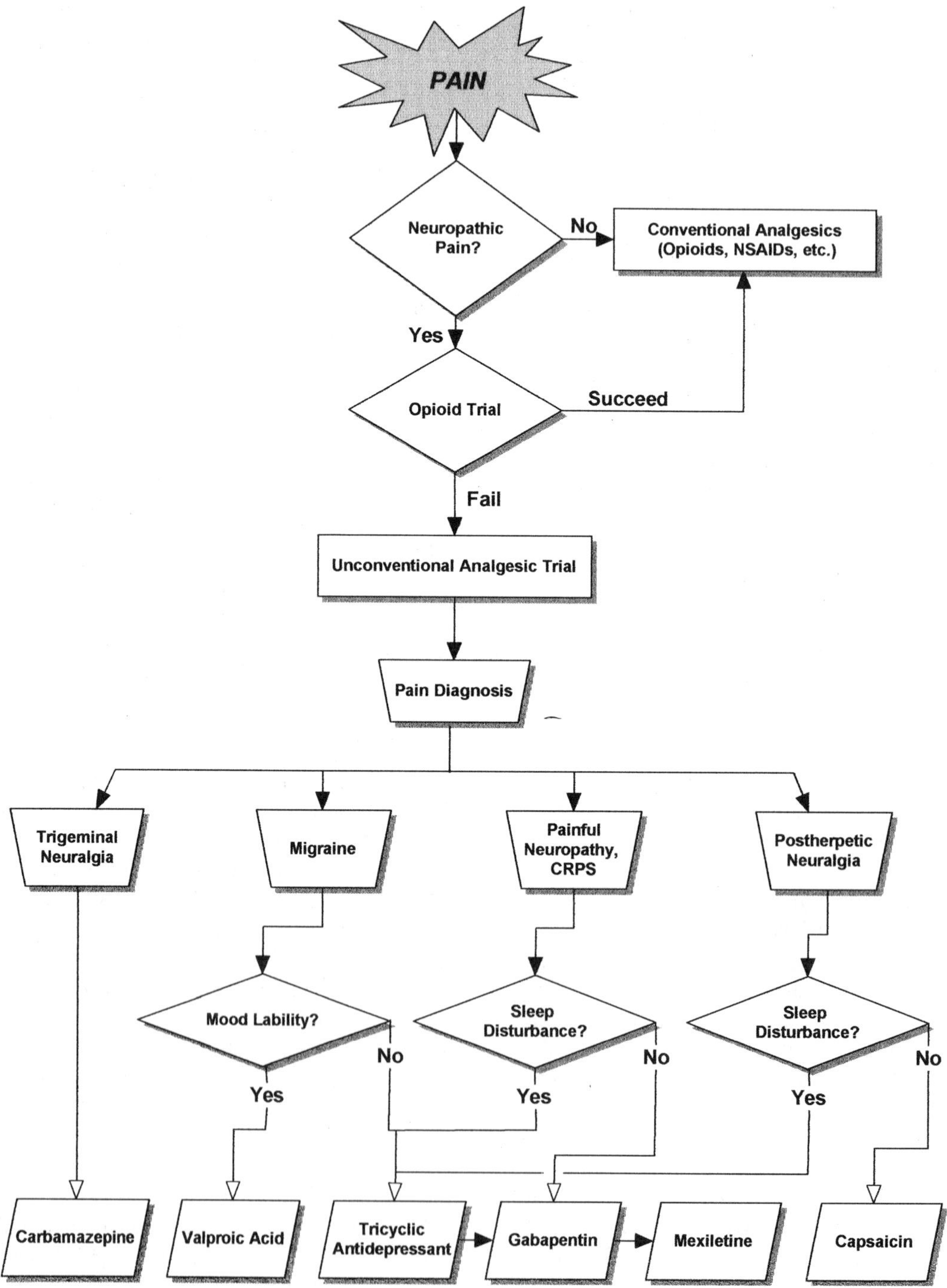

FIG. 13.4. An algorithm for the use of nonconventional analgesic drugs in various pediatric acute and chronic pain states.

by virtue of their membrane-stabilizing effects or their additive or synergistic enhancement of endogenous modulation of nociception in the CNS.

We are entering an era of new analgesic drug development by the pharmaceutical industry, and it is likely that in the next decade new compounds will be added to our armamentarium to fight pain in novel molecular ways. As our understanding of the molecular mechanisms of pain evolve, the category of unconventional analgesics will certainly expand.

REFERENCES

1. Henderson DJ, Withington BS, Wilson JA, et al. Perioperative dextromethorphan reduces postoperative pain after hysterectomy. *Anesth Analg* 1999;89:399–402.
2. McQuay HJ, Carroll D, Moore RA. Postoperative orthopedic pain—the effect of opioid premedication and local anaesthetic blocks. *Pain* 1988;33:291–295.
3. Bach S, Noreng MF, Tjellden NU. Phantom limb pain in amputees during the first 12 months following limb amputation after preoperative lumbar epidural blockade. *Pain* 1988;33:297–301.
4. Woolf CJ, Salter MW. Neuronal plasticity: increasing the gain in pain. *Science* 2000;288:1765–1769.
5. Woolf CJ, Mannion RJ. Neuropathic pain: aetiology, symptoms, mechanisms, and management. *Lancet* 1999;353:1959–1964.
6. Dellemijn P. Are opioids effective in relieving neuropathic pain? *Pain* 1999;80:453–462.
7. Sindrup SH, Jensen TS. Efficacy of pharmacological treatments of neuropathic pain: an update and effect related to mechanism of drug action. *Pain* 1999;83: 389–400.
8. Watson CPN. The treatment of neuropathic pain: antidepressants and opioids. *Clin J Pain* 2000;16:S49–S55.
9. Fishbain D. Evidence-based data on pain relief with antidepressants. *Ann Med* 2000;32:305–316.
10. Kingery WS. A critical review of controlled clinical trials for peripheral neuropathic pain and complex regional pain syndromes. *Pain* 1997;73:123–139.
11. Tremont-Lukats IW, Megeff C, Backonja M-M. Anticonvulsants for neuropathic pain syndromes: mechanisms of action and place in therapy. *Drugs* 2000;60: 1029–1052.
12. Brose WG, Cousins MJ. Subcutaneous lidocaine for treatment of neuropathic cancer pain. *Pain* 1991;45: 145–148.
13. Galer BS, Miller KV, Robotham MC. Response to intravenous lidocaine infusion differs based on clinical diagnosis and site of nervous system injury. *Neurology* 1993;43:1233–1235.
14. Murray KT, Barbey JT, Kopelman HA, et al. Mexiletine and tocainide: a comparison of antiarrhythmic efficacy, adverse effects, and predictive value of lidocaine testing. *Clin Pharmacol Ther* 1989;45:553–561.
15. Galer BS, Harle BS, Robotham MC. Response to intravenous lidocaine infusion predicts subsequent response to oral mexiletine: a prospective study. *J Pain Symptom Manage* 1996;12:161–167.
16. Chaplan SR, Bach FW, Shafer SL, et al. Prolonged alleviation of tactile allodynia by intravenous lidocaine in neuropathic rats. *Anesthesiology* 1995;83:775–785.
17. Dyck, JB, Wallace MS, Lu LQ, et al. Pharmacokinetics of lidocaine administered by computer-controlled infusion pump in humans. *Anesth Analg* 1995;80:S110.
18. Wallace MS, Dyck JB, Rossi SS, et al. Computer-controlled lidocaine infusion of the evaluation of neuropathic pain after peripheral nerve injury. *Pain* 1996;66: 69–77.
19. Schnider TW, Gaeta R, Brose WG, et al. Derivation and cross-validation of pharmacokinetic parameters for computer-controlled infusion of lidocaine in pain therapy. *Anesthesiology* 1996;84:1043–1050.
20. Wallace MS, Lee J, Sorkin L, et al. Intravenous lidocaine: effects on controlling pain after anti-GD2 antibody therapy in children with neuroblastoma—a report of a series. *Anesth Analg* 1997;85:794–796.
21. Lin YC, Sentivany-Collin S. The analgesic response to intravenous lidocaine in the treatment of mucositis pain. *Anesthesiology* 2000;93:A1258.
22. Dejgard A, Petersen P, Kastrup J. Mexiletine for treatment of chronic painful diabetic neuropathy. *Lancet* 1988;29:9–11.
23. Chabal C, Jacobson L, Mariano A, et al. The use of oral mexiletine for the treatment of pain after peripheral nerve injury. *Anesthesiology* 1992;76:513–517.
24. Kong K. Carbamazepine-induced hepatitis in a patient with cervical myelopathy. *Arch Phys Med Rehab* 1996; 77:305–6.
25. Loscher W. Valproate: a reappraisal of its pharmacodynamic properties and mechanism of action. *Prog Neurobiol* 1999;58:31–59.
26. AAP Committee on Drugs. Valproic acid: benefits and risks. *Pediatrics* 1982;70:316–319.
27. Mclean M. Gabapentin. *Epilepsia* 1995;36:S73–S86.
28. Andrews C, Fischer J. Gabapentin: a new agent for the management of epilepsy. *Ann Pharm* 1994;28:1188–96.
29. Bourgeois B. Antiepileptic drugs in pediatric practice. *Epilepsia* 1995;36:S34–S45.
30. Leiderman D, Garafalo E, LaMoreaux L. Gabapentin patients with absence seizures: two double-blind, placebo controlled studies. *Epilepsia* 1993;34[Suppl 6]:45.
31. Lee D, Steingard R, Cesena M, et al. Behavioral side effects of gabapentin in children. *Epilepsia* 1996;37:87–90.
32. Mellick G, Mellick L. Reflex sympathetic dystrophy treated with gabapentin. *Arch Phys Med Rehab* 1997; 78:98–105.
33. Robotham M, Harden N, Stacey B, et al. Gabapentin for the treatment of postherpetic neuralgia. *JAMA* 1998; 280:1837–1842.
34. Backonja M, Beydoun A, Edwards K, et al. Gabapentin for the symptomatic treatment of painful neuropathy in patients with diabetes mellitus. *JAMA* 1998;280: 1831–1836.
35. Wheeler DS, Vaux KK, Tam DA. Use of gabapentin in the treatment of childhood reflex sympathetic dystrophy. *Pediatr Neurol* 2000;22:220–221.
36. Bourgeois B. Antiepileptic drugs in pediatric practice. *Epilepsia* 1995;36:S34–S45.
37. Max M, Kishore-Kumar R, Schafer S, et al. Efficacy of desipramine in painful diabetic neuropathy: a placebo-controlled trial. *Pain* 1991;45:3–9.

38. Vrethem M, Boivie J, Arnqvist H, et al. A comparison of amitriptyline and maprotiline in the treatment of painful polyneuropathy in diabetics and nondiabetics. *Clin J Pain* 1997;13:313–323.
39. McQuay H, Tramer M, Nye B, et al. A systematic review of antidepressant in neuropathic pain. *Pain* 1996; 68:217–227.
40. Bowsher D. The effects of pre-emptive treatment of postherpetic neuralgia with amitriptyline: a randomized, double-blind, placebo-controlled trial. *J Pain Symptom Manage* 1997;13:327–331.
41. Kalso E, Tasmuth T, Neuvonen PJ. Amitriptyline effectively relieves neuropathic pain following treatment of breast cancer. *Pain* 1995;64:293–302.
42. Leijon G, Boivie J. Central post-stroke pain—a controlled trial of amitriptyline and carbamazepine. *Pain* 1989;36:27–36.
43. Ögren SO. Effects of antidepressant drugs on different receptors in the brain. *Eur J Pharmacol* 1981;70: 393–407.
44. Lavoie PA, Beauchamp G, Elie R. Tricyclic antidepressants inhibit voltage dependent calcium channel and Na^+-Ca^{2+} exchange in rat brain synaptosomes. *Can J Physiol Pharmacol* 1990;68:1414–1418.
45. Pancrazio JJ, Kamatchi GL, Roscoe AK, et al. Inhibition of neuronal Na^+ channels by antidepressant drugs. *J Pharmacol Exp Ther* 1998;284:208–214.
46. Reynolds IJ, Miller RJ. Tricyclic antidepressants block N-methyl-D-aspartate receptors: similarities to the action of zinc. *Br J Pharmacol* 1988;95:95–102.
47. Wilens T, Biederman J, Baldessarini RJ, et al. Cardiovascular effects of therapeutic doses of tricyclic antidepressants in children and adolescents. *J Am Acad Child Adolesc Psychiatry* 1996;35:1491–1501.
48. Varley C, McClellan J. Case study: two additional sudden deaths with tricyclic antidepressants. *J Am Academy Child Adolesc Psychiatry* 1997;36:390–394.
49. Collins J, Kerner J, Sentivany S, et al. Intravenous amitriptyline in pediatrics. *J Pain Symptom Manage* 1995;10:471–475.
50. Richeimer S, Bajwa Z, Kahraman S, et al. Utilization patterns of tricyclic antidepressants in a multidisciplinary pain clinic: a survey. *Clin J Pain* 1997;13:324–329.
51. Sindrup S, Gram L, Brosen K, et al. The selective serotonin reuptake inhibitor paroxetine is effective in the treatment of diabetic neuropathy symptoms. *Pain* 1990;42:135–144.
52. Markowitz JS, Patrick KS. Venlafaxine-tramadol similarities. *Med Hypotheses* 1998;51:167–168.
53. Lang E, Hord AH, Denson D. Venlafaxine hydrochloride (Effexor) relieves thermal hyperalgesia in rats with an experimental mononeuropathy. *Pain* 1998;68:151–155.
54. Schreiber S, Backer MM, Pick CG. The antinociceptive effect of venlafaxine in mice is mediated through opioid and adrenergic mechanisms. *Neurosci Lett* 1999;273: 85–88.
55. Ivani G, Bergendah, HT, Lampugnan E, et al., Plasma levels of clonidine following epidural bolus injection in children. *Acta Anaesthesiol Scand* 1998;42:306–311.
56. De Kock M, Crochet B, Morimont C, et al. Intravenous or epidural clonidine for intra- and postoperative analgesia. *Anesthesiology* 1993;79:525–531.
57. Zeigler D, Lyinch SA, Muir J, et al. Transdermal clonidine versus placebo in painful diabetic neuropathy. *Pain* 1992;48:403–408.
58. Byas-Smith MG, Max MB, Muir J, et al. Transdermal clonidine compared to placebo in painful diabetic neuropathy using two-stage 'enriched enrollment' design. *Pain* 1995;60:267–274.
59. Max MG, Schafer SC, Culnane M, et al. Association of pain relief with drug side-effects in postherpetic neuralgia: a single dose study of clonidine, codeine, ibuprofen, and placebo. *Clin Pharmacol Ther* 1988;43:363–371.
60. Maze M, Tranquilli W. Alpha-2 adrenoceptor agonists: defining the role in clinical anesthesia. *Anesthesiology* 1991;74:581–605.
61. Eisenach J, Kock M, Klimscha W. Alpha2-adrenergic agonists for regional anesthesia: a clinical review of clonidine. *Anesthesiology* 1996;85:655–674.
62. Motsch J, Bottiger B, Bach A, et al. Caudal clonidine and bupivacaine for combined epidural and general anaesthesia in children. *Acta Anaesthesiol Scand* 1997; 41:877–883.
63. Ivani G, Bergendahl H, Lampugnani E, et al. Plasma levels of clonidine following epidural bolus injection in children. *Acta Anaesthesiol Scand* 1998;42:306–311.
64. Jamali S, Monin S, Begon C, et al. Clonidine in pediatric caudal anesthesia. *Anesth Analg* 1994;78:663–666.
65. Klimscha W, Chiari A, Michalek-Saubere A, et al. The efficacy and safety of a clonidine/bupivacaine combination in caudal blockade for pediatric hernia repair. *Anesth Analg* 1998;86:54–61.
66. Robbins W. Clinical applications of capsaicinoids. *Clin J Pain* 2000;16:S86–S89.
67. McCleane G. Topical application of doxepin hydrochloride, capsaicin and a combination of both produces analgesia in chronic human neuropathic pain: a randomized, double-blind, placebo-controlled study. *Br J Clin Pharmacol* 2000;49:574–579.
68. Paice JA, Ferrans CE, Lashley FR, et al. Topical capsaicin in the management of HIV-associated peripheral neuropathy. *J Pain Symptom Manage* 2000;19:45–52.
69. Watson CPN, Evans RJ. The post-mastectomy pain syndrome and topical capsaicin: a randomized trial. *Pain* 1992;51:375–379.
70. Magnusson BM, Koskinen LD. In vitro percutaneous penetration of topically applied capsaicin in relation to in vivo sensation responses. *Int J Pharm* 2000;195:55–62.

14
Local Anesthetics

Myron Yaster, Joseph R. Tobin, and Sabine Kost-Byerly

Local anesthetics are drugs that reversibly block conduction of neural impulses along central and peripheral nerve pathways (1–10). To be effective, local anesthetics must be physically deposited, usually by needles or indwelling catheters, in the immediate vicinity of the nerves to be blocked (9,11–16). In this way, local anesthetics are unlike virtually all other drugs used in modern medicine, which, regardless of their means of entry into the body, are delivered to their site of action by a carrier, namely, the blood. Removal of local anesthetics from the neural tissue results in spontaneous and complete return of nerve conduction with no evidence of structural damage to nerve fibers as a result of the drug's effects (1–8,10).

For decades, children were considered poor candidates for regional (local) anesthetic techniques primarily because of their overwhelming fear of needles and because of the pain produced by needles in administering local anesthetics (4,8,11–16). Indeed, physicians saw little, if any, benefit of using local anesthetics in children. What was the sense of "sticking" a child (with a needle) twice—once with the local anesthetic and once for the procedure itself? Children were therefore unable to reap the benefits of these drugs and of regional anesthetic techniques in the management of their pain, despite the fact that regional blockade is often the most appropriate method of providing pain relief; this is particularly true for procedure-related pain, posttraumatic pain, and pain unresponsive to opioid therapy (17–22). Finally, local anesthetics can provide almost complete anesthesia in situations in which general anesthesia is neither possible nor practical, for example, newborn circumcision and procedure-related pain (23–25).

Procedure-related pain requires special attention (Chapter 36). It is pain that is inflicted on patients in the course of their medical or surgical treatment (26–29). It is also among the most difficult forms of pain to deal with by both the patient experiencing it and the health care professionals who must inflict it. Examples of procedure-related pain include insertion of an arterial or intravenous catheter (e.g., routine percutaneous intravenous access or cardiac catheterization), bone marrow aspiration, thoracostomy tube placement, lumbar puncture, and repair of minor surgical wounds (traumatic lacerations or deliberate incisions, e.g., before a cutdown for venous access). Unfortunately, the most frequent response of physicians to procedure-related pain is denial (26,30). This "turning away" is uniquely easy when dealing with pediatric patients because children can be physically restrained, are not routinely asked if they are in pain, and are usually unable to withdraw their consent. Fortunately, the appropriate use of local anesthesia can abolish much of this pain.

Additionally, because regional anesthesia produces profound analgesia with minimal physiologic alterations, it is increasingly being used in children as a component of intra- and postoperative pain management and posttraumatic pain management, and for pain that is difficult to treat with systemic narcotics (17–22). For example, children who cannot tolerate opioids because of opioid-induced ventilatory depression or who have become tolerant to the analgesic effects of opioids can be made completely pain free with the use of local anesthetic techniques. Prolonged analgesia can also be provided by administering local anesthetic agents continuously by way of indwelling catheters placed in the epidural, intrathecal, intercostal, intrapleural, or other spaces (Chapters 20 and 21). Indeed, because of these myriad benefits and our ability to overcome many of the technical difficulties that limited the use of local anesthetics in the past, local and regional anesthetic techniques have become an essential component in the armamentarium of managing childhood pain.

Thus, an understanding of the effects and uses of local anesthetics may be extremely helpful to physicians who treat children in pain. This chapter provides a physiologic, pharmacokinetic, and pharmacodynamic framework of the use of local anesthetic agents in children. The specific nerve blocks commonly used in pediatric pain management are discussed elsewhere in this book.

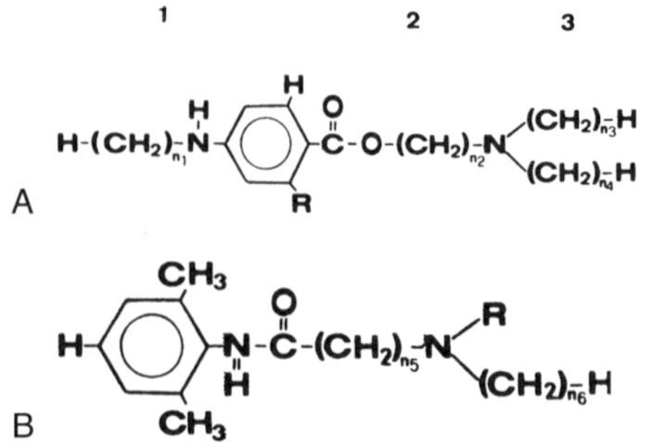

FIG. 14.1. General structure of local anesthetics. **A:** Ester (-COO-) agents. **B:** Amide (-CONH-) agents. 1, unsaturated (lipophilic) aromatic end; 2, intermediate (hydrocarbon) chain; 3, tertiary amine (hydrophilic) end. (From Dalens B. *Regional anesthesia in infants, children, and adolescents.* Baltimore: Williams & Wilkins, 1995, with permission.)

PHARMACOLOGY AND PHARMACOKINETICS OF LOCAL ANESTHETICS

Structure–Activity Relationships

All local anesthetics share a common chemical structure (1–8,10,31). They are all tertiary amines and weak bases. They are all composed of a lipophilic and a hydrophilic portion that are separated by a hydrocarbon chain (Fig. 14.1). The lipophilic portion is composed of an unsaturated aromatic ring, such as paraaminobenzoic acid, which is essential for the drug's anesthetic activity. The lipophilic portion is linked to its carbon chain either by an amide (-CONH-) or ester (-COO-) bond. The nature of this linkage is the basis for classifying the two major classes of local anesthetic agents used in clinical practice. They are either esters [e.g., tetracaine (Pontocaine), procaine (Novocain), chloroprocaine (Nesacaine), cocaine] or amides [lidocaine (Xylocaine), mepivacaine (Carbocaine), prilocaine, bupivacaine (Marcaine, Sensorcaine), ropivacaine (Naropin), L-bupivacaine or levobupivacaine (Chirocaine) (Tables 14.1 and 14.2; Fig. 14. 2). The final component of the molecule, the hydrophilic end, is a tertiary amine that confers on the molecule the properties of a weak base as well as its water solubility. Modifying the chemical structure of the local anesthetic molecule alters its intrinsic anesthetic potency, duration of action, rate of biodegradation, protein binding, and intrinsic toxicity. For example, adding a butyl group to the amine (hydrophilic) end of mepivacaine produces bupivacaine, a drug that is 35 times more lipid soluble and is three to four times more potent than the parent molecule (Fig. 14.2) (Tables 14.1 and 14.2). Additionally, this simple addition also yields a molecule that has a greater degree of protein binding and a longer duration of action. Similarly, substituting a propyl group for an ethyl group on the intermediate carbon chain of lidocaine produces etidocaine, a local anesthetic that is almost 50 times more lipid soluble and four to eight times more potent than the parent molecule. Etidocaine is also two to three times longer acting and better protein bound than lidocaine. Metabolism and biodegradation can also be affected by simple changes to the basic local anesthetic molecular structure. Adding a chlorine molecule to the aromatic ring (lipophilic end) of procaine produces chloroprocaine, a molecule that is

TABLE 14.1. *Comparative pharmacology of local anesthetics*

Classification	Toxic plasma concentration (μg/mL)	pKa	Fraction nonionized (%) pH 7.4	Protein binding (%)
Esters				
Procaine		8.9	3	6
Chloroprocaine		8.7	5	
Tetracaine		8.5	7	76
Amides				
Lidocaine	>5	7.9	25	64–70
Mepivacaine	>5	7.6	39	77
Bupivacaine	1.5	8.1	15	95
Ropivacaine	1.5	8.0	20	90–95
Etidocaine	1.5	7.7	33	94
Prilocaine	>5	7.9	24	55

pKa, pH at which ionized and nonionized concentrations of the drug are equal.

hydrolyzed by serum cholinesterase four times faster than its parent molecule procaine (Fig. 14.2). This rapid hydrolysis limits the duration of action and the systemic toxicity of chloroprocaine.

Several local anesthetics, such as bupivacaine, ropivacaine, and mepivacaine, exist in left- (S or L) and right- (D or R) handed configurations. The enantiomers may vary in their pharmacokinetics, pharmacodynamics, and, most important, their toxicity (Table 14.3). This is particularly important for bupivacaine and mepivacaine; their left-handed enantiomers are significantly less toxic than their right-handed counter parts (and their commercially available racemic mixtures) (Table 14.3) (32–34). Thus, an increasingly important feature in new local anesthetic drug development is the development of stereoselective enantiomers that are presumed to be less toxic than racemic mixtures. In fact, ropivacaine, a local anesthetic recently introduced into practice as a safer alternative to bupivacaine (see below) has been developed as a pure left-handed enantiomer (35,36).

Cellular Electrophysiology

In all excitable cells, ionic disequilibria across semipermeable membranes provide the potential energy for impulse conduction (37,38). For nerve cells, the most important ionic disequilibria are created and maintained by the sodium (Na^+)–potassium (K^+) pump (Fig. 14.3). This pump requires an energy-de-

TABLE 14.2. *Comparative pharmacology of local anesthetics*

Classification	Potency	Onset	Duration after infiltration (min)	Prolongation by epinephrine
Esters				
Procaine	1	Slow	30–60	Yes
Chloroprocaine	4	Rapid	30–45	Yes
Tetracaine	16	Slow	60–360	Yes
Amides				
Lidocaine	2	Rapid	60–90	Yes
Mepivacaine	2	Slow	60–120	Yes
Bupivacaine	16	Slow	150–360	No
Etidocaine	16	Slow	150–360	No
Ropivacaine	12	Intermediate	150–300	No
Prilocaine	2	Slow	60–120	Yes

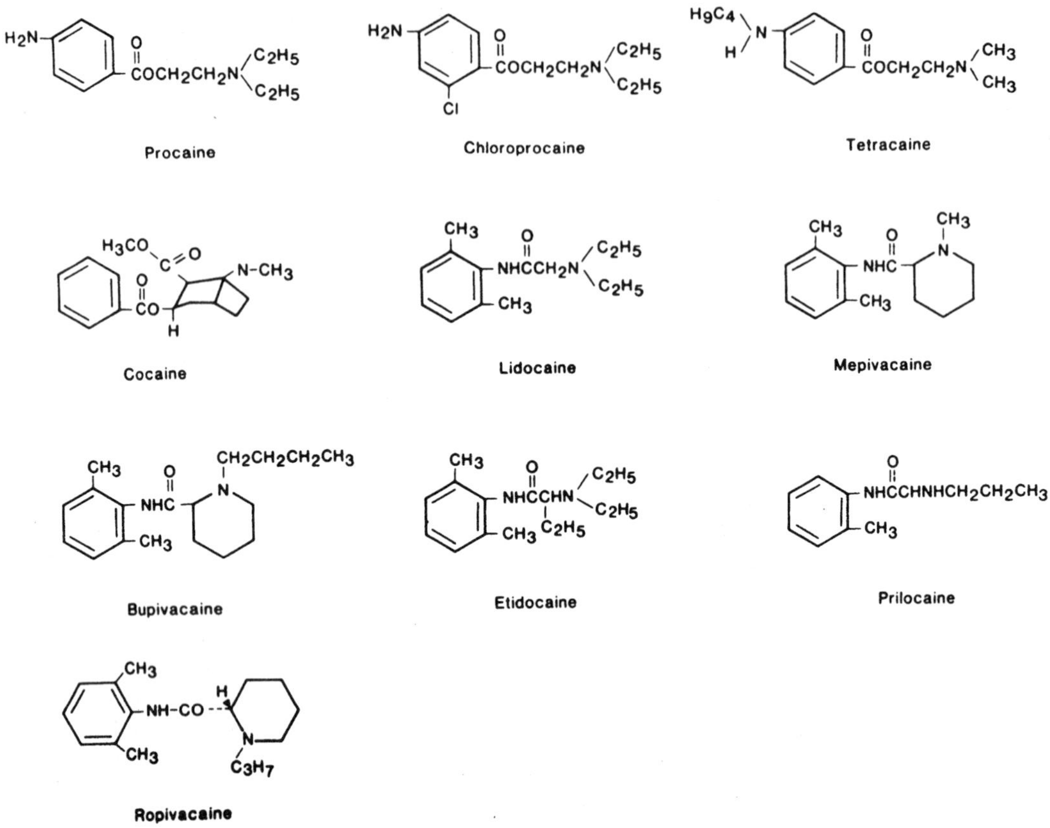

Procaine

Chloroprocaine

Tetracaine

Cocaine

Lidocaine

Mepivacaine

Bupivacaine

Etidocaine

Prilocaine

Ropivacaine

FIG. 14.2. Ester and amide local anesthetics. (From Stoelting RK. Local anesthetics. In: *Pharmacology and physiology in anesthetic practice*, 3rd Edition. Philadelphia: Lippincott Williams & Wilkins, 1999:158–181, with permission.)

pendent, membrane bound enzyme system, Na^+K^+ adenosine triphosphatase, which pumps three Na^+ ions of the cell for every two K^+ ions that enter (37). This results in a hyperpolarized outward current plus an inward leak current, which at equilibrium causes the interior of the cell to be negative in relationship to the exterior (Fig. 14.4). This difference in voltage across cell membranes is known as the resting mem-

TABLE 14.3. *Anesthetic duration and toxicity of local anesthetic isomers*

Drug	Duration	Toxicity
Etidocaine	S = R	S = R
Mepivacaine	S > R	S = R
Bupivacaine	S > R	S < R
Ropivacaine	S > R	S < R

S, left-handed enantiomer; R, right-handed enantiomer.

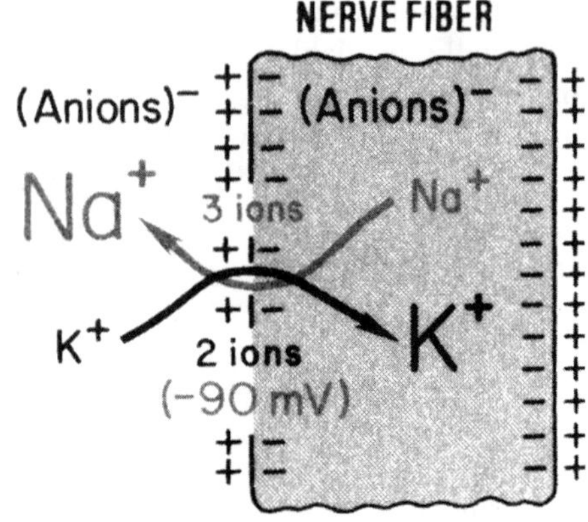

FIG. 14.3. Establishment of a resting membrane potential as a result of Na^+ and K^+ being pumped through the nerve membrane by the Na^+K^+ electrogenic pump, with three Na^+ ions passing outward through the membrane for each two K^+ ions passing inward. (From Guyton AC. *Textbook of medical physiology*. Philadelphia: WB Saunders, 1986:101–119, with permission.)

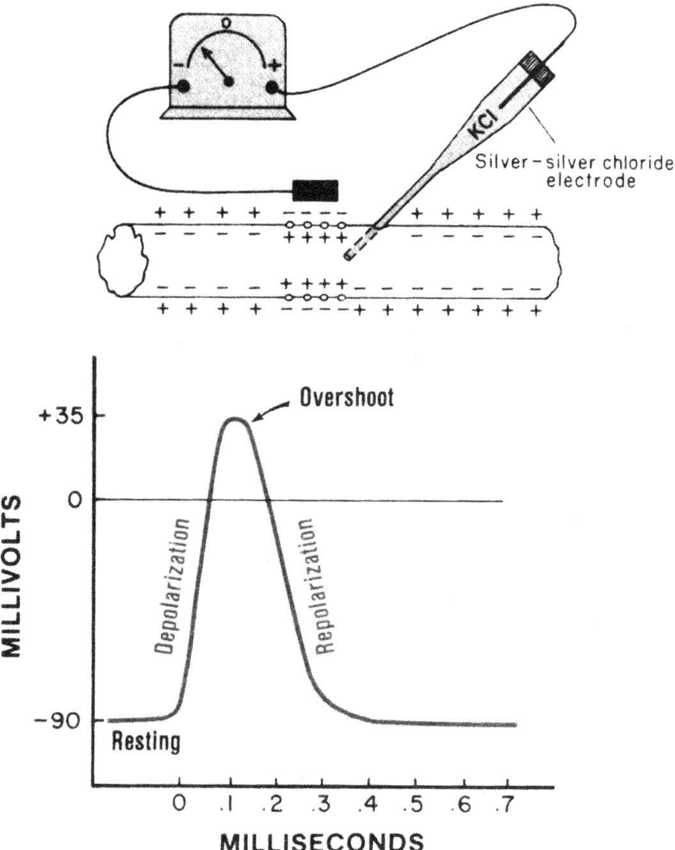

FIG. 14.4. A typical action potential recorded by a silver–silver chloride microelectrode. (From Guyton AC. *Textbook of medical physiology.* Philadelphia: WB Saunders, 1986:101–119, with permission.)

brane potential. An action potential is the rapid change in transmembrane potential followed by a return to the resting membrane potential. Propagation of the action potential along the entire length of a nerve axon is the basis of the signal-carrying ability of nerve cells.

Action potentials are conducted along nerve fibers by local current flow that produces depolarization of adjacent areas of the membrane. Conduction velocity is greatly increased by myelination, which results from the wrapping of Schwann cell membranes around the axon (Fig. 14.5). The lateral spaces between Schwann cells are referred to as the nodes of Ranvier. In nonmyelinated nerves, nerve impulses travel in a wave, much like a flame progressing down a fuse. In myelinated nerve, action potentials can only be generated at the nodes of Ranvier. Not only is conduction

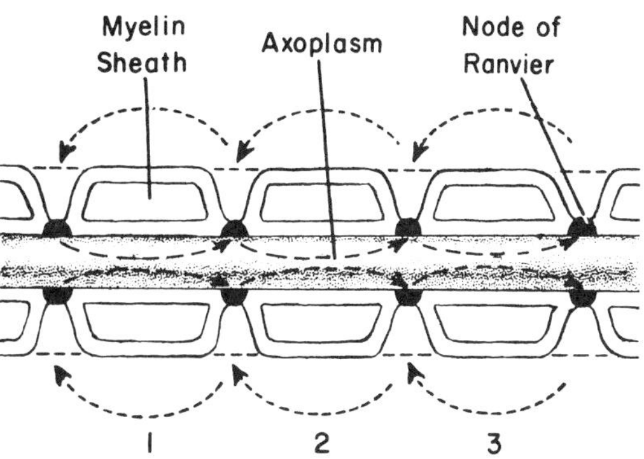

FIG. 14.5. Conduction along a myelinated axon. (From Guyton AC. *Textbook of medical physiology.* Philadelphia: WB Saunders, 1986:101–119, with permission.)

faster, it is metabolically more efficient because ion exchange occurs only at the nodes of Ranvier and less ion pumping is required to maintain the resting membrane potential.

During an action potential, voltage-gated Na^+ channels, or macromolecular "pores" in cell membranes, open briefly, allowing a small quantity of extracellular Na^+ to enter the cell. This depolarizes the plasma membrane. A more slowly developing outward current, usually of K^+ ions, helps to repolarize the membrane rapidly and restore electrical neutrality. Na^+ channels undergo transitions between being open, i.e., they are in ion-conducting states, and resting and inactivated (Fig. 14.6). The latter two states are nonconducting. Resting channels may activate to open ones, whereas inactivated channels must first undergo transition to the resting state. Local anesthetic molecules block neural transmission either by plugging the Na^+ channel (pore) and preventing ions from passing or by interfering with conformational changes that allow the channel to open (1,2,39,40). Thus, local anesthetics block impulse conduction through the inhibition of voltage-gated Na^+ channels, which prevents the achievement of a threshold potential that is necessary for generation of an action potential (41,42).

Local anesthetics do not alter the resting transmembrane potential or threshold potential of excitable membranes; rather, by blocking sodium permeability at specific ion-selective sodium channels, local anesthetics slow

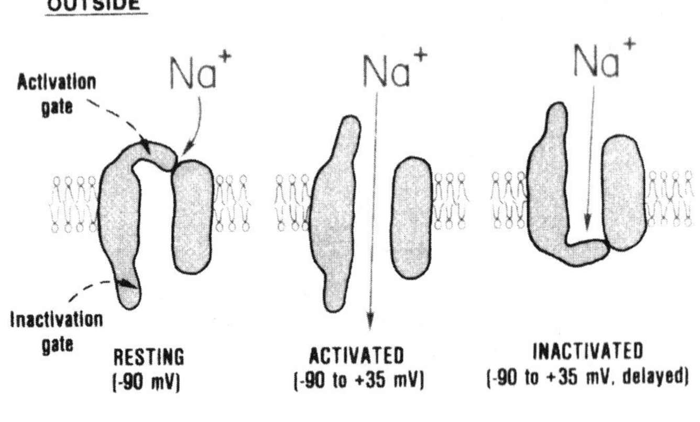

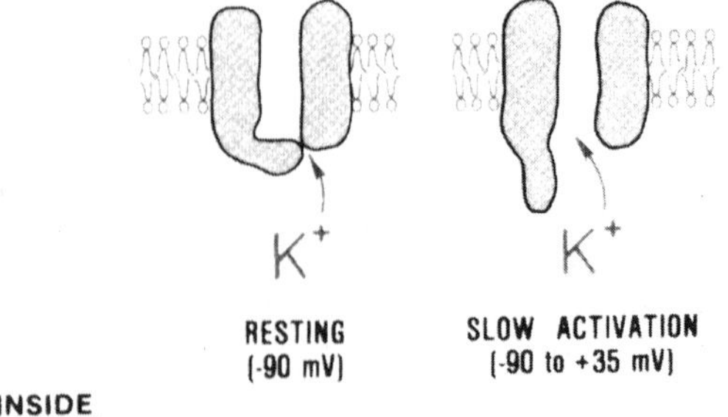

FIG. 14.6. Characteristics of the voltage-gated sodium and potassium channels, showing both activation and inactivation of the sodium channels but activation of the potassium channels only when the membrane potential is changed from the normal negative value to a positive value. (From Guyton AC. Membrane potentials and action potentials. In: Guyton AC, ed. *Textbook of medical physiology.* Philadelphia: Saunders, 1986:101–119, with permission.)

the rate of depolarization such that the threshold potential is not reached and an action potential cannot be propagated. Local anesthetics primarily block Na^+ channels that are in the inactivated state at specific sites located at both the intracellular and extracellular openings of the Na^+ channel (Fig. 14.7) (2). This prevents the Na^+ channel from changing to the resting or open state in response to nerve conduction (Figs. 14.6 and 14.7). Local anesthetic molecules gain access to the Na^+ channel only when they are in their activated or open state. Indeed, for this reason, a resting nerve is less sensitive to local anesthetic–induced conduction blockade than a nerve that is being repeatedly stimulated (see below).

As stated previously, local anesthetics are weak bases that exist in equilibrium between the neutral (B) and protonated charged (BH+) forms. The ratio of ionized B to nonionized BH+ molecules is defined by the Henderson–Hasselbach equation,

$$\frac{(BH+)}{(B)} = 10^{pKa-pH}$$

where pKa is the pH at which the ionized and nonionized concentrations of the drug are equal. Local anesthetics can inhibit Na^+ channels in both the ionized and nonionized forms. However, to reach the sodium channel, the local anesthetic must cross the nerve membrane, and it is primarily the nonionized (base) form of the drug that can do this. How much drug is available to cross the nerve membrane depends on the pKa of the drug and the pH of the fluid surrounding the nerve (Table 14.1) (1–3,31, 40). The pKa of a drug is defined as the pH at which half of the drug exists in the ionic form and the other half in the nonionized form. All local anesthetics are weak bases with a pKa greater than physiologic pH (7.4); indeed, the pKa for most local anesthetics lie between 7.7 and 9.1. Thus, these agents predominantly exist in the ionized (cationic) form in biologic fluids at physiologic pH. The lower the pKa of a drug, the more nonionized drug is available to cross the nerve membrane at physiologic pH. For example, 28% of lidocaine exists in the base (nonionized) form at pH 7.4 compared with only 2.5% for chloroprocaine because the pKa of these drugs are 7.9 and 9.0, respectively (Table 14.1). Acidosis and hypercarbia in the environment in which a local anesthetic is injected will further increase the ionized fraction of local anesthetic. This explains the poor analgesia that results when local anesthetics are infiltrated into infected or ischemic tissues, as might occur when local anesthetics are injected into traumatic lacerations before suturing.

After the local anesthetic is deposited near a nerve, it must diffuse from the nerve's outer surface its center. In large nerve roots, fibers are arranged in concentric layers, fibers that innervate the distal parts of the limb assume the core position, and fibers that innervate the proximal parts of the limb assume the outer portion (Fig. 14.8). Axons that reside in the outer layers of a nerve root will be anesthetized faster than axons in the core. Thus, when local anesthetics are deposited near a nerve trunk (e.g., axillary nerve block; Chapter 21), anesthesia spreads along the limb in a proximal (shoulder) to a distal (hand) direction (Figs. 14.8 and 14.9) (3). Finally, motor (myelinated) nerve fibers typically lay at the periphery of large nerve trunks and fibers, whereas sensory fibers are situated more centrally in the nerve. Thus, because of this anatomic arrangement, motor blockade typically occurs earlier than sensory blockade during peripheral nerve blocks (e.g., axillary or femoral nerve blockade; Chapter 21) (3).

Factors Affecting Neural Blockade

The minimal concentration of local anesthetic necessary to block impulse conduction along a given nerve fiber is called the C_m. Various factors affect C_m including fiber size and degree of myelination of the nerve to be blocked, pH, local calcium concentration, and the rate at which a nerve is stimulated. Each local anesthetic has a unique C_m, which reflects the differing potencies of each drug (Table 14.2). Relatively unmyelinated fibers, such as the Aδ and C fibers carry nociceptive information and have a lower C_m than heavily myelinated fibers that control muscle contrac-

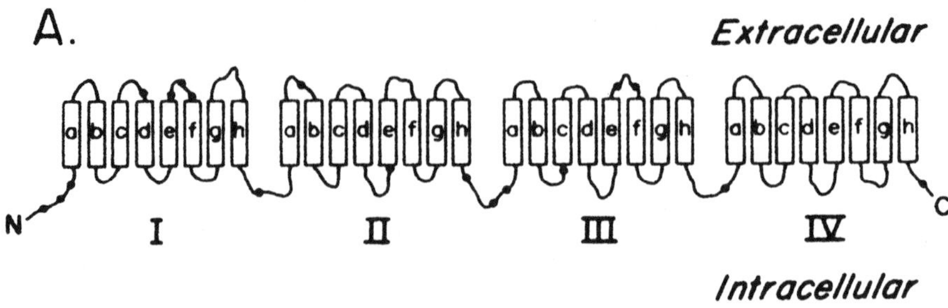

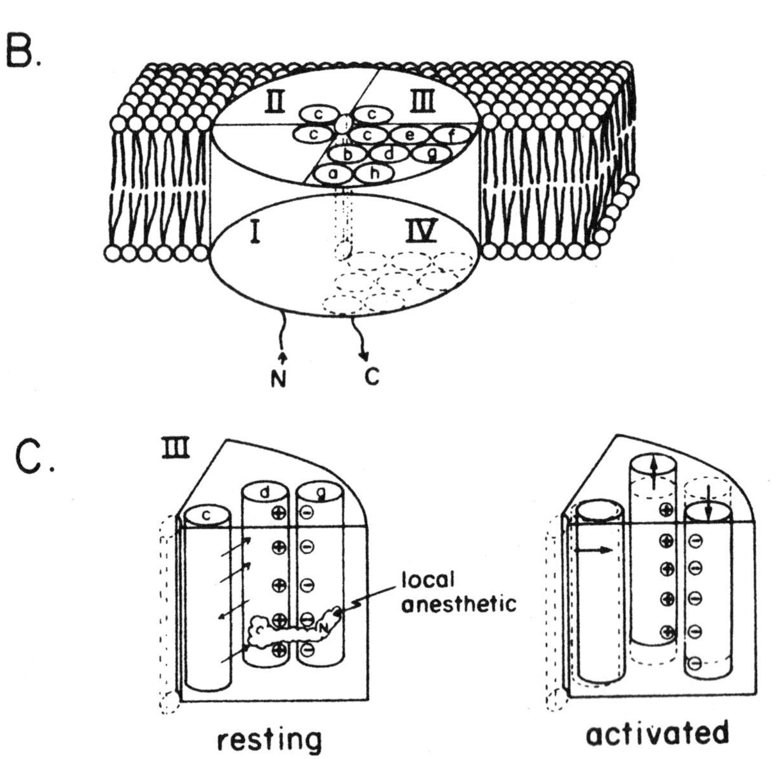

FIG. 14.7. A speculative model for the molecular mechanism of local anesthetic (LA) action. **A:** The primary sequence of the large subunit of the Na+ channel has four repeating domains (*I–IV*), each containing six to eight sequences of amino acids that probably form *a*-helical structures spanning the nerve membrane, denoted by the rectangles lettered *a* through *h*. **B:** Montal et al. have postulated that these helices packed together in approximately fourfold symmetry with the polar edges of the four *c* helices forming the lining of the ion pore, projecting through the center of the complex. For simplicity, only the extracellular (top) and intracellular (bottom, *dashed ellipses*) edges of the helices are shown in **B**. **C:** A stripped-down view of the quadrant III shows the postulated gating mechanism. Helix *d* is coupled to the pore-forming helix *c* and contains a series of basic amino acids that form a strip of positive charges. These charges are stabilized in the low dielectric milieu of the membrane interior by a strip of negative charges counterposed to them on helix *g*. Membrane depolarization activates the channel by pulling the *g* helix in, pushing the *d* helix out, thereby moving the *c* helix to open the channel pore. It has been speculated that a local anesthetic binds at a site near or on the gating helices, as drawn on the resting confrontation, and prevents these conformational changes. (From Butterworth JF, Strichartz GR. Molecular mechanisms of local anesthesia: a review. *Anesthesiology* 1990;72:711–734, with permission.)

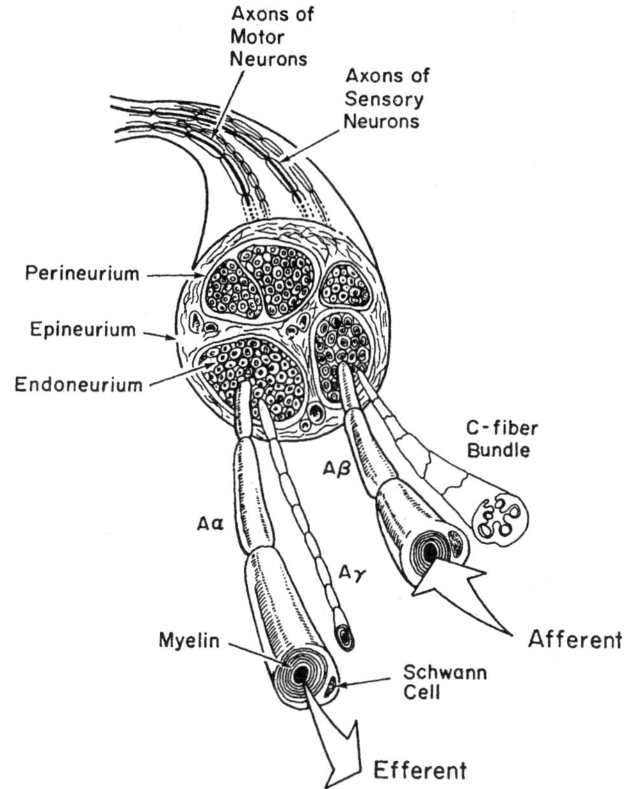

FIG. 14.8. Diagram of a peripheral nerve. The epineurium, with its easily permeable collagen fibers, is oriented along the long axis of the nerve. The perineurium is a discrete layer of cells, whereas the endoneurium is a delicate matrix of connective tissue embedding bundles of axons. Both afferent (sensory) and efferent (motor) axons are shown. Sympathetic efferent axons (not shown) are also present in mixed peripheral nerves. (From Tucker GT, Mather LE. Properties, absorption, and disposition of local anesthetic agents. In: Cousins MJ, Bridenbaugh PO, eds. *Neural blockade in clinical anesthesia and management of pain.* 3rd Edition. Philadelphia: Lippincott–Raven, 1998:55–95, with permission.)

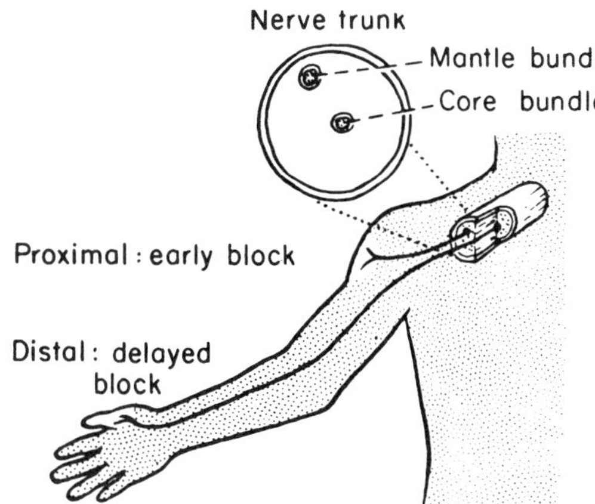

FIG. 14.9. Somatotopic distribution in peripheral nerve. Axons in large nerve trunks (e.g., axillary terminus of brachial plexus) are arranged so that the outer (mantle) fibers innervate the more proximal structures, and the inner (core) fibers, the more distal parts of a limb. With the local anesthetic diffusing inward down the mantle-to-core gradient, the analgesia salient sweeps down the limb in proximal-to-distal fashion. (From Tucker GT, Mather LE. Properties, absorption, and disposition of local anesthetic agents. In: Cousins MJ, Bridenbaugh PO, eds. *Neural blockade in clinical anesthesia and management of pain.* 3rd Edition. Philadelphia: Lippincott–Raven, 1998:55–95, with permission.)

TABLE 14.4. *Classification and characteristics of nerve fibers*

Fiber class	Subclass	Myelin	Function
A	α	++++	Motor proprioception
A	β	+++	Motor proprioception
A	γ	++	Muscle spindle
A	δ	+	Pain, temperature, light touch
B		+	Autonomic, efferents
C	s, C	–	Autonomic functions
C	d, γ, c	–	Pain, damaging temperature

tion (Table 14.4). Because of the lower C_m, less local anesthetic is necessary to block the transmission of pain than is required to produce muscle paralysis. Thus, one can block pain sensation and not block motor function by using dilute concentrations of local anesthetics. This is sometimes referred to as *differential nerve block*. In fact, concentrated local anesthetic solutions (e.g., 2% lidocaine versus 1.0%) increase the quality of sensory blockade only minimally. Conversely, a concentrated local anesthetic increases the incidence of motor blockade and systemic toxicity. To minimize this, concentrated solutions of local anesthetics can be diluted with preservative-free normal saline. Interestingly, when this is done in clinical practice, differential conduction blockade is often misinterpreted by patients as failure of the local anesthetic to produce adequate anesthesia because the patient may continue to perceive proprioception and light touch or have motor function although pain is completely blocked.

Furthermore, because the process of myelinization of the central nervous system (CNS) is not complete until approximately 18 months after birth, C_m may be reduced in younger children (43,44). Thus, newborns and infants may develop complete analgesia and even motor blockade when even dilute concentrations of local anesthetics are used. Finally, preganglionic B fibers of the autonomic nervous system are the most easily blocked of all nerve fibers, despite the fact that they are myelinated.

Other factors also influence the quality and duration of a nerve block, such as the addition of a vasoconstrictor to the anesthetic mixture, the use of mixtures of local anesthetics, and the site of drug administration. Vasoconstrictors, particularly epinephrine, are frequently added to local anesthetic solutions (2,45,46). Epinephrine decreases the rate of vascular absorption of local anesthetic from the site of administration, thereby increasing the time the local anesthetic is in contact with nerve fibers, particularly for drugs that are poorly lipid soluble such as lidocaine. This lengthens the duration of sensory blockade for lidocaine by almost 50% and decreases peak plasma local anesthetic concentrations by a third. More lipid-soluble agents such as bupivacaine, ropivacaine, and etidocaine are less affected by the addition of epinephrine (Table 14.2) (47).

By causing local vasoconstriction, epinephrine also reduces bleeding at sites of injury. Interestingly, epinephrine also improves the intensity of anesthesia and increases the effectiveness of dilute concentration of local anesthetics. Epinephrine-containing solutions should never be injected into areas supplied by end arteries, such as the penis or digits. Injection of an epinephrine-containing solution into these areas may lead to tissue ischemia or necrosis. Epinephrine is often added to local anesthetic solutions in concentrations of 5 to 10 μg/mL (1:200,000 to 1:100,000). Higher epinephrine concentrations offer no advantage in further reducing peak plasma local anesthetic concentrations and may in fact produce adverse systemic hemodynamic effects.

The onset and duration of action of a local anesthetic may also be affected by using mixtures of different local anesthetics and by the site of injection (48). Mixtures of local anesthetics allow the practitioner to combine drugs with rapid onset but short duration of action, such as chloroprocaine or lidocaine, with drugs with longer latencies and duration of action, such as bupivacaine or tetracaine (Table 14.2). The site of an injection also alters the duration of a nerve block based on the nerve's anatomy, differences in the rate of drug absorption, and the amount of drug deposited. Bupivacaine, for example, has a 4-hour duration when injected epidurally but a 10-hour duration when injected into the brachial plexus.

TOXICITY

Local anesthetics are weak drugs with a low margin of safety between the effective dose and the toxic dose. The systemic toxic effects of local anesthetics are determined by the total dose of drug administered, protein binding, the rapidity of absorption into the blood, and the site of injection. Toxicity primarily occurs by unintended intravenous administration or by accumulation of excessive amounts of drug administered either by repeated bolus dosing or by continuous infusion (49–51). This belies the idea of accepted maximal doses of these drugs because even small fractions of the accepted maximal doses of local anesthetics will produce toxic systemic effects if the local anesthetic is injected intra-arterially, intravenously, or into any highly vascular location (52). In general, peak absorption of local anesthetic depends on the site of the block because the site of injection influences the rate of plasma uptake by the vascularity of the tissues. The more vascular the site of injection, the more readily uptake can occur, and the more sudden and intense system toxic effects will be. The order of absorption from highest to lowest is (53–63):

intercostal, intrapleural, intratracheal → caudal/epidural → brachial plexus → distal peripheral → subcutaneous.

Peak local anesthetic blood levels are directly related to the total dosage of drug administered, regardless of the injection site or the volume of solution used (Chapters 20 and 21). Thus, the most dilute concentration of a local anesthetic should be used. Finally, to minimize the risk of accidental intravascular injection of local anesthetics, dosing should always be fractionated. Thus, if 12 mL of local anesthetic is to be injected, it is best to give four divided doses of 3 mL over 4 minutes rather than a single bolus of 12 mL over a minute. Additionally, low-dose epinephrine (5 μg/mL) is often added to local anesthetic solutions to serve as a marker (test dose) of intravascular injection because when administered intravascularly, it produces tachycardia (64). Unfortunately, the effectiveness of epinephrine as a marker of intravascular local anesthetic administration (tachycardia) may be inaccurate in children anesthetized with potent general anesthetics such as halothane (65,66). However, an electrocardiogram will reveal ST segment elevation and T wave changes within 20 seconds of intravenous injection (Fig. 14.10 (66).

Toxicity of local anesthetics can be divided by their manifestations in the cardiovascular system and the CNS. At recommended clinical doses (Table 14.5), local anesthetic plasma levels usually remain well below recognized toxic concentrations. A continuum of toxic effects exists and depends on the rapidity of rise and the total plasma concentration achieved after drug administration. Mild CNS side effects (tinnitus, light-headedness, dizziness, visual and auditory disturbances, restlessness, muscular twitching, fainting) occur at low plasma concentrations and severe side effects (seizures, coma, respiratory arrest) progress to cardiovascular collapse (arrhythmias, hypotension, cardiac arrest) as plasma levels increase.

After unintended intravascular injection, bupivacaine has been implicated in the production of ventricular arrhythmias and cardiovascular collapse unresponsive to resuscitative efforts and not preceded by signs of CNS toxicity. When equipotent local anesthetic doses are utilized, *in vivo* and *in vitro* laboratory studies indicate that bupivacaine may be more cardiotoxic than other local anesthetics such as lidocaine. Several studies in different species (sheep, cats, dogs, humans) have also suggested that the margin of safety between the onset of CNS toxicity and cardiovascular collapse is less for bupivacaine than for lido-

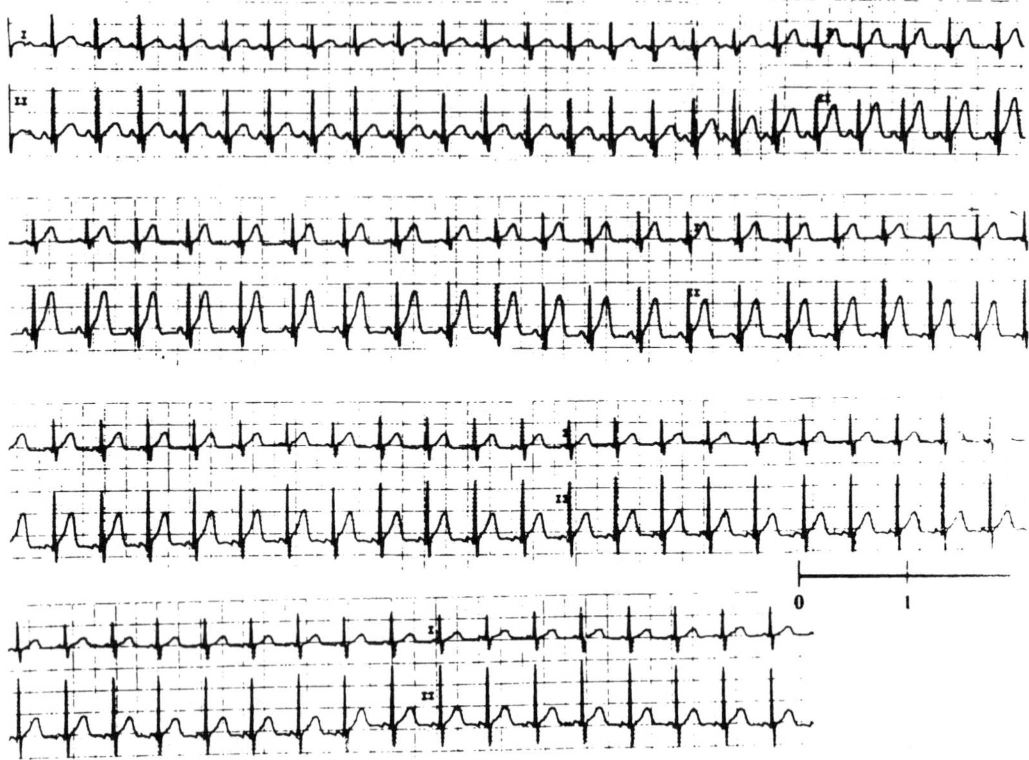

FIG. 14.10. Electrocardiographic changes associated with intravenous injection of local anesthetic and epinephrine 5 to10 μg/mL (1:200,000 to 1:100,000). Note the marked increase in the height of the T wave. (From Fisher QA, Shaffner DH, Yaster M. Detection of intravascular injection of regional anaesthetics in children. *Can J Anaesth* 1997;44:592–598, with permission.)

caine. Bupivacaine has a longer duration of action in both the nerve cell membrane and the entire cardiac conducting system than lidocaine because of its greater affinity for sodium channels. Because bupivacaine dissociates from the cardiac sodium channel more slowly than lidocaine, it slows conduction at lower heart rates (67). Slowing of the action potential in the Purkinje system leads to prolonged QRS and QT duration, which increases the likelihood of re-entrant rhythm that may be either ventricular or supraventricular with aberrant conduction (both wide complex). High-resolution ventricular epicardial mapping in rabbit hearts has provided the first direct evidence of re-entrant ventricular dysrhythmias via prolongation of ventricular effective refractory period and slowed conduction velocity in a dose- and use-dependent manner (68).

In addition to the direct effects of intravenous bupivacaine on the myocardium and conducting system, direct CNS mechanisms of bupivacaine-induced arrhythmias have been identified (69,70). Very small doses of bupivacaine administered intracerebrally or intraventricularly have produced the same cardiac arrhythmias seen with the administration of toxic doses intravenously (71–73). The mechanism for these CNS effects is thought to be blockade of GABA-ergic (γ-aminobutyric acid) neurons, which tonically inhibit the autonomic nervous system. This mechanism is postulated because of evidence of an intraventricularly administered GABA potentiator (midazolam) or peripheral autonomic ganglion blocker (hexamethonium) to terminate bupivacaine-induced dysrhythmias (74).

TABLE 14.5. *Suggested maximal doses of local anesthetics (mg/kg)*[a]

Drug (concentration)[b]	Spinal	Caudal/lumbar epidural	Maximal infusion (hr)	Peripheral[c]	Subcutaneous[c]
Esters					
Chloroprocaine 1.0% infiltration; 2%–3% epidural	NR	10–30[d]	30	8–10[d]	8–10[d]
Procaine	NR	NR		8–10[d]	8–10[d]
Tetracaine (0.5%–1.0%)	0.2–0.6[e]	NR		NR	NR
Amides					
Lidocaine (0.5%–2.0%) 0.5%–1.0% infiltration; 1%–2% peripheral epidural, subcutaneous; 5% spinal	1–2.5	5–7[d]	2–3	5–7[d]	5–7[d]
Bupivacaine (0.0625%–0.5%) 0.125%–0.5% infiltration; 0.25%–0.5% peripheral, epidural, subcutaneous	0.3–0.5	2–3[d]	0.4	2–3[d]	2–3[d]
Ropivacaine (0.2%, 0.5%, 0.75%, 1%) 0.2%–0.5% infiltration, peripheral, epidural, subcutaneous		2.5–4[d]	0.4–0.5	2.5–4[d]	2.5–4[d]
Levobupivacaine (0.25%, 0.5%, 0.75%) 0.125%–0.5% infiltration; 0.25%–0.5% peripheral, epidural, subcutaneous		2.5–4[d]	0.4	2.5–4[d]	2.5–4[d]
Etidocaine (0.5%–1%)	NR	3–4[d]		3–4[d]	3–4[d]
Prilocaine 0.5%–1% infiltration; 1%–1.5% peripheral; 2%–3% epidural	NR	5–7[d,f]		5–7[d,f]	5–7[d,f]

[a]These are suggested safe upper limits; direct intra-arterial or intravenous injection of even a fraction of these doses may result in systemic toxicity or death.
[b]Concentrations are in mg%; for example, a 1% solution contains 10 mg/mL.
[c]Epinephrine should never be added to local anesthetic solution administered in area of an end artery (e.g., penile nerve block).
[d]The higher dose is recommended only with the concomitant use of epinephrine 1:200,000.
[e]The minimal effective dose in children less than 10 kg is 1.5 to 2 mg.
[f]Total adult dose should not exceed 600 mg.
NR, not recommended.

Local anesthetics depress the maximal depolarization rate of the cardiac action potential. Bupivacaine-induced arrhythmias are particularly difficult to treat and include supraventricular tachycardia, atrioventricular heart block, ventricular tachycardia, premature ventricular contractions, and wide QRS complexes. Lidocaine is less toxic because its interactions with the cardiac sodium channel are characterized by "fast in–fast out," whereas for bupivacaine, it is "fast in–slow out." Indeed, one of the most important reasons for the development of ropivacaine and the pure enantiomer L form of bupivacaine (levobupivacaine) is their reduced cardiotoxicity.

The ventricular arrhythmias that precede the cardiovascular collapse seen after bupivacaine toxicity are more responsive to treatment with intravenous bretylium than with lidocaine (75). In anesthetized dogs, 20 mg/kg intravenous bretylium reverses bupivacaine-induced cardiac depression and elevates the threshold for ventricular tachycardia. Maxwell et al. (76) successfully treated two cases of bupivacaine-induced cardiac arrhythmias with intravenous phenytoin (Dilantin).

The plasma concentrations of local anesthetics that produce toxicity are specific for each drug used. Lidocaine (prilocaine and mepivacaine) produces CNS effects at plasma concentrations greater than 5 μg/mL. Conversely, bupivacaine and etidocaine produce toxicity at plasma concentrations of only 2 to 2.5 μg/mL. Hypercarbia may exacerbate CNS toxicity of local anesthetics by increasing cerebral blood flow. This may cause greater local anesthetic delivery to the brain and cause tighter binding of the ionized form of the drug to the sodium channel, prolonging toxic effects. Interestingly, cardiovascular and CNS toxicity has rarely been observed in children after local anesthetic administration. Convulsions have rarely been reported in children, although there are no significant differences in the sensitivity to the toxic effects of local anesthetics between newborn and adult animals. This may be owing to the concomitant use of sedatives, particularly the benzodiazepines, when performing nerve blocks in children. The benzodiazepines raise the seizure threshold and may mask or prevent the development of convulsions.

All local anesthetic agents except cocaine are potent peripheral vasodilators. At toxic concentrations, local anesthetics also directly depress the myocardium and its conduction system (77). These combined effects rapidly produce cardiovascular collapse and cardiac arrest. The treatment of toxic responses to local anesthetics is the same as for any emergency, namely, maintaining a patent *a*irway, ensuring adequate *b*reathing, and supporting *c*irculation (in other words, ABC). Patients who are seizing for even brief periods become acidotic and have ineffective ventilation (78,79). Thus, emergency airway and resuscitative equipment must be available for immediate use before the administration of any local anesthetic agent. Although true for all local anesthetic agents, bupivacaine-induced cardiovascular depression has been particularly difficult to treat and is considered more cardiac toxic than other local anesthetics. Bupivacaine toxicity has been frequently reported after intravenous regional anesthetic techniques (Bier blocks) and during anesthesia for labor and delivery, particularly when 0.75% (7.5 mg/mL) concentrations of bupivacaine were used. Like CNS toxicity, bupivacaine-induced cardiac toxicity occurs more frequently if the patient is hypercarbic, hypoxemic, or acidotic.

NEUROTOXICITY

Neurotoxicity from deposition of local anesthetics into the spinal or epidural space is a rare but devastating event (80,81). The spectrum of this neurotoxicity varies from pain in the lower back, buttocks, and posterior thighs (transient radicular irritation), to motor weakness, to partial or complete paralysis (cauda equina syndrome). Neurotoxicity has been attributed to faulty needle and local anesthetic sterilization techniques, antioxidants and preservatives, spinal microcatheter instrumentation, and the local anesthetics themselves, particularly lidocaine (80–82). When administered intrathecally in a 5% hyperbaric solution to adults in the lithotomy position, 5% hyperbaric lidocaine has been implicated in the development of transient radicular irritation (83,84). More dilute concentrations and alternative local anesthetics such as bupivacaine have not been implicated in this transient neurologic toxicity (85–87). Nevertheless, all local anesthetics have the potential to be neurotoxic, particularly in concentrations and doses larger than those used clinically. In histopathologic, electrophysiologic, behavioral, and neuronal cell models, lidocaine and tetracaine seem to have a greater potential for neurotoxicity than bupivacaine at clinically relevant concentrations.

ALLERGY

Drug allergy (allergic dermatitis, wheezing, hypotension) is uncommon with amide local anesthetics but does occur with the ester family of drugs. The ester-linked local anesthetics are metabolized into a known allergen, paraaminobenzoic acid, which is found in many suntan lotions. Patients with known allergies to suntan lotions may develop allergic dermatitis to ester local anesthetics. In our experience, however, local anesthetic allergy is extremely rare and often mistakenly attributed to adverse experiences occurring during dental anesthesia. In the dentist's office, many patients experience tachycardia and a sense of flushing and dizziness after nerve root infiltration with local anesthetics containing epinephrine. This is usually caused by direct intravascular injection of epinephrine or by rapid systemic absorption and does not mean that the patient is allergic to local anesthetics.

PHARMACOKINETICS

All the ester local anesthetics except cocaine are metabolized by plasma cholinesterase. The rate of hydrolysis is most rapid with chloroprocaine and longest with tetracaine. In fact, the rapidity of hydrolysis and the ubiquity of cholinesterase in the plasma limit the toxicity and the duration of action of ester local anesthetics. Conversely, because the cerebrospinal fluid does not contain cholinesterase, ester local anesthetics deposited in the subarachnoid space will last much longer than if administered in other parts of the body. Neonates and infants as old as 6 months of age have less than half of the adult levels of this plasma enzyme (88). Clearance may therefore be reduced and the effects of ester local anesthetics prolonged. In reality, this is only a theoretic concern. There is more than enough plasma cholinesterase to prevent the accumulation of ester-based local anesthetics, even in the neonate (89).

Amides, however, are metabolized in the liver in a much more complex and slow manner (90). The initial step in the metabolism of the amide local anesthetic is conversion of the amide base to aminocarboxylic acid and a cyclic aniline derivative. Complete metabolism requires further hydrolysis and *N*-dealkylation. This slow and complex metabolism means that sustained elevation of amide local anesthetic levels and systemic toxicity are more likely than with ester local anesthetics. Additionally, the amide local anesthetics are bound by plasma proteins, particularly α_1-acid glycoprotein (91). Alterations in the levels of these proteins may also lead to systemic toxicity. Prilocaine undergoes the most rapid metabolism, the metabolism of lidocaine and mepivacaine is of an intermediate level, and bupivacaine and etidocaine are the slowest to metabolize.

Neonates and young infants (younger than 3 months old) have reduced liver blood flow and immature metabolic degradation pathways. Thus, larger fractions of local anesthetics are unmetabolized and remain active in the plasma of infants, even when administered in doses (0.4 mg/kg per hour) that do not cause accumulation of local anesthetic in older children or adults. (49,92). In fact, in the neonate, more local anesthetic is excreted in the urine unchanged than in older patients. Furthermore, neonates and infants may be at increased risk of the toxic effects of amide local anesthetics because of lower levels of albumin and α_1-acid glycoproteins, which are proteins essential for drug binding (91). This leads to increased concentrations of free drug and potential toxicity, particularly with bupivacaine (93). Conversely, the larger volume of distribution at steady state found in the neonate for these (and other) drugs may confer some clinical protection by lowering plasma drug levels.

The metabolism of the amide local anesthetic prilocaine is unique in that it results in the production of oxidants (e.g., orthotoluidine) that can lead to the development of methemoglobinemia (94). When methemoglobin levels reach 3 to 5 g/dL, patients appear cyanotic and have a reduced oxygen-carrying capacity. This occurs in adults treated with prilocaine in doses greater than 600 mg (94,95). Because premature and full-term infants have decreased levels of methemoglobin reductase, they are more susceptible to developing methemoglobinemia. An additional factor rendering newborns more susceptible to methemoglobinemia is the relative ease by which fetal hemoglobin is oxidized compared with adult hemoglobin. Because of this, prilocaine cannot be recommended for use in neonates. Unfortunately, this may limit the use of an exciting new topical local anesthetic, lidocaine-prilocaine cream [EMLA (eutectic mixture of local anesthetics)] in the newborn because it contains prilocaine (24,96,97). Methemoglobinemia affects oxygen transport and can produce tissue hypoxia. Symptomatic patients can be treated with intravenous 1 to 2 mg/kg methylene blue administered over 5 minutes.

Finholt et al. (98) found that the volume of distribution, clearance, and elimination half-life of an intravenous 1- to 2-mg/kg bolus of lidocaine used to facilitate tracheal intubation or to treat arrhythmias in children older than 6 months are similar to those in adults (98). They recommend that lidocaine doses need not be altered based on age alone when lidocaine is administered intravenously. However, the elimination half-life of intravenously administered lidocaine in infants younger than 6 months is prolonged.

The intravenous administration of lidocaine even at recommended doses in children with right-to-left intracardiac shunts may produce systemic toxicity (99). Normally, approximately 60% to 80% of an intravenous lidocaine bolus is absorbed on the first pass through the lungs, then subsequently released over time (100). Indeed, the lungs are capable of extracting other local anesthetics, such as bupivacaine and prilocaine (101). In patients with right-to-left intracardiac shunts, venous blood enters the systemic circulation directly through the intracardiac defect, bypassing the lungs. Peak arterial concentrations of lidocaine would be expected to be higher and occur more rapidly. In fact, in lambs with right-to-left intracardiac shunts, lidocaine levels were double those of normal controls (102). These findings, however, were not duplicated in a human trial (103).

Uses of Local Anesthesia

As discussed in the introduction, local anesthetics are used primarily to treat pain as part of regional anesthetic techniques. These include topical application, local infiltration, peripheral nerve blocks, intravenous regional anesthesia (Bier blocks), epidural anesthesia, and spinal anesthesia. Because of differences in lipid solubility, protein binding, and spreading properties, not all local anesthetics can be used in all regional anesthetic techniques. Appropriate uses of local anesthetic agents for differing applications are listed in Table 14.6. These drugs are used less commonly to treat cardiac arrhythmias and increased intracranial pressure. Except for subcutaneous and topical routes of administration, regional anesthetic techniques are

TABLE 14.6. *Use of local anesthesia to produce regional anesthesia*

Classification	Topical	Local infiltration	Peripheral nerve block	Intravenous regional (Bier)	Epidural	Spinal
Esters						
Procaine	No	Yes	Yes	No	No	No
Chloroprocaine	No	Yes	Yes	Yes	Yes	No
Tetracaine	Yes	No	No	No	No	Yes
Cocaine	Yes	No	No	No	No	No
Benzocaine	Yes	No	No	No	No	No
Amides						
Lidocaine	Yes	Yes	Yes	Yes	Yes	Yes
Mepivacaine	No	Yes	Yes	No	Yes	No
Bupivacaine	No	Yes	Yes	No	Yes	Yes
Ropivacaine	No	Yes	Yes	No	Yes	Yes
Etidocaine	No	Yes	Yes	No	Yes	No
Prilocaine	No	Yes	Yes	Yes	No	No
Dibucaine	Yes	No	No	No	No	No

discussed elsewhere in this book (Chapters 20 and 21).

CHOICE OF LOCAL ANESTHETIC

The decision of which local anesthetic to use depends on multiple factors including route of administration (e.g., subcutaneous infiltration, peripheral nerve blockade, spinal or epidural blockade), onset time, duration of action, presence of a toxic metabolite, and/or presence of renal or liver disease. Where and how neural blockade is performed plays a very important role in the decision concerning local anesthetic use. Some local anesthetics such as dibucaine are effective only when applied topically; others are not. Similarly, some local anesthetics can be used intrathecally (e.g., tetracaine), and others cannot. Rarely does onset time influence this decision; most local anesthetics have a very rapid onset time, and onset time can be shortened in all local anesthetics by the addition of bicarbonate. In most clinical situations, the single most important issue in choosing a local anesthetic agent is the drug's duration of action, which can be short (approximately 30 minutes), intermediate (approximately 1 hour), or long (>90 minutes). Short-, intermediate-, and long-acting local anesthetics are differentiated in Table 14.2.

Local Ester Anesthetics

The ester-linked local anesthetics cocaine, procaine, tetracaine, and chloroprocaine are hydrolyzed at varying rates by plasma cholinesterase. All but cocaine are derivatives of paraaminobenzoic acid.

Cocaine

Cocaine is derived from the leaves of *Erythroxylon coca*, which is indigenous to Peru and Bolivia. The leaves have been chewed by the native population for centuries because of the ability of cocaine to produce a feeling of well-being and euphoria and to increase stamina to perform muscular work. It is a drug of abuse and can cause addiction. Cocaine stimulates the CNS and blocks the reuptake of catecholamines both centrally and peripherally. At low doses, it produces a sense of euphoria and mental alertness; at higher doses, it can produce convulsions, medullary depression, and respiratory failure. Cardiovascularly, it causes tachycardia, hypertension, and vasoconstriction. Indeed, it is the only local anesthetic that causes vasoconstriction; all others produce vasodilation. Toxic overdose can result in myocardial infarction, pulmonary edema, ventricular fibrillation, and death. Because of its vasoconstrictive properties, cocaine is commonly used to produce topical anesthesia on mucosal surfaces such as the mouth, nose, and throat.

Procaine and Chloroprocaine

Procaine (Novocaine) has a very short duration of action and a high pKa (8.9) and is highly ionized at physiologic pH. The plasma half-life is believed to be approximately 20 seconds. Hence, there is very little toxicity associated with this agent. Because of extremely limited protein binding, it has a short duration of action. Additionally, it has poor spreading and penetrating ability and is therefore rarely used in current practice. It does have antiarrhythmic properties and a congener, procainamide, has been developed as an effective oral antiarrhythmic agent. Chloroprocaine (Nesacaine) is a halogenated derivative of procaine that has pharmacologic properties similar to those of the parent molecule. It has a pKa of 9 and a rapid onset and short duration of action. It is available as a 1%, 2%, and 3% solution and can be used for infiltration anesthesia, peripheral nerve blockade, and epidural anesthesia. Onset time is rapid (5 to 10 minutes); it lasts for 45 minutes without epinephrine and 70 to 90 minutes with epinephrine. Systemic toxicity is very rare. Neurotoxicity has been reported with its intrathecal use and may be related to sodium bisulfite and methylparaben, antioxidants, and preservatives that were added to maintain its shelf life. Chloroprocaine containing the antioxidant disodium ethylenediaminetetraacetic acid has also been associated with transient, severe back pain after epidural administration (104). Nevertheless, because it is so rapidly metabolized by plasma cholinesterase, Tobias and O'Dell (105) reported its use in continuous epidural analgesia and anesthesia in neonates, a population susceptible to amide local anesthetic toxicity. Using a 3% chloroprocaine solution, these authors administered 1 to 1.5 mL/kg as an epidural bolus, followed by a continuous infusion of 1.5 mL/kg per hour.

Tetracaine

Tetracaine is a potent, long-acting ester local anesthetic primarily used in spinal anesthesia. It has a slow onset, very short plasma half-life, and long duration of action. Systemic toxicity is reported to be considerably higher than with procaine and 2-chloroprocaine, so it must be used cautiously when administered in peripheral nerve blocks (eyes) and topically on mucosal surfaces during endoscopy. When administered intrathecally, the adult dose varies from 5 to 20 mg and is mixed with either dextrose (hyperbaric), distilled water (hypobaric), or cerebrospinal fluid (isobaric). The baricity of the solution affects its spread. Because there is almost no cholinesterase in the cerebrospinal fluid, tetracaine will produce anesthesia lasting from 90 minutes to 4 hours depending on whether epinephrine is added to the solution. In children, the dose of spinal tetracaine is 0.2 to 0.4 mg/kg (106). In neonates, higher doses are required; typically, doses of 0.5 to 1.2 mg/kg are required to produce adequate anesthesia for surgery (107,108).

Benzocaine

Benzocaine is an ester local anesthetic with a pKa of 3.5 and pH in preparation between 4.5 and 6.0. It has a slow onset, short duration, and moderate toxicity. Benzocaine is a secondary amine, in contrast to all the other clinically used local anesthetics, which are tertiary amines. This limits the ability of the agent to pass through neural membranes. Consequently, its clinical use is limited to topical anesthesia. The estimated toxic dose is in the 200- to 300-mg range. Excessive use of benzocaine in children has been associated with methemoglobinemia.

Amide Local Anesthetics

Lidocaine

Lidocaine is the most commonly administered local anesthetic; it is effective when administered by infiltration and topical application and peripheral nerve, spinal, and epidural blockade. Lidocaine is rapidly active and lasts for 60 to 75 minutes when administered without epinephrine and 90 to 120 minutes when administered with epinephrine. The upper safe limit for lidocaine without epinephrine is 5 mg/kg (200 to 400 mg in adults) and 7 mg/kg (500 mg in adults) with epinephrine. Toxic symptoms occur when blood concentrations are greater than 5 μg/mL. Finally, lidocaine is the only local anesthetic that is used intravenously. Intravenous lidocaine is commonly used as an antiarrhythmic and as method of treating neuropathic pain. Neuropathic pain and the therapies for it are discussed in greater detail in Chapters 13 and 34 (109,110). In short, lidocaine is beneficial in the treatment of neuropathic pain states by blocking the conduction of sodium channels in peripheral and central neurons and thereby dampening both peripheral nociceptor sensitization and, ultimately, CNS hyperexcitability (109,110). An oral capsule form of lidocaine, mexiletine (Mexitil) is available and is commonly used in the treatment of arrhythmias and neuropathic pain that is alleviated by intravenous lidocaine (111,112). Finally, topical lidocaine, available as a patch (Lidoderm), is a promising new method of treating neuropathic pain and has been recently approved for this use by the U.S. Food and Drug Administration (113–115).

Bupivacaine

Bupivacaine is approximately four times more potent than lidocaine and is approximately twice as long acting. It has a slow onset of action, approximately 10 to 20 minutes, but has a duration of action of approximately 400 minutes. It is most commonly used in epidural, spinal, and nerve block anesthesia. Epinephrine does not reliably affect the duration of neural blockade but may decrease plasma uptake and help identify intravascular injection. Alkalinization with bicarbonate is equivocal and may result in precipitation. The upper safe limit for bupivacaine without epinephrine is 2 mg/kg (150 mg in adults) and 3 mg/kg (200 mg in adults) with epinephrine. The use of bupivacaine for major conduction block is associated with long-duration anesthesia, occasionally extending as long as 24 hours. As discussed in the section on toxicity above, it is the most toxic of all the local anesthetics and has been associated with considerable morbidity and mortality.

Ropivacaine and Levobupivacaine

These new local anesthetics are stereoselective enantiomers that are presumed to be less toxic than racemic mixtures. Both are equally potent with bupivacaine and have similar onset, duration, and qualities of analgesia. Of the two, ropivacaine has been more extensively studied in both children and adults (116–118). At lower concentrations, ropivacaine may produce less motor block than bupivacaine when administered at doses that produce comparable analgesia.

Subcutaneous Injection

Subcutaneous infiltration of the skin with a local anesthetic solution is the most commonly performed regional (local) anesthetic technique in pediatric practice. Local anesthetics, particularly lidocaine, are commonly injected subcutaneously before the performance of many painful medical and surgical procedures to minimize procedure-related pain. When used in this way, the local anesthetic agent blocks nerve conduction at the most terminal branches of the sensory nerves (Chapter 36).

Local anesthetic infiltration of traumatic lacerations requires special attention. Commonly, the wound is dirty and requires extensive scrubbing and irrigation. Should the local anesthetic be administered before cleansing, which would make cleansing painless, or after, to avoid introducing dirt and bacteria into the surrounding tissue? It is our practice to inject the local anesthetic through intact skin adjacent to the wound before the wound is cleaned. Alternatively, we block the peripheral nerve supplying the injured area more proximally because smaller amounts of local anesthetic are used, requiring fewer injections.

Because local anesthetics are manufactured at a pH of 4 to 5 and are administered by injection, they are in and of themselves painful. This pain can be minimized by using buffered anesthetic solutions and small needles (29,119,120). Buffering a local anesthetic solution, such as lidocaine, with a small amount of sodium bicarbonate (9 mL lidocaine combined with 1 mL bicarbonate, a 10:1 solution, or 1 mL bicarbonate with 29 mL bupivacaine) may make the injection painless and hasten the onset of analgesia (121). It may also shorten the duration of action (122). Adding too much bicarbonate will cause the local anesthetic to become less soluble and will precipitate from solution. Local anesthetics are not manufactured with buffer because the buffering affects their shelf life. Obviously, using small-gauge needles will affect the amount of pain produced when infiltrating local anesthetics. We use 26- to 30-gauge needles and inject the local anesthetic as soon as the needle punctures the skin. We do not aspirate first. Rather, we inject local anesthetics as the needle is advanced forward. Aspirating first is unnecessary because the amount of local anesthetic injected at each location is so small (0.1 to 0.2 mL) that even an intravascular injection would be inconsequential. Finally, the pain of drug administration can be further limited by using warm solutions that are injected slowly (123–125).

Lidocaine-Prilocaine Cream (EMLA)

A topical emulsion of lidocaine and prilocaine produces complete anesthesia of intact skin after application (24,126,127). Unfortunately, for best effect, this cream must be applied and covered with an occlusive dressing (such as clear plastic wrap) for 60 minutes before a procedure is performed. This limits its use unless the site is prepared well in advance of anticipated use. Furthermore, if the procedure is a venipuncture, multiple sites must be prepared in case one's initial attempt is unsuccessful. Unfortunately, the effectiveness of lidocaine-prilocaine cream (as with all other methods) for reducing pain depends on who makes the assessment. Soliman et al. (128) studied the effectiveness of EMLA compared with injected lidocaine for reducing the pain associated with venipuncture. Both an observer and a physician performing the procedure judged pain relief virtually complete in both groups. The children involved in the study were not as sanguine and were equally dissatisfied with both methods, particularly if the needle used for venipuncture was visible to them. Thus, despite the fact that two observers believed that the child was pain free, the child's cooperation with venipuncture did not improve. Therefore, it is not clear whether the delay involved in the use of this cream (60-minute wait for effect) is justified. Conversely, it may be more effective in children accustomed to frequent medical procedures (e.g., oncology patients) or for procedures in which the child cannot see the needle, such as lumbar puncture or bone marrow aspiration.

TAC Solution

For closure of lacerations, topical local anesthetics such as TAC [0.5% tetracaine, 1:2,000 adrenaline (epinephrine), and 11.8% cocaine) solution maybe used as a needleless alternative to local infiltration. TAC solution is an innovative method of topical anesthesia that avoids the use of a local anesthetic injection altogether (129–135). TAC is a local anesthetic solution applied directly to a laceration. The clear solution is made in the hospital pharmacy by mixing 60 mL 2% tetracaine with 120 mL 1:1,000 epinephrine and 28.32 g of cocaine, with normal saline added to bring the total volume to 240 mL. Because TAC is applied topically, it eliminates the need for an injection into the dirty wound edge and achieves anesthesia for both wound cleaning and suturing. It is most effective when used on lacerations of the face and scalp and less effective when used on extremity lacerations.

Because TAC contains epinephrine and cocaine, the only local anesthetic that is always a vasoconstrictor, it cannot be used in areas of the body supplied by end arteries, such as the digits, pinna, or nose. Furthermore, because of its cocaine content, inadvertent ingestion of the solution by patients can be catastrophic. Similarly, because cocaine is readily absorbed through mucosal surfaces, the use of TAC solution near mucous membranes should be avoided. Seizures have been reported even in children in whom the solution was applied properly to wound edges without a mucosal surface. Unfortunately, cocaine cannot be eliminated from the solution because solutions containing only tetracaine and epinephrine are much less effective in producing analgesia than solutions also containing cocaine (129,130).

Before administration, a history of allergy to paraaminobenzoic acid–containing suntan lotion or to local anesthetics should be obtained because both tetracaine and cocaine are ester local anesthetic agents. Typically, a 3-mL solution of TAC provides analgesia for a laceration approximately 3 cm long. Half of the solution is instilled directly into the wound and the other half is applied to a gauze pad held on the wound surface for 10 to 15 minutes. Failure to keep the TAC solution in contact with the wound surface for 10 to 15 minutes accounts for most inadequate blocks. In the 10% to 25% of patients in whom TAC is not completely effective, the subsequent injection of lidocaine is much less painful. Use of this topical preparation also avoids the swelling and distortion of the wound edges that may be caused by injected local anesthetic. Finally, gloves must be worn by all personnel coming into contact with TAC solution because it can cause vasoconstriction even in intact skin.

Iontophoresis

Iontophoresis is a method of transdermal administration of ionizable drugs in which the electrically charged components are propelled through the skin by an external electric field. Several drugs, such as lidocaine, corticosteroids, morphine, and fentanyl, can be delivered iontophoretically (136–139). This technique is not completely painless, and some younger children object to its use because of the tingling sensation of the electric current.

REFERENCES

1. Butterworth JF, Strichartz GR. Molecular mechanisms of local anesthesia: a review. *Anesthesiology* 1990;72: 711–734.
2. Strichartz GR. Neural physiology and local anesthetic action. In: Cousins MJ, Bridenbaugh PO, eds. *Neural blockade in clinical anesthesia and management of pain*. 3rd Edition. Philadelphia: Lippincott–Raven, 1998:35–54.
3. Tucker GT, Mather LE. Properties, absorption, and disposition of local anesthetic agents. In: Cousins MJ, Bridenbaugh PO, eds. *Neural blockade in clinical anesthesia and management of pain*. 3rd Edition. Philadelphia: Lippincott–Raven, 1998:55–95.
4. Dalens B. *Regional anesthesia in infants, children, and adolescents*. Baltimore: Williams & Wilkins, 1995.
5. Stoelting RK. Local anesthetics. In: *Pharmacology and physiology in anesthetic practice*, 3rd Edition. Philadelphia: Lippincott–Raven, 1999:158–181.
6. Catterall WA, Mackie K. Local anesthetics. In: Hardman JG, Limbird LE, eds. *Goodman and Gilman's the pharmacological basis of therapeutics*. New York: McGraw-Hill, 1996:331–348.
7. Tetzlaff JE. The pharmacology of local anesthetics. *Anesthesiol Clin North Am* 2000;18:217–33.
8. Wilder RT. Local anesthetics for the pediatric patient. *Pediatr Clin North Am* 2000;47:545–558.
9. Brown TC, Eyres RL, McDougall RJ. Local and regional anaesthesia in children. *Br J Anaesth* 1999;83: 65–77.
10. Wood M. Local anesthetic agents. In: Wood AJ, Wood M, eds. *Drugs and anesthesia: pharmacology for anesthesiologists*. Baltimore: Williams & Wilkins, 1990:319–346.
11. Yaster M, Maxwell LG. Pediatric regional anesthesia. *Anesthesiology* 1989;70:324–338.
12. Dalens B. Regional anesthesia in children. *Anesth Analg* 1989;68:654–672.
13. Rice LJ. Regional anesthesia and analgesia. In: Motoyama EK, Davis PJ, eds. *Anesthesia for infants and children*. St. Louis: Mosby Year Book, 1996:403–444.
14. Ross AK, Eck JB, Tobias JD. Pediatric regional anesthesia: beyond the caudal. *Anesth Analg* 2000;91: 16–26.
15. Sethna N. Regional anesthesia and analgesia. *Semin Perinatol* 1998;22:380–389.
16. Broadman LM, Rice LJ. Neural blockade for pediatric surgery. In: Cousins MJ, Bridenbaugh PO, eds. *Neural blockade in clinical anesthesia and management of pain*. 3rd Edition. Philadelphia: Lippincott–Raven, 1998:615–638.
17. Tobias JD. Anaesthetic management of the child with myotonic dystrophy: epidural anaesthesia as an alternative to general anaesthesia. *Paediatr Anaesth* 1995; 5:335–338.
18. Tobias JD, Lowe S, O'Dell N, et al. Continuous regional anaesthesia in infants. *Can J Anaesth* 1993;40: 1065–1068.
19. Yaster M, Tobin JR, Billett C, et al. Epidural analgesia in the management of severe vaso-occlusive sickle cell crisis. *Pediatrics* 1994;93:310–315.
20. Tobias JD. Continuous femoral nerve block to provide analgesia following femur fracture in a paediatric ICU population. *Anaesth Intensive Care* 1994;22:616–618.
21. Tobias JD, Haun SE, Helfaer M, et al. Use of continuous caudal block to relieve lower-extremity ischemia caused by vasculitis in a child with meningococcemia. *J Pediatr* 1989;115:1019–1021.
22. Anderson CT, Berde CB, Sethna NF, et al. Meningococcal purpura fulminans: treatment of vascular insufficiency in a 2-yr-old child with lumbar epidural sympathetic blockade. *Anesthesiology* 1989;71:463–464.
23. Maxwell LG, Yaster M, Wetzel RC, et al. Penile nerve block for newborn circumcision. *Obstet Gynecol* 1987; 70:415–419.
24. Taddio A, Ohlsson A, Einarson TR, et al. A systematic review of lidocaine-prilocaine cream (EMLA) in the treatment of acute pain in neonates. *Pediatrics* 1998; 101E1.
25. Stang HJ, Snellman LW, Condon LM, et al. Beyond dorsal penile nerve block: a more humane circumcision. *Pediatrics* 1997;100:E3.
26. Zeltzer LK, Jay SM, Fisher DM. The management of pain associated with pediatric procedures. *Pediatr Clin North Am* 1989;36:941–964.
27. McGrath PA, DeVeber LL. Helping children cope with painful procedures. *Am J Nurs* 1986;86:1278–1279.
28. McGrath PA, de Veber LL. The management of acute pain evoked by medical procedures in children with cancer. *J Pain Symptom Manage* 1986;1:145–150.
29. Yaster M, Krane EJ, Kaplan RF, et al. *Pediatric pain management and sedation handbook*. St. Louis: Mosby Year Book, 1997.
30. McGrath PJ, Unruh A. Medically caused pain. In: McGrath PJ, Unruh A, eds. *Pain in children and adolescents*. Amsterdam: Elsevier, 1987:133–142.
31. Covino BG, Wildsmith JA. Clinical pharmacology of local anesthetic agents. In: Cousins MJ, Bridenbaugh PO, eds. *Neural blockade in clinical anesthesia and management of pain*. 3rd Edition. Philadelphia: Lippincott–Raven, 1998:97–128.
32. Sarton E, Olofsen E, Romberg R, et al. Sex differences in morphine analgesia: an experimental study in healthy volunteers. *Anesthesiology* 2000;93:1245–1254.
33. Groen K, Mantel M, Zeijlmans PW, et al. Pharmacokinetics of the enantiomers of bupivacaine and mepivacaine after epidural administration of the racemates. *Anesth Analg* 1998;86:361–366.
34. Burm AG, Cohen IM, van Kleef JW, et al. Pharmacokinetics of the enantiomers of mepivacaine after intravenous administration of the racemate in volunteers. *Anesth Analg* 1997;84:85–89.

35. Arthur GR, Feldman HS, Covino BG. Comparative pharmacokinetics of bupivacaine and ropivacaine, a new amide local anesthetic. *Anesth Analg* 1988;67: 1053–1058.
36. Concepcion M, Arthur GR, Steele SM, et al. A new local anesthetic, ropivacaine. Its epidural effects in humans. *Anesth Analg* 1990;70:80–85.
37. Hille B. Introduction. In: Hille B, ed. *Ionic channels of excitable membranes*. Sunderland: Sinauer Associates, 1992:1–20.
38. Guyton AC. Membrane potentials and action potentials. In: Guyton AC, ed. *Textbook of medical physiology*. Philadelphia: Saunders, 1986:101–119.
39. Hille B. Mechanism of block. In: Hille B, ed. *Ionic channels of excitable membranes*. Sunderland: Sinauer Associates, 1992:390–422.
40. Bokesch PM, Raymond SA, Strichartz GR. Dependence of lidocaine potency on pH and PCO2. *Anesth Analg* 1987;66:9–17.
41. Hille B. Local anesthetics: hydrophilic and hydrophobic pathways for the drug-receptor reaction. *J Gen Physiol* 1977;69:497–515.
42. Hille B. The pH-dependent rate of action of local anesthetics on the node of Ranvier. *J Gen Physiol* 1977;69: 475–496.
43. Anand KJ, Hickey PR. Pain and its effects in the human neonate and fetus. *N Engl J Med* 1987;317: 1321–1329.
44. Fitzgerald M, Anand KJ. Developmental neuroanatomy and neurophysiology of pain. In: Schechter NL, Berde CB, Yaster M, eds. *Pain in infants, children, and adolescents*. Baltimore, MD: Williams & Wilkins, 1993:11–32.
45. Warner MA, Kunkel SE, Offord KO, et al. The effects of age, epinephrine, and operative site on duration of caudal analgesia in pediatric patients. *Anesth Analg* 1987;66:995–998.
46. Mather LE, Tucker GT, Murphy TM, et al. The effects of adding adrenaline to etidocaine and lignocaine in extradural anaesthesia II: pharmacokinetics. *Br J Anaesth* 1976;48:989–994.
47. Hurley RJ, Feldman HS, Latka C, et al. The effects of epinephrine on the anesthetic and hemodynamic properties of ropivacaine and bupivacaine after epidural administration in the dog. *Reg Anesth* 1991;16:303–308.
48. Seow LT, Lips FJ, Cousins MJ, et al. Lidocaine and bupivacaine mixtures for epidural blockade. *Anesthesiology* 1982;56:177–183.
49. Berde CB. Convulsions associated with pediatric regional anesthesia. *Anesth Analg* 1992;75:164–166.
50. Agarwal R, Gutlove DP, Lockhart CH. Seizures occurring in pediatric patients receiving continuous infusion of bupivacaine . *Anesth Analg* 1992;75:284–286.
51. McCloskey JJ, Haun SE, Deshpande JK. Bupivacaine toxicity secondary to continuous caudal epidural infusion in children . *Anesth Analg* 1992;75:287–290.
52. Moore DC, Bridenbaugh LD, Thompson GE, et al. Factors determining dosages of amide-type local anesthetic drugs. *Anesthesiology* 1977;47:263–268.
53. Desparmet J, Meistelman C, Barre J, et al. Continuous epidural infusion of bupivacaine for postoperative pain relief in children. *Anesthesiology* 1987;67:108–110.
54. Ecoffey C, Desparmet J, Berdeaux A, et al. Pharmacokinetics of lignocaine in children following caudal anaesthesia. *Br J Anaesth* 1984;56:1399–1402.
55. Ecoffey C, Desparmet J, Maury M, et al. Bupivacaine in children: pharmacokinetics following caudal anesthesia. *Anesthesiology* 1985;63:447–448.
56. Eyres RL, Bishop W, Oppenheim RC, et al. Plasma lignocaine concentrations following topical laryngeal application. *Anaesth Intensive Care* 1983;11:23–26.
57. Eyres RL, Kidd J, Oppenheim R, Brown TC. Local anaesthetic plasma levels in children. *Anaesth Intensive Care* 1978;6:243–247.
58. Tucker GT, Mather LE. Pharmacology of local anaesthetic agents. Pharmacokinetics of local anaesthetic agents. *Br J Anaesth* 1975;47[Suppl]:213–224.
59. Stayer SA, Pasquariello CA, Schwartz RE, et al. The safety of continuous pleural lignocaine after thoracotomy in children and adolescents. *Paediatr Anaesth* 1995;5:307–310.
60. Campbell RJ, Ilett KF, Dusci L. Plasma bupivacaine concentrations after axillary block in children. *Anaesth Intensive Care* 1986;14:343–346.
61. Tucker GT, Mather LE. Clinical pharmacokinetics of local anaesthetics. *Clin Pharmacokinet* 1979;4:241–278.
62. Smith T, Moratin P, Wulf H. Smaller children have greater bupivacaine plasma concentrations after ilioinguinal block. *Br J Anaesth* 1996;76:452–455.
63. Rothstein P, Arthur GR, Feldman HS, et al. Bupivacaine for intercostal nerve blocks in children: blood concentrations and pharmacokinetics. *Anesth Analg* 1986;65:625–632.
64. Moore DC, Batra MS. The components of an effective test dose prior to epidural block. *Anesthesiology* 1981; 55:693–696.
65. Desparmet J, Mateo J, Ecoffey C, et al. Efficacy of an epidural test dose in children anesthetized with halothane. *Anesthesiology* 1990;72:249–251.
66. Fisher QA, Shaffner DH, Yaster M. Detection of intravascular injection of regional anaesthetics in children. *Can J Anaesth* 1997;44:592–598.
67. Clarkson CW, Hondeghem LM. Mechanism for bupivacaine depression of cardiac conduction: fast block of sodium channels during the action potential with slow recovery from block during diastole. *Anesthesiology* 1985;62:396–405.
68. de La Coussaye JE, Brugada J, Allessie MA. Electrophysiologic and arrhythmogenic effects of bupivacaine. A study with high-resolution ventricular epicardial mapping in rabbit hearts. *Anesthesiology* 1992;77:132–141.
69. Riquelme CM, Bell B, Edwards J, et al. The influence of age on the cardiovascular toxicity of intravenous bupivacaine in young dogs. *Anaesth Intensive Care* 1987;15:436–439.
70. Moller R, Covino BG. Cardiac electrophysiologic properties of bupivacaine and lidocaine compared with those of ropivacaine, a new amide local anesthetic. *Anesthesiology* 1990;72:322–329.
71. Heavner JE. Cardiac dysrhythmias induced by infusion of local anesthetics into the lateral cerebral ventricle of cats. *Anesth Analg* 1986;65:133–138.
72. Thomas RD, Behbehani MM, Coyle DE, et al. Cardiovascular toxicity of local anesthetics: an alternative hypothesis. *Anesth Analg* 1986;65:444–450.
73. Bernards CM, Artru AA. Effect of intracerebroventricular picrotoxin and muscimol on intravenous bupivacaine toxicity. Evidence supporting central nervous system involvement in bupivacaine cardiovascular toxicity. *Anesthesiology* 1993;78:902–910.

74. Bernards CM, Artu AA. Hexamethonium and midazolam terminate dysrhythmias and hypertension caused by intracerebroventricular bupivacaine in rabbits. *Anesthesiology* 1991;74:89–96.
75. Kasten GW, Martin ST. Bupivacaine cardiovascular toxicity: comparison of treatment with bretylium and lidocaine. *Anesth Analg* 1985;64:911–916.
76. Maxwell LG, Martin LD, Yaster M. Bupivacaine-induced cardiac toxicity in neonates: successful treatment with intravenous phenytoin. *Anesthesiology* 1994;80:682–686.
77. Naguib M, Magboul MM, Samarkandi AH, et al. Adverse effects and drug interactions associated with local and regional anaesthesia. *Drug Saf* 1998;18:221–250.
78. Moore DC, Crawford RD, Scurlock JE. Severe hypoxia and acidosis following local anesthetic-induced convulsions. *Anesthesiology* 1980;53:259–260.
79. Moore DC, Bonica JJ. Convulsions and ventricular tachycardia from bupivacaine with epinephrine: successful resuscitation—congratulations! *Anesth Analg* 1985;64:844–846.
80. Horlocker TT. Complications of spinal and epidural anesthesia. *Anesthesiol Clin North Am* 2000;18: 461–485.
81. Horlocker TT, McGregor DG, Matsushige DK, et al. A retrospective review of 4767 consecutive spinal anesthetics: central nervous system complications. Perioperative Outcomes Group. *Anesth Analg* 1997;84:578–584.
82. Horlocker TT, McGregor DG, Matsushige DK, et al. Neurologic complications of 603 consecutive continuous spinal anesthetics using macrocatheter and microcatheter techniques. Perioperative Outcomes Group. *Anesth Analg* 1997;84:1063–1070.
83. Schneider M, Ettlin T, Kaufmann M, et al. Transient neurologic toxicity after hyperbaric subarachnoid anesthesia with 5% lidocaine. *Anesth Analg* 1993;76:1154–1157.
84. Hampl KF, Heinzmann-Wiedmer S, Luginbuehl I, et al. Transient neurologic symptoms after spinal anesthesia: a lower incidence with prilocaine and bupivacaine than with lidocaine. *Anesthesiology* 1998;88:629–633.
85. Hodgson PS, Neal JM, Pollock JE, et al. The neurotoxicity of drugs given intrathecally (spinal). *Anesth Analg* 1999;88:797–809.
86. Hodgson PS, Liu SS, Batra MS, et al. Procaine compared with lidocaine for incidence of transient neurologic symptoms. *Reg Anesth Pain Med* 2000;25: 218–222.
87. Liu SS, Ware PD, Allen HW, et al. Dose-response characteristics of spinal bupivacaine in volunteers. Clinical implications for ambulatory anesthesia. *Anesthesiology* 1996;85:729–736.
88. Zsigmond EK, Downs JR. Plasma cholinesterase activity in newborns and infants. *Can Anaesth Soc J* 1971;18:278–285.
89. Henderson K, Sethna NF, Berde CB. Continuous caudal anesthesia for inguinal hernia repair in former preterm infants. *J Clin Anesth* 1993;5:129–133.
90. Mihaly GW, Moore RG, Thomas J, et al. The pharmacokinetics and metabolism of the anilide local anaesthetics in neonates. I. Lignocaine. *Eur J Clin Pharmacol* 1978;13:143–152.
91. Lerman J, Strong HA, LeDez KM, et al. Effects of age on the serum concentration of alpha 1-acid glycoprotein and the binding of lidocaine in pediatric patients. *Clin Pharmacol Ther* 1989;46:219–225.
92. Larsson BA, Lonnqvist PA, Olsson GL. Plasma concentrations of bupivacaine in neonates after continuous epidural infusion. *Anesth Analg* 1997;84:501–505.
93. Luz G, Wieser C, Innerhofer P, et al. Free and total bupivacaine plasma concentrations after continuous epidural anaesthesia in infants and children. *Paediatr Anaesth* 1998;8:473–478.
94. Coleman MD, Coleman NA. Drug-induced methaemoglobinaemia. Treatment issues. *Drug Saf* 1996;14: 394–405.
95. Arens JF, Carrera AE. Methemoglobin levels following peridural anesthesia with prilocaine for vaginal deliveries. *Anesth Analg* 1970;49:219–222.
96. Taddio A, Shennan AT, Stevens B, et al. Safety of lidocaine-prilocaine cream in the treatment of preterm neonates. *J Pediatr* 1995;127:1002–1005.
97. Taddio A, Stevens B, Craig K, et al. Efficacy and safety of lidocaine-prilocaine cream for pain during circumcision . *N Engl J Med* 1997;336:1197–1201.
98. Finholt DA, Stirt JA, DiFazio CA, et al. Lidocaine pharmacokinetics in children during general anesthesia. *Anesth Analg* 1986;65:279–282.
99. Burrows FA, Lerman J, LeDez KM, et al. Alpha 1-acid glycoprotein and the binding of lidocaine in children with congenital heart disease. *Can J Anaesth* 1990;37: 883–888.
100. Jorfeldt L, Lewis DH, Lofstrom JB, et al. Lung uptake of lidocaine in man as influenced by anaesthesia, mepivacaine infusion or lung insufficiency. *Acta Anaesthesiol Scand* 1983;27:5–9.
101. Kietzmann D, Foth H, Geng WP, et al. Transpulmonary disposition of prilocaine, mepivacaine, and bupivacaine in humans in the course of epidural anaesthesia. *Acta Anaesthesiol Scand* 1995;39:885–890.
102. Bokesch PM, Castaneda AR, Ziemer G, et al. The influence of a right-to-left cardiac shunt on lidocaine pharmacokinetics. *Anesthesiology* 1987;67:739–744.
103. Burrows FA, Lerman J, LeDez KM, et al. Pharmacokinetics of lidocaine in children with congenital heart disease. Can J Anaesth 1991;38:196–200.
104. Stevens RA, Urmey WF, Urquhart BL, et al. Back pain after epidural anesthesia with chloroprocaine. *Anesthesiology* 1993;78:492–497.
105. Tobias JD, O'Dell N. Chloroprocaine for epidural anesthesia in infants and children. *AANA J* 1995;63: 131–135.
106. Rice LJ, DeMars PD, Whalen TV, et al. Duration of spinal anesthesia in infants less than one year of age. Comparison of three hyperbaric techniques. *Reg Anesth* 1994;19:325–329.
107. Abajian JC, Mellish RW, Browne AF, et al. Spinal anesthesia for surgery in the high-risk infant. *Anesth Analg* 1984;63:359–362.
108. Pietropaoli JA Jr, Keller MS, Smail DF, et al. Regional anesthesia in pediatric surgery: complications and postoperative comfort level in 174 children. *J Pediatr Surg* 1993;28:560–564.
109. Mao J, Chen LL. Systemic lidocaine for neuropathic pain relief. *Pain* 2000;87:7–17.
110. Abdi S, Lee DH, Chung JM. The anti-allodynic effects of amitriptyline, gabapentin, and lidocaine in a rat model of neuropathic pain. *Anesth Analg* 1998;87:1360–1366.
111. Jarvis B, Coukell AJ. Mexiletine. A review of its therapeutic use in painful diabetic neuropathy. *Drugs* 1998;56:691–707.

112. Galer BS, Harle J, Rowbotham MC. Response to intravenous lidocaine infusion predicts subsequent response to oral mexiletine: a prospective study. *J Pain Symptom Manage* 1996;12:161–167.
113. Devers A, Galer BS. Topical lidocaine patch relieves a variety of neuropathic pain conditions: an open-label study. *Clin J Pain* 2000;16:205–208.
114. Argoff CE. New analgesics for neuropathic pain: the lidocaine patch. *Clin J Pain* 2000;16[Suppl 2]:S62–S66.
115. Rowbotham MC, Davies PS, Verkempinck C, et al. Lidocaine patch: double-blind controlled study of a new treatment method for post-herpetic neuralgia. *Pain* 1996;65:39–44.
116. Kohane DS, Sankar WN, Shubina M, et al. Sciatic nerve blockade in infant, adolescent, and adult rats: a comparison of ropivacaine with bupivacaine. *Anesthesiology* 1998;89:1199–1208, discussion 10A.
117. Habre W, Bergesio R, Johnson C, et al. Pharmacokinetics of ropivacaine following caudal analgesia in children. *Paediatr Anaesth* 2000;10:143–147.
118. Wulf H, Peters C, Behnke H. The pharmacokinetics of caudal ropivacaine 0.2% in children. A study of infants aged less than 1 year and toddlers aged 1–5 years undergoing inguinal hernia repair. *Anaesthesia* 2000;55: 757–760.
119. Christoph RA, Buchanan L, Begalla K, et al. Pain reduction in local anesthetic administration through pH buffering. *Ann Emerg Med* 1988;17:117–120.
120. Orlinsky M, Hudson C, Chan L, et al. Pain comparison of unbuffered versus buffered lidocaine in local wound infiltration. *J Emerg Med* 1992;10:411–415.
121. McKay W, Morris R, Mushlin P. Sodium bicarbonate attenuates pain on skin infiltration with lidocaine, with or without epinephrine. *Anesth Analg* 1987;66:572–574.
122. Sinnott CJ, Garfield JM, Thalhammer JG, et al. Addition of sodium bicarbonate to lidocaine decreases the duration of peripheral nerve block in the rat. *Anesthesiology* 2000;93:1045–1052.
123. Serour F, Mandelberg A, Mori J. Slow injection of local anaesthetic will decrease pain during dorsal penile nerve block. *Acta Anaesthesiol Scand* 1998;42: 926–928.
124. Waldbillig DK, Quinn JV, Stiell IG, et al. Randomized double-blind controlled trial comparing room-temperature and heated lidocaine for digital nerve block. *Ann Emerg Med* 1995;26:677–681.
125. Fialkov JA, McDougall EP. Warmed local anesthetic reduces pain of infiltration. *Ann Plast Surg* 1996;36: 11–13.
126. Maunuksela EL, Korpela R. Double-blind evaluation of a lignocaine-prilocaine cream (EMLA) in children. Effect on the pain associated with venous cannulation. *Br J Anaesth* 1986;58:1242–1245.
127. Gajraj NM, Pennant JH, Watcha MF. Eutectic mixture of local anesthetics (EMLA) cream. *Anesth Analg* 1994;78:574–583.
128. Soliman IE, Broadman LM, Hannallah RS, et al. Comparison of the analgesic effects of EMLA (eutectic mixture of local anesthetics. to intradermal lidocaine infiltration prior to venous cannulation in unpremedicated children. *Anesthesiology* 1988;68: 804–806.
129. Blackburn PA, Butler KH, Hughes MJ, et al. Comparison of tetracaine-adrenaline-cocaine (TAC) with topical lidocaine-epinephrine (TLE): efficacy and cost. *Am J Emerg Med* 1995;13:315–317.
130. Ernst AA, Marvez-Valls E, Nick TG, et al. LAT (lidocaine-adrenaline-tetracaine. versus TAC (tetracaine-adrenaline-cocaine) for topical anesthesia in face and scalp lacerations. *Am J Emerg Med* 1995;13: 151–154.
131. Schilling CG, Bank DE, Borchert BA, et al. Tetracaine, epinephrine (adrenalin), and cocaine (TAC) versus lidocaine, epinephrine, and tetracaine (LET) for anesthesia of lacerations in children. *Ann Emerg Med* 1995;25:203–208.
132. Ernst AA, Marvez E, Nick TG, et al. Lidocaine adrenaline tetracaine gel versus tetracaine adrenaline cocaine gel for topical anesthesia in linear scalp and facial lacerations in children aged 5 to 17 years. *Pediatrics* 1995;95:255–258.
133. Anderson AB, Colecchi C, Baronoski R, et al. Local anesthesia in pediatric patients: topical TAC versus lidocaine. *Ann Emerg Med* 1990;19:519–522.
134. Hegenbarth MA, Altieri MF, Hawk WH, et al. Comparison of topical tetracaine, adrenaline, and cocaine anesthesia with lidocaine infiltration for repair of lacerations in children. *Ann Emerg Med* 1990;19: 63–67.
135. Smith GA, Strausbaugh SD, Harbeck-Weber C, et al. Comparison of topical anesthetics without cocaine to tetracaine-adrenaline-cocaine and lidocaine infiltration during repair of lacerations: bupivacaine-norepinephrine is an effective new topical anesthetic agent. *Pediatrics* 1996;97:301–307.
136. Zempsky WT, Ashburn MA. Iontophoresis: noninvasive drug delivery. *Am J Anesthesiol* 1998;25:158–162.
137. Ashburn MA, Gauthier M, Love G, et al. Iontophoretic administration of 2% lidocaine HCl and 1:100,000 epinephrine in humans. *Clin J Pain* 1997;13:22–26.
138. Ashburn MA, Streisand J, Zhang J, et al. The iontophoresis of fentanyl citrate in humans. *Anesthesiology* 1995;82:1146–1153.
139. Ashburn MA, Stephen RL, Ackerman E, et al. Iontophoretic delivery of morphine for postoperative analgesia. *J Pain Symptom Manage* 1992;7:27–33.

15

Psychiatric Assessment and Management of Pediatric Pain

Lu Ann Sifford

Multidimensional concepts of pain emphasize the physiologic, sensory, cognitive, behavioral, affective, and sociocultural factors that contribute to a patient's pain experience (1). Children's perception of and communication of pain reflect all these factors as well as their developmental level and previous pain experience. The assessment and medical management of pain in children are discussed elsewhere in this text. In this chapter, we consider psychiatric methods useful in the treatment of pain in children. Optimal pain management is interdisciplinary and involves collaboration with other physicians and practitioners from multiple disciplines including nursing, physical and occupational therapy, psychology, social services, child life, and pastoral care. Psychiatric participation can play a vital role in the assessment and treatment of the many underlying contributions to pediatric pain. The psychiatrist's unique role in the care of a child with pain is to diagnose and treat comorbid psychiatric conditions that may complicate the treatment of pain. Patients with pain frequently suffer from depression, anxiety, and other psychiatric disorders that are often not recognized or are undertreated. These disorders can adversely influence the intensity or duration of pain and undermine the child's behavior and coping strategies.

When a child experiences pain with no identifiable physical cause or pain does not respond adequately to medical treatment, a psychiatrist is often consulted to determine whether the symptoms are primarily psychologic in nature. Somatization is the experience and expression of psychologic distress in the form of pain or other physical symptoms. Although somatization is the hallmark of somatoform disorders, psychosomatic symptoms can also be part of the clinical presentation of other psychiatric disorders including mood, anxiety, and adjustment disorders. The diagnosis and treatment of psychosomatic pain are discussed elsewhere in this volume.

Like all unpleasant experiences, pain can have emotional consequences. In addition, the circumstances surrounding the pain including the nature of the illness or injury can result in emotional distress. Psychiatric consultation may be requested to assess the psychologic reactions to a painful illness, injury, or medical procedure. Reaction to a painful event can range from normal fear, anxiety, or sadness to the development of a psychiatric disorder such as posttraumatic stress disorder (PTSD). Children who have psychologic factors that exacerbate pain or interfere with its treatment may benefit from psychiatric intervention, whether or not they meet diagnostic criteria for a psychiatric disorder.

Psychiatric participation in pain management involves the use of pharmacologic as well as nonpharmacologic interventions to address pain and associated symptoms. The psychiatric consultant should fully evaluate pain and the adequacy of medical management. Adequate relief of pain often results in the disappearance of symptoms attributed to a psychiatric disorder. Psychologic variables such as the meaning of pain, fear of death, anxious or depressed mood, and coping strategies can all contribute to the experience of pain (1,2). Psychologic techniques effective in both acute procedure-related pain and chronic or recurrent pain include education, relaxation therapy, distraction, hypnosis, biofeedback, cognitive-behavioral therapy, and family therapy (3,4).

GENERAL CONSIDERATIONS IN THE ASSESSMENT OF PEDIATRIC PAIN PATIENTS

The diagnostic evaluation of a child with pain should include assessment of the psychologic, social, cognitive, educational, and medical factors that contribute to the clinical presentation (5). Psychiatric assessment of children with pain is complicated because the expression of pain and emotional distress vary with developmental age. Pain, depression, fear, and anxiety are manifested primarily behaviorally in preschool children. Until children can adequately describe their pain and emotions verbally, behavioral observations and parental report must be relied on to assess a child's pain and emotional state. Behavioral observations are problematic because the manifestations of pain, anxiety, and depression may be indistinguishable from each other. Further, behavioral responses vary with development; behavior that is normal for a preschool child may be a symptom of severe emotional problems in an older child.

When a child is able to provide a self-report, a description of symptoms should be obtained from the child. There is often little agreement between children and their parents in the symptoms reported or their severity; thus, the child and parents should be interviewed separately whenever possible (1,6–8). This is particularly important when treating symptoms of depression and anxiety. Pain and symptoms of depression or anxiety may be experienced differently in different settings. Therefore, information from schools or day care centers may be desirable in children with chronic or recurrent pain.

In addition to obtaining the history from the child and parents, evaluation requires a careful review of the medical record and consultation with the treating medical team. Previous pain treatments and their perceived effectiveness should be reviewed. When medical treatment is thought to be ineffective, it is important to determine whether this is owing to an inadequate therapeutic trial, intolerable adverse effects, or noncompliance. Multiple factors can influence compliance, such as the meaning of medication to the parent or child, misunderstanding of administration, or poor patient cooperation. Education or implementation of a behavioral modification program for the child may improve compliance with the treatment regimen. A careful history of the onset of psychologic symptoms in relation to pain, medical illness, or medications may suggest that these symptoms are secondary to the medical condition or medications.

DEPRESSION IN CHILDREN WITH PAIN

Depression in children with pain can be a direct result of a medical condition, medication side effects, or a response to the stresses associated with the diagnosis and treatment of their medical condition. Pain and other debilitating symptoms such as nausea and vomiting can result in feelings of despair and an inability to cope. Symptoms of depression often resolve with pain relief. Even acknowledging the existence of pain and an attempt to relieve it often lead to an improvement in depressive symptoms. Therefore, *the first step in the evaluation and treatment of depressive symptoms in a child is to ensure that optimal pain relief is provided.*

Depression in patients with a painful medical illness or injury is often underdiagnosed and untreated (9,10). Appropriate treatment depends on the recognition of symptoms of depression by the primary health care provider; however, this recognition can be very difficult in a child with pain. Even when depression is identified, it may go untreated (11,12). Many clinicians believe that if depression is an understandable response to a painful illness, injury, or stressful situation, it is an appropriate reaction and therefore does not require treatment. An important role for the psychiatrist in the treatment of children with pain is to educate staff to evaluate children for symptoms of depression or anxiety at regular medical visits.

Once depressive symptoms have been identified, the child psychiatrist should be consulted to clarify the diagnosis and provide treatment recommendations. Depressed mood may be a temporary emotional state or a symptom of a clinical syndrome. Major depressive disorder (MDD) and adjustment disorder are common diagnoses for patients with significant depressive symptoms. Other depressive disorders that should be considered include dysthymic disorder, mood disorder owing to a general medical condition, or substance-induced mood disorder.

DIFFERENTIAL DIAGNOSIS OF DEPRESSED MOOD

Depressed Mood in Response to Negative Events

Depressed mood or sadness in response to the experience of a painful medical condition or hospitalization should be differentiated from a depressive disorder. In children with a medical illness, hospitalization and physical limitations can result in disruption of family and peer relationships. As part of their reaction to a medical illness or hospitalization, many children experience symptoms such as feelings of sadness, anxiety, sleep difficulties, or mild behavioral problems. Parents and children usually regard this as a normal response to the illness or injury, and these symptoms typically resolve rapidly with improvement in the child's pain or physical symptoms. For children with chronic illnesses, these symptoms can recur in response to negative events experienced during the course of the illness. For example, many children and adolescents experience symptoms of depression during hospitalization, which disappear when they are discharged.

Supportive therapy or interventions to support coping are often helpful. These normal responses usually resolve within a few weeks. Prolonged sadness or atypical symptoms such as excessive guilt, suicidal ideation or preoccupation with death, feelings of worthlessness, or marked impairment in functioning suggest a depressive disorder.

Major Depressive Disorder

A diagnosis of major depressive episode, as defined by the *Diagnostic and Statistical Manual of Mental Disorders, Fourth Edition* (*DSM-IV*), requires depressed mood or a loss of interest in nearly all activities for a period of at least 2 weeks. Children or adolescents may present with an irritable rather than depressed mood. At least four additional symptoms must be present including disturbances in appetite, sleep, concentration, psychomotor activity or energy level, feelings of worthlessness or guilt, or recurrent thoughts of death or suicidal ideation. To meet the standard definition, symptoms must result in impairment in functioning and not be attributed to a medical illness, medications, or bereavement (13).

There are few developmental variations in the core features of MDD. Most evidence suggests that children are less likely than adults to experience weight loss or hypersomnia (14). Developmental changes in other symptoms of depression are not well documented; however, there is little doubt that the expression of mood varies according to developmental level. Nonverbal behaviors and parental report in preschool children are important because children may lack verbal and cognitive skills to describe their mood. Preschool children may exhibit social withdrawal, apathy, failure to thrive, or increasing frequency of tantrums. As language skills develop, children are better able to describe their feelings. Children may use many different terms to describe depressed mood such as "sad," "blue," "bored", "down," or "bummed." Children may describe themselves in negative terms such as dumb or worthless. Signs of depression include frequent crying, irritability, school difficulties, social withdrawal, and a loss of interest and pleasure in many usual childhood activities.

Children may also exhibit pain or other somatic complaints (15).

Evaluation of depression in a child with pain is further complicated by the overlap of symptoms of depression and many medical illnesses. Some symptoms of depression such as fatigue and disturbances of sleep or appetite may be owing to medical illness or treatment side effects. Focus on the psychologic symptoms of depression (anhedonia, dysphoria, guilt, poor self-esteem, hopelessness, and suicidal ideation or preoccupation with death) rather than somatic symptoms may help in the diagnosis of depression.

Pain and somatic complaints can also be symptoms of depressive disorders (15–17). Children presenting with pain may deny any awareness of depression or may not communicate their depressed mood to the physician. Some children do not have the ability to identify or communicate their emotional state, whereas others may deny symptoms or attribute their depression to pain because of the stigma associated with psychiatric conditions. The clinician may have to rely on the parents for assessment of depression; however, parents may also be more likely to identify somatic complaints than depression in their children.

Although symptom overlap makes it more difficult to diagnose major depression in patients with a painful medical condition, the two frequently coexist. Adults with chronic pain have an increased prevalence of depressive disorders, and patients with major depression have increased complaints of pain (18). Depression interacts with chronic pain to increase morbidity and can result in increased pain intensity and less ability to use coping strategies. In adults, pain has been associated with increased suicide risk (9,19). There are fewer studies of the relationship between pain and psychiatric comorbidity in children and adolescents; however, preliminary studies support a similar association between chronic pain and affective disorders (6,20). The relationship between acute pain and depressive symptoms is less clear. Stressful life events have been shown to precipitate depression (15,21,22). An acute painful episode could, therefore, precipitate a major depressive episode in susceptible individuals.

Dysthymic Disorder

Dysthymic disorder is a chronic depression of insufficient severity to meet the criteria for a major depressive episode. Symptoms must persist for at least 1 year in children and adolescents to meet diagnostic criteria for this disorder according to *DSM-IV* (13). The diagnosis of dysthymic disorder in a medically ill child poses the same challenges that complicate the diagnosis of major depression.

Mood Disorder Owing to a General Medical Condition and Substance-Induced Mood Disorders

The occurrence of depressive symptoms caused by the direct physiologic effects of a medical illness is classified as a mood disorder owing to a general medical condition (13). It is often difficult to assess whether depression is caused by the illness itself or the patient's reaction to the disease. Medical conditions known to cause depressive symptoms include endocrine and neurologic disorders, porphyria, and cancer (23). Symptoms improve with treatment of the underlying medical condition, but psychiatric intervention may be necessary.

There are many medications that are associated with depression; however, very few have been shown to have a direct causal effect. A diagnosis of substance-induced mood disorder is given when there is a temporal relationship between the onset of the medication and symptoms of depression (13). In a medically ill patient, this is complicated because depression could also be owing to the illness itself or a psychologic reaction to the illness. Medications reported to cause depressive symptoms include steroids, oral contraceptives, benzodiazepines, opioids, histamine receptor antagonists (cimetidine and ranitidine), antihypertensive medications (reserpine, methyldopa, and propanolol), chemotherapeutic agents (vincristine, vinblastine, procarbazine, L-asparaginase, and interferon), and some antibiotics such as amphotericin B (24).

Adjustment Disorder

Adjustment disorder with depressed mood is one of the most common diagnoses made by consultation–liaison psychiatrists in hospitalized children. Adjustment disorder is diagnosed when a child has significant depressive symptoms that develop after an identifiable stressor (13). A painful illness, injury, and hospitalization are examples of stressful events that can precipitate an adjustment disorder. Although symptoms are not of sufficient severity or duration to meet diagnostic criteria for a mood disorder, children may experience significant distress.

TREATMENT OF DEPRESSION

Children with symptoms of depression that are thought to contribute significantly to pain, distress, or interfere with functioning should be treated regardless of whether they meet diagnostic criteria for a MDD. Practice parameters for the assessment and treatment of children and adolescents with depressive disorders published by the American Academy of Child and Adolescent Psychiatry provides a comprehensive review of the literature and treatment guidelines for children with depressive disorders (25).

Although there are few published studies on the management of depression in children with pain or medical illnesses, it is clear that pain and any medical conditions should be treated. If depressive symptoms are thought to be secondary to a medication, it should be discontinued or the dose reduced if possible. If the child's medical condition requires continued treatment, there may be other medications with comparable pharmacologic activity that do not cause depression.

Treatment should begin with psychotherapy for children with mild to moderate depression. If there is no improvement in 6 to 12 weeks, a trial of antidepressants is indicated. Children who are unable to participate in therapy or who present with severe depression may benefit from antidepressants from the beginning of therapy (25,26). Psychotherapy, particularly cognitive-behavioral therapy, has been shown to be effective in children with major depression (27,28). However, children with depression and pain may have other stresses inherent in a medical illness such as coping with hospitalization, grief, fear of pain, or worry about imagined causes of pain that should be considered. Various psychotherapeutic techniques are used in treating children with pain. Crisis intervention, short-term therapy, education, group therapy, hypnosis, cognitive-behavioral therapy, play therapy, family therapy, parental counseling, and supportive therapy may be used. Treatment of depression in a child with pain often requires a combined approach. The psychotherapeutic approach should be selected based on the needs of the child. For example, a child with depressive symptoms and pain owing to injuries from repeated child abuse requires very different treatment than a child whose symptoms are owing to terminal cancer. Because children are influenced by their parents and environment, it is necessary to work extensively with the family. For children with chronic pain, this may involve helping parents to avoid reinforcing pain behaviors and improve compliance with the medical management. Parents of a child who had a serious accident, such as a burn, may need help coping with their own feelings of guilt and grief so that they are able to help their child cope. Interdisciplinary care conferences are often helpful to develop a comprehensive treatment plan and coordinate care. Nursing, child life, physical and occupational therapy, social services, psychology, and pastoral care are often invaluable in helping children and their families cope with pain and depression. It is crucial, however, to define the roles of each clinician carefully. Care conferences also provide the psychiatrist an opportunity to assess the attitudes and behavior of the medical staff toward the child and intervene if it is thought they contribute to the child's pain or depression.

PHARMACOTHERAPY

Use of psychotropic medications by child psychiatrists has increased in the 1990s. There has been an increase in the use of selective serotonin reuptake inhibitors (SSRIs) compared with tricyclic antidepressants (TCAs) and an increase in polypharmacy (29,30). Fluoxetine and sertraline are among the top ten most commonly prescribed medications used off-label in pediatric patients (31). Most psychopharmacologic agents approved for use by the U.S. Food and Drug Administration have not been tested and approved for use in children (32). Although the Food and Drug Administration mandates that the manufacturers must not market or promote medications for a use not approved, physicians are free to prescribe a drug for any purposes they deem appropriate, and such off-label use is a standard part of pediatric practice (33). As a result, product monographs and guidelines published in the *Physicians' Desk Reference* cannot be relied on for information on safety, efficacy, adverse effects, or appropriate doses of most medications in children. The primary reason for inadequate labeling is the lack of valid research data in pediatrics. There is growing concern about this increased use of psychotropic medications in children and the need for further research and improved labeling of drugs used in treating psychiatric illness in children (31,34–36). There is a similar lack of information on the effectiveness of many psychologic interventions in children (27). Clearly, more research is needed to determine the most effective treatments for children with psychiatric illnesses (Table 15.1A–C).

Clinicians must, therefore, base their treatment decisions on downward extrapolation of adult studies or case reports and small pilot studies in children. Parents and children (when developmentally appropriate) should be informed about the disorder and the available treatment alternatives in terms of efficacy and potential risks and benefits (37). Many parents are very well educated and become concerned about disclaimers in the *Physicians' Desk Reference* regarding safety and effectiveness not having been established in pediatric patients. Therefore, it is prudent to inform the parents of the labeling issues as well as the evidence in the literature for safe and effective use. Medications should be considered as part of a broader treatment plan that encompasses all aspects of a child's life, and should be integrated into a treatment plan as an adjunct to other psychologic interventions. Identification of target symptoms and assessment of risks and benefits are essential for effective use of medications.

Antidepressants

SSRIs have become a first-line treatment for depressed children and adolescents requiring pharmacotherapy (25,38,39). In comparison to TCAs, SSRIs are safer in overdose situations, have more benign side effects, and greater ease of administration, which may increase compliance with treatment. SSRIs have been shown effective in adults with MDD. Although most studies of antidepressants have found no difference from placebo in the acute treatment of MDD (40,41), fluoxetine has recently been demonstrated to be effective in children ages 7 to 17 (42). There are also ongoing studies that suggest that SSRIs may be effective in treating MDD in children (43). Developmental factors may influence the response to medications in children (44). For example, children metabolize some medications faster than adults (45). In addition, the serotonergic system matures earlier than the central noradrenergic system, which may explain the increased effectiveness of SSRIs compared with standard TCAs in children.

Pharmacologic management of depression in a child with a painful illness requires careful consideration of the underlying medical illness, drug interactions, and contraindications. The primary side effects of the SSRIs are abdominal distress and headache. This can pose potential problems for children who present with chronic or recurrent abdominal pain or headache. There are no studies to determine whether these children are more sensitive to these adverse effects or whether pain complaints improve with resolution of depressive symptoms.

TABLE 15.1A. *Selective serotonin reuptake inhibitors*

Adverse effects: The most common adverse effects are gastrointestinal (dyspepsia, nausea, emesis, diarrhea, or decreased appetite), headache, sedation or activation (nervousness, anxiety, restlessness, agitation, or insomnia), sexual dysfunction. Children may be more likely to develop behavioral activation.
Withdrawal symptoms: Common physical symptoms include dizziness, lightheadedness, nausea, fatigue, headache, and sensory and sleep disturbance. Psychologic symptoms reported are anxiety, irritability, and tearfulness.

Drug	Labeled indications[a]	Dose[b]	Available forms	CYP interactions
Citalopram (Celexa)	Adults: depression Pediatrics: safety and effectiveness not established	Initial dose: 10–20 mg p.o. daily Dose range: 10–40 mg/d Maximal dose: 60 mg/d	Tablets: 20 mg scored, 40 mg scored Oral solution: 10 mg/5 mL (peppermint flavor) Parenteral: none	Metabolism: 3A4, 2C19 Inhibits: 1A2 (w), 2C19 (w), 2D6 (w)
Fluoxetine (Prozac, Sarafem)	Adults: depression, OCD, bulimia nervosa, premenstrual dysphoric disorder Pediatrics: safety and effectiveness has not been established	Initial dose: 5–10 mg p.o. each morning Dose range: 20–60 mg/d Maximal dose: 80 mg/d	Capsules: Prozac 10, 20, 40 mg Tablets: Prozac 10 mg scored, Serafem 10, 20 mg Oral solution: Prozac 20 mg/5 mL (mint flavor) Parenteral: none	Metabolism: 3A4, 2C9*, 2D6 Inhibits: 3A4 (p), 2D6 (p), 1A2 (m), 2C19 (m)
Fluvoxamine (Luvox)	Adults: OCD Pediatrics: OCD in children 8 yr and older	Initial dose: 12.5–25 mg p.o. q.h.s. Dose range: 25–100 mg b.i.d. Maximal dose: 200 mg/d (300 mg in adults)	Tablets: 25 mg, 50 mg scored, 100 mg scored Oral solution: none Parenteral: none	Metabolism: 3A4, 2D6 Inhibits: 1A2 (p), 3A4 (p), 2C9 (m), 2C19 (m), 2D6 (w)
Paroxetine (Paxil, Paxil CR)	Adults: depression, OCD, panic disorder, social phobia Pediatrics: safety and effectiveness not established	Initial dose: paroxetine 10–20 mg (usually in the morning), paroxetine (controlled release) 12.5 mg Dose range: 10–60 mg/d Maximal dose: paroxetine 60 mg; paroxetine (controlled release) 62.5 mg	Tablets: 10 mg, 20 mg scored, 30 mg, 40 mg Controlled-release tablets: 12.5, 25 mg Oral suspension: 10 mg/5 mL (orange flavored)	Metabolism: 2D6* Inhibits: 2D6 (p), 1A2 (w), 3A4 (w), 2C9 (w), 2C19 (w)
Sertraline (Zoloft)	Adults: depression, OCD, panic disorder, posttraumatic stress disorder Pediatrics: OCD in children 6 years and older	Initial dose: 12.5–25 mg daily Dose range: 25–200 mg Maximal dose: 200 mg	Tablet: 25, 50, and 100 mg scored Oral concentrate: 20 mg/mL (menthol scent) Parenteral: none	Metabolism: 3A4*, 2C9, 2C19, 2D6 Inhibits: 2C19 (m), 1A2 (w), 3A4 (w), 2C9 (w), 2D6 (w)

TABLE 15.1B. *Tricyclic antidepressants*

Adverse effects: Sedation and postural hypotension are common, particularly at the beginning of treatment. Anticholinergic effects include dry mouth, urinary retention, constipation, blurred vision, tachycardia, and memory dysfunction. Anticholinergic effects are more common in children taking tertiary amines (imipramine, amitryptyline, and clomipramine) than secondary amines (nortriptyline and desipramine). Sedation and postural hypotension are also common. Weight gain can occur with prolonged use. TCAs commonly produce a benign increase in heart rate. Several cases of sudden death have been reported in prepubertal children taking tricyclic antidepressants.
Monitor: Electrocardiogram and vital signs should be obtained at baseline. Vital signs and electrocardiograms should be repeated when the daily dose is more than 2.5 mg/kg per day (or for nortriptyline 1.0 mg/kg per day) and after each increase of 50 to 100 mg/d. Suggested limits: electrocardiogram (PR, 0.2 seconds; QRS, 0.12 seconds, or 130% of baseline; QTc, 0.48 seconds); heart rate, 110 to 130 (children), 110 to 120 (adolescents); blood pressure, 120/80 (children), 140/90 (adolescents). Plasma drug concentrations should be monitored routinely. Plasma levels do not always correlate with clinical effectiveness.
Withdrawal: Anticholinergic withdrawal results in a flu-like syndrome with gastrointestinal symptoms (nausea cramps, vomiting), headache, muscle aches, and lethargy.

Drug	Labeled indications[a]	Dose[b]	Available forms	CYP interactions
Amitriptyline (Elavil)	Adults: depression Pediatrics: depression in patients 12 years and older	Initial dose: 10–25 mg/d or 1 mg/kg per day given in 3 divided doses Dose range: 2–5 mg/kg per day (adult dose range: 150–300 mg/d) Maximal dose: 5 mg/kg per day or 300 mg, whichever is less; doses >3 mg/kg per day require close monitoring (manufacturer recommends 10 mg t.i.d. and 20 mg q.h.s. as the initial dose for adolescents)	Tablets: 10, 25, 50, 75, 100, 150 mg Oral suspension: none Parenteral: 10 mg/mL	Metabolism: 1A2, 3A4, 2C9, 2C19, 2D6 Inhibits: 2D6 (m)
Clomipramine (Anafranil)	Adult: OCD Pediatric: approved for the treatment of OCD in children 10 years and older	Initial dose: 25 mg p.o. q.h.s. Dose range: 2–3 mg/kg per day administered in divided doses; 50–200 mg/d administered in divided doses (adult dose range: 150–250 mg/d) Maximal dose: 3 mg/kg or 200 mg, whichever is less	Capsules: 25, 50, 75 mg Oral solution: none Parenteral: none	Metabolism: 1A2, 3A4, 2C9, 2C19, 2D6 Inhibits: 2D6 (m)

Desipramine[c] (Norpramin, Petrofrane)	Adult: depression Pediatric: desipramine is not recommended for use in children; safety and efficacy have not been established	Initial dose: 10–25 mg Dose range: 1–5 mg/kg per day administered in divided doses, monitor carefully in doses >3 mg/kg per day (adult dose range: 150–300 mg/d) Maximal dose: children, 5 mg/kg per day; adolescents, 5 mg/kg or 150 mg, whichever is less (manufacturer recommends 25–100 mg/d for adolescents; in more severely ill patients, dose can be gradually increased to 150 mg/d)	Tablets: 10, 25, 50, 75, 100, 150 mg Oral solution: none Parenteral: none	Metabolism: 1A2, 2D6* Inhibits: 2D6 (m)
Imipramine (Tofranil)	Adults: depression Pediatrics: approved for the treatment of depression in adolescents; indicated for the treatment of enuresis in children older than 6 yr	Initial dose: 10–25 mg q.h.s. Dose range: 2–5 mg/kg per day; children should be closely monitored when receiving doses >3 mg/kg per day (adult dose range: 150–300 mg/d) Maximal dose: children, 5 mg/kg per day or 200 mg, whichever is smaller; adolescents, 100 mg/d; adults, 300 mg	Imipramine tablets: 10, 25, 50 mg Oral solution: none Parenteral: 12.5 mg/mL Imipramine pamoate, sustained release capsules: 75, 100, 125, 150 mg	Metabolism: 1A2*, 3A4, 2C9, 2C19, 2D6 Inhibits: 2D6 (m)
Nortriptyline (Aventyl, Pamelor)	Adults: depression Pediatric: approved for the treatment of depression in adolescents	Initial dose: 10 mg Dose range: 1–3 mg/kg per day; children should be monitored closely when receiving doses >1 mg/kg/d; adult dose range: 50–150 mg/d Maximal dose: 2.5 mg/kg or 150 mg/d (manufacturer recommends 30–50 mg/d for adolescents)	Capsules: 10, 25, 50, 75 mg Oral solution: 10 mg/5 mL Parenteral: none	Metabolism: 2D6* Inhibits: 3A4, 2C9, 2C19, 2D6

TABLE 15.1C. *Benzodiazepines*

Adverse effects: Sedation or fatigue occurs most frequently. Motor incoordination, lethargy, cognitive dulling or confusion, and anterograde amnesia occur with higher doses. Behavioral disinhibition (irritability, oppositional behavior, lability, increased activity) may occur. Tolerance and dependence have been reported in adults.
Withdrawal: Common symptoms include insomnia, anxiety, jitteriness, palpitations, tremulousness, muscle twitching, nausea, sweating, heightened sensitivity to light and sound, perceptual disturbances, and depersonalization or concentration difficulties. Severe withdrawal symptoms, including delirium, psychotic symptoms, or seizures, are usually limited to adults taking excessive doses for an extended period.

Drug	Labeled indications[a]	Dose[b]	Available forms	CYP interactions
Lorazepam (Ativan)	Adults: anxiety disorders, preanesthetic sedation, status epilepticus Pediatric: anxiety in children 12 years and older (lorazepam administered intravenously or intramuscularly is not recommended in patients younger than 18 yr of age)	Initial dose: 0.05 mg/kg administered every 4–8 hr Dose range: 0.02–0.09 mg/kg every 4–8 hr (usual adult dose: 2–6 mg/d) Maximal dose: depends on body weight and tolerance (usual maximal oral dose for adults is 10 mg/d or 4 mg/dose; usual maximal intravenous dose for adults is 2 mg) Peak response: amnestic response, 60–90 min (oral); 15–20 min (intravenous); 60 min (sublingual)	Tablets: 0.5-mg white, 5-sided; 1-mg white, 5-sided; 2-mg white, 5-sided Injection: 2 mg/mL: 4 mg/mL Oral solution: lorazepam Intensol: 2 mg/mL	Not involved in metabolism interactions via CYP enzymes

Every effort has been made to ensure that the information in this table is accurate and reflects current practice. However, the reader is urged to check the current literature and package inserts for changes in indications, doses, drug interactions, and adverse effects. Doses are guidelines only, taken from the available literature and manufacturer's package inserts. Because of the lack of definitive research on the treatment of children, it is often necessary to treat children based on guidelines for adults. Dose adjustments in children should be undertaken carefully, taking into account their lower body weight and differences in metabolism. Doses must be individualized based on clinical response and adverse effects.

[a]Most medications have more extensive therapeutic uses. Please refer to the current literature for guidelines on off-label uses in pediatrics.

[b]Dose may vary based on clinical indication, age, and weight of the patient. Dose should be individualized and titrated based on clinical response and adverse effects.

[c]Desipramine has been associated with sudden death in prepubertal children. A causal relationship has not been established, however, clinical practice favors the use of another tricyclic as a first choice.

[*]Primary CYP enzyme involved in the metabolism, where known; (w), weak; (m), moderate; (p), potent; CYP, cytochrome P; p.o., orally; OCD, obsessive-compulsive disorder; q.h.s., every night (at bedtime); b.i.d., twice daily; t.i.d., three times daily.

In addition, children with pain may have medical conditions requiring treatment with medications that can interact with SSRIs. Amitriptyline, nortriptyline, imipramine, desipramine, clomipramine, and doxepin have all been reported useful in the treatment of neuropathic and headache pain syndromes (1,6). The use of psychotropics for the treatment of pain is detailed in Chapter 13. When a child or adolescent is being treated with a TCA for pain and also requires pharmacologic management of depression, the question becomes whether to increase the TCA to a therapeutic level for the treatment of depression or add an SSRI to the TCA. TCAs have been shown effective in adults; however, controlled studies in children and adolescents have failed to demonstrate efficacy in the treatment of depression (8,46). Several explanations have been proposed including small sample sizes, high placebo responses, poor study design, and developmental differences between children and adults (8). If there is a difference in effectiveness in response to TCAs based on maturation of the noradrenergic system, it is not known at what age TCAs should be expected to work. TCAs vary in their norepinephrine reuptake and serotonin reuptake blocking effects, and relatively few TCAs have been adequately studied in children. If serotonergic agents are effective in the treatment of depression in children and noradrenergic agents are not, TCAs such as clomipramine, which are more serotonergic, should be considered to treat both pain and depression in children.

From a practical clinical standpoint, because of the lack of demonstrated efficacy and the reported sudden deaths occurring in children treated with desipramine and imipramine, it may be best to add an SSRI when treating a child for depression who is already receiving a TCA for pain. However, SSRIs can significantly increase the plasma level of TCAs via competitive inhibition of the cytochrome P-450 2D6. Therefore, plasma levels of TCAs should be monitored closely, and an electrocardiogram (ECG) obtained regularly to assess cardiotoxicity.

Selective Serotonin Reuptake Inhibitors

SSRIs currently available in the United States include fluoxetine, sertraline, paroxetine, fluvoxamine, and citalopram. Currently, only fluvoxamine and sertraline have Food and Drug Administration–approved indications for use in children. Both are approved for the treatment of obsessive-compulsive disorder in children. Fluvoxamine is indicated in children 8 years of age and sertraline at 6 years of age. Although obsessive-compulsive disorder is the only psychiatric disorder for which pediatric use of SSRIs have been approved, off-label use in children based on adults studies is extensive (39).

The potentially broad range of indications, relatively benign adverse effects, ease of administration, and low lethality after overdose have contributed to the increased use of SSRIs in both adults and children. SSRIs are clearly effective in a variety of conditions in adults including MDD, obsessive-compulsive disorder, panic disorder, social phobia, PTSD, bulimia nervosa, and premenstrual syndrome (47,48). There are very few double-blind, placebo-controlled studies that document the effectiveness of SSRIs in children. Preliminary studies suggest that SSRIs may be effective for the treatment of obsessive-compulsive disorder, depression, and selective mutism in children and adolescents (49).

All the SSRIs appear to be equally efficacious for the treatment of anxiety and depression (50). The time to onset of the antidepressant effect is the same for all SSRIs, and they share similar adverse effects. When selecting an SSRI, a history of an effective response in the patient or family members should be considered. Other considerations are the elimination half-life, extent of protein binding, and potential drug interactions. Although the literature emphasizes the similarities among the medications, individuals vary in their clinical responses as well as adverse effects from one to another. Therefore, if a child does not tolerate or respond to one medication, a trial with another SSRI is indicated.

Adverse Effects

The adverse effects of SSRIs are dose dependent and may subside with time (25,39, 51,52). The most common adverse effects reported in adults are associated with the central or autonomic nervous system, gastrointestinal symptoms, and sexual dysfunction (48,52). Central nervous system activation may result in complaints of anxiety, agitation, jitteriness, or insomnia. Behavioral activation, which consists of motor restlessness, excitement, irritability, disinhibition, or silliness, may be particularly common in children (52). Mania and hypomania resulting from any of the SSRIs have been reported in children and adolescents (53). Further studies to determine the clinical course in these children are needed. However, clinicians should monitor closely for worsening behavioral problems in children treated with SSRIs. Activation may interfere with sleep, and it may be helpful to take the dose earlier in the day. Paradoxically, some patients become sedated on SSRIs. When this occurs, the medication should be administered at night. Other neurologic adverse effects such as headache and tremor have been reported. Autonomic effects include dry mouth, excessive perspiration, and weight changes. The most common gastrointestinal symptoms are nausea, diarrhea, and anorexia. Administering the medication with meals may help reduce stomach upset. Gastrointestinal symptoms tend to diminish over the first month of treatment. Infrequent adverse effects associated with the use of SSRIs include the syndrome of inappropriate antidiuretic hormone secretion, extrapyramidal effects, and bleeding complications (54).

Increases in suicidal or violent behavior have been anecdotally associated with fluoxetine in adults. There have also been case reports of self-injurious behavior in children and adolescents treated with fluoxetine (52). Subsequent reviews found no evidence to support the notion that SSRIs trigger emergent suicidal ideation above rates normally associated with depression. In fact, SSRIs generally reduce the risk of suicide in depressed adults (55). Clinical studies of SSRIs in aggressive and violent behavior have been more limited, but findings seem to suggest that SSRIs reduce aggression (56). There was considerable press coverage of increased violence and suicidal ideation with SSRIs, particularly fluoxetine, and many parents are very frightened about the prospect of using these medications. Often adolescents or family members do not bring up these concerns but are very anxious about the use of these medications. It is, therefore, important to address this concern when informing family members about more routine adverse effects.

Overdose

One of the major advantages of SSRIs is their safety in overdose (52,57). Deaths as a result of ingestions solely of SSRIs are extremely rare. Ingestions of as much as 30 times the usual daily dose result in mild or no symptoms in adults. Drowsiness, tremor, nausea, and vomiting typically result from larger ingestions. More serious symptoms such as decreased consciousness, seizures, or ECG changes may occur at very high doses [>75 times the usual dose (58)]. There is some concern that citalopram may be more likely to result in fatalities when taken in large overdoses than the other SSRIs and therefore should be avoided in patients likely to take overdoses (59).

Selective Serotonin Reuptake Inhibitor Discontinuation

Rapid discontinuation of an SSRI may result in withdrawal symptoms (55,60). The most common physical symptoms include dizziness, lightheadedness, nausea and vomiting, fatigue, lethargy, aches and chills, headache, and sensory or sleep disturbances. Increased anxiety, irritability and crying spells may also occur. These symptoms have been reported with all SSRIs but occur most frequently with rapid tapering of paroxetine and fluvoxamine because of their relatively short half-life and nonlinear pharmacokinetics (61). SSRIs are not drugs of abuse, and families should be reassured that symptoms of withdrawal do not indicate that the child is addicted to the medication. Withdrawal symptoms most often begin within 1 to 10 days and can occur after as few as 6 to 8 weeks of treatment (26,62). Drugs with shorter half-lives should be tapered slowly. Fluoxetine does not require tapering because of its long half-life and that of its active metabolite. It may, therefore, be a good choice when compliance is a concern.

Drug Interactions

Clinicians should be aware that SSRIs could result in clinically important drug interactions when administered with other agents metabolized by the cytochrome P-450 isoenzymes. Alteration in hepatic metabolism owing to isoenzyme induction or inhibition is of particular concern. The result of these interactions is either accumulation of the drug, leading to toxicity, or decreased plasma concentrations, causing reduced efficacy. These interactions are most significant with medications that have a narrow therapeutic index such as TCAs, theophylline, antiepileptics, and type IC antiarrhythmics. SSRIs inhibit the metabolism of many medications; however, other medications may also result in increased or decreased levels of SSRIs through inhibition or induction of cytochrome P-450 isoenzymes.

Clinically important isoenzymes include CYP1A2, CYP3A3 and CYP3A4 (CYP3A3/4), CYP2D6, and CYP2C9 and CYP2C19 (52,63–65). Drugs that interact with these isoenzymes can inhibit, induce, or have no effect on metabolism. Induction of metabolism requires days to start and stop; however, inhibition occurs immediately. When an active drug is metabolized to an inactive metabolite, inhibition can result in increased drug levels and potential toxicity. Alternatively, if the therapeutic effect depends on conversion to an active metabolite, then inhibition of metabolism results in decreased levels of the effective component and decreased clinical effect. For example, codeine's analgesic properties are dependent on metabolism by CYP2D6 to the active metabolite morphine. Inhibition may, therefore, result in inadequate analgesia.

The SSRIs have variable influences on individual CYP450 isoenzymes. SSRIs are both substrates and inhibitors of CYP2D6. The degree of inhibition *in vitro* from most potent to least is paroxetine, fluoxetine, sertraline, fluvoxamine, and citalopram (66). Paroxetine, fluoxetine, and its metabolite norfluoxetine are potent inhibitors of CYP2D6. Sertraline, fluvoxamine, and citalopram are weak inhibitors of CYP2D6 and therefore less likely to result in significant drug interactions when combined with substrates of CYP2D6. The CYP2D6 isoenzyme is responsible for the hydroxylation of the TCAs and is involved in the metabolism of many other antidepressants (paroxetine, fluoxetine, venlafaxine), many antipsychotics, several antiarrhythmic agents (encainide, mexiletine, flecainide), and chlorpheniramine. Many beta-blockers (including propanolol) accumulate in the presence of inhibitors of CYP2D6, causing increased risk of bradycardia and hypotension. Physicians seeking to avoid such an interaction may decide to use atenolol or nadolol, beta-blockers that do not undergo hepatic metabolism and therefore are not affected by SSRIs (67).

Codeine is metabolized by CYP2D6 to morphine. If this enzyme is inhibited, the analgesic efficacy may be diminished. Reduced production of metabolites by inhibition of CYP2D6 may also result in diminished analgesic effectiveness of hydrocodone, oxycodone, and tramadol (67).

SSRIs vary in their effects on other cytochromes, including CYP1A1/2, CYP2C9 and CYP2C10, CYP2C19, and CYP3A4/5 (66). CYP3A3/4 metabolizes many medications that may be important in treating a child with a painful medical illness (68). CYP3A4 is inhibited by fluoxetine, fluvoxamine, and, to a lesser extent, sertraline. Coadministration with the triazolobenzodiazepines (triazolam, alprazolam, and midazolam) may result in increased levels of the benzodiazepine. The dose of these anxiolytics should be reduced and the patient monitored for signs of toxicity when coadministered with medications that inhibit CYP3A4. Alternatively, the patient may be treated with a benzodiazepine that is eliminated by glucuronidation (lorazepam, oxazepam, or temazepam), thus avoiding the potential interaction. Other medications that may require dose reduction and clinical monitoring for toxicity when used with medication that inhibit CYP3A4 include TCAs, carbamazepine, cyclosporin A, calcium channel blockers (diltiazem, nifedipine, verapamil), lidocaine, opioids, and dextromethorphan (68). Fluvoxamine and fluoxetine should not be used in combination with astemizole (Hismanal), cisapride (Propulsid), or terfenadine (Seldane, no longer available in the United States) because increased levels are associated with QT prolongation and torsade de pointes, which can be fatal.

Fluvoxamine is the only SSRI that is a potent inhibitor of CYP1A2 and CYP2C9 (69). When combined with substrates of CYP1A2, such as theophylline, caffeine, ropivacaine, haloperidol, clozapine, olanzapine, amitriptyline, clomipramine, and imipramine, fluvoxamine may increase levels of these medications (68). Inhibition of CYP450 A9 results in increased levels of warfarin and phenytoin. Fluoxetine, paroxetine, sertraline, and citalopram have little or no effect of CYP2C9 activity (70). Fluvoxamine is also a potent inhibitor of CYP2C19 (71). Fluoxetine is a moderate inhibitor of CYP2C19 (72). Drugs that inhibit CYP2C19 have the potential to cause drug interactions with substrates of CYP2C19 such as clozapine, diazepam, some anticonvulsants and antidepressants, propanolol, and nonsteroidal anti-inflammatory agents.

The risk of drug interactions increases with the number of drugs taken by a patient concomitantly. Such interactions, when caused by competitive enzyme inhibition, increase with higher concentrations of the medications. In addition, drugs do not necessarily produce similar interactions in all people.

Variability in the activity or expression of certain cytochrome P-450 isoenzymes, including CYP2D6 (lacking in 5% to 10% of whites) and CYP2C19 (with slow enzymatic activity in 3% to 5% of whites and approximately 20% of Japanese and Chinese), contributes to these differences (62). Therefore, it is always prudent to start at a low level and increase the dose slowly. Information based on the cytochrome P-450–mediated drug interactions may be used to anticipate possible drug interactions or make rational choices in choosing one drug over another in a selected patient. Recent reviews of cytochrome P-450–mediated drug interactions may be found elsewhere (63–65,67). Information on cytochrome P-450–based drug interactions is expanding rapidly. Therefore, before combining medications, it is important to review the most recent literature. Internet websites are also available that provide current charts of cytochrome P-450 drug interactions.

http://www.dml.georgetown.edu/depts/pharmacology/clinlist.html

American College of Clinical Pharmacology: Drugs and Cytochrome P450 Isoenzymes (http://www.accp.com/p450.html)

Clinically Used Drugs Metabolized by Cytochrome P-450

Further clinical research is needed on the metabolic pathways of commonly used medications and their drug interactions. However, these drug interactions are only one criterion in rational drug selection. Other drug interactions that should be considered include interference with absorption, protein binding, or additive adverse effects. Because SSRIs are highly protein bound, consideration must be given to their interactions with other medications that are highly protein bound such as warfarin, digoxin, anticonvulsants, and cisplatin. Fluvoxamine and citalopram are less protein bound and therefore are better choices for patients taking these medications (73).

Serotonin Syndrome

Interaction of SSRIs with other serotonergic medications may induce serotonin syndrome. This syndrome results from a precipitous increase in central nervous system concentration of serotonin and manifests with cognitive-behavioral changes (confusion, restlessness, agitation), neuromuscular abnormalities (incoordination, dizziness, myoclonus, tremor, hyperreflexia, rigidity), and autonomic nervous system dysfunction (diaphoresis, hyperthermia, hypertension or hypotension, tachycardia, nausea, vomiting, diarrhea) (74). This is a serious and sometimes fatal reaction. Concurrent administration of SSRIs and monoamine oxidase inhibitors) should be avoided. Combined use results in profound serotonin syndrome owing both to inhibition of metabolism of serotonin by the monoamine oxidase and inhibition of serotonin reuptake by the SSRI. Serotonin syndrome can also result from any drug combination that increases serotonin through inhibition of its reuptake, increased release or synthesis, or direct stimulation of serotonin receptors. Several medications exhibit significant serotonin reuptake inhibition including nefazodone, trazodone, amitriptyline, clomipramine, imipramine, venlafaxine, dextromethorphan, meperidine, pentazocine, amphetamine, and cocaine. Other medications that may enhance serotonergic activity include lithium, tryptophan, buspirone, *Hypericum perforatum* (St. John's wort), dextromethorphan, tryptophan, zolmitriptan, sumatriptan, sibutramine, rizatriptan, and naratriptan (74). Coadministration of serotonergic drugs should be undertaken with caution and careful clinical monitoring.

Serotonin syndrome can also occur when the metabolism of an SSRI is impaired through cytochrome P-450–based drug interactions. This in not often of clinical significance because patients tolerate a broad range of SSRI concentrations. However, serotonin syndrome has been described in a child owing to inhibition of sertraline metabolism by erythromycin (75).

Tricyclic Antidepressants

Tricyclic antidepressants are no longer the first-line treatment of childhood depression or anxiety disorders. Studies of TCAs have not shown significant benefit over placebo in the treatment of depression. Also, there have been rare occurrences of sudden death in children treated with therapeutic doses of TCAs. Six cases (five boys ages 8, 8, 9, 9, and 14 years and one 12-year-old girl) of unexplained death have been reported in children treated with standard doses of desipramine (76,77). One death was reported in a 7-year-old boy receiving imipramine (6 mg/kg) and thioridazine (76). The risk of sudden death in children ages 5 to 14 years treated with desipramine may be increased by a factor of two to three beyond that occurring naturally in the general population (4.2 deaths per million per year) (78). However, it has not been clearly established whether or how TCAs contributed to the deaths. It has been suggested that these deaths may be related to cardiac arrhythmias, and TCAs (especially desipramine) may increase the vulnerability to arrhythmias (79–81). As a consequence of these deaths, there has been concern about the safety of TCAs, particularly desipramine, in children.

Before Initiation

A careful review for possible cardiac symptoms such as chest pain, shortness of breath, palpitations, dizziness, or syncopal episodes should be obtained. TCA treatment should be considered very carefully in children with a family history of arrhythmias, premature cardiac disease, conduction defects, unexplained fainting, or sudden death (82). Baseline ECG, heart rate, and blood pressure should be obtained. If there are abnormalities, a pediatric cardiologist should be consulted. Parents should be informed of the possible association of TCAs with sudden death. TCAs lower the seizure threshold; therefore, it is important to inquire about a history of seizures (26,82). Whether children are included in these discussions depends on their age and ability to understand the risks and benefits of medications.

Monitoring

Treatment should be initiated with small doses and increased gradually. The suggested initial dose is 10 to 25 mg per day or 0.5 mg/kg per day imipramine or its equivalent (83–85). Divided doses are used in prepubertal children because they metabolize TCAs more rapidly. ECGs should be rechecked after reaching a dose of 1.0 mg/kg per day nortriptyline or 2.5 mg/kg per day imipramine. Serial ECGs are recommended with each dose increase of 50 to 100 mg per day thereafter (46,86). The dose should be increased until a clinical response or maximal dosage is achieved. The maximal dosage for amitriptyline, desipramine, and imipramine is 5 mg/kg or 300 mg per day. Nortriptyline has a maximal dosage of 2.5 mg/kg or 150 mg per day (86). The dosage should be reduced or the drug discontinued if the following parameters are reached or exceeded: PR interval, 0.2 seconds; QRS interval, 0.12 seconds or 130% of baseline; QTC, 0.48 seconds; resting heart rate 110 to 130 beats per minute (children) or 110 to 120 beats per minute (adolescents); and blood pressure, 120/80 mm Hg (children) or 140/90 mm Hg (adolescents) (46,86). Excessive weight gain has been reported, and, therefore, weight should be monitored in patients taking TCAs.

Adverse Effects

Common adverse effects of TCAs include anticholinergic symptoms such as dry mouth, constipation, urinary retention, blurred vision, tremor, orthostatic hypotension, and tachycardia. Asymptomatic cardiovascular effects include increases in pulse, diastolic blood pressure, and prolongation of the PR, QRS, and QT intervals (86). Drowsiness may also occur, particularly at the beginning of treatment. Many symptoms are transitory and can be minimized by increasing the dose gradually. Educating the children and their families about the possibility of these adverse effects and how to manage them may help the children adjust to the medications and improve compliance. For example, sugarless beverages and gum may help alleviate the dry mouth and prevent weight gain associated with the use of TCAs. Anticholinergic symptoms are more severe with tertiary amines (amitriptyline, imipramine, clomipramine) than with secondary amines (nortriptyline, desipramine).

Overdose

TCAs can be lethal when taken in an accidental or intentional overdose (87). Parents should be informed of this risk and medications kept away from young children and potentially suicidal individuals.

Tricyclic Antidepressant Discontinuation

Medications should be continued for 4 to 6 months after improvement in symptoms. TCAs should be tapered over a 2- to 3-week period (83,85). Abrupt discontinuation from moderate or high doses results in anticholinergic rebound. This presents as a flu-like syndrome with gastrointestinal distress, headache, and lethargy.

Drug Interactions

Most adverse interactions with TCAs result from additive sedative or anticholinergic effects. In addition, medications that inhibit or induce hepatic enzymes may alter plasma levels of TCAs.

ANXIETY IN CHILDREN WITH PAIN

As is the case for depression, a strong correlation exists between pain and anxiety (3,17,88). Pain contributes to increased anxiety, which in turn may lead to increased pain. A patient in pain may present with symptoms of anxiety that subside once the pain is controlled. Anxiety may be a temporary response to a new or fearful situation, a symptom resulting from an underlying physical condition, a side effect of medications, or a symptom of an anxiety disorder. Anxiety is a component of many psychiatric disorders and occurs with increasing frequency in chronically ill patients. Anxiety disorders have been shown to be associated with high levels of somatic preoccupation. Common anxiety disorders of children include separation anxiety, social phobia, and generalized anxiety disorder. These children may present with somatic symptoms such as fatigue, muscle tension, headaches, and abdominal or chest pain.

Anxiety may also be secondary to the stress of hospitalization or medical procedures. Previous painful experiences during medical procedures may result in increased anticipatory anxiety for subsequent procedures and symptoms of a stress disorder; therefore, adequate pain management for initial procedures should be a priority. Anxiety disorders that may result from painful injury or illness include PTSD, acute stress disorder, and adjustment disorders. Specific phobias may stem from past painful experiences or complicate the evaluation and treatment of a painful condition.

Anxiety Symptoms Resulting from Painful Events

Psychiatric consultation is often requested to evaluate and treat psychologic sequelae of an acute painful event. Many serious childhood illnesses or their treatments may result in acute pain. Pain may accompany a variety of traumatic events such as physical or sexual abuse, burns, motor vehicle accidents, and accidental or intentional gunshot wounds. The response may be very different if the injury was accidentally or purposely self-inflicted, it occurred in a natural disaster, or it resulted from a violent attack. Emotional recovery may be complicated by grief or survival guilt.

The child's response to pain may be further complicated by stresses imposed by hospitalization. Children may be required to undergo diagnostic evaluations, such as computed tomography or magnetic resonance scans, which, even if not painful, may be very frightening. In addition, children are often required to interact with many unfamiliar health care professionals and endure significant alterations in their daily routine or separation from their parents or siblings. These changes can cause significant stress for children and their families in addition to the already present stress of coping with pain. Reactions to these stresses can vary from a normal response to a psychiatric disorder such as PTSD.

Differential Diagnosis of Anxiety Symptoms After a Painful Event

Normal Response

Anxiety is often a normal response to pain or fearful situations. Many children have fears associated with medical staff and hospitals that are transient and do not interfere with functioning. Often, this anxiety is the result of past painful experiences; however, other fears such as fear of strangers or separation may contribute to the anxiety in a child with pain. These children usually respond well to cognitive preparation and reassurance when facing the anxiety-provoking situation. Efforts should be made to minimize painful procedures and provide optimal analgesia or sedation when needed. Nonpharmacologic techniques should be used whenever possible to help children cope with the stress of medical examinations and treatments.

Adjustment Disorder

Adjustment disorders may present with anxiety symptoms as well as other emotional or behavioral responses. The adjustment disorders are classified according to the predominant symptoms: adjustment disorder with depressed mood, with anxiety, with mixed anxiety and depressed mood, with disturbance of conduct, with mixed disturbance of emotions and conduct, and unspecified (13). These symptoms may occur after a painful illness or injury. The symptoms are thought to be in excess of the expected reaction and cause significant distress of disturbance in functioning, yet they do not meet diagnostic criteria for another psychiatric disorder. Symptoms must occur within 3 months of the stressor and must not persist for more than 6 months after the stressor. This is a common diagnosis applied to children in the hospital by consultation–liaison physicians. Psychologic treatments such as education, play therapy, support, cognitive-behavioral therapy, and family therapy are usually sufficient. A short course of benzodiazepines may occasionally be needed.

Posttraumatic Stress Disorder

Recent studies have documented posttraumatic symptoms after painful accidents, medical illness, and treatment in adults. Children and adolescents have also been shown to be at risk for the development of stress reactions. PTSD symptoms have been shown in children treated for cancer, burns, and motor vehicle accidents (89–95). Children and adolescents treated for cancer may have even higher rates of PTSD than adults (89,96). A child's reaction may be related more to the trauma associated with the medical procedures required than the diagnosis of cancer itself. It is increasingly evident that severe illness or its treatment may cause posttraumatic symptoms. However, the relationship between pain and PTSD is unclear. PTSD in serious illness or injury may be related to the threat of death; however, the contribution of pain to the development of PTSD has not been determined.

PTSD is a pervasive anxiety disorder that follows exposure to an extremely traumatic event (13). The trauma must involve experiencing or witnessing an event capable of causing death, injury, or threat to physical integrity. The initial response includes intense fear, horror, or helplessness. In children, this may be expressed by agitation or disorganized behavior. Revisions in the definition of a traumatic event in the *DSM-IV* no longer require that the traumatic event be outside the realm of normal human experience; therefore, stress reactions to medical illnesses and painful accidents may meet diagnostic criteria for PTSD that were excluded in *DSM-III*. Children's ability to perceive threats of death depends on their developmental age. Younger children who are unable to understand that death is a permanent state may experience a potentially fatal event very differently than older children or adults. Painful traumatic events affecting children include sexual or physical abuse, physical injuries, or medical illnesses including diagnostic or therapeutic procedures.

Symptoms of PTSD are classified into three categories: (a) intrusive re-experiencing of the traumatic event, (b) avoidance of stimuli associated with the event or numbing, and (c) persistence symptoms of hyperarousal. Symptoms must cause significant distress or impairment in functioning and persist longer than 1 month. Diagnosis of PTSD in both children and adults requires at least one symptom of re-experiencing, three symptoms of avoidance or numbing, and two symptoms of increased arousal (13). Clinical presentation varies with developmental age (97). Adolescents may present with symptoms very similar to adults; however, presentation may be very different in younger children.

Re-experiencing symptoms may involve intrusive recollections, recurrent frightening dreams, intrusive thoughts about the event, flashbacks, and psychologic distress or physical reactivity with exposure to cues that symbolize the traumatic event. Preschool children may re-enact the trauma through play. Repetitive dreams are uncommon before 5 years of age (98). School-age children may express symptoms through nightmares, play, drawings, or re-enactment of the trauma. There is increasing awareness of hallucinations occurring in traumatized children that are conceptualized as part of the dissociative symptoms that occur in the context of PTSD (99,100).

Avoidance or emotional numbing is indicated by efforts to avoid places, activities, conversations, and thoughts or feelings that are reminders of the trauma. A child may also display amnesia for aspects of the trauma, decreased interest in normal activities, feelings of detachment from others, and restricted emotions or a sense of a foreshortened future. Young children may experience more avoidance behavior (90). This is likely related to children's inability to understand or express these symptoms. For example, questions about a foreshortened future are meaningless to children with a limited concept of time. Children may also express belief in omens that were warning signs predicting future trauma or display a restricted range of affect, social withdrawal, and loss of developmental skills.

Sleep disturbances, irritability or angry outbursts, poor concentration, hypervigilance, and exaggerated startle are symptoms of increased arousal. Chronic hyperarousal frequently causes somatic complaints such as fatigue, headache, muscle tension, or abdominal pain. Sleep disturbances may be especially common in children. Preschool children may present primarily with symptoms of anxiety. For example, separation anxiety or new fears may develop. Regressive behaviors or loss of developmental skills may also occur.

Although there is no question that even very young children are affected by trauma, there is not a clear consensus on the presentation of PTSD at different developmental levels. There is ongoing controversy about the appropriateness of using *DSM-IV* criteria to diagnose PTSD in children (97). Many children exhibit several PTSD symptoms but do not meet diagnostic criteria according to *DSM-IV*. Adjustment disorder should be considered in the differential diagnosis for children who do not meet diagnostic criteria for PTSD and whose impairment is disproportionate to the stressor. Other stress reactions such as acute stress disorder or phobic avoidance may be the focus of treatment. On a practical level, children with symptoms that impair functioning should be treated whether or not they meet full *DSM-IV* criteria.

Acute Stress Disorder

Acute stress disorder was introduced in *DSM-IV* to document the long-described acute stress response (13). Acute stress disorder is conceptually similar to PTSD in that it includes re-experiencing, avoidance, and symptoms of increased arousal after a traumatic event. Acute stress disorder occurs within 4 weeks of the trauma, lasts between 2 days and 4 weeks, and has a stronger emphasis on dissociative symptoms than does PTSD. Dissociative symptoms include (a) a subjective sense of numbing, detachment, or an absence of emotional responsiveness, (b) a reduction of awareness of surroundings, (c) depersonalization, (d) derealization, and (e) an inability to recall important aspects of the trauma. The diagnosis requires at least three of these symptoms either while experiencing the trauma or after the event. A major rationale for the diagnosis is to identify individuals at risk of developing chronic PTSD who may benefit from early treatment.

Risk Factors for the Development of Posttraumatic Stress Disorder

Little is known about the course of stress disorders and what leads to the development of chronic (lasting longer that 3 months) PTSD. Not everyone who experiences trauma develops PTSD, and a number of factors may affect the outcome.

The type, duration, and frequency of trauma typically influence the course of PTSD. Trauma is classified as type I when a child experiences a single event (for example, rape or an accident) or type II when the child experiences repeated trauma (chronic child abuse, repeated medical procedures) (98). Reaction to repeated injury is different from the reaction to a single event. Children who experience type II trauma are more likely to demonstrate massive denial, dissociation, numbing, or personality problems (101). The likelihood of developing PTSD also depends on the type of painful event (102). For example, the rate of PTSD after a rape or aggravated assault is highly relative to other painful traumatic events (103,104).

The perception of life threat correlates with PTSD symptoms in adults and has been hypothesized as important in children exposed to trauma. However, appreciation of a traumatic event as life threatening may be dependent on the developmental level of the child. The role of children's appraisal of life threat and posttraumatic stress symptoms were evaluated in children with a potentially fatal illness or therapy, such as bone marrow transplantation (105,106). Although the appreciation of the threat to their lives posed by their illness increased with age, there was no significant association between the appreciation of life threat and symptoms of PTSD. Children's subjective appraisal of threat to life has been shown to be associated with symptoms of PTSD in other studies (107–109). Thus, further research is needed on the understanding of life threat and its contribution to PTSD symptoms in relation to developmental age. Because the most frequent cause of pain in pediatric cancer is treatment related, perhaps PTSD symptoms in pediatric cancer are related more to pain than life threat.

Individual characteristics of the child may influence the development of PTSD. A preexisting psychiatric disorder has been shown to contribute to the development of PTSD (110). A child's temperament or psychologic health before the trauma, the age at the time of trauma, the unique meaning of the event, history of pain or traumatic events, and coping resources have all been suggested to influence how children cope with a traumatic event (97,110).

Environmental influences such as family functioning and social support may also mitigate the impact of trauma (93,111). A parent's reactions are likely to have a significant influence on the child's symptoms, especially for younger children. A severe medical illness or injury may be traumatic to both children and their parents, and parents may develop PTSD symptoms (105,112–115). Consistent with this idea are studies showing that children and adolescents are more likely to be diagnosed with PTSD when their mothers also have PTSD (109,114–117).

Treatment of Acute Stress Disorder

The rationale for psychiatric treatment soon after a traumatic event is to decrease symptoms of anxiety and prevent the development of chronic PTSD. Although psychologic intervention soon after a trauma seems appropriate, there is actually little evidence to document the effectiveness of this early intervention (118,119). Stress debriefing has been used shortly after trauma, particularly in cases in which children have witnessed traumatic violent events such as school shootings. This is less frequently used after an individual is exposed to trauma; however, psychiatric consultation may help a child or family cope when a child has been in a painful traumatic event, such as a road accident in which a sibling was killed, a traumatic amputation, or a shooting.

Early psychologic intervention may be requested primarily because of the traumatic nature of the injury rather than symptoms in the child. In these cases, the consultation may be sought by staff because of their sense of helplessness and to master vicariously the trauma encountered by the child. It is hoped that early treatment may be more efficacious and prevent the development of a chronic disorder.

Psychologic debriefing involves a mechanism for discussing the event and responses to it, clarifying misconceptions, providing support, and promoting adaptive coping strategies. Although often perceived as helpful by the victims, there is little evidence that debriefing is effective in helping the psychologic recovery of those exposed to trauma (102). There is some evidence that debriefing may actually worsen the outcome in some cases (120). Few studies of early interventions in children exist. In a community disaster, communication immediately after the event was the intervention that children reported was most helpful to them (102). Children communicated verbally, physically, and through their artwork. Further research is needed to determine which psychologic interventions are most effective for children exposed to a traumatic event.

Until research has determined whether these methods are effective, it seems justified to provide intervention after a major trauma, particularly in children with early signs or risk factors. The interventions should be tailored to facilitate coping based on the nature of the traumatic events and a diagnostic assessment of the child and family. It is important to consider factors that may influence outcome, including coping styles, previous trauma, a history of psychologic morbidity, and dissociation related to the trauma. Separation and loss of friends and family members may be additional stressors that require different interventions or timing. Early intervention often involves education about the possible reactions to traumatic events, support, and careful efforts to facilitate information processing of the original stressful event in a safe, structured setting. Working with the family is essential because anxiety in the parents may increase the child's distress (121). The child's distress can in turn reinforce the sense of helplessness and distress in the parents. Further, parents serve as role models for children's coping abilities. Teaching parents interventions, such as distraction or breathing exercises, may also be helpful. Occasionally, parents may benefit from a referral to a mental health professional for further evaluation and treatment of their own stress reactions. Collaboration with medical staff is necessary to avoid re-experiencing trauma and to fully prepare a child for potentially traumatic procedures when necessary. Benzodiazepines may be helpful for acute symptoms unresponsive to psychologic interventions.

Pharmacologic Management of Acute Stress Disorder

Benzodiazepines

Benzodiazepines effectively treat acute anxiety symptoms that occur shortly after a trauma. The benzodiazepines are rapidly effective and generally well tolerated. However, whether early administration of benzodiazepines after a trauma prevents the development of PTSD is controversial (122,123). Benzodiazepines may be beneficial to treat target symptoms of anxiety and insomnia for a brief period. It has been hypothesized that benzodiazepines may also help prevent PTSD by reducing anxiety, thereby facilitating mental processing of the traumatic event or preventing changes in the noradrenergic system typically associated with stress. However, contrary to expectation, benzodiazepines administered shortly after trauma failed to show a major effect on the course of PTSD (123).

The benzodiazepines are useful for reducing phobic behavior, anticipatory anxiety, and sleep difficulties. For patients whose anxiety is acute and related to specific stressors, use is directed at reduction of acute symptoms. Prolonged use is generally not recommended (83,87). The choice of which benzodiazepine to use depends primarily on the half-life, rate of absorption and distribution, and potential drug interactions.

Lorazepam is frequently used in pediatric patients, although the *Physicians' Desk Reference* indicates that safety and effectiveness are not established in children younger than 12 years of age. Lorazepam (Ativan), oxazepam (Serax), and the hypnotic triazolam (Restoril) are metabolized by direct conjugation and do not have active metabolites. Unlike the other benzodiazepines that are oxidized by the liver, these drugs are not affected by medications that inhibit cytochrome P-450 enzymes. The recommended dose of lorazepam is 0.05 mg/kg/dose every 4 to 8 hours with a range of 0.02 to 0.1 mg/kg (124, 125). In medically ill or very young children, it is best to start at very low doses to avoid oversedation. An oral dose is absorbed at an intermediate rate with effect in approximately 60 minutes. The onset of effect after intravenous administration is between 15 to 30 minutes. Lorazepam is rapidly absorbed from the oral mucosa and can also be administered sublingually (126). The half-life in adults ranges from 10 to 16 hours. The half-life is similar in older children; however, newborns have a prolonged excretion of the drug (mean half-life of 40 hours). When being discontinued, the dose should be tapered gradually to avoid withdrawal symptoms. Withdrawal typically occurs within 2 to 3 days.

Adverse Effects

The most common adverse effects are due to central nervous system depression (83,87). Benzodiazepines often produce sedation, fatigue, and difficulty concentrating. They can cause confusion, lack of coordination, and visual disturbances and are associated with dependence and withdrawal. Anterograde amnesia may occur, especially with the short-acting benzodiazepines. There is little evidence on the impact of long-term use of benzodiazepines. However, given the possible impact on memory and the deleterious effects of central nervous system depression on learning, these medications should be used cautiously in children. Episodes of disinhibition and behavioral dyscontrol have been reported in children and adolescents (85).

Overdose

The most common symptoms include ataxia, lethargy, coma, and respiratory depression (127). Most recover with supportive care and activated charcoal.

Discontinuation

Discontinuation of benzodiazepines can result in withdrawal symptoms, rebound symptoms, or relapse or recurrence of the symptoms for which the benzodiazepines were prescribed (83,85). Common withdrawal symptoms include jitteriness, anxiety, palpitations, tachycardia, muscle cramps, insomnia, nightmares, nausea, and heightened sensitivity to light or sound. Seizures can occur rarely. Withdrawal symptoms may occur after only 4 to 8 weeks of administration or even within 2 to 3 days in patients treated with drugs with a shorter half-life such as lorazepam or alprazolam. Rebound anxiety is the experience of symptoms of anxiety that are more intense than baseline symptoms. These symptoms typically occur a few days after discontinuing the medications and last as long as 72 hours. The original anxiety symptoms usually recur over longer periods.

Antidepressants

A recent study of acute stress disorder in pediatric burn patients suggests that low-dose imipramine (1 mg/kg) may reduce acute stress disorder symptoms (128). Nightmares, flashbacks, symptoms of hyperarousal, and frequent crying were the most common symptoms reported. These symptoms remitted or decreased in intensity in the majority of children treated with imipramine. These children were also receiving additional medications for the management of pain, pruritus, and anxiety. Anxiety was managed with 0.03 mg/kg lorazepam every 4 to 6 hours. It is not clear how imipramine interacted with these other medications to mitigate the symptoms of acute stress disorder. Imipramine should be used with care owing to the association of sudden death with the use of TCAs. Although all cases of sudden death occurred with doses of greater than 3 mg/kg, careful monitoring of blood levels and ECGs is recommended.

Treatment Of Posttraumatic Stress Disorder

PTSD can develop into a chronic condition with symptoms occurring years after the traumatic event (103). Individuals who spontaneously recover usually do so within the first 3 months. Patients with more numerous and severe symptoms in the acute phase are more likely to develop chronic PTSD (129,130). Persistent physical impairment may slow recovery from PTSD (130,131). Individuals with PTSD are more likely to have almost any other psychiatric disorder, including depressive disorders, anxiety disorders, phobias, substance abuse, and somatization disorders (103). The prevalence of somatization is particularly high in those with PTSD, suggesting the importance of the evaluation for PTSD in patients with chronic or recurrent pain (132,133). Most individuals with PTSD have at least one other psychiatric disorder; therefore, treatment planning should take into consideration the possibility of additional diagnoses.

Various psychologic treatments have been described in the treatment of PTSD; however, there is little empiric research documenting the effectiveness (134). Exposure, anxiety management, cognitive behavioral management, and education are considered the most useful psychotherapeutic techniques (135, 136). In children, this involves a direct exploration of the trauma, instructing the child and parents in relaxation techniques, education and correction of misattribution about the trauma, and behavioral management programs for maladaptive behaviors. The most common element of effective treatment is exposure to traumatic memories, emotions, and thoughts. Through exposure, the cycle of avoiding memories and feelings is broken and the anxiety eventually decreases. The patient acquires an understanding of the trauma as well as a sense of mastery and control over the memories. Exposure-based therapies include desensitization, eye movement desensitization and reprocessing, and flooding. Eye movement desensitization is a relatively new technique that has been proposed as a treatment for PTSD (137). It involves individuals making saccadic eye movements while imaging the traumatic event. Although promising, the effectiveness remains controversial, and there are no studies on its use in children with PTSD. Children who do not respond to psychotherapy or who have severe symptoms may require a combination of medications and psychotherapy.

Pharmacologic Management of Posttraumatic Stress Disorder

There are few studies on the use of medications in the treatment of PTSD in children (97,111). Extrapolating from studies in adults, it seems reasonable to use medications to modulate symptoms of PTSD sufficiently to allow the patient to engage in and benefit from exposure-based therapies. Several different types of drugs have been studied in the treatment of PTSD in adults including antidepressants, anxiolytics, and mood stabilizers (138). Comorbid conditions tend to occur in both children and adults with PTSD. In children, these are frequently attention deficit hyperactivity disorder, other anxiety disorders, brief psychotic disorders, suicidal ideation, and a trend toward depressive disorders (110). Comorbid conditions and target symptoms should be considered in selecting medications. Despite the lack of definitive studies, SSRIs are often recommended as an initial medication (139,140).

Specific Phobia

A specific phobia is defined as a marked or persistent fear of a specific object or situation (13). Predisposing factors for the development of a specific phobia may include a traumatic event (141–143). In the medical setting, needle or blood phobias may develop after painful procedures such as injections or venipunctures (144). Anxiety can generalize after painful events to include all medical staff or even a medical building. Other phobias that may be a focus of clinical attention include claustrophobic responses to magnetic resonance imaging or computed tomography scanners or to closed bedside curtains. In general, these phobias respond to psychologic interventions such as education, cognitive behavioral therapy, relaxation training, progressive desensitization, and family therapy. In some cases, the fear is so intense that the child cannot focus on psychologic interventions or there is insufficient time to work with a child before a diagnostic evaluation. It is important to avoid traumatizing a child with a phobia by forced exposure to a feared situation. Occasionally, a feared procedure can be delayed until there is time to prepare the child; however, benzodiazepines or even conscious sedation may be necessary in other cases.

Other Causes of Anxiety Symptoms

Anxiety symptoms can occur in a variety of medical conditions including endocrine, cardiovascular, respiratory, metabolic, and neurologic conditions (13). Anxiety symptoms may also occur owing to the administration or withdrawal of particular medications. A thorough assessment should be done to rule out the diagnosis of an anxiety disorder caused by a medical condition or medication. Because untreated pain can result in considerable anxiety, it is important to assure that pain is optimally treated.

Anxiety disorders or symptoms of anxiety are commonly reported in children with chronic or recurrent pain (145,146). Several primary anxiety disorders are associated with pain complaints including generalized panic disorder, generalized anxiety disorders, chronic PTSD, and separation anxiety disorder (19,147). These anxiety disorders may coexist in children with a painful injury or medical condition. Treatment of anxiety is important in children both with and without a medical explanation for their pain. Treatment may not eliminate pain complaints but will usually help control anxiety that interacts to increase pain. Cognitive-behavioral therapy may be effective, and pharmacologic intervention may be tried after initiating psychosocial treatments. SSRIs, benzodiazepines, or buspirone may be effective; however, there is little research on the pharmacologic management of anxiety disorders in children other than obsessive-compulsive disorder (148). Anxiety disorders are often associated with multiple somatic complaints. The evaluation and treatment of somatization is discussed further elsewhere in this text.

CONCLUSION

Pain has profound impact on levels of emotional distress, and, clearly, psychologic factors such as depression and anxiety can intensify pain. A comprehensive evaluation of children in pain and optimal pain control is essential. Interdisciplinary collaboration helps ensure that both the physical disorder and complicating psychosocial factors are appropriately evaluated and treated. Psychiatric involvement in the treatment of children with pain is an integral part of a comprehensive multidisciplinary approach. Psychiatrists offer unique expertise in evaluating the multiple factors that mediate a child's perception of and response to pain. Children with symptoms of depression or anxiety that are thought to contribute significantly to pain or interfere with functioning should be treated regardless of whether they meet diagnostic criteria for a psychiatric disorder. Various psychotherapeutic techniques are used including crises intervention, brief psychotherapy, cognitive-behavioral therapy, supportive therapy, education, relaxation or distraction, hypnosis, play therapy, group therapy, family therapy, and parental counseling. Treatment often requires a combined approach based on the needs of the child. Psychotherapeutic medications can be a very helpful addition to the treatment plan. Pharmacologic management requires careful consideration of the underlying medical illness, potential drug interactions, and contraindications. Because of a lack of controlled studies in children, the physician must often extrapolate from information on the treatment of adults. Further research is required to identify and document optimal psychiatric treatment for children with painful conditions.

REFERENCES

1. Gil K, Edens J, Wilson J, et al. Coping strategies and laboratory pain in children with sickle cell disease. *Ann Behav Med* 1997;19:22–29.
2. Speigel D. Cancer and depression. *Br J Psychiatry Suppl* 1996;30:109–119.
3. Cardona L. Behavioral approaches to pain and anxiety in the pediatric patient. *Child Adolesc Psychiatr Clin North Am* 1994;3:449–464.
4. Kuttner L. Mind-body methods of pain management. *Child Adolesc Psychiatr Clin North Am* 1997;6: 783–796.
5. AACAP. Practice parameter for the psychiatric assessment of children and adolescents. *J Am Acad Child Adolesc Psychiatry* 1997;36:4S–20S.
6. Egger H, Angold A, Costello E. Headaches and psychopathology in children and adolescents. *J Am Acad Child Adolescent Psychiatry* 1998;37:951–958.
7. Canning E. Mental disorders in chronically ill children: case identification and parent-child discrepancy. *Psychosom Med* 1994;56:104–108.
8. Birmaher B, Ryan N, Williamson D, et al. Childhood and adolescent depression: a review of the past 10 years. Part II. *J Am Acad Child Adolesc Psychiatry* 1996;35:1575–1583.
9. Magni G, Rigatti-Luchini S, Fracca F, et al. Suicidality in chronic abdominal pain: an analysis of the Hispanic Health and Nutrition Examination Survey (HHANES). *Pain* 1998;76:137–144.
10. Porter S, Fein J, Ginsburg K. Depression screening in adolescents with somatic complaints presenting to the

emergency department. *Ann Emerg Med* 1997;29: 141–145.

11. Puura K, Almqvist F, Tamminen T, et al. Children with symptoms of depression—what do adults see? *J Child Psychol Psychiatry* 1998;39:577–585.
12. Cassidy L, Jellinek M. Approaches to recognition and management of childhood psychiatric disorders in pediatric primary care. *Pediatr Clin North Am* 1998;45: 1037–1052.
13. American Psychiatric Association. *Diagnostic and statistical manual of mental disorders, 4th edition (DSM-IV)*. Washington, DC: American Psychiatric Association, 1994.
14. Kovacs M. Presentation and course of major depressive disorder during childhood and later years of the lifespan. *J Am Acad Child Adolesc Psychiatry* 1996; 35:705–715.
15. Birmaher B, Ryan N, Williamson D, et al. Child and adolescent depression: a review of the past 10 years. Part I. *J Am Acad Child Adolesc Psychiatry* 1996;35: 1427–1439.
16. De Wester J. Recognizing and treating the patient with somatic manifestations of depression. *J Fam Pract* 1996;43:S3–15.
17. Sifford L. Psychiatric assessment of the child with pain. *Child Adolesc Psychiatr Clin North Am* 1997;6: 745–781.
18. Ruoff G. Depression in the patient with chronic pain. *J Fam Pract* 1996;43:S25–33.
19. Von Korff M, Simon G. The relationship between pain and depression. *Br J Psychiatry Suppl* 1996;30: 101–108.
20. Varni J, Rapoff M, Waldron S, et al. Chronic pain and emotional distress in children and adolescents. *J Dev Behav Pediatr* 1996;17:154–161.
21. Williamson D, Birmaher B, Frank E, et al. Nature of life events and difficulties in depressed adolescents. *J Am Child Adolesc Psychiatry* 1998;37:1049–1057.
22. Shalev A, Freedman S, Peri T, et al. Prospective study of posttraumatic stress disorder and depression following trauma. *Am J Psychiatry* 1998;155:630–637.
23. Jellinek M, Snyder J. Depression and suicide in children and adolescents. *Pediatr Rev* 1998;19:255–264.
24. Rouchell A, Pounds R, Tierney J. Depression. In: Rundell J, Wise M, eds. *Textbook of consultation—liaison psychiatry*. Washington, DC: American Psychiatric Press, 1996:310–345.
25. AACAP. Practice parameters for the assessment and treatment of children and adolescents with depressive disorders. *J Am Acad Child Adolesc Psychiatry* 1998; 37:63S–83S.
26. Birmaher B. Should we use antidepressant medications for children and adolescents with depressive disorders? *Psychopharmacol Bull* 1998;34:35–39.
27. Reinecke M, Ryan N, DuBois D. Cognitive-behavioral therapy of depression and depressive symptoms during adolescence: a review and meta-analysis. *J Am Acad Child Adolesc Psychiatry* 1998;37:26–34.
28. Clarke G, Rhode P, Lewinsohn P, et al. Cognitive-behavioral treatment of adolescent depression: efficacy of acute group treatment and booster sessions. *J Am Acad Child Adolesc Psychiatry* 1999;38:272–279.
29. Safer D. Changing patterns of psychotropic medication prescribed by child psychiatrists in the 1990s. *J Child Adolesc Psychopharmacol* 1997;7:267–274.
30. Olfson M, Marcus S, Pincus H, et al. Antidepressant prescribing practices of outpatient psychiatrists. *Arch Gen Psychiatry* 1998;55:310–316.
31. Walkup J, Cruz K, Kane S, et al. The future of pediatric psychopharmacology. *Pediatr Clin North Am* 1998;45:1265–1278.
32. Laughren T. Regulatory Issues in pediatric psychopharmacology. *J Am Acad Child Adolesc Psychiatry* 1996;35:1276–1282.
33. Committee on Drugs. *Unapproved uses of approved drugs, the package insert, and the Food and Drug Administration: subject review.* Pediatrics 1996;98: 143–145.
34. Vitello B, Jensen P. Medication development and testing in children and adolescents. Current problems, future directions. *Arch Gen Psychiatry* 1997;54:871–876.
35. Riddle M, Labellarte M, Walkup J. Pediatric psychopharmacology: problems and prospects. *J Child Adolesc Psychopharmacol* 1998;82:87–97.
36. Riddle M, Subramaniam G, Walkup J. Efficacy of psychiatric medications in children and adolescents. *Psychiatr Clin North Am Ann Drug Ther* 1998;5: 269–285.
37. Jensen P. Ethical and pragmatic issues in the use of psychotropic agents in young children. *Can J Psychiatry* 1998;43:585–588.
38. Hughes C, Emslie G, Crimson M, et al. Depression TTCPoMToCM. The Texas Children's Medication Algorithm Project: report of the Texas Conference Panel on Medication Treatment of Childhood Major Depressive Disorder. *J Am Acad Child Adoles. Psychiatry* 1999;38:1442–1454.
39. Labellarte M, Walkup J, Riddle M. The new antidepressants: selective serotonin reuptake inhibitors. *Pediatr Clin North Am* 1998;45:1137–1155.
40. Mandoki M, Tapia M, Tapia M, et al. Venlafaxine in the treatment of children and adolescents with major depression. *Psychopharmacol Bull* 1997;33:149–154.
41. Martin A, Kaufman J, Charney D. Pharmacotherapy of early-onset depression. *Child Adolesc Clin North Am* 2000;9:135–157.
42. Emslie G, Rush A, Weinberg W, et al. A double-blind, randomized, placebo-controlled trial of fluoxetine in children and adolescents with depression. *Arch Gen Psychiatry* 1997;54:1031–1037.
43. Ryan N, Varma D. Child and adolescent mood disorders—experience with serotonin based therapies. *Biol Psychiatry* 1998;44:336–340.
44. Toysyali M, Greenhill L. Child and adolescent psychopharmacology: important developmental issues. *Pediatr Clin North Am* 1998;45:1021–1035
45. Rudorfer M, Potter W. Metabolism of tricyclic antidepressants. *Cell Mol Neurobiol* 1999;19:373–409.
46. Daly J, Wilens T. The use of tricyclic antidepressants in children and adolescents. *Pediatr Clin North Am* 1998; 45:1123–1135.
47. Stahl S. Mergers and acquisitions among psychotropics: antidepressant takeover of anxiety may now be complete. *J Clin Psychiatry* 1999;60:282–283.
48. Dunner D, Greden J, Greist J, et al. Serotonin: the first decade. *J Clin Psychiatry* 1999;17:4–52.
49. Emslie G, Walkup J, Pliszka S, et al. Nontricyclic antidepressants: current trends in children and adolescents. *J Am Acad Child Adolesc Psychiatry* 1999;38: 517–528.

50. Nurnberg H, Thompson P, Hensley P. Antidepressant medication change in a clinical treatment setting: a comparison of the effectiveness of selective serotonin reuptake inhibitors. *J Clin Psychiatry* 1999;60:574–579.
51. Zajecka J, Amsterdam J, Quitkin F, et al. Changes in adverse events reported by patients during 6 months of fluoxetine therapy. *J Clin Psychiatry* 1999;60:389–394.
52. Leonard H, March J, Rickler K, et al. Pharmacology of the selective serotonin reuptake inhibitors in children and adolescents. *J Am Acad Child Adolesc Psychiatry* 1997;36:725–736.
53. Go F, Malley E, Birmaher B, et al. Manic behaviors associated with fluoxetine in three 12- to 18-year-olds with obsessive-compulsive disorder. *J Child Adolesc Psychopharmacol* 1998;8:73–80.
54. Goldberg R. Selective serotonin reuptake inhibitors: infrequent medical adverse effects. *Arch Fam Med* 1998;7:78–84.
55. Tollefson G, Rosenbaum J. Selective serotonin reuptake inhibitors. In: Schatzberg A, Nemeroff C, eds. *The American Psychiatric Press textbook of pharmacology*, 2nd ed. Washington, DC: American Psychiatric Press, 1998:219—237.
56. Fuller R. The influence of fluoxetine on aggressive behavior. *Neuropsychopharmacology* 1996;14:77–81.
57. Phillips S, Brent J, Kulig K, et al. Fluoxetine verses tricyclic antidepressants: a prospective multicenter study of antidepressant drug overdoses. The antidepressant study group. *J Emerg Med* 1997;15:439–445.
58. Barbey J, Roose S. SSRI safety in overdose. *J Clin Psychiatry* 1998;59:42–48.
59. Edwards J, Anderson I. Systematic review and guide to selection of selective serotonin reuptake inhibitors. *Drugs* 1999;57:507–533.
60. Zajecka J, Tracy K, Mitchell S. Discontinuation symptoms after treatment with serotonin reuptake inhibitors: a literature review. *J Clin Psychiatry* 1997;58: 291–297.
61. Goldstein B, Goodnick P. Selective serotonin reuptake inhibitors in the treatment of affective disorders: III. Tolerability, safety and pharmacoeconomics. *J Psychopharmacol* 1998;12:S55–S87.
62. Goodnick P, Goldstein B. Selective serotonin reuptake inhibitors in affective disorders: basic pharmacology. *J Psychopharmacol* 1998;12:S5–S20.
63. Oesterheld J, Shader R. Cytochromes: a primer for child and adolescent psychiatrists. *J Am Child Adolesc Psychiatry* 1998;37:447–450.
64. Ten Eick A, Nakamura H, Reed M. Drug-drug interactions in pediatric psychopharmacology. *Pediatr Clin North Am* 1998;45:1233–1264.
65. Flockhart D, Osterheld J. Cytochrome P450-mediated drug interactions. *Child Adolescent Psychiatr Clin North Am* 2000;9:43–76.
66. Sproute B, Naranjo C, Bremner K, et al. Selective serotonin reuptake inhibitors and CNS drug interactions: a critical review of the evidence. *Clin Pharmacokinet* 1997;33:454–471.
67. Virani A, Mailis A, Shapiro L, et al. Drug interaction in human pain: pharmacotherapy. *Pain* 1997;73:3–13.
68. Bertz R, Granneman G. Use of in vitro and in vivo data to estimate the likelihood of metabolic pharmacokinetic interactions. *Drug Interactions* 1997;32:211–258.
69. Schmider J, Greenblett D, Von Moltke L, et al. Inhibition of CYP2C9 by selective serotonin inhibitors in vitro: studies of phenytoin p-hydroxylation. *Br J Clin Pharmacol* 1997;44:495–498.
70. Hemeryck A, De Vriendt C, Belpaire F. Inhibition of CYP2C9 by selective serotonin inhibitors: in vitro studies with tolbutamide and (S)-warfarin using human liver microsomes. *Eur J Clin Pharmacol* 1999; 54:947–951.
71. Olesen O. Fluvoxamine-clozapine drug interaction: inhibition in vitro of five isoforms involved in clozapine metabolism. *J Clin Psychopharmacol* 2000;20:35–42.
72. Jeppensen U, Gram L, Vistisen K, et al. Dose-dependent inhibition of CYP1A2, CYP2C19 and CYP2D6 by citalopram, fluoxetine, fluvoxamine and paroxetine. *Eur J Clin Pharmacol* 1996;51:73–78.
73. DeVane C, Sallee F. Serotonin selective reuptake inhibitors in child and adolescent psychopharmacology: a review of published experience. *J Clin Psychiatry* 1996;57:55–66.
74. Lane R, Baldwin D. Selective serotonin reuptake inhibitor-induced serotonin syndrome: review. *J Clin Psychopharmacol* 1997;17:208–221.
75. Lee DO, Lee CD. Serotonin syndrome in a child associated with erythromycin and sertraline. *Pharmacotherapy* 1999;19:894–896.
76. Varley C, McClellan J. Case study: two additional sudden deaths with tricyclic antidepressants. *J Am Acad Child Adolesc Psychiatry* 1997;36:390–394.
77. Popper C, Ziminitzky B. Sudden death putatively related to desipramine treatment in youth: a fifth case and a review of speculative mechanisms. *J Child Adolesc Psychopharmacol* 1995;5:283–300.
78. Biederman J, Thisted R, Greenhill L, et al. Estimation of the association between desipramine and the risk of sudden death in 5 to 14 year old children. *J Clin Psychiatry* 1995;56:87–93.
79. Mezzacappa E, Steingard R, Kindlon D, et al. Tricyclic antidepressants and cardia autonomic control in children and adolescents. *J Am Acad Child Adolesc Psychiatry* 1998;37:52–59.
80. Walsh B, Greenhill L, Giardina E, et al. Effects of desipramine on autonomic input to the heart. *J Am Child Adolesc Psychiatry* 1999;38:1186–1192.
81. Waslick B, Walsh B, Greenhill L, et al. Cardiovascular effects of desipramine in children and adults during exercise testing. *J Am Acad Child Adolesc Psychiatry* 1999;38:179–186.
82. Dulcan M, Bregman J, Weller E, et al. Treatment of childhood and adolescent disorders. In: Schatzberg A, Nemeroff C. *The American Psychiatric Press textbook of psychopharmacology*, 2nd ed. Washington, DC: American Psychiatric Press, 1998: 803–850.
83. Birmaher B, Yelovich A, Renaud J. Pharmacologic treatment for children and adolescents with anxiety disorders. *Pediatr Clin North Am* 1998;45:1187–1204.
84. Spencer T, Wilens T, Biederman J. Psychotropic medication for children and adolescents. *Child Adolesc Psychiatr Clin North Am* 1995;4:97–121.
85. Velosa J, Riddle M. Pharmacologic treatment of anxiety disorders in children and adolescents. *Child Adolesc Psychiatr Clin North Am* 2000;9:119–133.
86. Wilens T, Biederman J, Baldessarini R, et al. Cardiovascular effects of therapeutic doses of tricyclic antidepressants in children and adolescents. *J Am Acad Child Adolesc Psychiatry* 1996;35:1491–1501.

87. Bernstein G, Perwien A. Anxiety disorders. *Child Adolesc Psychiatr Clin North Am* 1995;4:305–322.
88. Green W, Kowalik S. Psychopharmacologic treatment of pan and anxiety in the pediatric patient. *Child Adolesc Psychiatr Clin North Am* 1995;3:465–483.
89. Stuber M, Christakis D, Houskamp B, et al. Posttraumatic symptoms in childhood leukemia survivors and their parents. *Psychosomatics* 1996;37:254–261.
90. Landolt M, Boehler U, Schwager C, et al. Post-traumatic stress disorder in paediatric patients and their parents: an exploratory study. *J Pediatr Child Health* 1998;34:539–543.
91. Butler R, Rizzi L, Handwerger B. The assessment of posttraumatic stress disorder in pediatric cancer patients and survivors. *J Pediatr Psychol* 1996;21: 499–504.
92. Gardner G, August C, Githens J. Psychological issues in bone marrow transplantation. *Pediatrics* 1997;60: 625–631.
93. Butler R, Rizzi L, Handwerger B. Brief report: the assessment of posttraumatic stress disorder in pediatric cancer patients. *J Pediatr Psychol* 1996;21:499–504.
94. Stuber M, Kazak A, Meeske K, et al. Is posttraumatic stress a viable model for understanding responses to childhood cancer? *Child Adolesc Psychiatr Clin N Am* 1998;7:169–182.
95. Digallo A, Barton J, Parry-Jones W. Road traffic accidents: early psychological consequences in children and adolescents. *Br J Psychiatry* 1997;170:358–362.
96. Pelcovitz D, Libov B, Mandel F, et al. Posttraumatic stress disorder and family functioning in adolescent cancer. *J Trauma Stress* 1998;11:205–221.
97. AACAP. Practice parameters for the assessment and treatment of children and adolescents with posttraumatic stress disorder. *J Am Acad Child Adolesc Psychiatry* 1998;37:4S–26S.
98. Terr L. Childhood traumas: an outline and overview. *Am J Psychiatry* 1991;148:10–20.
99. Kaufman J, Birmaher B, Clayton S, et al. Case study: trauma-related hallucinations. *J Am Acad Child Adolesc Psychiatry* 1997;36:1602–1605.
100. Gavin L, Roesler T. Posttraumatic distress in children and families after intubation. *Pediatr Emerg Care* 1997;13:222–224.
101. Wintgens A, Boileau B, Robaey P. Posttraumatic stress symptoms and medical procedures in children. *Can J Psychiatry* 1997;42:611–616.
102. Allen S, Dlugokinski E, Cohen L, et al. Assessing the impact of a traumatic community event of children and assisting with their healing. *Psychiatr Ann* 1999;29: 93–98.
103. Solomon S, Davidson J. Trauma: prevalence, impairment, service use and cost. *J Clin Psychiatry* 1997;58: 5–11.
104. Foa E, Meadows E. Psychological treatments for posttraumatic stress disorder: a critical review. *Annu Rev Psychol* 1997;48:449–480.
105. Stuber M, Nader K, Houskamp B, et al. Appraisal of life threat and acute trauma responses in pediatric bone marrow transplant patients. *J Traum Stress* 1996;9: 673–686.
106. Stuber M, Meeske K, Gonzalez S, et al. Posttraumatic stress in childhood cancer survivors I: the role of appraisal. *Psychooncology* 1994;3:305–312.
107. Stallard P, Velleman R, Baldwin S. Prospective study of post-traumatic stress disorder in children involved in road traffic accidents. *BMJ* 1998;317:1619–1623.
108. Stuber M, Kazak A, Meeske K, et al. Predictors of posttraumatic stress symptoms in childhood cancer survivors. *Pediatrics* 1997;100:958–964.
109. Barakat L, Kazak A, Meadows A, et al. Families surviving childhood cancer: a comparison of posttraumatic stress symptoms with families of healthy children. *J Pediatr Psychol* 1997;22:843–859.
110. Famularo R, Fenton T, Kinscherff R, et al. Psychiatric comorbidity in childhood post traumatic stress disorder. *Child Abuse Neglect* 1996;20:953–961.
111. Pfefferbaum B. Posttraumatic stress disorder in children: a review of the past 10 years. *J Am Acad Child Adolesc Psychiatry* 1997;36:1503–1511.
112. Rizzone L, Stoddard F, Murphy J, et al. Posttraumatic stress disorder in mothers of children and adolescents with burns. *J Burn Care Rehabil* 1994;15:158–163.
113. Kazak A, Stuber M, Barakat L, et al. Predicting posttraumatic stress symptom in mothers and fathers of survivors of childhood cancers. *J Am Acad Child Adolesc Psychiatry* 1998;37:823–831.
114. de Vries A, Kassam-Adams N, Cnaan A, et al. Looking beyond the physical injury: posttraumatic stress disorder in children and parents after pediatric traffic injury. *Pediatrics* 1999;104:1293–1299.
115. Fukunishi I. Posttraumatic stress symptoms and depression in mothers of children with severe burn injuries. *Psychol Rep* 1998; 83:331–335.
116. Famularo R, Fenton T, Kinscherff R, et al. Maternal and child posttraumatic stress disorder in cases of child maltreatment. *Child Abuse Neglect* 1994;18:27–37.
117. Pelcovitz D, Goldenberg B, Kaplan S, et al. Posttraumatic stress disorder in mothers of pediatric cancer survivors. *Psychosomatics* 1996;37:116–126.
118. Bryant R, Harvey A, Dang S, et al. Treatment of acute stress disorder: a comparison of cognitive-behavioral therapy and supportive counseling. *J Consult Clin Psychol* 1998;66:862–866.
119. Foa E, Meadows E. Psychosocial treatments for posttraumatic stress disorder: a critical review. *Annu Rev Psychol* 1997;48:449–480.
120. Bisson J, Jenkins P, Alexander J, et al. Randomized controlled trial of psychological debriefing for victims of acute burn trauma. *Br J Psychiatry* 1997;171: 78–81.
121. Kazak A, Barakat L. Brief report: parenting stress and quality of life during treatment for childhood leukemia predicts child and parent adjustment after treatment ends. *J Pediatr Psychol* 1997;22:749–758.
122. Mellman T, Byers P, Augenstein J. Pilot evaluation of hypnotic medication during acute traumatic stress response. *J Traum Stress* 1998;11:563–569.
123. Gelpin E, Bonne O, Peri T, et al. Treatment of recent trauma survivors with benzodiazepines. *J Clin Psychiatry* 1996;57:390–394.
124. McCall J, Fisher C, Warden G, et al. Lorazepam given the night before surgery reduces preoperative anxiety in children undergoing reconstructive burn surgery. *J Burn Care Rehabil* 1999;20:151–154.
125. Henry D, Burwinkle J, Klutman N. Determination of sedative and amnestic doses of lorazepam in children. *Clin Pharm* 1991;10:625–628.
126. Yager J, Seshia S. Sublingual lorazepam in childhood serial seizures. *Am J Dis Child* 1988;142:931–932.

127. Wiley C, Wiley J. Pediatric benzodiazepine ingestion resulting in hospitalization. *J Toxicol Clin Toxicol* 1998;36:227–231.
128. Robert R, Blakeney P, Villarreal C, et al. Imipramine treatment in pediatric burn patients with symptoms of acute stress disorder: a pilot study. *J Am Acad Child Adolesc Psychiatry* 1999;38:873–882.
129. Mayou R, Bryant B, Duthie R. Psychiatric consequences of road traffic accidents. *BMJ* 1993;307: 647–651.
130. Blanchard E, Hickling E, Vollmer A, et al. Short-term follow-up of posttraumatic stress disorder in motor vehicle accidents. *Behav Res Ther* 1995;11:360–377.
131. Kuch K, Cox B, Evans R, et al. Phobias, panic and pain in 55 survivors of road vehicle accidents. *J Anxiety Disord* 1994;8:181–187.
132. Baker D, Mendenhall C, Simbartl L, et al. Relationship between posttraumatic stress disorder and self-reported physical symptoms in Persian Gulf war veterans. *Arch Intern Med* 1997;157:2076–2078.
133. Geisser M, Roth R, Bachman J, et al. The relationship between symptoms of post-traumatic stress disorder and pain, affective disturbance and disability among patients with accident and non-accident related pain. *Pain* 1996;66:207–214.
134. Goenjian A, Karayan I, Pynoos R, et al. Outcome of psychotherapy among early adolescents after trauma. *Am J Psychiatry* 1997;154:536–542.
135. Foa E, Davidson J, Frances A. The expert consensus guideline series: treatment of posttraumatic stress disorder. *J Clin Psychiatry* 1999;60:6–33.
136. March J, Amaya-Jackson L, Murray M, et al. Cognitive-behavioral psychotherapy for children and adolescents with posttraumatic stress disorder after a single-incident stressor. *J Am Acad Child Adolesc Psychiatry* 1998; 37:585–593.
137. Shapiro F. Eye movement desensitization and reprocessing (EMDR) and the anxiety disorders: clinical and research implications of an integrated psychotherapy treatment. *J Anxiety Disord* 1999;13:35–65.
138. Davidson J. Biologic therapies for posttraumatic stress disorder: an overview. *J Clin Psychiatry* 1997;58: 29–32.
139. Davidson J, Connor K. Management of posttraumatic stress disorder: diagnostic and therapeutic issues. *J Clin Psychiatry* 1999;60:33–38.
140. series. Tecg. Treatment of posttraumatic stress disorder. The expert consensus panels for PTSD. *J Clin Psychiatry* 1999;60:3–76.
141. Fyers A. Current approaches to the etiology and pathophysicology of specific phobias. *Biol Psychiatry* 1998; 44:1295–1304.
142. King N, Eleona G, Ollendick T. *Etiology of childhood phobias: current status of Rachman's three pathways theory.* Behav Res Ther 1998;36:297–309.
143. Townend E, Dimigen G, Fung D. A clinical study of child dental anxiety. *Behav Res Ther* 2000;38:31–46.
144. Kleinknecht R. Acquisition of blood, injury, and needle fears and phobias. *Behav Res Ther* 1994;32:817–823.
145. Scharff L. Recurrent abdominal pain in children: a review of psychological factors and treatment. *Clin Psychol Rev* 1997;17:145–166.
146. Hyams J, Burke G, Davis P, et al. Abdominal pain and irritable bowel syndrome in adolescents: a community based study. *J Pediatr* 1996;129:220–226.
147. Roy-Byrne P. Generalized anxiety and mixed anxiety-depression: association with disability and health care utilization. *J Clin Psychiatry* 1996;57:86–91.
148. AACAP. Practice parameters for the assessment and treatment of children and adolescents with anxiety disorders. *J Am Acad Child Adolesc Psychiatry* 1997;36: 69S–84S.

16

Assessment and Management of Somatoform Pain Disorders

Stephen R. King

Health care providers and parents alike are familiar with children's complaints of illness or pain for which no apparent cause can be found. In community samples, between 25% and 44% of children and adolescents report recent histories of somatic complaints such as stomach aches and headaches (1,2). Most of these symptoms are transient and not indicative of any serious illness and do not lead to significant restrictions of activity. It is quite normal, however, for children to experience psychologic stress in response to illness and injury. Increases in depression, anxiety, and irritability, as well as changes in or reduction of normal activity, are understandable and adaptive. The psychologic response becomes maladaptive when it is out of proportion to the seriousness of the illness or injury and causes significant impairment in social, occupational, or other important areas of functioning. The psychiatric term for this kind of response is somatization disorder. Within the *Diagnostic and Statistical Manual of Mental Disorders, Fourth Edition* (*DSM-IV*) category of somatoform disorders, there are several conditions that involve maladaptive pain responses. These include somatization disorder, undifferentiated somatization disorder, pain disorder, somatoform disorder not otherwise specified, and conversion disorder (3). These conditions differ mainly on the basis of the number, severity, and duration of physical symptoms. Somatization disorder involves multiple symptoms of at least 6 months' duration, some of which may or may not include pain. Undifferentiated somatization disorder may be diagnosed when the number of symptoms required for somatization disorder is not met. In pain disorder, the predominant focus of clinical attention is the pain itself, and psychologic factors are judged to have an important role in its onset, severity, exacerbation, or maintenance. Conversion disorder involves symptoms or deficits affecting voluntary motor or sensory functioning whose onset has been judged to be associated with psychologic stressors or conflicts; essentially the conflict has been "converted" into a physical symptom. The distinction among these disorders is not always clear, especially as they pertain to a pediatric population. Etiologically, all may be related to some stress or conflict, and in all, a preexisting medically verifiable illness may be either a predisposing factor or a modeling agent for the symptom. Pain is a subjective experience in which psychologic, environmental, and physiologic factors are believed to play a role (4), and there is no one-to-one relationship between the extent of tissue involvement and the degree of pain. Chronic pain in particular is thought to be heavily influenced by nonorganic factors, including previous pain experience, culture, gender, and temperament (5).

Besides their common psychologic origins, the other element that most of these disorders have in common is their chronicity. Somatization disorder and pain disorder can be diagnosed only after they have been present at least 6 months.

EPIDEMIOLOGY

Prevalence of recurrent pain without apparent organic cause is very common among children and adolescents. Campo et al. (6) found that almost 3% of 11 to 15 year olds attending a general pediatric service had frequent complaints of pain and frequent pain-related doctor visits. Other studies have shown that complaints of recurrent pain may be as high as 15% at any given time within a general pediatric population (7). The number of cases that meet criteria for somatoform disorder is much smaller. Epidemiologic surveys using the *DSM-IV* criteria have not been done but might be expected to yield very low numbers of positive cases because of the symptom and duration requirements. Some authors have questioned whether the *DSM-IV* criteria for somatoform disorders are clinically and developmentally appropriate for children (8), but there is little argument that children do have somatoform conditions.

Somatoform disorders, however defined, tend to affect girls more than boys, with ratios between 3:1 and 6:1 reported (6,9,10). Somatoform symptoms have rarely been reported in children younger than 5 years of age, and the only available study that reported the race of patients found blacks and Hispanics to be overrepresented (11). There is some evidence that lower socioeconomic status is associated with a higher incidence of somatoform disorders and pain syndromes (12).

RISK FACTORS

The most frequently cited factor in the development of somatoform disorder in children is stress. In a study of 105 pediatric patients who were diagnosed as having conversion disorders, Maloney (13) reported that 97% of them had experienced major family crises before the onset of the conversion symptoms, and 60% of this group were also experiencing unresolved grief reaction. Both of these percentages were significantly higher than those of matched psychiatric controls. The most common conversion symptoms among patients in this study were abdominal pain and syncope. Although girls outnumbered boys, the difference was not significant. Pillay and Lalloo (14) also reported that family-related stressors, such as marital discord, recent divorce or separation, or the birth of a sibling, were present in the majority (95%) of their patients who were diagnosed with psychogenic pain disorder. Likewise, stressful events within the family, school, or peer relationships were found in 89% of the cases of child and adolescent conversion disorder reported by Siegel and Barthel (11). Other studies have cited school-related stress and long-term family problems as precipitating factors (15,16).

Despite the findings of the studies cited above, the presence of stress in and of itself is not a very useful clinical predictor of somatoform pain because stress is not specific to somatoform disorders. Rather, it is contributory to a host of psychiatric disturbances and medical conditions as well. For example, in one widely cited study of childhood conversion symptoms, 97% of those with the diagnosis had experienced some family stress, but this was also true of 92% of the psychiatric controls (13).

Conversely, some stressors seem to be somewhat more specific to somatoform disorders. One of these is the recent death of a close relative, which may be more than twice as likely to predict a somatoform reaction than another form of psychiatric reaction in the child (13). Clinically, a pain symptom that is similar to one experienced in the recently deceased may be a positive indicator of a somatoform process.

Another specific stressor that may be implicated in the development of somatoform pain disorder is a history of physical or sexual abuse. Eisendrath and colleagues (17) found that a history of physical abuse significantly discriminated patients who had psychogenic abdominal pain from those with inflammatory bowel disease or Crohn disease. Other authors have reported a higher frequency of pain symptoms and other somatic symptoms in sexually abused children than in psychiatric controls (18). Studies of fibromyalgia, a chronic and painful muscular condition that is clearly worsened by psychologic stress, have identified a history of sexual abuse as one of the major triggers of the condition (19,20).

Modeling is often cited as a mechanism by which the child may develop pain symptoms. From a social learning perspective, modeling may be seen as a learned coping response that elicits reinforcers such as attention or special care similar to those that have been given to the family member on whom the symptoms were modeled. From a dynamic perspective, modeling may serve as a way of identifying with or communicating with the ill or deceased family member. Studies of conversion symptoms and unexplained pain symptoms in children have identified personal models for symptoms in more than 50% of the cases (4,14), and one study discusses the phenomenon of self-modeling in adolescents, in which patients with organic disorders in full remission re-experience the symptoms after periods of stress (21). The author notes that the organic and nonorganic factors are particularly difficult to sort out in these cases.

Early theories of conversion hysteria assumed that an underlying hysterical personality style was the root of the disorder. Research on adults has provided little empiric support for this theory (12). Psychologic studies of children have been limited by their inability to distinguish stable personality traits from state characteristics related to the distress of the disorder itself. The so-called *la belle indifference* which is characteristic of the hysterical personality style has not been found to be a reliable diagnostic sign in childhood conversion disorders (11). Temperamental differences in children have been found to be related to pain tolerance (22), but the relationship of temperament to somatoform pain has not been examined.

Although no particular personality style has been linked to the development of somatoform disorders, they may be more likely to occur when another psychiatric condition is present or when there has been a history of psychiatric problems. The comorbidity of somatoform disorders with other psychiatric conditions was investigated by Livingston et al. (23). They reviewed 95 consecutive admissions to a child psychiatry inpatient service. Eight patients were diagnosed as having somatization disorder, and all of them carried at least one other diagnosis as well. Volkmar and associates (9) reported that 50% of their patients with conversion disorder had previously been in psychiatric treatment for other problems. More recent studies have shown a strong link between somatic complaints and psychiatric problems. For example, Egger at al. (24) found that girls with anxiety disorders were five times more likely to report somatic complaints such as stomach aches and musculoskeletal pains than girls with no psychiatric complaints, whereas headaches and muscle pains were overrepresented in depressed boys. In a prospective study of the relationship of somatic complaints and psychopathology, Zwaigenbaum et al. (25) reported that children with multiple somatic complaints were at significantly higher risk than controls for the development of major depression when seen 4 years later. Other studies (26–31) suggest that there is also a higher incidence of psychiatric disorders in close relatives of patients with somatoform disturbances. Modeling, family stress caused by the psychiatric disturbance, and biologic predisposition have all been proposed as possible explanatory mechanisms for these findings.

Because somatoform disorders are often thought to result from an individual's inability to verbally express conflict or affect, some researchers have investigated the possibility that the symptoms may reflect deficits in left hemisphere functioning. The overall results of early studies in this area, which were reviewed by Shapiro and Rosenfeld (32), are inconclusive and often contradictory, although some research does support the hypothesis (33). Shapiro and Rosenfeld point out that in their own clinical sample of children with somatoform disorders 75% had some kind of learning, cognitive, or neurologic problem and that their perceptual accuracy scores on the Rorschach test were lower than average, possibly another indicator of subtle neuropsychologic deficit. Further investigations of the neuropsychologic correlates of somatoform disorders are necessary to clarify these relationships.

ASSESSMENT

Adequate assessment of pain that has the potential of becoming maladaptive involves approaching the problem from a biopsychosocial perspective. All relevant factors that may be contributing to the pain symptoms should be considered, and this should be communicated to the patient at the very beginning of the assessment process. This avoids the resistance and resentment that often greet the clinician when a psychiatric explanation is offered after all the medical possibilities have been exhausted. Because abdominal pain, headaches, chest pain, and limb pain are the most common pain complaints associated with somatoform disorders in children, the clinician should be especially aware of the possibility of nonmedical factors when these symptoms are present. Thus, the psychosocial history becomes at least as important as the physical examination and other medical procedures. The patient and the family should be questioned about a history of psychiatric disturbances, recent stresses, and deaths or serious illnesses in the family that may serve as models. The use of a structured pain interview, such as the Children's Comprehensive Pain Questionnaire (34), may facilitate the gathering of such information.

When talking to patients and families about nonmedical factors involved in pain, the physician should explain that stress, life changes, poor school performance, and the like may affect the way in which symptoms are perceived or tolerated and that part of the treatment may involve dealing with some of these factors. Discussion of these factors as causal should be avoided because this may give the patient the impression that physical causes are not being considered.

An excellent way to assess some of the stress and environmental factors associated with pain is to have the child keep a pain diary. The simplest type requires the child to keep a daily record of when pain begins and ends. Location and intensity of the pain are noted as well. Ratings of intensity should be meaningful to the child and developmentally appropriate. Younger children may find it helpful to use numbers that correspond to facial representations of pain intensity (Chapter 7). Older children may prefer a numerical scale in which 0, for example, corresponds to "no pain," and 10 corresponds to "the worst pain I can imagine." Asking the child to create metaphors that convey the levels of intensity (e.g., "it's like fire," "it's like a big knot that gets tighter and tighter") may aid in developing an appropriate record-keeping system. Other items in the diary may include recording what the patient did to alleviate the pain and what activities were missed because of the pain. McGrath (34) described a number of different approaches to the creation of a pain diary, including the use of visual analog scales, and the interested reader is referred to this volume for further information.

Use of the pain diary yields many benefits for patient and physician alike. It serves as a baseline against which the efficacy of subsequent interventions may be assessed. It also helps to assess the patient's and family's motivation for other nonmedical interventions. Information gathered from the diary may help differentiate organic from nonorganic factors. For example, description and location of pain sites may be more vague and changeable in somatoform than disease-based pain. Somatoform pain may be more likely to lead to avoidance of unpleasant activities, whereas organic pain generally affects all activity (32). Finally, the very act of keeping the diary may reduce or, in some cases, eliminate the symptoms. Controlled studies of the effectiveness of a symptom diary for pain reduction have not been reported, but the phenomenon has been observed clinically. Some patients report that keeping the diary made them realize that the pain or its frequency was not as severe as previously thought. It is thought that keeping track of the symptoms may give the patient a sense of control over them, which, in turn, may lead to reduction in the symptoms themselves.

If the physician has ordered medical tests or prescribed medical treatment, the effectiveness of these interventions should be assessed at a follow-up visit. The symptom diary should be reviewed at this time. In many instances, the physician will sense that the interventions thus far introduced are having a beneficial effect or that medical tests have offered a reasonable alternative hypothesis that may be pursued, including consultation from another medical specialty. If neither of these situations is present, it is a good time to think about psychiatric or psychologic consultation. The purpose of such consultation is twofold: first, to rule out any psychiatric or behavioral disturbance that may be contributing to the pain condition and second, to help develop a treatment plan. A psychologic consultation may include formal psychologic and intelligence testing, which may help reveal dynamics, coping style, learning disabilities, and other factors that may be relevant to treatment, but the psychological tests cannot in themselves be relied on to make a diagnosis.

TREATMENT

There has been very little systematic study of the treatment of children who have been formally diagnosed with somatoform pain disorders. Psychotherapy and family counseling are often mentioned as the treatments of choice, although further specifics such as types of therapy or counseling, expected length of treatment, and success rates are typically lacking. One exception to this trend is a study of psychogenic pain disorder that noted that 76% of the patients showed symptom remission after short-term psychotherapy, but the usefulness of this study is limited by the lack of a control group (14).

Conversely, there is an extensive and growing literature on the treatment of pain conditions in which psychogenic and nonorganic factors may play a prominent role, including recurrent pain syndromes and idiopathic pain disorders. Many of these treatment approaches may be appropriate to the treatment of cases that carry a formal psychiatric diagnosis as well because both etiologically and symptomatically, these disorders may be more alike than different.

Because the approach to assessment of pain should be multidimensional, so should the treatment. This may include the judicious use of medication, even when it is thought that there is a significant psychogenic component. The physician does not have to offer an organic explanation of the pain to justify a medical treatment. Mild analgesics, for example, may be helpful in changing the child's perception of the pain, although they are not likely by themselves to eliminate the syndrome. Antidepressant medications have demonstrated usefulness in reducing pain (36,37), and the adjunctive use of these medications may be indicated for older children and adolescents, especially when there is suspicion of coexisting depression. The interested reader is referred to Sifford's detailed review (Chapter 15) of medications for psychiatric conditions in which pain may be a symptom. A recent review of the use of antidepressants in the treatment of adult psychogenic pain disorder suggests that they are effective (38), and there are some clinical reports of their effectiveness in the treatment of recurrent pain syndromes in children (34).

Psychotherapy is a nonpharmacologic intervention that can be helpful in both general and specific ways. Although there has been little research on the use of psychotherapy as a major intervention, there are clearly clinical situations that warrant its use. When pain is related to the loss or death of a loved one, for example, supportive therapy can help the child feel less isolated and more understood, which can have a general therapeutic effect. Psychodynamic therapy, which proceeds from the assumption that the somatic symptom is a conscious expression of an unconscious conflict or feeling, may be an appropriate treatment when the suspected source of the pain is a deep-seated psychologic conflict, such as guilt feelings over having been sexually abused. The therapist's role is to help the child identify the source of the conflict and to understand why it is being expressed somatically. The therapist interprets the meaning of the child's symptoms, as well as resistance and other behavior within the therapy itself. For young children, interpretation of the child's play may take place as well. Development of a trusting relationship between therapist and patient is a vital part of the treatment. Because psychotherapy can be time-consuming and expensive and requires a significant commitment from the family and the child, it should only be considered as a treatment when there are clear indications for its need.

When there is an assumption that the child's pain symptoms are brought on or maintained by pathologic family dynamics, family therapy may be the treatment of choice. For example, in a high-conflict family that suppresses the open expression of conflict, the child's somatic complaint may serve as an expression of that conflict and a way of getting help. Minuchin et al. (39) identified a number of family characteristics that, along with physiologic vulnerability, predispose some family members to developing psychosomatic problems. These factors are enmeshment, overprotectiveness, rigidity, and lack of conflict resolution. The so-called psychosomatic family resists change and growth. If a crisis or other event threatens to throw the family into conflict or otherwise upset the status quo, the child's symptoms emerge or worsen, refocusing the family on the sick child. Therapy is directed toward changing these characteristics. Techniques include challenging, relabeling of symptoms, and supporting of differentiation and independence in the identified patient. Treatment studies on diabetic and anorectic patients have shown symptom improvement (40–42). Studies using family therapy as a treatment for somatoform pain disorders have not been done, but the dynamics and treatment would be the same. Again, family therapy is expensive and time-consuming, and treatment should be directed at families in which there is suspicion of significant dysfunction. The more common situation in which a basically healthy family member is inadvertently reinforcing pain behavior can be handled through more direct educational and behavioral approaches.

Behavioral approaches to pain relief differ from psychotherapy not only in their methods but in their underlying assumptions. In the behavioral view, there is no underlying psychopathology but only pain behavior that is maintained by particular contingencies in the environment. If the therapist's analysis of pain behavior reveals that there are contingencies (e.g., school avoidance, extra attention) that are reinforcing the pain behavior, then behavioral intervention may be appropriate, regardless of the cause of the pain. Most behavioral approaches to pain control that have been applied to the treatment of pain in chronic illnesses, such as sickle cell disease and juvenile rheumatoid arthritis, are thus equally applicable to the treatment of somatoform pain.

The most basic behavioral approach to pain control involves a combination of rewarding adaptive coping behavior and ignoring pain behavior. This may include frequent praise for maintaining normal activity while minimizing discussion of the pain (43). A more elaborate protocol might involve the dispensing of activity reinforcers or tangible rewards to the child for maintaining complaint-free periods or otherwise engaging in appropriate behavior. Case reports of the successful application of shaping (graduated reinforcement) and extinction (ignoring and time out) to problems of recurrent abdominal pain, idiopathic headache, and conversion paralysis have been reported in the behavioral literature (44–46). Negative reinforcement involving removal of an aversive condition (e.g., no television or reading for pleasure) when the desired behavior (e.g., no complaints of pain) is achieved has also been found successful (47).

Cognitive-behavioral approaches to treatment also focus on behavioral change but emphasize the patient's cognitions, perceptions, and beliefs as exercising an essential role in effecting behavior change. According to the cognitive-behavioral view, it is not the stimulus itself to which the subject responds, but the individual's perception or interpretation of the stimulus. Treatment focuses on changing the child's perception of the stimulus rather than manipulating the contingencies in the environment. Such an approach is naturally suited to the treatment of pain because pain behavior is as much the result of attitudes and beliefs as it is of tissue damage or external contingencies. Cognitive behavioral techniques have been shown clinically effective in treatment of various pain syndromes, including recurrent abdominal pain and recurrent headache, in which psychologic factors are believed to play a significant role (48,49).

A general cognitive approach that has been used extensively in pain management protocols for children involves the teaching of self-regulation skills, which include progressive relaxation, guided imagery, and meditative breathing. These techniques have been successfully used in the control of such diverse pain problems as arthritis pain (50), headache pain (51), recurrent abdominal pain (48), and procedure pain in the treatment of cancer (52). They can be taught easily and adapted to the situation and personality of the child. An added psychologic advantage is that the child feels he or she is actively doing something to control the pain. As part of a multistrategy treatment approach, these techniques have reportedly been successful in management of somatoform pain on pediatric wards (32), although no results of controlled studies have been reported.

Hypnosis is a self-regulatory strategy that has become increasingly utilized in pain management programs in recent years. Broadly defined, hypnosis is an altered state of awareness in which an individual develops a heightened concentration on or responsiveness to certain ideas or images that will aid in achieving a desired effect. Children are particularly good subjects for hypnosis because of their ability to move in and out of imaginative states. The effectiveness of hypnosis in controlling procedure pain and pain associated with acute and chronic diseases has been well documented (53–57) (Chapter 18).

There are few formal studies regarding the use of hypnosis as a treatment for psychogenic or nonorganic pain. Kohen and colleagues (58) reported that 53% of pediatric patients who presented with pain as the primary symptom achieved complete remission of pain after an average of fewer than three sessions of hypnosis. Other studies (59,60) report that hypnosis has been successful in the treatment of somatoform disturbances with and without pain. In no cases was symptom substitution reported.

Biofeedback is another self-regulatory technique that uses increased self-awareness as a means of effecting behavior change. The biofeedback apparatus provides visual or auditory feedback of changes in activities such as muscle tension, heart rate, and blood pressure that the patient would not normally be aware of. In a typical pain reduction protocol, the patient first goes through a series of relaxation exercises, which is followed by training on the biofeedback equipment in which he or she learns what kinds of cognitive strategies are most associated with reductions in autonomic arousal. In the biofeedback treatment of headache, for example, the patient may observe that anticipatory anxiety is associated with contractions of the muscles in the forehead, whereas use of guided imagery has a relaxing effect. Controlled studies of biofeedback have shown that it is effective in the treatment of pediatric migraine (61) and muscle tension headache (62). There have also been case reports of its usefulness in treating other recurrent pains (34). A recent study by Allen and Shriver (63) demonstrated that the effect of biofeedback is enhanced when parents become actively involved in the treatment by helping to reinforce appropriate pain-related behavior. Although studies on the use of biofeedback in treating somatoform pain have not been done, this mode of treatment may be particularly well suited for children with these symptoms. Biofeedback is generally perceived as a physical rather than a psychologic treatment and thus may help overcome the initial resistance to psychologic interventions that many children have. Conversely, a good deal of interaction between therapist and patient occurs in the biofeedback sessions, and this may serve as a nonthreatening way of beginning a therapeutic alliance for further work. Some clinicians believe that a two-stage process of treatment of somatoform disorders, i.e., symptom removal followed by psychotherapy, may be very effective (32), and biofeedback or hypnosis may be an ideal way of providing that first stage.

SUMMARY AND DIRECTIONS FOR FUTURE RESEARCH

Children who develop somatic symptoms that represent something other than organic pathology have long challenged and frustrated clinicians and researchers alike. Pain has been a particularly difficult symptom to understand and treat because of its idiosyncratic and highly subjective nature. The long-held view that somatic symptoms are either organic or psychogenic has given way to a view that symptoms are multidetermined. The current diagnostic criteria for somatoform disorders largely reflect this view.

Stress, loss, modeling, prior psychiatric and physical illness, family communication style, and neuropsychologic abnormalities have all been hypothesized as possible factors contributing to the development of somatoform disorders. To date, very little research has been done to validate these hypotheses. Studies of treatment of somatoform pain and conversion symptoms are likewise lacking, although behavioral and psychologic treatments of other recurrent pain conditions have proved quite successful and may hold promise for the treatment of somatoform pain conditions as well.

As Fritz et al. (8) pointed out, the *DSM-IV* categories for somatoform disorders are more appropriate for adults than for children. Relatively few children meet the formal diagnostic criteria for somatoform disorder, but there are many children who have chronic pain with multiple causes. Future research, using larger samples and multiple interventions, should target this heterogeneous group of patients to determine what individual or combined treatments might offer the greatest relief. The contribution of variables of interest, such as learning style, temperament, and family dynamics, could be assessed as well.

Pain, no matter what its cause, is what hurts. Whether the result of a traumatic injury, a chronic medical illness, or a complex set of environmental, biologic, and psychologic circumstances, any pain that interferes with the normal activity of the child deserves adequate attention and treatment. Much of what constitutes adequate attention and treatment of somatoform pain remains unknown, but the reformulation of the problem in biopsychosocial terms as well as contributions from other areas of pain research raise the hope that better understanding of this most complex and fascinating phenomenon will continue in the years ahead.

REFERENCES

1. Garber J, Walker LS, Zeman J. Somatization symptoms in a community sample of children and adolescents: further validation of the children's somatization inventory. *Psychol Assess* 1991;3:588–595.
2. Taylor DC, Szatmari P, Boyle MH, et al. Somatization and the vocabulary of everyday bodily experiences and concerns: a community study of adolescents. *J Am Acad Child Adolesc Psychiatry* 1996;35:491–499.
3. American Psychiatric Association. *Diagnostic and statistical manual of mental disorders, fourth edition.* Washington, DC: American Psychiatric Association, 1994.
4. Melzack R, Wall PD. Pain mechanisms: a new theory. *Science* 1965;150:971–978.
5. McGrath PA. Psychological aspects of pain perception. In: Schechter NL, Berde C, Yaster M, eds. *Pain in infants, children, and adolescents.* Baltimore, MD: Williams & Wilkins, 1993:39–63.
6. Campo JV, Jansen-McWilliams L, Comer D, et al. Somatization in pediatric primary care: association with psychopathology, functional impairment and use of services. *J Am Acad Child Adolesc Psychiatry* 1999;38: 1093–1101.
7. Maddison TC. Recurrent pain in children. *Med J Aust* 1977;1:708–710.
8. Fritz GK, Fritsch S, Hagino O. Somatoform disorders in children and adolescents: a review of the past 10 years. *J Am Acad Child Adolesc Psychiatry* 1997;36:1329–1338.
9. Volkmar FR, Poll J, Lewis M. Conversion reactions in childhood and adolescence. *J Am Acad Child Psychiatry* 1984;23:424–430.
10. Offord DR, Boyle MH, Szatmari P, et al. Ontario Child Health Study II: six-month prevalence of disorder and rates of service utilization. *Arch Gen Psychiatry* 1987;44:832–836.
11. Siegel M, Barthel RP. Conversion disorders on a child psychiatry service. *Psychosomatics* 1986;27:201–204.
12. France RD, Krishnan KRR, Houpt J, et al. Personality and chronic pain. In: France RD, Krishnan KRR, eds. *Chronic pain.* Washington, DC: American Psychiatric Press, 1988:419–435.
13. Maloney MJ. Diagnosing hysterical conversion reactions in children. *J Pediatr* 1980;97:1016–1020.

14. Pillay AL, Lalloo M. Psychogenic pain disorder in children. *S Afr Med J* 1989;76:195–196.
15. Levine MD, Rapoport LA. Recurrent abdominal pain in school children: the loneliness of the long distance physician. *Pediatr Clin North Am* 1984;31:969–991.
16. Kennedy WA. School phobia: rapid treatment of fifty cases. *J Abnorm Psychol* 1965;70:285–289.
17. Eisendrath SJ, Way LW, Ostroff JW, et al. Identification of psychogenic abdominal pain. *Psychosomatics* 1986; 27:705–712.
18. Livingston R. Sexually and physically abused children. *J Am Acad Child Adolesc Psychiatry* 1987;26:413–415.
19. Goldberg RT, Pachas WN, Keith D. Relationship between traumatic events in childhood and chronic pain. *Disabil Rehabil* 1999;21:23–30.
20. Epstein SA, Kay G, Clauw D, et al. Psychiatric disorders in patients with fibromyalgia: a multi-center investigation. *Psychosomatics* 1999;40:57–63.
21. Friedman SB. Conversion symptoms in adolescents. *Pediatr Clin North Am* 1975;20:873–882.
22. Schechter NL. Pain and pain control in children. *Curr Probl Pediatr* 1985;15:1–67.
23. Livingston R, Taylor JL, Crawford SL. A study of somatic complaints and psychiatric diagnosis in children. *J Am Acad Child Adolesc Psychiatry* 1988;27:185–187.
24. Egger HL, Costello EJ, Alaatin E, et al. Somatic complaints and psychopathology in children and adolescents: stomach aches, musculoskeletal pains and headaches. *J Am Acad Child Adolesc Psychiatry* 1999; 38:852–860.
25. Zwaigenbaum L, Szatmaari P, Boyle MH, et al. Highly somatizing young adolescents and the risk of depression. *Pediatrics* 1999;103:1203–1209.
26. Routh DK, Ernst AR. Somatization disorder in relatives of children and adolescents with functional abdominal pain. *J Pediatr Psychol* 1984;9:427–437.
27. Slater E. The 35th Mosley lecture. *J Ment Sci* 1961;107:359–381.
28. Bohman M, Cloninger CR, VonKnorring A, et al. An adoption study of somatoform disorders III. *Arch Gen Psychiatry* 1984;41:872–878.
29. Cloninger CR, Sigvardsson S, VonKnorring A, et al. An adoption study of somatoform disorders II. *Arch Gen Psychiatry* 1984;41:863–871.
30. Sigvardsson S, VonKnorring A, Bohman M, et al. An adoption study of somatoform disorders I. *Arch Gen Psychiatry* 1984;41:853–859.
31. Kreichman AM. Siblings with somatoform disorders in childhood and adolescence. *J Am Acad Child Adolesc Psychiatry* 1987;26:226–231.
32. Shapiro EG, Rosenfeld AA. *The somatizing child: diagnosis and treatment of conversion and somatization disorders*. New York: Springer-Verlag, 1987.
33. Min SK, Lee BO. Laterality in somatization. *Psychosom Med* 1997;59:236–240.
34. McGrath PA. *Pain in children: nature, assessment and treatment*. New York: Guilford, 1990.
35. Michels PJ, Adams AB, McBride P. Chronic pain. *J Fam Pract* 1983;17:591–610.
36. Botney M, Fields HL. Amitriptyline potentiates morphine analgesia by a direct action on the central nervous system. *Ann Neurol* 1983;13:160–164.
37. Egger H, Angold A, Costello E. Headaches and psychopathology in children and adolescents. *J Am Acad Child Adolesc Psychiatry* 1998;37:951–958.
38. Fishbain DA, Cutler RB, Rosomoff HL, et al. Do antidepressants have an analgesic effect in psychogenic pain and somatoform pain disorders?: a meta-analysis. *Psychosom Med* 1998;60:503–509.
39. Minuchin S, Baker L, Rosman BL, et al. A conceptual model of psychosomatic illness in children. *Arch Gen Psychiatry* 1975;32:1031–1038.
40. Forsander G, Persson B, Sundelin J, et al. Metabolic control in children with insulin-dependent diabetes mellitus 5 years after diagnosis: early detection of patients at risk for poor metabolic control. *Acta Paediatr* 1998; 87:857–864.
41. Eisler I, Dare C, Russell GF, et al. Family and individual therapy in anorexia nervosa: a 5 year follow-up. *Arch Gen Psychiatry* 1997;54:1025–1030.
42. Robin AL, Gilroy M, Dennis AB. Treatment of eating disorders in children and adolescents. *Clin Psychol Rev* 1998;18:421–446.
43. Masek BJ, Russo DC, Varni JW. Behavioral approaches to the management of chronic pain in children. *Pediatr Clin North Am* 1984;31:949–968.
44. Sank LI, Biglan A. Operant treatment of a case of recurrent abdominal pain in a 10 year old boy. *Behav Ther* 1974; 5:677–681.
45. Miller AJ, Kratochwill TR. Reduction of frequent stomachache complaints by time out. *Behav Ther* 1979;10: 211–218.
46. Klonoff EA, Moore DJ. "Conversion reactions" in adolescents: a biofeedback based operant approach. *J Behav Ther Exp Psychiatry* 1986;17:179–184.
47. Campo JV, Negrini BJ. Case study: negative reinforcement and behavioral management of conversion disorder. *J Am Acad Child Adolesc Psychiatry* 2000;39:787–790.
48. Scharff L. Recurrent abdominal pain in children: a review of psychological factors and treatment. *Clin Psychol Rev* 1997;17:145–166.
49. Sanders MR, Shepherd RW, Cleghorn G, et al. The treatment of recurrent abdominal pain in children: a controlled comparison of cognitive-behavioral family intervention and standard pediatric care. *J Consult Clin Psychol* 1994;62:306–314.
50. Varni JW. Behavioral medicine in hemophilic arthritic pain management: two case studies. *Arch Phys Med Rehabil* 1981;62:183–187.
51. Richter IL, McGrath PJ, Humphreys PJ, et al. Cognitive and relaxation treatment of paediatric migraine. *Pain* 1986;25:195–203.
52. Dahlquist LM, Gil KM, Armstrong FD, et al. Behavioral management of children's distress during chemotherapy. *J Behav Ther Exp Psychiatry* 1985;16:325–329.
53. Kuttner L, Bowman M, Teasdale M. Psychological treatment of distress, pain and anxiety for young children with cancer. *Dev Behav Pediatr* 1988;9:374–381.
54. McGrath PA, DeVeber LL. Helping children cope with painful procedures. *Am J Nurs* 1986;86:1278–1279.
55. Zeltzer LK, Dash J, Holland JP. Hypnotically induced pain control in sickle cell anemia. *Pediatrics* 1979;64:533–536.
56. LeBaron S, Hilgard JR. *Hypnotherapy of pain in children with cancer*. Los Altos, CA: Wm. Kaufmann, 1984.
57. Wilson JJ, Gil KM. The efficacy of psychological and pharmacological interventions for the treatment of chronic disease-related and non-disease related pain. *Clin Psychol Rev* 1996;16:573–597.
58. Kohen DP, Olness KN, Colwell SO, et al. The use of re-

laxation-mental imagery (self-hypnosis) in the management of 505 pediatric behavioral encounters. *Dev Behav Pediatr* 1984;5:21–25.
59. Williams DT, Hirsch G. The somatizing disorders: somatoform disorders, factitious disorders and malingering. In: Kestenbaum CJ, Williams DT, eds. *Handbook of clinical assessment of children and adolescents (vol II)*. New York: New York University Press, 1988:743–768.
60. Williams DJ, Singh M. Hypnosis as a facilitating therapeutic adjunct in child psychiatry. J Am Acad Child Psychiatry 1976;15:326–342.
61. Fentress DW, Masek BJ, Mehegan JE, et al. Biofeedback and relaxation response training in the treatment of pediatric migraine. *Dev Med Child Neurol* 1986;28:139–146.
62. Attanasio V, Andrasek F, Blanchard EB, et al. Behavioral treatment of pediatric tension headache. Paper presented at the annual meeting of the Association for the Advancement of Behavior Therapy, Philadelphia, 1984.
63. Allen KD, Shriver MD. Role of parent-mediated pain behavior management strategies in biofeedback treatment of childhood migraines. *Behav Ther* 1998;29:477–490.

17

Psychologic and Behavioral Treatment of Pain in Children and Adolescents

Patrick J. McGrath, Bruce Dick, and Anita M. Unruh

This chapter reviews psychologic and behavioral strategies (other than hypnosis) used in the treatment of pediatric pain. A standardized approach is used in discussing each strategy. This includes (a) a brief description of the psychologic or behavioral intervention including a discussion of the mechanism of action of the strategy, (b) the pain problems for which the strategy is used, (c) the advantages and disadvantages of the method, and (d) how to implement the strategy and the best sources of additional information about the approach. Before we begin a discussion of specific strategies, some general concepts should be discussed.

There is an unfortunate tendency in some circles to believe that psychologic methods are morally or ethically better than medical, especially pharmacologic, methods. Although there are advantages and disadvantages of every pain-control method in terms of effectiveness, side effects, and costs, no one method is morally or ethically better than another. In some situations, the negative view of pharmacologic treatment takes the form of an irrational fear of addiction. Indeed, 60% of first-year medical students reported they would be moderately to extremely concerned about addiction if a family member were given morphine for pain (1). We have found that mothers often fear addiction to acetaminophen used for relief of pain from surgery (2). In fact, there is no danger of addiction if a drug is administered for pain relief. In other situations, the fear is that the child will learn to solve all life's problems with drugs. There is absolutely no evidence that this will occur in response to the appropriate use of drugs (3). These prejudices against pharmaceutical methods sometimes deprive children of appropriate interventions for their pain.

A second common, but false, belief is that if a psychologic treatment is effective, there must have been a psychologic problem causing the pain. Another version of this belief is that psychologic strategies will only be effective if there is a psychologic cause of the pain. This is a logical flaw best illustrated by an analogous example. Postoperative pain can often be alleviated with morphine. However, postoperative pain is not caused by morphine deprivation but by surgical trauma. Psychologic methods of pain management can be effective with pain from a known physical or psychologic cause or pain from unknown causes.

Formal psychologic treatments should often be used in conjunction with medical methods (4), although circumstances may exist when specific types of cotherapy are not advised. Informal psychologic interventions accompany every medical intervention. This cannot be avoided because all medical acts are embedded in a psychologic context. Health professionals cannot choose to avoid using psychology to treat pain. Our choice is whether to use psychology in a conscious, constructive fashion or to leave the psychologic aspect of our interventions to chance.

A third false belief is that the amount of pain can be accurately predicted from the extent of tissue damage and that the impact of pain can be predicted from the degree of pain. The underlying disease/disorder causing the pain, the pain itself, the disability, and the handicap that may result from pain are each separate planes of experience with varied causes (5). The amount of pain does not necessarily predict the degree of disability or handicap that may result.

Finally, it is necessary to think of pain, disability, and handicap as distinct phenomena that may be independent. Disability refers to the specific behaviors that a child is prevented from engaging in, whereas handicap is a change in social role (5). Although most people usually think of disability and handicap as flowing inevitably from the severity of pain, this is clearly not the case. We all know of children with quite severe pain who were able to function with little disability or handicap. Similarly, some children with significant disability (for example, inability to run) substitute one set of activities for their previous activities and show little disruption of their social roles (in terms of friends, family, and school). Other children with the same disability have major disruptions in their social roles (handicap).

Disability and handicap may also contribute to pain. For example, a child who takes to his or her bed because of limb pain from complex regional pain syndrome type I and misses school may become depressed and anxious about returning to school and have significant disuse of his or her limb. He or she may be in a great deal more pain than if he or she had maintained a somewhat modified regular routine.

The factors causing pain may not be the same as those influencing disability and handicap. For example, social and psychologic factors may initiate and maintain disability or handicap even if the cause of the pain is specifically organic.

We now discuss psychologic and behavioral strategies in pain management. Table 17.1 provides an overview of the strategies that will be discussed.

GOOD CLINICAL PAIN PRACTICE

Description

Good clinical pain practice includes a number of standard procedures that lead to pain reduction. We are including them here because they are important and are often not seen to be directly effective and are often assumed to be in place. There are several critical principles to be considered in the maintenance of good clinical pain practice for a child.

TABLE 17.1. *Psychologic and behavioral pain management strategies*

Treatment method	Empirically supported for use with	Not yet empirically supported but often used for
Muscle relaxation	Migraine, tension headache, procedure pain	Cancer pain, chronic pain, postoperative pain
Biofeedback alone (without relaxation)		Migraine, tension headache
Cognitive-behavioral methods	Headache, procedure pain	Recurrent abdominal pain, disease-related pain (e.g., cancer, juvenile rheumatoid arthritis, sickle cell disease, fibromyalgia)
Operant techniques	Chronic pain with handicap	Procedure pain
Group therapy		Any pain problem for which psychologic treatment is indicated
Exercise therapy		Complex regional pain syndrome, juvenile fibromyalgia, musculoskeletal pain
Art and play therapies		Children with serious social handicaps because of chronic pain or extreme fear of procedural pain
Family therapy		Children handicapped by pain
Problem solving		All pain problems
Modeling, role-playing, behavioral rehearsal		All pain problems

1. Generally, only the child with pain can really tell how much pain is being experienced. This follows from the International Association for the Study of Pain's definition of pain (6) that emphasizes that pain is subjective. If a child says he or she is in pain, then, unless we have very good evidence to the contrary, we should believe the child. It follows that when self-report is available, it is the gold standard for pain measurement. Often self-report is not available, and behavior must be used as the prime indicator of pain. However, it is necessary to use developmentally appropriate measures and to ensure that the measure is appropriate to the type of pain that the child is experiencing. In particular, longer lasting pain results in less obvious pain behaviors than does pain that lasts a short time (7).

2. Whenever pain is likely to occur, it should be measured and targeted for intervention. Pain should be routinely measured in children after surgery. Indeed, a survey by Johnston and associates (C. C. Johnston et al., unpublished) suggests that pain should be measured in all hospitalized children. They found that children who were in the hospital and did not have surgery were as likely to have pain as those who did have surgery. Pain measurement could and should become part of the vital signs assessment that is routine in hospitals.

3. It is better to prevent pain than to treat it once it occurs. Prevention is better than treatment for humanitarian, physiologic, and medical reasons (8–10). Pain may activate physiologic, biochemical, and cellular processes that change the response to future pain. This central neural plasticity or central sensitization may cause previously nonpainful stimuli to be painful or may enhance the response to painful stimuli (10). As a result, unnecessary needle procedures and surgeries should be avoided, and pain should always be treated before it emerges.

4. When possible, parents should accompany children undergoing painful procedures. Although some children may be somewhat more disruptive with their parents present, almost all children indicate that they prefer having a parent present to help them cope with pain (11,12). If parents are given specific instructions on what they should do to help their child during the procedure, they can significantly reduce the distress that their child feels (11,13,14).

5. Children should be given developmentally appropriate explanations of what is going to happen to them. Explanations should be geared to a child's level, using language that the child understands. In addition, children should never be lied to or tricked into a painful experience. Deceiving children will likely increase their anxiety as they will never be sure when the next procedure might occur.

There is little research to determine how good clinical pain practice increases coping with pain or how it may reduce pain. The trust engendered by such a milieu may reduce anxiety, and specific aspects of the milieu may control aspects of the pain experience. Avoiding unnecessary painful procedures and treating pain may assist by reducing sensitization. Increased use of pain medicine appears to be a result of appropriate routine measurement of pain (11,15).

Advantages and Disadvantages

There are no disadvantages to good clinical pain practice. The major advantages accrue to the patient in terms of increased comfort. However, the health care practitioner may also benefit considerably from reduced stress from seeing children suffer and a sense of accomplishment as pain is well managed.

Implementation And Further Information

Implementation depends on a combination of factors including education of staff; appropriate institutional policies and procedures (such as routine measurement of pain as part of quality assurance), sufficient staff time (e.g., to be able to explain procedures to children), and appropriate physical facilities to accommodate parents). Several sources of information can be consulted for help in implementing a therapeutic milieu. These include books such as this volume and those by McGrath and Finley (16) and the *Sourcebook of Pediatric Pain* website (http://is.dal.ca/>painsrc/).

MUSCLE RELAXATION

Description

Several different types of muscle relaxation are used to help children with pain, including tension relaxation, suggestion relaxation, mini-relaxation, and differential relaxation. Jacobson (17) first described relaxation, using extensive training in a tension-relaxation style of relaxation training to treat a variety of disorders including different pain disorders. Schultz and Luthe (18) introduced autogenic training, which consisted of suggestions of heaviness and warmth and positioning of the body to produce relaxation. Finally, Benson (19,20) popularized a version of Eastern breathing techniques that induce relaxation.

Muscle relaxation using the tension-relaxation method requires the alternate tension of muscle groups. Typically, instructions are given to tense and hold a muscle group for 5 to 10 seconds, to notice the feeling of tension in the muscles, and then to release the tension and relax the muscle group. Often these instructions are combined with suggestions of relaxation, heaviness, and warmth and images of relaxing situations. The muscle groups used vary, and it is not clear that any specific muscle groupings are better than any other.

The heart of the suggestion method of relaxation is repeated suggestions of calmness, relaxation, heaviness, and warmth. These are often combined with pleasant imagery of being relaxed. The suggestion method of relaxation is similar to the tension-relaxation method without the tension.

Mini-relaxation is a very brief relaxation exercise similar to Benson's (19) relaxation response. In mini-relaxation, deep breathing is used to trigger relaxation throughout the body. Typically, five slow, deep breaths are accompanied by suggestions of calmness and relaxation.

Differential relaxation refers to learning to relax one part of the body while maintaining sufficient tension in other parts of the body. For example, an adolescent with migraine might learn to relax her jaw and shoulders while maintaining tension in her arms and trunk necessary for her to continue with her class work. Differential relaxation is often taught subsequent to complete relaxation, using either the tension-relaxation method or the suggestion method. The mechanisms of action of relaxation training are not known. There are several possibilities:

1. reduction of muscle tension causing decrease in ischemic pain,
2. changes in brain chemistry, particularly serotonin metabolism,
3. induction of feelings of control,
4. reduction of autonomic reactivity,
5. distraction.

No clear data indicate that one mechanism is the most important.

Problems Appropriate for Relaxation

Relaxation has been demonstrated effective in the treatment of migraine and muscle contraction headaches (21). Procedure pain can be effectively reduced by a combination of procedures including relaxation (22). Relaxation may also be useful in reducing distress from cancer pain, chronic pain, and postoperative pain, although there are no studies to demonstrate this.

Advantages and Disadvantages

Most people find learning and performing relaxation exercises quite pleasant. There are few negative side effects of relaxation training. A small number of very anxious children or adolescents may feel out of control when relaxation starts to take effect. Relaxation training taught by a psychologist may be quite expensive. Costs can be reduced by using minimal therapist contact methods (23–25) or group methods. Relaxation has no direct analgesic effect and can only reduce pain by changing stress or anxiety. Thus, relaxation may be inappropriately used as a substitute for analgesic therapy (26).

Implementation and Further Information

Cautela and Groden (27) created a detailed manual for teaching professionals how to teach children to relax. *Help Yourself* (24) is a patient manual that includes a relaxation tape. This program has been shown to be effective in the treatment of migraine headache in adolescents (28) and adults (29). The corresponding professional manual (25) guides the health care professional in implementing the program. McCaffery and Beebe (26) have an excellent chapter on the implementation of relaxation (although not focused on children).

BIOFEEDBACK: TEMPERATURE, ELECTROMYOGRAPHY, ELECTROENCEPHALOGRAPHY, TEMPORAL PULSE

Description

Biofeedback consists of the measurement and control of a physiologic response usually not thought to be under voluntary control. The physiologic response is amplified or transformed so that the response can be monitored and understood by the patient. The patient then attempts to modify the response. Types of biofeedback include finger temperature biofeedback, α-electroencephalography biofeedback, muscle electromyography biofeedback, and temporal pulse biofeedback. Both physiologic and psychologic explanations for the mechanism of the action of biofeedback have been suggested. Psychologic explanations are couched in terms of increasing sense of control and mastery and resulting changes in self-efficacy (30). Physiologic explanations are based on specific physiologic changes caused by the biofeedback. For example, electromyography biofeedback is thought to be effective because of a reduction in muscle tension; temperature biofeedback is thought to be effective because it induces relaxation and a sense of self-control.

Problems Appropriate for Biofeedback

Biofeedback is used to treat migraine and muscle contraction headache in children and adolescents (31). Biofeedback is also used as a method to teach relaxation. The review of Holden et al. (32) of the use of biofeedback methods in pediatric headache treatment concluded that these methods fall into the "probably efficacious" category because of a lack of well-designed studies that used biofeedback alone and did not include relaxation.

Advantages and Disadvantages

Attanasio and colleagues (31) outlined the advantages and disadvantages of using biofeedback with children. The advantages of using biofeedback with children, compared with adults, are that children are more enthusiastic about the procedure and have a quick rate of learning. They are less skeptical about being able to self-regulate and have fewer experiences of treatment failure. Children are usually eager to practice with home-training devices. The increased psychophysiologic lability of children might also be an advantage by increasing the opportunity to cause physiologic changes and thus learn biofeedback. Disadvantages also include the short attention span of children, the tendency of some children to engage in off-task behavior during sessions, anxiety about the equipment and the discomfort from removal of sensors, and the difficulty of some children in understanding the treatment rationale. The authors also note that emotional problems and scheduling difficulties may interfere with treatment.

Biofeedback requires trained instructors and specialized equipment.

Implementation

Culbert et al. (33) reported patient and parent feedback data that show high levels of satisfaction with biofeedback with children. They provide an excellent review of basic clinical techniques, biofeedback equipment, and relevant developmental issues in using biofeedback with children. Their review also lists a number of disorders to which biofeedback methods have been applied including headache, reflex sympathetic dystrophy, juvenile rheumatoid arthritis, and fibromyalgia.

COGNITIVE-BEHAVIORAL METHODS

Description

Cognitive-behavioral methods include distraction, imagery, and transformation. Distraction refers to anything that takes attention away from the painful situation. Imagery involves the use of vivid, usually visual, representations of pleasant scenes or actions. Imagery is a type of deliberate directed daydreaming. Transformation is the attempt to change the evaluation of an event or sensation from being horrible or awful to being irritating or unfortunate. All these techniques are designed to modify or change the frequency of unwanted thoughts and behaviors that result from pain. For example, as pain increases so may a child's levels of anxiety, hopelessness, and anger leading to pain behaviors that can be disruptive to the child and the child's caregivers. These behaviors could include withdrawal, depression, avoidance, or acting out. By intervening at the level of thinking, these techniques aim to influence and modify feelings experienced and behaviors displayed by a child in pain.

For children younger than 8 years of age, the typical approach is to teach the parents to implement the program in collaboration with the child. Older children and adolescents may implement the program themselves. However, there is emerging evidence that involving the parents leads to better outcomes (34).

The mechanisms of action of the various cognitive-behavioral methods have not been well delineated. In the case of acute pain, such as pain from an injection, cognitive methods appear to function predominantly as distracters. Given previous research showing pain's effects on attentional processing (35), it follows that distracters may give a pain sufferer something on which to focus attention. Giving a pain sufferer something on which to focus attention may facilitate the person's ability to switch attention away from pain. Distracters may reduce anxiety before an injection and the affective aspect of pain and thus reduce the overall distress. In the case of longer lasting pain, cognitive methods may act primarily to reduce negative evaluations of the situation.

Problems Appropriate for Cognitive-Behavioral Methods

Cognitive methods have been used for both acute pain such as needle pain (L. Miller and P. J. McGrath, unpublished data) and longer lasting pain such as headache (36). Powers (22) reviewed research on cognitive-behavioral methods employed to treat procedure-related pain (such as lumbar puncture and bone marrow aspirations) and found that these methods met all criteria for categorization as "well-established." In a review by Janicke and Finney (37), cognitive behavioral therapy was reported to fall into the category of a "probably efficacious" therapy for treating recurrent abdominal pain. These authors noted that more well-designed studies are required to clarify the efficacy of cognitive methods with recurrent abdominal pain. Walco et al. (38) identified cognitive-behavioral strategies as promising techniques for use with disease-related pain (such as cancer pain, juvenile rheumatoid arthritis, sickle cell disease, and fibromyalgia) but called for the development of treatment protocols and controlled studies to clarify the effectiveness of these strategies.

Advantages and Disadvantages

Cognitive methods are effective with children older than 8 or 9 years of age because these children are able to self-initiate and maintain their use of these strategies. Children who are younger will require a coach, who may be a parent or health care professional, to implement cognitive strategies. Children younger than 8 or 9 years of age will find it very difficult if not impossible to use these strategies without their coach to prompt them (39,40). Cognitive methods may appeal more to patients who use metacognitive thinking (willingly think about how they think).

Implementation and Further Information

Implementation of cognitive methods requires a trained therapist or a detailed instruction manual. *Help Yourself*, which includes a patient manual (24) and a professional handbook (25) to teach cognitive interventions, has been shown effective in the treatment of migraine headache. McCaffery and Beebe (26) provide an excellent review of some cognitive methods as applied to pain. A promising cognitive-behavioral therapy model for inpatient pain management in adolescents who are significantly handicapped by their pain is also being successfully used that incorporates group and family therapy principles (41). This model emphasizes the importance of taking family and other social factors into account in cognitive-behavioral therapy.

OPERANT TECHNIQUES

Description

Operant methods include positive reinforcement, punishment, and extinction. Operant methods for pain management were developed and initially evaluated for adults with chronic pain by Fordyce (42). Operant strategies do not target pain *per se* but pain behavior, such as complaining of pain or grimacing. In addition, the target behavior can be disability, such as time in bed or handicap (e.g. failure to attend school).

Positive reinforcement occurs when a behavior is followed by a pleasant or positive event. This tends to increase the probability of the behavior. Extinction is the withdrawal of reinforcement for a behavior. It should usually be accompanied by differential reinforcement of other, alternative, appropriate behavior.

Negative reinforcement refers to the removal of a negative event when the desired behavior is produced. Negative reinforcement increases the probability of the target behavior occurring.

Punishment is the following of an event by an unpleasant or negative event. Punishment and negative reinforcement as a treatment of pain are rarely if ever indicated because these negative techniques lead to withdrawal from the situation or avoidance of the punisher. Moreover, punishment can result in aggressive behavior toward the punisher or an increase in pain behavior.

Most operant practitioners believe that operant methods are effective because of operant conditioning, the strengthening of patterns of behavior because of their effect. Behaviors followed by positive or pleasurable events increase; behaviors followed by removal of positive events or by negative events decrease. Others have argued that operant methods have their impact by changing patients' conceptualization of their pain and by changing patients' self-efficacy (30).

Problems Appropriate for Operant Methods

Operant methods with adults have been well studied in chronic pain with handicap and shown to be effective. These methods have been less widely studied with children, but there is some evidence of effectiveness (34,43,44). Chronic pain with handicap is the most common problem for which operant methods are used. Operant methods may also be used with procedure pain. Janicke and Finney (37) reviewed a number of therapies for recurrent abdominal pain and found that operant methods were not proven effective in treating this problem.

Advantages and Disadvantages

In some circumstances (especially when extinguishing pain behavior), operant methods may give the impression that the health professional is uncaring. In addition, because they appear so simple, operant methods may be misused. Of particular concern is that operant methods may be effectively used to discourage children from confiding their problems to their parents or other adults. This problem may be obviated by the use of positive methods that reinforce normal activities despite pain (reducing disability) rather than focus on the reduction of pain complaints.

Operant techniques are probably best used in combination with other techniques to directly reduce the pain. For example, Allen and Shriver (34) found that operant techniques implemented by parents that primarily target disability and handicap can significantly improve the results obtained from biofeedback treatment of pediatric headache.

Implementation and Further Information

The people implementing operant methods must be thoroughly trained. Although operant methods appear to be simple, they require comprehensive understanding for their proper use. Fordyce's (42) book on operant methods remains an excellent primer.

GROUP THERAPY

Description

Group therapy simply refers to a psychologic or psychoeducational therapy delivered in a group. The type of therapy may be of any variety, including cognitive-behavioral, behavioral, psychoanalytic, and experiential.

In addition to the specific mode of action of the therapeutic intervention (e.g., relaxation, problem solving, psychotherapy), group therapy can use peer pressure, social support, and modeling by peers to increase the power of the treatment and compliance to treatment. In addition, groups may engender a sense of power or control that can positively benefit coping with pain.

Problems Appropriate for Group Therapy

Any pain problem for which psychologic therapy is indicated (e.g., headache, chronic pain, sickle-cell pain, or even procedure pain) may be appropriate for group therapy. There are, however, few data on group therapy for pain with children and adolescents.

Advantages and Disadvantages

Group therapy costs less than individual treatment and may be more effective. The sense of shared experience may be particularly helpful for adolescents who may feel isolated or different because of their pain problem. Scheduling difficulties and finding enough children of similar age with similar problems are often difficult to manage. Finally, some people are too shy to participate in group therapy.

Peer support groups are another form of group therapy. There are no data on the effectiveness of these methods in pediatric pain, but they may be helpful for some individuals. The development of the worldwide web provides another alternative for social support groups, but there are few evaluative data available on this application.

Implementation and Further Information

Adolescent girls are the most likely targets for group therapy because they are more likely than any other group or adolescent boys to suffer chronic or recurrent pain, and, thus, organizing a group is more feasible. In addition, adolescent girls may be more ready psychologically to participate in a group. Pain groups for childhood headache have been discussed (44). The classic book by Yalom (46) remains an excellent primer on group methods.

EXERCISE THERAPY

Description

Exercise therapy typically consists of the use of physical rehabilitation methods employed in physical and occupational therapy. These programs involve the use of exercise aimed at increasing flexibility, mobility, and fitness. These aims are targeted through the use of personal exercise programs employing methods such as stretching, hydrotherapy, aerobic exercise, exercise aimed at improving coordination of movement, weight-bearing exercises, and functional activities (e.g., handwriting). Although exercise therapy usually involves a program personalized to the patient, the administration of exercise therapy has been carried out in both individual and group therapy situations. These programs are often carried out in a health care setting by multidisciplinary teams of therapists and are aimed at generalizing the methods to the patient's everyday home routine.

The mechanism of action of this therapy has not been clearly explained. Some researchers have suggested that exercise produces endorphins or other pain-related mediators working through a variety of physiologic factors (e.g., increased blood flow, hormonal shifts) may play an important role (47). Increased fitness and self-esteem related to improved physical ability may also underlie the success of this method in many cases.

Problems Appropriate for Exercise Therapy

Research has suggested the efficacy of exercise therapy for children and adolescents with complex regional pain syndrome (47), juvenile fibromyalgia, and musculoskeletal pain. Almost any kind of pain condition that is exacerbated by decreased fitness and mobility is appropriate for this type of therapy because it can be paced to whatever level is appropriate for the patient's physical and psychologic needs. Unfortunately, good data are not yet available to demonstrate the effectiveness.

Advantages and Disadvantages

This type of therapy is aimed at helping patients generalize exercise skills to their individual daily routines. Although the initial costs of such programs can be considerable, the long-term costs, once incorporated into daily routines, are minimal. Patient progress can be easily monitored through brief follow-up visits. Exercise therapy is also easily tailored to individual needs and is relatively simple to learn and carry out with minimal specialized equipment requirements.

Implementation and Further Information

Exercise therapy may involve the participation of multidisciplinary teams of health care professionals (including physical therapists, occupational therapists, psychologists, nurses, and physicians). Early stages of these programs involve supervised exercise program personalization and practice, which proceed with the goal of helping patients perform their individual program independently. Sherry and colleagues (47) have reported remarkable results in a clinical series with children with complex regional pain syndrome.

ART AND PLAY

Description

The use of art or play with children may take many forms, but it generally occurs in a permissive, therapeutic environment in which the child is allowed to express feelings and concerns through the medium of art or play. Crayons, markers, paints, puppets, and dolls are used. The therapeutic use of art or play by child life workers, occupational therapists, or nurses should be distinguished from art of play *therapy* conducted by a trained art or play therapist. The former commonly takes place in the routine preparation of children for surgery or other painful procedures. It is meant as a psychoeducational or didactic technique in which expression is encouraged and misinformation may be detected and corrected. One or two sessions are common, but children with repeated exposure to aversive procedures may engage in frequent use of art or play to express their feelings.

Art or play therapy, in contrast, refers to a therapeutic endeavor in which a relationship with a trained therapist is fostered and conflicts are uncovered and resolved. Therapy is usually undertaken with disturbed children and may continue for several months.

Mechanism of Action

When art or play is used therapeutically, dispelling fears, providing information, distraction and role-playing of coping appear to be important. It is thought that uncovering and working through conflicts may be important in art or play therapy.

Problems Appropriate for Therapeutic Play or Art or Play or Art Therapy

Art and play are used to help children with a variety of pain problems to express themselves and to reduce medical fears. Art or play therapy is used with children who have serious social handicaps because of chronic pain or extreme fear of procedure pain.

Advantages and Disadvantages

Because play and art are natural media for children, these methods may encourage expression when traditional verbal methods are unsuccessful. Therapeutic art and play are widely used and often helpful.

Art or play therapy is expensive, and no data indicate that these therapies are effective. A tendency may exist to overinterpret children's play or art and posit a psychologic cause of pain when none exists.

Implementation and Further Information

Materials and a sensitive child life worker or nurse with the time and patience to encourage expression are all that are needed for art or play to be used therapeutically. Indeed, with minimal instruction, most parents can use play or art therapeutically.

For art or play therapy, a trained play or art therapist is required. Landgarten and Lubbers (48) wrote a clear text on clinical art therapy. There are no data supporting the use of play or art therapy in chronic pain and, as far as we know, no ongoing studies in this area.

FAMILY THERAPY

Description

Family therapy is a wide-ranging term that may include behavioral family therapy, systemic family therapy, or structural family therapy. The presumed mechanisms of action vary with the specific form of family therapy used. From a behavioral perspective, family therapy is designed to encourage the family to support healthy behavior and reduce support for pain behavior on the part of the identified patient. This may include resolving family conflicts that may cause stress or reduce the ability to cope. Using a systems model (49), family therapists have delineated common aspects of psychosomatic families. According to this model, the most outstanding feature of such families is the enmeshed system in which they operate. In these families, relationships are characterized by constant intrusion into each others' lives, weak boundaries between members, and extreme proximity. Personal autonomy is subjugated to demands for family loyalty. Typically, such families are child oriented and overprotective and focus an abnormal amount of attention on the child's psychologic and physiologic functioning. If symptoms such as pain appear, possibly as a function of intense somatic concerns within the family, members tend to mobilize in an attempt to protect the child, thus rewarding the behavior. Both pain and handicap may become absorbed into the family system, and the illness becomes the child's "identity card." The family system serves to maintain the pain and handicap.

The objective of family therapy in such cases is to increase the child's sense of autonomy and independence and to challenge the enmeshed family system.

Problems Appropriate for Family Therapy

The problems for which family therapy are appropriate have not been well delineated. It is probably only appropriate in situations in which a child is handicapped by pain. There have been few good evaluations of the effect of family therapy on pain. Allen and Shriver (34) have shown that very brief behavior instructions to parents enhanced the effect of biofeedback in migraine.

Advantages and Disadvantages

Family therapy of the traditional sort is expensive because it requires a trained mental health specialist interacting with the family for eight to 30 or more sessions. No properly designed studies evaluate the effectiveness of more traditional family therapy for children with pain. Very brief interventions in which parents are instructed how to interact with their children in pain may enhance the effectiveness of treatment.

Implementation and Further Information

Family therapy requires a therapist with graduate training in family therapy techniques. Several well-accepted family therapy texts have been published (49,50). One therapy model that incorporates aspects of family therapy in a pain management program for adolescents has shown promise (41). There is, at this time, general agreement that involving families in treatment is very helpful. However, there are only limited data showing that specific treatments are effective (34).

PROBLEM SOLVING

Description

Problem solving consists of defining the problem, brainstorming possible solutions, listing the advantages and disadvantages of each potential solution, appraising the best solution, implementing the plan to deal with the problem, and reviewing the effectiveness of the chosen solution.

The exact mechanism of action of problem solving has not been completely delineated. Two types of mechanisms likely operate. In some situations, problem solving will lead to the discovery of the trigger or cause of the pain or the way of eliminating a known trigger or cause. In other situations, problem solving can be used to replace unrealistic negative thoughts ("catastrophizing") by generating specific useful coping strategies.

Problems Appropriate for Problem Solving

Any pain for which the cause or trigger can be mitigated or eliminated can be treated with problem solving. In addition, pain that can be managed with better coping strategies can still be helped by problem solving.

Advantages and Disadvantages

Problem solving is a generic skill that is useful for a broad range of problems. Anecdotal reports suggest that a positive side effect of problem solving is a feeling of being able to confront new situations not related to the situations confronted in original training. Problem solving is a difficult skill to learn. In particular, it is difficult to learn how to generalize problem solving to different situations and to use it without prompting. There are no published studies at present that evaluate the use of problem solving in pediatric pain problems.

Implementation and Further Information

The steps involved in problem solving are brainstorming, listing advantages and disadvantages, appraisal, choosing the optimal solution, implementation, and review. *Help Yourself* (24,25) reviews the application of problem solving to treatment of migraine headaches.

MODELING, ROLE-PLAYING, AND BEHAVIORAL REHEARSAL

Description

Modeling is a behavior portrayed to a child for the child to learn that behavior. Modeling can be taught by a live model or by a videotape and can use people, cartoon characters, or puppets. Not only can different methods of modeling be used but also different types of models. Mastery models refer to models who cope without any evidence of fear or anxiety. Coping models are those who evidence anxiety but overcome the anxiety to cope with the stressor. Modeling, role-playing, and behavioral rehearsal are usually used to increase adaptive and decrease maladaptive coping strategies in children and adolescents with pain.

Role-playing and behavioral rehearsal involve pretending to be in a situation and practicing what to do. Repeated role-playing and rehearsal can lead to overlearning a behavior and increasing skill at enacting the behavior, increased confidence in being able to execute the behavior, and reduced anxiety. These methods are used to implement coping skills.

Modeling, role-playing, and behavioral rehearsal appear to function by reducing anxiety (perhaps by desensitization), teaching skills, and increasing self-confidence in the ability to perform the behavior.

Problems Appropriate for Modeling, Role-Playing, and Behavioral Rehearsal

Modeling, role-playing, and behavioral rehearsal can be used in teaching any technique useful for coping with pain. For example, a film might teach a child to relax during a needle procedure in which the child models the behavior, role-plays, and rehearses the skill.

Advantages and Disadvantages

Modeling, role-playing, and behavioral rehearsal have a very wide range of uses and are excellent teaching methods. These methods require a skilled therapist to direct the child and sufficient time to teach the child. The basic psychology of modeling, role-playing, and behavioral rehearsal is well worked out (51). However, little evaluation of the effectiveness of these methods in teaching pain-management skills has been done.

Implementation

Modeling, role-playing, and behavioral rehearsal as applied to pain management are described in *Help Yourself* (24,25) and in the work of Meichenbaum and Deffenbacher (51) with stress inoculation training.

DISCUSSION

Psychologic methods of pain relief for children and adolescents are not as widely used and understood as they might be. Some of these methods, such as relaxation training and cognitive strategies, are highly specialized and used generally only by psychologists or other mental health professionals. A serious limitation to the widespread use of these psychologic techniques of pain control is the high cost of implementing them. This shortcoming is being overcome by the development and validation of minimal therapist contact programs (23,24,36) that enable any health professional to deliver these specialized techniques, with a reduced investment of professional time.

A more difficult barrier to overcome is the failure of many health professionals to realize that psychologic techniques of pain management are ideally suited as combined therapies or sole therapy for a variety of pain problems. Moreover, psychologic therapies are appropriate for pain that is not psychologically caused.

The only areas in which there is a reasonable body of research on psychologic methods for pain management in children and adolescents is in the use of cognitive-behavioral techniques applied to headache and applied to procedures. Other styles of therapy and other pain problems, especially disease-related pain, have not been investigated (38).

Psychologic methods pervade all health care and will be used deliberately either effectively or clumsily and ineffectively. Although psychologists are usually better trained in intensive individual therapy, it is the responsibility of all health professionals to learn to apply psychologic methods of pain control. Moreover, information technologies such as the worldwide web provide opportunities to increase access to psychologic treatment methods. Children and adolescents in pain need psychologic and behavioral treatments to help them with their pain.

ACKNOWLEDGMENT

Dr. McGrath is supported by a Distinguished Scientist Award of the Canadian Institutes of Health Research. Mr. Dick is supported by an IWK Grace Health Centre Graduate Research Scholarship and a Dalhousie University Graduate Fellowship. Dr. Unruh's research is supported by the Social Sciences and Humanities Research Council.

REFERENCES

1. Weissman DE, Dahl JL. Attitudes about cancer pain: a survey of Wisconsin's first-year medical students. *J Pain Symptom Manage* 1990;5:345–349.
2. Forward SP, Brown TL, McGrath PJ. Mothers' attitudes and behavior toward medicating children's pain. *Pain* 1996;67:469–474.
3. McGrath PJ, Unruh AM. *Pain in children and adolescents*. Amsterdam: Elsevier, 1987.
4. Holroyd KA, Cordingley GE, Pingel JD, et al. Enhancing the effectiveness of abortive therapy: a controlled evaluation of self-management training. *Headache* 1989;29:148–153.
5. World Health Organization. *International classification of impairments, disabilities and handicaps*. Geneva: World Health Organization, 1980.
6. Mersky H, Bogduk N. *Classification of chronic pain: descriptions of chronic pain syndromes and definitions of pain terms*. Seattle: IASP Press, 1994.
7. Chambers CT, Reid GJ, McGrath PJ, et al. Development and preliminary validation of a postoperative pain measure for parents. *Pain* 1996;68:307–313.
8. Anand KJS, Sippell WG, Aynsley-Green A. A randomised trial of fentanyl anaesthesia in preterm neonates undergoing surgery: effects on the stress response. *Lancet* 1987;1:243–247.
9. Platt MPW, Aynsley-Green A, Anand KJS. The ontogeny of the stress response and its implications for pediatric practice. In: Tyler D, Krane E, eds. *Advances in pain research and therapy, volume 15. Pediatric pain*. New York: Raven Press, 1990:123–136.
10. Woolf CJ. Recent advances in pathophysiology of acute pain. *Br J Anaesth* 1989;63:139–146.
11. Ross DM, Ross CA. *Childhood pain: current issues, research and management*. Baltimore: Urban & Schwarzenberg, 1988.
12. Gonzalez JC, Routh DK, Saab PG, et al. Effects of parent presence on children's reactions to injections: behavioral, physiological and subjective aspects. *J Pediatr Psychol* 1989;14:449–462.
13. Bauchner H, Vinci R, Bak S, et al. Parents and procedures: a randomized controlled trial. *Pediatrics* 1996; 98:861–867.
14. Blount RL, Bachanas PJ, Powers SW, et al. Training children to cope and parents to coach them during routine immunizations: effects on child, parent and staff behaviors. *Behav Ther* 1992;23:689–705.
15. Stevens B. Development and testing of a pediatric pain management sheet. *Pediatr Nurs* 1990;16:543–548.
16. Finley GA, McGrath PJ. *Measurement of pain in infants and children*. Seattle: IASP Press, 1998.
17. Jacobson E. *You must relax*. New York: McGraw-Hill, 1957.
18. Schultz JH, Luthe W. *Autogenic training: a psychophysiologic approach to psychotherapy*. New York: Grune & Stratton, 1959.
19. Benson H. *The relaxation response*. New York: Times Books, 1975.
20. Benson H. *Beyond the relaxation response*. New York: Times Books, 1984.
21. McGrath P, Larsson B. Headache in children and adolescents. *Child Adolesc Psychiatr Clin North Am* 1997; 6:843–861.
22. Powers SW. Empirically supported treatments in pediatric psychology: procedure-related pain. *J Pediatr Psychol* 1999;24:131–145.
23. Burke EJ, Andrasik F. Home- vs. clinic-based biofeedback treatment for pediatric migraine: results of treatment through one-year follow-up. *Headache* 1990;29: 434–440.
24. McGrath PJ, Cunningham SJ, Lascelles JJ, et al. *Help yourself: a program for treating migraine headaches* [patient manual and audiotape]. Ottawa: University of Ottawa Press, 1990.
25. McGrath PJ, Cunningham SJ, Lascelles JJ, et al. *Help yourself: a program for treating migraine headaches* [professional handbook]. Ottawa: University of Ottawa Press, 1990.
26. McCaffery M, Beebe A. *Pain: clinical manual for nursing practice*. St. Louis: Mosby, 1989.
27. Cautela JR, Groden J. *Relaxation: a comprehensive manual for adults, children, and children with special needs*. Champaign, IL: Research Press, 1978.
28. McGrath PJ, Humphreys P, Keene D, et al. The efficacy and efficiency of a self-administered treatment for adolescent migraine. *Pain* 1989;49:321–324.
29. Richardson GM, McGrath PJ. Cognitive-behavioral therapy for migraine headaches: a minimal therapist-contact approach versus a clinic-based approach. *Headache* 1990;29:352–357.
30. Blanchard EB, Andrasik F. *Management of chronic headaches: a psychological approach*. New York: Pergamon Press, 1985.
31. Attanasio V, Andrasik F, Burke EJ, et al. Clinical issues in utilizing biofeedback with children. *Clin Biofeedback Health* 1985;8:134–141.
32. Holden EW, Deichmann MM, Levy JD. Empirically supported treatments in pediatric psychology: recurrent pediatric headache. *J Pediatr Psychol* 1999;24:91–109.
33. Culbert TP, Kajander RL, Reaney JB. Biofeedback with children and adolescents: Clinical observations and patient perspectives. *J Dev Behav Pediatr* 1996;17: 342–350.
34. Allen KD, Shriver MD. Role of parent-mediated pain behavior management strategies in biofeedback treatment of childhood migraines. *Behav Ther* 1998;29: 477–490.
35. Eccleston C. Chronic pain and attention: a cognitive approach. *Br J Clin Psychol* 1994;33:535–547.
36. Richter I, McGrath PJ, Humphreys PJ, et al. Cognitive and relaxation treatment of pediatric migraine. *Pain* 1986;25:195–203.
37. Janicke DM, Finney JW. Empirically supported treatments in pediatric psychology: recurrent abdominal pain. *J Pediatr Psychol* 1999;24:115–127.
38. Walco GA, Sterling CM, Conte PM, et al. Empirically supported treatments in pediatric psychology: disease-related pain. *J Pediatr Psychol* 1999;24:155–167.
39. McGrath PJ, Craig KD. Developmental and psychological factors in pediatric pain. *Pediatr Clin North Am* 1989;36:823–836.
40. Hobbs SA, Moguin LE, Tyroler M, et al. Cognitive behavior therapy with children: has clinical utility been demonstrated? *Psychol Bull* 1980;87:147–165.
41. Elliott EA, Connell H. Family cognitive behavioral pain management for adolescents: a process model to guide decisions and interventions. Poster session presented at the International Symposium on Paediatric Pain, London, 2000.

42. Fordyce WE. *Behavioral methods for chronic pain and illness*. St. Louis: Mosby, 1976.
43. Sank LI, Biglan A. Operant treatment of a case of recurrent abdominal pain in a 10-year-old boy. *Behav Ther* 1974;5:677–681.
44. Minuchin S, Baker L, Rosman B, et al. A conceptual model of psychosomatic illness in children: family organization and family therapy. *Arch Gen Psychiatry* 1975;32:1031–1038.
45. Engel JM, Rapoff MA. A component analysis of relaxation training for children with vascular, muscle contraction, and mixed-headache disorder. In: Tyler D, Krane E, eds. *Advances in pain research and therapy, volume 15. Pediatric pain*. New York: Raven Press, 1990:273–290.
46. Yalom ID. *The theory and practice of groups*. New York: Basic Books, 1970.
47. Sherry DD, Wallace CA, Kelley C, et al. Short- and long-term outcomes of children with complex regional pain syndrome type I treated with exercise therapy. *Clin J Pain* 1999;15:218–223.
48. Landgarten HB, Lubbers D. *Adult art psychotherapy: issues and applications*. New York: Brunner/Mazel, 1999.
49. Minuchin S. *Families and family therapy*. Cambridge: Harvard University Press, 1974.
50. Goldenberg I, Goldenberg H. *Family therapy: an overview*. Monterey, CA: Brooks Cole, 1985.
51. Meichenbaum D, Deffenbacher JL. Stress inoculation training. *Counsel Psychol* 1988;16:69–90.

18

Hypnotherapy and Imagery for Managing Children's Pain

Leora Kuttner and Richard Solomon

Over the past 25 years, hypnosis[1] has been creatively adapted to help children through acute painful experiences in the emergency room (1–3), through procedures associated with cancer such as bone marrow aspirations and lumbar punctures (4–13), and with post-operative pain (14,15). In more chronic and persistent conditions, it has been successfully used for children with sickle cell disease (16,17), burns (18–22), and tension and migraine headaches (23,24). Research reviews consistently conclude that hypnosis works to help children in pain (25–28) and should be thought of as an essential component of any comprehensive approach to pain management for children.

Hypnosis, as well as other behavioral pain control methods such as deep breathing and distraction, can be easily integrated into medical and nursing interventions to improve outcome. It provides an enhanced way to cope, heightens the child's sense of safety, comfort, self-esteem, and control and may reduce the need for pain medication. Indeed, hypnosis is a uniquely valuable tool for managing pain (29–31). As Barber and Adrian (29) stated: "No other psychological tool that I know of is so efficacious in creating comfort out of discomfort with none of the adverse side effects associated with medical treatments of comparable efficacy." Children in pain do not require lengthy inductions because they are often already in a heightened state of awareness and, as such, highly suggestible (32). Often only seconds of time are required. Thus, hypnosis should be common in the armamentarium of pediatric professionals, introduced early in the treatment process, and not be used as a therapy of last resort.

This chapter reviews what the pediatric professional needs to know about the nature of hypnosis, how it works, and how it can be applied to children of different ages. Key components of the hypnotherapeutic approach are described with case examples that detail the ways in which hypnosis can facilitate pain control for children. Finally, important resources for professionals to learn the skills of hypnotherapy are listed.

WHAT IS HYPNOSIS?

Hypnosis is an altered state of consciousness utilizing intensified attention within a relaxed physical state to achieve a trance state that is different from both the normal waking state and any of the stages of sleep. It resembles, but is not identical to, various meditative states with its narrowly focused attention, primary process thinking, and ego receptivity (33). In a trance, attention is narrowed, focused, and absorbed, allowing perceptions and sensations to be enhanced, modified, or changed. All humans and children especially have this natural capacity to use an internal

[1]The term *hypnosis* is used throughout the chapter because it has historical value, offers a set of clear and distinct techniques, and has been the term most associated with research. Other terms such as relaxation and mental imagery, cyberphysiologic approaches, mind-body techniques can arguably be used interchangeably.

imaginative process to affect broad physiologic changes. The characteristics of a trance include the temporary suspension of critical judgment (30), the rapid assimilation of internal or external data (34), and the capacity to make an incongruent feeling or idea congruent, otherwise referred to as trance logic (35). *Hypnotherapy* is the treatment modality in which a patient in this altered state of consciousness can be treated with a range of different methods such as direct or indirect suggestion, hypnoanalgesia (suggestions for analgesia), or amnesia. For children facing painful experiences, hypnotherapy can induce a change in the child's perception of pain that appears to bypass the child's conscious effort. This process suits the apparent involuntary nature of pain. Hypnosis differs from behavioral-cognitive techniques, such as *distraction*, in which attention is primarily focused on external objects, thus retaining strong reality contact in contrast to inner imaginal process of hypnosis to maximize coping.

Although hypnosis offers an important coping skill to children, the ultimate form of hypnosis is *self-hypnosis*, which gives control directly to the child to engage in this process whenever and wherever the need arises. In the management of many chronic habit problems or pain conditions, the child's self-management is crucial to long-term success, underlining the requirement that hypnosis be taught early on, at the time of diagnosis, because it empowers the child's coping capacity during the vicissitudes of therapy. The ability to modulate pain and increase comfort furthers the child's sense of independence and self-sufficiency (36,37). Hypnosis can reduce feelings of helplessness and depression and decreases reliance on medication and hospital staff (38). Consequently, hypnosis can be adapted to suit the child with chronic and recurring pain as well as acute pain.

THEORETICAL RATIONALE: HOW DOES HYPNOSIS MODIFY PAIN?

Hypnosis produces powerful reductions in both clinical and experimental perceptions of pain (4,30,31,39,40). Although the mechanisms of hypnotic analgesia are not completely understood, the scientific evidence suggests that hypnosis works in a complex way that requires both psychologic and physiologic mechanisms for a full explanation.

Theorists supporting psychologic explanations contend that response to suggestion can be explained in terms of social role enactments, contextual demands, and coping strategies (41–43). Indeed, the psychologic goal of hypnosis is to use the power of suggestion to shift the child from the relatively passive or helpless state of directly experiencing anxiety and pain, to a state of coping, empowerment, and control. Helping the child, in a context of nurturing support, to focus attention on a more pleasant alternative often reduces pain perception. When the child can reduce anxiety and no longer resists or fights the pain, this further alters his or her perception of pain. In this more cognitive-behavioral model, the clinician's task is to recognize that the child is "entranced with his or her pain" and help modify the child's fixed preoccupation by shifting attention to alleviate suffering.

Conversely, theories that focus on the dissociation aspect of the hypnotic process assert that pain is masked from overt awareness by an amnesia-like barrier between dissociated streams of consciousness (30,44). Pain is registered by the body and by covert awareness during hypnotic analgesia, yet the nature of dissociation separates this perception and experience from consciousness. This theory may explain the hypnotherapist's ability to help the child reduce pain by suggesting and achieving alternative experiences, such as pain sensations becoming more distant, or changing in character from, for example, burning to a more pleasant tingling.

Physiologic explanations for hypnosis propose that hypnotic analgesia can inhibit incoming sensations at the spinal cord level. The gate control theory of pain of Melzack and Wall (45,46) provides the theoretic framework for understanding how this mechanism works. The brain in its altered state of consciousness is maintained to exert a downward influence on the central nervous system modulating the "gates" at the dorsal horn of the spinal cord and altering pain perception or reception at the central nervous system level. Recent research strongly suggests that spinal reflex mechanisms can indeed be inhibited by hypnotic analgesia (47), although the precise mechanism is unknown. One proposed mechanism, that hypnosis is the natural way of releasing endorphins and enkephalins, has not yet been supported by research (40,48–50). Barber and Mayer (40) found that hypnotic analgesia for experimental pain is not reversed by the administration of naloxone hydrochloride. Finer and Terenius (50) reported that patients experiencing hypnotic analgesia showed no increase in endorphin levels in contrast to the elevated endorphin levels in patients experiencing acupuncture.

MEDICAL CONSIDERATIONS

Hypnosis and related behavioral methods should be an integral part of any comprehensive medical approach for children facing predictably painful or anxiety-producing medical procedures. Despite advances in pain management, many children still experience hospitalization and the prospect of medical procedures as very frightening. Anxiety increases the reports and intensity of pain. Hypnosis, along with child life intervention, is the treatment of choice for anxiety associated with pain or the threat of pain inherent in hospital procedures. Recent advances in pediatric medical approaches, including especially the use of conscious sedation for medical procedures, have lulled physicians and other health care practitioners into believing that so-called time-consuming ancillary approaches like hypnosis are not needed. Quite to the contrary, hypnosis can and should be used along with advanced medical approaches like conscious sedation. Additional medical benefits of hypnosis include possible reduction in the dosage and frequency of medication owing to a reduction in both pain and anxiety. In fact, conscious sedation and rapidly acting anesthetics are very time-consuming and expensive in terms of the need for equipment, medication, and personnel and may have serious, even fatal, side effects (51). Hypnotherapeutic approaches are comparatively quicker and less expensive and have no side effects. Therefore, when the child or adolescent can use hypnosis effectively to reduce or eliminate pain, these approaches should be the treatment of choice. What typically limits the use of hypnotherapy is the lack of systematic training of health professionals (see below).

Once trained, physicians, nurses, psychologists, social workers, child life workers, and other pediatric professionals can use hypnosis in any medical setting where pain and/or anxiety are routine features of medical care.

In the *emergency department*, children often arrive in pain. The hectic atmosphere of the emergency department, the sudden dislocation from the familiar, parents' anxiety, and the child's fear of the unknown all contribute to the child's anxiety. There is often a prejudice among emergency department staff that there is not enough time to address these issues, that "the child will have to be held down to be sutured," but the skillful and incisive use of pediatric hypnosis can be especially effective here, particularly for children as young as 3 or 4 years of age. Hypnosis can meet the child's need for a sense of control, the parents' need to feel trust in emergency department staff, and staff's need to convince the family that suturing a wound can be painless. There are few things as reassuring as a medical professional arriving on the scene to teach the child ways that they can help themselves through a frightening situation by using breathing, relaxation, and their own imagination. Within minutes, the tenor of the situation can change to become manageable.

In the *outpatient office setting*, the use of breathing, distraction, bubble blowing, and hypnosis has been shown to be effective in helping children through the pain of multiple immunizations (52,53). Hypnotic suggestions that children will easily enter anesthesia and comfortably reawaken from surgical procedures should routinely be incorporated into *pre- and postoperative settings*. As part of hospital-wide policies for the care of children in pain, *in-patient units* all over the country are now expected to make pain the "fifth vital sign" and incorporate behavioral approaches into pediatric pain management protocols. Finally, even in the *intensive care unit* where high technology dominates, hypnosis can introduce an element of self-control, changing a child's focus from respirators, powerful medications, and constant procedures, to a favorite place or favorite activity that may soothe and comfort her.

Clearly, then, hypnotic analgesia should be used routinely as a pain management method in any number of medical settings. There are, however, contraindications that health professionals should be aware of because hypnosis can have medical costs as well as benefits. One cost can be the underdiagnosis and undertreatment by a patient skilled in hypnotic pain control, typically children or teens accustomed to dealing with ongoing or severe chronic pain. In the pediatric medical setting, pain has great signal value as a guide to both diagnosis and treatment. The best assessments include the child's self-report. Covering up important symptoms with hypnosis can mislead assessments. Headaches can indicate tumors and stomach aches Crohn disease or ulcerative colitis. Use of hypnosis can delay diagnosis. Therefore, it is important that diagnostic information from the child's pain be thoroughly evaluated before the therapeutic use of hypnosis is begun. Hypnotherapy should also be used cautiously with children who are emotionally fragile or seriously disturbed and never used with children who are psychotic. Beyond these few contraindications, hypnosis is quite safe.

HYPNOSIS WITH CHILDREN

Hypnosis is highly rewarding to use with children. It capitalizes on the child's developmental needs and their prolific imaginations as the agents of change (1–4,7,31,53–56). For a successful outcome, the clinician needs to enter the child's world cognitively, emotionally, and imaginatively. This exercise can be creative and enjoyable for both the clinician and the child. Cognitively, children are concrete thinkers whose imaginations thrive on favorite activities, themes, and places. They want to believe that their "brain switches can turn off pain" or that discomfort will lessen as they walk through "Candyland." Emotionally, children facing painful experiences seek adults they can trust to help them maintain autonomy, control, and even mastery in the face of challenging circumstances. As the examples below demonstrate, when introducing children to hypnotic techniques, it is best to use the child's own language to address the pain through suggestions for sensation alteration and increasing comfort. When children discover that an unpleasant and painful experience improves when they use their hypnotic imaginations, the feeling of mastery is exhilarating. The only limits to the ways that hypnosis can be used to reduce pain are the limits of the clinician's creativity.

Hypnosis with the Preschool-Age Child

Research has recently extended to children as young as 3 years who have been found capable of transforming their sensations and relieving pain during taxing medical procedures (7,52). Hypnosis with preschool-age children is a somewhat different phenomenon than with the school-age child and adolescent. Children under the age of 6 move fluidly between the world of fantasy and reality. This is the age of imaginary playmates and the spontaneous playing out of fears or concerns (55). Consequently, children younger than 6 years of age are a greater challenge to work with hypnotically. They require an informal, activity-based method during which the child is free to move around. The clinician needs to be engaging and informal, using a style and tone of voice quite unlike the quiet, soothing tone commonly used with adults or adolescents (54).

Hypnosis with preschool-age children is so different that it is not strictly accurate to refer to the experience as true hypnosis. A better term is *protohypnosis* (57) or *imaginative involvement* (31,53,57). The effects of positively directing a young child's imagination can be rapid and powerful, creating partial anesthesia or sensation alteration within a few minutes (31). Props such as puppets, bubbles, music, or a favorite story can also be helpful in promoting and maintaining the child's trance experience (3,7,53,61).

For the younger child, closing the eyes is invariably associated with going to sleep—something that no alert or anxious preschoolers will willingly do or should be expected to do, particularly in hospital. With children younger than 6 years of age, the hypnotic trance can occur with the eyes open. During hypnosis, the child's gaze often becomes more fixed—a sign of greater absorption. These children are often unfamiliar with the concept of relaxing, and so instructions to relax maybe meaningless to them.

Inviting a 3-year-old child to enter a hypnotic trance before a minor surgical procedure might be stated as follows:

> Let's pretend you're a fluffy bunny, just as cuddly as your bunny at home. As you snuggle under the sheet, you can make your own bed right here and begin to feel safe and comfortable. Your Mom will rub your back so that the fur on your bunny back will feel so good that your back will begin to go to sleep and you won't be bothered by the washing...

Whenever therapeutic methods are used with children and teens, it is essential to correctly gauge their emotional and cognitive age, so that the imagery, language, and style of the hypnotic experience is consonant with the child, and not confusing or boring. Chronologic age may not always be an accurate measure because anxiety and pain tend to make a child regress. Consequently, the clinician must be creative and sensitive, observe the child closely during the trance, and respond to the changes in the child. This can become more challenging if hypnosis is being used to modify pain perception during a medical procedure. Under these conditions, the clinician must simultaneously coordinate with the team and pace the child. The goal is to maximize the child's coping ability during the more painful part of the medical procedure, through suggestion, heightened absorption, and imagery (6,7,53,61).

Hypnosis with the School-Age Child and Adolescent

Children, particularly those of school age, have a heightened capacity for hypnosis. The peak of hypnotizability is from 8 to 12 years of age (57). Children and adolescents (whose trances more closely resemble those of adults) can absorb themselves into the hypnotic trance far more easily and rapidly than adults. Most children 6 years of age or older are able to sit or lie still, attend, respond to verbal direction, and become easily hypnotized. They are able to close their eyes and follow the process of relaxing and releasing muscle tension around the painful site.

Children will often report their own spontaneous elaborations after their hypnotic trances that reveal the degree to which the child made the trance his or her own relevant experience.

Using the child's own experiences, enthusiasms, or interests makes the experience more attractive and absorbing. Gathering this information from the child, parent, or nurse and using it in the trance experience improve cooperation and make hypnosis more successful. A useful question to ask is: "What helped in the past when you were in pain?" or "What did you do or think about that helped the pain settle?" This information can then be woven into a relevant and absorbing imaginative experience for the child (54,61,62).

For example, creating a hypnotic trance for a school-age child who loves pizza and is about to undergo a painful or distressing procedure can be as simple as saying the following:

> Because you love pizza so much, I've got an interesting proposal for you—while your nurse puts the nasogastric tube down your nose, we'll go on an amazing bike ride to the magic pizza mountain. All you'll need to do is get yourself comfortable...that's it. Now close your eyes so you can see better.... Good. Nod your head when you've got your gear on and you're on your speedy bike... Can you see the track ahead?... We're ready to explore this scrump-

tious mountain, and while we whiz through the cheese, you may be amazed to notice how little the tube bothers you...

In the above example, the clinician's participation in creating an alternate experience counters the anticipated distress and build up of tension and resistance in the child.

Role of the Parent During Hypnosis

When children face anxiety provoking and/or painful procedures, they naturally look to their parents as their most reliable ally. Involving parents in the hypnotherapy training process for pain control with their child is essential. Parents are often intrigued by the hypnotic process and are frequently highly motivated to be coaches for their children (61,62). Some parents may have used hypnosis or relaxation during pregnancy and delivery and may as a result be more receptive and experienced. Others may be fearful because of either religious beliefs or experience with theatrical hypnotic displays. Parents should be reassured that this is a therapeutic process in which the child's own capacities are being developed and used to his or her benefit. The child will be able to remember everything afterward, often feeling good about the experience. Explanations that hypnosis "feels like" daydreaming are often helpful to parents and help to demystify the process. Parents are often interested in the use of hypnosis, particularly if it means less reliance on pain medication.

Parents should thus be encouraged to be present during hypnosis, which often comforts and reassures the child. Remember, parents of children in pain are often distressed and need to comfort their child. It is thus rarely justifiable to separate parents from their children. In the exceptional case that the parent is not acting in the child's best interests or the parent's anxiety is overwhelming the child, separation is justified. Generally, parents can be directed to be allies and play a useful part of the hypnotic process (58).

In fact, many parents wish to be an active participant in easing their child's pain and distress, to learn to actively guide or coach their child using the hypnotic process (61,62). Far from being dangerous, our experience is that parents will use their new skills wisely and judiciously. This has been most evident with children facing recurrent painful procedures, such as intravenous lines and spinal taps, and with children in chronic severe pain such as in Crohn disease or during bone marrow transplantation. In these situations, parents recognize the value of using hypnosis to reduce anticipatory anxiety and increase comfort and are highly motivated to make it work. Training needs to be provided by a health professional skilled in hypnosis. Because it is a highly specific situation, parents learn within in one or two trials, often modeling the clinician. Parents will frequently practice at home with their child. When given support by the nursing and medical team, parents together with the child will demonstrate their new skills, creating an effective trance during the medical procedure in the clinic or hospital (61,62).

COMPONENTS OF HYPNOSIS

Stages of the Hypnotic Process

Preinduction Talk

Before hypnosis can be used to induce analgesia, the clinician must make contact with the child in an age-appropriate manner and create the alliance that will make the hypnotherapy possible. Knowing the child's dislikes, fears, interests, hopes, and areas of skill and comfort helps to fine-tune the induction and hypnotic process. If time is pressing, parents can be helpful in quickly relaying information, for example, the child's favorite sport. Next, it is important to explore the child's past experiences with pain and empathize with their distress in facing a painful experience. Explaining, in understandable language, why the procedure or painful experience is necessary is a way to gain the child's trust. Then offer the child a trick or new way to cope with the procedure or experience. Because most children do not know what hypnosis is, the clinician should provide a brief age-appropriate explanation. Here is an example appropriate for a child 6 to 8 years old:

By focusing on what you truly want to do, like playing with your kitty cats in your imagination, you will be having a nicer experience than just being here in the clinic. Your brain will not notice the procedure nearly as much because you're having fun with your cats and will be more comfortable.... I will be there with you, helping, and before you know it, the procedure will all be over and done.

Induction

Induction is the process by which the child is led into a hypnotic trance. The process focuses on narrowing attention and leading the child into greater attentional absorption so that the child settles into an altered state of consciousness. Once in a trance, the therapeutic work can occur, such as providing suggestions, creating dissociation from the pain, and other beneficial methods.

Various induction techniques are available such as visual and auditory imagery, eye fixation, and ideomotor techniques (31). Some useful examples for children in pain follow.

Visual Imagery Induction

Imagine your favorite place.... I'm not sure exactly where it is, but you know it very very well.... It's a place where you like to be and you feel comfortable and happy. You may want to close your eyes so you can see it more clearly. Take your time so that you can smell the smells, see all the things, feel what it's like there and hear the sounds. When you're at your favorite place, let me know, by wiggling your finger...

Ideomotor Induction

Ideomotor inductions involve using movement to help the child induce a trance. These types of inductions are particularly useful in promoting the idea that the child can gain control over the pain.

Put your arms straight out in front of you so that they are about 10 inches apart. There's a powerful magnet pulling your arms together.... Just let it happen...allow your arms come together...watch it happen. When they touch together, it's a signal to your body to let go...close your eyes and immediately become more comfortable.... Take a deep breath in.... As you let your breath out, you can already experience that your body is not nearly as bothered by the pain...

Relaxation

Relaxation as part of hypnosis is generally only helpful with children older than 6 years of age. It is not a critical component of a child's trance and may be impossible and counterproductive to attain for the child in acute pain. For the child in traction or with a chronic illness, however, relaxation can ease muscle rigidity and tension and promote well-being. General or progressive relaxation or relaxation specific to the painful site can be used.

In a pre- or postoperative situation with a young child for whom sleep is desirable, but in which the direct suggestion of sleep would be met with resistance, the teddy bear or favorite toy technique is useful.

What does your bear do when he goes sleep? You hold him how he likes to be held. Let him get comfortable. Pat him.... Is he getting sleepy? Let his head get comfortable.... Pat his tummy nicely.... Let his arms get sleepy and comfortable. Now the bear is feeling sleepy all over...so cozy...so comfortable...so easy...

Hypnotic Suggestions

Hypnotic suggestions for pain reduction should promote distancing or dissociation from the physical and psychologic trauma. Techniques can range from distraction to suggestions for direct hypnoanalgesia such as the "magic glove" or the "pain switch" [for a video example, see *No Fears, No Tears* (61)]. Distancing suggestions move the pain away from the child or transfer the pain to another part of the body, such as a hand that can be shaken to dispel the pain.

Hypnoanalgesia: The Pain Switch

The idea that the brain controls the body needs to be explained to the child in a way that he or she can best understand.

The nerves send their pain message directly to the brain where it is interpreted and understood.

> The brain then sends these messages back to the body. We can focus attention on the switches that control the incoming pain messages and turn them down, so that our bodies receive a dimmer pain message and feel less pain. Now concentrate, find the switch in your brain that goes to the part of your body that is hurting...nod your head when you've found it...notice what color it is and type of switch and turn your pain switch down...notch by notch...at each notch you'll notice slightly less pain...it's very interesting...continue going as far down as you want so you'll be comfortable...

Elaborations could include more details about the switch and descriptions of the changing sensation of pain as the switch is turned down. The criterion for success is that the child feels a significant difference between the switched-off area and a complementary nonaffected area. This can be tested with a sterile needle or pencil point. The goal is not the removal of pain but the diminution of pain and the subsequent feeling of power over the pain. This technique is particularly useful for children with chronic or recurrent pain problems.

EXAMPLES OF HYPNOSIS FOR THE CHILD IN PAIN

Children in Acute Pain

Fractures

A child in pain often spontaneously moves into a hypnotic trance with narrowed absorption and attention to the pain. The clinician's task is to recognize that the child is entranced with his or her pain and help modify the child's fixed preoccupation shifting attention to alleviate suffering.

> A 4-year-old girl with a fractured femur was admitted to the emergency department. She was screaming with pain and seemed very anxious. After codeine was administered, the clinician helped focus her attention by asking her to tell where the pain was and where it was not. Pointing to her abdomen, the clinician asked "Does it hurt here?" The child said "no." "How about here?" (pointing to her hip). "No." "Good," said the clinician, "then it hurts here and here" (pointing to her left femur and knee) "but not here and here" (pointing to her tummy and hip). The clinician continued to ask and focus the child on where the pain was, noting the greater areas where the pain was not present. She concluded with "That's good! In a few minutes you'll notice that it'll be hurting even less in your knee and leg."

It was not necessary to give the child a hypnotic induction because the child was already in an altered state of consciousness. The therapeutic work was to sustain the trance and redirect the child's attention to the limits of the pain, so that she no longer felt overwhelmed. Her panic and anxiety were reduced by providing boundaries to the pain sensation that she feared was endless. This heightened receptivity to suggestion and altered states of awareness occur most often in acute pain and trauma cases and often in the emergency department of hospitals (1). The recognition of this receptive state can greatly facilitate care and treatment in these situations.

Burns

Hypnosis is regarded as a potent tool to break the vicious cycle between the patient's emotional response to a burn and the destructive physiologic sequelae (18–22). The following hypnotic induction was given while burn dressing was applied to an 8-year-old boy who scorched his hand on a hot plate.

> Let's use your brain to help your hand feel better. Close your eyes, and then take a big breath in...and out.... Now walk down three steps outside and nod your head when you can see the big bucket of snow at the bottom of the stair. You know how wonderfully cold and soft snow feels.... Put that sore hand of yours straight into the snow now.... Can you feel the cooling? Your hand feels cool and much more comfortable.... You'll probably feel the pain begin to ease as the cold takes the heat out of your hand...

This example is used to show how the approach might be modified for a 4-year-old boy. Note that the style of the hypnotic trance is more interactive and action oriented, and the language is simple.

> Let's pretend there's a bucket of snow here.... You know what snow looks like, don't you?... What does it feel like?... That's right! Take that

> hand you put on the hot plate and now put it into this bucket of cold cold snow. It's fluffy and soft too, isn't it?... How else does it feel? Can you feel that it makes that hand go so so cold that you can hardly feel anything.... That feels good.... When the hand is feeling the cold so that is more comfortable, you nod your head to let me know...

The choice of language is often critical to guiding the child's experience. Wherever possible, use the child's own words for his or her pain, including sensory and affective adjectives. In the previous example, referring to the child's hand as "the" hand in contrast to "your" hand, encourages some distance or dissociation for the child from his painful hand. With the younger child's blurred boundaries between reality and fantasy, it may be harder to sustain the therapeutic trance, particularly if a painful medical procedure is being performed (7,54). These taxing situations demand even greater flexibility of the clinician to move with the child, as he or she enters, exits, and re-enters the therapeutic trance state during times of anxiety or uncertainty.

Children Facing Procedural Pain: Lumbar Puncture and Bone Marrow Aspiration

A 14-year-old boy had a relapse of leukemia and again faced multiple invasive procedures (lumbar punctures and bone marrow aspirations). He did not want sedation or anesthesia because they made him feel "too weird." The patient was a very large adolescent and could not be easily forced to do anything against his will. So, when he became resistant to almost any requests made by medical staff for cooperation, the staff consulted psychologic services.

After exploring the dire need for the procedures, the patient's feelings about his relapse, having to go through procedures repeatedly, and how difficult all that must be, the therapist was able to form an alliance with the patient. Eventually, the idea of self-regulation was introduced as a scientifically proven way to help with the pain of procedures. Adolescents enjoy the appeal to their newly emerging abstract thinking abilities. The evidence was convincing, and the patient wanted to use breathing relaxation and mental imagery to cope with what he now understood were truly necessary procedures. He was suggestible and used deep breathing, counting, and progressive muscle relaxation as his induction. He enjoyed going to a favorite place for imagery and used turning off the pain switches for his hypnoanalgesic suggestions. He was very good at relaxing himself and readily entered an altered state of consciousness. After impressive initial successes, he became proud of his ability to practically sleep through painful procedures!

Children with Chronic, Recurrent Pain

Most children are highly motivated to get rid of pain. This is particularly true for the child with a chronic illness. Hypnosis can play an important part in conjunction with other therapies in empowering the child in chronic or recurrent pain, and diminishing the grip of familiar pain that limits the child's activity. Hypnosis has been effective, for example, in the treatment and management of rheumatoid arthritis, Crohn disease, and juvenile migraine and tension headaches (23,24).

> A 10-year-old boy with occasional migraine headaches and more frequent mild headaches reported that his medication was not reliable in easing his pain and discomfort. He was keen to do something to help himself. The boy's ambition was to be an ambulance man. His mother reported that he would play for hours constructing rescues and resuscitation with his toys. It was suggested to him that he might like to experience what happens to the pain in his head when he goes on a rescue mission using his imagination. He was led through a fantasy rescue, the details of which he was invited to complete. It was also suggested that the closer he came to saving his patients from death and disaster, the less head pain he would feel. After 7 minutes, the boy reported that he had saved the man from the roof of the house and that his head felt fine again. The session was audiotaped, and the boy took the tape home to use when he needed it or until he became proficient in doing "rescue missions" on his own. His metaphor of saving the man from the roof

of the house echoed saving himself from the pain in his body's roof—his head. He has made good progress in controlling his headaches.

TRAINING FOR PROFESSIONALS

The practice of hypnosis requires training and experience. There are several excellent resources designed for the pediatric professional to learn the skills. In terms of written resources, Olness' book (31) remains the premier reference in the field. Workshops are regularly provided by the Canadian Clinical Hypnosis Societies in the various provinces and by the American Society of Clinical Hypnosis in the different states. The Society of Developmental and Behavioral Pediatrics offers an annual 3-day intensive pediatric hypnosis course. In a recent evaluation, participants in that course indicated an overwhelming positive response to the value of that course and subsequent increased practice satisfaction from use of the skills taught in the course (59). (For further information about training, contact the Society for Behavioral Pediatrics, 241 East Gravers Lane, Philadelphia, PA 19118 or The American Society of Clinical Hypnosis, 2250 E. Devon Avenue, Suite 336, Des Plaines, IL 60018.) Recently, Solomon et al. developed and then evaluated their seminar called "Pediatric Pain Management: A Professional Course." The evaluation showed that pediatric professionals taking the 2-day seminar increased their knowledge related to cognitive-behavioral pain management strategies (including hypnosis) and acquired specific skills for their implementation in clinical settings (60). In addition, the seminar includes a children's book written specifically for the course by Fred Rogers (of the well-known children's TV show "Mr. Rogers' Neighborhood") and a special module that pediatric professionals can use to teach children and parents relaxation and mental imagery skills in small group settings. Satisfaction with the course was overwhelmingly positive. (For more information, contact Richard Solomon, M.D., University of Michigan, Department of Pediatrics and Communicable Diseases, 300 North Ingalls Building, Room 6D16, Ann Arbor, MI 48109-0456.)

CONCLUSION

Despite important advances in the knowledge of pediatric pain management, children's anxiety and pain are still undertreated both in in-patient and out-patient settings. Time pressures and heavy workloads impede the implementation of effective behavioral techniques such as hypnosis. The most commonly raised objection from medical and nursing staff to the use of hypnosis is "I don't have time." This comment is based on the outdated idea of hypnosis as a lengthy process of induction, relaxation, and suggestion. We have learned a great deal about how rapidly patients in pain respond to hypnosis. The benefits, which include a better relationship between clinician and child, far outweigh the time and effort required.

Another widely held belief is that with effective pain medications, behavioral approaches such as hypnosis have become less important. For children and their parents, the treatment of fear and anxiety is just as important the treatment of pain. For anxiety, hypnosis is the modality of choice. So, take a deep breath, relax, and imagine how much better children will feel when you add hypnosis to your approach to children who face painful medical procedures. The only limits to hypnosis are the limits of the child's imaginative capacity and the clinician's' ability to understand and capitalize on that imagination.

REFERENCES

1. Kohen DP. Applications of relaxation/mental imagery (self-hypnosis) in pediatric emergencies. *Int J Clin Exp Hypn* 1986;34:283–294.
2. Kohen DP, Olness K. Child hypnotherapy: uses of therapeutic communication and self-regulation for common pediatric situations. *Pediatr Basics* 1987;April:1–10.
3. Kuttner L. Helpful strategies in working with preschool children in pediatric practice. *Pediatr Ann* 1991;20:120–127.
4. Zeltzer L, LeBaron S. Hypnotic and nonhypnotic techniques for the reduction of pain and anxiety during painful procedures in children and adolescents with cancer. *Behav Pediatr* 1982;101:1032–1035.
5. Kellerman J, Zeltzer L, Ellenberg L, et al. Adolescents

with cancer: hypnosis for the reduction of the acute pain and anxiety associated with medical procedures. *J Adolesc Health Care* 1983;4:85–90.
6. Kuttner L, Bowman M, Teasdale M. Psychological treatment of distress, pain and anxiety for young children with cancer. *J Dev Behav Pediatr* 1988;9:374–381.
7. Kuttner L. Management of young children's acute pain and anxiety during invasive medical procedures. *Pediatrician* 1989;16:39–44.
8. Ellis JA, Spanos NP. Cognitive-behavioral interventions for children's distress during bone marrow aspirations and lumbar punctures: a critical review. *J Pain Symptom Manage* 1994;9:96–108.
9. Genuis ML. The use of hypnosis in helping cancer patients control anxiety, pain, and emesis: a review of recent empirical studies. *Am J Clin Hypn* 1995;37: 316–325.
10. Smith JT, Barabasz A, Barabasz M. Comparison of hypnosis and distraction in severely ill children undergoing painful medical procedures. *J Counsel Psychol* 1996;43:187–195.
11. Steggles S, Damore-Petingola S, Maxwell J, et al. Hypnosis for children and adolescents with cancer: an annotated bibliography, 1985–1995. *J Pediatr Oncol Nurs* 1997;14:27–32.
12. Liossi C, Hatira P. Clinical hypnosis versus cognitive behavioral training for pain management with pediatric cancer patients undergoing bone marrow aspirations. *Int J Clin Exp Hypn* 1999;47:104–116.
13. Powers SW. Empirically supported treatments in pediatric psychology: procedure-related pain. *J Pediatr Psychol* 1999;24:131–145.
14. Lambert SA. The effects of hypnosis/guided imagery on the postoperative course of children. *Dev Behav Pediatr* 1996;17:307–310.
15. Rapkin DA, Straubing M, Holroyd JC. Guided imagery, hypnosis and recovery from head and neck cancer surgery: an exploratory study. *Int J Clin Exp Hypn* 1991;39:215–226.
16. Dinges DF, Whitehouse WG, Orne EC, et al. Self-hypnosis training as an adjunctive treatment in the management of pain associated with sickle cell disease. *Int J Clin Exp Hypn* 1997;45:417–432.
17. Zeltzer L, Dash J, Holland JP. Hypnotically induced pain control in sickle cell anemia. *Pediatrics* 1979;64: 533–536.
18. Van der Does AJW, Van Dyck R, Spijker RE. Hypnosis and pain in patients with severe burns: a pilot study. *Burns* 1988;14:399–404.
19. Patterson DR, Questad KA, Boltwood MD. Hypnotherapy as a treatment for pain in patients with burns: Research and clinical considerations. *J Burn Care Rehab* 1987;8:263–268.
20. Ewin DM. Emergency room hypnosis for the burned patient. *Am J Clin Hypn* 1986;29:7–12.
21. Berstein NR. Management of burned children with the aid of hypnosis. *J Child Psychol Psychiatry* 1963;4:93.
22. Bonham A. Procedural pain in children with burns. Part 2: nursing management of children in pain. *Int J Trauma Nurs* 1996;2:74–77.
23. Olness K, MacDonald J, Uden D. Prospective study comparing propanolol, placebo and hypnosis in management of juvenile migraine. *Pediatrics* 1987;79: 593–597.
24. Smith MS, Womack WM. Stress management techniques in childhood and adolescence. *Clin Pediatr* 1987;11:581–585.
25. Chaves JF. Recent advances in the application of hypnosis to pain management. *Am J Clin Hypn* 1994;37: 117–129.
26. Vessey JA, Carlson KL. Nonpharmacological interventions to use with children in pain. *Issues Comprehens Pediatr Nurs* 1996;19:169–182.
27. Tan SY, Leucht CA. Cognitive-behavioral therapy for clinical pain control: a 15-year update and its relationship to hypnosis. *Int J Clin Exp Hypn* 1997;45:396–416.
28. Kuttner L. Mind-body methods of pain management. *Child Adolesc Psychiatr Clin North Am* 1997;6: 783–796.
29. Barber J, Adrian C. *Psychological approaches to the management of pain*. New York: Brunner/Mazel, 1982.
30. Hilgard ER, Hilgard JR. *Hypnosis in the relief of pain*. New York: Brunner/Mazel, 1994.
31. Olness K. *Hypnosis and hypnotherapy with children*. New York: Guilford Press, 1996.
32. Barber J. Rapid induction analgesia: a clinical report. *Am J Clin Hypn* 1977;19:138–147.
33. Fromm E. The nature of hypnosis and other altered states of consciousness: an ego psychological theory. In: Fromm E, Shor RE, eds. *Hypnosis: developments in research and new perspectives*, 2nd ed. Hawthorne, NY: Aldine, 1979.
34. Orne MT. The nature of hypnosis: artifact and essence. *J Abnorm Soc Psychol* 1959;58:277–299.
35. Speigel H, Spiegel D. *Trance and treatment: clinical uses of hypnosis*. New York: Basic Books, 1978.
36. Olness K. The use of self-hypnosis in the treatment of childhood nocturnal enuresis. A report on 40 patients. *Clin Pediatr (Phila)* 1975;14:273–275, 278–279.
37. Kohen DP, Botts P. Relaxation/mental imagery (self-hypnosis) in Tourette's syndrome: experience with four children. *Am J Clin Hypn* 1987;4:227–237.
38. Kohen DP. Application of relaxation/mental imagery (self-hypnosis) to the management of asthma: report of behavioral outcomes of a two-year prospective controlled study. *Am J Clin Hypn* 1986;28:196(abst).
39. Zeltzer LK, Fanurik D, LeBaron S. The cold pressor pain paradigm in children: feasibility of an intervention model (part II). *Pain* 1989;37:305–313.
40. Barber J, Mayer D. Evaluation of the efficacy and neural mechanisms of a hypnotic analgesia procedure in experimental and clinical dental pain. *Pain* 1977;4:41–48.
41. Barber TX, Wilson SC. Hypnosis, suggestions, and altered states of consciousness: experimental evaluation of the new cognitive-behavioral theory and the traditional trance-state theory of 'hypnosis'. *Ann N Y Acad Sci* 1977;296:34–47.
42. Coe WC, Sarbin TR. Hypnosis from the standpoint of a contextualist. *Ann N Y Acad Sci* 1977;296:2–13.
43. Spanos NP. Hypnotic behavior: a social-psychological interpretation of amnesia, analgesia, and 'trance logic'. *Behav Brain Sci* 1986;9:440–467.
44. Hilgard ER. *Divided consciousness: multiple controls in human thought and action*. New York: John Wiley & Sons, 1977.
45. Melzack R, Wall PD. Pain mechanisms: a new theory. *Science* 1965;150:971–979.
46. Melzack R, Wall PD. *The challenge of pain*. London: Penguin Books, 1988.
47. Crawford JH, Knebel T, Vendemia JMC. The nature of

hypnotic analgesia: neurophysiological foundation and evidence. *Contemp Hypn* 1998;15:22–33.
48. Goldstein A, Hilgard E. Lack of influence of the morphine antagonist naloxone on hypnotic analgesia. *Proc Natl Acad Sci U S A* 1975;72:2041–2043.
49. Olness K. Hypnotherapy: a cyberphysiologic strategy in pain management. *Pediatr Clin North Am* 1989;36: 873–884.
50. Finer B, Terenius L. Endorphin involvements during hypnotic analgesia in chronic pain patients. Paper presented at the Third World Congress on Pain of the International Association for the Study of Pain, Edinburgh, Scotland, August 4–11, 1981.
51. Parke TJ, Stevens JE, Rice AS, et al. Metabolic acidosis and fatal myocardial failure after propofol infusion in children: five case reports. *BMJ* 1992;305: 613–616.
52. Felt BT, Mollen E, Diaz S, et al. Behavioral interventions reduce infant distress at immunization. *Arch Pediatr Adolesc Med* 2000;154:719–24.
53. Sugarman LI. Hypnosis in a primary care practice: developing skills for the "new morbidities." *J Dev Behav Pediatr* 1996;17:300–305.
54. Kuttner L. Favorite stories: a hypnotic pain-reduction technique for children in acute pain. *Am J Clin Hypn* 1988;30:289–295.
55. Olness K. Hypnosis in pediatric practice. *Curr Probl Pediatr* 1981;12:1–47.
56. Lee LH, Olness KN. Effects of self-induced mental imagery on autonomic reactivity in children. *J Dev Behav Pediatr* 1996;17:323–327.
55. Fraiberg, SH. *The magic years*. New York: Scribner's Sons, 1959.
56. Hilgard JR. *Personality and hypnosis: a study of imaginative involvement*. Chicago. The University of Chicago Press, 1979.
57. Morgan AH, Hilgard JR. The Stanford hypnotic scale for children. *Am J Clin Hypn* 1979;21:78–85.
58. Gardner GG. Parents: obstacles or allies in child hypnotherapy? *Am J Clin Hypn* 1974;17:44–49.
59. Mize WL. Clinical training in self-regulation and practical pediatric hypnosis: what pediatricians want pediatricians to know. *J Dev Behav Pediatr* 1996;17:317–322.
60. Solomon RS, Walco GA, Robinson MR. Pediatric pain management: program description and preliminary evaluation results of a professional course. *J Dev Behav Pediatr* 1998;19:193–195.
61. Kuttner L. *No fears, no tears: children with cancer coping with pain* [videotape and manual]. Boston: Fanlight Productions, 1986.
62. Kuttner L. *No fears, no tears—13 years later* [videotape]. Boston: Fanlight Productions, 1998.

19

Neurosurgical Procedures for the Treatment of Pediatric Pain

Jodi L. Smith and Joseph R. Madsen

Pediatricians have been slow to realize the possibilities of pain-relieving operations; it has perhaps been too easy simply to give more narcotics and overlook suffering in a child who is less articulate about his or her complaints than an adult. Likewise, neurosurgeons have been slow to apply standard procedures to the pain problems of childhood. Yet it is a rewarding experience indeed to witness the return of smiles, laughter, appetite, ambulation, and hope in a child who has been bedridden, withdrawn, and obviously miserable despite heavy sedation, even if this is only for a few weeks or months (1).

The use of neurosurgical procedures to relieve pain in children has not received the attention that it deserves. The promise of medical treatment of pain has led to the neglect of classically established surgical procedures. In addition, practitioners have focused primarily on pain relief in adults; the special needs of children in pain have not been addressed.

Currently, neurosurgical procedures for pain relief are available for patients of all ages. These procedures are reserved typically for pain that is refractory to other less invasive, nonsurgical modalities or in which there is intolerance of side effects. Unfortunately, their application to pediatric patients has been extremely underutilized. Classic neurosurgical operations for pain relief have included neuroablative procedures, which alleviate pain by surgically interrupting pain pathways, and neurostimulation procedures, which relieve pain through electrical stimulation of peripheral nerves or the central nervous system. Such procedures were fairly common in the past. However, with the increased availability of more sophisticated medical options for pain control, the demand for neurosurgical pain procedures declined. Despite this, neurosurgical techniques continue to be developed for the treatment of chronic pain in adults; these include induction of lesions at the dorsal root entry zone (DREZ lesioning), placement of epidural and intrathecal catheters for intraspinal infusion of narcotics and local anesthetics, and the implantation of deep brain and spinal epidural stimulators for electrical stimulation of the central nervous system and peripheral nerves, respectively. Such procedures are able to provide successful pain relief without unwanted side effects and complications.

In contrast to the widespread involvement of neurosurgeons in the treatment of chronic pain in adults, there has been little, if any, involvement of neurosurgeons in alleviating pediatric pain. This likely results, at least in part, from the fact that the clinical importance of pediatric pain has been emphasized only recently. Unlike adults, young children often are nonverbal and are unable to articulate their pain, and it has been assumed that children do not experience pain to the same degree as adults. This, in turn, has led to inadequate management of pain in the pediatric population. In addition, there are currently no neurosurgeons who specialize in the treatment of pediatric pain. Likewise, there are no neurosurgeons who specialize in the treatment of pain and also have specific pediatric neurosurgical expertise. Moreover, studies demonstrating the effectiveness of particular pain procedures in the pediatric age group are currently lacking. Despite the obvious deficiency of neurosurgical approaches to the treatment of pediatric pain, neurosurgical procedures are available for the relief of chronic pain in the pediatric population. The purpose of this chapter is to highlight some of these procedures and to discuss their utility in treating painful disorders in children.

DECOMPRESSIVE SURGERY

Neurosurgical methods for the management of pediatric pain are similar to those currently used to alleviate pain in adults. These include neuroablative operations such as anterolateral cordotomy, myelotomy, and DREZ lesioning; placement of epidural and intrathecal catheters for intraspinal infusion of narcotics and local anesthetics; and the implantation of spinal epidural stimulators for electrical stimulation of peripheral nerves. However, before discussing these options, it is important to point out that other, less traditional neurosurgical procedures (e.g., decompressive surgery) also can be effective in alleviating intractable excess pain in children. This is particularly evident in the following two patients with malignant tumors whose severe pain responded to decompressive surgery.

Case 1. A 10-year-old girl with metastatic osteogenic sarcoma and malignant pleural effusion presented with severe bilateral lower extremity pain and paresis. An epidural catheter was placed and tunneled subcutaneously for treatment with epidural narcotics at home. Unfortunately, her pain worsened, and eventually she became refractory to increasing doses of epidural narcotics. Moreover, her lower extremity paresis began to worsen during the epidural narcotic infusions, and she developed intermittent quadriparesis. A magnetic resonance imaging scan was performed that revealed an epidural fluid collection and epidural tumor extending diffusely throughout the spinal cord, especially in the upper cervical and lower lumbar regions. The family initially refused decompressive surgery for the purpose of preserving neurologic function, but they consented to surgery for palliation of the pain. Consequently, she underwent cervical and lumbar decompressive laminectomies for removal of epidural tumor and evacuation of epidural fluid that was infected with fungus. Postoperatively, she had a dramatic improvement in her pain, which was controlled adequately at home with low-dose oral morphine. She died approximately 3 weeks later.

Case 2. A 16-year-old boy presented with thoracic radiculopathy and was found to have a rare malignant melanotic schwannoma in the epidural space at the T11 level. He initially underwent an extradural decompression and stabilization with Harrington rods. However, he subsequently presented with severe bilateral lower extremity pain, which was so excruciating that doses of intravenous morphine sufficient to cause apnea were unable to relieve the pain. In addition, he had decreased leg strength and worsening of his bladder function. An emergency myelogram was performed that demonstrated a complete block at the T11 level. He subsequently underwent re-exploration and resection of intradural tumor. Postoperatively, his pain remained well controlled on oral pain medication until his death from disease progression roughly 1 year later.

In both cases, the neurosurgical service was consulted regarding whether an ablative surgical procedure, such as a rhizotomy, would be appropriate for pain palliation. Instead, decompressive surgeries were performed; these were no more invasive than an ablation procedure, but were just as effective in relieving the pain.

NEUROABLATIVE PROCEDURES

Central Nervous System

Ablative procedures such as rhizotomy, cordotomy, and myelotomy have been employed for more than 50 years to alleviate intractable excess pain. Currently, there are three main types of neurosurgical ablative procedures involving the central nervous system that are used to treat medically refractory pain (Fig. 19.1): (a) selective anterolateral

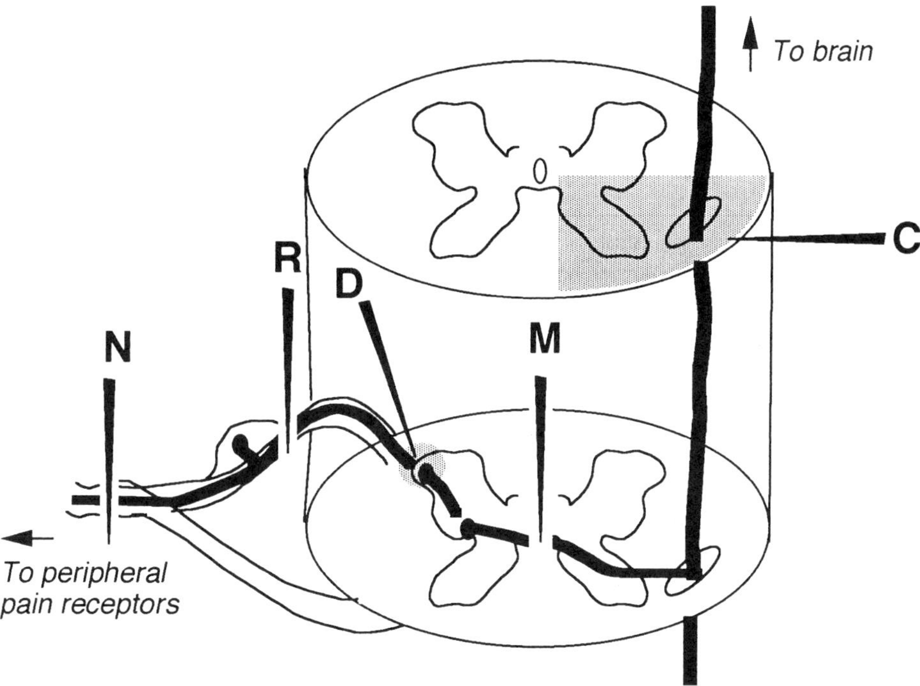

FIG. 19.1. Ablative procedures to interrupt principal pain pathways. *N*, neurectomy (division of a peripheral nerve); *R*, rhizotomy (division of a dorsal root); *D*, dorsal root entry zone (DREZ, lesion in the substantia gelatinosa); *M*, myelotomy (midline interruption of crossing fibers in the anterior commissure); *C*, cordotomy (ablation of the lateral spinothalamic tract).

cordotomy, (b) myelotomy, and (c) DREZ lesions. Ablative procedures produce their effects by surgically interrupting specific afferent pain fibers without injuring adjacent functional neural tissues. Benefits of ablative procedures include elimination of unremitting pain resulting either from malignancy or from peripheral nerve deafferentation. Limitations of such procedures include failure to eliminate central deafferentation pain and the generation of unwanted adverse effects such as motor weakness, deafferentation dysesthesias, intractable deafferentation pain, dorsal column dysfunction, and respiratory and bladder dysfunction. Such side effects can result either from disruption of motor pathways, other sensory pathways, or pain inhibitory pathways from the brainstem that are adjacent to and not clearly demarcated from ascending pain pathways or from maladaptive regeneration of the lesioned afferent pain fibers. Today, such techniques have been improved to provide successful pain relief while minimizing the aforementioned side effects and complications.

Selective Anterolateral Cordotomy

Selective anterolateral cordotomy is the operation by which the lateral spinothalamic tract is surgically interrupted, either by percutaneous or open technique, for the relief of somatic pain below the level of the mandible. This has proven useful as a short-term method for relieving pain in patients with malignant disease as well as in some patients with painful nonmalignant conditions that are intractable. When selecting patients for cordotomy, it is necessary to determine the particular type of pain. The lateral spinothalamic tract mediates pain that is sharp or lancinating. This pain is alleviated by selective anterolateral cordotomy in at least 90% of patients. The major contraindication of both percutaneous and open surgical procedures is severe pulmonary dysfunction. Additionally, a cordotomy can exacerbate or delay the recovery of neurologic deficits of recent onset, such as paresis or rectal and bladder incontinence. These effects, however, are usually temporary.

Percutaneous cordotomy is easier and often is tolerated better than open surgical cordotomy. Because the risks are reduced significantly and the results are comparable, percutaneous cordotomy is currently the procedure of choice for adults (2–4). However, the surgical risks that lead to avoidance of open procedures in debilitated, often elderly, cancer patients would be significantly reduced in pediatric patients.

The complication rate of percutaneous cordotomy is relatively low. Ipsilateral hemiparesis appears in a small number of patients. This typically lasts a few days to a few weeks; rarely is it a permanent deficit. Ataxia lasting only few hours is observed in approximately one of five patients and is probably the most common complication. Intermittent bladder catheterization is required postoperatively in roughly 10% of cases, typically in patients with preoperative bladder dysfunction. Postcordotomy dysesthetic syndromes (burning pain over the entire area that was made analgesic) are rare, probably occurring in fewer than 1% of patients.

Immediately after the cordotomy, more than 90% of patients consider themselves to be pain free or comfortable enough that no analgesics are necessary. By the end of 3 months, successful pain relief is reduced to approximately 85%. By 1 year, at least some pain returns to approximately 40% of patients. By 2 years, an average of 60% of patients no longer have complete pain relief. The gradual loss of pain suppression is accompanied by increased sensory function at progressively more caudal spinal cord levels, presumably reflecting plasticity of neural function. The greater neural plasticity in very young patients may lead to exaggerated demonstration of this phenomenon.

Myelotomy

Myelotomy, like selective anterior cordotomy, involves the surgical interruption of the spinothalamic tract for the relief of somatic pain. The goal of this operation, which was first described by Armour (5) in 1927, is to lesion the decussating spinothalamic fibers that travel in the anterior commissure and subserve pain perception bilaterally. In theory, this operation should produce symmetric analgesia bilaterally with pain relief restricted to those areas where sensation has been altered. Unfortunately, this theoretically attractive operation has not been as effective as predicted on anatomic grounds. Most neurosurgeons now agree that the typical open longitudinal midline myelotomy provides only a temporary loss of pain and temperature sensation in a girdle area that corresponds to the level of the cord incision.

At present, there are no reliable criteria for selecting patients who might benefit from myelotomy for pain control. This procedure can be useful in the management of bilateral pelvic and peroneal pain because the surgical alternative, bilateral cordotomy, carries a greater risk of bladder dysfunction. The utility of myelotomy in treating pain in children is unknown.

Dorsal Root Entry Zone Lesions

In 1976, Nashold et al. (6) described a procedure for treating pain that resulted in the focal destruction of the DREZ (i.e., the mediolateral aspect of the dorsal rootlets and Rexed laminae I and II of the dorsal horn of the spinal cord). Surgical lesioning of this area, the so-called DREZ procedure, abolishes pain conduction from peripheral nerves without damaging other sensory nerve fibers. Since 1976, the DREZ procedure has been used successfully to treat intractable excess pain resulting from brachial or sacral plexus avulsion, paraplegia, herpes, cancer, and limb amputation. In addition, DREZ radiofrequency lesions in the nucleus caudalis of the trigeminal system have been successful in relieving intractable facial pain.

The most common and most successful application of the DREZ procedure is for reduction of deafferentation pain that is observed after brachial plexus avulsion, especially in young motorcycle riders. At present, there are more than 100 patients reported in this category, with many of them having had more than a 5-year follow-up period, and the overall success rate approaches 85% (7). Because some of these patients are teenagers, the experience gained can be applied directly to the adolescent age group and probably be extended to the pediatric age group as well.

Besides the deafferentation pain that follows brachial or sacral plexus avulsion, the DREZ procedure has also been successful in relieving other types of intractable excess pain including postparaplegic pain, postamputation (i.e., phantom limb) pain, postherpetic neuralgia, and facial pain. With regard to postparaplegic pain, certain characteristics are helpful in predicting patients likely to have a successful outcome from the DREZ procedure. For example, 74% of patients with pain caudal to the level of injury and 90% of those with unilateral pain report good results, whereas only 20% of those with diffuse pain and 38% of those with burning pain obtain good results (8). Regarding pain that occurs after limb amputation, this can either be the result of stump or phantom limb pain. Although the DREZ procedure is highly effective in relieving phantom limb pain, stump pain responds less well to this type of treatment (9). This therapy may be useful in the treatment of children who require limb amputations for osteogenic sarcomas or other types of extremity tumors.

Previous studies have shown that patients with postherpetic neuralgia involving the spinal nerves have a good response to treatment with the DREZ procedure; however, as pointed out by Friedman and Bullitt (10), the effectiveness of this procedure is relatively short-lived. In their study, 91% of 32 patients had immediate pain relief. By 6 months, 53% of them continued to have good pain relief, but by 18 months, only 25% of patients were reporting good pain relief. Patients with intractable facial pain may also benefit from DREZ radiofrequency lesions in the nucleus caudalis of the trigeminal system. Bernard et al. (11) documented 18 patients who underwent this procedure to ameliorate medically intractable facial pain from a variety of origins. Ninety percent of these patients had satisfactory pain relief during the immediate postoperative period, and 58% still had good pain relief at the time of follow-up. In this study, the best long-term results were observed in patients with postherpetic neuralgia. There was a 71% success rate in patients who underwent the nucleus caudalis DREZ procedure for treatment of their facial pain. In another study (12), five patients with intractable facial pain caused by cancer were treated with the nucleus caudalis DREZ procedure, and all five of them had substantial pain relief shortly after surgery. Long-term follow-up revealed that two of these patients continued to have a significant improvement in their pain and activity level, whereas the remaining three patients had less pain than preoperatively but were still limited in their activity. This procedure seems promising for children with facial sarcomas who have intractable facial pain after tumor resection.

Peripheral Nervous System

Ablative procedures involving the peripheral nervous system can also be employed to alleviate intractable excess pain from a variety of causes. Such procedures produce their effects by surgical ablation of peripheral, spinal, cranial, or sympathetic nerves. Currently, there are several types of ablative procedures involving the peripheral nervous system that are available to treat medically refractory pain including peripheral neurectomy, spinal dorsal rhizotomy, sympathectomy, trigeminal gangliolysis, and cranial sensory nerve rhizotomy.

Peripheral Neurectomy

Peripheral neurectomy, a procedure in which part of one or more peripheral branches of the cranial or spinal nerves is resected, was the original neurosurgical ablative procedure performed for the treatment of chronic pain. Currently, however, peripheral nerve resection is rarely used in the management of patients with chronic pain. There are three main advantages of this procedure: (a) the ease of the operation, (b) the low morbidity associated with the procedure, and (c) the predictable loss of function, i.e., complete anesthesia in the territory of the sectioned nerve. Despite this, numerous disadvantages clearly outweigh the advantages. First, with the exception of the trigeminal nerve and a few of the cutaneous nerves of the extremities, most peripheral nerves are mixed; therefore, a peripheral neurectomy results in loss of both sensory and motor function, with the loss of motor function often lasting longer than the sensory loss. Second, peripheral neurectomy results in the loss of all sensory modalities, not just pain and temperature sensation as in a selective anterior cordotomy. Thus, patients are at risk of skin and joint complications from lack of sensation. Third, adjacent intact sensory nerves frequently sprout into the denervated areas resulting in a circumferential decrease in the region of anesthesia. Such regeneration is a significant complicating factor, especially in young patients who have a long expected survival. Fourth, resection of the trigeminal nerve can result in the development of anesthesia dolorosa, a pain syndrome in which patients experience a painful numbness in the anesthetic regions after trigeminal nerve ablative procedures. The pain is typically described as an intense, constant burning type of pain that mainly affects the ipsilateral eye and mouth and is not triggerable. Finally, partial or complete transection of a peripheral nerve can result in the formation of a traumatic neuroma, a nodular mass of regenerating axons and Schwann cells that forms at the end of a proximal nerve stump, reflecting reactive hyperplasia during attempted regeneration. Not all neuromas are painful, but some produce pain that is worse than the original pain.

Today, there are very few indications for peripheral neurectomies in the management of medically refractory pain. The most common application is in the treatment of patients with intractable trigeminal neuralgia who have failed percutaneous gangliolysis (a procedure that produces longer pain relief with less sensory loss and has just as low a morbidity rate as peripheral neurectomy) and who are not candidates for an intracranial procedure. Such patients can undergo resection of branches of the trigeminal nerve, including the supraorbital, infraorbital, and mandibular nerves, in an attempt to gain pain relief by inducing anesthesia in the facial areas innervated by these nerves. Other patients that might benefit from peripheral neurectomy are amputees with pain resulting from a stump neuroma. Such an operation might provide relief from the distressing stump pain if the pain is caused by pressure on the neuroma.

Spinal Dorsal Rhizotomy

Spinal dorsal rhizotomy was first described in 1889 by Abbe (13). Since its first description, many neurosurgeons have performed this operation with success. The procedure has two main advantages: (a) it avoids muscle paralysis by sparing motor fibers and (b) it produces total anesthesia in a defined region of the body. A total dorsal rhizotomy to a functional limb should not be performed because the complete sectioning of all dorsal roots to an extremity results in the loss of γ and proprioceptive afferent fibers, rendering the limb functionally useless. However, this is not a concern in the rostralmost four cervical, thoracic, and rostralmost two lumbar nerves in which motor loss usually does not produce a clinically significant deficit. Moreover, paravertebral nerve blocks with a local anesthetic can be performed preoperatively to ascertain specifically which regions of the body will be anesthetized by the procedure. Patients with cancer pain tend to achieve the best results, and cancer pain in any region of the body can be treated by dorsal rhizotomy, although pain in the thoracoabdominal region is the type that is treated most commonly. In contrast, dorsal rhizotomy is not useful for treating intractable excess pain resulting from nonmalignant disease such as postthoracotomy pain, postherpetic neuralgia, and postparaplegic pain (14).

Sympathectomy

Surgical sympathectomy for the treatment of pain involves three principal sites of denervation: the limbs, the heart, and the abdominal viscera. To determine the potential effectiveness of a surgical sympathectomy in treating a particular type of pain, a temporary pharmacologic sympathetic blockade can be performed before surgery. Sympathectomy of the limb is successful in treating painful ischemic states such as Raynaud phenomenon and other chronic pain disorders such as causalgia and Sudeck atrophy.

Another painful disorder that frequently is treated successfully, at least in the short-term by surgical sympathectomy, is reflex sympathetic dystrophy. Specifically, reflex sympathetic dystrophy is a sympathetically maintained, chronic pain disorder that may occur as a consequence of a fracture or crush injury to a limb or from repetitive occupational microtrauma. The following signs and symptoms occur in the affected limb: (a) burning, deep musculoskeletal pain, (b) hyperalgesia to light touch, (c) vasomotor changes such as skin discoloration and marked coldness of skin in response to exposure to cold, (d) trophic changes involving skin, hair, and fingernails, and (e) muscle weakness and atrophy/dystrophy. Sympathetic blocks, pharmacologic sympathectomy, and surgical sympathectomy provide only short-term pain relief because of the invariable return of increased sympathetic tone and associated symptoms in the affected limb. In contrast, aggressive physical therapy combined with either intermittent epidural infusions of local anesthetics (e.g., bupivacaine) and narcotic agents (e.g., fentanyl or morphine) or the continuous epidural infusion of α_2 agonist agents (e.g., clonidine hydrochloride) by means of a surgically implanted epidural catheter and programmable infusion pump can provide long-term pain relief. Similarly, epidural spinal stimulators and peripheral nerve stimulators with implanted electrodes and programmable generators lead to good long-term pain relief and control of vasomotor changes. Regardless of the type of neurosurgical procedure selected to treat this chronic pain disorder, the single most important consideration for a good outcome is early and aggressive therapy.

Rhizotomy/Gangliolysis

Percutaneous trigeminal rhizotomy is considered by many to be the initial surgical procedure of choice for treatment of most patients with trigeminal neuralgia (i.e., tic douloureux). It is best accomplished with a radiofrequency lesion or the injection of anhydrous glycerol and results in a more selective and less dense sensory loss than a peripheral neurectomy. Facial pain resulting from cancer can be successfully treated by rhizotomy of the cranial sensory nerves—the trigeminal, nervous intermedius, and glossopharyngeal; however, these procedures are less commonly indicated for facial pain resulting from other causes. When such patients fail medical management, they should initially undergo gangliolysis or suboccipital craniotomy for microvascular decompression of the involved cranial nerve. Only when microvascular decompression has failed should rhizotomy be considered because rhizotomy can result in postoperative paresthesias and anesthesia dolorosa. Unfortunately, rhizotomy is not an appropriate operation for the treatment of atypical facial pain, which is the type of facial pain commonly observed in children.

ELECTRICAL STIMULATION

Electrical stimulation of both central and peripheral nervous systems can be employed to treat intractable excess pain resulting from diverse causes. For example, transcutaneous electrical nerve stimulation (TENS) is a method for stimulating nerves through electrodes applied to the skin; it is effective for the symptomatic treatment of both acute and chronic pain. It is relatively inexpensive and easy to use and it has no serious side effects or complications. The best results are obtained when the TENS unit is used as a part of multimodal therapy.

Electrical stimulation of the peripheral nerves using implanted devices has been used for more than 20 years to treat some types of medically refractory pain. In contrast to classic ablative neurosurgical procedures that relieve pain by reducing sensory input, electrical stimulation relieves pain by augmenting afferent impulses. Stimulating electrodes can be implanted under local anesthesia, and the optimal location of the electrodes can be confirmed intraoperatively by test stimulation or the application of neurophysiologic monitoring. Patient selection is critical for this technique to be successful. In particular, the pain must result from an injury to the nervous system or from tissue damage in the painful area, and the patient must derive some pain relief either from TENS in the painful area or, if the underlying peripheral nerve is superficial enough, from transcutaneous stimulation of this nerve. Patients likely to benefit from such treatment include those with posttraumatic neuropathy, neuroma pain, reflex sympathetic dystrophy, or causalgia. In such patients, including children, electrical stimulation of the affected nerve(s) proximal to the injury can provide lasting pain relief.

Electrical stimulation of the dorsal columns of the spinal cord can also be used to alleviate some types of pain. This is achieved by the production of paresthesias in the painful body part. Such stimulation is delivered by means of flat electrodes that are surgically implanted just posterior to the dorsal columns during laminectomy and then connected to a neurostimulator. Electrical stimulation of the spinal cord can also be supplied by epidurally placed, flexible wire electrodes that can be inserted through a Tuohy needle into the epidural space without performing a laminectomy. Both techniques can be performed under local anesthesia, which enables assessment of the patient's response to stimulation during the procedure. The electrodes can then be manipulated until stimulation is maximally sensed in the area of pain before implanting the system. In addition, an extension of epidurally placed electrodes may be left externalized to perform stimulation trials before committing the patient to a permanent implant. If stimulation does not produce adequate pain relief, the electrodes can be removed easily.

As with other types of electrical stimulation for pain relief, appropriate patient selection is essential for obtaining good long-term results with both dorsal column and epidural spinal stimulation. These procedures typically are reserved for patients whose pain is refractory to other types of therapies. Such patients include those with phantom limb and stump pain, painful peripheral neuropathies, postherpetic neuralgia, spinal cord lesions with circumscribed segmental pain, ischemic pain, pain from multiple sclerosis, chronic sciatica, chronic low back and radicular leg pain (failed back surgery syndrome), and sympathetically maintained pain (reflex sympathetic dystrophy). For many of these patients, effective alternative treatment is not available, and the nondestructive nature of dorsal column or epidural spinal stimulation makes these procedures quite attractive. The main disadvantage is the relatively high cost of the equipment and its implantation. Partial relief of pain with a TENS unit, although helpful in predicting those individuals likely to achieve a good result from dorsal column or epidural spinal stimulation, cannot be relied on solely as a way of selecting patients for this procedure. Moreover, patients must have a somatic type of pain diagnosis with evidence of tissue damage or neurologic dysfunction that explains the location of their pain because pain that is poorly defined, diffuse, and multifocal rarely responds to dorsal column or epidural spinal stimulation. Retrospectively, pain resulting from malignant disease, plexus or root avulsion, and paraplegia, as well as pain referred only to the low back and coccygeal areas, has responded poorly to electrical stimulation of the spinal cord.

Potential complications associated with implantation of epidural and dorsal column spinal stimulators include skin erosion, infection (especially in patients who have undergone extended trial stimulation with exteriorized electrodes), electrical system failure manifested as abrupt cessation of paresthesias owing to lead breakage, change of paresthesias secondary to electrode migration, and intensity changes of paresthesias associated with changes of body position. Results obtained from dorsal column and epidural spinal stimulators are comparable with at least 50% of patients achieving pain relief from spinal stimulation (15).

INTRASPINAL INFUSION OF NARCOTIC AND LOCAL ANESTHETIC AGENTS

Narcotic and local anesthetic agents can be administered either epidurally or intrathecally for the treatment of pain secondary to malignancy, acute severe perioperative or posttraumatic pain, and chronic benign pain syndromes. In fact, the introduction of intraspinal narcotic analgesia has led to a substantial decrease in the number of neuroablative pain procedures currently being performed. Narcotic analgesics act directly on regions of the brain and spinal cord that contain high concentrations of specific opiate receptors (16). These regions include the limbic system, periaqueductal gray matter, medial thalamic nuclei, hypothalamus, spinoreticular tracts, substantia gelatinosa, spinal trigeminal nucleus, nucleus tractus solitarius, and vagus nerve. Intraspinal narcotics produce selective analgesia without affecting nonnociceptive sensory modalities and motor or autonomic reflexes.

Effective long-term pain control can be achieved by the intraspinal infusion of narcotic agents such as fentanyl, morphine, and meperidine, local anesthetic agents such as bupivacaine, and α_2 agonists such as clonidine hydrochloride. Such infusions can be accomplished intermittently either by percutaneous puncture or by a surgically implanted epidural or subarachnoid catheter and a subcutaneous injection port or manually activated pump. Intraspinal infusions can also be given continuously by a surgically implanted epidural or subarachnoid catheter and a programmable infusion pump with reservoir (17). Patients likely to benefit from intraspinal narcotic infusion are those with severe pain of malignant or nonmalignant origin who are currently achieving some, but not completely adequate, pain control from oral or parenteral narcotic medication. Before implanting a permanent infusion system, patients are given a trial dose by means of a percutaneously placed lumbar subarachnoid catheter or lumbar puncture. This should provide at least a 50% reduction in pain, without side effects, for roughly 8 to 24 hours when 0.5 to 1.0 mg morphine is administered intrathecally or when 5 to 10 mg is administered epidurally (17). Trial candidates who demonstrate this type of response can be expected to achieve successful pain control with intraspinal narcotic delivery from a permanent infusion system.

The use of intraspinal narcotic infusion for treatment of intractable cancer pain is associated with a sustained reduction in the reported level of pain and also with a decrease in oral and parenteral narcotic usage (18). This, in turn, results in improved quality of life. Some types of pain have been shown to be more responsive to this method of pain control. For example, somatic pain tends to respond more effectively than visceral pain, nociceptive pain is more responsive than neuropathic pain, and continuous pain is more responsive than intermittent pain induced by activity (19). In addition, infusion of intraspinal narcotics can also be effective in treating chronic noncancer pain such as severe refractory central pain resulting from spinal cord injury. Potential complications of this type of pain treatment include infection of the infusion system requiring removal and administration of appropriate antibiotics, malfunction of the delivery system secondary to occlusion or migration of the catheter, inversion of an infusion pump in the subcutaneous pocket making refilling of the pump impossible without manual or surgical repositioning, skin breakdown over the subcutaneous pocket containing the infusion pump, and drug-related problems such as pruritus, nausea, urinary retention, and respiratory depression (16). Moreover, tolerance to the particular narcotic agent being infused can occur, requiring escalation of the narcotic dose to achieve the same analgesic effect over time. In fact, dose escalation can be observed in as many as 60% of patients receiving intraspinal narcotics (20). However, this does not seem to limit the value of this treatment because high escalating doses are frequently well tolerated and additional pain control can be achieved by changing narcotic agents or combining drugs.

CONCLUSION

The use of neurosurgical procedures in pediatric patients has the potential to alleviate significant suffering in a previously silenced population. Once again, we must recognize that children are not simply small adults; their presentation of symptoms and their response to treatment are unique. We must increase awareness and dialogue about these issues among all pediatric caregivers to accomplish the goal of alleviating intractable excess pain in children.

REFERENCES

1. Matson DM. *Neurosurgery of infancy and childhood*, 2nd ed. Springfield, IL: Charles C Thomas, 1969:847.
2. Rosomoff HL, et al. Percutaneous radiofrequency cervical cordotomy: technique. *J Neurosurg* 1965;23:639–644.
3. Mullan J. Percutaneous cordotomy. *J Neurosurg* 1971; 35:360.
4. Tasker RR. Percutaneous cervical cordotomy. In: Schmidek HH, Sweet WH, eds. *Operative neurosurgical techniques: indications, methods, and results*, 2nd ed. Orlando, FL: Grune & Stratton, 1988:1191–1205.
5. Armour D. Surgery of the spinal cord and its membranes. *Lancet* 1927;1:691.
6. Nashold BS Jr, et al. In: Bonica JJ, et al. eds. *Advances in pain research and therapy, volume 1*. New York: Raven Press, 1976:959–963.
7. Friedman AH, Nashold BS Jr, Bronec PR. Dorsal root entry zone lesions for the treatment of brachial plexus avulsion injuries: a follow-up study. *Neurosurgery* 1988; 22:369–373.
8. Friedman AH, Nashold BS Jr. DREZ lesions for relief of pain related to spinal cord injury. *J Neurosurg* 1986;65:465–469.
9. Saris SC, Iaccono RP, Nashold BS Jr. DREZ lesions for relief of post-amputation pain. *J Neurosurg* 1985;62: 72–76.
10. Friedman AH, Bullitt E. Dorsal root entry zone lesions in the treatment of pain following brachial plexus avulsion, spinal cord injury, and herpes zoster. *Appl Neurophysiol* 1988;51:164–169.
11. Bernard EJ, Nashold BS Jr, Caputi F, et al. Nucleus caudalis DREZ lesions for facial pain. *Br J Neurosurg* 1987;1:81–92.
12. Rossitch E Jr, Zeidman SM, Nashold BS Jr. Nucleus caudalis DREZ for facial pain due to cancer. *Br J Neurosurg* 1989;3:45–50.
13. Abbe R. A contribution to the surgery of the spine. *Med Rec (NY)* 1889;35:149.
14. Onofrio BM, Campa HK. Evaluation of rhizotomy. Review of 12 years' experience. *J Neurosurg* 1972;36: 751–755.
15. Urban, BJ. Percutaneous spinal epidural stimulation for pain relief. In: Wilkins RH, Rengachary SS, eds. *Neurosurgery*, 2nd ed. New York: McGraw-Hill, 1996: 4015–4019.
16. Gorecki JP. Intraspinal infusion of narcotic drugs. In: Wilkins RH, Rengachary SS, eds. *Neurosurgery*, 2nd ed. New York: McGraw-Hill, 1996:4009–4014.
17. Waldman SD. Implantable drug delivery systems: practical considerations. *J Pain Symptom Manage* 1990;5: 169–174.
18. Hassenbusch SJ, Pillary PK, Magdinec M, et al. Constant infusion morphine for intractable cancer pain using an implanted pump. *J Neurosurg* 1990;73:405–409.
19. Abram SE. Advances in chronic pain management since gate control. *Reg Anesth* 1993;18:66–81.
20. Onofrio BM, Yaksh TL. Long-term pain relief produced by intrathecal morphine infusion in 53 patients. *J Neurosurg* 1990;72:200–209.

20

Central Blocks in Children and Adolescents

Joëlle F. Desparmet, Richard A. Hardart, and Myron Yaster

The treatment and alleviation of pain are a basic human right that exists regardless of age (1–4). Unfortunately, even when their pain is obvious, children frequently receive no or inadequate treatment for pain and for painful procedures (5). We now know that all children, even the critically ill, respond to noxious stimuli with biochemical and physiologic stress responses that if untreated can lead to increased patient morbidity and mortality (6,7). Effective pain management produces myriad patient benefits including reduced morbidity and mortality, early mobilization, and shortened hospital stay (8–10). Pain management has therefore become an essential component of modern pediatric, anesthetic, and surgical practice.

Weak analgesics with antipyretic properties (e.g., acetaminophen, ibuprofen) and opioids (e.g., codeine, morphine) are the mainstays of pediatric pain therapy. For more difficult to treat pain, continuous central or spinal analgesia, local anesthetics administered either alone or in combination with opioids, α_2 agonists, or other drugs are often used (11). Spinal analgesia, either subarachnoid (*intrathecal*) or epidural, provides profound analgesia with minimal systemic side effects (e.g., sedation, respiratory depression) by blocking nociceptive impulses from entering the central nervous system (12–21). Indeed, in pediatric practice, epidural analgesia has become the most commonly performed regional anesthetic technique for the intra- and postoperative management of patients with urologic, orthopedic, and general surgical procedures below the T-4 dermatomal level (nipple line). It is also used in the management of pain in patients with vascular insufficiency secondary to intense vasoconstriction (e.g., purpura fulminans), sickle cell vaso-occlusive crisis, and cancer unresponsive to parenteral and enteral opioids (12,22–25).

This chapter discusses the anatomy, physiology, basic science, pharmacology, side effects, and clinical applications of intrathecal and epidural analgesia in the management of acute and chronic pain in children.

ANATOMY

The spinal cord is protected by both the bony vertebral column and three connective tissue coverings that comprise the meninges: the pia, arachnoid, and dura maters (Fig. 20.1). The spinal cord itself is covered by the pia mater, a highly vascular membrane, which together lie in a sac filled with cerebrospinal fluid (CSF). This sac is composed of two layers: an inner layer called the arachnoid mater, which is in contact with the CSF, and an outer layer called the dura mater, which is in contact with extradural fat, blood vessels, and connective tissues. The dura and arachnoid maters can be punctured with a needle or catheter to allow diagnostic sampling of CSF (a spinal tap) or the administration of drugs directly into the CSF. The latter is called an *intrathecal*, *subarachnoid*, or *spinal* injection.

CSF is an ultrafiltrate of blood plasma with which it is in hydrostatic and osmotic equilibrium. It is a clear and colorless fluid that bathes and surrounds the brain, spinal cord, and spinal nerve roots. Drugs directly deposited into the CSF have a very profound effect on nerve transmission within the central nervous system. Beyond the dura mater is the epidural space, the external limit of which is the liga-

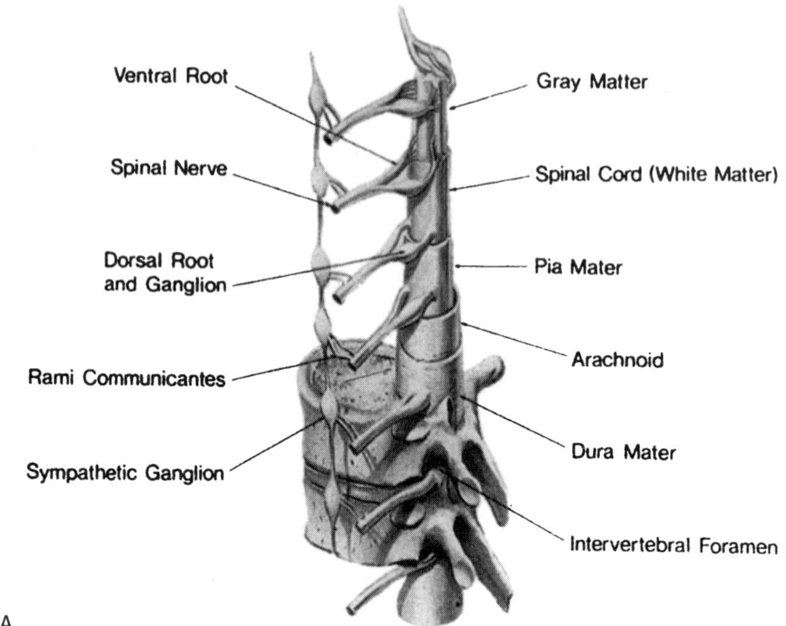
Ventral Root
Spinal Nerve
Dorsal Root and Ganglion
Rami Communicantes
Sympathetic Ganglion
Gray Matter
Spinal Cord (White Matter)
Pia Mater
Arachnoid
Dura Mater
Intervertebral Foramen
A

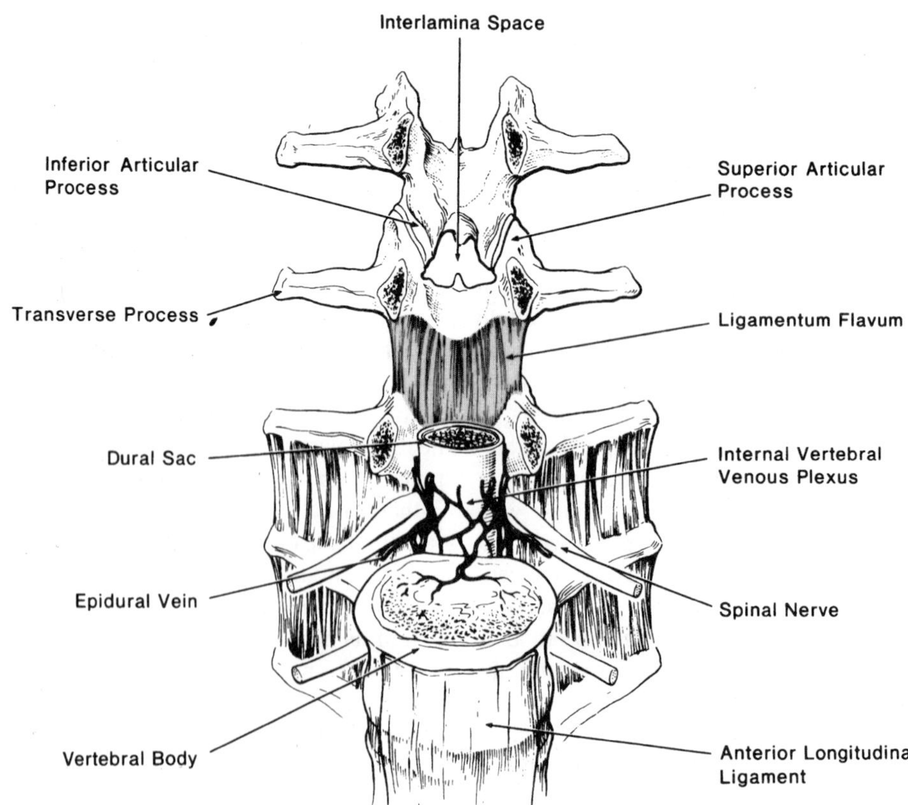
Interlamina Space
Inferior Articular Process
Superior Articular Process
Transverse Process
Ligamentum Flavum
Dural Sac
Internal Vertebral Venous Plexus
Epidural Vein
Spinal Nerve
Vertebral Body
Anterior Longitudinal Ligament
B

mentum flavum ("the yellow ligament"). The epidural space extends from the foramen magnum, where the dura is fused to the base of the skull, to the sacral hiatus, which is covered by the sacrococcygeal ligament. The epidural space is filled with fat, nerve roots, blood vessels (arteries and a venous plexus), connective tissue, and lymphatics (Fig. 20.1).

The spinal nerve roots arise from the spinal cord and emerge from the spinal canal through the vertebral foramina. They pass through the CSF and the dura as they exit the canal. As nerves enter and exit the spinal cord into the epidural space, they are enclosed by a short cuff of meninges. Within this cuff is a blind pocket of spinal fluid that is separated from the epidural space by greatly thinned dura. This region provides easy passage of drugs into the spinal fluid, and the efficacy of epidural blockade depends in part on diffusion of drug across the dura into the spinal fluid in this area. Spinal roots serve motor, sensory, and autonomic functions. Sensory afferent impulses can be blocked or modified at the roots or cord.

The spinal cord and its coverings lie within the vertebral column. This column consists of 33 vertebrae, has four curves, and is bound together by several ligaments that give it stability and elasticity. The cervical and lumbar curves are convex anteriorly, whereas the thoracic and sacral curves are convex posteriorly (Fig. 20.2). The curves affect the spread of centrally administered drugs. The vertebrae are numbered in a descending fashion by region. Thus, of the five lumbar vertebrae, the most cephalic (or closest to the skull) is the first and is numbered L-1, whereas the one most caudad or distant and closest to the sacrum is the fifth or L-5.

Relative anatomic differences of the spinal column exist between children and adults. The flexibility of the spine and the absence of lumbar lordosis make spinal or epidural techniques easier in children than in adults. The relationship of the termination of the spinal cord and the dural sac to the bony spine presents some concern. At birth, the spinal cord ends at L-3 and the dura mater at S-3. As the child grows, the bony structures grow more than the contents of the spinal canal, and the cord and dural sac rise to reach their adult height (L-l and S-2, respectively) by the end of the first year of life (Fig. 20.3). In the older child and adult, needle entry into the subarachnoid or epidural space is most commonly performed in the lumbar region (lumbar puncture) at a level below the termination of the spinal cord, usually between the L-3 and L-4 or L-4 and L-5 vertebrae. This needle insertion level is chosen to prevent accidental injury to the spinal cord if the needle is advanced too far forward. Thus, infants are at greater risk of an injury to the spinal cord during lumbar punctures at the L3-4 level because in these patients the spinal cord ends at L-3 (rather than L-1).

Finally, the sacrum of a child is flat, and, in most cases, the bony landmarks are readily seen and palpable. The wide sacral hiatus overlying the uncalcified sacrococcygeal ligament provides easy access to the epidural space. In fact, entry into the epidural space at this level is the most common form of epidural analgesia in young children and is referred to as a *caudal* block. In newborns and infants, the sacrum is composed mostly of cartilage and

FIG. 20.1. A: The spinal cord and its related structures. (From Bridenbaugh PO, Greene NM, Brull SJ. Spinal (subarachnoid) neural blockade. In: Cousins MJ, Bridenbaugh PO, eds. *Neural blockade in clinical anesthesia and management of pain.* Philadelphia: Lippincott–Raven Publishers, 1998:203–241, with permission.) **B:** An anterior view demonstrates the relationship between the epidural space, dura, arachnoid, and pia membranes. Note the large number of veins that are in continuity with the veins draining the vertebral body. (From Macintosh RR. *Lumbar puncture and spinal analgesia.* Edinburgh: E & S Livingstone, 1957. Reprinted in Cousins MJ, Veering BT. Epidural neural blockade. In: Cousins MJ, Bridenbaugh PO, eds. *Neural blockade in clinical anesthesia and management of pain.* Philadelphia: Lippincott–Raven Publishers, 1998:243–321.)

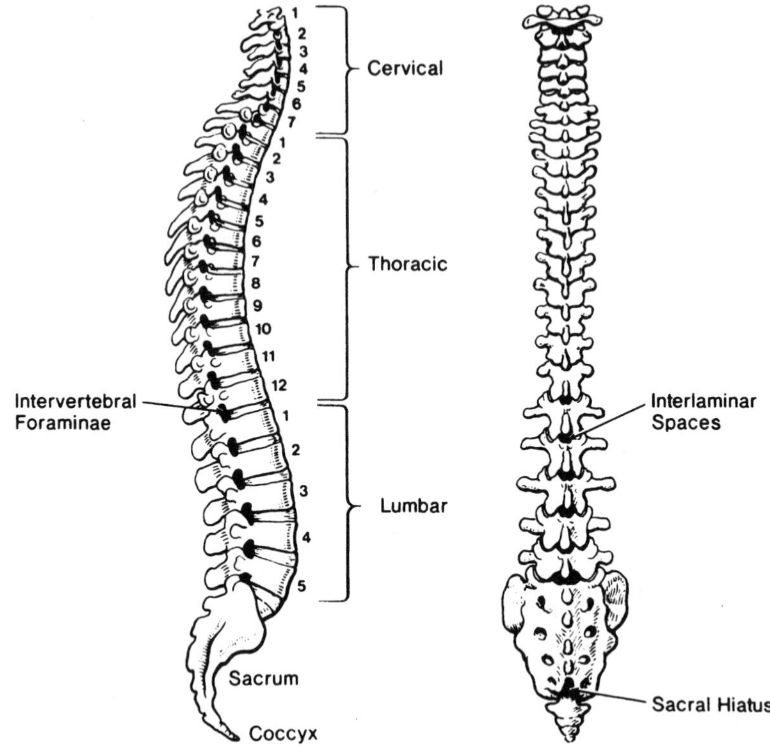

FIG. 20.2. Vertebral column, lateral **(left)** and posterior **(right)** views illustrate curvatures and intralaminar spaces. (From Bridenbaugh PO, Greene NM, Brull SJ. Spinal (subarachnoid) neural blockade. In: Cousins MJ, Bridenbaugh PO, eds. *Neural blockade in clinical anesthesia and management of pain.* Philadelphia: Lippincott–Raven Publishers, 1998:203–241, with permission.)

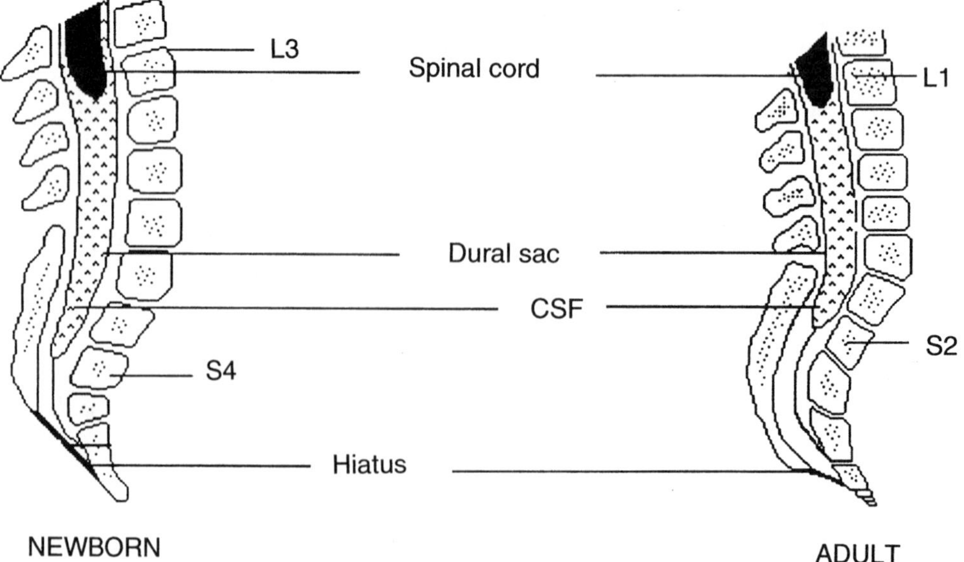

FIG. 20.3. Anatomic differences between the spine of children and adults. The spine is straighter and more supple in children, and the dural sac and spinal cord are situated lower in the spine.

soft bony tissue. Not surprisingly, cases of bone and even rectal punctures have been reported when a caudal approach to the epidural space was attempted. Another consideration in caudal anatomy is the presence of sacral bony anomalies. One should examine the sacrum and the overlying soft tissue before performing a caudal block to detect such anomalies. Special attention should be paid to dimples cephalad to the coccyx, hair patches, pigmented lesions, or fistulous tracks. Any of these findings can be a marker of spinal dysraphism (26). In addition, anomalies in the position of the dural sac reflection can occur in as many as 10% of the population. This can result in an inadvertent dural puncture.

The midline structures of the posterior vertebral column are the most important landmarks for identifying and entering the epidural space at either the lumbar or thoracic level. The spinous processes are the obvious landmarks, indicating both the midline and spinal levels. In the lumbar region, the spinous processes are short and broad with a slight downward angle. In the thoracic region, the spinous processes become longer and thinner with a pronounced downward angle. Skin and loose subcutaneous fat cover the spinous processes. The supraspinous ligament connects the tips of the spinous processes. Fibrous tissue fills the interspace and joins the processes together. At the inner border of the bony spinal canal, the tough ligamentum flavum joins the interior margins of the lamina. The epidural space is just inside the ligamentum flavum. This space is filled with loose fat, blood vessels, and nerve roots as they exit the spinal canal. The distance from the skin to the epidural space is age dependent and increases with age. At birth, this distance is only 6 mm and only 10 to 12 mm at 1 year of age (27–30). Eyres and colleagues (31) estimated that the distance from the skin to the epidural space is approximately 1 mm/kg, whereas Ecoffey et al. (32) reported that the skin to epidural distance ranges from 10 to 18 mm at the lumbar level and 7 to 14 mm at the thoracic level in infants younger than 3 years of age. Thus, when epidural needles are inserted in young children, short needles (5 cm versus 8 to 12 cm) will greatly facilitate success. As patients age, the distance between the skin and epidural space increases in length and can be greater than 8 to 12 cm in adults.

PHYSIOLOGIC CONSIDERATIONS OF CENTRAL BLOCKADE

With currently available drugs (opioids, local anesthetics, α_2 agonists, tramadol, ketamine), spinal or epidural blockade can result in analgesia with or without sympathetic or somatic blockade, respiratory depression, or sedation. Local anesthetics produce analgesia with little risk of sedation or respiratory depression but with a high potential of somatic and, in older children, sympathetic blockade. Opioids, tramadol, and α_2 agonists, conversely, have little possibility of producing sympathetic or somatic blockade but a high likelihood of producing respiratory depression and/or sedation (33–36).

In adults, there is ample evidence of improved postoperative pulmonary function, favorable changes in bowel recovery after abdominal surgery, reduced hypercoagulability and graft thromboses after peripheral vascular surgery, and fewer thromboembolic complications after total joint arthroplasty in patients treated with epidural analgesia. These studies have reinforced the view that perioperative epidural neuraxial blockade not only provides superior analgesia but also attenuates postoperative morbidity and mortality (37–41). There are no such studies in children. To better understand why epidural and spinal analgesia is so effective and salutary, we discuss the physiologic effects of neural blockade system by system.

Nervous System Responses to Neural Blockade

Local anesthetics interrupt nerve impulse transmission regardless of function by blocking sodium permeability at specific ion-selective sodium channels, thereby preventing propagation of action potentials (Chapter 14)

(42). To reach the sodium channel, the local anesthetic must cross the nerve's outer surface to reach the nerve's center. Thicker, more myelinated fibers are therefore more difficult to block, and thinner, less myelinated fibers are easier to block. Thus, relatively unmyelinated fibers, such as the Aδ and C fibers, which carry nociceptive afferent information and sympathetic outflow are easier to block than the heavily myelinated fibers that control muscle contraction (Chapter 14). Motor blockade after epidural or spinal blockade is annoying but rarely life threatening. Sympathetic blockade is potentially very dangerous.

The sympathetic nervous system runs the length of the thoracic spine and is integral in the control of blood pressure and perfusion. In simple terms, stimulation of the sympathetic nervous system produces the "fight-or-flight" response: arterial and venous vasoconstriction, mydriasis, sweating, and increased heart rate, blood pressure, and myocardial contractility. Blockade of the sympathetic nervous system, or *sympathectomy*, results in hypotension secondary to arterial and venous vasodilation. The loss of venous tone results in pooling of blood in large capacitance (venous) vessels, loss of venous return to the right heart, and decreased cardiac output. Normally, sudden changes in venous tone are compensated for by the baroreceptors that reflexively increase vascular tone peripherally and the heart rate centrally. High blockade (T2-4) prevents not only peripheral vasoconstriction but also reflex tachycardia.

Sympathetic control of the central and peripheral vasculature resides at spinal levels T-1 to L-2. Cardiac sympathetic fibers reside at T1-4, and peripheral, vasoconstrictor fibers are located at T1-L2. Thus, high blockade (above T-4) can result in bradycardia, hypotension, and cardiovascular collapse, whereas low blockade results in vascular dilation in the pelvis and lower limbs. Complete sympathetic blockade occurs when local anesthetics reach the cervical (or higher) dermatomes, most commonly as the result of inadvertent intrathecal administration of a large dose of local anesthetics. This event, which is often called a *total spinal*, requires immediate control of the airway and breathing because of the loss of brainstem control of both the circulation and breathing.

Cardiovascular Responses to Epidural Blockade

Interestingly, the hemodynamic response to sympathetic blockade is age dependent. In adults, the predominant response to sympathetic blockade is profound hypotension and bradycardia. The severity of this response is dependent on the patient's intravascular volume status. Hypovolemia exaggerates this response and fluid loading mitigates it. Unlike adults, children younger than 8 years of age show little or no change in blood pressure after epidural or intrathecal administration of local anesthetics, even when the block achieved reaches high thoracic levels (43,44). Furthermore, fluid loading before a regional technique in children younger than 8 years is not required if the patient has a normal circulating blood volume. Why hypotension is so rare is unclear, but a number of hypotheses have been proposed to explain this phenomenon. Children may pool less blood in the blocked area of the body because of a smaller lower extremity to body surface ratio than that of adults. Alternatively, there may be less baseline sympathetic tone in children compared with adults.

Respiratory Response to Epidural Blockade

Both respiratory drive and function can be affected by regional anesthetic techniques. Local anesthetics, by blocking motor efferents to respiratory muscles, can cause apnea, even in a fully conscious patient. Obviously, when this occurs, support of airway and breathing is mandatory. Several analgesics commonly administered in the spinal and epidural space can affect respiratory control in the brainstem. Opioid analgesics depress respiratory drive whether they reach the brainstem via the bloodstream or the CSF. Spinal administration, either intrathecally or epidurally, directly places an opioid agonist into the CSF, which bathes the receptor sites in the spinal cord (substantia gelatinosa) and brain. This "backdoor" to the receptor significantly reduces the amount of agonist needed to relieve pain (45). After spinal administration, opioids are absorbed by the epidural veins and redistributed to the systemic circulation where they are metabolized and excreted. Hydrophilic agents, such as morphine, cross the dura more slowly than more lipid-soluble agents such as fentanyl or meperidine (46). This physicochemical property is responsible for the more prolonged duration of action of spinal morphine and its relatively slow onset of action after epidural administration (47–49). Regardless of their lipophilicity, intrathecally administered opioids can produce respiratory depression (50–52). Indeed, many clinicians believe that spinally administered lipophilic opioids such as sufentanil may be less likely than morphine to migrate rostrally in the CSF and be less likely to cause delayed respiratory depression. Although this may be true for epidural opioid administration, it is not true for intrathecally administered opioids (50,53). Local anesthetics, by blocking the brainstem respiratory centers and the reticular activating system, can cause respiratory depression, although this is a general, not a specific, effect.

Hormonal Response to Epidural Blockade

As in adults, spinally administered local anesthetics block the stress response to intraoperative surgical stimuli in children. Surgical stress is associated with a variety of changes in endocrine and metabolic function. Stress hormones such as epinephrine, norepinephrine, cortisol, glucagon, insulin, and growth hormone are released, resulting in gluconeogenesis, glycogenolysis, and protein break down (negative nitrogen balance). The mechanism by which central blockade abolishes or diminishes these responses is probably related to blockade of either afferent or efferent pathways or both. Opioids are less effective than local anesthetics in blocking the stress response, indicating that pain relief *per se* is not as important as neural blockade. In children, it is unclear how important the reduction in the stress response is and whether this leads to improvement in morbidity and mortality.

CENTRAL BLOCKADE

Caudal Epidural Block

The caudal approach to the epidural space is the most frequently used technique in pediatric clinical practice because it is simple, reliable, easy to perform, and safe (14,16,21). The epidural space is easier to access in children at the level of the sacrococcygeal ligament than at the lumbar spine, and needle insertion at this level of the back has a reduced risk of causing direct spinal cord trauma. The caudal approach to the epidural space can be used for either single or, when using a catheter, multiple or continuous drug dosing. Nevertheless, many practitioners prefer the lumbar approach to the epidural space when placing an indwelling catheter because they fear serious systemic and local infection after continuous caudal blockade. Obviously, this fear is of greatest concern in non–toilet-trained, young patients because the entry site of the caudal catheter lies within the child's diaper. Fortunately, this fear of infection either does not exist, or if it does, is extremely rare. Kost-Byerly et al. (54), in a study of 170 patients, reported that despite the potential for urofecal contamination, serious systemic and local infection after 72 hours of continuous caudal blockade did not occur.

Success in this deceptively easy technique is dependent on the anesthesiologist's knowledge of the anatomic, physiologic, pharmacologic, and psychologic differences related to the child's size and stage of development. Proper patient selection using history, the planned surgical procedure, and a physical examination of the sacrum increases the likelihood of successful block.

Anatomy and Superficial Landmarks

The sacral hiatus is a bony opening in the sacrum resulting from the failure of the laminae of the last sacral vertebra to fuse. It allows access to the sacral canal from below. It is bounded laterally by the sacral cornua, superiorly by the median sacral ridge and inferiorly by the coccyx. The opening is roofed by a thin ligament, the sacrococcygeal ligament, fatty tissue, and skin. The sacral hiatus is situated at the third angle of an equilateral triangle whose two other angles are the posterior superior iliac spines (Fig. 20.4). When locating the hiatus, one first locates the posterior, superior iliac spines on each side of the top of the sacrum. Imagining the third angle of an equi-

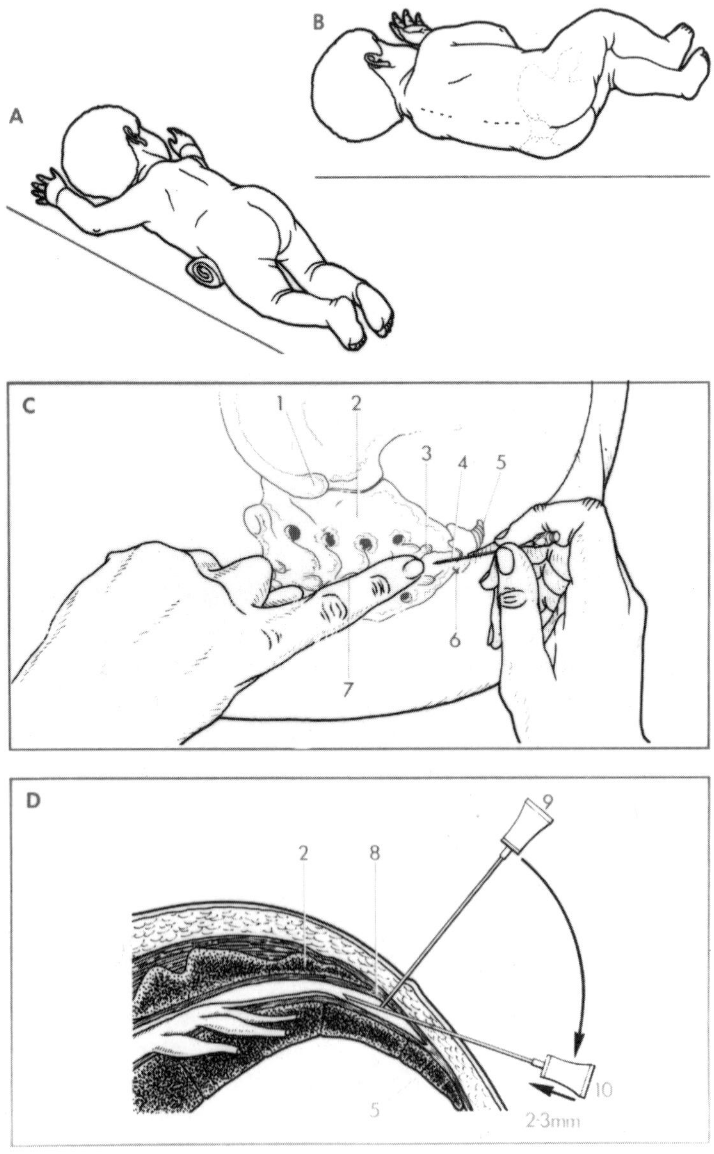

FIG. 20.4. Caudal anatomy and insertion technique. Patients can be placed in a prone **(A)** or lateral decubitus **(B)** position. **C:** The anatomy of the sacrum is depicted. Note that the needle is inserted at the top of the gluteal fold in the sacral hiatus. *1*, posterior, superior iliac crest; *2*, sacrum; *3*, sacral horns or sacral cornua; *4*, sacral hiatus; *5*, coccyx; *6*, sacrococcygeal ligament; *7*, midline. **D:** The needle punctures the sacrococcygeal ligament (*8*) at a 30- to 75-degree angle (*9*). Once through the ligament, the needle is flattened and advanced 1 to 2 mm (*10*). (From Dalens B. *Anesthesie locoregionale de la naissance a l'age adulte.* Paris: Editions Pradel, 1993:186, with permission.)

lateral triangle, one should be able to palpate the twin sacral cornua and between them, a midline depression just above the coccyx. The tip of the index finger fits almost perfectly in this small, round depression. When moving the finger slowly from side to side, the sacral cornua can be felt on each side. It is important to note that in the lateral position, the soft tissues of the buttocks sag dependently and can cause one to misjudge the midline. Instead, use only the bony landmarks to indicate the proper position for needle puncture.

The other important landmark when performing a caudal is an imaginary line going through the two S-2 foramina that are immediately below and medial to the posterior superior iliac spines. This is the upper limit above which the inserted needle should not pass. It is at the S-2 level that the dural sac ends. Advancing the needle above this point risks an accidental dural puncture (spinal tap). Finally, the infant's and young child's (younger than 8 years of age) epidural space offers less resistance to the cephalad spread of injected drugs and to the advancement of a catheter. Indeed, epidural catheters placed at the caudal insertion site can be threaded to the thoracic region, which allows narrower bands of segmental anesthesia with reduced volumes of administered drugs (55–57). Placement can be verified using nonionic contrast medium if the catheter is not radiopaque (58,59).

Single-Dose ("Shot") Caudal Epidural Injection

Because most children are afraid of needles in the abstract and in the pain they produce in the concrete, virtually all central blocks are performed in either anesthetized or heavily sedated patients (14,16,21,60,61). Obviously, any deeply sedated or anesthetized patient requires monitoring of respiratory and hemodynamic functions while consciousness is altered (62–65). Additionally, we believe that these patients require intravenous access as well, both for the delivery of drugs to maintain sedation and as means of rescuing patients who develop sedation-induced complications. These sedation- (and local anesthetic–) induced complications include laryngospasm, respiratory depression, and cardiovascular collapse (62–65).

Once the child is asleep and all vital signs are stable, the child is placed gently on his or her side and the sacral hiatus is located. Then, using a scrupulous aseptic technique (skin preparation with an iodine or chlorhexidine solution and sterile boundary drapes, gloves, needles, and catheters), the hiatus is punctured with a short-bevel, 1.5-in., 22-gauge spinal puncture needle at a 30- to 75-degree angle with the skin (Fig. 20.4). Typically, the site for needle insertion is slightly caudad to the sacral cornua with a goal of advancing the needle just under the bony ridge at the superior margin of the hiatus. Even in newborns and small children, a distinct "give" or "pop" is felt when the sacrococcygeal ligament is punctured. It is not necessary to advance the needle farther into the sacral canal. In babies, the distance from the sacral hiatus to the dural sac is no more than 1 to 1.5 cm. Advancing the needle may result in puncturing the sacral bone straight through to the rectum or puncturing the dural sac, producing a spinal tap. In older children, once the sacrococcygeal ligament has been punctured, the needle hub can be depressed toward the skin surface and the needle advanced 0.5 cm farther into the canal (Fig. 20.4). Advancing the needle slightly makes stabilizing the needle easier.

Needle stabilization is accomplished by bracing the back of the nondominant hand against the patient's buttock and sacrum and holding the needle hub firmly with a pencil or pincer grip. Needle placement is then checked by aspirating gently with a syringe for blood or CSF. Using a slip tip syringe rather that a Luer-Lok syringe will decrease the chance of inadvertent movement of the needle. If blood or clear liquid is aspirated, the needle should be withdrawn and the procedure started again. The inability to aspirate fluid does not ensure that the needle is not in a blood vessel or the dural sac. To detect intravascular entry, low-dose epinephrine (5 μg/mL) is often added to local anesthetic solutions to serve as a marker (test dose) of intravascular injection (66–68). Unfortunately, in anesthetized children, intravenous epinephrine does not consistently produce tachycardia, even with atropine pretreatment (69,70). However, it does produce ST segment elevation and T-wave changes within 20 seconds of administration, making electrocardiographic analysis a reasonable method of intravascular detection (Chapter 14) (70–73).

In awake patients, the test dose also serves to detect direct intrathecal injection of the anesthetic solution. One to 3 mL of local anesthetic administered in the epidural space produces minimal effects. However, when administered intrathecally, rapid, profound motor and sensory blockade ensues. Obviously, these effects are difficult to detect in an anesthetized or heavily sedated patient. After negative testing, the remainder of the dose is fractionated to minimize local anesthetic–induced toxicity.

Continuous Caudal Epidural Catheters

Continuous epidural blockade or intermittent bolus dosing can be achieved by placing a catheter in the epidural space. This can be achieved by puncturing the sacrococcygeal ligament with a regular 20- to 22-gauge intravenous catheter and then advancing the catheter to the hub (1 to 5 cm). Alternatively, a specific epidural catheter can be passed through a needle. When using the latter approach, a standard 19- or 20-gauge epidural catheter is passed through a short, 5-cm, 17- or 18-gauge Tuohy or Crawford needle (depending on the brand of catheter used). Smaller diameter catheters (21 to 24 gauge) are available but often kink and are harder to inject because of their increased resistance. Short-length needles offer more control than standard adult, 10-cm needles. Epidural catheters introduced by the caudal route can be advanced in the epidural space to levels as high as the high thoracic spine. This is especially true in young children (younger than 8 to10 years of age) because the fatty tissue contained in the epidural space at that age is thin and loose (55,56). Some clinicians have more success with this technique than others.

Access to the sacral canal is achieved in the same way as with a single-shot caudal injection. The relatively blunt Tuohy or Crawford needles produce a more pronounced "give" or "pop" on entering the epidural space than sharper needles. After piercing the sacrococcygeal ligament, the needle hub is depressed toward the skin, and the needle is advanced 3 to 5 mm. Saline can be injected to demonstrate that the needle is in a potential space, presumably the sacral canal. Resistance suggests malposition of the introducer needle, and the procedure should be restarted. One should also observe the soft tissue at the level of the needle tip to rule out subcutaneous infiltration. Almost effortless injection suggests the proper position of the introducer, and the clinician should proceed with catheter insertion.

Before inserting the catheter, the clinician must decide, based on the surgical plan, at which spinal level to place the catheter. Without breaking sterile technique, the catheter tip is placed at the desired position with the catheter extending back along the skin to the introducer. Using the marks on the catheter, the clinician notes the length of catheter insertion required to achieve the desired spinal level. The catheter is then inserted with little resistance until the desired depth is reached. When the desired position is achieved, the introducer is removed with care not to disturb the catheter position. If resistance is met at the point where the catheter leaves the introducer, the clinician may depress the hub of the introducer to improve the alignment of the catheter cephalad in the sacral canal. If the catheter will not pass easily, it is not in the correct position and the procedure should be repeated. Note that the catheter should never be pulled back through the introducer needle because of the possibility of transection by the introducer's sharp edge. The resulting transected or *sequestered* section of catheter will need to be removed surgically (74). To avoid this problem, one should remove the introducer and the catheter together as a single unit.

Once the catheter is in the desired position, it should be tested in the same manner as the needle for the single-shot technique. The catheter is first tested by aspirating for CSF or blood. Then, an epinephrine-containing solution is injected to detect intravascular injection (68,70). If aspiration or the test dose is suggestive of intravascular or intrathecal injection, the catheter can be withdrawn 1 to 2 cm back into the epidural space. After repositioning the epidural catheter, the process of testing for placement is repeated. If on retesting the catheter is intravascular or intrathecal, we believe that it is best to remove the catheter. If properly placed, the desired dose should be administered with continued attention to the possibility of intravascular injection and the possible signs and complications thereof. The catheter must be secured with a transparent dressing such as Tegaderm (3M Health Care, St. Paul, MN, U.S.A.) or OpSite (Smith & Nephew Richards, Memphis, TN, U.S.A.) that allows daily examination of the puncture site. To minimize the risk of fecal or urinary soiling, we carefully affix the dressing in the crease of the buttocks and reinforce the edges of the dressing, particularly the lower edge with waterproof tape.

The epidural catheter insertion site should be inspected daily for evidence of local infection and to ensure that the overlying dressing is intact. Infection is very rare but can occur. Like all invasive catheters, colonization occurs from skin flora that tracks along the catheter (75). A mild erythema occasionally occurs at the site of catheter insertion when catheters have been left in place for several days. This erythema must be differentiated from cellulitis. The development of cellulitis and/or an epidural abscess is a medical emergency requiring immediate medical and surgical intervention. The signs and symptoms of an epidural abscess are similar to those of an epidural hematoma (Table 20.1). Unlike patients with an epidural hematoma, patients with epidural abscess are often febrile and have other signs of infection including an elevated white blood cell count and erythrocyte sedimentation rate. Although there may be no connection between skin erythema and cellulitis, it is our practice to remove epidural catheters in any patient who develops skin erythema. Furthermore, we often treat this skin erythema with topical antibiotics. Finally, epidural catheters should be removed in any patient in whom there is a fever of unknown origin or who develops systemic sepsis.

When inspecting the epidural insertion site, a collection of fluid is occasionally detected pooling between the skin and the clear occlusive dressing. In most cases, this is edema fluid leaking through the insertion site hole from the surrounding subcutaneous tissue or back flow from the epidural infusion. It is not CSF. It usually does not require any special treatment except for reinforcing or changing the dressing.

Because of the proximity of the sacrococcygeal ligament to the anus, there is always a potential for fecal contamination, particularly if the catheter is required to produce analgesia for extended periods. If a catheter is contaminated by fecal or urinary soiling, we remove it.

In general, if epidural anesthesia is planned for more than 3 days, it is advisable to tunnel the exit site of the catheter away from the anus (Fig. 20.5) (12). This technique, which can also be used for long-term lumbar or thoracic

TABLE 20.1. *Differentiation of epidural abscess and hematoma*

Sign or symptom	Abscess	Hematoma
Fever	✔	✗
Localized back pain	✔	✔
Localized tenderness	✔	✔
Radicular pain	✔	✔
Paraplegía	✔	✔
Sensory loss	✔	✔
Urinary and fecal retention	✔	✔
Incontinence	✔	✔
Defect on myelography	✔	✔
Localized lesion on magnetic resonance imaging	✔	✔

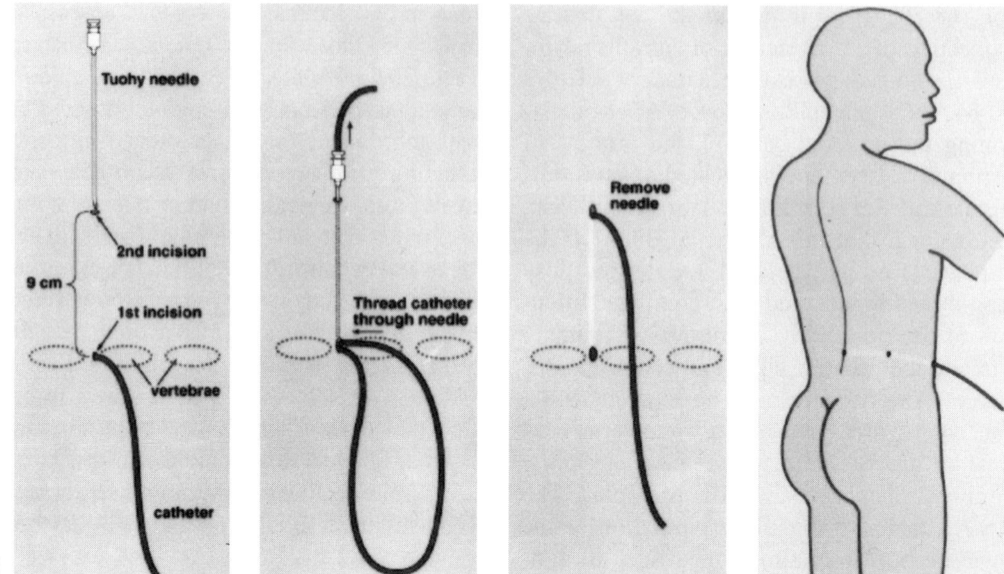

FIG. 20.5. Tunneling an epidural catheter. **A:** A 19-gauge epidural catheter is inserted into the lumbar or thoracic epidural space through a 17-gauge Tuohy needle and threaded 3 to 6 cm into the epidural space; a 2-mm horizontal incision is made at the catheter exit site. **B:** The Tuohy needle is reinserted 9-cm lateral to the initial entry site, and the tip is brought out through the previous incision. **C:** The catheter is threaded retrograde through the Tuohy needle, and the Tuohy needle is removed, allowing the catheter to exit the skin distally from the insertion site over the spine. **D:** Steps 2 to 4 are repeated another one to two times to bring the catheter exit site to the anterior abdominal or thoracic wall. (From Aram L, Krane EJ, Kozloski LJ, et al. Tunneled epidural catheters for prolonged analgesia in pediatric patients. *Anesth Analg* 2001;19:1432–1438, with permission.)

epidurals, is similar to routine placement until the catheter is properly positioned. Before removing the introducer, the catheter is tested for intravascular/intrathecal injection as above. If the tests are reassuring, a 5-cm Tuohy or Crawford needle is inserted into the subcutaneous tissue 4 cm superior and lateral to the caudal insertion site. This needle is advanced toward the caudal introducer and should be made to exit the subcutaneous tissue through the hole made by the introducer. The introducer is then removed, taking care not to disturb the catheter position. Now, the catheter is threaded retrograde through the tunneling needle and the tunneling needle is removed. Pay attention to the original insertion site. The catheter can kink or protrude. Using gentle massage and, sometimes, gentle traction on the exiting catheter, it should be made to lie flat under the skin. These catheters can be maintained for weeks with proper care and monitoring.

Drugs and Drug Dosing

The single-shot technique can provide analgesia even to low thoracic levels both during surgery and for 4 to 6 hours postoperatively. Because in pediatric surgery the technique is usually combined with general anesthesia, the focus of drug choice is long duration of action, not rapid onset. Consequently, longer acting agents like bupivacaine and ropivacaine are more commonly used than lidocaine. The volume of the local anesthetic may be as important as the actual amount of drug administered. A small volume of concentrated drug will not spread through the epidural space in the same way as a large volume of dilute drug even though the actual dose might be the same. There are specific concentrations of local anesthetics that have been found to provide both adequate density of blockade and adequate spread through the epidural space. Doses are chosen by adjusting the volumes of theses acceptable solutions.

Table 20.2 shows doses used by different authors depending on the level of analgesia desired. Factors that clearly affect the required dose include age, weight, and height. Many formulas have been proposed to calculate as precisely as possible the dose required for different levels of sensory blockade (76–80). There is, however, considerable variability from patient to patient. Because of this variability, one cannot predict precisely the response to a given dose in a given patient even when widely accepted formulas are used.

When 0.25% bupivacaine without epinephrine is administered in a caudal block, most children can walk without evidence of residual motor or sympathetic block and can be discharged home within 1 to 2 hours of the caudal block (81). Less concentrated bupivacaine may not provide adequate analgesia (82–84). The addition of opioids such as hydromorphone, morphine, or fentanyl or α_2 agonists such as clonidine will significantly increase the duration of analgesia produced by an epidural.

Continuous caudal epidural infusions can be effective for pain from the chest down, depending on how high the catheter threads and/or the drug and drug volume administered. Threading high catheters from a caudal insertion becomes more difficult with age. In infants, it is relatively easy to advance the catheter to thoracic levels. Consequently, pain from high abdominal or thoracic procedures can be treated with caudal epidurals in infants. With increasing age, caudal epidural catheters are more reliable for abdominal, perineal, or lower extremity procedures. Contraindications are similar to those for the single-shot technique. Complications can include migration of the catheter tip into a vessel or the thecal sac, epidural hematoma or abscess, nerve root palsy, and, if the catheter breaks, a foreign body in the epidural space (74).

Continuous infusions of local anesthetics either alone or in combination with opioids, α_2 agonists, and other adjuvants are discussed in the section on continuous lumbar and thoracic epidural analgesia. It is important to note that just as with intermittent caudal epidural dosing, strict attention must be paid to drug concentration and infusion rates to avoid the administration of toxic doses of drug (85,86).

TABLE 20.2. *Volumes of local anesthetic (0.25% bupivacaine or 0.2% ropivacaine) for single-dose caudal block*

Volume (mL/kg)	Dermatomal level
0.5	Sacral
0.75	T-12 (inguinal)
1	Lower thoracic
1.25	Mid to high thoracic

Indications, Contraindications, and Complications

Single-dose caudal blockade produces analgesia that lasts for 4 to 12 hours (87,88). Continuous techniques using indwelling catheters can last for days to months (12). Complications, which are rare, are primarily caused by injection directly into the bloodstream or by an equivalent route such as intraosseous injection. Neurologic complications after single-shot caudal injections have not been reported in children. Conversely, because respiratory depression after caudal injection of opioids has been reported, children receiving opioids by that route should be closely monitored (51). Contraindications are few and include infection at the site of puncture, acquired or congenital coagulation disorders, progressive neurologic disease (more from a medicolegal point of view than from added risk), and bone anomalies because of the risk of underlying malposition of the dural sac and the spinal cord.

Other Approaches to the Epidural Space

The effects of epidural analgesia are the same regardless of how and where (caudal, lumbar, or thoracic) the epidural injection is administered. There is, therefore, broad overlap between the techniques, testing, and complications associated with these catheters. Lumbar and thoracic epidural catheters are routinely placed in anesthetized children. Although there are theoretic reasons to suggest that this increases the risk of neurologic injury, all the longitudinal studies published to date have confirmed the safety of these techniques. Indeed, one could presume an increased risk of neurologic injury if insertion of an epidural catheter were attempted in a moving and uncooperative child (89). In a study that demonstrated the utility of epidural analgesia in the treatment of sickle cell vaso-occlusive crisis, the only accidental dural puncture occurred in a patient who was not sedated (24). The following discussions of lumbar and thoracic epidural catheters focus on the technical differences, referring for similarities to the above discussion of caudal epidural catheters and on drug dosing.

LUMBAR EPIDURAL BLOCK

The Landmarks

As already discussed, the position of the spinal cord and its enveloping structures is age dependent. In babies and newborns, the cord lies low in the vertebral canal, making it especially important to locate the correct vertebral interspace. The L3-4 interspace used for the lumbar approach is identified by a line joining the posterior superior spines of the iliac bones. This interspace should always be located first and serves as a landmark for other lumbar and sacral interspaces. Interspaces above or below the L3-4 interspace are located by counting up or down. In the same way, T-3 is located by finding the roots of the scapular spines and T-7 by locating the inferior angle of the scapula. The anatomic structures that the needle crosses as the needle punctures skin, subcutaneous fat, and ligaments are the same as in adults but are much softer and easier to penetrate. Thus, in smaller children, caution and a slow, deliberate approach should be exercised at all times to avoid accidental needle puncture of the dura.

The Epidural Technique

As in caudal blocks, most children are anesthetized or heavily sedated before the procedure and the same precautions should be used as discussed above. Once the child has been turned on his or her side, the knees are brought as close to the chest as possible without hindering respiratory function. If possible, an assistant should stand on the other side of the child and keep the child's knees in the appropriate position during the procedure. Sterile technique is observed.

It is preferable for the anesthesiologist to sit so that the back of the child is positioned at eye level. This helps to keep the needle in a direction perpendicular to the axis of the spine and minimizes failures caused by a lateral course of the needle. Like the Crawford needle used for caudal insertion, short, 5-cm, 17- or 18-gauge Tuohy or Weiss needles are available for pediatric lumbar or thoracic epidural insertion. Through these needles, 19- or 20-gauge epidural catheters can be inserted, usually no more than 3 to 5 cm beyond the tip of the needle. Catheters are made of many different materials and are available in either styletted or nonstyletted forms. In our experience, nylon and polyamide catheters are less likely to kink and are easier to thread than Teflon catheters.

There are several accepted techniques for identifying the epidural space. Each depends on a change in the resistance to infusing some liquid or gas. The ligaments that join the spinous processes are firm and will not easily accept infiltration with air or saline. The epidural space, in contrast, is a potential space that readily accommodates infusion of liquid or air. It is, therefore, the loss of the resistance to injection that alerts the clinician that the needle has entered the epidural space.

In one technique, the right hand of the anesthesiologist holds a saline-filled syringe connected to the Tuohy needle. The needle is inserted in the chosen interspace until the needle engages the supraspinous ligament. The right hand then keeps a constant pressure on the plunger but does not advance the needle. When engaged in the ligaments, the saline will not inject despite moderate pressure on the plunger. Alternatively, a microdrip infusion set can be used to identify the epidural space (28). The back of the left hand lies on the child's back, and the left fingers direct and advance the needle and syringe. The needle travels through the soft supraspinous ligament, then the interspinous ligament, which becomes progressively harder, and finally the firm ligamentum flavum. Even in babies, a loss of resistance to injection is distinctly felt when the ligamentum flavum is crossed.

In another technique, a syringe with 2 mL of air is attached to the Tuohy needle. Once the supraspinous ligament is engaged, tapping the syringe plunger produces a bounce. None of the air will be injected. The needle is then advanced a millimeter at a time until a tap causes air to be injected instead of bouncing back, indicating that the epidural space has been entered. Unfortunately, there have been several reports of circulatory collapse from a venous air embolism using this technique (90,91). Because of this, Berde and Sethna (92) have advocated the avoidance of this technique.

The short bevel of the pediatric size needle is small enough to fit in the epidural space even in babies, and the catheter should have no problem entering the epidural space. If there is resistance when the catheter reaches the tip of the needle, however, it could mean that the bevel is lying partly in the ligamentum flavum; attempts to force the catheter in should be avoided. It is preferable to withdraw the needle and catheter together and try again, this time slowly advancing the needle 1 to 2 mm farther after the loss of resistance. In all cases, once the catheter is in place, proper position should be checked by gentle aspiration as well as by administering a test dose as described for caudal epidural catheters.

If an infusion is started, great care must be given to ensure that there can be no confusion as to what is injected into the catheter. All entry ports to the infusion lines must be labeled, indicating that they lead to the epidural catheter.

Thoracic Epidural Catheters

Because the volume of local anesthetic solution required to produce analgesia is directly related to the distance of the catheter tip to the innervation of the site required for analgesia, caudal and lumbar epidural catheters may not provide adequate analgesia for abdominal or thoracic pain. Thus, it is desirable to have the epidural catheter tip at the spinal level that corresponds to the patient's pain. For chest pain or surgery, that means having the catheter tip at thoracic levels. As discussed previously, frequently in young children, a catheter placed by the caudal approach can be threaded up to high thoracic levels (55,56). Because of the technical difficulties involved in placing catheters directly at thoracic levels, the caudal approach is our preference, although there are many who advocate thoracic placement even in the very young (93).

In older children and adolescents, it certainly is practical to place catheters at thoracic levels. The thoracic technique is similar to the lumbar technique with some important distinctions. Most important, the spinal cord spans the thoracic region and can, therefore, be injured by placing a needle too deeply. It is wise to exercise particular caution when using this approach. The ligamentous anatomy of the thoracic spine is the same as the lumbar spine. The spinous processes are longer and slant sharply downward. In addition, the interspaces are narrower. The angle of the introducer needle, therefore, needs to be cephalad and precise.

Because the vertebral processes are more slanted at thoracic level, a paramedian rather than a midline approach to the interspace is sometimes necessary. This technique is not discussed here.

Drugs and Drug Dosage

Various drugs, drug dosages, volumes, and concentrations have been used. The most common choices involve a mixture of local anesthetics and opioids. Increasingly in Europe the α_2 agonist clonidine is also being added (37,94–98).

The choice of drug(s) is based on the patient's age and size, the underlying medical condition, and the margin of safety. Most of the pharmacokinetic modeling and dosing guidelines used in pediatric anesthesia and analgesia have been based on single doses of local anesthetic administered in the operating room setting (31,99–102). When multiple doses or continuous infusions are used, the use of operating room dosing has resulted in seizures and cardiovascular collapse (85,103). To avoid this, Berde (86) suggested that epidural bupivacaine infusions be limited to 0.4 to 0.5 mg/kg per hour. In infants younger than 2 months of age, this dose should be reduced by 30%. When a more dense block is required, Tobias and O'Dell (104) have recommended the use of 2% to 3% chloroprocaine. This ester class local anesthetic is broken down by plasma cholinesterase (Chapter 14) and does not accumulate to the same degree that amide local anesthetics do. Conversely, Yaster and colleagues (105,106) use lidocaine in concentrations ranging from 3 to 5 mg/mL rather than bupivacaine and employ daily monitoring of lidocaine blood levels to avoid systemic toxicity.

Opioids can be administered alone, in combination with a local anesthetic, or in combination with a local anesthetic and/or clonidine. The most commonly used opioids are fentanyl, morphine, and hydromorphone. Epidural fentanyl is administered in dose of 0.5 to 1 μg/kg per hour. Higher doses result in unacceptable pruritus. When combined with local anesthetic or given by infusion, epidural morphine is administered in doses of 4 to 8 μg/kg per hour. When administered in bolus doses, 30 μg/kg morphine is administered every 8 to 12 hours. Hydromorphone is less potent in the epidural space than when it is given intravenously. Intravenously hydromorphone is five times more potent than morphine. Epidurally, it is only two to three times as potent (107,108). We administer epidural hydromorphone in doses of 3 to 4 μg/kg per hour.

Neuroaxial-administered opioids have several common side effects, including pruritus, urinary retention, and nausea and vomiting. The least common and most important side effect is respiratory depression. The hallmark of impending respiratory depression after neuroaxial opioid administration is increasing sedation and decreasing depth, not necessarily rate, of respiration. Respiratory depression occurs rapidly with hydrophobic opioids such as fentanyl and sufentanil and slowly with hydrophilic agents such as morphine and hydromorphone (51,109–111). The hydrophilic agents induce respiratory depression more slowly because the rostral spread of opioid is delayed. Conversely, the hydrophilic agents are more potent analgesics than the hydrophobic opioids because of better binding of these opioids to the receptors in the spinal cord adjacent to the area in which the drug is administered. Finally, opioid-induced side effects can be antagonized without affecting analgesia by administering very low doses of naloxone by continuous intravenous infusions. Typically, doses of 0.25 to 1 μg/kg per hour are used.

Drugs and dosing of the most commonly used local anesthetics and opioids are listed in Tables 20.3 through 20.6. Ropivacaine or L-bupivacaine can be substituted for bupivacaine in these tables (112,113).

Because of the enormous individual variations in pain perception, fixed doses and time intervals make little sense in the rational treatment of pain. Continuous epidural infusions can provide steady analgesic levels but are not a panacea because the perception and intensity of pain are not constant. For example, a postoperative patient may be very comfortable resting in bed and may require little adjustment in pain management. This same patient may experience excruciating pain when coughing, voiding, or getting out of bed. Thus, rational pain management requires some form of titration to effect whenever any analgesic therapy is administered. To give patients, and in some cases parents and nurses, some measure of control over their or their children's pain therapy, demand analgesia or patient-controlled analgesia (PCA) devices

TABLE 20.3. *Bupivacaine[a] + opioid continuous low lumbar epidural infusion orders*

Site of pain	Bupivacaine (mg/mL)	Fentanyl (μg/mL)	Hydromorphone (μg/mL)	Morphine (μg/mL)	Continuous infusion (mL/kg/hr)	Drug delivered
Below the umbilicus (T-10)	1.0	2–2.5			0.2–0.3	B: 0.2–0.3 mg/kg/hr F: 0.4–0.75 μg/kg/hr
Below the umbilicus (T-10)	1.0		10		0.2–0.3	B: 0.2–0.3 mg/kg/hr H: 2–3 μg/kg/hr
Below the umbilicus (T-10)	1.0			20–30	0.2–0.3	B: 0.2–0.3 mg/kg/hr M: 4–9 μg/kg/hr
Above the umbilicus (T-10)	1.0	2–2.5			0.3–0.4	B: 0.3–0.4 mg/kg/hr F: 0.6–1.0 μg/kg/hr
Above the umbilicus (T-10)	1.0		10		0.3–0.4	B: 0.3–0.4 mg/kg/hr H: 3–4 μg/kg/hr
Above the umbilicus (T-10)	1.0			20	0.3–0.4	B: 0.3–0.4 mg/kg/hr M: 6–8 μg/kg/hr

[a]Note ropivacaine or L-bupivacaine can be substituted for bupivacaine in this table.
B, bupivacaine; F, fentanyl; H, hydromorphone; M, morphine.

TABLE 20.4. *Continuous lidocaine + fentanyl epidural infusion*

Weight (kg)	Lidocaine (mg/mL)	Fentanyl (μg/mL)	Dose (mL/kg/hr)	Drug delivered
<4	1 (0.1%)	None	1	L: 1 mg/kg/hr
<20	3 (0.3%)	1	0.5	L: 1.5 mg/kg/hr F: 0.5 μg/kg/hr
>20[a]	5 (0.5%)	1.5	0.3	L: 1.5 mg/kg/hr F: 0.45 μg/kg/hr

[a]Maximal dose: 14 to 16 mL/hr.
L, lidocaine; F, fentanyl.

TABLE 20.5. *Continuous lidocaine + morphine epidural infusion*

Weight (kg)	Lidocaine (mg/mL)	Morphine (μg/mL)	Dose (mL/kg/hr)	Drug delivered
<4	1 (0.1%)	None	1	L: 1 mg/kg/hr
<20	3 (0.3%)	10	0.5	L: 1.5 mg/kg/hr M: 5 μg/kg/hr
>20	5 (0.5%)	15	0.3	L: 1.5 mg/kg/hr M: 4.5 μg/kg/hr

[a]Maximal dose: 14 to 16 mL/hr.
L, lidocaine; M, morphine.

TABLE 20.6. *Continuous lidocaine + hydromorphone epidural infusion*

Weight (kg)	Lidocaine (mg/mL)	Hydromorphone (μg/mL)	Dose (mL/kg/hr)	Drug delivered
<4	1 (0.1%)	None	1	L: 1 mg/kg/hr
<20	3 (0.3%)	8	0.5	L: 1.5 mg/kg/hr H: 4 μg/kg/hr
>20[a]	5 (0.5%)	13	0.3	L: 1.5 mg/kg/hr H: 3.9 μg/kg/hr

[a]Maximal dose: 14 to 16 mL/h.
L, lidocaine; H, hydromorphone.

have been developed (114–117). These are microprocessor-driven pumps with a button that the patient presses to self-administer a small dose of opioid. Although most typically used intravenously, patient controlled-epidural analgesia is a very effective method of pain control (118,119).

PCA devices allow patients to administer small amounts of an analgesic whenever they feel a need for more pain relief. The dose of drug, number of boluses per hour, and the time interval between boluses (the *lock-out period*) are programmed into the equipment by the pain service physician to allow maximal patient flexibility and a sense of control with minimal risk of overdose. Generally, because older patients know that if they have severe pain, they can obtain relief immediately, many prefer dosing regimens that result in mild to moderate pain in exchange for fewer side effects such as nausea or pruritus.

The PCA pump computer stores within its memory how many boluses the patient has received as well as how many attempts that the patient has made at receiving boluses. This allows the physician to evaluate how well the patient understands the use of the pump and provides information to program the pump more efficiently. In epidural PCA, continuous "background" infusions are used in addition to self-administered boluses. It is also useful to realize that the time needed for a bolus dose to effect change is longer with epidural compared with intravenous drug administration. Thus, the lock-out period is longer, usually 15 minutes compared with 5 to 8 minutes for intravenous PCA.

PCA requires a patient with enough intelligence and manual dexterity and strength to operate the pump. Thus, it was initially limited to adolescents and teenagers, but the lower age limit of those in whom this treatment modality can be used continues to fall. In fact, it has been our experience that any child able to play a video game can operate a PCA pump (ages 5 to 6 years). Allowing parents or nurses to initiate a PCA bolus is controversial. Monitto et al. (120) recently demonstrated that nurses and parents can be empowered to initiate intravenous PCA boluses and to use this technology safely in children younger than even 1 year of age. In this study, the incidence of common opioid-induced side effects is similar to that observed in older patients (120). Difficulties with PCA include its increased costs, patient age limitations, and the bureaucratic (physician, nursing, and pharmacy) obstacles (protocols, education, storage arrangements) that must be overcome before its implementation. Contraindications to the use of patient controlled analgesia include inability to push the bolus button (weakness, arm restraints), inability to understand how to use the machine, and a patient's (or parent's) desire not to assume responsibility for his/her own care.

Doses of the most commonly used local anesthetic bupivacaine and an opioid in epidural PCA are listed in Table 20.7. When administering bupivacaine and an opioid, the maximal amount of drug a patient can receive per hour is 0.4 mg/kg bupivacaine and *either* 0.8 to 1.0 μg/kg fentanyl *or* 4 μg/kg hydromorphone *or* 8 μg/kg morphine. Ropivacaine

TABLE 20.7. *Bupivacaine + opioid patient-controlled analgesia low lumbar epidural infusion orders*

Bupivacaine (mg/mL)	Fentanyl (μg/mL)	Hydromorphone (μg/mL)	Morphine (μg/mL)	Continuous infusion (mL/kg/hr)	Bolus dose (mL/dose)	Bolus/hr	Drug delivered
1.0	2–2.5			0.2	0.1	0	B: 0.2 mg/kg/hr F: 0.4–0.5 μg/kg/hr
1.0		10		0.2	0.1	0	B: 0.2 mg/kg/hr H: 2 μg/kg/hr
1.0			20	0.2	0.1	0	B: 0.2 mg/kg/hr M: 4 μg/kg/hr
1.0	2–2.5			0.2	0.1	1	B: 0.3 mg/kg/hr F: 0.6–0.75 μg/kg/hr
1.0		10		0.2	0.1	1	B: 0.3 mg/kg/hr H: 3 μg/kg/hr
1.0			20	0.2	0.1	1	B: 0.3 mg/kg/hr M: 6 μg/kg/hr
1.0	2–2.5			0.2	0.1	2	B: 0.4 mg/kg/hr F: 0.8–1.0 μg/kg/hr
1.0		10		0.2	0.1	2	B: 0.4 mg/kg/hr H: 4 μg/kg/hr
1.0			20	0.2	0.1	2	B: 0.4 mg/kg/hr M: 8 μg/kg/hr

[a]Note ropivacaine or L-bupivacaine can be substituted for bupivacaine in this table.
B, bupivacaine; F, fentanyl; H, hydromorphone; M, morphine.

or L-bupivacaine can be substituted for bupivacaine in these tables.

Lidocaine and an opioid can also be given via epidural PCA (Table 20.8). The maximal hourly dose of lidocaine is 2 mg/kg. The maximal hourly opioid dose is *either* 0.8 to 1.0 μg/kg fentanyl *or* 4 μg/kg hydromorphone *or* 8 μg/kg morphine.

SPINAL BLOCKADE

Although pediatric spinal anesthesia and analgesia were first described at the turn of the 20th century, it fell into disrepute because of the fear of inducing paralysis, the greater suitability and safety of general anesthesia, and the high incidence of postdural headache

TABLE 20.8. *Lidocaine + opioid patient-controlled analgesia low lumbar epidural infusion orders*

Lidocaine (mg/mL)	Fentanyl (μg/mL)	Hydromorphone (μg/mL)	Morphine (μg/mL)	Continuous infusion (mL/kg/hr)	Bolus dose (mL/dose)	Bolus/hr	Drug delivered
5.0	2–2.5			0.2	0.1	0	L: 1 mg/kg/hr F: 0.4–0.5 μg/kg/hr
5.0		10		0.2	0.1	0	L: 1 mg/kg/hr H: 2 μg/kg/hr
5.0			20	0.2	0.1	0	L: 1 mg/kg/hr M: 4 μg/kg/hr
5.0	2–2.5			0.2	0.1	1	L: 1.5 mg/kg/hr F: 0.6–0.75 μg/kg/hr
5.0		10		0.2	0.1	1	L: 1.5 mg/kg/hr H: 3 μg/kg/hr
5.0			20	0.2	0.1	1	L: 1.5 mg/kg/hr M: 6 μg/kg/hr
5.0	2–2.5			0.2	0.1	2	L: 2 mg/kg/hr F: 0.8–1.0 μg/kg/hr
5.0		10		0.2	0.1	2	L: 2 mg/kg/hr H: 4 μg/kg/hr
5.0			20	0.2	0.1	2	L: 2 mg/kg/hr M: 8 μg/kg/hr

L, lidocaine; F, fentanyl; H, hydromorphone; M, morphine.

in this age group compared with older patients (21,121–123). The exact incidence of postdural puncture headache in children is unknown. One report of pediatric oncology patients found very few headaches after spinal puncture (124), and another study found headaches to be rare in children younger than 13 years of age but common in older children (125). The resurgence of this anesthetic technique is largely owing to the belief, popularized by Abajian et al., that the high risk of postanesthesia apnea in patients born prematurely can be reduced or eliminated in children who are anesthetized with spinal anesthetics (126–130).

Technique

A spinal block (or tap) can be performed with the child in either a sitting position or lying on his or her side in a slightly head-up position. Regardless of the position chosen, the back is arched and the neck is kept in a neutral position. Flexing the head has resulted in airway obstruction and hypoxemia (131). After infiltrating the overlying skin with a skin wheal of local anesthetic (1% lidocaine) or applying a topical anesthetic [lidocaine-prilocaine (EMLA) cream], a 22-, 25-, or 26-gauge, styletted spinal needle is introduced at the L4-5 or L5-S1 interspace and is advanced slowly until it punctures the dura. In infants, CSF is found at a depth of 10 to 15 mm from the skin. Once identified, a 1-mL syringe filled with the local anesthetic is attached to the needle hub and the solution injected over a period of 15 to 20 seconds. At the end of the injection, some CSF should be aspirated into the syringe, mixed with the solution left in the hub, and reinjected to ensure that the total dose has been given. This amount of local anesthetic injected by barbotage may seem small, but it can represent a large fraction of the total drug dose administered. Indeed, disregarding it could result in low or inadequate levels of analgesia. After local anesthetic administration, the patient is placed in the supine position. It is important not to lift the patient's legs above the level of the head (e.g., in placing an electrocautery pad) because this may result in a "total" spinal (132).

Drugs and Drug Dose

The most commonly used local anesthetics are hyperbaric 0.5% to 1% tetracaine in 5% dextrose (hyperbaric), 5% lidocaine in 7.5% dextrose (hyperbaric), and 0.25% to 0.5% bupivacaine, with (hyperbaric) or without (isobaric) 8.25% dextrose (127,133). Epinephrine is often added to prolong the duration of neural blockade. The proportional dose of local anesthetic required to produce a subarachnoid block is higher in neonates compared with older children and adults. The resulting anesthesia is also more short-lived. Hyperbaric tetracaine is administered in doses ranging from 0.2 to 1 mg/kg; the higher doses in newborns and the lower doses in older children. Bupivacaine is administered in doses ranging from 0.6 to 0.8 mg/kg in newborns and 0.2 to 0.4 mg/kg in older children. Lidocaine is administered in doses of 1 to 3 mg/kg. Because lidocaine may induce a transient radicular neuropathy, it is no longer routinely used (134,135).

Indications, Contraindications, and Complications

As in all anesthetic techniques, spinal anesthesia and analgesia have benefits and disadvantages. It is primarily indicated for short procedures of the lower abdomen in premature and ex-premature infants, such as inguinal hernia repair. It is also indicated for children in whom it would be preferable to avoid general anesthesia, such as children with respiratory disabilities or progressive muscular disease. Because spinal hemorrhage is a rare but disastrous complication, spinals are contraindicated in newborns with inadequate coagulation and children with acquired or congenital bleeding disorders. Infection at the puncture site, unstable hemodynamic status, and difficult airways are also relative contraindications. Complications include total spinal anesthesia, postdural puncture headache, backache, and neurologic sequelae (cauda equina syndrome).

In unusual circumstances, catheters can be placed in the intrathecal space for the treatment of longer term pain syndromes. Continuous spinal infusions can take advantage of the extremely high potency of intrathecal analgesics. Implanted intrathecal infusion pumps can carry enough drug for weeks of analgesia without any external catheters or pumps (136,137).

CONCLUSION

Regional anesthesia is an additional tool in the management of acute and chronic pain in children. It is not indicated for all children and under all circumstances. Risks and benefits should be carefully weighed before conducting any anesthesia technique. This axiom becomes particularly true with regional anesthesia in children in whom ease of execution and relative absence of side effects can lull the operator into thinking that the technique is devoid of complications. Moreover, in some cases, its superiority over other analgesia techniques has not yet been demonstrated in sufficiently large groups of patients. Nonetheless, when indicated and conducted with care, regional anesthesia provides safe and effective pain relief in children of all ages.

REFERENCES

1. Schechter NL, Berde CB, Yaster M. *Pain in infants, children, and adolescents*. Baltimore: Williams & Wilkins, 1993.
2. Yaster M, Krane EJ, Kaplan RF, et al. *Pediatric pain management and sedation handbook*. St. Louis: Mosby Year Book, 1997.
3. Agency for Health Care Policy and Research. *Clinical practice guidelines: acute pain management in infants, children, and adolescents: operative and medical procedures*. Rockville, MD: U.S. Department of Health and Human Services, 1992.
4. Agency for Health Care Policy and Research. *Clinical practice guidelines: acute pain management: operative or medical procedures and trauma*. Rockville, MD: U.S. Department of Health and Human Resources, 1992.
5. Schechter NL. The undertreatment of pain in children: an overview. *Pediatr Clin North Am* 1989;36:781–794.
6. Anand KJ, Sippell WG, Aynsley-Green A. Randomised trial of fentanyl anaesthesia in preterm babies undergoing surgery: effects on the stress response. *Lancet* 1987;1:62–66.
7. Anand KJ, Hickey PR. Halothane-morphine compared with high-dose sufentanil for anesthesia and postoperative analgesia in neonatal cardiac surgery. *N Engl J Med* 1992;326:1–9.
8. Rodgers A, Walker N, Schug S, et al. Reduction of postoperative mortality and morbidity with epidural or spinal anaesthesia: results from overview of randomised trials. *BMJ* 2000;321:1493.
9. Dahl JB, Kehlet H. The value of pre-emptive analgesia in the treatment of postoperative pain. *Br J Anaesth* 1993;70:434–439.
10. Liu S, Carpenter RL, Neal JM. Epidural anesthesia and analgesia. Their role in postoperative outcome. *Anesthesiology* 1995;82:1474–1506.
11. McGrath PA. Development of the World Health Organization guidelines on cancer pain relief and palliative care in children. *J Pain Symptom Manage* 1996;12: 87–92.
12. Aram L, Krane EJ, Kozloski LJ, et al. Tunneled epidural catheters for prolonged analgesia in pediatric patients. *Anesth Analg* 2001;92:1432–1438.
13. Berde CB, Sethna NF, Levin L, et al. Regional analgesia on pediatric medical and surgical wards. *Intensive Care Med* 1989;15[Suppl 1]:S40–S43.
14. Dalens B, Hasnaoui A. Caudal anesthesia in pediatric surgery: success rate and adverse effects in 750 consecutive patients. *Anesth Analg* 1989;68:83–89.
15. Dalens B, Tanguy A, Haberer JP. Lumbar epidural anesthesia for operative and postoperative pain relief in infants and young children. *Anesth Analg* 1986;65: 1069–1073.
16. Dalens B. Regional anesthesia in children. *Anesth Analg* 1989;68:654–672.
17. Giaufre E, Dalens B, Gombert A. Epidemiology and morbidity of regional anesthesia in children: a one-year prospective survey of the French-Language Society of Pediatric Anesthesiologists. *Anesth Analg* 1996; 83:904–912.
18. Ross AK, Eck JB, Tobias JD. Pediatric regional anesthesia: beyond the caudal. *Anesth Analg* 2000;91:16–26.
19. Sethna N. Regional anesthesia and analgesia. *Semin Perinatol* 1998;22:380–389.
20. Yaster M, Maxwell LG, Nicholas EJ. Local anesthetics in the management of acute pain in children: a primer for the non-anesthesiologist. *Compr Ther* 1991;17: 27–35.
21. Yaster M, Maxwell LG. Pediatric regional anesthesia. *Anesthesiology* 1989;70:324–338.
22 Anderson CT, Berde CB, Sethna NF, et al. Meningococcal purpura fulminans: treatment of vascular insufficiency in a 2-yr-old child with lumbar epidural sympathetic blockade. *Anesthesiology* 1989;71:463–464.
23. Collins JJ, Grier HE, Sethna NF, et al. Regional anesthesia for pain associated with terminal pediatric malignancy. *Pain* 1996;65:63–69.
24. Yaster M, Tobin JR, Billett C, et al. Epidural analgesia in the management of severe vaso-occlusive sickle cell crisis. *Pediatrics* 1994;93:310–315.
25. Golianu B, Krane EJ, Galloway KS, et al. Pediatric acute pain management. *Pediatr Clin North Am* 2000; 47:559–587.
26. Heij HA, Nievelstein RA, de Zwart I, et al. Abnormal anatomy of the lumbosacral region imaged by magnetic resonance in children with anorectal malformations. *Arch Dis Child* 1996;74:441–444.
27. Yamashita M. Mathematical formulae for assessing

the depth of the epidural space in children. *Anaesthesia* 1997;52:94–95.

28. Yamashita M. Airless identification of the epidural space in infants and children. *Anesth Analg* 1994;78:610.
29. Bosenberg AT, Gouws E. Skin-epidural distance in children. *Anaesthesia* 1995;50:895–897.
30. Hasan MA, Howard RF, Lloyd-Thomas AR. Depth of epidural space in children. *Anaesthesia* 1994;49: 1085–1087.
31. Eyres RL, Hastings C, Brown TC, et al. Plasma bupivacaine concentrations following lumbar epidural anaesthesia in children. *Anaesth Intensive Care* 1986; 14:131–134.
32. Ecoffey C, Dubousset AM, Samii K. Lumbar and thoracic epidural anesthesia for urologic and upper abdominal surgery in infants and children. *Anesthesiology* 1986;65:87–90.
33. Ozcengiz D, Gunduz M, Ozbek H, et al. Comparison of caudal morphine and tramadol for postoperative pain control in children undergoing inguinal herniorrhaphy. *Paediatr Anaesth* 2001;11:459–464.
34. Zenz M, Zenner D. Tramadol or ketamine for caudal analgesia? *Br J Anaesth* 2000;85:805–807.
35. Scott DA, Blake D, Buckland M, et al. A comparison of epidural ropivacaine infusion alone and in combination with 1, 2, and 4 microg/mL fentanyl for seventy-two hours of postoperative analgesia after major abdominal surgery. *Anesth Analg* 1999;88:857–864.
36. Luz G, Innerhofer P, Oswald E, et al. Comparison of clonidine 1 microgram kg-1 with morphine 30 micrograms kg-1 for post-operative caudal analgesia in children. *Eur J Anaesthesiol* 1999;16:42–46.
37. Curatolo M, Petersen-Felix S, Scaramozzino P, et al. Epidural fentanyl, adrenaline and clonidine as adjuvants to local anaesthetics for surgical analgesia: meta-analyses of analgesia and side-effects. *Acta Anaesthesiol Scand* 1998;42:910–920.
38. Jorgensen H, Wetterslev J, Moiniche S, et al. Epidural local anaesthetics versus opioid-based analgesic regimens on postoperative gastrointestinal paralysis, PONV and pain after abdominal surgery. *Cochrane Database Syst Rev* 2000;4:CD001893.
39. Rosenfeld BA, Beattie C, Christopherson R, et al. The effects of different anesthetic regimens on fibrinolysis and the development of postoperative arterial thrombosis. Perioperative Ischemia Randomized Anesthesia Trial Study Group. *Anesthesiology* 1993;79:435–443.
40. Christopherson R, Beattie C, Frank SM, et al. Perioperative morbidity in patients randomized to epidural or general anesthesia for lower extremity vascular surgery. Perioperative Ischemia Randomized Anesthesia Trial Study Group. *Anesthesiology* 1993;79:422–434.
41. Parker SD, Breslow MJ, Frank SM, et al. Catecholamine and cortisol responses to lower extremity revascularization: correlation with outcome variables. Perioperative Ischemia Randomized Anesthesia Trial Study Group. *Crit Care Med* 1995;23:1954–1961.
42. Strichartz GR. Neural physiology and local anesthetic action. In: Cousins MJ, Bridenbaugh PO, eds. *Neural blockade in clinical anesthesia and management of pain*. Philadelphia: Lippincott–Raven, 1998:35–54.
43. Dohi S, Naito H, Takahashi T. Age-related changes in blood pressure and duration of motor block in spinal anesthesia. *Anesthesiology* 1979;50:319–323.
44. Payen D, Ecoffey C, Carli P, et al. Pulsed Doppler ascending aortic, carotid, brachial, and femoral artery blood flows during caudal anesthesia in infants. *Anesthesiology* 1987;67:681–685.
45. Yaksh TL. Pharmacology and mechanisms of opioid analgesic activity. *Acta Anaesthesiol Scand* 1997;41: 94–111.
46. Etches RC, Sandler AN, Daley MD. Respiratory depression and spinal opioids. *Can J Anaesth* 1989;36: 165–185.
47. Cousins MJ, Mather LE. Intrathecal and epidural administration of opioids. *Anesthesiology* 1984;61: 276–310.
48. Sabbe MB, Yaksh TL. Pharmacology of spinal opioids. *J Pain Symptom Manage* 1990;5:191–203.
49. Yaksh TL. The spinal pharmacology of acutely and chronically administered opioids. *J Pain Symptom Manage* 1992;7:356–361.
50. Swenson JD, Owen J, Lamoreaux W, et al. The effect of distance from injection site to the brainstem using spinal sufentanil. *Reg Anesth Pain Med* 2001;26:306–309.
51. Attia J, Ecoffey C, Sandouk P, et al. Epidural morphine in children: pharmacokinetics and CO2 sensitivity. *Anesthesiology* 1986;65:590–594.
52. Nichols DG, Yaster M, Lynn AM, et al. Disposition and respiratory effects of intrathecal morphine in children. *Anesthesiology* 1993;79:733–8; discussion 25A.
53. Eisenach JC. Lipid soluble opioids do move in cerebrospinal fluid. *Reg Anesth Pain Med* 2001;26:296–297.
54. Kost-Byerly S, Tobin JR, Greenberg RS, et al. Bacterial colonization and infection rate of continuous epidural catheters in children. *Anesth Analg* 1998;86:712–716.
55. Bosenberg AT, Bland BA, Schulte-Steinberg O, et al. Thoracic epidural anesthesia via caudal route in infants. *Anesthesiology* 1988;69:265–269.
56. Gunter JB, Eng C. Thoracic epidural anesthesia via the caudal approach in children. *Anesthesiology* 1992;76: 935–938.
57. Rasch DK, Webster DE, Pollard TG, et al. Lumbar and thoracic epidural analgesia via the caudal approach for postoperative pain relief in infants and children. *Can J Anaesth* 1990;37:359–362.
58. Marquort H, Grenzer G, Schroeder U. Routine postoperative epidural analgesia. X-ray control of epidural catheter position and prevention of the spread of epidural contrast media. *Anaesthesist* 1993;42:501–508.
59. van Niekerk J, Bax-Vermeire BM, Geurts JW, et al. Epidurography in premature infants. *Anaesthesia* 1990;45:722–725.
60. Rice LJ. Regional anesthesia and analgesia. In: Motoyama EK, Davis PJ, eds. *Anesthesia for infants and children*. St. Louis: Mosby Year Book, 1996:403–444.
61. Broadman LM, Rice LJ. Neural blockade for pediatric surgery. In: Cousins MJ, Bridenbaugh PO, eds. *Neural blockade in clinical anesthesia and management of pain*. Philadelphia: Lippincott–Raven Publishers, 1998: 615–638.
62. American Academy of Pediatric Dentistry. Guidelines for the elective use of pharmacologic conscious sedation and deep sedation in pediatric dental patients. *Pediatr Dent* 1993;15:297–301.
63. American Academy of Pediatrics Committee on Drugs. Guidelines for monitoring and management of pediatric patients during and after sedation for diagnostic and therapeutic procedures. *Pediatrics* 1992;89: 1110–1115.

64. Guidelines for the elective use of conscious sedation, deep sedation, and general anesthesia in pediatric patients. Committee on drugs. Section on anesthesiology. *Pediatrics* 1985;76:317–321.
65. Cote CJ, Karl HW, Notterman DA, et al. Adverse sedation events in pediatrics: analysis of medications used for sedation. *Pediatrics* 2000;106:633–644.
66. Moore DC, Batra MS. The components of an effective test dose prior to epidural block. *Anesthesiology* 1981; 55:693–696.
67. Abraham RA, Harris AP, Maxwell LG, et al. The efficacy of 1.5% lidocaine with 7.5% dextrose and epinephrine as an epidural test dose for obstetrics. *Anesthesiology* 1986;64:116–119.
68. Tobias JD. Caudal epidural block: a review of test dosing and recognition of systemic injection in children. *Anesth Analg* 2001;93:1156–1161.
69. Desparmet J, Mateo J, Ecoffey C, et al. Efficacy of an epidural test dose in children anesthetized with halothane. *Anesthesiology* 1990;72:249–251.
70. Fisher QA, Shaffner DH, Yaster M. Detection of intravascular injection of regional anaesthetics in children. *Can J Anaesth* 1997;44:592–598.
71. Tanaka M, Nishikawa T. Evaluating T-wave amplitude as a guide for detecting intravascular injection of a test dose in anesthetized children. *Anesth Analg* 1999;88: 754–758.
72. Tanaka M, Nishikawa T. The efficacy of a simulated intravascular test dose in sevoflurane-anesthetized children: a dose-response study. *Anesth Analg* 1999; 89:632–637.
73. Tanaka M, Kimura T, Goyagi T, et al. Evaluating hemodynamic and T wave criteria of simulated intravascular test doses using bupivacaine or isoproterenol in anesthetized children. *Anesth Analg* 2000;91:567–572.
74. Lenox WC, Kost-Byerly S, Shipley R, et al. Pediatric caudal epidural catheter sequestration: an unusual complication. *Anesthesiology* 1995;83:1112–1114.
75. Bjornson HS, Colley R, Bower RH, et al. Association between microorganism growth at the catheter insertion site and colonization of the catheter in patients receiving total parenteral nutrition. *Surgery* 1982;92:720–727.
76. Takasaki M, Dohi S, Kawabata Y, et al. Dosage of lidocaine for caudal anesthesia in infants and children. *Anesthesiology* 1977;47:527–529.
77. Schulte-Steinberg O, Rahlfs VW. Spread of extradural analgesia following caudal injection in children. A statistical study. *Br J Anaesth* 1977;49:1027–1034.
78. Melman E, Penuelas JA, Marrufo J. Regional anesthesia in children. *Anesth Analg* 1975;54:387–390.
79. Busoni P, Andreuccetti T. The spread of caudal analgesia in children: a mathematical model. *Anaesth Intensive Care* 1986;14:140–144.
80. McGown RG. Caudal analgesia in children. Five hundred cases for procedures below the diaphragm. *Anaesthesia* 1982;37:806–818.
81. Saint-Raymond S, O'Donovan F, Ecoffey C. Criteria of recovery from caudal anesthesia in children. *Cah Anesthesiol* 1990;38:246–248.
82. Wolf AR, Valley RD, Fear DW, et al. Bupivacaine for caudal analgesia in infants and children: the optimal effective concentration. *Anesthesiology* 1988;69: 102–106.
83. Gunter JB, Dunn CM, Bennie JB, et al. Optimum concentration of bupivacaine for combined caudal—general anesthesia in children. *Anesthesiology* 1991;75: 57–61.
84. Malviya S, Fear DW, Roy WL, et al. Adequacy of caudal analgesia in children after penoscrotal and inguinal surgery using 0.5 or 1.0 ml.kg-1 bupivacaine 0.125%. *Can J Anaesth* 1992;39:449–453.
85. McCloskey JJ, Haun SE, Deshpande JK. Bupivacaine toxicity secondary to continuous caudal epidural infusion in children. *Anesth Analg* 1992;75:287–290.
86. Berde CB. Convulsions associated with pediatric regional anesthesia. *Anesth Analg* 1992;75:164–166.
87. Fisher QA, McComiskey CM, Hill JL, et al. Postoperative voiding interval and duration of analgesia following peripheral or caudal nerve blocks in children. *Anesth Analg* 1993;76:173–177.
88. Warner MA, Kunkel SE, Offord KO, et al. The effects of age, epinephrine, and operative site on duration of caudal analgesia in pediatric patients. *Anesth Analg* 1987;66:995–998.
89. Krane EJ, Dalens BJ, Murat I, et al. The safety of epidurals placed during general anesthesia. *Reg Anesth Pain Med* 1998;23:433–438.
90. Schwartz N, Eisenkraft JB. Probable venous air embolism during epidural placement in an infant. *Anesth Analg* 1993;76:1136–1138.
91. Guinard JP, Borboen M. Probable venous air embolism during caudal anesthesia in a child. *Anesth Analg* 1993;76:1134–1135.
92. Sethna NF, Berde CB. Venous air embolism during identification of the epidural space in children. *Anesth Analg* 1993;76:925–927.
93. Tobias JD, Lowe S, O'Dell N, et al. Thoracic epidural anaesthesia in infants and children. *Can J Anaesth* 1993;40:879–882.
94. Bernard JM, Kick O, Bonnet F. Comparison of intravenous and epidural clonidine for postoperative patient-controlled analgesia. *Anesth Analg* 1995;81:706–712.
95. Carabine UA, Milligan KR, Moore J. Extradural clonidine and bupivacaine for postoperative analgesia. *Br J Anaesth* 1992;68:132–135.
96. Constant I, Gall O, Gouyet L, et al. Addition of clonidine or fentanyl to local anaesthetics prolongs the duration of surgical analgesia after single shot caudal block in children. *Br J Anaesth* 1998;80:294–298.
97. Cook B, Grubb DJ, Aldridge LA, et al. Comparison of the effects of adrenaline, clonidine and ketamine on the duration of caudal analgesia produced by bupivacaine in children. *Br J Anaesth* 1995;75:698–701.
98. Delaunay L, Leppert C, Dechaubry V, et al. Epidural clonidine decreases postoperative requirements for epidural fentanyl. *Reg Anesth* 1993;18:176–180.
99. Ecoffey C, Desparmet J, Maury M, et al. Bupivacaine in children: pharmacokinetics following caudal anesthesia. *Anesthesiology* 1985;63:447–448.
100. Ecoffey C, Desparmet J, Berdeaux A, et al. Pharmacokinetics of lignocaine in children following caudal anaesthesia. *Br J Anaesth* 1984;56:1399–1402.
101. Eyres RL, Kidd J, Oppenheim R, et al. Local anaesthetic plasma levels in children. *Anaesth Intensive Care* 1978;6:243–247.
102. Eyres RL, Bishop W, Oppenheim RC, et al. Plasma bupivacaine concentrations in children during caudal epidural analgesia. *Anaesth Intensive Care* 1983;11: 20–22.
103. Maxwell LG, Martin LD, Yaster M. Bupivacaine-in-

duced cardiac toxicity in neonates: successful treatment with intravenous phenytoin. *Anesthesiology* 1994;80:682–686.
104. Tobias JD, O'Dell N. Chloroprocaine for epidural anesthesia in infants and children. *AANA J* 1995;63: 131–135.
105. Yaster M, Andresini J, Krane EJ. Epidural analgesia. In: Yaster M, Krane EJ, Kaplan RF, et al., eds. *Pediatric pain management and sedation handbook.* St. Louis: Mosby Year Book, 1997:113–146.
106. Yaster M, Kost-Byerly S, Maxwell LG. The management of pain in sickle cell disease. *Pediatr Clin North Am* 2000;47:699–710.
107. Chaplan SR, Duncan SR, Brodsky JB, et al. Morphine and hydromorphone epidural analgesia. A prospective, randomized comparison. *Anesthesiology* 1992;77: 1090–1094.
108. Brodsky JB, Chaplan SR, Brose WG, et al. Continuous epidural hydromorphone for postthoracotomy pain relief. *Ann Thorac Surg* 1990;50:888–893.
109. Karl HW, Tyler DC, Krane EJ. Respiratory depression after low-dose caudal morphine. *Can J Anaesth* 1996; 43:1065–1067.
110. Krane EJ. Delayed respiratory depression in a child after caudal epidural morphine. *Anesth Analg* 1988;67: 79–82.
111. Krane EJ, Tyler DC, Jacobson LE. The dose response of caudal morphine in children. *Anesthesiology* 1989;71:48–52.
112. McCann ME, Sethna NF, Mazoit JX, et al. The pharmacokinetics of epidural ropivacaine in infants and young children. *Anesth Analg* 2001;93:893–897.
113. Collins JJ, Grier HE, Kinney HC, et al. Control of severe pain in children with terminal malignancy. *J Pediatr* 1995;126:653–657.
114. Yaster M, Billett C, Monitto C. Intravenous patient controlled analgesia. In: Yaster M, Krane EJ, Kaplan RF, et al., eds. *Pediatric pain management and sedation handbook.* St. Louis: Mosby Year Book, 1997: 89–112.
115. Schechter NL, Berrien FB, Katz SM. The use of patient-controlled analgesia in adolescents with sickle cell pain crisis: a preliminary report. *J Pain Symptom Manage* 1988;3:109–113.
116. Lehmann KA. New developments in patient-controlled postoperative analgesia. *Ann Med* 1995;27:271–282.
117. Berde CB, Lehn BM, Yee JD, et al. Patient-controlled analgesia in children and adolescents: a randomized, prospective comparison with intramuscular administration of morphine for postoperative analgesia. *J Pediatr* 1991;118:460–466.
118. Lejus C, Schwoerer D, Furic I, et al. Fentanyl versus sufentanil: plasma concentrations during continuous epidural postoperative infusion in children. *Br J Anaesth* 2000;85:615–617.
119. Caudle CL, Freid EB, Bailey AG, et al. Epidural fentanyl infusion with patient-controlled epidural analgesia for postoperative analgesia in children. *J Pediatr Surg* 1993;28:554–559.
120. Monitto CL, Greenberg RS, Kost-Byerly S, et al. The safety and efficacy of parent-/nurse-controlled analgesia in patients less than six years of age. *Anesth Analg* 2000;91:573–579.
121. Tourtellotte WW, Henderson WG, Tucker RP, et al. A randomized, double-blind clinical trial comparing the 22 versus 26 gauge needle in the production of the post-lumbar puncture syndrome in normal individuals. *Headache* 1972;12:73–78.
122. Atabaki S, Ochsenschlager D. Post-lumbar puncture headache and backache in pediatrics: a case series and demonstration of magnetic resonance imaging findings. *Arch Pediatr Adolesc Med* 1999;153:770–773.
123. Geurts JW, Haanschoten MC, van Wijk R, et al. Post-dural puncture headache in young patients. A comparative study between the use of 0.52 mm (25-gauge) and 0.33 mm (29-gauge) spinal needles. *Acta Anaesthesiol Scand* 1990;34:350–353.
124. Bolder PM. Postlumbar puncture headache in pediatric oncology patients. *Anesthesiology* 1986;65:696–698.
125. Berkowitz S, Green BA. Spinal anesthesia in children: report based on 350 patients under 13 years of age. *Anesthesiology* 1950;12:376–379.
126. Liu LM, Cote CJ, Goudsouzian NG, et al. Life-threatening apnea in infants recovering from anesthesia. *Anesthesiology* 1983;59:506–510.
127. Abajian JC, Mellish RW, Browne AF, et al. Spinal anesthesia for surgery in the high-risk infant. *Anesth Analg* 1984;63:359–362.
128. Sartorelli KH, Abajian JC, Kreutz JM, et al. Improved outcome utilizing spinal anesthesia in high-risk infants. *J Pediatr Surg* 1992;27:1022–1025.
129. William JM, Stoddart PA, Williams SA, et al. Post-operative recovery after inguinal herniotomy in ex-premature infants: comparison between sevoflurane and spinal anaesthesia. *Br J Anaesth* 2001;86:366–371.
130. Somri M, Gaitini L, Vaida S, et al. Postoperative outcome in high-risk infants undergoing herniorrhaphy: comparison between spinal and general anaesthesia. *Anaesthesia* 1998;53:762–766.
131. Gleason CA, Martin RJ, Anderson JV, et al. Optimal position for a spinal tap in preterm infants. *Pediatrics* 1983;71:31–35.
132. Bailey A, Valley R, Bigler R. High spinal anesthesia in an infant. *Anesthesiology* 1989;70:560.
133. Mahe V, Ecoffey C. Spinal anesthesia with isobaric bupivacaine in infants. *Anesthesiology* 1988;68: 601–603.
134. Hodgson PS, Neal JM, Pollock JE, et al. The neurotoxicity of drugs given intrathecally (spinal). *Anesth Analg* 1999;88:797–809.
135. Schneider M, Ettlin T, Kaufmann M, et al. Transient neurologic toxicity after hyperbaric subarachnoid anesthesia with 5% lidocaine. *Anesth Analg* 1993;76: 1154–1157.
136. Sethna NF, Berde CB. Continuous subarachnoid analgesia in two adolescents with severe scoliosis and impaired pulmonary function. *Reg Anesth* 1991;16: 333–336.
137. Berde CB, Sethna NF, Conrad LS, et al. Subarachnoid bupivacaine analgesia for seven months for a patient with a spinal cord tumor. *Anesthesiology* 1990;72: 1094–1096.

21

Peripheral Nerve Blockade in the Management of Postoperative Pain in Children

Bernard Dalens

Postoperative pain management has produced a large number of publications during the past decade. Therefore, it is not surprising that the concept of pain management has at the same time evolved considerably. Originally, the main problem was the identification of pain. Thus, considerable efforts were made to evaluate pain at different ages and in various circumstances. Then, the question was to identify the agents and techniques suitable for providing reliable and safe pain relief. Currently, the tools are here to both evaluate pain and provide complete analgesia in surgical patients. The problem remaining is the adequate application to avoid peaks and valleys while maintaining a steady-state level of analgesia. As well, expectations of the parents and the children have changed over the years; full analgesia is no more deemed sufficient. A high degree of comfort and well-being is now expected. The most minor adverse effects of analgesia that were long considered as normal or inevitable are now unacceptable.

As the expectations of parents and children of pain management have changed considerably, so too has the attitude of practitioners. Pain relief is now considered an essential objective of pediatric anesthesia care, and the postoperative condition of children has been improved in almost an exponential way in recent years. However, although pain relief is now considered as a patient's elementary right, new limitations interfere with patient care. The main limitations are the economic pressures to reduce hospital stay and monitoring of the patients as well as to restrict the use of sophisticated drugs and devices and the morbidity of analgesia techniques, which is not negligible (1,2). Adverse effects of treatments aiming at saving the lives of patients or, at least, improving their physical status can be considered acceptable. However, complications that can occasionally be life threatening are not acceptable for techniques aimed at just improving the comfort of the patients. Furthermore, some techniques of analgesia can even hide early symptoms of surgical complications, thus worsening the surgical outcome. Even though pain cannot (and must not) be considered as an early symptom of a compartment syndrome that should have been recognized long before its late occurrence, some surgeons are reluctant to have many of their patients adequately treated for postoperative pain. Thus, efficacy is not the only parameter to be considered; safety is certainly as important.

After the rediscovery of regional anesthetic techniques for pediatric patients 25 years ago, central block procedures, especially caudal anesthesia, have gained widespread acceptance owing to their extraordinary efficacy and apparent simplicity. However, many complications, mostly minor but sometimes severe, especially with catheter techniques, have limited regional techniques and initiated a shift toward more peripheral techniques. Peripheral nerve blocks, nerve trunk blocks, and compartment space blocks have been extensively evaluated in children. Although they are not yet properly taught in many academic institutions, their many advantages are now well acknowledged (3), while concomitantly their safety, especially the fear of delayed and definitive nerve lesions, has been established (4). New developments in continuous techniques with catheter placement along nerve paths and fascial planes open new ways to long-lasting and more limited postoperative pain management. These techniques will, in many cases, replace both catheter techniques in central blocks and intravenous or subcutaneous techniques of patient-controlled anesthesia with opioids.

The objective of this chapter is to describe the most suitable techniques of peripheral nerve blockade, their indications and limitations, the strategy of their use either alone or in combination with other analgesia techniques (multimodal analgesia), and the monitoring of the patients.

RATIONALE FOR USE OF PERIPHERAL NERVE BLOCKADE IN THE MANAGEMENT OF POSTOPERATIVE PAIN

Components of Postoperative Pain and Comparative Efficacy of Techniques of Analgesia

Postsurgery pain is multifactorial. The main causes are

1. skin and muscle incisions, surgical handling of fascias, damage to periosteum and bones (somatic pain),
2. ischemia of mesenteric vessels and digestive spasms (visceral pain),
3. local inflammatory disorders and spinal reflexes (inflammation and neural plasticity),
4. postoperative care, e.g., joint mobilizations, wound dressings, venipunctures (procedural pain and pain on mobilization).

Postoperative pain is a persistent pain that depends not only on central sensitization (5,6) but also on inputs from peripheral sources such as damaged tissues (7,8). Consequently, prevention and treatment of this type of pain should target not only central sensitization, as do narcotics, but also peripheral sources of pathology for as long as these sources are active. This objective can only be reliably achieved by blocking peripheral nociceptive inputs. This is easily ensured by peripheral nerve blockade with either a single-shot or a continuous technique (depending on the expected duration of peripheral inputs). In clinical practice, parenteral opioids and regional anesthetic techniques are equally effective for postoperative pain at rest, whereas only regional anesthetic techniques are effective for pain in the mobilization of patients, procedural pain, prevention of inflammatory disorders, and neural plasticity (9).

Selection of the Best Strategy for Postoperative Analgesia

General Considerations

Although pain is essentially an individual perception and feeling, it is possible to evaluate preoperatively the expected duration and intensity of postoperative pain within acceptable limits for most patients. This is the case at least for elective surgery with the same surgical technique by the same surgeon. In addition, the context significantly influences the techniques used by introducing particular limitations or offering better access to specialized monitoring of the patient. Schematically, the anesthesiologist may be facing three different situations:

1. elective surgery on ambulatory patients (outpatient surgery),
2. elective surgery on same-day (not yet hospitalized) surgical patients who will be admitted to the hospital after surgery
3. emergency surgery or surgery on patients whose physical status is not stabilized or in whom evolving disorders might develop postoperatively.

Outpatient Surgery

Outpatient surgery requires minimally invasive anesthesia, i.e., avoidance of long-lasting agents prone to impair vital functions, especially respiratory and neurologic ones. Currently, the quality of pain relief at home after day-case surgery is not satisfactory in a number of patients, mainly owing to pain despite standard analgesic medications (10–13). Whenever applicable, depending on the site of surgery, a regional anesthesia with local anesthetics only or with the addition of a safe adjuvant (such as clonidine) would be the most effective and safest choice. Intra- and postoperative analgesia is ensured by the same technique, the effects of which are limited to the supplied dermatomes. In most cases, general anesthesia can be lightened, avoiding the use of narcotics and muscle relaxants. Spontaneous breathing can be maintained with or without tracheal intubation. The decision to use a central block procedure (such as a caudal anesthesia) or a peripheral nerve block depends on the location of the surgical field. Whenever possible, a more limited technique is preferable because it requires fewer drugs, is less prone to yield complications, and is better tolerated by the child.

Hospitalized Patients

Patients undergoing major surgery with a planned hospital stay usually require long-lasting analgesia techniques. If they are expected to experience only pain at rest, which is commonly the case after abdominal and urologic surgeries, regional anesthetic procedures (mainly epidural anesthesia) and administration of parenteral narcotics (especially as patient-controlled analgesia) are almost equally effective (14–16). The choice then depends on the local protocols, the quality of postoperative monitoring, and the expectations of the patients and their families because both techniques have drawbacks. Conversely, if pain on mobilization (thoracic surgery, orthopedic procedures) or procedural pain (wound dressings, mobilization of drainages) is expected, parenteral narcotics are not adequate, and regional block procedures are the best choice (17). The decision to use a central block procedure with long-lasting additives (such as morphine) or catheter placement and a peripheral nerve block, also with additives or catheter placement, should depend only on the site of surgery. Currently, only central block procedures are appropriately taught, whereas most residents and anesthesiologists are not adequately trained in peripheral nerve block procedures. This is no longer acceptable because the morbidity of peripheral nerve blocks is consistently less than that of central block procedures (4) and that of parenteral narcotic use.

Emergency Procedures and Patients Prone to Neurologic Complications

Patients undergoing emergency procedures and/or those whose physical status is not stabilized require special attention. Although the basic considerations of pain management itself are the same as for elective surgery, related factors have to be considered. Parenteral narcotics have central effects other than pain relief. These include sedation and respiratory depression that may be detrimental and impair clinical monitoring of patients whose cerebral, hemodynamic, or respiratory status is not stabilized (18,19). Conversely, regional block procedures may require a positioning of the patient, which may be very painful itself or may aggravate actual lesions. There may also be legal implications in the case of neurologic lesions that were not fully evaluated (and documented, preferably in the presence of a witness or by a neurologist) before the performance of the block procedure. Conversely, owing to a more limited action, regional block procedures represent the best strategy for providing analgesia in most patients: they may allow surgery without requiring general anesthesia and do not impair the vital functions of the patients, especially cerebral functions and consciousness.

Principles of Selection of a Peripheral Nerve Block Technique: Single-Shot, Addition of Adjuvants, or Catheter Technique

Peripheral nerve blocks aiming for postoperative pain relief are performed with local anesthetics. In many surgical procedures, a single-shot nerve block is appropriate in terms of both morbidity and duration of analgesia (20–22). The most commonly used local anesthetics are presented in Table 21.1. Lidocaine and mepivacaine are recommended for surgery involving soft tissues, removal of implants, and reduction of noncomplicated fractures. Most single-shot peripheral nerve blocks procedures are applicable to ambulatory patients. Persistence of sensory blockade does not preclude hospital discharge with competent parents, provided motor blockade, if any, has partially recovered. In this case, the potential dangers of delayed identification of a compartment syndrome are minimal, even in the absence of adequate monitoring (which obviously is not recommended), as was reported in two children given continuous epidural infusion of local anesthetics with opioids (23). Motor blockade is poorly tolerated by children, especially infants and young children; it should be avoided when not required for the success of the surgery. Occasionally, motor blockade can result from an unwanted spread of the local anesthetic solution to distant nerves or anatomic spaces. This can happen with ilioinguinal/iliohypogastric nerve blocks where the local anesthetics can reach the ipsilateral femoral nerve. This precludes hospital discharge owing to lower limb motor blockade (see below). Epidural and even subarachnoidal spread of the local anesthetic can occur after a lumbar plexus block. Parents and patients should be advised that these side effects are not frequent and have no detrimental consequences, provided the block procedure is performed in an operating room environment by a trained anesthesiologist.

Long-lasting local anesthetics such as racemic bupivacaine, ropivacaine, or levobupivacaine (24–27) should be selected when longer lasting postoperative pain is expected. Although they do not systematically preclude outpatient surgery, they require adequate monitoring by either the nurses or the parents. The duration of pain relief can exceed 12 hours, sometimes even 18 hours. Precautions should be taken with boisterous children to avoid trauma to anesthetized areas. If there is a possibility that a compartment syndrome is developing, the hemodynamic status of the relevant limb should be carefully monitored. This is best done with hourly evaluations of the temperature and recoloration time of the limb and the mobility of the toes or fingers.

Depending on the surgery, postoperative pain may not be fully prevented or treated by single-shot procedures with either short- or long-lasting local anesthetics only. Concomitant administration of adjuvants may be of great help to prolong the overall duration of analgesia. Apart from epinephrine (see below), clonidine at doses ranging from 1 to 2

TABLE 21.1. *Commonly used local anesthetics for peripheral nerve blocks*

Local anesthetic	Usual concentration (%)	Usual doses (mg/kg)	Maximal[a] dose (plain) (mg/kg)	Maximal[a] dose with epinephrine (mg/kg)	Latency (min)	Duration of effects (hr)
Aminoesters						
Chloroprocaine	2–3	≤7	10	10	7–15	0.5–1
Aminoamide						
Lidocaine	0.5–2	≤5	7.5	10	5–15	0.75–2
Mepivacaine	0.5–1.5	≤7	8	10	5–15	1–1.25
Bupivacaine	0.25–0.5	≤2	2.5	3	15–30	2.5–6[b]
Ropivacaine	0.2–1	≤3	3.5	Not used	5–12	2.5–4[b]
Levobupivacaine	0.25–0.5	≤3.5	4.5	4.5	15–30	2.5–6[b]

[a]Maximal doses are debatable and, in practice, irrelevant; toxicity results from peak plasma concentration of the free unbound form, not from the total dose injected. The maximum doses mentioned in this table are safe when given as single injections, whereas they might or might not be safe after multiple previous injections (or continuous infusion), especially with long-lasting local anesthetics (bupivacaine and probably ropivacaine and levobupivacaine).

[b]May last more than 12, even 18, hours after some block procedures (especially sciatic nerve block).

μg/mL is the most commonly used adjuvant (28). Although no large series of pediatric patients given a peripheral block has been yet published, this addition consistently prolongs the duration of analgesia (29–31) without precluding hospital discharge. This is based on the experience with caudal and epidural anesthesia (32). Part, if not all, of the efficacy is owing to the vasoactive effect on the vessels supplying the nerves (see above). They should not be administered at close proximity to terminal arteries (penile, pudendal, digital nerve, or intraorbital blocks). Occasionally, sensory blockade may last more than 18, even 24, hours, especially after sciatic nerve blocks. Hospital discharge may be debatable in these cases, especially if there is a possibility that a compartment syndrome could develop at home. Basically, any patient at risk of compartment syndrome should be kept under close supervision by trained nursing staff. Temperature and coloration of the limb (or toes), recoloration time, and sensory and motor functions must be systematically and regularly checked, whether or not a nerve block has been performed. Pain is not an early symptom but a late complication, and the diagnosis must be established long before its occurrence, even in a patient deprived of analgesia. If the local conditions are such that a compartment block is highly probable, then the most logical approach would be to continuously measure the pressure in the relevant compartment(s) by inserting an intravenous cannula connected to a pressure manometer (as that used for an arterial line). Alternatively, preventive fasciotomies should be considered.

If long-lasting pain relief is mandatory, placement of a reinjection catheter along the nerve path or within a fascial compartment traversed by the nerve to be blocked (33–36) is probably the most suitable and safest technique. This is the case, although the technique is new with few data available in the literature, especially in pediatric patients. This fascinating technique for hospitalized patients requires that specifically designed devices allowing both nerve stimulation (sheathed needles) and catheter placement are available. It also ensures that appropriate monitoring of the patient is guaranteed, especially with boisterous children and with patients at risk of developing a compartment syndrome, e.g., under a plaster cast.

Multimodal Pain Management Strategies

Because of their efficacy, peripheral nerve blocks provide adequate analgesia in supplied areas for most operations. There are, however, circumstances in which combining different therapeutic approaches for relieving pain results in better efficacy with fewer side effects (37,38). This is especially true when extended or distant lesions are involved. Performing several nerve blocks at the same time may result in systemic toxicity. However, relieving the main source of pain by performing a single nerve block (with or without catheter technique) is safe and can easily be completed by the administration of rather small doses of enteral/parenteral nonsteroidal anti-inflammatory drugs, peripheral analgesics, or narcotics. The adverse effects of both techniques would be considerably reduced, whereas their synergistic effects would result in excellent pain relief. The different aspects of multimodal analgesia are developed in another chapter of this textbook.

ANATOMIC, PHARMACOLOGIC, AND PHYSIOLOGIC CONSIDERATIONS

Structure of Peripheral Nerves

Peripheral nerves are made up of bundles (fascicles) of myelinated and/or unmyelinated nerve fibers ensheathed within connective tissue. Unmyelinated or C fibers consist of small-caliber axons surrounded by a sheath of flat cells resting on a basement membrane, the Schwann cell sheath. This basement membrane is tightly attached to the axonal membrane (axolemma) with which it forms the neurilemma or endoneural sheath. These fibers convey slow pain stimuli to the dorsal horn of the spinal cord.

Myelinated fibers have an additional sheath interposed between the neurolemma and the

Schwann cell sheath—the myelin sheath with regular interruptions, the nodes of Ranvier, where the axonal membrane (axolemma) is directly exposed to the extracellular milieu (39). The nodes of Ranvier enable the saltatory propagation of action potentials (40), thus speeding up nerve transmission as compared with C fibers (see chapter 14). Myelinated fibers are divided according to their diameters, which influence the rate of impulse transmission. A fibers are myelinated rapid conduction fibers. B fibers, myelinated slow conduction fibers, correspond to the preganglionic sympathetic efferent fibers). Efferent A fibers are further subdivided into three groups: A fibers that supply motor innervation to the skeletal muscles, A fibers that supply the extrafusal muscle fibers, and A fibers that supply the intrafusal muscle fibers. Afferent A fibers mainly consist of A fibers that convey impulses from the peripheral encapsulated receptors and A fibers that convey the impulses from various peripheral receptors including nociceptors.

Nerve trunks can be formed by a single type of nerve fibers (pure sensory or motor nerves). Usually they are made of several types of fibers organized as fascicles that are surrounded by their own sheath (41), the *perineurium*, formed by several concentric layers of collagen tissue (Fig. 21.1). Within this sheath, each individual fiber is surrounded by nonneuronal glial cells that form the *endoneurium*. The entire nerve is surrounded by a sheath of connective tissue and tightly joined cells called the *epineurium*, which plays a role as a blood–nerve barrier. The motor fibers (myelinated) typically lie at the periphery, whereas the sensory fibers are situated at the center of the nerve. Because of this arrangement, motor blockade occurs earlier than sensory blockade during peripheral nerve blocks.

These nerve envelopes are not fully differentiated at birth. Myelinization is not fully achieved until the twelfth year of life (42,43). Lack of myelin favors penetration of local anesthetics, a process further enhanced by the reduced size of nerve fibers and the shorter distance between successive nodes of Ranvier. As a consequence, nerve blockade occurs earlier and is more complete, even with administration of diluted solutions of local anesthetics in infants and young children. Ad-

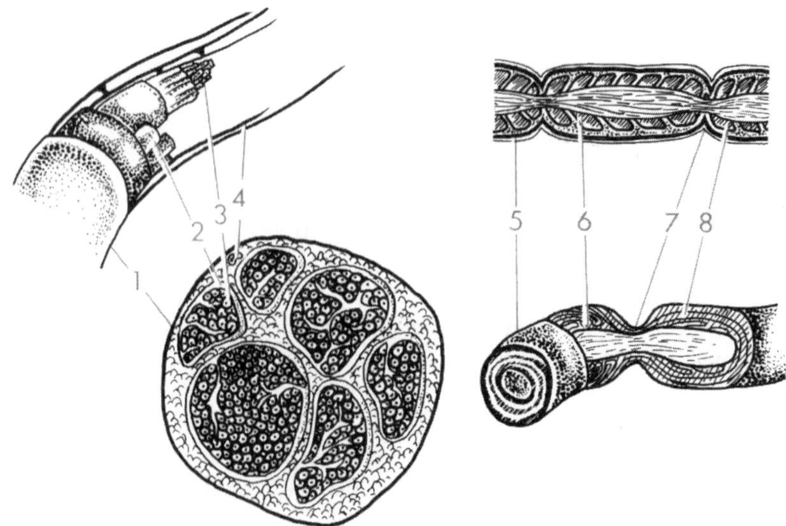

FIG. 21.1. Typical structure of a mixed peripheral nerve. *1*, epineurium; *2*, perineurium; *3*, endoneurium; *4*, arteriole; *5*, Schwann cell sheath; *6*, axolemma; *7*, node of Ranvier; *8*, myelin sheath.

ditionally, the nerve envelopes (epineurium, perineurium) are loosely attached to underlying nerve structures. This favors the spread of local anesthetics along the nerve path and improves the quality of nerve blockade in young patients.

The different nerve coverings, made of connective tissue, have both sensory (nervi nervorum) and vascular (vasa nervorum) supplies (44–47). The vessels, accompanied by C fibers, ramify and anastomose with each other to form an intraneural vascular plexus arranged in four planes parallel to the long axis of the nerve. This vascular network plays a considerable role in the local anesthetic absorption that is greater at the center (well vascularized) than at the periphery of the nerve. After a nerve block, functional recovery occurs earlier in central, mainly sensory, fascicles (which were the last to be blocked) than in peripheral ones, which are mostly motor.

Pharmacologic Considerations

Local Anesthetics

The most commonly used local anesthetics are listed in Table 21.1. Their main pharmacologic characteristics are detailed elsewhere in this textbook. Several properties have to be kept in mind when performing a peripheral nerve block in infants and children. Their local availability depends on the three following factors:

1. their local spread from the site of injection, which is often considerable in infants along nerve paths within the so-called perineural sheaths,
2. their fixation at the local binding sites such as surface proteins and lipids, especially myelin (43,48), which is scarce in infants,
3. the local vascularity on which their systemic absorption depends.

The pharmacodynamic effects depend on the permeability of nerve envelopes. In infants, the endoneurium is loose and easily traversed by local anesthetics in both directions, and therefore nerve blockade develops early and is comparatively shorter lasting than in older children. During the growth of children, there is an enrichment of the endoneurium with connective tissues that makes it less permeable. Consequently, the latency and duration of all local anesthetics increase with age.

Maximal "safe" doses of local anesthetics are rather imprecise because toxic levels of local anesthetics are not clearly established, even in adults. From anecdotal case reports in adults, these maximal safe doses are believed to range from 8 to 10 mg/kg for lidocaine and mepivacaine, 2.5 to 3 mg/kg for bupivacaine, and probably more than 4 mg/kg for ropivacaine and levobupivacaine. After injection of such doses, peak plasma concentrations range from 3 to 5 μg/mL for lidocaine and mepivacaine and 0.5 to 1 μg/kg for bupivacaine (49,50); however, they are not known for ropivacaine. It should be kept in mind that the toxic form of any local anesthetic is the free, unbound form that is difficult to measure and does not correlate with the total concentration.

Additives

Epinephrine is the most commonly used α-adrenergic agonist, usually in concentrations ranging from 1:200,000 to 1:400,000. Its addition to local anesthetics with no intrinsic vasoconstrictive properties offers several advantages: vascular absorption, thus hazards of systemic toxicity are decreased; duration of short-acting local anesthetics (lidocaine and mepivacaine) is consistently prolonged; and accidental intravenous injection can be immediately identified (within 20 seconds) on the electrocardiographic tracings where it results in ST segment elevation, T-wave changes (51–54), and/or occasional heart rate changes. Because ropivacaine has intrinsic vasoconstrictive properties, the addition of epinephrine offers no advantage and might even be detrimental; early detection of inadvertent intravenous injection is not possible unless a test dose with a solution containing epinephrine (or isoproterenal) was previously given, which would significantly complicate the block procedure. The same does not apply to levobupivacaine, but few data are available on this agent.

Clonidine, an α_2-adrenergic agonist, has recently been introduced in clinical practice as a safe additive to local anesthetics suitable for central and peripheral blocks (55–58). Administered in doses ranging from 1 to 3 μg/kg, clonidine consistently increases (usually by a factor of 2) both the intensity and duration of nerve blockade with no perceptible hemodynamic effects in children. After epidural administration and peripheral nerve blocks, the peak plasma concentration of lidocaine, and probably of other local anesthetics also, is significantly reduced (58).

Sodium bicarbonate has been added to different local anesthetics with the aim of increasing their nonionized form, thus improving cell membranes crossing and shortening the latency. However, the clinical relevance of this adjuvant remains controversial (59,60), and in no case does this addition affect the quality of postoperative analgesia.

Peripheral administration of *opioids* along nerve paths and plexuses has led to contradictory results, and the pharmacologic basis of such administration is debatable. In the current state of scientific knowledge, addition of narcotics to local solutions used for peripheral nerve blocks is not recommended in children.

Physiologic and Psychologic Considerations

Entering the operating theater is a stressful experience for any patient but more so for infants and children who in many cases cannot cope with their anxiety. Additionally, children are facing specific limitations. They do not acquire their complete body image until the tenth year of age. They have not mastered language or communication tools nor have much experience of pain to allow them to make comparisons. Therefore, for them, pain is felt more like an "all or none" phenomenon than a perception that can be described in precise terms. Most of the time, they cannot grasp the concept of paresthesia or that of differential blockade (touch is different from pain). For these reasons, nerve trunks and perineural spaces should be located using physical means independent of the child's cooperation (electrical stimulation or loss of resistance technique, depending on the selected technique). Most children do not want to be conscious during surgery and regional block procedures. Light general anesthesia is commonly accepted in pediatrics and has proved to be safe in large series of patients (4). Regional anesthesia is a technique of analgesia, not anesthesia, in pediatrics, and its advantages and inconveniences have to be compared with other available techniques of analgesia, i.e., parenteral opioids.

A pain-free postoperative course has very positive psychologic effects on the patient, his/her family, and the nursing/medical staff. Early wound dressings are free of pain and well accepted, and the first hours after completion of surgery are usually very quiet. However, peripheral nerve blockade may result in adverse psychologic reactions: young children poorly tolerate persistent motor blockade and even the absence of all sensory perception may be considered unacceptable. This anxiety can be attenuated by providing detailed explanations preoperatively to the child and his or her family and by ensuring pleasant environmental conditions postoperatively. In any case, highly concentrated anesthetic solutions aimed at providing motor blockade have to be restricted to patients undergoing surgery in which complete motor blockade is absolutely necessary; in any other circumstances, motor blockade should be avoided by using diluted solutions.

SAFETY ISSUES, CONTRAINDICATIONS, AND COMPLICATIONS

Contraindications to Peripheral Nerve Blockade

General contraindications (61) to peripheral nerve blockade are few. They mainly include infection at the puncture site and allergy to local anesthetics, which is a very rare condition in pediatrics. Bleeding disorders or patients on anticoagulant therapy may represent relative contraindications, mainly for block procedures in which inadvertent vascular penetration is a risk. Degenerative axonal diseases have long been considered as absolute contraindications to performing any regional block procedure, although no data support the hypothesis that such techniques could be an aggravating factor. However, no data support the hypothesis that performing a block is safe and, in cases of medicolegal implications, the anesthesiologist will have to prove that the block performed could not have negatively influenced the course of the illness, which is impossible. Therefore, with such patients, it is often preferable to avoid any form of regional anesthesia unless a written informed consent is obtained, preferably after complete neurologic examination by a pediatric neurologist.

As previously mentioned, patients at risk of compartment syndrome require adequate monitoring of the hemodynamics of the relevant limb (temperature, color, recoloration time). If this clinical monitoring is not available, performing a regional block would be imprudent and must be contraindicated. Parental refusal and severe psychoneurotic disorders should also be considered as contraindications. Specific contraindications are mentioned with the description of the relevant technique.

Conditions for Safe Performance of a Peripheral Nerve Block

Peripheral nerve block procedures are anesthetic techniques; consequently, all the safety rules applicable to the anesthetic management of pediatric patients must apply when a peripheral nerve block is planned (22,61): The block procedure must be performed by a trained and experienced anesthesiologist in an environment that offers all the usual monitoring and resuscitation equipment commonly available in an operating theater, using the same precautions and monitoring as recommended for managing patients under general anesthesia.

Previous establishment of an intravenous line is essential (62), and (automated) control of electrocardiographic tracings, blood pressure, and respiratory rate is the minimal monitoring required. Pulse oximetry, control of body temperature, and, whenever available, measurement of tidal volume and end-tidal CO_2 are mandatory, especially when general anesthesia is concomitantly used in young children. Vital signs, the agents, doses, and techniques used should be recorded on a complete anesthesia chart. Sound selection of local anesthetics and adjuvants and the use of adequate and specifically designed devices (e.g., insulated and noninsulated needles, catheters) are essential.

The technique of injection of the local anesthetic must follow the now well-established safety precautions (Table 21.2). The distribution of anesthesia must be evaluated and the results reported on the anesthesia chart. Adequate monitoring of the patient is necessary both intra- and postoperatively. Patients given single-shot nerve blocks are eligible for outpatient surgery, but hospital discharge should only be permitted when motor function is at least partially restored. Patients at risk of compartment syndrome require specific monitoring of the hemodynamic status of the relevant limb, as previously described. Patients with long-lasting blockade, especially with the catheter technique, require regular evaluation of the distribution of analgesia and sterility of the dressing protecting the catheter.

Sound Selection of Block Needles and Catheters

The devices required for a regional block are rather simple but specific (Table 21.3). Needles specifically designed to perform the relevant technique in children are necessary (22,61). Local infiltrations and field blocks can be safely performed using standard intramuscular needles (21 to 23 gauge and 30 to 55 mm long). Intradermal wheals can be performed with a short (no more than 30 mm long) and thin (25 to 27 gauge) intradermic needle. Compartment and fascial plane blocks (e.g., fascia iliaca compartment block, penile block via the subpubic space, rectus sheath

TABLE 21.2. *Safety precautions for the selection and performance of a peripheral nerve block procedure*

1. When several techniques are suitable, select the safest approach.
2. Obtain informed consent from the parents (even in an emergency, whenever possible).
3. Warn the patient and family about a possible failure of the technique and explain the alternatives that could be used.
4. Select patients carefully, on an individual basis: obtain detailed medical records and family history, perform a preoperative physical examination; when appropriate, obtain complementary (biologic, radiologic) examination or advice or consult other physicians (e.g., neurologist, cardiologist).
5. Apply the safety protocol before and during injection of the anesthetic solution:
   a. Perform an aspiration test before any injection.
   b. Evaluate the effects of a 1–2 mL test dose containing 1 μg/kg epinephrine (or 0.1 μg/kg isoproterenol) on the electrocardiogram tracings and blood pressure.
   c. Inject the local anesthetic at a slow rate (<10 mL/min).
   d. Verify that usual resistance is being felt throughout the injection procedure.
   e. Repeat aspiration during injection (every 5 mL at least) and before each reinjection (when a reinjection catheter is maintained in place).
6. Maintain detailed anesthetic records on a chart (vital signs, techniques and drugs used, stages of surgery, any other relevant information).
7. Maintain a detailed postoperative record: evaluate the distribution of anesthesia, indicate adverse effects and drugs administered, evaluate the return of motor and sensory functions.
8. Monitor respiration and pulse oxymetry of patients given epidural/intrathecal narcotics, preferably in specialized units, for 24 hours. The same postoperative supervision is recommended for interpleural and intercostal nerve blocks.

block) require using a short-bevel needle for precise localization of the corresponding fascial plane, especially where there are several successive fascial planes (63,64). When long-lasting blockade is sought for postoperative pain relief, a larger short-bevel needle that allows insertion of a reinjection catheter if necessary should be used. Although epidural catheters are suitable, their insertion at the inner surface of a facial plane (which is often tightly adherent to underlying structure) is difficult, sometimes almost impossible. Therefore, catheters with a metallic guide are mandatory and considerably facilitate the technique (Fig. 21.2).

Localization of plexuses and mixed nerves should not be performed by seeking paresthesia with standard intramuscular needles because of the danger of direct nerve damage (65,66). Instead, it should be performed by eliciting muscle twitches in supplied territories with a nerve stimulator delivering adequate current intensities, usually in the range of 0.5 to 1 mA. An appropriate electrical stimulus can depolarize a nerve fiber (without damaging it) and initiate an action potential coupled with ionic flux through different membrane channels.

Three factors are essential: (a) the intensity of the electric current with the minimal value, the rheobase, (b) the application time of the electric current measured by the chronaxy, the minimal time necessary to initiate an action

TABLE 21.3. *Recommended needles for local infiltrations and peripheral nerve blocks*

Block procedure	Recommended device	Alternate device
Intradermal wheals	Intradermal needles (25–27 gauge, 25–30 mm long)	None
Local infiltration and field blocks	Standard intramuscular needles (21–23 gauge, 30–55 mm long)	None
Compartments and fascial plane blocks (fascia iliaca, penile, rectus sheath blocks)	Short (30–55 mm) and short bevel (45–55 degree) needles	Epidural needles (intercostal block), neonatal spinal needle
Mixed trunk nerve and plexus blocks	Insulated 21–23 gauge short bevel needles of appropriate length connected to a nerve stimulator (0.5–1 mA)	Unsheathed needles with the same characteristics connected to a nerve stimulator (0.5–1 mA)

A

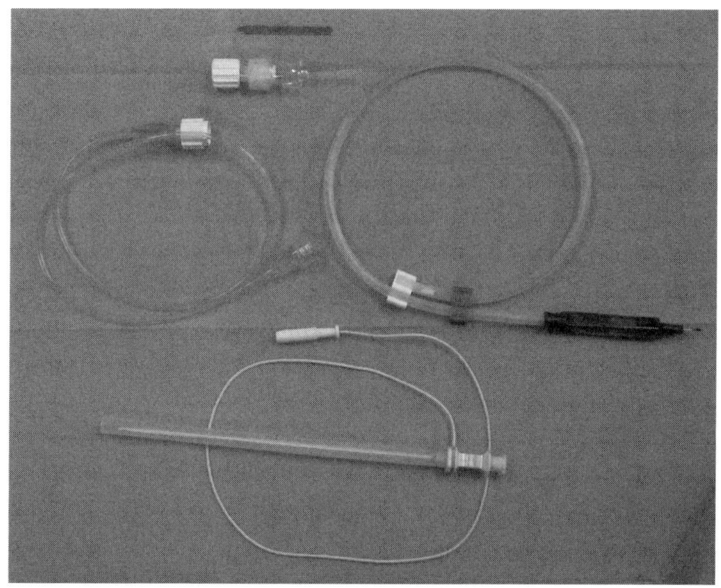

B

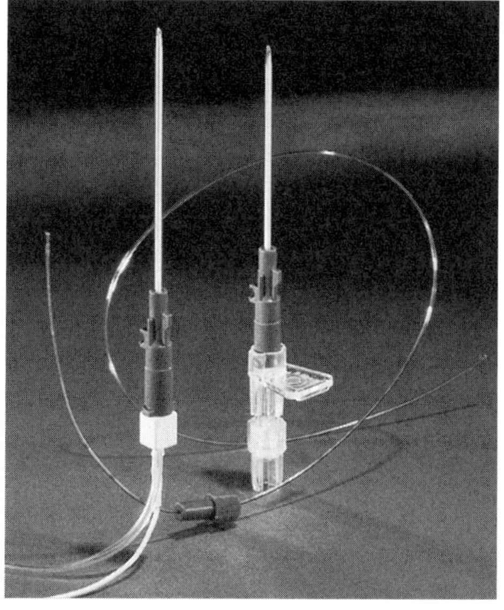

FIG. 21.2. Typical sets for catheter placement along nerve paths and fascial planes. **A:** Set from Pajunk includes a small lancet (for skin puncture point incision), an insulated needle, a catheter with a removable metallic guide (for easy insertion following the Seldinger technique), an extension line for connection to an infusion pump. **B:** Set from Braun (Melsungen, Germany) includes an insulated metallic needle (to be connected with a nerve stimulator) with a cannula and a catheter to be inserted through the cannula after removal of the metallic needle.

potential when a direct current twice the intensity of the rheobase is applied, and (c) the distance between the electrical source and the nerve fiber (transmitted intensity of the electric current is inversely proportional to the square of the distance).

Each nerve fiber has a specific chronaxy that is inversely proportional to its degree of myelination. Because the sensory fibers are less myelinated than the motor fibers, their chronaxy is higher, and, by calibrating the nerve stimulator, it is easy to selectively depolarize the motor fibers (thereby eliciting muscle twitches) without depolarizing sensory fibers (i.e., without eliciting paresthesia or pain).

Although a block procedure can be achieved with unsheathed, short-bevel needles connected to the nerve stimulator (67), using insulated, short-bevel needles is considerably safer and more effective. For most peripheral nerve block procedures, a needle 35 mm long is appropriate; sciatic nerve blocks and direct lumbar plexus blocks require longer needles (as long as 180 mm) in large patients.

From a practical point of view, the nerve stimulator should be connected to a conductive needle, the tip of which acts as the cathode (negative polarity), the anode (positive pole) being connected to the skin electrode, preferably placed distally over the relevant nerve path. The intensity of delivered current is adjusted to 1.5 to 2 mA during the progression of the block needle toward the nerve. When twitches are elicited, this intensity is decreased (to not less than 0.5 mA to avoid any insertion too close to the nerve). Twitches must still be present when the needle is free of any pressure or movement. When this is obtained, the injection of the local anesthetic can be performed following the usual safety protocols. To avoid any misinterpretations, one should take into account only the muscle contractions produced by the stimulation of the nerve at a distance from the site of puncture.

Long-lasting pain relief can be easily obtained if a reinjection catheter is introduced close to the plexus nerves, along a nerve path or within the relevant compartment of a compartment block. When a continuous block procedure is planned, the equipment must be selected carefully. Several devices are available, none of which is currently entirely satisfactory. Continuous compartment blocks (e.g., fascia iliaca compartment block, intercostal nerve block, intrapleural block) require precise identification of the relevant fascial plane and catheter placement. This can be done with an epidural needle through which an appropriately sized epidural catheter can be inserted. Insertion is easier, and it is preferable that a reinforced catheter be used. An alternative method is to use an over-the-needle cannula that is carefully inserted through the relevant fascia (to avoid damaging the tip of the cannula). The blunt, short-bevel needle is then removed. Depending on the location and the desired duration of the block, either the cannula is used as a reinjection catheter or a true catheter is inserted through the lumen of the cannula, which is then removed. Leakage is not unusual when the cannula is removed, but this can usually be fixed by applying a slightly compressive dressing.

Insertion of a catheter along a mixed nerve path requires accurate location of this nerve using a nerve stimulator and an insulated needle. However, most currently available needles do not allow catheter placement. Pajunk (Geisingen, Germany) has released several sets that include an insulated needle, a catheter, and a metallic guide. The technique consists of locating the nerve path as usual, then introducing the metallic wire through the needle to place its tip 1 to 3 cm ahead of the tip of the block needle, then removing the needle, and pushing the catheter over the guide. An alternative is to use the same over-the-needle cannula as for continuous compartment blocks and then connecting the blunt metallic needle to the nerve stimulator. When the nerve is located, the needle is removed while the cannula is tightly maintained in place. Next, a catheter (preferably reinforced) is inserted through the cannula, and the cannula is removed. Both techniques are rather complicated and expensive; furthermore, the progression of the catheter cannot easily be controlled. Nonetheless, this "blunt" placement (as for continuous epidural anesthesia) is clinically successful in most cases. The main problems are not related to a failed technique but rather to the difficulty of protecting the catheter from accidental removal by a pain-free and very active child.

A stimulating catheter has been developed to improve the technique. This catheter tip can deliver an electrical current (when connected to a nerve stimulator) and should be inserted bluntly, as previously described. Then, it is connected to the nerve stimulator to check whether twitches are elicited; if they are, then the block needle is removed, a new control is made, and the anesthetic solution is injected. This (expensive) device offers the possibility of checking the positioning of the catheter hours or days after its insertion in case of delayed failure of the block. The nerve stimulator can be reconnected to the catheter, and, if no twitches are obtained, the catheter is slowly removed until twitches appear again: then a bolus dose is injected, and the infusion line is re-established. This sophisticated device is very interesting from a theoretic point of view, but its practical value in pediatric practice remains to be verified. This is because most of the time, when a catheter-related problem occurs, it is not a slight displacement in an immobile patient but a complete withdrawal by a very active child.

Complications

Performing a peripheral nerve block may result in several complications (Table 21.4), most of which are avoidable by learning the correct technique, using an appropriate device, and applying the basic safety rules.

Complications Owing to the Block Needle

Because block needles are used blindly, they may damage a nerve trunk, especially when the wrong needle is used or when it is imprudently inserted (4,65,66). Vascular lesions may lead to a compressive hematoma. Other tissue lesions such as arterial wounds (68–70) and pneumothorax [especially after interpleural (71), intercostal, stellate ganglion, interscalene, and paravertebral blocks] can be produced by attempted peripheral nerve blocks, the presenting symptoms of which can be delayed by several hours (69).

Complications of the Technique of Nerve or Space Location

Several adverse effects, both minor and major, have been reported. These include electrical burns (use of an inappropriate nerve stimulator) and nerve damage while seeking paresthesia (4,65,66).

Complications of Catheters

Use of peripherally inserted catheters is a recent technique; no complications have been yet reported. However, from experience with epidural catheters, several complications can be expected, such as misplacement, kinking, knotting, and rupture. Leakage around the puncture point is not unusual, as is inadvertent removal. There is also a danger of bacterial contamination. Malfunctioning of infusion pumps may also result in unsatisfactory blockade or true complication.

TABLE 21.4. *Complications of peripheral nerve blockade*

Complications related to the device used
Block needle
Direct trauma to nerve trunks
Vascular damage and potentially compressive hematoma
Technique of nerve/space location
Electrical burns
Nerve trauma while seeking for paresthesias
Catheters
Misplacement
Kinking, knotting, rupture
Secondary migration or withdrawal
Complications due to a faulty technique
Bacterial contamination
Unsafe technique of injection: nerve compression
Injection in the wrong space
Block failure
Inappropriate distribution of anesthesia
Complications owing to the local anesthetic solution
Local toxicity
Use of wrong solution (permanent neurologic damage)
Transient (or long-lasting) neurologic complications with intrathecal use of lidocaine
Complications owing to preservatives, antioxidants, or epinephrine
Systemic toxicity
Neurologic toxicity (seizures, vascular collapse, respiratory arrest)
Cardiac toxicity with bupivacaine mainly (arrhythmias, major vascular collapse)
Allergy
Masking complications where pain can be a warning symptom (compartment syndrome)
Complications owing to adjuvants
Epinephrine
Ischemic disorders
Necrosis (close to terminal arteries)
Clonidine
Sedation

Local and Systemic Toxicity of the Local Anesthetic

Use of wrong solutions (72) or additives (73,74) can lead to definitive neurologic damage that is entirely avoidable. A very effective way to avoid syringe mismatches is to use a specific cart for regional block procedures. Repeated injections of highly concentrated local anesthetics may also result in local myotoxicity (75). Systemic toxicity can result from inadvertent intravascular injection of local anesthetics or from an excessive dose. It may involve the central nervous system, the heart, and the metabolism of hemoglobinemia (methemoglobinemia), although allergic reactions are rare. Several additives in local anesthetic solutions may also produce complications. For example, epinephrine may result in gangrene when injected close to terminal arteries. Clonidine may produce significant sedation, although respiratory depression or severe hypotension is rare in infants and children. Moderate hypotension with or without bradycardia may occur occasionally with large clonidine doses in adolescents or in patients with abnormal vascular regulation, such as patients with renal disease receiving antihypertensive therapies.

Overall Incidence of Complications of Peripheral Nerve Blocks in Children

The above-mentioned list of potential complications of peripheral nerve blockade could give the impression that these regional anesthetic techniques are hazardous. Although few data are available, there is now scientific evidence that the overall incidence of complications during and after peripheral nerve blockade is extremely low. This is contrary to what was commonly believed for many years. The Australian Incident Monitoring Study (72) collected 2,000 claims involving 160 pediatric patients given a regional block procedure. These claims involved 83 epidurals, 42 spinals, four intravenous regional anesthetics, three ophthalmic blocks, 14 local infiltrations, and 14 brachial plexus blocks. Giving details, the authors found that the largest single cause of complications was circulatory problems and that 24 complications resulted from drug errors (including ten "wrong" drugs and 14 "inappropriate uses"). In a 1-year prospective study involving 85,412 pediatric anesthesia cases including 24,409 regional anesthesia (15,013 central and 9,396 peripheral blocks), 23 adverse effects, all minor, were reported; all occurred during central blocks, i.e., none during peripheral nerve blocks (4). In practice, the danger of complications during and after peripheral nerve blockade is low, even extremely low, provided the safety precautions are followed. They compare favorably with central block procedures (although their complication rate is low, especially when compared with the rate reported in adults).

TECHNICAL CONSIDERATIONS

Upper Extremity Blocks

Regional Anatomy

The sensory and motor supply of the upper limbs depends on the brachial plexus that is formed by the union of the ventral rami of the fifth cervical to first thoracic spinal nerve. It is enclosed in a perineurovascular sheath derived from the deep cervical fascia and is carried distally as the limb develops. The perineurovascular space surrounding the brachial plexus nerves is not continuous but is divided into two compartments at the level of the coracoid process of the scapula. Therefore, supraclavicular approaches (within the interscalene space) and axillary approaches to the brachial plexus do not result in the same distribution of anesthesia.

Supraclavicular Brachial Plexus Blocks

Supraclavicular blocks are selected when axillary blocks are not applicable (local lesions at the site of injection, positioning of the patient unsuitable) or not appropriate (insufficient supplied territory). Because the brachial plexus is situated within the extended interscalene space, it can be blocked at various levels, and many techniques have been described. Three basic approaches have been used and reported in children: Winnie's interscalene (76), perisubclavian (77), and paras-

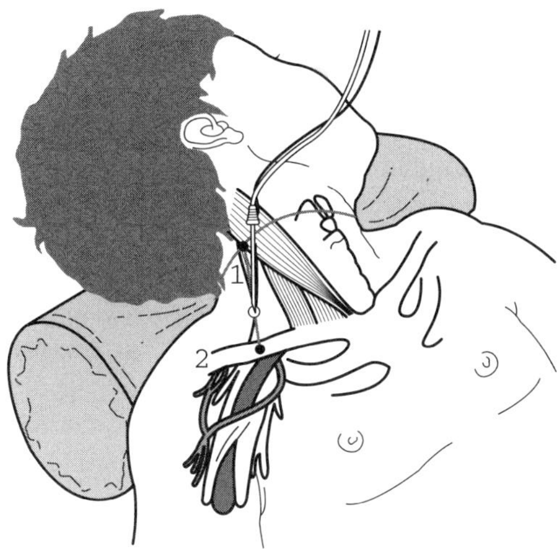

FIG. 21.3. Parascalene approach to the brachial plexus. *1*, skin projection of the C-6 transverse process (Chassaignac tubercle); *2*, clavicle.

calene approaches (78). Only the last (parascalene) approach has proved to be safe in children (78,79) and is described here.

The technique consists of penetrating the interscalene space at a distance from the apical pleura and following an insertion route that would avoid encountering the great vessels of the neck, the vagus and phrenic nerves, the stellate ganglion, and the epidural and subarachnoid spaces. The patient is placed supine with a rolled sheet under the shoulders to extend the neck and stretch the brachial plexus components (Fig. 21.3). The arm is extended along the chest wall and the head turned toward the contralateral side. The landmarks are the skin projection of the transverse process of C-6 in the interscalene groove, at the level of the cricoid cartilage, and the midpoint of the upper border of the clavicle (Fig. 21.3). The needle, connected to a nerve stimulator, is inserted perpendicularly to the skin at the union of the lower third with the upper two-thirds of the line joining the two landmarks until muscle twitches are elicited in the upper limb. An appropriate volume of local anesthetic is then injected (Table 21.5).

A catheter can be introduced within the interscalene space through the lumen of the block needle when long-lasting anesthesia is desired (80); the length of catheter introduced should not exceed 2 to 3 cm and precautions have to be taken to avoid bacterial contamination and secondary dislodgment. The anesthetized area is that area supplied with both the infra- and supraclavicular branches of the brachial plexus. The lower branches of the cervical plexus are blocked in more than 50% of procedures. Almost no adverse effects result from this procedure, although occasionally Horner syndrome may occur in fewer than 5% of patients.

Axillary Blocks

Axillary approaches to the brachial plexus are the most commonly used in pediatric pa-

TABLE 21.5. *Usual recommended volume of local anesthetic for most common peripheral nerve block procedures*

Approach	2–10 kg	15 kg	20 kg	25 kg	30 kg	40 kg	50 kg	≥60 kg
Supraclavicular	1 mL/kg	12.5 mL	15 mL	17.5 mL	20 mL	22.5 mL	25 mL	30 mL
Axillary	0.5 mL/kg	7.5 mL	10 mL	10 mL	12.5 mL	15 mL	17.5 mL	20 mL
Lumbar plexus (psoas compartment)	1 mL/kg	15 mL	20 mL	20 mL	20 mL	20 mL	20 mL	20 mL
Femoral (specific)	0.7 mL/kg	8 mL	12 mL	15 mL	15 mL	17.5 mL	20 mL	25 mL
Fascia iliaca and three-in-one	1 mL/kg	12.5 mL	15 mL	17.5 mL	20 mL	22.5 mL	25 mL	30 mL
Proximal sciatic	1 mL/kg	15 mL	17.5 mL	20 mL	22.5 mL	25 mL	27.5 mL	30 mL
Popliteal	0.3–0.5 mL/kg	5 mL	6.5 mL	8 mL	10 mL	12 mL	12 mL	12 mL

tients and should be considered first because they are virtually free of all complications. Accidental or deliberate arterial puncture is the most common complication. This technique is particularly recommended for anesthesia of the forearm and hand. Several techniques have been described that are all applicable to children. Suitable sites of puncture are shown in Figure 21.4, and most authors recommend inserting a needle at a 45-degree angle to the skin, pointing toward the chest, at the upper edge of the axillary artery (22,61). The needle is advanced until it penetrates the perineurovascular sheath. A characteristic "click" is usually obtained.

With the classic technique of the axillary block, the radial aspect of the forearm, which is supplied by the musculocutaneous nerve, remains unanesthetized in approximately 40% of procedures. To overcome this problem, the author recommends using a puncture site where the lower border of the pectoralis major muscle and the coracobrachialis muscle cross. The block needle is advanced perpendicularly to the skin, pointing toward the lower border of the humerus against which the axillary artery is immobilized by finger pressure (Fig. 21.4). The needle is advanced until twitches are elicited. Alternatively, a needle can be advanced until arterial pulses are transmitted to the needle. Recommended volumes of anesthetic solutions are listed in Table 21.5. Placement of a reinjection catheter is possible and often easier than at supraclavicular levels, but dressing and prevention of accidental removal with arm movements are difficult.

Intravenous Regional Anesthesia (Bier Block)

Intravenous regional anesthesia or Bier block allows intraoperative analgesia of the limb (usually the upper extremity), distal to an inflated tourniquet (Fig. 21.5). The technique is occasionally recommended for a short-duration orthopedic procedure (setting a fracture of the forearm) in pediatric patients (81). Contraindications include extensive wounds, ischemic disorders, unstable fractures, convulsive disorders, septicemia, cardiac dysrhythmia, hypovolemia, and sickle cell disease. The technique consists of inserting an intravenous cannula in a superficial

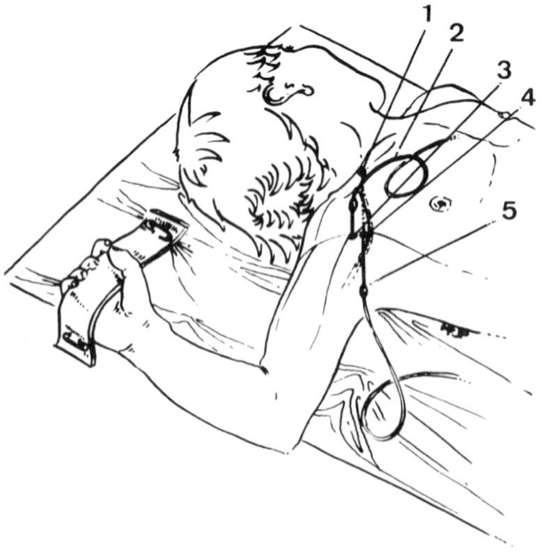

FIG. 21.4. Usual techniques of axillary blocks. *1*, midpoint of the clavicle; *2*, the author's axillary approach; *3*, crossing of the coracobrachialis muscle with the pectoralis major; *4*, axillary artery; *5*, classic axillary approach.

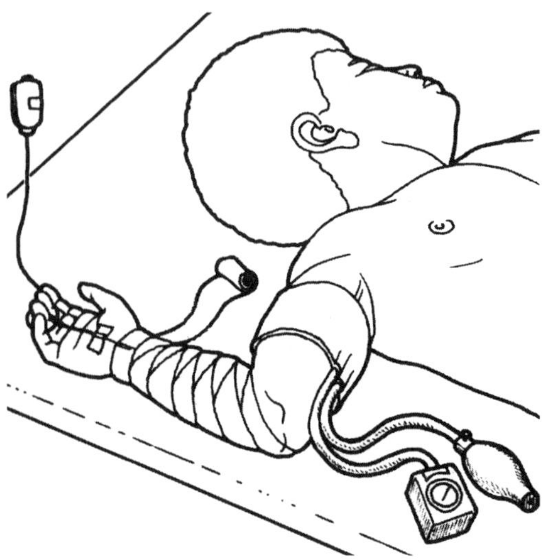

FIG. 21.5. Technique of intravenous regional anesthesia (Bier block).

vein close to the site of surgery. The limb is then exsanguinated, classically with an Esmarch bandage. A tourniquet is placed proximally on the arm and inflated to at least twice the systolic pressure. The Esmarch bandage is then removed and 1 mL/kg (not exceeding 40 mL) of 0.25% to 0.5% plain lidocaine is injected. Ten minutes later, a second tourniquet is placed just distal to the first one (i.e., over an anesthetized area) and inflated to the same pressure values. The first tourniquet is then deflated, and the surgery can begin. Whatever the circumstances, the second tourniquet must not be deflated and removed before 20 minutes and no later than 90 minutes. The drawbacks of this technique are many. Tourniquets are very poorly tolerated by children, and pain returns within seconds after the removal of the tourniquet at the end of the procedure. The quality of analgesia depends on the degree of exsanguination of the limb, and patchy analgesia can result. This is not accepted by children, will make surgery impossible in most cases, and is not uncommon. Accidental deflation of the tourniquet results in systemic toxicity, and fatalities have been reported in children (82). Therefore, the technique of intravenous regional anesthesia should not be recommended for routine use in children, and it should even be contraindicated for lower limb procedures.

Lower Extremity Blocks

Regional Anatomy

The lower extremities are supplied by two separate plexuses, the lumbar and sacral plexuses.

The lumbar plexus innervates the anterior aspect of the leg. Formed by the union of the ventral rami of the first four lumbar spinal nerves, the lumbar plexus lies within the substance of the psoas muscle in a fascial plane limited by the dorsal and the ventral part of the psoas, the "psoas compartment" (83).

The sacral plexus supplies the posterior aspect of the leg; it is formed by the union of the ventral rami of the fifth lumbar to the fourth sacral spinal nerves. It lies on the anterior aspect of the piriformis muscle, behind the posterior wall of the pelvic cavity.

Lumbar Plexus Nerve Blocks

Direct Lumbar Plexus Blocks (Psoas Compartment Blocks)

The lumbar plexus can be approached with the patient in the semiprone position, with the side to be blocked uppermost. Two puncture sites are suitable (Fig. 21.6): (a) the middle of a line extending from the fifth lumbar spine to the posterior iliac spine (84) (modified Chayen technique) or (b) the cross-section of the line joining the two iliac crests with a perpendicular line joining the posterior iliac spine (84,85) (Winnie technique). In practice, the site of puncture as described by Winnie is slightly too lateral, and, therefore, it is recommended to displace it more medially by 1 to 2 cm depending on the patient's age. The block needle is connected to a nerve stimulator and is inserted perpendicularly to the skin until twitches are elicited in the thigh (quadriceps muscle) or leg. Recommended volumes of anesthetic solutions are listed in Table 21.5. When long-lasting pain relief is sought, a catheter can be inserted within the psoas compartment, using an appropriate device (Fig. 21.7). The distribution of anesthesia involves the territory supplied by all lumbar plexus nerves and occasionally by a part of that supplied by the sacral plexus. In some patients, the local anesthetic spreads to the epidural or even the subarachnoid space; therefore, doses of local anesthetics acceptable for epidural anesthesia should only be administered during these procedures to avoid complications. This side effect occurs less often with the newly available block needles, probably owing to a better design of their tip. Placement of a reinjection catheter (86) allows effective continuous (postoperative pain relief) or discontinuous (early joint mobilization) analgesia with fewer limitations than with epidural catheters. For continuous infusion, 5 mL per hour of 0.125% bupivacaine or 0.2% ropiva-

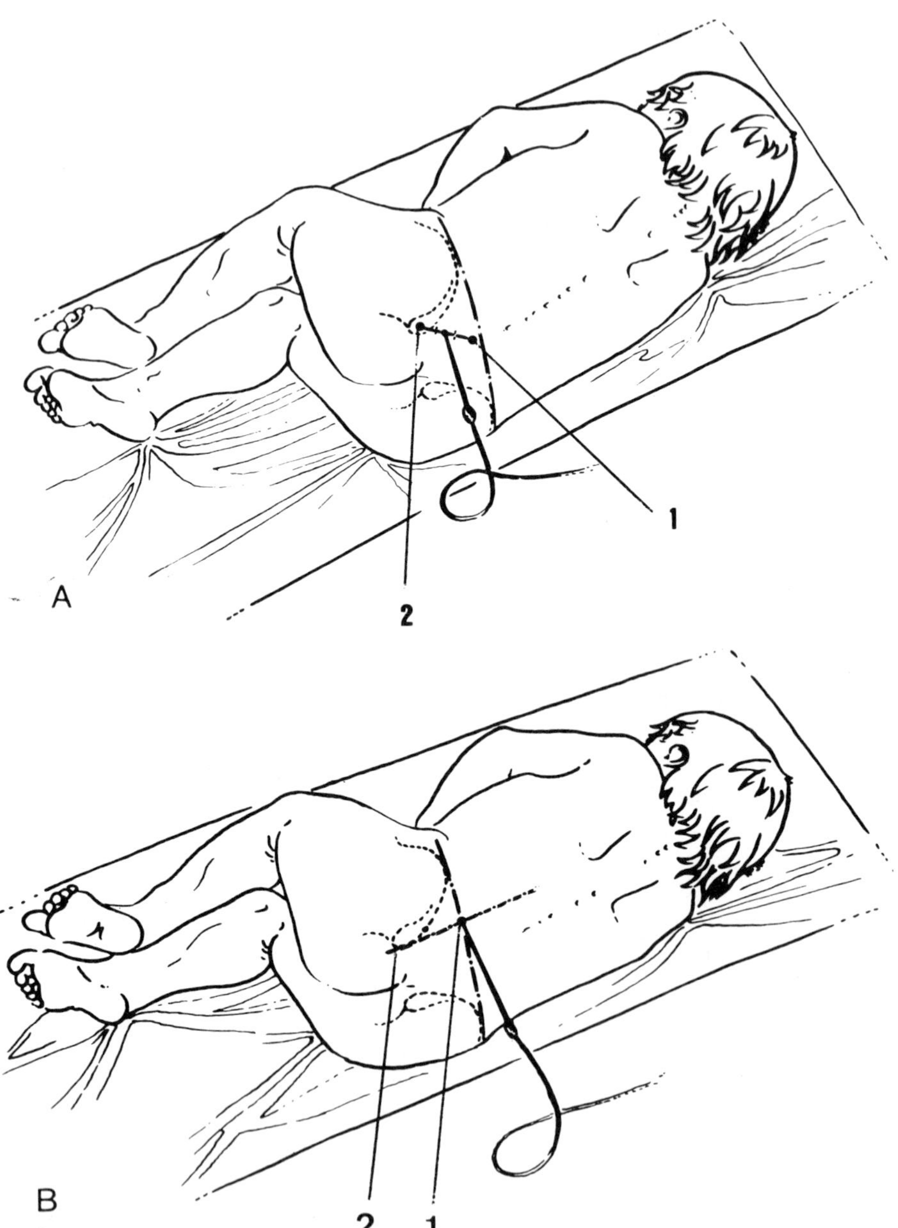

FIG. 21.6. Lumbar plexus block. **A:** Psoas compartment block (modified from Chayen D, Nathan H, Chayen M. The psoas compartment block. *Anesthesiology* 1976;45:95–99). *1*, spinous process of the fifth lumbar vertebra; *2*, posterior superior iliac spine. **B:** Winnie technique (85). *1*, intercristal line; *2*, posterior superior iliac spine.

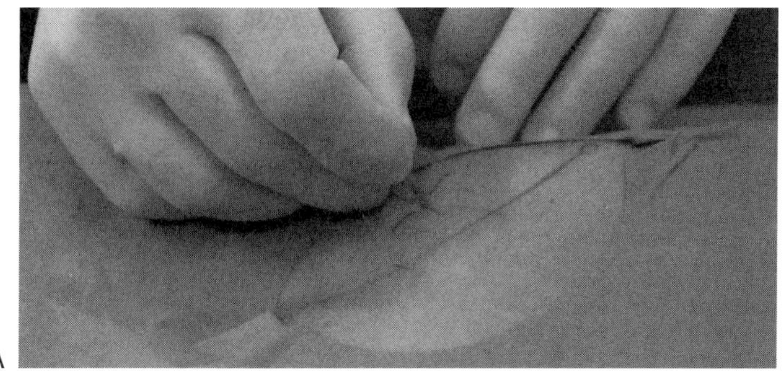

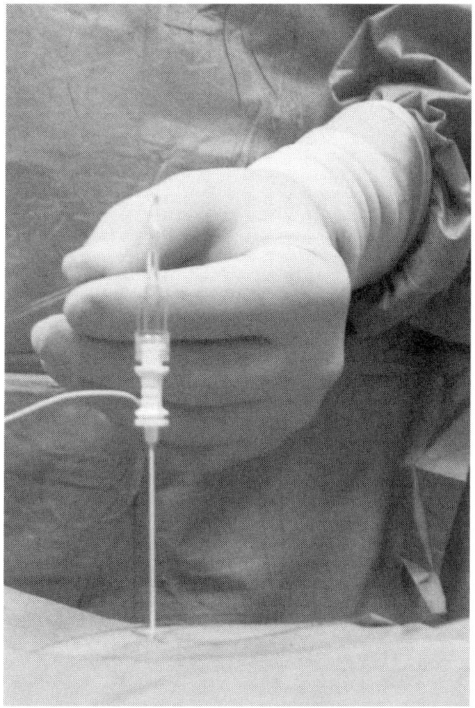

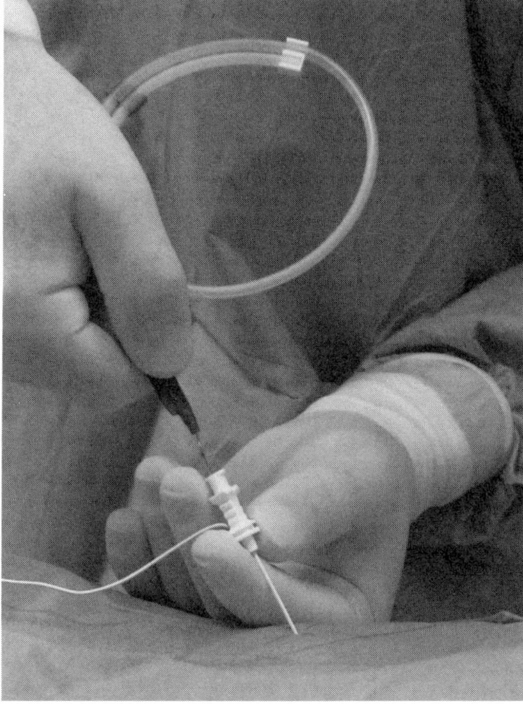

FIG. 21.7. Continuous fascia iliaca compartment block. **A:** Forehole. **B:** Introduction of the block needle at right angles to the skin. **C:** Introduction of the catheter with its metallic guidewire into the lumen of the block needle. (*Continued*).

caine in children weighing more than 30 kg usually provides excellent analgesia; this dose can be adjusted by titration later.

Because of the insertion route, this technique may threaten the pelvic content if performed without sufficient precautions; additionally, there is a danger of epidural spread of the anesthetic solution. For these reasons, indications of direct lumbar plexus block should be restricted to unilateral surgeries of significant importance involving the hip, femur bone and thigh, and knee. The lumbar plexus block can be an alternative to epidural anesthesia in cases in which fascia iliaca compartment or femoral nerve blocks are not deemed appropriate.

Specific Femoral Nerve Block

Femoral nerve block (87–89) is the easiest technique of peripheral nerve blockade with virtually no adverse effects. The technique is

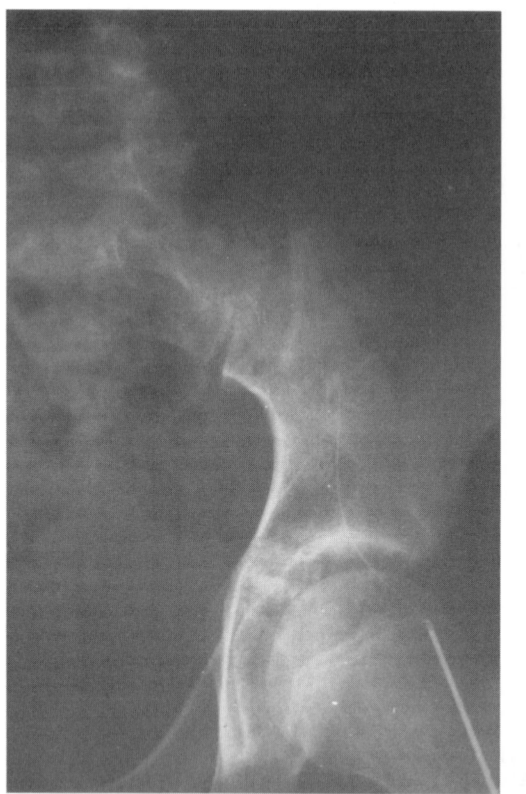

D

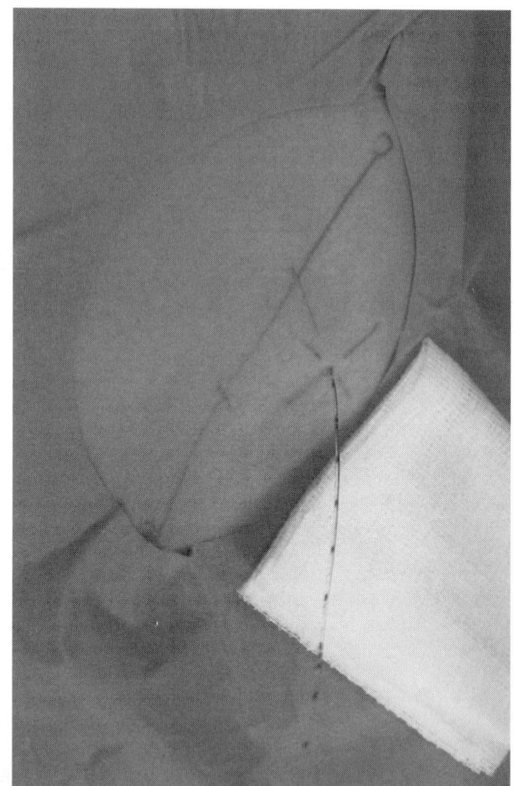

E

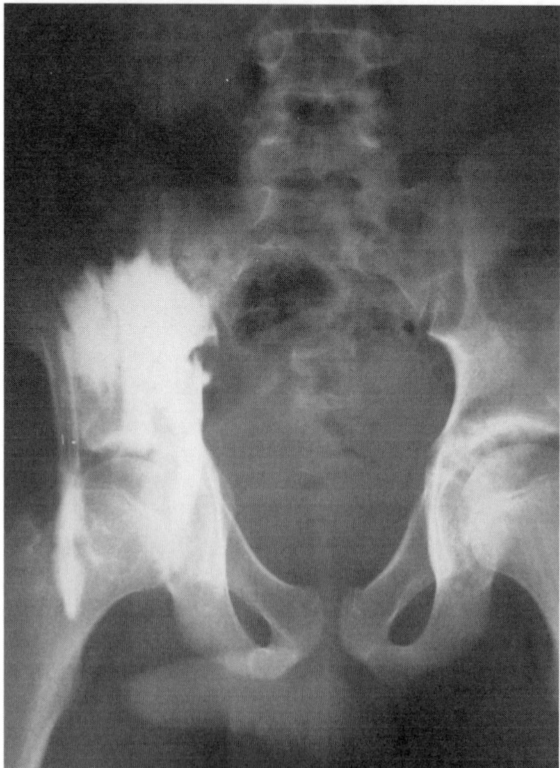

F

FIG. 21.7. (*Continued*). **D:** Control x-ray shows the right positioning of the catheter with the metallic guidewire still inside its lumen. **E:** External view of the catheter emerging from the site of puncture. **F:** Spread of the local anesthetic (with contrast material) along the inner aspect of the fascia iliaca.

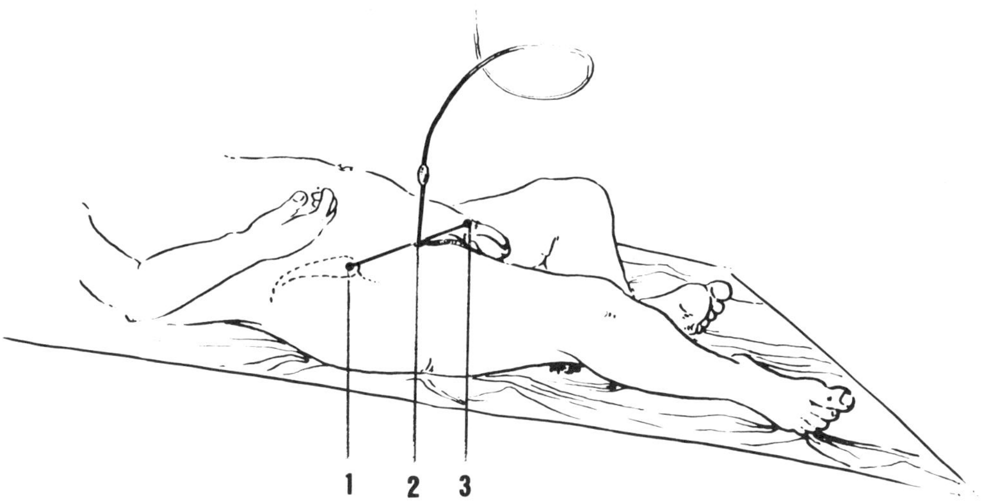

FIG. 21.8. Femoral nerve block. *1*, anterior superior iliac spine; *2*, femoral artery; *3*, spine of the pubic bone (pubic spine).

performed with the child in the supine position. The site of puncture lies 0.5 to 1 cm below the inguinal ligament and lateral to the femoral artery. The needle, preferably connected to a nerve stimulator, is inserted perpendicularly to the skin until twitches are elicited in the quadriceps muscle (Fig. 21.8). Recommended volumes of anesthetic solutions are listed in Table 21.5. The anesthetized area includes the upper aspect of the thigh, the medial aspect of the leg, and the periosteum of the femur. The main indication of this block is pain relief after a femoral shaft fracture, providing excellent analgesia for the application of traction as well as for the necessary and usually painful manipulations of the leg that occur during radiologic examinations. Prolonged analgesia can be obtained by maintaining along the femoral nerve path a plastic cannula or introducing a reinjection through the block needle (90,91).

"Three-in-One" and Fascia Iliaca Compartment Block

The "three-in-one" block (92) consists of injecting the anesthetic solution close to the femoral nerve and forcing it cephalad toward the lumbar plexus. The three-in-one block requires the same position and landmarks as for the classic femoral nerve blocks. Instead of being inserted vertically, the needle is advanced rostrally at a 30-degree (or less) angle to the skin until either paresthesia or muscle twitches are elicited while firm finger pressure is applied on the femoral artery to force the anesthetic upward, toward the lumbar plexus. The success rate is variable: the femoral nerve is almost constantly blocked, whereas the lateral cutaneous and obturator nerves remain unblocked in most children.

Because the lumbar plexus lies within the psoas muscle, all its branches run a significant part of their course at the inner part of the fascia iliaca that encloses both the psoas and iliacus muscles. Thus, injecting sufficient amounts of local anesthetics just below the fascia iliaca should result in blocking all lumbar plexus nerves as a result of the diffusion of the anesthetic solution at the inner surface of the fascia. The same landmarks and position that are used for a femoral nerve block are suitable. A short-bevel needle is inserted perpendicularly to the skin, 0.5 to 1 cm below the union of the lateral with the two medial thirds of the skin projection of the inguinal ligament (93). A first give (with loss of resistance if gentle pressure is exerted on the barrel of a syringe) is felt as the tip of the needle crosses the fascia lata, and then a second one occurs as the fascia iliaca is pierced. After aspirating for blood, the anesthetic solution is then injected. The femoral nerve is almost constantly blocked, whereas the lateral cutaneous nerve is blocked in more than 90% of patients and the obturator nerve in more than 80% of patients. Recommended volumes of anesthetic solutions are listed in Table 21.5. The anesthetized area also includes areas supplied by upper branches of the lumbar plexus in more than 75% of procedures. The fascia iliaca compartment block is extremely easy to perform and safe, and introducing a catheter below the fascia iliaca allows continuous or discontinuous infusion of local anesthetics that permits long-lasting or intermittent analgesia (e.g., for wound dressings, joint mobilization). Continuous infusions are usually performed using 0.125% bupivacaine or 0.2% ropivacaine at rates ranging from 5 to 10 mL per hour; more concentrated solutions and larger infusion volumes can occasionally be administered without significantly increasing the danger of systemic toxicity.

Lateral Cutaneous Nerve Block

The lateral cutaneous nerve block is usually performed to complement a specific femoral nerve block or as the sole block for performing a muscle biopsy. With the patient in the dorsal recumbent position, the needle is inserted perpendicularly to the skin 1 cm below the junction of the lateral one-fourth and the medial three-fourths of the inguinal ligament (94) until it crosses the fascia lata with a characteristic give. Then two-thirds of the local anesthetic are injected in a fan-shaped manner almost parallel to the skin. The needle is then withdrawn, and the remaining solution is injected superficial to the fascia lata. Brown and Dickens (95) recommend inserting the needle above the inguinal ligament, just medially to the anterosuperior iliac spine, until a loss of resistance is felt as the needle enters the canal within which the nerve runs. The recommended volume of local anesthetic is 0.3 mL/kg to a maximum of 10 mL.

Sciatic Nerve Blocks

Sciatic nerve blocks are recommended for operations on the lower leg, including the ventral and lateral aspects of the leg and its periosteum as well as for the foot (94,96). Indeed, there are no contraindications to the use of this nerve block, and the sensory blockade achieved is of comparatively long duration. If bupivacaine is used, analgesia exceeding 12 hours is the rule rather than the exception. Proximal approaches are easier to perform but require long needles and greater doses of local anesthetics. A popliteal approach is technically slightly more difficult to perform but requires less local anesthetic, provides longer lasting analgesia after a single injection of local anesthetic, and allows easier insertion of a reinjection catheter that is easier to dress and maintain in place.

Proximal Sciatic Nerve Blocks

Three proximal approaches are suitable for sciatic nerve blockade. The posterior approach is performed with the child lying on the contralateral side, with the thighs flexed by 90 degrees (Fig. 21.9A). The insulated needle of appropriate size is attached to a peripheral nerve stimulator and inserted perpendicularly to the skin at the midpoint of the line joining the caudal end of the coccyx with the greater trochanter of the femur. It is advanced toward the ischial tuberosity until twitches are elicited in the foot. Anterior approaches were described for use in adult patients in the dorsal recumbent position (97–99). They can be used in children but are more difficult than posterior approaches and may result in complications, such as penetration of the femoral vessels by the block needle. Lateral approaches, equally effective and virtually free of complications, are performed with the patient lying in the supine position (Fig. 21.9B) (96,100,101). The technique consists of inserting the needle horizontally, 1 to 3 cm below the lateral skin projection of the greater trochanter, aiming at passing immediately below the lower border of the femur until twitches are elicited in the foot. Recommended volumes of anesthetic solutions for

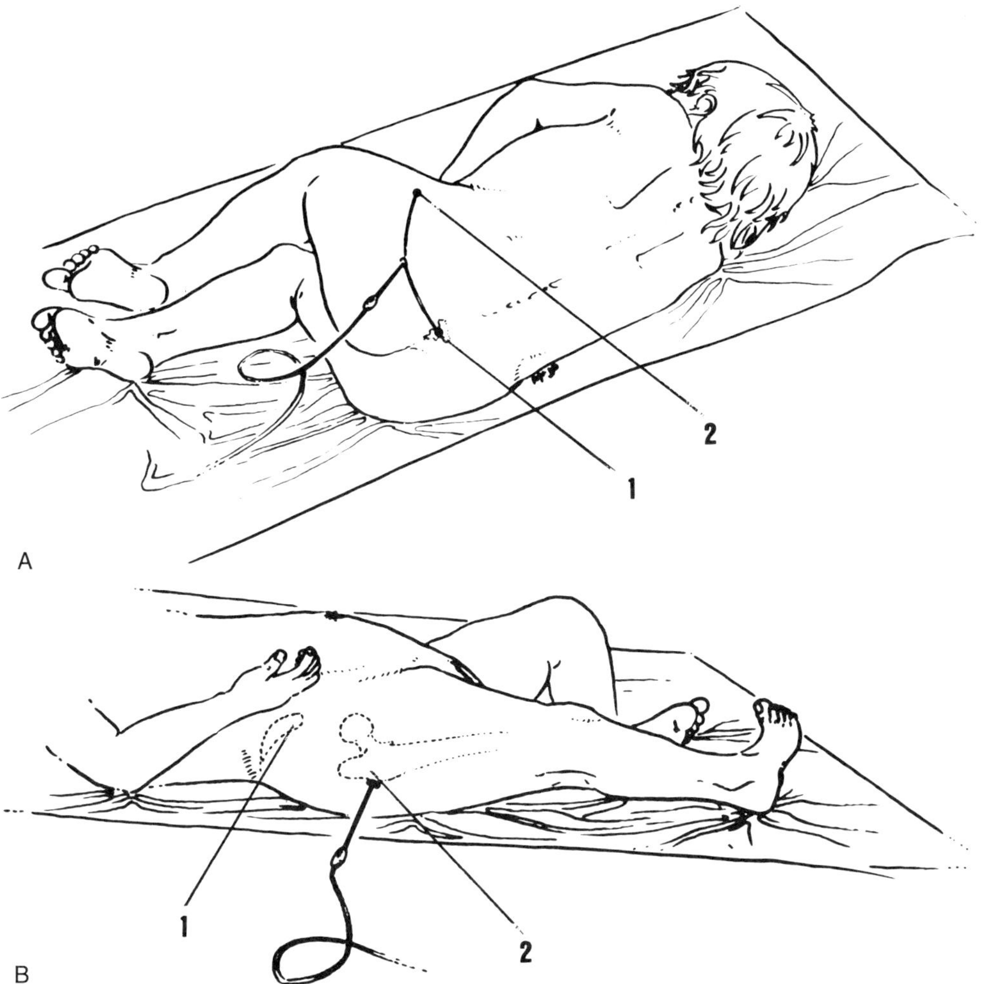

FIG. 21.9. Sciatic nerve blocks. **A:** Posterior approach. *1*, caudal extremity of the coccyx; *2*, greater trochanter of the femur. **B:** Lateral approach. *1*, anterior superior iliac spine; *2*, greater trochanter of the femur.

these blocks are listed in Table 21.5. Using an appropriate device, a catheter can be inserted along the sciatic nerve path, mainly during the lateral approach, to provide long-lasting analgesia (Fig. 21.10). The dressing of the catheter should be very carefully done to avoid secondary displacement, which often occurs inadvertently during lower limb movements.

The distribution of anesthesia is identical to either of these techniques and includes the area supplied by the sciatic nerve and its terminal branches and, in almost all patients, the dorsal part of the thigh that is supplied by the posterior femoral cutaneous nerve of the thigh.

Sacral Nerve Blocks in the Popliteal Fossa

The sciatic nerve and its division branches can be approached at knee level using a single-injection technique because of the presence of a common epineural sheath for these nerves in the popliteal fossa (102). Several techniques have been described (103–105). The simplest one consists of placing the child in a prone or semiprone position, with the

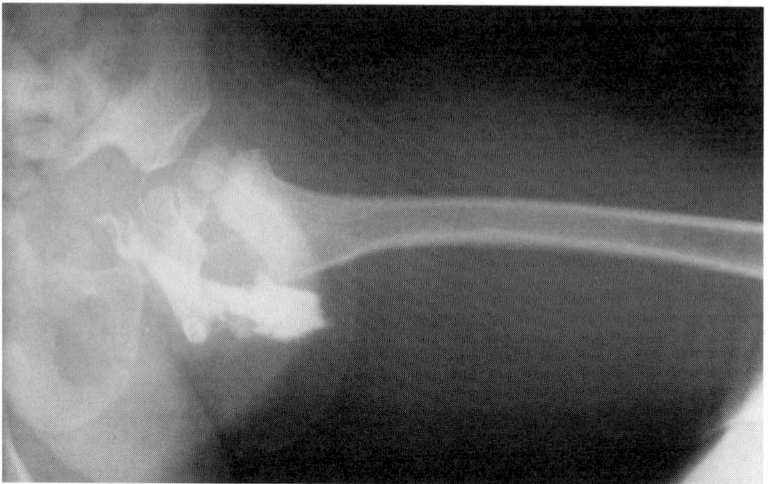

FIG. 21.10. Catheter placement along the sciatic nerve path (lateral approach to the sciatic nerve) and typical spread of the injected solution.

limb to be blocked uppermost, and the legs flexed at a 30-degree angle to make the limits of the popliteal fossa more apparent. The landmarks are the upper angle of the popliteal fossa, the popliteal artery (optional), and the horizontal skin crease of the knee joint. The bisecting line is drawn down to its crossing with the skin crease line. The puncture site lies 0.5 to 1 cm lateral to the bisecting line of the upper angle (and lateral to the popliteal artery), at the junction of its upper fourth with the lower three-fourths (Fig. 21.11A). The needle is inserted at a 45- to 60-degree angle to the skin until twitches are elicited in the foot. The nerves lie below the popliteal membrane, the piercing of which can be identified by a characteristic click that can even be sought by a loss-of-resistance technique. Recommended volumes of anesthetic solutions are listed in Table 21.5. A reinjection catheter can be easily introduced for providing long-lasting pain relief (especially after clubfoot surgery) (Fig. 21.11B).

Trunk Nerve Blocks

Penile Nerve Block

Penile nerve block provides excellent analgesia that lasts for 12 hours or more after penile surgery (except for penoscrotal hypospadias repair) (106,107) with 0.5% bupivacaine. This block is particularly useful for circumcision, whether performed in the newborn or older patient. In older children, the effectiveness of the penile nerve block compares favorably with other techniques such as caudal or topical anesthesia (108). Additionally, penile nerve blocks can be easily repeated if necessary. Alternatively, lidocaine jelly can be repeatedly applied to the surgical wound to provide prolonged analgesia for circumcision (108), but the technique is less reliable and can result in redness and blistering of the foreskin (109). Ring blocks (Fig. 21.12A) can also be alternatively used and are even preferred to the dorsal penile nerve block by some authors (110).

Several techniques have been described in children. Some are potentially dangerous, but approaching the nerves via the subpubic space is easy, safe, and remarkably effective (107,111,112). With the patient lying supine, the block needle is inserted through the two layers of the fascia superficialis (Fig. 21.12B), immediately below the symphysis pubis, 0.5 to 1 cm lateral to the midline (one injection for each side). Because the penis is supplied by terminal arteries, epinephrine

A 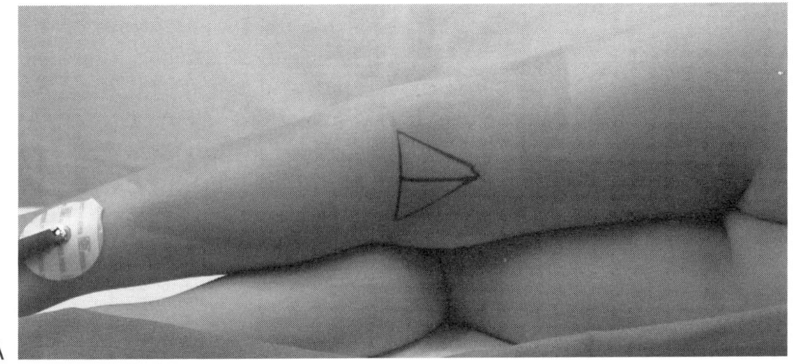

B 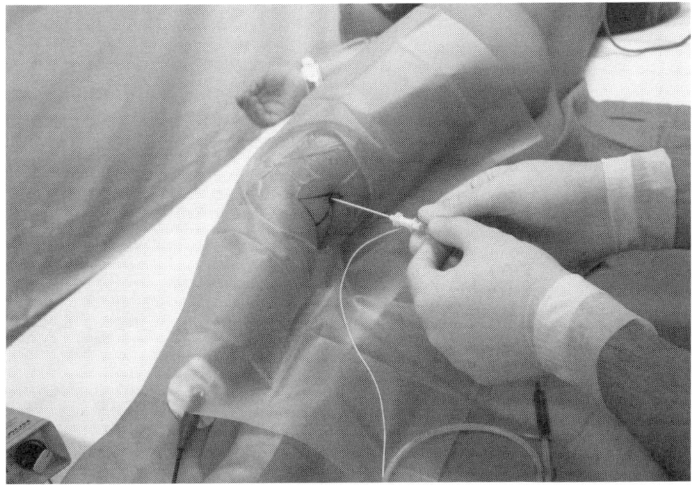

FIG. 21.11. Popliteal block. **A:** Landmarks. **B:** Puncture technique with catheter placement through the insulated block needle.

must not be added to the anesthetic solution. Alternatively, a subcutaneous ring of local anesthetic at the base of the penis can provide consistent analgesia (113). However, rather large amounts of local anesthetic are necessary (2 mg/kg bupivacaine), and inadequate analgesia is reported in as many as 20% of patients. Topical anesthesia has been recommended as an alternative to penile blocks for urethral meatotomy (114) or neonatal circumcision (115).

Ilioinguinal and Iliohypogastric Nerve Blocks

The ilioinguinal and iliohypogastric nerve blocks provide pain relief for operations performed in the inguinal region, such as orchiopexy and inguinal herniorrhaphy (116). Both nerves derive from L-1 and supply the cutaneous sensory innervation of the scrotum, the root of the penis, and the area above the inguinal ligament. Iliohypogastric and ilioinguinal nerve block provides adequate ipsilateral analgesia for intra- and postoperative pain relief of most operations in the inguinal region (e.g., herniorrhaphy, orchidopexy, hydrocele) including emergency procedures (e.g., strangulated hernia with intestinal obstruction).

The block procedure can be achieved with a single-puncture technique with the patient lying in the dorsal recumbent position. The landmarks are the umbilicus and the anterosuperior iliac spine. The puncture site lies at the

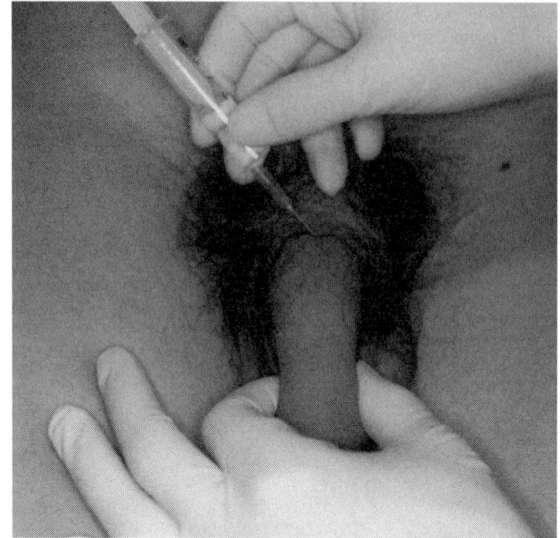

A

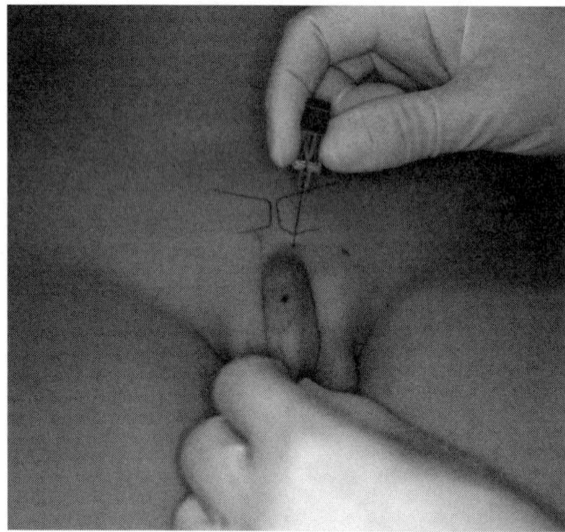

B

FIG. 21.12. Penile blocks. **A:** Ring block in an adolescent. **B:** Penile bloc via the subpubic space (infant).

union of the lateral one-fourth with the medial three-fourths of the line joining the anterosuperior iliac spine to the umbilicus. A short (2.5 to 3 cm) and short-bevel needle is introduced at a 45- to 60-degree angle to the skin pointing toward the midpoint of the inguinal ligament until the external aponeurosis of the external oblique muscle is pierced (often with some difficulty) with a clearly identifiable give (Fig. 21.13). Then, a single injection of 0.3 to 0.4 mL/kg of 0.25% to 0.5% bupivacaine (to a maximum of 10 mL) is made in a fan-shaped manner. The success rate of this technique is high, more than 95%, and the distribution of anesthesia involves the areas supplied by the medial branch of the iliohypogastric nerve, the ilioinguinal nerve, and the genital branch of the genitofemoral nerve. The same quality of blockade can be obtained by infiltrating the cord intraoperatively; however, the first stage of the surgery, until exposure of the cord, requires additional analgesia (usually intravenous opioids) or a consistent deepening of anesthesia.

The technique has no specific contraindications, although one colonic puncture has been reported (117), and no real complications. Undesired nerve block, mainly femoral nerve blocks that may prevent discharge from the hospital for those scheduled for outpatient surgery, is not unusual (118–120). This is a result of the spread of large volumes of local anesthetics at the inner surface of the different fascial planes sought when the classic approach is used (121). A study involving

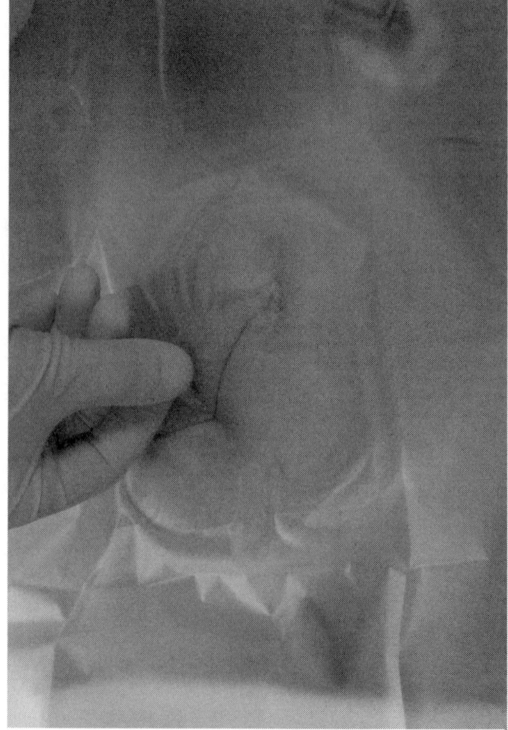

FIG. 21.13. Ilioinguinal/iliohypogastric nerve block (single-injection technique).

30 pediatric patients divided into two groups found unexpectedly high plasma bupivacaine concentrations (without clinical signs of toxicity) in patients weighing 10 to 15 kg, thus causing the authors to recommend not injecting more than 1.25 mg/kg in infants (122). Ropivacaine might improve the safety of the block procedure, but no data are currently available, and this agent is not approved for use for this indication.

Paraumbilical or Rectus Sheath Block

The rectus sheath or paraumbilical block (123–125) provides excellent analgesia of the periumbilical area (supplied by the tenth intercostal nerve), which makes it an ideal block for the repair of umbilical hernias and hernias of the linea alba. The child is placed in the supine position. The landmarks are the umbilicus and the lateral borders of the rectus abdominis muscles (or the line drawn 2 cm lateral to the linea alba on each side). The puncture sites, one per side, are located at the crossing of the outer border of the muscle with the horizontal line passing over the center of the umbilicus (Fig. 21.14). A short and short-bevel needle is then inserted obliquely, pointing to the upper border of the umbilicus at a 60-degree angle to the skin until it pierces (with difficulty) the rectus sheath with a characteristic give. A 0.2 mL/kg-volume of 0.5% bupivacaine, either plain or with 1/200,000 epinephrine, is injected. When the needle is withdrawn, injection of 0.5 to 1 mL of the solution subcutaneously would still improve the quality of analgesia. The same technique is repeated on the other side. This technique is virtually free of complications if the use of sharp needles is avoided, and its success rate is extremely high.

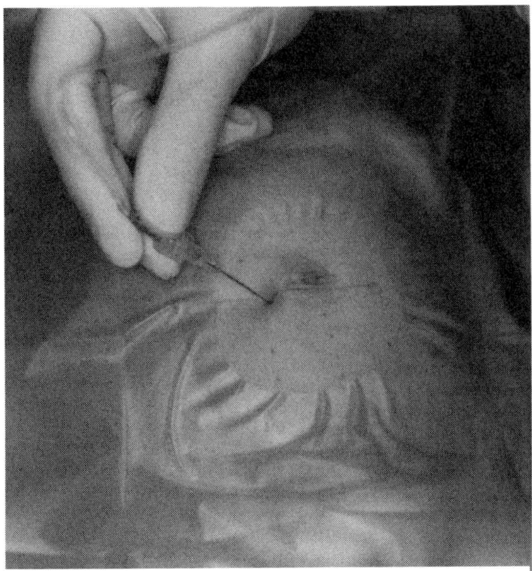

FIG. 21.14. Periumbilical or rectus sheath block.

Intercostal Nerve Blocks

Intercostal nerve blocks can provide excellent analgesia of the chest and abdominal walls, especially for patients with rib fractures or after thoracotomy, liver transplantation, and pleural drainage. Single-shot injections provide 4 to 10 hours of pain relief, particularly if a long-lasting local anesthetic such as bupivacaine is used. Continuous analgesia with indwelling intercostal catheters is also possible (126,127). Intercostal nerve blocks should not be used in spontaneously breathing children with impaired blood–gas exchange. In addition, these patients are not eligible for outpatient surgery because they would require intensive medical observation owing to the danger of clinically delayed pneumothorax.

The safest approach is via the midaxillary line with the child lying semiprone using a short (30 mm), short-bevel, and not too thin (24-gauge or higher) needle; 22-gauge Tuohy needles are excellent. It is mandatory to interpose an extension line between the syringe and the needle. The needle is introduced immediately below the lower border of the rib at an 80-degree angle to the chest, pointing cephalad, so as to pass just below the rib while continuous pressure is exerted on the plunger (Fig. 21.15). Once the skin has been pierced, it has been recommended to redirect the needle dorsally to decrease the danger of pleural damage (128). Entry into the intercostal space is identified by a clear loss of resistance: the progression of the needle is stopped and 1 mL of 0.125 to 0.25% bupivacaine with 1:400,000

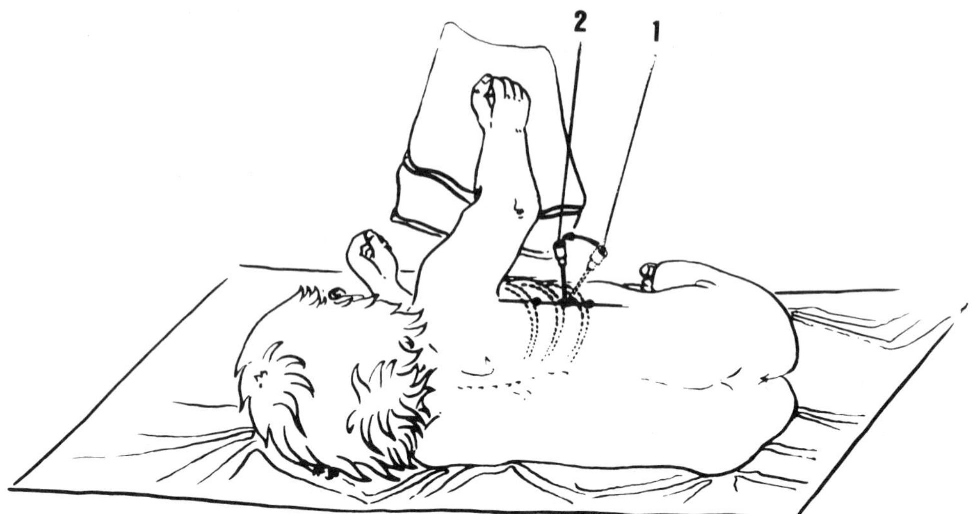

FIG. 21.15. Intercostal nerve block. *1*, insertion of the needle until it contacts the lower border of the upper rib; *2*, redirection of the needle and insertion into the intercostal space.

epinephrine is injected following the safety protocols. This provides long-lasting (8 to 18 hours) analgesia. To obtain adequate distribution of anesthesia, several adjacent intercostal spaces have to be blocked, which increases the dangers of complications.

Vascular absorption from the intercostal space is rapid, almost equivalent to an intravenous injection (129). Thus, only diluted local anesthetics must be administered, and the total dose of bupivacaine should not exceed 2 mg/kg. Great attention must also be paid to the total dose of epinephrine, which must not exceed 4 μg/kg. Ropivacaine will probably replace bupivacaine in the future because of its lower systemic toxicity and intrinsic vasoactive properties, which makes the use of epinephrine irrelevant.

A catheter can be introduced in the intercostal space supplying the center of the area to be anesthetized. When large volumes of local anesthetic are injected, distant intercostal spaces (even contralateral ones) can be reached, thus providing adequate prolongation of pain relief with a single injection in a number of patients. However, a detrimental spread to adjacent paravertebral spaces and to the epidural space can also occur. Regardless of the technique used or the volume injected, all children given an intercostal nerve block must be admitted to the intensive care unit for careful monitoring of respiratory function and delayed pneumothorax.

Thoracic Paravertebral Block

The thoracic paravertebral space extends laterally to the vertebral bodies of thoracic vertebrae. The spinal nerves run a significant part of their course in this paravertebral space where they can be easily blocked (130–133) with a single-injection technique, a safer alternative to intercostal nerve blockade, which requires several punctures.

The technique is performed with the patient in the semiprone position, with the side to be blocked uppermost. Usually, the spinous and transverse processes of T7-9 (T4-6 in case of thoracotomy) are identified, and the puncture site is marked 1 to 2 cm lateral to the T-8 spinous process (Fig. 21.16). The same equipment required for an epidural anesthesia is used: a Tuohy needle, loss-of-resistance (LOR) syringe, and epidural catheter. The needle is inserted perpendicularly to the skin, the stylet is then removed and the LOR syringe is connected before the needle is forwarded while exerting continuous pressure on

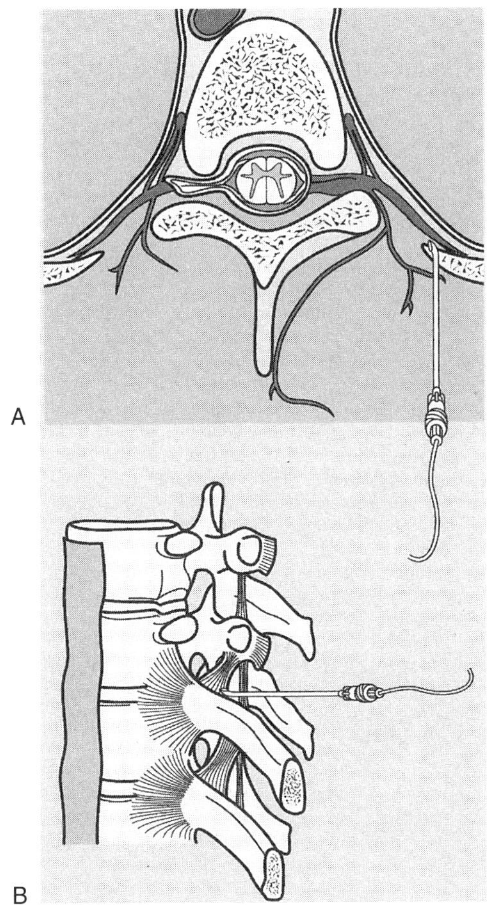

FIG. 21.16. Thoracic paraveretbral space block. **A:** Cross section. **B:** Lateral view.

the plunger of the LOR syringe until it contacts the transverse process. The needle is then "walked" upward along the surface of the transverse process until it passes just above its cranial border, pierces the costotransverse ligament, and enters the paravertebral space with a typical loss of resistance. The epidural catheter is then inserted for 2 to 3 cm (this may require some patience and several attempts) and then securely taped.

The recommended local anesthetic is 0.25% bupivacaine administered at a starting dose of 0.5 mL/kg, followed by repeated injections (same dose) or a continuous infusion of the same local anesthetic at a rate of 0.25 mL/kg per hour. Continuous infusion provides better pain relief than intermittent injections while plasma concentrations remain rather low, for both lidocaine and bupivacaine, at least in adults (134). The spread of the local anesthetic is not uniform so that when contrast material is added to the solution, one can see either a cloud-like and ill-defined spread surrounding the puncture site or a well-delineated laterovertebral longitudinal spread from T-12 to T-6 or above. Even with the cloud-like spread, at least five spinal nerves are blocked, which is usually appropriate. The technique compares favorably with continuous interpleural anesthesia (135). Its failure rate is low and complications are rare (132).

Other Techniques

With the notable exception of dental blocks, nerve blocks involving the nerves supplying the head and/or the neck are not commonly performed in children. Interpleural blocks have been studied, yet their indications remain unclear; their efficacy is debatable and their safety questionable. Topical anesthesia can be effective for postoperative pain relief and is still underutilized. Sprays of local anesthetics can provide analgesia for the tonsillar bed after tonsillectomy (42); the technique is safe if the concentration of lidocaine does not exceed 2% to avoid paralysis of the pharynx, swallowing disorders, and systemic toxicity. Infiltration of muscles and deep fascial wound layers with long-acting local anesthetics at the completion of surgery have been recommended for postoperative pain relief, but as yet has not gained wide acceptance in pediatric practice.

CONCLUSION

Managing postoperative pain in children requires a rational approach that maximizes patient comfort and safety. At one time, it was believed by some that children neither experienced pain nor remembered pain to the same extent that adults do. Additionally, children were considered unsuitable candidates for regional anesthesia because of a perception that performing blocks in children was technically too difficult and because of the exaggerated fear of needles that most children have. We now know that none of this is true.

In managing postoperative pain, several treatment strategies can be envisaged, of which the use of peripheral nerve blockade is one of the most effective and easily manageable. The ability to insert reinjection catheters along nerve paths dramatically improves the flexibility of these techniques. It provides prolonged and limited analgesia with low doses of local anesthetics and has fewer adverse effects and limitations than both central block procedures and systemic administrations of opioids. It provides better comfort for the patient with early ambulation and joint mobilization. Additionally, when these techniques are truly integrated in the pain prevention strategy plan, they not only relieve pain but also prevent pain before it starts. Obviously, prevention is always better than having to treat the myriad negative psychologic and physiologic effects that pain can cause.

REFERENCES

1. Tsui SL, Irwin MG, Wong CM, et al. An audit of the safety of an acute pain service. *Anaesthesia* 1997;52: 1042–1047.
2. Chen PP, Ma M, Chan S, et al. Incident reporting in acute pain management. *Anaesthesia* 1998;53:730–735.
3. Ross AK, Eck JB, Tobias JD. Pediatric regional anesthesia: beyond the caudal. *Anesth Analg* 2000;91:16–26.
4. Giaufré E, Dalens B, Gombert A. Epidemiology and morbidity of regional anesthesia in children—a one-year prospective survey of the French-Language Society of Pediatric Anesthesiologists (ADARPEF). *Anesth Analg* 1996;83:904–912.
5. Hayes C, Molloy AR. Neuropathic pain in the perioperative period. *Int Anesthesiol Clin* 1997;35:67–81.
6. Sorkin LS, Wallace MS. Acute pain mechanisms. *Surg Clin North Am* 1999;79:213–229.
7. Treede RD. Peripheral acute pain mechanisms. *Ann Med* 1995;27:213–216.
8. Coderre TJ, Katz J. Peripheral and central hyperexcitability: differential signs and symptoms in persistent pain. *Behav Brain Sci* 1997;20:404–419.
9. Gentili ME, Mazoit JX, Samii K, et al. The effect of a sciatic nerve block on the development of inflammation in carrageenan injected rats. *Anesth Analg* 1999; 89:979–984.
10. Rawal N, Hylander J, Nydahl PA, et al. Survey of postoperative analgesia following ambulatory surgery. *Acta Anaesthesiol Scand* 1997;41:1017–1022.
11. Kotiniemi LH, Ryhanen PT, Valanne J, et al. Postoperative symptoms at home following day-case surgery in children: a multicentre survey of 551 children. *Anaesthesia* 1997;52:963–969.
12. Beauregard L, Pomp A, Choiniere M. Severity and impact of pain after day-surgery. *Can J Anaesth* 1998;45: 304–311.
13. Grenier B, Dubreuil M, Siao D, et al. Paediatric day case anaesthesia: estimate of its quality at home. *Paediatr Anaesth* 1998;8:485–489.
14. Bray RJ, Woodhams AM, Vallis CJ, et al. A double-blind comparison of morphine infusion and patient controlled analgesia in children. *Paediatr Anaesth* 1996;6:121–127.
15. Lejus C, Roussière G, Testa S, et al. Postoperative extradural analgesia in children: comparison of morphine with fentanyl. *Br J Anaesth* 1994;72:156–159.
16. Mann C, Pouzeratte Y, Boccara G, et al. Comparison of intravenous or epidural patient-controlled analgesia in the elderly after major abdominal surgery. *Anesthesiology* 2000;92:433–441.
17. Moon MR, Luchette FA, Gibson SW, et al. Prospective, randomized comparison of epidural versus parenteral opioid analgesia in thoracic trauma. *Ann Surg* 1999;229:684–691.
18. Kart T, Christrup LL, Rasmussen M. Recommended use of morphine in neonates, infants and children based on a literature review: part 1—pharmacokinetics. *Paediatr Anesth* 1997;7:5–11.
19. Kart T, Christrup LL, Rasmussen M. Recommended use of morphine in neonates, infants and children based on a literature review: part 2—clinical use. *Paediatr Anesth* 1997;7:93–101.
20. Tobias JD, Mencio GA. Popliteal fossa block for postoperative analgesia after foot surgery in infants and children. *J Pediatr Orthop* 1999;19:511–514.
21. Peng PW, Chan VW. Local and regional block in postoperative pain control. *Surg Clin North Am* 1999;79: 345–370.
22. Dalens BJ. Regional anesthesia in children. In: Miller R, ed. *Anesthesia, volume 1*, 5th ed. New York: Churchill-Livingstone, 2000:1549–1585.
23. Dunwoody JM, Reichert CC, Brown KL. Compartment syndrome associated with bupivacaine and fentanyl epidural analgesia in pediatric orthopaedics. *J Pediatr Orthop* 1997;17:285–288.
24. Fanelli G, Casati A, Beccaria P, et al. A double-blind comparison of ropivacaine, bupivacaine, and mepivacaine during sciatic and femoral nerve blockade. *Anesth Analg* 1998;87:597–600.
25. Bertini L, Tagariello V, Mancini S, et al. 0.75% and 0.5% ropivacaine for axillary brachial plexus block: a clinical comparison with 0.5% bupivacaine. *Reg Anesth Pain Med* 1999;24:514–518.
26. Vaghadia H, Chan V, Ganapathy S, et al. A multicentre trial of ropivacaine 7.5 mg x ml(-1) vs bupivacaine 5 mg x ml(-1) for supra clavicular brachial plexus anesthesia. *Can J Anaesth* 1999;46:946–951.
27. Gunter JB, Gregg T, Varughese AM, et al. Levobupivacaine for ilioinguinal/iliohypogastric nerve block in children. *Anesth Analg* 1999;89:647–649.
28. Nishina K, Mikawa K, Shiga M, et al. Clonidine in paediatric anaesthesia. *Paediatr Anaesth* 1999;9:187–202.
29. Bernard JM, Macaire P. Dose-range effects of clonidine added to lidocaine for brachial plexus block. *Anesthesiology* 1997;87:277–284.
30. Reinhart DJ, Wang W, Stagg KS, et al. Postoperative

analgesia after peripheral nerve block for podiatric surgery: clinical efficacy and chemical stability of lidocaine alone versus lidocaine plus clonidine. *Anesth Analg* 1996;83:760–765.

31. Singelyn FJ, Dangoisse M, Bartholomee S, et al. Adding clonidine to mepivacaine prolongs the duration of anesthesia and analgesia after axillary brachial plexus block. *Reg Anesth* 1992;17:148–150.
32. Klimscha W, Chiari A, Michalek-Sauberer A, et al. The efficacy and safety of a clonidine/bupivacaine combination in caudal blockade for pediatric hernia repair. *Anesth Analg* 1998;86:54–61.
33. Mezzatesta JP, Scott DA, Schweitzer SA, et al. Continuous axillary brachial plexus block for postoperative pain relief. Intermittent bolus versus continuous infusion. *Reg Anesth* 1997;22:357–362.
34. Singelyn FJ, Aye F, Gouverneur JM. Continuous popliteal sciatic nerve block: an original technique to provide postoperative analgesia after foot surgery. *Anesth Analg* 1997;84:383–386.
35. Ebert B, Ganser J. Die axillare Plexuskatheterblockade im Kindes- und Jugendalter. [Axillary plexus catheter block in childhood and adolescence]. *Handchir Mikrochir Plast Chir* 1997;29:303–306.
36. Ganapathy S, Wasserman RA, Watson JT, et al. Modified continuous femoral three-in-one block for postoperative pain after total knee arthroplasty. *Anesth Analg* 1999;89:1197–202.
37. Kehlet H. Acute pain control and accelerated postoperative surgical recovery. *Surg Clin North Am* 1999;79: 431–443.
38. Filos KS, Lehmann KA. Current concepts and practice in postoperative pain management: need for a change? *Eur Surg Res* 1999;31:97–107.
39. Landon DN, Williams PL. Ultrastructure of the node of Ranvier. *Nature* 1963;199:575–577.
40. Stämpfli R. Saltatory conduction in nerves. *Physiol Rev* 1954;34:101–112.
41. Thomas PK. The connective tissue of peripheral nerve: an electron microscope study. *J Anat* 1963;97:35–44.
42. Carpenter MB. Development and histogenesis of the nervous system. In: Carpenter MB, ed. *Human neuroanatomy*, 7th ed. Baltimore: Williams & Wilkins, 1976:49.
43. Benzon HT, Strichartz GR, Gisen AJ, et al. Developmental neurophysiology of mammalian peripheral nerves and age-related differential sensitivity to local anesthetics. *Br J Anaesth* 1988;61:754– 760.
44. Sauer SK, Bove GM, Averbeck B, et al. Rat peripheral nerve components release calcitonin gene-related peptide and prostaglandin E2 in response to noxious stimuli: evidence that nervi nervorum are nociceptors. *Neuroscience* 1999;92:319–325.
45. Parke WW, Watanabe R. The intrinsic vasculature of the lumbosacral spinal nerve roots. *Spine* 1985;10:508–515.
46. Mackenzie ML, Allt G. The vasa nervorum: microcorrosion casts for scanning electron. *Acta Anat (Basel)* 1989;136:319–324.
47. Amenta F, Mione MC, Napoleone P. The autonomic innervation of the vasa nervorum. *J Neural Transm* 1983;58:291–297.
48. Rosenberg PH, Kytta J, Alila A. Absorption of bupivacaine, etidocaine, lidocaine and ropivacaine into N-heptane, rat sciatic nerve, and human extradural subcutaneous fat. *Br J Anaesth* 1986;58:310–314.
49. Mazoit JX, Denson DD, Samii K. Pharmacokinetics of bupivacaine following caudal anesthesia in infants. *Anesthesiology* 1988;68:387–391.
50. Dalens BJ, Mazoit JX. Adverse effects of regional anaesthesia in children. *Drug Saf* 1998;19:251–268.
51. Freid EB, Bailey AG, Valley RD. Electrocardiographic and hemodynamic changes associated with unintentional intravascular injection of bupivacaine with epinephrine in infants. *Anesthesiology* 1993;79:394–398.
52. Fisher QA, Shaffner DH, Yaster M. Detection of intravascular injection of regional anaesthetics in children. *Can J Anaesth* 1997;44:592–598.
53. Tanaka M, Nishikawa T. Evaluating T-wave amplitude as a guide for detecting intravascular injection of a test dose in anesthetized children. *Anesth Analg* 1998;86: 952–957.
54. Kozek-Langenecker SA, Marhofer P, Jonas K, et al. Cardiovascular criteria for epidural test dosing in sevoflurane- and halothane-anesthetized children. *Anesth Analg* 2000;90:579–583.
55. Singelyn FJ, Dangoisse M, Bartholomee S, et al. Adding clonidine to mepivacaine prolongs the duration of anesthesia and analgesia after axillary brachial plexus block. *Reg Anesth* 1992;17:148–150.
56. Reinhart DJ, Wang W, Stagg KS, et al. Postoperative analgesia after peripheral nerve block for podiatric surgery: clinical efficacy and chemical stability of lidocaine alone versus lidocaine plus clonidine. *Anesth Analg* 1996;83:760–765.
57. Bernard JM, Macaire P. Dose-range effects of clonidine added to lidocaine for brachial plexus block. *Anesthesiology* 1997;87:277–284.
58. Mazoit JX, Benhamou D, Veillette Y, et al. Clonidine and or adrenaline decrease lidocaine plasma peak concentration after epidural injection. *Br J Clin Pharmacol* 1996;42:242–245.
59. Curatolo M, Petersen-Felix S, Arendt-Nielsen L, et al. Adding sodium bicarbonate to lidocaine enhances the depth of epidural blockade. *Anesth Analg* 1998;86: 341–347.
60. Chow MYH, Sia ATH, Koay CK, et al. Alkalinization of lidocaine does not hasten the onset of axillary brachial plexus block. *Anesth Analg* 1998;86:566–568.
61. Dalens BJ, ed. *Regional anesthesia in infants, children and adolescents*. London: Williams & Wilkins, 1995.
62. Eyres RL. Local anesthetic agents in infancy. *Paediatr Anesth* 1995;5:213–218.
63. Sparks CJ, Rudkin GE, Agiomea K, et al. Inguinal field block for adult inguinal hernia repair using a short-bevel needle. Description and clinical experience in Solomon Islands and an Australian teaching hospital. *Anaesth Intensive Care* 1995;23:143–148.
64. Scott RA, Jakeman CM, Perry SR, et al. Peribulbar anesthesia and needle length. *J R Soc Med* 1995;88: 594P.
65. Selander D, Edshage S, Wolff T. Paraesthesia or no paraesthesia. *Acta Anesthesiol Scand* 1979;23:27–33.
66. Chambers WA. Peripheral nerve damage and regional anesthesia. *Br J Anaesth* 1992;69:429–430.
67. Bosenberg AT. Lower limb nerve blocks in children using unsheathed needles and a nerve stimulator. *Anesthesia* 1995;50:206–210.
68. Zipkin M, Backus WW, Scott B, et al. False aneurysm of the axillary artery following brachial plexus block. *J Clin Anesth* 1991;3:143–145.

69. Vohra A, Tolhurst Cleaver CL. Delayed vascular puncture following axillary brachial plexus sheath cannulation. *Anaesthesia* 1992;47:814.
70. Kaplan R, Schiff-Keren B, Alt E. Aortic dissection as a complication of celiac plexus block. *Anesthesiology* 1995;83:632–635.
71. Stromskag KE, Minor B, Steen PA. Side effects and complications related to interpleural analgesia: an update. *Acta Anesthesiol Scand* 1990;34:473–477.
72. Fox MA, Webb RK, Singleton R, et al. The Australian Incident Monitoring Study. Problems with regional anaesthesia: an analysis of 2000 incident reports. *Anaesth Intensive Care* 1993;21:646–649.
73. Denton J, Schreiner RL, Pearson J. Circumcision complication: reaction to treatment of local hemorrhage with topical epinephrine in high concentration. *Clin Pediatr* 1978;17:285–286.
74. Sara CA, Lowry CJ. A complication of circumcision and dorsal nerve block of the penis. *Anaesth Intensive Care* 1984;13:79–85.
75. Hogan Q, Dotson R, Erickson S, et al. Local anesthetic myotoxicity: a case and review. *Anesthesiology* 1994; 80:942–947.
76. Winnie AP. Interscalene brachial plexus block. *Anesth Analg* 1970;49:455–466.
77. Winnie AP, Collins VJ. The subclavian perivascular technique of brachial plexus anesthesia. *Anesthesiology* 1964;25:353–363.
78. Dalens B, Vanneuville G, Tanguy A. A new parascalene approach to the brachial plexus in children: comparison with the supraclavicular approach. *Anesth Analg* 1987;66:1264–1271.
79. McNeely JK, Hoffman GM, Eckert JE. Postoperative pain relief in children from the parascalene injection technique. *Reg Anesth* 1991;16:20–22.
80. Monzo E, Baeza C, Sanchez ML, et al. Bloqueo paraescalenico continuo en la cirugia del hombro [Continuous parascalene block for shoulder surgery]. *Rev Esp Anestesiol Reanim* 1998;45:377–383.
81. Bratt HD, Eyres RL, Cole WG. Randomized double-blind trial of low and moderate-dose lidocaine regional anesthesia for forearm fractures in childhood. *J Pediatr Orthop* 1996;16:660–663.
82. Heath M. Deaths after intravenous regional anaesthesias. *Br Med J (Clin Res Ed)* 1982;285:913–914.
83. Chayen D, Nathan H, Chayen M. The psoas compartment block. *Anesthesiology* 1976;45:95–99.
84. Dalens B, Tanguy A, Vanneuville G. Lumbar plexus block in children—a comparison of two procedures in 50 patients. *Anesth Analg* 1988;67:750–758.
85. Winnie AP. Regional anesthesia. *Surg Clin North Am* 1975;55:861–892.
86. Chudinov A, Berkenstadt H, Salai M, et al. Continuous psoas compartment block for anesthesia and perioperative analgesia in patients with hip fractures. *Reg Anesth Pain Med* 1999;24:563–568.
87. Tondare AS, Nadkami AV. Femoral nerve block for fractured shaft of femur. *Can Anaesth Soc J* 1982;29: 270–271.
88. Khoo ST, Brown TCK. Femoral nerve block—the anatomical basis for a single injection technique. *Anaesth Intensive Care* 1983;11:40–42.
89. Ronchi L, Rosenbaum D, Athouel A, et al. Femoral nerve blockade in children using bupivacaine. *Anesthesiology* 1989;70:622–624.
90. Johnson CM. Continuous femoral nerve blockade for analgesia in children with femoral fractures. *Anaesth Intensive Care* 1994;22:281–283.
91. Tobias JD. Continuous femoral nerve block to provide analgesia following femur fracture in a paediatric ICU population. *Anaesth Intensive Care* 1994;22:616–618.
92. Winnie AP, Ramamurthy S, Durrani Z. The inguinal paravascular technic of lumbar plexus anesthesia: the "3-in-1" block. *Anesth Analg* 1973;52:989–996.
93. Dalens B, Vanneuville G, Tanguy A. Comparison of the fascia iliaca compartment block with the 3-in-1 block in children. *Anesth Analg* 1989;69:705–713.
94. McNicol LR. Lower limb blocks for children—lateral cutaneous and femoral nerve blocks for postoperative pain relief in paediatric practice. *Anesthesia* 1986;41: 27–31.
95. Brown TC, Dickens DR. A new approach to lateral cutaneous nerve of thigh block. *Anaesth Intensive Care* 1986;14:126–127.
96. Dalens B, Tanguy A, Vanneuville G. Sciatic verve blocks in children: comparison of the posterior, anterior, and lateral approaches in 180 pediatric patients. *Anesth Analg* 1990;70:131–137.
97. McNicol LR. Sciatic nerve block for children—sciatic nerve block by the anterior approach for postoperative pain relief. *Anaesthesia* 1985;40:410–414.
98. Beck GP. Anterior approach to sciatic verve block. *Anesthesiology* 1963;24:222–224.
99. Magora F, Pessachovitch B, Shoham I. Sciatic nerve block by the anterior approach for operations on the lower extremity. *Br J Anaesth* 1974;46:121–123.
100. Ichiyanagi K. Sciatic verve block: lateral approach with the patient supine. *Anesthesiology* 1959;20:601–604.
101. Guardini R, Waldron BA, Wallace WA. Sciatic verve block: a new lateral approach. *Acta Anaesthesiol Scand* 1985;29:515–519.
102. Vloka JD, Hadzic A, Lesser JB, et al. A common epineural sheath for the nerves in the popliteal fossa and its possible implications for sciatic nerve block. *Anesth Analg* 1997;84:387–390.
103. Kempthorne PM, Brown TC. Nerve blocks around the knee in children. *Anaesth Intensive Care* 1984;12: 14–17.
104. Konrad C, Johr M. Blockade of the sciatic nerve in the popliteal fossa: a system for standardization in children. *Anesth Analg* 1998;87:1256–1258.
105. Tobias JD, Mencio GA. Popliteal fossa block for postoperative analgesia after foot surgery in infants and children. *J Pediatr Orthop* 1999;19:511–514.
106. Maxwell LG, Yaster M, Wetzel RC, et al. Penile nerve block for newborn circumcision. *Obstet Gynecol* 1987;70:415–419.
107. Dalens B, Vanneuville G, Dechelotte P. Penile block via the subpubic space in 100 children. *Anesth Analg* 1989;69:41–45.
108. Tree-Trakarn T, Pirayavaraporn S. Postoperative pain relief for circumcision in children: comparison among morphine, nerve block, and topical analgesia. *Anesthesiology* 1985;62:519–522.
109. Holliday MA, Pinckert TL, Kiernan SC, et al. Dorsal penile nerve block vs topical placebo for circumcision in low-birth-weight neonates. *Arch Pediatr Adolesc Med* 1999;153:476–480.
110. Lander J, Brady-Fryer B, Metcalfe JB, et al. Comparison of ring block, dorsal penile nerve block, and topi-

cal anesthesia for neonatal circumcision: a randomized controlled trial. *JAMA* 1997;278:2157–2162.
111. Fontaine P, Dittberner D, Scheltema KE. The safety of dorsal penile nerve block for neonatal circumcision. *J Fam Pract* 1994;39:243–248.
112. Ishigooka M, Yaguchi H, Hashimoto T, et al. Penile block via subpubic space for children who underwent superficial operation of the penis. *Urol Int* 1994;53:147–149.
113. Irwin MG, Cheng W. Comparison of subcutaneous ring block of the penis with caudal epidural block for post-circumcision analgesia in children. *Anaesth Intensive Care* 1996;24:365–367.
114. Cartwright PC, Snow BW, McNees DC. Urethral meatotomy in the office using topical EMLA cream for anesthesia. *J Urol* 1996;156:857–858; discussion 858–859.
115. Maxwell LG, Yaster M, Wetzel RC, et al. Penile nerve block for newborn circumcision. *Obstet Gynecol* 1987;70:415–419.
116. Markham SJ, Tomlinson J, Hain WR. Ilioinguinal nerve block in children. A comparison with caudal block for intra and postoperative analgesia. *Anaesthesia* 1986;41:1098–1103.
117. Johr M, Sossai R. Colonic puncture during ilioinguinal nerve block in a child. *Anesth Analg* 1999;88: 1051–1052.
118. Greig JD, McArdle CS. Transient femoral nerve palsy complicating preoperative ilioinguinal nerve blockade for inguinal herniorrhaphy. *Br J Surg* 1994;81:1829.
119. Notaras MJ. Transient femoral nerve palsy complicating preoperative ilioinguinal nerve blockade inguinal for herniorrhaphy. *Br J Surg* 1995;82:854.
120. Leng SA. Transient femoral nerve palsy after ilioinguinal nerve block. *Anaesth Intensive Care* 1997;25:92.
121. Rosario DJ, Jacob S, Luntley J, et al. Mechanism of femoral nerve palsy complicating percutaneous ilioinguinal field block. *Br J Anaesth* 1997;78:314–316.
122. Smith T, Moratin P, Wulf H. Smaller children have greater bupivacaine plasma concentrations after ilioinguinal block. *Br J Anaesth* 1996;76:452–455.
123. Muir J, Ferguson S. The rectus sheath block—well worth remembering. *Anaesthesia* 1996;51:893–894.
124. Ferguson S, Thomas V, Lewis I. The rectus sheath block in paediatric anesthesia: new indications for an old technique? *Paediatr Anaesth* 1996;6:463–466.
125. Courrèges P, Poddevin F, Lecoutre D. Para-umbilical block: a new concept for regional anesthesia in children. *Paediatr Anaesth* 1997;7:211–214.
126. Downs CS, Cooper MG. Continuous extrapleural intercostal nerve block for post thoracotomy analgesia in children. *Anaesth Intensive Care* 1997;25:390–397.
127. Karmakar MM, Critchley L. Continuous extrapleural intercostal nerve block for post thoracotomy analgesia in children. *Anaesth Intensive Care* 1998;26:115–116.
128. Shelly MP, Park GR. Intercostal nerve blockade for children. *Anesthesia* 1987;42:541–544.
129. Rothstein P, Arthur GR, Feldman HS, et al. Bupivacaine for intercostal nerve blocks in children: blood concentrations and pharmacokinetics. *Anesth Analg* 1986;65:625–632.
130. Lönnqvist PA. Continuous paravertebral block in children. Initial experience. *Anesthesia* 1992;47:607–609.
131. Karmakar MK, Booker PD, Franks R, et al. Continuous extrapleural paravertebral infusion of bupivacaine for post-thoracotomy analgesia in young infants. *Br J Anaesth* 1996;76:811–815.
132. Richardson J, Lonnqvist PA. Thoracic paravertebral block. *Br J Anaesth* 1998;81:230–238.
133. Saito T, Den S, Tanuma K, et al. Anatomical bases for paravertebral anesthetic block: fluid communication between the thoracic and lumbar paravertebral regions. *Surg Radiol Anat* 1999;21:359–363.
134. Catala E, Casas JI, Unzueta MC, et al. Continuous infusion is superior to bolus doses with thoracic paravertebral blocks after thoracotomies. *J Cardiothorac Vasc Anesth* 1996;10:586–568.
135. Lönnqvist PA, Hesser U. Radiological and clinical distribution of thoracic paravertebral blockade in infants and children. *Paediatr Anaesth* 1993;3:83–87.

22

Regional Anesthetic Techniques for Chronic Pain Management in Children

Robert T. Wilder

MANAGEMENT IN CHILDREN

This chapter examines the role of regional neural blockade in common pediatric chronic and recurrent pain syndromes. Included herein are categories of long-standing pain in children in which the pain has considerable adverse influence on the child's daily functions and prevents the child from assuming normal roles irrespective of child's coping ability. An attempt has been made to use an evidence-based approach to the use of regional anesthesia in these settings, but there are often no prospective trials of regional anesthesia in the pediatric age range for these problems. Of necessity, therefore, there has to be extrapolation from the adult literature, where it exists. Additionally, the experience of the author and colleagues is included.

Although it has long been widely recognized that an interdisciplinary approach is necessary for effective management of complex pain syndromes in adults (1), such an approach came later to the management of childhood pain (2). In 1986, an interdisciplinary pediatric pain clinic and pain consultation program was organized at Children's Hospital, Boston, with an infrastructure similar to interdisciplinary adult pain clinics. This service encompasses all subspecialties of pediatric medicine, psychology, anesthesiology, surgery, and physical therapy (3). Regional neural blockade is clearly only one facet of multimodal diagnostic and therapeutic approaches to these complex pain problems. It may be used in the assessment of the source of the pain, as an aid in diagnosis, and for the treatment of chronic pain.

Advantages of Regional Analgesia

Regional neural blockade is effective when medications applied to nerves selectively and reversibly interrupt sympathetic, visceral, and/or somatic neural nociceptive transmission. To the extent that peripheral nociceptive input is contributing to the chronic pain syndrome, such application may be therapeutic. Generally, regional anesthesia is used as a therapeutic option when systemic therapies either have failed to provide adequate analgesia or have excessive, uncontrolled side effects. An effort is made to reduce undesirable effects of regional techniques by manipulating drug dose and site of application and by using combinations of medications to provide additive or synergistic pain control. Low concentrations of some local anesthetic drugs preferentially interrupt the transmission of pain sensation with considerable preservation of motor and other sensory functions. Neuraxial use of opioids or α_2 agonists without local anesthetics can provide excellent analgesia while preserving sympathetic, sensory, and motor function. In some locations, e.g., the lumbar and cervicothoracic sympathetic chains, sympathetic nerve transmission can be blocked by local anesthetics in isolation from somatic nerves. In sympathetically mediated pain states, repeated intermittent injections or short-term continuous infusions of a local anesthetic agent can produce analgesia lasting, for unexplained reasons, far longer than the expected pharmacologic duration of action of the drug. In complex pain conditions involving multiple pain pathways such as cancer or recurrent sickle cell crisis, combinations of medications are administered via indwelling catheters. For more prolonged pain control, chemical neurolytic agents may be used for permanent destruction of pain conducting pathways in the terminally ill child.

Regional anesthetic techniques are also performed for diagnostic purposes. They may selectively block specific neural transmission pathways to allow determination of the origin of the pain and to potentially differentiate sympathetically mediated pain, somatically mediated pain, and central pain states.

Finally, regional anesthetic techniques with local anesthetics may be used for prognostic effects. They allow the patient to experience the effects of loss neural function that result from a permanent neurolytic block or neurosurgical ablative procedure, including numbness and such potential side effects as loss of motor or sphincter function.

General Techniques for Pediatric Regional Nerve Blocks

The basic requisites for successful and safe performance of regional neural blockade in infants and children are similar to those for neural blockade in adults (4). The physician performing such blocks should start with a thorough independent evaluation including review of child's medical history, physical examination, and previous treatments. These lead to a proper understanding the possible mechanism(s) of the child's pain. No invasive procedures should be attempted without parental consent and, if the child is old enough to understand, his or her assent. If the child is very young or if consciousness is altered owing to disease process or medication, then the parent(s) guided by the health care team caring for the child must make the appropriate decision. Meticulous attention must be paid to psychologic preparation of the child and parent(s) for the neural blockade. It behooves the physician to explain carefully how the block is performed and what is expected from neural blockade. This includes what it will feel like after the procedure, such as numbness from sensory block or weakness from motor block, as well as possible complications, failures, and limitations. Thus, it is crucial to discuss with older children and their parent(s) the various risks, consequences, and alternatives to the recommended procedure to allow informed choice.

Performance of a regional anesthetic technique in a child requires either proficiency in the same or at least expertise in the same technique in adults and an appreciation for the specific differences in pediatric anatomy, physiology, and pharmacology. Often required, as well, is the ability to perform sedation or general anesthesia safely in pediatric patients; this is often required because regional neural blockade techniques require needles that children may find quite frightening and generally dislike. This dictates observance of an appropriate n.p.o. (nothing by mouth) period for major nerve blockade or general anesthesia and an assistant whose sole job is the administration of the sedation or general anesthesia, and immediate availability of full resuscitative drugs and equipment. A peripheral nerve stimulator may be useful as an aid for successful location of nerve(s) when the child's cooperation is difficult to obtain in the presence of mental disability, heavy sedation, or general anesthesia (5). Fluoroscopic guidance can be helpful in correct placement of a needle in a variety of circumstances. Fluoroscopy turns a blind procedure into one in which the location of the needle is accurately known. It is useful whenever nerves are not easily accessible such as blocks of the lumbar sympathetic chain or celiac plexus. Fluoroscopy can also help if there is abnormal anatomy (6), distorted anatomy owing to previous surgery (7), or disease processes (e.g., cancer), or poor anatomic landmarks (e.g., obesity). It is required when the precise location of a neural target is essential for permanent destruction (chemical neurolysis). Basically all the principles of neural blockade in adult chronic pain management should be observed with appropriate modifications and meticulous attention to their limitations as applied to children (8).

Regional techniques in children are usually performed using either intravenous sedation or general anesthesia. Many children have a fear of needles and may not adequately lie still to allow safe placement of a block needle. Figure 22.1 demonstrates this fear and dislike. The child has been told that the injection will hurt "like a little bee sting." Note the size of the bees in relation to the size of the child. The syringe is the black object towering over her. The decision to employ sedation or general anesthesia is dependent on the developmental maturity and anxiety of the child. The older, more cooperative child can be rendered comfortable and unaware yet responsive to verbal communication for the safe conduct of regional technique. Such a technique permits assessment of paresthesia and the effect of a local anesthetic test dose. This minimizes the risk of inadvertent needle placement into intravascular and subarachnoid spaces. When general anesthesia is required, signs of misplaced local anesthetic may not be apparent until emergence from anesthesia; however, sedation may not be a safe option in an infant or younger child or any child with severe anxiety, nausea, intractable pain, or severe illness. In these circumstances, general anesthesia may be preferred. This assures an immobile child with a secured airway, so that undivided attention may be directed toward the conduct of the block. As noted above, correct placement of the needle may be aided by use of a nerve stimulator or fluoroscopy with an image intensifier. As an example, central neuraxial catheters, either epidural or intrathecal, for chronic administration of local anesthetics, α_2 agonists, and/or opioids may be safely placed in the anesthetized child under the guidance of an image intensifier and with the position confirmed by contrast epidurography or myelography. Such a strategy provides

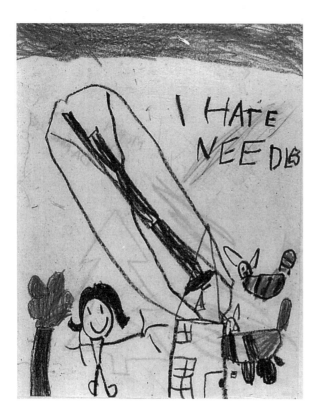

FIG. 22.1. Drawing by a patient indicating her dislike of needles. She was told that it will hurt like "a little bee sting." Note the size of the bees in relation to the size of the patient in the drawing.

the greatest safety and ensures the highest rate of successful placement of the catheter, particularly in an otherwise uncooperative patient and may spare the child another procedure.

Because of the frequent need for sedation or general anesthesia and the requirement for fluoroscopy to ensure optimal needle placement, it is often preferable to use continuous catheter techniques in children and adolescents who might otherwise, as adults, receive a course of repeated injections. In addition to reducing the risk of exposure to anesthesia and radiation, continuous techniques also allow a less anxious, more cooperative child who is better able to fully participate in his or her care. When using continuous infusions of local anesthetics, it is important to understand the pharmacokinetics of local anesthetics in the pediatric population to avoid overdose (9–11). Our experience demonstrates that bupivacaine at rates not greater than 0.4 to 0.5 mg/kg per hour do not cause accumulation or systemic toxicity (11).

Indications for neural blockade in children are essentially the same as in adults. Blocks are employed for diagnosis, therapy, or as an adjunct to other therapies. Their justification, patient selection, and the decision to apply specific blocks in specific pain conditions are discussed under the different pain syndrome sections.

COMPLEX REGIONAL PAIN SYNDROME (REFLEX SYMPATHETIC DYSTROPHY)

Complex regional pain syndrome (CRPS) is a syndrome of chronic neuropathic pain in association with signs and symptoms of autonomic dysfunction. Using the International Association for the Study of Pain definition, CRPS requires the presence of regional pain and sensory changes after a noxious event. Further, the pain is associated with findings such as abnormal skin color, temperature change, abnormal sudomotor activity, or edema. The combination of these findings exceeds their expected magnitude in response to known physical damage during and after the inciting event (12). Clinical criteria for this syndrome have been defined requiring at least two neuropathic pain descriptors and two physical signs of autonomic dysfunction (Table 22.1) (13). Figure 22.2 shows a typical adolescent with CRPS. What triggers the pathophysiologic process of CRPS is poorly understood. The sympathetic nervous system has traditionally been implicated in the maintenance of the pain, although recent work questions this premise (14). Other names CRPS type I include reflex sympathetic dystrophy (RSD), Sudeck atrophy, shoulder-hand syndrome, posttraumatic pain syndrome, and others. Causalgia, which has the same clinical profile but occurs after injury to a named nerve, is properly referred to as CRPS type II.

The exact incidence of CRPS in children is unknown. It was previously thought to be exclusively a disease of adults because many of the older large series included no one younger than 16 years of age. Over the past decade, however, several studies of CRPS in children have been reported (13,15,16). They imply that CRPS in children is probably not as rare as previously thought but that it is often not diagnosed or treated appropriately.

The demographics of CRPS in childhood are different from those in adults. CRPS in

TABLE 22.1. *Signs and symptoms of complex regional pain syndrome*

Neuropathic descriptors	Signs of autonomic dysfunction
Burning	Cyanosis
Dysesthesia	Mottling
Paresthesia	Hyperhydrosis
Mechanical allodynia	Extremity cooler than contralateral by 3°C
Hyperalgesia to cold	Edema

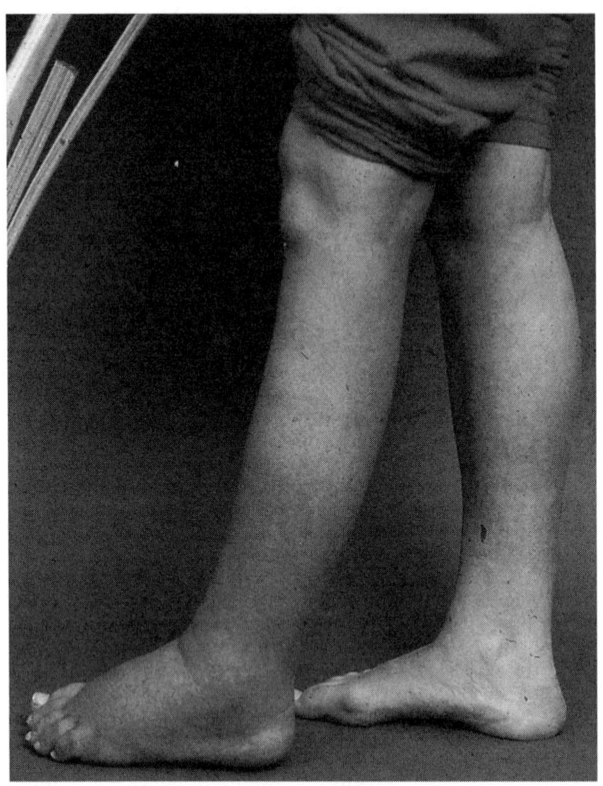

FIG. 22.2. A typical adolescent patient with complex regional pain syndrome of the lower extremity. Note the edema and color change.

adults occurs more often in the upper extremities (17). The ratio of males to females varies between studies, although there is probably a slight preponderance of females overall. In childhood and adolescence, it is seen predominantly in females (M:F = 1:6) and in the lower extremities (lower:upper = 5:1) (18). It tends to occur in highly stressed adolescents who are involved in competitive sports, often from an early age. In their series of 70 children and adolescents with CRPS, Wilder et al. (13) reported that 60 were involved in competitive sports, often of an individual nature. The injuries antecedent to CRPS were most commonly minor sprain, twists, or overuse injuries. Although most of the patients began medical treatment for their injury soon afterward (mean, 10 days), the diagnosis of CRPS was not made until an average of 11 months after the injury. Therapy instituted at that point followed an algorithm that stressed physical therapy, transcutaneous electrical nerve stimulation, and cognitive and behavioral pain management techniques. Neural blockade was reserved for patients not progressing after an adequate trial of the above regimen who required blockade to initiate physical therapy or who developed progressive physical disability on the above regimen.

Because the exact cause of CRPS is not clear, the primary objective of treatment is mobilization of the involved limb actively and passively in regular, aggressive physical therapy (19). Such therapy is crucial to strengthen and restore muscle and joint function. All other treatments are primarily supportive measures designed to attenuate or abolish the pain to facilitate the primary objective: to prevent atrophy and restore normal function. Figure 22.3 demonstrates this concept. Sympathetic and somatic nerve blocks are only part of the multidisciplinary treatment algorithm. They should be used as a means of providing pain relief to facilitate physical therapy, gen-

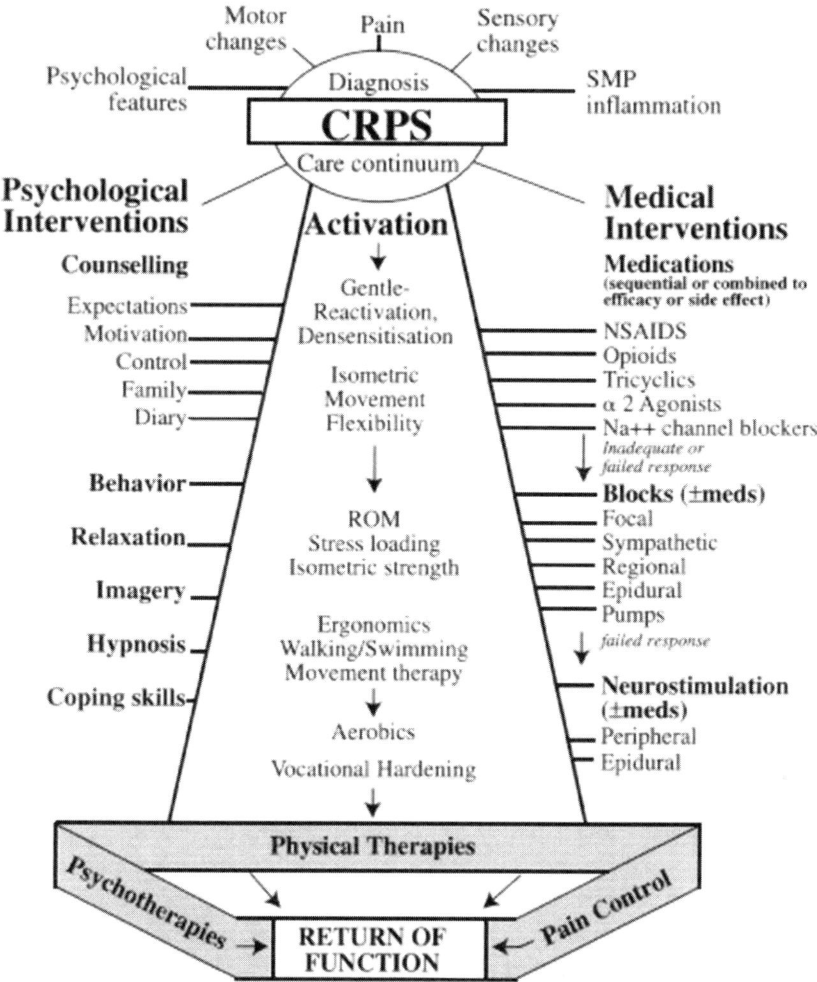

FIG. 22.3. Essential levels of physical therapy governed by progress that is limited only by the degree of pain and successful treatment of pain by using the different pharmacologic or interventional modalities. *CRPS*, complex regional pain syndrome. (From Stanton-Hicks M, Baron R, Boas R, et al. Complex regional pain syndromes: guidelines for therapy. *Clin J Pain* 1998;14:155–166, with permission.)

erally after trials of neuropathic pain medications. It is important to realize that this algorithm was generated by a consensus conference and that there are no controlled studies demonstrating its efficacy. Steroids and nonsteroidal anti-inflammatory drugs are reported to be effective with variable results primarily for an underlying inflammatory condition (20). Transcutaneous electrical nerve stimulation is simple, noninvasive, and acceptable to most children as a means to control pain, but efficacy is inconsistent (13,21). Psychologic counseling is an integral part of the therapy for most children at our clinic to evaluate family dynamics and underlying psychologic factors that may contribute to the genesis or maintenance of CRPS. After initial psychologic evaluation, stress reduction and relaxation techniques, with or without biofeedback, are taught to the patient while additional psychotherapy is provided as needed on an individualized basis (22–24). Tricyclic antidepressants and anticonvulsants have been shown to be useful in the treatment of other forms of neuropathic pain and appear to be quite helpful in this syndrome as well (25). Steroids have also been used with reported success (25,26). Sympathetic nerve interruption with local anesthetics may either reduce or abolish pain in some patients and improve regional blood flow to the limb. In severe cases, adequate pain alleviation is only relieved with somatic nerve blockade.

Sympathetic Blockade

Intermittent or continuous sympathetic blockade may be indicated for the treatment of CRPS that is unresponsive to conservative measures of vigorous physical therapy and adjuvant therapy. If pain is completely alleviated and the autonomic changes reversed by sympathetic blockade, this is indicative of sympathetically mediated pain. If the pain is only partially reduced after the blockade, then the possibility exists that the sympathetically mediated pain is only one component or the condition is advanced. Nevertheless, even partial pain relief may encourage the patient to use the affected limb and participate effectively in a rehabilitation program. Olsson et al. (15) described a technique for predicting who will have a positive response to sympathetic blockade. Phentolamine, a presynaptic α_1 and postsynaptic α_2 receptor blocker, is infused intravenously until the patient develops signs of α blockade such as tachycardia, decreased blood pressure, or stuffy nose. Those who experience a dramatic decrease in their pain are likely to benefit from sympathetic blocks.

For CRPS of the upper extremities, selective intermittent cervicothoracic (stellate) ganglion blockade is performed. The landmarks and technique for the anterior paratracheal approach is similar to that used in adults (27). For children younger than 10 years of age, we usually use general anesthesia because this procedure is more frightening than painful. The safety and success of this block require the child to be completely immobile. We maintain spontaneous respiration with halothane or isoflurane during the procedure because even a small quantity of local anesthetic injected into the cervical subarachnoid space can cause a total spinal block, which may be readily discerned by the sudden cessation of regular respiration. For cooperative and older children, we prefer conscious sedation to preserve the child's cooperation during the procedure.

The landmarks, vital structures near the stellate ganglion, and technique are illustrated in Figure 22.4. A 22- or 23-gauge, blunt, short-bevel needle is appropriate at all ages. After standard sterile preparation, draping, and cutaneous infiltration of local anesthetic, the carotid artery and jugular vein are retracted laterally, and the needle is advanced in a coronal plane until it contacts the anterior tubercle of sixth cervical vertebra. The needle should be attached to a saline-filled syringe via flexible tubing to identify loss of resistance anterior to the longus colli and prevertebral fascia and to confirm lack of blood return. Subsequently, 1% lidocaine plain solution is given in four to six increments of 0.1 mL each to test for intravascular effect. If the needle is in the vertebral artery, the most feared complication, even a few milligrams of lidocaine can cause grand

FIG. 22.4. Block of the cervicothoracic or the stellate ganglion. **A:** General disposition (deep plane); **B:** Transverse section; **C:** cutaneous landmarks; **D:** puncture technique; **E:** needle orientation (transverse section at C-6 level). *1*, longus colli muscle; *2*, middle cervical ganglion; *3*, vertebral body and transverse process of C-6; *4*, cervicothoracic (stellate) ganglion; *5*, esophagus; *6*, trachea; *7*, apical pleura; *8*, brachial plexus; *9*, tubercle of the first rib; *10*, anterior scalene muscle; *11*, anterior ramus of C-7 root; *12*, vertebral artery; *13*, neck of the first rib; *14*, first thoracic ganglion; *15*, subclavian artery; *16*, cardiac branch; *17*, subclavian loop; *18*, inferior thyroid veins; *19*, inferior thyroid arteries; *20*, components of the brachial plexus; *21*, Chassaignac tubercle; *22*, common carotid artery; *23*, internal jugular vein; *24*, vagus nerve (X); *25*, sternocleidomastoid muscle; *26*, thyroid. (From Dalens B. *Regional anesthesia in infants, children, and adolescents.* London: Williams & Wilkins Waverly Europe; 1995, with permission.)

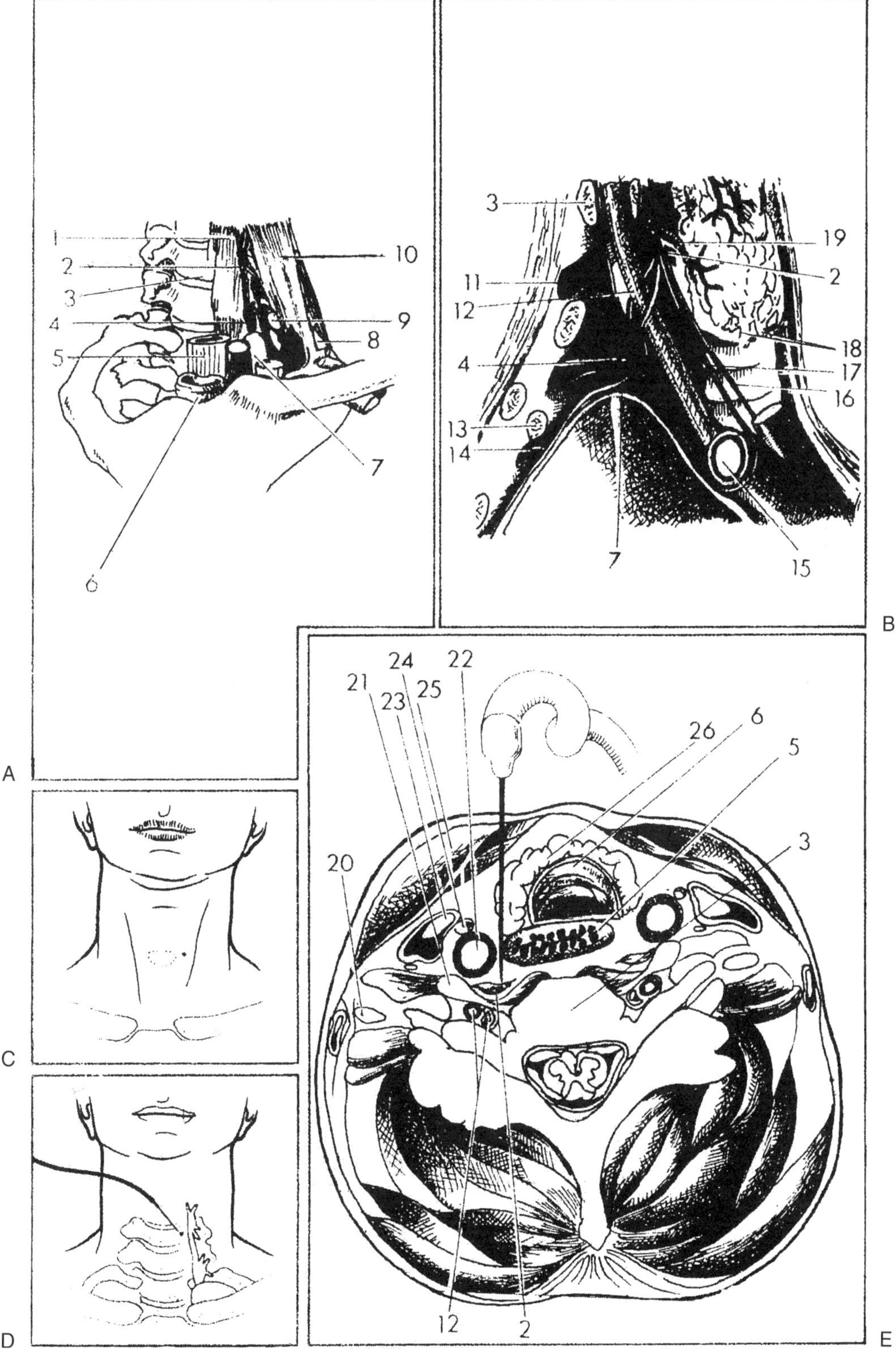
1
2
3
4
5
6
7
8
9
10
A
3
19
2
11
12
18
4
17
16
13
14
7
15
B
C
D
24
22
21
23
25
26
6
5
20
3
12
2
E

mal seizures. The patient is instructed not to speak but rather to answer questions regarding symptoms of systemic effect with finger signals for yes or no. It is useful to have an assistant change syringes and inject the solutions. After successful test-dosing, we slowly inject 0.2 mL/kg of 0.25% plain bupivacaine solution to a maximum of 14 mL (28).

Continuous sympathetic blockade is preferable for children who require repeated general anesthetic for the performance of stellate blockade. In addition to the factors listed in the introduction, the postoperative sedation will interfere with active physical therapy during the immediate post-block pain-free period, and the success rate may not be the same with repeated blocks. There are numerous techniques employed in adults for continuous stellate ganglion blockade via an indwelling catheter placed either by an anterior approach for stellate block (29,30) or by brachial plexus blockade (31). The disadvantages of the former technique are inconvenience and easy dislodgement of the catheter with neck movements. The latter technique is associated with upper extremity somatic nerve blockade that may hinder active physical therapy. Reiestad et al. (32) reported the use of interpleural technique for control of CRPS pain of the upper extremities in adults. The interpleural stellate sympathetic blockade is associated with intercostal nerve blockade and slight, if any, brachial plexus blockade.

The technique of percutaneous interpleural catheter placement in children is similar to that described in adults (32). The procedure is performed in the lateral decubitus position with the affected side nondependent. The interpleural space is identified in a spontaneously breathing child who is either awake or anesthetized with an inhalational agent. The catheter is introduced in the fourth intercostal space, and, under fluoroscopic guidance, it is directed cephalad and posterior until the catheter tip reaches T1-2 vertebral body. The catheter position is confirmed with the injection of radiocontrast agent (Omnipaque 180). A chest x-ray should be taken a few hours after the procedure to rule out pneumothorax. The child is hospitalized and the catheter is injected twice a day with bupivacaine solution. Before each injection, the child is placed in the lateral decubitus position with the affected side up and the head down approximately 15 degrees to favor cephalad pooling of the injected solution. The catheter is aspirated for air and blood before slow administration of 0.8 mL/kg of 0.25% plain bupivacaine solution over 10 minutes. The child is observed for 30 minutes for any adverse effects and evidence of successful sympathetic blockade (e.g., ipsilateral Horner signs, change in the skin color and temperature of the extremity).

For the treatment of CRPS of the lower extremities, continuous lumbar paravertebral sympathetic blockade is preferable for much the same reasons stated in upper extremity sympathetic blockade. Continuous lumbar epidural blockade also has advantages over continuous epidural blockade: (a) selective sympathetic blockade confirms that the pain is sympathetically mediated and (b) selective sympathetic blockade preserves protective reflexes and does not interfere with bowel and bladder function, ambulation, or cooperation with active physical therapy.

For lumbar sympathetic blockade, passage of the needle can be more painful than for stellate blockade, but less patient cooperation is required. Therefore, heavier sedation and analgesia can be used and is desirable.

The patient is placed in the lateral decubitus position with the affected side up. After standard sterile preparation, drape, and subcutaneous infiltration of local anesthetic, an 18-gauge Tuohy epidural needle 12 cm in length is used. The needle is introduced approximately 4 to 5 cm lateral to the second or third lumbar spinous process, just lateral to the edge of the erector spinae muscles (33). Figure 22.5 demonstrates the landmarks and correct needle placement. The needle is advanced anteromedially until contact is made with the lateral border of the vertebral body. Further advancement is made slowly under the guidance of the image intensifier to position the needle tip at the anteromedial border of the vertebral body where the sympathetic chain lies. With fluoroscopy, the needle tip should appear to lie anterior to

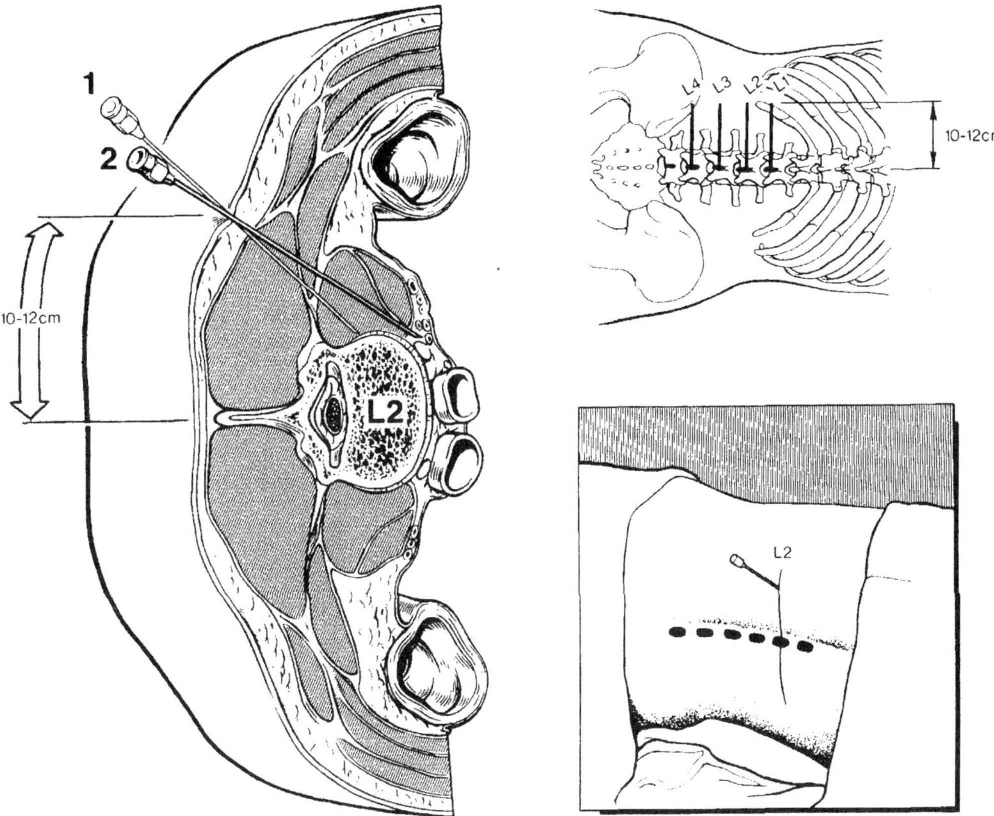

FIG. 22.5. Lumbar sympathetic block landmarks and technique. The author prefers a single needle at L_3 rather than L_2 using large volumes of local anesthetic (1 mL/kg to a maximum of 30 mL) to ensure spread to all the lumbar sympathetic ganglia. The needle is placed as shown by needle *1*. It is then walked off the vertebral body such that the tip ends up in front of the vertebral body on both posterior–anterior and lateral views as shown by *2*. (From Breivik H, Cousins MJ, Löfström JB. Sympathetic neural blockade of upper and lower extremity. In: Cousins MJ, Bridenbaugh PO, eds. *Neural blockade in clinical anesthesia and management of pain*, 3rd ed. Philadelphia: Lippincott–Raven Publishers, 1998:411–447, with permission.)

the vertebral body on both anteroposterior and lateral views. Often loss of resistance is felt as the needle pierces the psoas fascia. Correct needle placement should be confirmed with an injection of radiocontrast solution (Omnipaque 180). Fluoroscopy should then demonstrate linear spread of the solution in the prevertebral space both in the anteroposterior and lateral views (Fig. 22.6). A 20-gauge epidural catheter is passed through the Tuohy needle and advanced 3 to 4 cm past the end of the needle, and the needle is withdrawn. Passage of the catheter may require gentle pressure, but it should not be forced too vigorously. The catheter is secured using a transparent sterile dressing over the entry site and waterproof plastic tape. A gauze dressing and foam tape are placed over it, and the catheter is wound around to the anterior abdominal wall and attached to an injection port. After test-dosing, effective sympathetic blockade is confirmed by rise in skin temperature, loss of sweating, and vasodilation. Continuous blockade is then maintained by infusion of 0.1% to 0.25% bupivacaine at a dose not exceeding 0.4 to 0.5 mg/kg per hour for 5 to 10 days. The patient requires twice-daily vis-

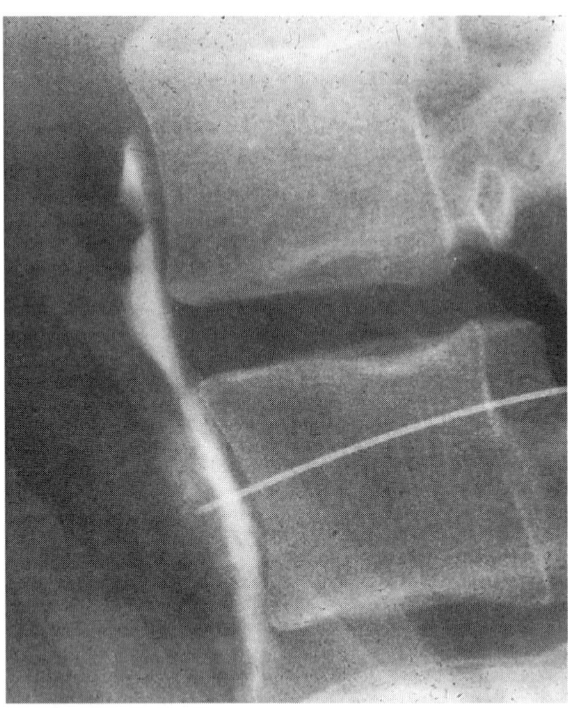

FIG. 22.6. Radiograph shows the linear spread of contrast in the prevertebral space indicating appropriate placement of a lumbar sympathetic block.

its by a pain treatment physician for assessment of the effectiveness of the blockade and presence of side effects. Readjustment of the infusion rate may be required to minimize the potential side effects that may result from prolonged infusion such as somatic nerve blockade owing to diffusion of the local anesthetic over time. Patients should be cared for on a hospital ward where the nurses are familiar with the presentation and treatment of CRPS. The nursing care plan for patients on continuous infusion of local anesthetic requires hourly observation for early detection of signs and symptoms of local anesthetic systemic toxicity or subarachnoid catheter migration.

Complications of lumbar sympathetic blockade are very rare if strict adherence to proper technique is observed and the correct placement of the needle is performed with image-intensifier guidance. Potential complications are puncture of the great vessels, kidney, or ureter, subarachnoid injection, perforation of an intervertebral disc, and damage of a somatic nerve (27). After successful placement of the sympathetic block, the patient must make an effort to participate in physical therapy to derive maximal benefit from the pain relief.

Continuous Epidural Block

Some patients with CRPS do not experience pain relief from sympathetic block. For these children, a continuous epidural block may be useful. The goal is to decrease the level of pain sufficiently to allow physical therapy to proceed. A dense motor or sensory block will interfere with physical therapy and is not desirable. Often, therefore, use of local anesthetic alone is less effective than the combination of local anesthetic with an opioid, clonidine (34), or both. When placing the epidural catheter, it is important to remember that it may be required for 7 to 10 days of therapy. Therefore, meticulous sterile technique including mask, gown, and gloves is appropriate. It may also be beneficial to tunnel the catheter. This may be easily accomplished with a second 3.5-in. Tuohy or Crawford needle. While the original needle remains in the ligament protecting the epidural catheter, make a 2-mm incision on either side of it using a no. 11 blade. Starting laterally, tunnel the second needle to bring the tip out into the incision. Remove the original needle from the ligament and off the catheter. Then thread the catheter through the second needle. When the second needle is withdrawn, the catheter should lie completely below the skin. A single horizontal mattress stitch of 4-0 Vicryl may be useful to close the incision, but often a single Steri-Strip will suffice.

One potential problem with epidural analgesia for CRPS is the development of tachyphylaxis or tolerance to local anesthetic. This has been reported (35) and has also been seen in several patients at Children's Hospital, Boston. Despite radiographic documentation of correct catheter placement, local anesthetic solutions become less effective over time. This appears to occur most rapidly in patients with only partial pain relief. Sensitization of the dorsal horn is believed to play a role (35). Addition of an opioid or clonidine to the local anesthetic may decrease or prevent this problem.

Neurolytic and Surgical Lumbar Sympathectomy

Lumbar sympathectomy with a neurolytic agent and surgery is rarely used in children both because they usually respond to more conservative measures and because the potential for permanent neural damage is unacceptable in young patients with a long life expectancy. Surgical lumbar sympathectomy can result in unacceptable sympathetic dysfunction in the pelvic organs. In 14 years of treating children with CRPS, the pain management physicians at Children's Hospital, Boston, had to resort to phenol lumbar sympathetic blockade on two occasions and to a surgical lumbar sympathectomy in one child. In all cases, these procedures were performed to improve circulation to a limb threatened by ischemia and unresolving infection, not for pain management.

Intravenous Regional Sympathetic Blockade

Intravenous regional sympathetic block (IVRSB) (i.e., Bier block) has also been used for the management of CRPS. Various sympatholytic and other therapeutic agents have been used. Guanethidine IVRSB has been shown in several double-blind trials to be ineffective for the treatment of CRPS (25,36–38). There is also an unacceptably high incidence of side effects with guanethidine (36). IVRSB has been shown to be effective with bretylium in open-label and prospective blinded trials (39,40). Ketorolac has also been used in intravenous regional blocks. Success has been reported in open label (41) and retrospective (42) trials. No prospective blinded trial has been performed, and gastritis has been reported as a complication of this technique (43). There is also a single report that clonidine can be effective in IVRSB (44). Given several reports of the efficacy of transdermal (45,46) and epidural clonidine (34) in CRPS, the addition of clonidine may be recommended pending further data. Finally, methylprednisolone, which has been used for years as an oral agent for CRPS, was also used in one uncontrolled, open-label trial for CRPS (47). The patients received an IVRSB using lidocaine and methylprednisolone. While the limb was anesthetized, the affected joints were manipulated in a progressive, controlled fashion. Physiotherapy was used thereafter. Although 91% of patients had good or moderate results, it is unclear whether the beneficial effect is from local or systemic effects of the steroids or it may even be unrelated to the steroids. The benefit may have been derived from the manipulation and physiotherapy alone.

Spinal Cord Stimulators

Spinal cord stimulators have been used with reported success for CRPS (48). An advantage of spinal cord stimulation is that it is nondestructive and fully reversible. The patient can, and should, undergo a trial using percutaneous leads before final implantation of the stimulator. Complications can include infection, movement, and breakage of the leads. The battery will wear out in 2 to 5 years, depending on frequency of use, requiring replacement of the stimulator.

MYOFASCIAL PAIN SYNDROMES

Musculoskeletal pain is common in children as well as in adults. Myofascial pain involving single or multiple muscle groups is not uncommon in childhood and early adulthood and is frequently unrecognized (49). Any skeletal muscle in the body can develop myofascial pain. Myofascial pain starts as a neuromuscular dysfunction and can produce dystrophic changes in the muscles. The precise pathophysiologic process is not clear. Repeated wear and tear of a muscle and its tendinous, fascial, and bony attachments may predispose the muscles for myofascial pain when subjected to stress and muscle loading. The injured muscle develops a painful, hyperirritable spot called a myofascial trigger point. A myofascial pain syndrome in a single muscle presents with characteristic local pain pattern, trigger points, and referred pain. The pain usually follows a history of muscular strain and is associated with muscle weakness and limitation of movement but no atrophy. These features constitute the basis for clinical diagnosis of myofascial pain syndrome (50). The afflicted muscle can be identified by the feel of a taut muscle band caused by spasm and the presence of a tender spot that evokes referred pain and autonomic hyperactivity if palpated. The trigger point may not be readily evident in chronic myofascial pain syndromes.

Each acute single-muscle myofascial pain syndrome is recognized by its unique pattern of referred pain and the trigger point. Because every skeletal muscle can potentially develop myofascial trigger pain, these syndromes are categorized by the region of the body to which referred pain is relayed. Extensive classification of various referred pain patterns and location of trigger points for the most commonly occurring myofascial pain syndromes are well described by Travell and Simons (51).

In children, temporomandibular joint dysfunction with myofascial pain is a common and well-studied clinical disorder (52,53). In one study, 35% of the children exhibited associated reactive depression (52). The treatment involves localized heat application, muscle relaxants, nonsteroidal anti-inflammatory drugs, occlusion adjustment by oral surgeon, and supportive psychotherapy.

Other acute and chronic myofascial pain syndromes are also relatively common in childhood. They are similar to adult syndromes and probably occur more frequently than previously recognized (49,54,55). Myofascial pain has been reported in a child as young as 5 years of age. As in adult myofascial pain syndromes, if the acute phase of the syndrome is missed or the underlying perpetuating cause is not dealt with, the pain can become chronic owing to persistent muscle spasm and eventually become more resistant to treatment. This can further lead to secondary emotional and physical dysfunction. Specific musculoskeletal pain disorders are increasingly recognized in children and adolescents. As increasing numbers of children and adolescents are participating in organized sports, mounting number of sports-related injuries are reported. Overuse injuries appear to occur in children as frequently, if not more so, as in adults. Inadequate preparation, poor training, and instability of the rapidly growing musculoskeletal system are major predisposing factors to these injuries (56).

Treatment

The specific treatment of myofascial pain is dependent on identification of the muscle or muscle group involved and locating of the trigger points. The therapy could be ineffective if underlying causes sustaining the hyperirritability of the muscle are not corrected. Such perpetuating factors include improper use, poor nutrition, infections, and emotional stress.

Stretch-and-Spray Technique

The patient is placed in a relaxed posture. A vapor coolant spray (e.g., Fluori-Methane, Gebauer Company, Cleveland, OH, U.S.A.) is applied to the skin in sweeps parallel to the affected muscle fibers to inactivate the trigger points. After application of the vapor coolant, the muscle is allowed to gradually and passively stretch. With repeated applications, the muscle is stretched to its full length. Next, the skin is warmed with hot moist packs and repeated active stretching of the muscle to full range of motion without excess loading is carried out by the patient (57).

Trigger Point Injection

The purpose of the injection is to disrupt and inactivate the trigger points. The use of a local anesthetic such as 0.5% procaine, 1% lidocaine, or 0.25% bupivacaine can attenuate the pain associated with stimulation of the trigger points and postinjection discomfort. The taut band of muscle is immobilized between two fingers, and the needle is rapidly advanced to transfix the trigger point, which is confirmed by triggering sudden severe referred pain. Immediately after the injection, a hot moist pack is applied to minimize the postinjection pain. A few minutes later, the muscle is stretched passively and then actively through its full range of the motion. A series of injections may be required to obtain a long-lasting effect, particularly with chronic myofascial pain.

Younger children do not appreciate injections and may not cooperate to allow successful trigger point injection. The injection *per se* can initiate emotional distress that may maintain the myofascial pain. Therefore, other modalities should be tried before needling. These may include spray and stretch, nonsteroidal anti-inflammatory drugs, muscle relaxants, transcutaneous electrical nerve stimulation, muscle stretch exercise, and cognitive and behavioral pain management techniques such as distraction and relaxation with or without biofeedback.

SICKLE CELL CRISIS PAIN

The worst pain experienced by patients with sickle cell anemia is that of vaso-occlusive crisis (VOC). VOC can develop in any tissue, in any body part, involve many areas of the body, and may last for weeks (58). It can develop spontaneously or be precipitated by febrile illness, dehydration, trauma, exposure to cold, and emotional upset. Musculoskeletal pain is the most common and painful manifestation of VOC in children older than 2 years of age. The abdomen is the second most common site of sickle cell pain crisis.

The standard treatment of the VOC has been adequate analgesia, oxygenation, and hydration. Correction of the precipitating factors is crucial for halting the sickling process. During a severe acute painful crisis, the treatment consists of systemic opioids such as morphine or hydromorphone (Dilaudid) by continuous infusion or by patient-controlled analgesic infusion pump. Nonsteroidal anti-inflammatory drugs such as ketorolac may also be useful if the patient's renal function is not compromised by the sickle cell disease.

Most moderate to severe painful crises can be managed with the above-mentioned treatment. However, a small number of patients in severe acute pain crisis are intolerant to opioid therapy owing to distressing pruritus, nausea and emesis, excessive sedation, or respiratory depression. Respiratory acidosis or hypoxemia owing to hypoventilation can perpetuate the sickling of the red blood cells. For these patients, central or peripheral neural blockade should be considered. Regional techniques block the transmission of the neural activity along the somatic and/or sympathetic nerves, thereby decreasing the nociception input from the periphery without the risk of central depression. This technique is of benefit for localized painful crisis (Table 22.2). Epidural blocks have been shown to be effective in controlling the pain of VOC (59,60). Occasionally, it may be necessary to use two epidural catheters, lumbar and thoracic, to control generalized VOC pain unresponsive to systemic opioids. A continuous infusion of a diluted local anesthetic (e.g., 0.1% or 0.125% bupivacaine) with or without an opioid is administered. The combined rate of the infusions should not exceed 0.4 to 0.5 mg/kg per hour of bupivacaine to prevent systemic toxicity (11).

TABLE 22.2. *Techniques of regional analgesia with local anesthetics*

Site of pain	Location of pain	Regional analgesic technique
Thigh, anterior and anteromedial and anterolateral aspects	Unilateral	Three-in-one block, fascia iliaca compartment block
Thigh, posterior aspect; leg and foot or lower extremity	Unilateral	Lumbar epidural analgesia or lumbar paravertebral somatic block
Pelvic	—	Lumbar epidural analgesia
Upper extremity	Unilateral	Brachial plexus analgesia
Upper extremity	Bilateral	Cervical epidural analgesia
Abdomen and thoracic	—	Thoracic epidural analgesia

CYSTIC FIBROSIS

Cystic fibrosis is a disorder of exocrine function leading to intestinal malabsorption, recurrent pulmonary infections, disorders in sweating, and possible late diabetes mellitus. These patients require repeated hospitalizations and continual aggressive pulmonary toilet including bronchodilators, antibiotics, chest physiotherapy, and voluntary coughing of their thick secretions (61).

These patients may have chronic and recurrent pain as a consequence of metabolic derangements and therapy, particularly in the advanced stages of the disease (62–67). The chest is the most common source of the pain experienced by these patients. Most chest pain is musculoskeletal owing to pulled or torn intercostal muscles, and costochondritis, with pleuritis, pneumothorax, and rib fracture also reported as causes of chest pain (67). Multiple rib fracture pain can be severe enough to precipitate respiratory decompensation in patients with limited respiratory reserve, necessitating ventilatory support. Thoracic epidural analgesia with combination of diluted local anesthetic and opioid (e.g., 0.1% bupivacaine and 2 μg/mL fentanyl) has been successfully used to treat this pain over periods of 7 to 14 days.

A few patients may experience abdominal pain resulting from chronic and recurrent pancreatitis. Headaches and facial pains are among the most common chronic pain in patients with cystic fibrosis. The main etiologic factors are hypercarbia or hypoxia, migraine, and sinusitis (67). Occasionally, unilateral headache may follow surgical clean out of the frontal sinuses owing to injury of the supraorbital nerve and may require repeated nerve blocks to alleviate the headache.

Patients with cystic fibrosis also present to the surgical suite for a variety of procedures including lobectomies, cholecystectomies, splenorenal shunts, and appendectomies. Many of these episodes can be managed well with systemic opioids supplemented with a nonsteroidal anti-inflammatory drug (e.g., ketorolac). In advanced stages, these patients are at high risk of life-threatening respiratory complications after thoracic and upper abdominal procedures. Both incisional pain and the opioid therapy can further worsen the already impaired respiratory function of the patient with cystic fibrosis. Pain causes the patient to splint, which hampers deep breathing and coughing. Opioid may cause respiratory depression and shallow respiration. Therefore, regional anesthesia is frequently offered for peripheral surgery and combined continuous epidural analgesia with general anesthesia for torso surgery and postoperative pain control. Thoracic epidural is thought to be helpful after lung transplant to enhance good pulmonary hygiene (68). The objectives of the anesthetic management are to control pain effectively, allow extubation of the trachea at the end of the surgery, and avoid opioid analgesia to avert adverse effects on pulmonary mechanics (69–72).

CANCER PAIN

Cancer pain in children is common. It may be the presenting and most distressing cancer symptom and has been reported to persist for a long time before initiation of the cancer therapy (73). Pain is also a major symptom in children with advanced cancer. The precise prevalence of pediatric cancer pain has not been studied. One prospective study by the Pediatric Branch of the National Cancer Institute over a 6-month period demonstrated that some degree of pain was experience by approximately 50% of the inpatient and 25% of the outpatient children with cancer (74).

Most of the pharmacologic principles of management of the cancer pain in adults are applicable to children; however, the success of the analgesic therapy also depends on understanding the pediatric patient and the different types of childhood malignancy and their clinical course. As in adults, each child's pain syndrome is the result of a combination of causes and unique to that individual child (Table 22.3). Treatment-related pain is preponderant among all children with cancer followed by tumor-related and procedure-related pain. In addition to knowing the cause, it is necessary to identify the probable mechanism of pain in a particular patient to select the most appropriate therapy.

Pain as a symptom of childhood malignancy usually lasts for a short period because most tumors are amenable to cancer therapy. Chronic pain associated with malignant disease is rare and occurs in fewer than 5% of the children (75). The painful terminal stage in children is very often short because once the tumor becomes unresponsive to cancer therapy, it rapidly terminates the child's life.

The control of childhood cancer pain has been managed primarily by the pediatric oncology team (oncologists, primary care nurse) in collaboration with a radiation therapist, a psychologist/psychiatrist, play therapist, social workers, physical therapist, and pastoral workers. The recent evolving of pediatric interdisciplinary pain services has presented an opportunity for a pediatric anesthesiologist to become an active and valuable member of the team (3).

TABLE 22.3. *Disease and treatment-related pain syndromes in children with cancer*

- Pain associated with tumor infiltration
  - Bone pain
    - Leukemia and lymphoma, particularly intractable to treatment, can invade the bone marrow and infiltrate the periosteum producing pain in the long bones, back, sternum, pelvis, or skull
    - Primary tumors of the bones, particularly osteogenic sarcoma and Ewing sarcoma; metastatic tumors such as sarcomas and neuroblastomas
  - Nerve pain
    - Compression or infiltration of peripheral nerves, roots, plexuses, cranial nerves, and spinal cord
  - Headache
    - May be owing to rise in intracranial pressure, hemorrhage, meningeal infiltration (leukemic and lymphoma), parenchymal brain metastases (osteosarcoma, soft-tissue sarcomas) and metabolic changes
  - Visceral pain
    - Liver and spleen may be enlarged and painful in children with leukemia or lymphoma; intra-abdominal and retroperitoneal solid tumors (lymphoma, Wilms, neuroblastoma, rhabdomyosarcoma, hepatoblastoma) may produce pain owing to visceral stretch
- Pain associated with cancer therapy
  - Painful procedure
    - Bone marrow aspiration and biopsy, lumbar puncture/post-lumbar puncture headaches, venipuncture, Port-a-cath access, and intravenous catheter placement
  - Postoperative pain
    - Incision pain from a surgical procedure (e.g, thoracotomy, laparotomy); phantom pain or other neuropathic pain after amputation or limb-sparing procedures for osteogenic or Ewing sarcoma
  - Pain after chemotherapy or radiation therapy
    - Painful peripheral neuropathy after vincristine; bone pain owing to osteoporosis of long bones and vertebrae after prolonged steroid therapy; radiation-induced fibrosis around major nerves and exacerbated painful neuropathies after chemotherapy and tumor-damaged nerves; mucositis or esophageal ulceration associated with chemotherapy, irradiation, or infection; hemorrhagic cystitis; herpes zoster

Adapted from Berde CB, Anand KS, Sethna NF. Pediatric pain management. In: Gregory GA, ed. *Pediatric anesthesia.* New York: Churchill-Livingstone, 1989;716–717; and Miser AW, Jiser JS. The treatment of cancer pain in children. *Pediatr Clin Am* 1990; 36:4,979–998.

Rationale for Regional Techniques

Regional analgesia has been less commonly used in pediatric patients with cancer than for adults for several reasons. Childhood malignancies intractable to standard cancer therapy often spread rapidly and may produce diffuse pain usually not amenable to local and regional neural blockade. Systemic opioid therapy remains the most important means for pediatric cancer pain control and is effective in most situations. Even in far-advanced childhood malignancy, chemotherapy and radiation therapy can, in many cases, offer adequate analgesia by shrinking the tumor. Nevertheless, despite the use of these therapies, many children with terminal malignancy do not experience adequate analgesia. Wolfe et al. (76) reported that pain management was successful in only 27% of children dying of cancer at Children's Hospital, Boston. For many children, the answer is more optimal use of opioids, together with adjuvant medications. Regional analgesia has been used in a minority of patients with severe pain. Typical indications for this intervention have included limiting side effects of opioids, neuropathic pain unresponsive to either rapid escalation of opioids or massive opioid infusions, analgesia for thoracocenteses for the drainage of malignant pleural effusions, and instillation of intrapleural chemotherapy (77). Another common use of regional anesthesia in pediatric patients with cancer is for the relief of postoperative pain (78). Finally, although limb-sparing operations have largely replaced amputation for sarcomas, amputation is necessary on occasion (79). This can be associated with a high incidence of phantom pain (80). Use of perioperative regional anesthesia for amputation may be able to decrease this distressing symptom (81).

The most commonly used regional techniques in pediatric patients with cancer are central neuraxial blocks, either epidural or subarachnoid. Either can be safely and effectively performed using an indwelling catheter for the management of chronic pain. When an epidural or subarachnoid catheter is inserted percutaneously, the tip of the catheter is placed close to the dermatome of pain origin using fluoroscopic guidance. For chronic pain control, the catheter should be tunneled subcutaneously to a skin exit away from the entry site of the vertebral interspace using the technique described above in the section on CRPS (Fig. 22.7). The externalized catheters are connected to a small portable infusion pump. Securing the catheter in a subcutaneous tunnel at the time of the initial placement minimizes the risk of infection, allows ease of skin care, and

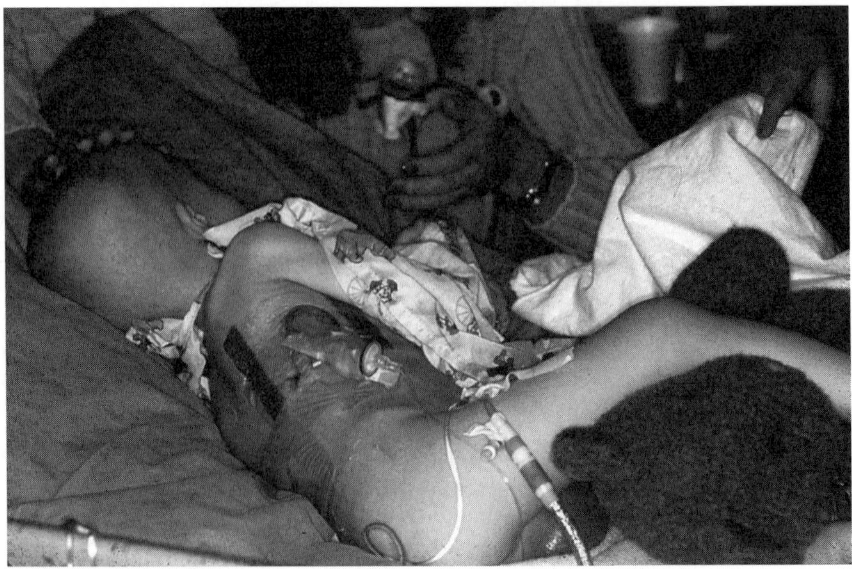

FIG. 22.7. An oncology patient with a tunneled epidural catheter for prolonged analgesia.

prevents dislodgement of the catheter in long-term therapy (82). Overall, an externalized catheter is probably more appropriate than an implanted pump for most pediatric patients with cancer. An externalized catheter can usually be maintained for the few weeks required for these patients. Also, local anesthetic is usually required in addition to neuraxial opioid for optimal pain control (83,84). This can be difficult to administer using an implanted pump because of the large volumes required. Nonetheless, implanted pumps have been successfully used in pediatric patients (85).

Although neuraxial catheters are highly effective in the treatment of intractable pain in appropriately selected patients (77), complications are not uncommon (86,87). These range from minor infections at the skin entry site, mechanical malfunction, and dural puncture headache through epidural abscess (88) and paraplegia (87). Use of fluoroscopy to guide placement of the catheter and tunneling the catheter subcutaneously may reduce the risk of complications.

Children who have become resistant to enormous doses of systemic opioids may experience withdrawal symptoms if the systemic opioids are rapidly withdrawn after starting neuraxial opioids (83). Some children who have developed tolerance to massive administration of systemic opioids require large doses of epidural or subarachnoid opioids for analgesia. The addition of spinal or epidural local anesthetic infusion provides rapid pain control with reversal of respiratory depression and drowsiness. Tolerance to epidural and subarachnoid opioids and local anesthetic has been variable. One patient received subarachnoid analgesia for 7 months with bupivacaine (7). It is now practical and safe to continue epidural and subarachnoid infusions at home for prolonged lengths of time providing care is maintained through close liaison with home nursing providers (77).

Clonidine is now approved for epidural use in the management of cancer pain in adults. There is a strong literature for its efficacy administered both intrathecally (89,90) and epidurally (91,92) for this indication. Although not approved for pediatric use, there is a case report of epidural clonidine use in the treatment of pain from left pelvic chondrosarcoma in a 10-year-old girl (93). There are also several studies on acute epidural or caudal use demonstrating safety and efficacy in pediatric patients (94–98).

Contraindications for Central Neural Blockade

Thrombocytopenia leading to coagulation disorders is frequent in advanced cancer owing to bone marrow suppression by chemotherapy or by metastatic infiltration by the tumor. The placement of indwelling epidural and subarachnoid catheters should be carried out immediately after correction of the coagulation deficiency by platelet transfusion.

Septicemia is an absolute contraindication because of the risk for colonization microorganisms around foreign bodies. Strafford et al. (88) reported a case in which the catheters was left *in situ* despite known septicemia because pain control in this dying patient was thought to be paramount. The patient developed an epidural infection requiring decompressive laminectomy. In general, indwelling catheters should be removed from the neural axis if patient develops fever and sepsis.

Other Regional Techniques

In addition to central neuraxial blocks, other regional techniques have been applied to pediatric oncology patients. There are two case reports of celiac plexus block. One was used in a 3-year-old boy with severe abdominal pain from an unresectable hepatoblastoma. This child had a history of severe bronchopulmonary dysplasia resulting from prematurity (born at 25 weeks postconceptional age). Systemic opioids adequate to treat his pain caused severe respiratory depression. Celiac plexus blockade with ethanol was performed under general anesthesia and with computed tomographic guidance. After the block, the child was completely free of pain, discharged home without analgesics, and remained comfortable and was able to sleep well until he died of progressive renal failure 9 weeks after the celiac plexus block (99). The other was performed for a 7-year-old boy with abdominal pain secondary to a recurrent adrenal neuroblastoma. After neurolytic celiac plexus blockade, he experienced control of his abdominal pain for almost 3 months (100). This modality is underutilized and should be considered for children with pain caused by upper abdominal malignancy. It is a good alternative to thoracic spinal or epidural analgesia for visceral pain because it provides excellent analgesia without the need for specialized nursing care.

Cooper et al. (101) also described using an intrascalene brachial plexus catheter for a 6-year-old patient with osteosarcoma of the humerus. This was causing severe neuropathic pain that was poorly controlled with opioids despite respiratory depression.

REFERENCES

1. Bonica JJ. *The management of pain*. Philadelphia: Lea & Febiger, 1953.
2. Berde CB, Anand KJS, Sethna NF. Pediatric pain management. In: Gregory G, ed. *Pediatric anesthesia*. New York: Churchill-Livingstone, 1989:715–717.
3. Berde C, Sethna NF, Masek B, et al. Pediatric pain clinics: recommendations for their development. *Pediatrician* 1989;16:94–102.
4. Sethna NF, Berde CB. Pediatric regional anesthesia. In: Gregory G, ed. *Pediatric anesthesia*. New York: Churchill-Livingstone, 1989:647–651.
5. Bosenberg AT. Lower limb nerve blocks in children using unsheathed needles and a nerve stimulator. *Anaesthesia* 1995;50:206–210.
6. Cooper MG, Sethna NF. Epidural analgesia in patients with congenital lumbosacral spinal anomalies. *Anesthesiology* 1991;75:370–374.
7. Berde CB, Sethna NF, Conrad LS, et al. Subarachnoid bupivacaine analgesia for seven months for a patient with a spinal cord tumor. *Anesthesiology* 1990;72: 1094–1096.
8. Bonica JJ. Neural blockade in the interdisciplinary pain clinic. In: Cousins MJ, Bridenbaugh PO, eds. *Neural blockade in clinical anesthesia and management of pain*. Philadelphia: JB Lippincott, 1988.
9. Agarwal R, Gutlove DP, Lockhart CH. Seizures occurring in pediatric patients receiving continuous infusion of bupivacaine. *Anesth Analg* 1992;75:284–286.
10. McCloskey JJ, Haun SE, Deshpande JK. Bupivacaine toxicity secondary to continuous caudal epidural infusion in children. *Anesth Analg* 1992;75:287–290.
11. Berde CB. Convulsions associated with pediatric regional anesthesia. *Anesth Analg* 1992;75:164–166.
12. Stanton-Hicks M, Janig W, Hassenbusch S, et al. Reflex sympathetic dystrophy: changing concepts and taxonomy. *Pain* 1995;63:127–133.
13. Wilder RT, Berde CB, Wolohan M, et al. Reflex sympathetic dystrophy in children. Clinical characteristics and follow-up of seventy patients. *J Bone Joint Surg Am* 1992;74A:910–919.
14. Ribbers GM, Geurts AC, Rijken RA, et al. Axillary brachial plexus blockade for the reflex sympathetic dystrophy syndrome. *Int J Rehabil Res* 1997;20:371–380.
15. Olsson GL, Arnér S, Hirsch G. Reflex sympathetic dystrophy in children. In: Tyler DC, Krane EJ, eds. *Pediatric pain, volume 15*. New York: Raven Press, 1990: 323–331.
16. Stanton RP, Malcolm JR, Wesdock KA, et al. Reflex sympathetic dystrophy in children: an orthopedic perspective. *Orthopedics* 1993;16:773–779.
17. Schwartzman RJ, Kerrigan J. The movement disorder of reflex sympathetic dystrophy. *Neurology* 1990;40: 57–61.
18. Wilder RT. Reflex sympathetic dystrophy in children and adolescents: differences from adults. In: Jänig W, Stanton-Hicks M, eds. *Reflex sympathetic dystrophy: a reappraisal, volume 6*. Seattle: IASP Press, 1995:67–77.
19. Stanton-Hicks M, Baron R, Boas R, et al. Complex regional pain syndromes: guidelines for therapy. *Clin J Pain* 1998;14:155–166.
20. Glick EN. Reflex dystrophy (algoneurodystrophy): results of treatment by corticosteroids. *Rheumatol Phys Med* 1973;12:84–88.
21. Robaina FJ, Rodriguez JL, de Vera JA, et al. Transcutaneous electrical nerve stimulation and spinal cord stimulation for pain relief in reflex sympathetic dystrophy. *Stereotact Funct Neurosurg* 1989;52:53–62.
22. Grunert BK, Devine CA, Sanger JR, et al. Thermal self-regulation for pain control in reflex sympathetic dystrophy syndrome. *J Hand Surg [Am]* 1990;15:615–618.
23. Barowsky EI, Zweig JB, Moskowitz J. Thermal biofeedback in the treatment of symptoms associated with reflex sympathetic dystrophy. *J Child Neurol* 1987;2:229–232.
24. Gainer MJ. Hypnotherapy for reflex sympathetic dystrophy. *Am J Clin Hypn* 1992;34:227–232.
25. Kingery WS. A critical review of controlled clinical trials for peripheral neuropathic pain and complex regional pain syndromes. *Pain* 1997;73:123–139.
26. Christensen K, Jensen EM, Noer I. The reflex dystrophy syndrome response to treatment with systemic corticosteroids. *Acta Chir Scand* 1982;148:653–655.
27. Breivik H, Cousins MJ, Löfström JB. Sympathetic neural blockade of upper and lower extremity. In: Cousins MJ, Bridenbaugh PO, eds. *Neural blockade in clinical anesthesia and management of pain*, 3rd ed. Philadelphia: Lippincott–Raven Publishers, 1998: 411–447.
28. Lunn R, Sethna N, Berde C, et al. Stellate ganglion blockade in infants and children. *Anesthesiology* 1989; 71:A1023.
29. Linson MA, Leffert R, Todd DP. The treatment of upper extremity reflex sympathetic dystrophy with prolonged continuous stellate ganglion blockade. *J Hand Surg [Am]* 1983;8:153–159.
30. Todd DP. Prolonged stellate block in treatment of reflex sympathetic dystrophy. *Agressologie* 1991;32: 281–282.

31. Gibbons JJ, Wilson PR, Lamer TJ, et al. Interscalene blocks for chronic upper extremity pain. *Clin J Pain* 1992;8:264–269.
32. Reiestad F, McIlvaine WB, Kvalheim L, et al. Interpleural analgesia in treatment of upper extremity reflex sympathetic dystrophy. *Anesth Analg* 1989;69:671–673.
33. Berde CB, Sethna NF, Micheli LJ. A technique for continuous lumbar sympathetic blockade for severe reflex sympathetic dystrophy in children and adolescents. *Anesth Analg* 1988;67:S4.
34. Rauck RL, Eisenach JC, Jackson K, et al. Epidural clonidine treatment for refractory reflex sympathetic dystrophy. *Anesthesiology* 1993;79:1163–1169.
35. Maneksha FR, Mirza H, Poppers PJ. Complex regional pain syndrome (CRPS) with resistance to local anesthetic block: a case report. *J Clin Anesth* 2000;12: 67–71.
36. Jadad AR, Carroll D, Glynn CJ, et al. Intravenous regional sympathetic blockade for pain relief in reflex sympathetic dystrophy: a systematic review and a randomized, double-blind crossover study. *J Pain Symptom Manage* 1995;10:13–20.
37. Ramamurthy S, Hoffman J. Intravenous regional guanethidine in the treatment of reflex sympathetic dystrophy/causalgia: a randomized, double-blind study. Guanethidine Study Group. *Anesth Analg* 1995;81: 718–723.
38. Kaplan R, Claudio M, Kepes E, et al. Intravenous guanethidine in patients with reflex sympathetic dystrophy. *Acta Anaesthesiol Scand* 1996;40:1216–1222.
39. Ford SR, Forrest WH, Eltherington L. The treatment of reflex sympathetic dystrophy with intravenous regional bretylium. *Anesthesiology* 1988;68:137–140.
40. Hord AH, Rooks MD, Stephens BO, et al. Intravenous regional bretylium and lidocaine for treatment of reflex sympathetic dystrophy: a randomized, double-blind study. *Anesth Analg* 1992;74:818–821.
41. Vanos DN, Ramamurthy S, Hoffman J. Intravenous regional block using ketorolac: preliminary results in the treatment of reflex sympathetic dystrophy. *Anesth Analg* 1992;74:139–141.
42. Connelly NR, Reuben S, Brull SJ. Intravenous regional anesthesia with ketorolac-lidocaine for the management of sympathetically-mediated pain. *Yale J Biol Med* 1995;68:95–99.
43. Litman SJ, Vitkun SA, Poppers PJ. Gastric irritation after ketorolac Bier block for treating reflex sympathetic dystrophy. *J Clin Anesth* 1994;6:526–527.
44. Gintautas J, Housny W, Kraynack BJ. Successful treatment of reflex sympathetic dystrophy by bier block with lidocaine and clonidine. *Proc West Pharmacol Soc* 1999;42:101.
45. Kirkpatrick AF, Derasari M. Transdermal clonidine: treating reflex sympathetic dystrophy. *Reg Anesth* 1993;18:140–141.
46. Davis KD, Treede RD, Raja SN, et al. Topical application of clonidine relieves hyperalgesia in patients with sympathetically maintained pain. *Pain* 1991;47: 309–317.
47. Zyluk A. Results of the treatment of posttraumatic reflex sympathetic dystrophy of the upper extremity with regional intravenous blocks of methylprednisolone and lidocaine. *Acta Orthop Belg* 1998;64: 452–456.
48. Calvillo O, Racz G, Didie J, et al. Neuroaugmentation in the treatment of complex regional pain syndrome of the upper extremity. *Acta Orthop Belg* 1998;64:57–63.
49. Bates T, Grunwaldt E. Myofascial pain in childhood. *J Pediatr* 1958;53:198–209.
50. Travell J. Myofascial trigger points: clinical view. In: Bonica JJ, Albe-Fessard D, eds. *Advances in pain research and therapy, volume 1*. New York: Raven Press, 1976.
51. Travell JG, Simons DG. *Myofascial pain and dysfunction: the trigger point Manual*. Baltimore: Williams & Wilkins, 1983.
52. Belfer ML, Kaban LB. Temporomandibular joint dysfunction with facial pain in children. *Pediatrics* 1982;69:546–547.
53. Cooper BC, Alleva M, Cooper DL, et al. Myofacial pain dysfunction: analysis of 476 patients. *Laryngoscope* 1986;96:1099–1106.
54. Fine PG. Myofascial trigger point pain in children. *J Pediatr* 1987;111:547–548.
55. Aftimos S. Myofascial pain in children. *N Z Med J* 1989;102:440–441.
56. Micheli LJ. Overuse injuries in children's sports: the growth factor. *Orthop Clin North Am* 1983;14:337–360.
57. Simons DG. Myofascial pain syndromes. In: Basmajian JV, Kirby L, eds. *Foundation of physical medicine and rehabilitation*. Baltimore: Williams & Wilkins, 1984:209–215.
58. Powers DR. Natural history of sickle-cell disease-the first 10 years. *Semin Hematol* 1975;12:267.
59. Yaster M, Tobin JR, Billett C, et al. Epidural analgesia in the management of severe vaso-occlusive sickle cell crisis. *Pediatrics* 1994;93:310–315.
60. Tobias JD. Indications and application of epidural anesthesia in a pediatric population outside the perioperative period. *Clin Pediatr (Phila)* 1993;32:81–85.
61. Davis P. Cystic fibrosis. *Semin Respir Med* 1985;6: 261–270.
62. Ross J, Gamble J, Schultz A, et al. Back pain and spinal deformity in cystic fibrosis. *Am J Dis Child* 1987;141:1313–1316.
63. Mitchell EA, Elliott RB. Spontaneous fracture of the sternum in a youth with cystic fibrosis. *J Pediatr* 1980;97:789–790.
64. Rush PJ, Shore A, Coblentz C, et al. The musculoskeletal manifestations of cystic fibrosis. *Semin Arthritis Rheum* 1986;15:213–225.
65. MacLusky I, McLaughlin FJ, Levison H. Cystic fibrosis: part II. *Curr Probl Pediatr* 1985;15:1–39.
66. MacLusky I, McLaughlin FJ, Levison H. Cystic fibrosis: part I. *Curr Probl Pediatr* 1985;15:1–49.
67. Ravilly S, Robinson W, Suresh S, et al. Chronic pain in cystic fibrosis. *Pediatrics* 1996;98:741–747.
68. Lillehei CW, Mayer JE, Shamberger RC, et al. Pediatric lung transplantation and "lessons from Green Surgery." *Ann Thorac Surg* 1999;68:S25–S27.
69. Kang SB. Continuous thoracic epidural anesthesia for biliary tract surgery and for postoperative pain relief in a patient with cystic fibrosis. *Anesth Analg* 1982; 61:793–795.
70. Bruce DL, Gerken MV, Lyon GD. Postcholecystectomy pain relief by intrapleural bupivacaine in patients with cystic fibrosis. *Anesth Analg* 1987;66:1187–1189.
71. Edelman DS. Laparoscopic cholecystectomy under continuous epidural anesthesia in patients with cystic fibrosis. *Am J Dis Child* 1991;145:723–724.

72. Kaukuntla HK, Amer KM, Honeybourne D, et al. Extrapleural bronchial artery ligation for life-threatening hemoptysis in cystic fibrosis—a case report. *Angiology* 2000;51:787–792.
73. Miser AW, Dothage JA, Wesley M, et al. The prevalence of pain in a pediatric and young adult cancer population. *Pain* 1987;29:73–83.
74. Miser AW, McCalla J, Dothage JA, et al. Pain as a presenting symptom in children and young adults with newly diagnosed malignancy. *Pain* 1987;29:85–90.
75. Miser AW, Miser JS. The treatment of cancer pain in children. *Pediatr Clin North Am* 1989;36:979–999.
76. Wolfe J, Grier HE, Klar N, et al. Symptoms and suffering at the end of life in children with cancer. *N Engl J Med* 2000;342:326–333.
77. Collins JJ, Grier HE, Sethna NF, et al. Regional anesthesia for pain associated with terminal pediatric malignancy. *Pain* 1996;65:63–69.
78. Tobias JD, Oakes L, Rao B. Continuous epidural anesthesia for postoperative analgesia in the pediatric oncology patient. *Am J Pediatr Hematol Oncol* 1992;14:216–221.
79. Merimsky O, Kollender Y, Inbar M, et al. Palliative major amputation and quality of life in cancer patients. *Acta Oncol* 1997;36:151–157.
80. Krane EJ, Heller LB. The prevalence of phantom sensation and pain in pediatric amputees. *J Pain Symptom Manage* 1995;10:21–29.
81. Bach S, Noreng JF, Tjellden NU. Phantom limb pain in amputees during the first 12 months following limb amputation after preoperative lumbar epidural blockade. *Pain* 1988;33:297–301.
82. Berde CB. Regional analgesia in the management of chronic pain in childhood. *J Pain Symptom Manage* 1989;4:232–237.
83. Tanelian DL, Cousins MJ. Failure of epidural opioid to control cancer pain in a patient previously treated with massive doses of intravenous opioid. *Pain* 1989;36:359–362.
84. Du Pen SL, Kharasch ED, Williams A, et al. Chronic epidural bupivacaine–opioid infusion in intractable cancer pain. *Pain* 1992;49:293–300.
85. Galloway K, Staats PS, Bowers DC. Intrathecal analgesia for children with cancer via implanted infusion pumps. *Med Pediatr Oncol* 2000;34:265–267.
86. Nitescu P, Sjoberg M, Appelgren L, et al. Complications of intrathecal opioids and bupivacaine in the treatment of "refractory" cancer pain. *Clin J Pain* 1995;11:45–62.
87. Appelgren L, Nordborg C, Sjoberg M, et al. Spinal epidural metastasis: implications for spinal analgesia to treat "refractory" cancer pain. *J Pain Symptom Manage* 1997;13:25–42.
88. Strafford MA, Wilder RT, Berde CB. The risk of infection from epidural analgesia in children: a review of 1620 cases. *Anesth Analg* 1995;80:234–238.
89. van Essen EJ, Bovill JG, Ploeger EJ, et al. Intrathecal morphine and clonidine for control of intractable cancer pain. A case report. *Acta Anaesthesiol Belg* 1988;39:109–112.
90. Coombs DW, Saunders RL, Fratkin JD, et al. Continuous intrathecal hydromorphone and clonidine for intractable cancer pain. *J Neurosurg* 1986;64:890–894.
91. Eisenach JC, Rauck RL, Buzzanell C, et al. Epidural clonidine analgesia for intractable cancer pain: phase I. *Anesthesiology* 1989;71:647–652.
92. Eisenach JC, DuPen S, Dubois M, et al. Epidural clonidine analgesia for intractable cancer pain. The Epidural Clonidine Study Group. *Pain* 1995;61:391–399.
93. Queinnec MC, Esteve M, Vedrenne J. Positive effect of regional analgesia (RA) in terminal stage paediatric chondrosarcoma: a case report and the review of the literature. *Pain* 1999;83:383–385.
94. Luz G, Innerhofer P, Oswald E, et al. Comparison of clonidine 1 microgram kg-1 with morphine 30 micrograms kg-1 for post-operative caudal analgesia in children. *Eur J Anaesthesiol* 1999;16:42–46.
95. Lee JJ, Rubin AP. Comparison of a bupivacaine-clonidine mixture with plain bupivacaine for caudal analgesia in children. *Br J Anaesth* 1994;72:258–262.
96. Jamali S, Monin S, Begon C, et al. Clonidine in pediatric caudal anesthesia. *Anesth Analg* 1994;78:663–666.
97. Ivani G, Mattioli G, Rega M, et al. Clonidine-mepivacaine mixture vs plain mepivacaine in paediatric surgery. *Paediatr Anaesth* 1996;6:111–114.
98. Klimscha W, Chiari A, Michalek-Sauberer A, et al. The efficacy and safety of a clonidine/bupivacaine combination in caudal blockade for pediatric hernia repair. *Anesth Analg* 1998;86:54–61.
99. Berde CB, Sethna NF, Fisher DE, et al. Celiac plexus blockade for a 3-year-old boy with hepatoblastoma and refractory pain. *Pediatrics* 1990;86:779–781.
100. Staats PS, Kost-Byerly S. Celiac plexus blockade in a 7-year-old child with neuroblastoma. *J Pain Symptom Manage* 1995;10:321–324.
101. Cooper MG, Keneally JP, Kinchington D. Continuous brachial plexus neural blockade in a child with intractable cancer pain. *J Pain Symptom Manage* 1994;9:277–281.
102. Dalens B. *Regional anesthesia in infants, children, and adolescents.* London: Williams & Wilkins Waverly Europe; 1995.

23

Nursing Management of the Child in Pain

Marion E. Broome and Myra M. Huth

Research indicates that pain is a priority and a frequently encountered nursing problem and focus of intervention for children in health care settings (1). Pain management is one of the 433 interventions identified as a critical nursing function in The Nursing Intervention Classification System (2). When children are in health care settings such as ambulatory clinics and inpatient units and in the home, nurses are the professionals who have the most frequent and closest contact. This places nurses in a unique and central position to advance pain management with children through nurse-initiated interventions, research, and theory development (3).

Many advances in health care professionals' awareness of assessment and effective management of children's pain have taken place over the past quarter century. Various age-appropriate tools are available to assist nurses to assess pain in infants, children, and adolescents. However, research continues to document inconsistent or lack of use of these tools by nurses. Inadequate pain assessment leads to inaccurate selection of pharmacologic and nonpharmacologic interventions for a child (3,4). Recent research reveals that children and adolescents who undergo both inpatient and outpatient surgeries continue to report moderate to severe levels of pain, even after receiving analgesics (5–10).

This chapter presents a model of pain management that can be used by practicing nurses, researchers, and nursing students to assess, intervene, and evaluate infant, child, and adolescent pain across settings. The empiric literature examining nursing assessment, interventions, and outcomes over the past decade are highlighted and recommendations for future research and nursing practice are presented.

A MODEL OF NURSES' PAIN MANAGEMENT PRACTICE

In the early 1990s, the Agency for Health Care Policy and Research published acute and cancer pain clinical practice guidelines to be used by health care professionals in clinical sites (11–13). The guidelines were meant to direct clinical practice; however, the length of the guidelines and a disjointed approach that did not provide specific guidance left nurses wondering how to implement them. The Nursing Pain Management Model, used to organize this chapter, was originally derived from the Model of a Theory of Acute Pain Management (3) (Fig. 23.1). The model has been adapted to provide nurses with clear practice guidelines that help them to make decisions to reduce acute, chronic, and recurrent pediatric pain in a variety of settings.

The model consists of four levels that build on one another and when implemented should result in satisfactory pain reduction (Fig. 23.1). The first level of the model depicts *the nurse's characteristics and setting*, both of which influence the pain management process. The second level, *initial pain assessment*, incorporates the pain history, current pain level, developmental level, coping strategies, and cultural background of the infant or child. *Therapeutic interventions*, the third level, comprise child–parent support, analgesic administration, and comfort measures. The fourth level presents information related

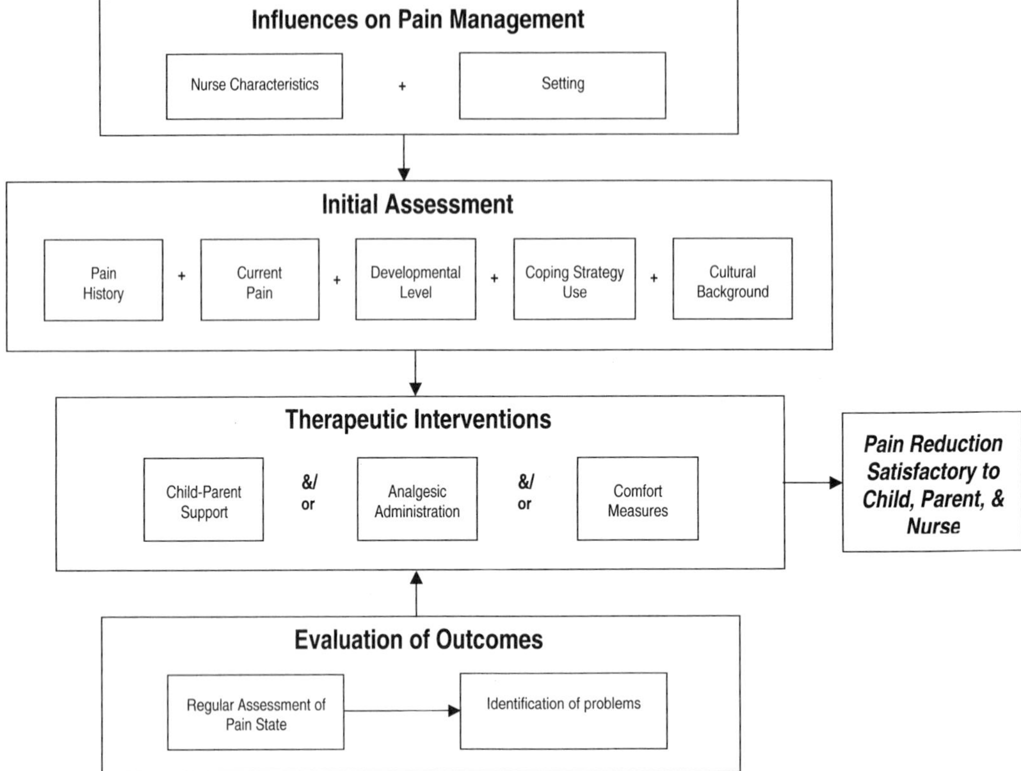

FIG. 23.1. Nursing pain management model. (Adapted from Huth MM, Moore SM. Prescriptive theory of acute pain management in infants and children. *J Soc Pediatr Nurs* 1998;3:23–32, with permission.)

to the *need for ongoing assessment of pain and physiologic states* that guides the nurse in the identification of problems such as inadequate pain relief, behavioral distress, unacceptable physiologic paremeters, and side effects, indicating that further therapeutic intervention is needed.

INFLUENCES ON PAIN MANAGEMENT

Nurse Characteristics

Nurses have a responsibility as patient advocates to ensure adequate pain management. Research indicates that nurses' characteristics such as knowledge, experience, beliefs about pain, and accountability all influence how they manage a child's pain (14).

Knowledge and Experience

Intuitively, professionals think that a person's knowledge and experience determine his or her ability to manage children's pain. However, systematic surveys about the pain management knowledge of pediatric nurses provide a different perspective. These surveys report that nurses often have a poor understanding of the pharmacologic principles of common analgesics. Nurses lack knowledge about the appropriate doses (15–18), routes of administration (15,16), frequency of administration (15,16,19), types of analgesics selected given the medical diagnosis (16,17), side effects (18), and opioids (18). In one survey, physicians also lacked knowledge regarding the appropriate doses of analgesics (16). A survey administered to pediatric and adult bone marrow transplant nurses found that the mean correct response to knowledge items was average (79%), although nurses had a high level of pain assessment knowledge (18).

Nurses' past experiences with pain management can affect their current pain management practice. Studies have found that pediatric nurses use past experience as a basis for making present or future pain management decisions (20) and that they learn how to assess pain "on the job" from more experienced nurses (21,22). One study found that nurses with more than 10 years of experience were less likely to administer analgesics (19), whereas others found no relationship or difference between nurses' knowledge and years of experience (18,21).

Attitudes and Beliefs

Attitudes and personal beliefs about pain and pain relief influence nurses' pain management practices. Many nurses still hold misconceptions about analgesic administration and report concern about the risk of respiratory depression (15,17,18), addiction to narcotics (15,23), and fear of medicating infants experiencing pain (16). Attitudes and beliefs toward analgesics transcend continents because nurses in the Netherlands also report negative feelings toward analgesics and postpone giving them as long as possible (20).

In one study, both nurses and physicians identified that nurses were more likely to wait longer before remedicating a child (16). Other surveys report that nurses believe that children feel less pain than adults (17), attribute more pain to vocal children who express their pain, and are more likely to administer nonopioid analgesics to children who vocalize their pain (19).

Margolius and colleagues (24) found significantly high correlations between nursing education level and beliefs related to pain ($r = 0.52$) and between nursing education level and perception of effective pain management ($r = 0.31$). These findings suggest that the nurses providing direct care, the ones with the least education, were found to hold the most misconceptions about effective pain management and the least likely to question existing pain management practices.

Some surveys report more positive findings about nurses' beliefs and attitudes regarding children's pain management. In one study, most pediatric nurses believed that pain assessment is an essential first step for alleviating children's pain, that accurate documentation leads to more effective pain management, and that nurses can make a difference in how children cope with painful situations (25). Most of the nurses in this study strongly disagreed that children do not need analgesics as often as adults do, that they become addicted to narcotics more easily, and that if they are asleep, they are pain free.

There seems to be a gradual shift occurring in pediatric nurses' beliefs and attitudes about analgesics, pain assessment, and pain management practices as evidenced by some of the most recent surveys (18,25,26). However, the answers of nurses on surveys about their pain management attitudes and beliefs have not always coincided with actual practice (16, 25,27,28).

Past Pain

Past pain experiences shape how a child interprets and responds to a painful experience; therefore, it is logical to think that a nurse's personal experience with pain will also influence his/her pain management practices. Research reveals that nurses' personal pain experience, either their own or their child's, influences their pain medication administration practices (27–30). In their study, Seymour et al. (29) found that almost every nurse reported that they reflected on their own pain experiences in an effort to understand and imagine an infant's pain. Intensive care nurses who reported a personal pain experience selected more pain indicators in a critically ill child than nurses who did not report a personal pain experience (30). The role of experience as a factor seems to be an important one that affects pain management and clearly needs further study.

Accountability

The public and the Joint Commission on Accreditation of Healthcare Organizations are mandating that health care professionals be accountable for the care that they deliver. Better access to information has given parents a greater understanding of what is realistic to expect in the care that their child receives. Findings extrapolated from some of the studies reviewed suggest that accountability for reducing pain is not always nurses' first priority.

Some investigators report that nurses postpone administering analgesics as long as possible (16,20). In one qualitative study, nurses expressed frustration about managing bladder spasms; however, they did not try other pain interventions in an attempt to manage the pain (23). In the same study, symptoms such as fever were given priority over managing pain.

The literature reports, however, that some nurses are concerned about providing adequate pain control and do view it as their professional responsibility (29). These nurses considered teaching parents how to manage their infant's pain with comfort measures and distraction as part of their professional responsibility and as an aid to their own assessments.

Clear and concise documentation of the actions that a nurse takes when a child is in pain is one way to demonstrate accountable and responsible practice. Yet, research reveals documented pain assessments and interventions are unsystematic and inconsistently done, do not reflect children's reports, and rarely contain nurses' observations (25,31,32). Advances in nursing pain control have occurred in the past 30 years, but until children's pain is assessed more consistently and treated more vigorously using multimodal interventions, nurses are not accepting accountability for providing an environment for satisfactory pain reduction.

The Setting

Work-related factors such as workload, pain policies, and colleagues influence nurses' pain management process. If practice environments are such that nurses are unable to adequately assess, therapeutically intervene, and evaluate outcomes, pain management is compromised.

Workload

Efforts to control rising health care costs as well as the nursing shortage have resulted in fewer professional nurses, and personnel with less training are being used for health care delivery. One common criticism of this approach is the presumption that the quality of care provided to the child and family will decline. In a qualitative study, Hamers et al. (20) reported that the administration of analgesics was highly dependent on a nurse's workload and time. This is an important finding and one that is often discussed in anecdotal reports by nurses; however, to date there is no research that investigates nurse–staffing ratios at the unit level on pain management practices.

Pain Policies and Practice

Pain guidelines from federal agencies (e.g., Agency for Health Care Policy and Research) have little impact unless they are implemented in clinical practice. Pain policies, protocols, and standards of care need to reflect the organization's commitment to high-quality care and regulation of pain management. Pain management based on policies and protocols can assist nurses in decision making, leaving less room for indecision and doubt (14). For instance, in one survey, 40% (n = 80) of pediatric nurses reported that the lack of a protocol or a standing order in the institution inhibited their use of lidocaine-prilocaine cream [EMLA (eutectic mixture of local anesthetics)] for venipuncture and intravenous catheter insertion (33). Interestingly, Joyce et al. (32) reported that a pain flow sheet was not used by nurses according to the protocols derived from the Agency for Health Care Policy and Research guidelines despite a formal in-service and self-study program. Findings indicated that not one child had a documented pain assessment every 2 hours for the first 24 postoperative hours.

These two opposing results indicate further research is needed on the influences of policy on pain management practice.

Colleagues and Health Care Professionals

Collegial consultation and support are an essential component of the unit milieu and influence nurses' pain management practices. Results of one survey indicate that 89% of 27 pediatric critical care nurses learned about pain management from their current work environment (34). Other studies also confirm that pain management techniques are learned from more experienced nurses (21,22). These findings would suggest that institution-wide and unit-based programs related to pain management should remain a top priority.

INITIAL ASSESSMENT

Assessment, the crucial first step in managing pain, includes measuring a child's pain, but it also involves gathering data from other sources and making a clinical decision. Pain is multidimensional and includes sensory, affective, cognitive, behavioral, sociocultural, and physiologic dimensions. Thus, all aspects require an initial assessment. The depth of initial assessment data will vary depending on the setting and frequency of the child's visits. For example, children seen yearly or more often in a primary care setting can have their initial pain assessment data updated by asking the child and parent about pain experiences since the last visit, new coping strategies used to help with pain, and developmental and cultural changes. For infants and children with a chronic painful illness who are undergoing hospitalization, a comprehensive initial nursing assessment could be made available through the primary health care professional's office (35) or from the hospital's pain management program if the child has been referred. The initial nursing pain assessment of a child admitted to a day surgery unit for his/her first surgery and hospitalization would be different from that done in inpatient settings. In the latter case, an assessment of all five factors (e.g., coping, culture) is necessary because these aspects have not been previously assessed. The nursing history provides nurses with initial data on development, culture, and past coping strategies. Despite the setting, an initial assessment of only current pain is inappropriate and provides insufficient data for the nurse to base decisions on which therapeutic interventions are needed for pain reduction. Pain management is a continuous and ongoing process that needs to result in satisfactory pain reduction.

Pain History

The acute pain management guidelines recommend that health care professionals obtain a pain history at the time of admission (11,12). Obtaining a pain history is not just relegated to physicians but should be an integral part of nursing practice because nurses are the "front-line" managers of pediatric pain. Documentation of a child's past pain experiences, perception of pain, usual pain behaviors, the words that a child uses to express hurt, and previously effective treatments optimizes pain management (3). Beyer and colleagues (35) suggest that an interview format or a therapeutic play session for a younger child is ideally suited to obtaining information about pain because they are informal and nonthreatening atmospheres. None of the nursing studies reviewed for this chapter included a pain history as part of the assessment process; however, several can be found in pain references (3,11–13).

Current Pain

As discussed in other chapters, current pain intensity should be assessed with a child self-report, which is the gold standard of pain measurement by an age-appropriate, reliable, and valid pain tool. Infant or young child behavior can be assessed with behavioral pain tools coupled with a parent report. A current pain assessment also includes the location, quality, and duration of pain.

Most research on infants describes the physiologic and behavioral indicators that nurses use to assess pain. Facial expressions, body movements, vocalizations, sleep/wake states, physiologic measures, affect, and self-comfort behaviors were the common indicators of infant pain that nurses used (21,22,26,36,37). Other key cues included data in notes and nurses' judgment about data in notes, consolability, cry types and characteristics, and the infant's interaction with others (21,22). Only two studies identified the parents' views of the infant's comfort as pertinent to the nurse's pain assessment (29,37). One study found that the use of only infant behaviors to assess pain was not sufficient to encourage nurses to administer a pain medication (37). Standardized infant pain measures were not generally used in the studies reviewed, but they may be impractical and unfeasible for use in a clinical setting because they often require observer training or equipment for assessment, coding, and analysis (38).

There is strong evidence provided in the literature that nurses are not using pain rating scales specifically developed for children. Between 27% and 66% of respondents identified that they or their institution were not using any tools to assess pain in children (25,31, 39,40). A recent investigation found that when nurses used self-report pain tools, 47% used the numeric rating scale (41). Other studies found between 20% and 52% of pain assessments were done using a word descriptor scale, 27% a behavioral observation scale, 47% an infant pain scale (even though children were 3 to 6 years old), and 1% to 18% a "happy-sad face" tool (31,32,41).

Like the infant population, children's pain is commonly assessed informally, without the use of a pain tool. In the studies reviewed, most nurses (70% to 97%) used the child's verbal expression to assess pain, either through crying, verbal expression of pain, or request for medication (41–43). Some studies reported that 49% to 98% of nurses assessed a child's pain by observing the child's behavior (30,31,41). Physiologic changes were also used by 60% to 80% of nurses (30,31,41,42).

Physiologic measures such as heart rate, blood pressure, respiratory rate, transcutaneous oxygen, palmar sweating, vagal tone, and endorphin concentration provide information about general distress levels, but they are not sensitive or specific indicators of children's pain (3,5,11,12). Therefore, physiologic measures should be used only as adjuncts to self-report and behavior. As the previous research indicates, current assessments done by nurses are limited to the sensory dimension of pain. Because pain has both sensory and affective components, both should be assessed so that appropriate interventions can be implemented (35).

Documentation of pain assessment is an indirect method of determining the frequency and consistency of pain assessments. Results show that nurses are not consistently assessing pain in children. For example, in one study, 42% of charts reviewed across all three shifts did not reflect any pain assessment (25). Similarly, no child had a documented assessment of pain every 2 hours during the first 24 hours after surgery (32). One study reported that the intensity and duration of pain were documented by only 35% of nurses and quality of pain by fewer (23%) (31). In contrast to the previous chart reviews, 60% of nurses reported that they assessed pain in children every 1 to 2 hours before and after analgesics were given, and 15% reported that they assessed pain every 3 to 4 hours before and after procedures (41).

Developmental Level

Cognitive and psychosocial development affects the child's perception, behavioral response, and communication about pain (44). Therefore, the child's ability to communicate and cope with pain is influenced by his or her developmental level. Assessment of the child's language and personal-social development must occur for effective intervention. In the studies reviewed, nurses did not formally assess or document the child's developmental level, although assessments may have been done informally. An initial developmental assessment that is documented communicates vital information to all nurses caring for a child and further guides their choice of therapeutic intervention.

There is a paucity of research that explores pain assessment in children who are cognitively impaired, and the research that is available indicates that nurses have difficulty assessing their pain. In a study by Fanurik et al. (45), more than half of the assessments of a cognitively impaired child's ability to use a numerical rating scale by preoperative nurses were found to be inaccurate. In another related study, 48% (n = 20) of parents reported that health care professionals had difficulty assessing and treating their cognitively impaired child's pain, and 26% (n = 11) said that their child's pain level was underestimated and therefore undertreated (46). Health care professionals may have difficulty assessing the pain of children with a cognitive or communication impairment based on observation because of their behavioral abnormalities or facial grimacing (46). In cases in which a child is unable to provide a reliable self-report, a parent is a good alternative because they know and understand best their child's usual behaviors.

Coping Strategy Use

Coping strategies are behavioral and cognitive efforts that the infant or child uses to assist in managing stress or anxiety (47). The use of coping strategies is also affected by cognitive development, and the child's frequency of use changes with age (48). Children use increasingly more strategies, combinations of strategies, and shift from passive methods of coping with pain to cognitive strategies as they age (49,50). Assessment and documentation of the infant's or child's coping strategies from a child and/or parent report are necessary for effective intervention. There was no study in the literature that reported that the child's use of coping with pain was assessed.

Cultural Background

Culture is recognized as an important factor in shaping experiences and responses to pain for the individual, family, and nurse (51). A documented cultural history therefore is imperative for holistic and comprehensive pain management. A person's culture influences the understanding of the meaning of the illness or pain; responses; attitudes toward health, illness, and treatment; and expectations from others (35). Differences have been reported in various ethnic groups of children's experience of pain (52,53). The research of Beyer et al. (53) is one illustration of a deliberate attempt to design a culturally sensitive and developmentally based sensory pain instrument for children.

Hart (54) administered a questionnaire assessing culture and self-reported practices to 548 pediatric nurses from four children's hospitals. Nurses reported that cultural assessments were not routinely performed beyond that for the admission intake form. However, 65% of the respondents indicated that they experienced problems that they believed were related to cultural differences at least once per week. Fifty-five percent reported they would use a cultural assessment form every time a patient was admitted but were willing to only spend 15 minutes or less obtaining cultural information along with the routine admission.

THERAPEUTIC NURSING INTERVENTIONS

Various nursing interventions are used to manage children's pain. These interventions are defined as any treatments, based on the clinical judgment and knowledge that a nurse demonstrates to enhance child outcomes (2). Nursing interventions include both direct and indirect care, as well as both nurse- and physician-initiated treatments that nurses are responsible for implementing and evaluating.

When a nurse chooses to intervene during a child's pain experience, the management is based on a previous or current assessment of the pain using an established assessment tool and contextual cues. To be effective, interventions must be clearly linked to an assessment. Interventions must also be tailored to the individual child and family, e.g., they must be developmentally appropriate and culturally sensitive. Finally, timely evaluation of the effectiveness of the intervention must be conducted so that adjustments can be made and progress toward specified outcomes continues.

The choice of nursing interventions varies based on the setting. Infants and children scheduled for immunizations do not receive analgesics before immunization but should receive child-parent support and age-appropriate comfort measures. Conversely, a preschooler recovering from open-heart surgery in the intensive care unit should receive child–parent support, analgesic administration, and comfort measures. The choice of comfort measures should be based on the child's developmental level, past pain experiences, and use of successful past coping strategies during painful experiences.

The nursing interventions listed in Table 23.1 provide a nurse with a wide repertoire of options. The interventions listed are only selected examples and are not an exhaustive list. Nursing interventions for the child in pain can be classified into three major categories: child–parent support, administration of therapeutic treatments including analgesia and adjuvants, and provision of comfort measures (2). Given the focus of this chapter, only those interventions that are nurse implemented and evaluated are discussed.

Child and Parental Support

Pain is a very stressful experience for both a child and parents and, in turn, often becomes stressful for the health care provider who is providing a therapeutic treatment that has some degree of discomfort associated with it. Nurses are frequently the health care provider and traditionally have been responsible for educating parents and children about pain management to increase their knowledge and abilities (55). There are various ways to support both children who will be experiencing pain and their parents. Pain education should be multifocal and should include preparation of both the child and parents about what to expect during the medical event as well as how the child might feel and respond. Nurses also implement both pharmacologic and nonpharmacologic strategies to reduce pain perception and increase comfort (56).

Preparation of Child and Parent for Pain

The overall purpose of preparing children and parents for a painful experience is to provide them with knowledge and skills that will enable them to effectively deal with pain. Yap (57) described four purposes of preparation for children and parents: (a) to transmit information to decrease stress by increasing cognitive control and decreasing uncertainty, (b) encourage emotional expression so that feelings can be recognized and validated and social support can be provided to buffer stress, (c) develop trust between the child, parents, and health care provider, and (d) teach coping strategies such

TABLE 23.1. *Nursing interventions for managing children's pain*

Intervention (2)	Examples	Source
Child and parental support		
Preparation		
Parent education	*A child in pain: how to help, what to do*	Ref. 92
Sensory/procedural information	*Pain, pain, go away* (booklet)	Ref. 91
Parent presence	Parkland Memorial Hospital guidelines	Refs. 59, 93
Anxiety reduction	Breathing exercises	Refs. 91, 94
Therapeutic treatments		
Analgesic administration	AHCPR guidelines	Refs. 11–13
Comfort measures		
Calming technique	Swaddling, rocking	Ref. 95
Distraction	Blowing bubbles, counting backwards, kaleidescope	Refs. 96, 97
Relaxation	Progressive relaxation, simple relaxation	Refs. 98, 99

AHCPR, Agency for Health Care Policy and Research.

as relaxation, self-talk, and imagery. Most of the preparation literature related to painful events is based on procedural studies (Chapter 31). Few studies have examined the preparation of the child and parents for postoperative surgical pain, but those that did found that simple education techniques alone are not sufficient to affect outcomes. In a study of 93 children 8 to 18 years of age who were undergoing a spinal fusion and who were randomized to receive standard care or a standardized educational program, there were no significant differences in the location, quality, or intensity of pain experienced over 4 postoperative days (55). In another study (M. Huth, M. Broome, K. Mussato, et al., unpublished observation, 2002), 51 parents of children having cardiovascular surgery were randomly assigned to a group for preparation using a booklet about pain assessment and management. Although parents who received the parent assessment and management booklet did increase their knowledge about pain, in general, there were few significant differences in the treatment and control groups related to postoperative pain outcomes. In both studies, parents were highly satisfied with the education that they received. Influencing pain outcomes requires a multidimensional approach to managing pain, including analgesics, the use of comfort measures by both parents and staff, and education. Yet, in actual practice, the information that parents want and need to receive about pain management continues to be inadequate, and children are still suffering unnecessarily (35,46,58).

Encouraging Parental Presence

Supporting parental presence when a child is in pain is a critical area in which nurses can be very proactive (59). With few exceptions, most institutions have not developed guidelines for family presence or discussed the appropriate role that parents can play when their child is in pain. This lack of guideline development is likely a reflection of the ambivalence on the part of many health care professionals to actively involve parents when a child is in pain (59).

Nurses and physicians vary in their acceptance, or encouragement, of parental presence during painful procedures. The type of painful procedure influences the attitudes of health care providers. Bauchner et al. (60) reported that 66% of physicians and nurses in the emergency department preferred parents be present during treatment of lacerations, whereas only 14% agreed to their being present during lumbar punctures. Some health care providers, especially those who primarily care for adult patients, believe that seeing a child in pain makes the parents and physician nervous, upsets the child, or results in parents interfering with a procedure (59).

In studies of parents in the emergency department, most parents (90%) said they wanted to be present when their child experienced a painful procedure (60,61). The majority believed that their child wanted them there and that their presence would calm the child. They were also interested in knowing what the physician was doing. Parents reported they had to be proactive about being present because only half of the parents choosing to stay had been asked to do so by a health care provider.

It is difficult to understand why health care professionals would not want a parent present when a child is in pain. Many health care professionals have observed on occasion that some children, especially those who are younger, seem more distressed when their parents are present. They then infer that the child is "trying to get attention" or "experiencing more pain" than if the parents were not present. In reality, children often use those active coping behaviors that health care professionals label distress to signal parents to help them (62). Further, researchers have demonstrated that parents can learn effective ways to help their child cope with a painful procedure (63–66).

There have been various studies conducted on the effects of parental presence on children's response to painful procedures, in which investigators have examined children's responses during dental treatment, immunizations, venipuncture, lumbar punctures, and bone marrow aspirations. In general, studies have found that younger children are more distressed when their parent is present (67, 68), whereas others found parental presence had little effect on children (69,70). Child distress increases during a procedure when developmentally inappropriate amounts of control over the procedure are given to the child (71), when the physician distracts a parent with social talk (72), when parents do not focus their attention on the child (63,72), or when the parent is a "cheerleader or overinvolved" (62,71). Child distress decreases when the physician interacts directly with the child (71) or when parents use simple distraction and focused coping skills (63–65,73).

We now know that some things that parents do during painful procedures are more helpful than others, and it is the responsibility of the health care professional to teach parents how to be most supportive with their child. These "parenting behaviors for pain" do not come naturally, although some parents learn useful strategies from trial and error.

Analgesic Administration

There is overwhelming evidence that appropriate use of analgesics works to effectively reduce pain perception in children (Chapters 11–13). Systematic studies of the effectiveness of analgesics in reducing children's pain have increased dramatically over the past decade. In a review of 41 prospective studies of pharmacologic interventions for children in pain reported in the literature from 1987 to 1995, Maikler (74) found that various analgesic options (e.g., morphine, lidocaine-prilocaine cream) have all been found efficacious in reducing children's pain during procedures and the postoperative period. Other studies, however, report that analgesics are still underutilized by health care providers (39,75).

Some progress has been made in nurses' knowledge of and attitudes about the administration of analgesics in the past decade. In 1990, McCaffery and Ferrell (76) found that almost half of 456 nurses surveyed failed to increase the dose of an opioid when the last dose administered was insufficient. In another study comparing nurses' decision making for adult and pediatric patients in pain, exaggerated fears of respiratory depression and denial of children's ability to feel pain affected nurses' choices about analgesia administration (17). In a study by Pederson and Parran (18), the use of opioids was the area identified most commonly about which nurses needed more information. This is likely a reflection of the lack of integration of pain and pharmacology into many undergraduate curricula until very recently. Other studies have documented that even when nurses (and other health care providers) hold positive perceptions about pain management, their actual choices of pain medications reflect a lack of knowledge about analgesia (15,16,77).

Part of the answer to suboptimal pain management practices may lie in differences in judgments about pain that nurses make when compared with self-reports of patients. Nurses' ratings have been consistently lower across studies. In one of the few studies that examined how these differences in assessment might be reflected in actual practice, Weldon et al. (78) compared differences in the amount of analgesics received by the child postoperatively based on who controlled the administration of the patient-controlled analgesia. They reported that nurses not only rated the children's pain significantly lower than the children did but also administered significantly less analgesics over a 3-day period than the children did themselves.

It may be that, although increased educational efforts and pain management standards developed by hospitals in the past decade have made it difficult for nurses to hold negative attitudes about the need for pain management, they have not changed their actual practices. Although benchmarking and report cards giving physicians feedback about their practices related to medical outcomes are frequently used (79), nurses are not usually provided such feedback about their interventions with patients. Another major issue related to the appropriate use of analgesics, especially for those children needing aggressive pain management and ongoing monitoring, is assurance of patient safety and the constraints that nurses face related to this in today's practice world. Inpatient units often are not adequately staffed to provide monitoring according to standards. In one report of a quality management project on conscious sedation, Ross and Fochtman (80) described the threats to the nurse's ability to monitor patient status during conscious sedation procedures owing to competing demands in their patient load. The average procedure took 69 minutes for recovery and even longer in ambulatory settings. This need for vigilant monitoring, in light of average patient loads and high acuity levels, is sometimes unrealistic and often results in less than optimal pain management for the child.

Comfort Measures

In a recent review analyzing published review articles on the use of nonpharmacologic strategies for pediatric pain management, Lambert (81) described and categorized comfort measures reported in the literature. Some of these interventions require more interaction on the part of the child than others. Those that are passive in nature include physical touch, the use of heat/cold, transcutaneous electrical nerve stimulation, and sucrose and sucking (82). Others require more active participation on the part of the child and include distraction, relaxation, simple imagery, and hypnosis. In general, these interventions have been found effective in reducing a child's pain response as measured by pain behaviors, self-report, and parent report (81,82). These techniques are most effective when they require the use of multiple senses including auditory, visual, tactile, and kinesthetic (82) and when the child and parent work together (63,72).

There has been a dramatic increase in the interest in and use of distraction with patients in both acute and chronic care in which pain is experienced. Nurses often use distraction with children during acutely painful procedures, as do parents. Distraction is considered the simplest of the three interventions and most commonly used by nurses. In 1996, McCarthy et al. (83) surveyed 47 pediatric oncology and bone marrow transplant centers, and 80% reported using all three techniques, along with information and reinforcement, routinely. Nurses were the providers most often responsible for implementing the interventions in the survey. Yet, the setting in which nurses work affects the implementation of these strategies, with nurses in busy inpatient wards reporting less consistent use. In a descriptive, exploratory study of 54 nurses, Pederson and Harbaugh (84) described patterns of use of five different nonpharmacologic techniques including distraction, breathing, relaxation, imagery, and changing perceptions of stimuli. These nurses reported a lack of time and heavy workload that precluded their use of these techniques with children. They most often employed the techniques during procedures, and nurses perceived parents to be helpful.

Many pain experts recommend that parents be encouraged to use nonpharmacologic strategies with their child. Yet, these are not always simple techniques or known by parents intuitively (55). Studies (58,83) report that parents do not spontaneously know how to employ nonpharmacologic techniques; therefore, it is incumbent on nurses to teach parents. There are various resources that nurses can access to learn the techniques and then teach them to parents (Table 23.1). Research indicates that when nurses are taught how to use nonpharmacologic strategies (66), they not only increase their knowledge of and comfort with them but report increased use of the strategies 2 months later. Again, however, having time to use and evaluate the use of the techniques is crucial. On inpatient units or in clinics where nurses have heavy workloads, it will be more difficult for nurses to implement what they know. The use of and teaching of these techniques take time.

EVALUATION OF OUTCOMES OF PAIN MANAGEMENT

Despite the setting, evaluation of the infant's or child's pain and coping should occur every hour until pain is controlled or the infant or child is discharged. When initial interventions are ineffective, nurses should provide further child–parent support, consider further analgesic administration, and add comfort measures. Traditionally, many nurses wait until the child or parent reports pain or requests more medication before further interventions are offered. In this model, evaluation of outcomes is a continuous process until pain reduction occurs (3).

The primary focus of measurement of outcomes for pain management should be the child and, in some cases, the parent. Outcome assessment focuses on examining changes in patients' health status as a result of interventions provided in health care settings (85). Outcome measures must be feasible (e.g., easy to use, using cost-effective techniques), sensitive to changes that result from a nurse's intervention, and influenced by a minimum of other confounding factors (86). Both short- and long-term outcomes should be measured. Short-term outcomes (e.g., pain intensity) are often easier to document and demonstrate changes in because the patient is usually more accessible and there are fewer confounding factors than for long-term outcomes. Given that, even with the most aggressive pain management approaches, not every child's pain can be prevented or completely eradicated, and the overall goal for managing pain should be to increase the child's and parents' satisfaction with pain reduction (Fig. 23.1).

Although there are few outcomes of pain management that are related solely to nursing interventions, there are several outcome variables that are considered nursing sensitive (85,86). Examples of both short- and long-term outcomes related to pain management in children with chronic pain are found in Table 23.2. Having nurses document that what they do is effective (or even influential) in patient outcomes related to pain; nurses who provide direct care must document what, when, and how they intervene with a child in pain and evaluate the effectiveness of their intervention.

There are various measures that nurses can use to evaluate outcomes for the infant or child in pain (Table 23.3). Some of these measures are more appropriate for some populations of children with pain (e.g., chronic versus postoperative), and some are more feasible (e.g., time for administration, scoring requirements) than others. There is now a body of studies that have reported implementing institutional strategies and nursing care techniques that have improved nurses' practices related to assessment, administration of analgesics, and use of comfort measures (31,34,38,39,55). However, all these studies use multimodal approaches and a purposive, multidisciplinary team approach to improving pain care. These approaches included not only educating nurses about pain assessment and

TABLE 23.2. *Examples of outcome variables for selected nursing-sensitive outcome categories for a child in pain with sickle cell disease*

Outcome category (85)	Example of outcome variables
Physiologic	Sleep
Functional	School attendance
Behavioral	Coping strategies during vaso-occlusive episodes
Knowledge	Understanding of new analgesic regimes
Home functioning	Ability to complete assigned chores
Family strain	Parental stress
Symptom control	Number of vaso-occlusive events
Quality of life	Health quality of life
Goal attainment	Able to play soccer season
Patient satisfaction	Child/parent satisfaction with pain management
Utilization of service	Emergency department visits
Nursing diagnosis resolution	Increased comfort
Psychosocial	Self-efficacy

TABLE 23.3. *Outcome measures of effective nursing pain assessment and management practices*

Outcome (100)	Measures	Sources
Sleep	Nursing Child Assessment Sleep/Activity Record	Ref. 101
Parent attitudes about pain and medication	Medication Attitude Questionnaire	Ref. 102
Coping with pain	Pediatric Coping Strategies Scale	Ref. 103
Pain level Sensory	VAS; Baker-Wong FACES Scale; Adolescent Pediatric Pain Tool; OUCHER	Refs. 53, 104, 105
Affective	Facial Affective Scale	Ref. 106
Pain: disruptive effects	School absenteeism, pain diaries, VAS	Ref. 107

VAS, visual analog scale.

management but written and published standards of care, interdisciplinary rounds, use of standardized tools, inclusion of parents, chart audits to evaluate outcomes, and feedback to individual nurses about their care.

RECOMMENDATIONS FOR NURSING PRACTICE AND RESEARCH

Appropriate, efficient, and effective pain assessment and management strategies that improve physical and emotional outcomes for children and that are satisfying to both child and parents remain a top priority in nursing (1,3). All nurses, regardless of setting or role, should play an active role in meeting this priority. For instance, nurse educators must continue to integrate content into the undergraduate and graduate curricula that addresses pain management for patients across the lifespan, including neonates and children. They must structure clinical experiences in outpatient, inpatient, and community settings for students that will provide many opportunities to reinforce the principles of pain management learned in the classroom.

In practice at the bedside, nurses should be held accountable for safe and effective pain management through the application of the most up-to-date knowledge and skills in pain assessment and management. This requires each nurse to have a sound working knowledge of which reliable and valid assessment tools are available. The institution must provide the resources to implement adequate pain practices, including materials to assess pain in children and the time to implement them. Although pharmacologic and nonpharmacologic tools to treat the overwhelming majority of pain experienced by children are available, those strategies are not always employed in inpatient, clinic, and community settings. Nurses should receive ongoing instruction in both standard and innovative techniques for pediatric pain management and then be held accountable for using them. This would require regular audits of patient charts and evaluation of cases at nursing rounds. This ongoing evaluation would facilitate nurses' learning via the case method, a proven educational strategy for clinicians. An institution truly interested in improving pain care must focus more attention on supporting nurses in their efforts to improve pain management for children.

There remains much research to be done testing both pharmacologic and nonpharmacologic interventions. These studies should evaluate the effectiveness of selected analgesics for various pain experiences, as well as examine characteristics of the individual that influence analgesic administration and efficacy. The realities of implementing and evaluating nonpharmacologic intervention studies are well documented in the literature (83,88). Researchers have already documented the difficulties involved in recruiting a true control group (e.g., refusing standard care) and how expensive some intervention studies can be when an "objective intervener" is required.

The use of parents as coaches is an important area in which research has demonstrated some promising effects (72,89). Many health care professionals, however, remain uncomfortable with parents being present and discourage it, especially during invasive procedures when children are most distressed (59). Additional research is needed to test individualized approaches to using nonpharmacologic strategies with children. The reality is that children and parents, even those who do agree to be in a research study, will modify and tailor an intervention to fit their needs. Researchers need to know more about how this is done and what the true effects are on outcomes.

Greater institutional commitment that supports better practices related to pain management should be systematically evaluated. An example of one such commitment is in place at Boston Children's Hospital (M. Curley, personal communication, 2002). The Center for Nursing Excellence sponsored a 2-day retreat with three nursing pain experts, the hospital pain team, and staff from throughout the hospital. Consensus was reached by all regarding the selection of several evidence-based pain assessment tools that would be implemented throughout the institution. Evaluation of the implementation, consisting of baseline and follow-up data on documentation of assessments, was conducted 6 months later. Although such an evaluation is time-consuming and confounding variables were noted, such initiatives are necessary if pain practices are to improve.

Nursing, medical, and psychologic sciences have developed a body of knowledge over the past two decades that has improved the care of children in pain to a marked degree. Some parents are satisfied with the way their child's pain is managed in inpatient settings. However, a significant number of children who are hospitalized still does not receive adequate pain management (5–10,90). Nurses are the gatekeepers of children's pain, especially in inpatient settings. Nurses can enhance, through education and anticipatory guidance, a child's and the parents' understanding of his or her pain experience, accurately and continually assessing the child's pain, and then, working with physicians and other health care professionals, employ state-of-the-art strategies to manage pain effectively. It is only through teamwork between the nurse, physician, parents, and child that all children can be promised a satisfactory reduction in pain (3).

REFERENCES

1. Broome ME, Woodring B, O'Connor-Von S. Research priorities for the nursing of children and their families: a Delphi study. *J Pediatr Nurs* 1996;11:281–287.
2. McCloskey JC, Bulechek GM, eds. *Iowa Intervention Project: nursing intervention classification (NIC)*, 2nd ed. St. Louis: Mosby Year Book, 2000.
3. Huth MM, Moore SM. Prescriptive theory of acute pain management in infants and children. *J Soc Pediatr Nurs* 1998;3:23–32.
4. McGrath PA. Pain in the pediatric patient: practical aspects of assessment. *Pediatr Ann* 1995;24:126–138.
5. Gauthier J, Finley G, McGrath P. Children's self-report of postoperative pain intensity and treatment threshold: determining the adequacy of medication. *Clin J Pain* 1998;14:116–120.
6. Gillies ML, Smith LN, Parry-Jones WLI. Postoperative pain assessment and management in adolescents. *Pain* 1999;79:207–215.
7. Hultcrantz E, Linder A, Markström A. Tonsillectomy or tonsillotomy? A randomized study comparing postoperative pain and long-term effects. *Int J Pediatr Otorhinolaryngol* 1999;51:171–176.
8. Romsing J, Hertel S, Møller-Sonnergaard J, et al. Postoperative pain in Danish children: self-report measures of pain intensity. *J Pediatr Nurs* 1996;11:119–124.
9. Tesler MD, Wilkie DJ, Holzemer WL, et al. Postoperative analgesics for children and adolescents: prescription and administration. *J Pain Symptom Mange* 1994; 9:85–95.
10. Warnock FF, Lander J. Pain progression, intensity and outcomes following tonsillectomy. *Pain* 1998;75:37–45.
11. Acute Pain Management Guideline Panel. *Acute pain management in infants, children, and adolescents: operative and medical procedures. Quick reference guide for clinicians* (AHCPR pub. no. 92-0020). Rockville, MD: Agency for Health Care Policy and Research, Public Health Service, U.S. Department of Health and Human Services, 1992.
12. Acute Pain Management Guideline Panel. *Acute pain management: Operative or medical procedures and trauma. Clinical practice guideline* (AHCPR pub. no. 92-0020). Rockville, MD: Agency for Health Care Policy and Research, Public Health Service, U.S. Department of Health and Human Services, 1992.
13. Jacox A, Carr DB, Payne R, et al. *Management of cancer pain. Clinical practice guideline no. 9* (AHCPR pub. no. 94-0592). Rockville, MD: Agency for Health Care Policy and Research, U.S. Department of Health and Human Services, 1994.
14. Abu-Saad HH, Hamers JPH. Decision-making and paediatric pain: a review. *J Adv Nurs* 1997;26:946–952.

15. Schmidt K, Eland J, Weiler K. Pediatric cancer pain management: a survey of nurses' knowledge. *J Pediatr Oncol Nurs* 1994;11:4–12.
16. Read JV. Perceptions of nurses and physicians regarding pain management of pediatric emergency room patients. *Pediatr Nurs* 1994;20:314–318.
17. Gonzalez JC, Routh DK, Armstrong FD. Differential medication of child versus adult postoperative patients: the effect of nurses' assumptions. *Child Health Care* 1993;22:47– 59.
18. Pederson C, Parran L. Bone marrow transplant nurses' knowledge, beliefs, and attitudes regarding pain management. *Oncol Nurs Forum* 1997;24:1563–1571.
19. Hamers JPH, Abu-Saad HH, van den Hout MA, et al. The influence of children's vocal expressions, age, medical diagnosis and information obtained form parents on nurses' pain assessments and decisions regarding interventions. *Pain* 1996;65:53–61.
20. Hamers JPH, Abu-Saad HH, Halfens RJG, et al. Factors influencing nurses' pain assessment and interventions in children. *J Adv Nurs* 1994;20:853–860.
21. Fuller BF, Conner DA. The influence of length of pediatric nursing experience on key cues used to assess infant pain. *J Pediatr Nurs* 1997;12:155–168.
22. Fuller B, Thomson M, Conner DA, et al. Relationship of cues to assessed infant pain level. *Clin Nurs Res* 1996;5:43–66.
23. Woodgate R, Kristjanson LJ. A young child's pain: how parents and nurses `take care.' *Int J Nurs Stud* 1996;33:271–284.
24. Margolius FR, Hudson KA, Michel Y. Beliefs and perceptions about children in pain: a survey. *Pediatr Nurs* 1995;21:111–115.
25. Jacob E, Puntillo KA. Pain in hospitalized children: pediatric nurses' beliefs and practices. *J Pediatr Nurs* 1999;14:379–390.
26. McCain GC, Morwessel NJ. Pediatric nurses' knowledge and practice related to infant pain. *Issues Compr Pediatr Nurs* 1995;18:277–286.
27. Burokas L. Factors affecting nurses' decisions to medicate pediatric patients after surgery. *Heart Lung* 1985; 14:373–379.
28. Gadish HS, Gonzalez JL, Hayes JS. Factors affecting nurses' decisions to administer pediatric pain medication postoperatively. *J Pediatr Nurs* 1988;3:383–390.
29. Seymour E, Fuller BF, Pedersen-Gallegos L, et al. Modes of thought, feeling, and action in infant pain assessment by pediatric nurses. *J Pediatr Nurs* 1997; 12:32–50.
30. Coffman S, Alvarez Y, Pyngolil M, et al. Nursing assessment and management of pain in critically ill children. *Heart Lung* 1997;26:221–228.
31. Salanterä S, Lauri S, Salmi TT, et al. Nursing activities and outcomes of care in the assessment, management, and documentation of children's pain. *J Pediatr Nurs* 1999;14:408–415.
32. Joyce BA, Keck JF, Gerkensmeyer JE. Evaluating the implementation of a pain management flow sheet. *J Pediatr Nurs* 1999;14:304–312.
33. May K, Britt R, Newman MM. Pediatric registered nurse usage and perception of EMLA. *J Soc Pediatr Nurs* 1999;4:105–112.
34. Pederson C, Bjerke T. Pediatric pain management: A research-based clinical pathway. *Dimens Crit Care Nurs* 1999;18:42–51.
35. Beyer JE, Platt AE, Kinney TR, et al. Practice guidelines for the assessment of children with sickle cell pain. *J Soc Pediatr Nurs* 1999;4:61–73.
36. Howard VA, Thurber FW. The interpretation of infant pain: physiological and behavioral indicators used by NICU nurses. *J Pediatr Nurs* 1998;13:164–174.
37. Hudson-Barr DC, Duffey MA, Holditch-Davis D, et al. Pediatric nurses' use of behaviors to make medication administration decisions in infants recovering from surgery. *Res Nurs Health* 1998;21:3–13.
38. Stevens B, Koren G. Evidence-based pain management for infants. *Curr Opin Pediatr* 1998;10:203–207.
39. Broome ME, Richtsmeier A, Maikler V, et al. Pediatric pain practices: a national survey of health professionals. *J Pain Symptom Manage* 1996;11:312–320.
40. Colwell C, Clark L, Perkins R. Postoperative use of pediatric pain scales: children's self-report versus nurse assessment of pain intensity and affect. *J Pediatr Nurs* 1996;11:375–382.
41. Jacob E, Puntillo KA. A survey of nursing practice in the assessment and management of pain in children. *Pediatr Nurs* 1999;25:278–286.
42. Caty S, Tourigny J, Koren I. Assessment and management of children's pain in community hospitals. *J Adv Nurs* 1995;22:638–645.
43. Rheiner J, Megel ME, Hiatt M, et al. Nurses' assessments and management of pain in children having orthopedic surgery. *Issues Compr Pediatr Nurs* 1998;21:1–18.
44. Harbeck C, Peterson L. Elephants dancing in my head: a developmental approach to children's concepts of specific pains. *Child Dev* 1992;63:138–149.
45. Fanurik D, Koh JL, Harrison RD, et al. Pain assessment in children with cognitive impairment: an exploration of self-report skills. *Clin Nurs Res* 1998;7:103–124.
46. Fanurik D, Koh JL, Schmitz ML, et al. Children with cognitive impairment: parent report of pain and coping. *Dev Behav Pediatr* 1999;20:228–234.
47. Lazarus R. Stress, coping and illness. In: Friedman H, ed. *Personality and disease*. New York: John Wiley & Sons, 1990:97–120.
48. Ryan-Wenger N. Coping behavior in children: methods of measurement for research and clinical practice. *J Pediatr Nurs* 1994;9:183–195.
49. Ryan N. Stress coping strategies identified from school age children's perspectives. *Res Nurs Health* 1989;12:111–121.
50. Sharrer V, Ryan-Wenger N. A longitudinal study of age and gender differences of stressors and coping strategies in school-aged children. *J Pediatr Health Care* 1995;9:123–130.
51. Bernstein BA, Pachter LM. Cultural considerations in children's pain. In: Schechter NL, Berde CB, Yaster M, eds. *Pain in infants, children, and adolescents*. Baltimore: Williams & Wilkins, 1993:113–122.
52. Pfefferbaum B, Adams J, Aceves J. The influence of culture on pain in Anglo and Hispanic children with cancer. *J Am Acad Child Adolesc Psychiatry* 1990;29: 642–647.
53. Beyer J, Villarruel A, Denyes M. *The Oucher: user's manual and technical report*. Kansas City, MO: School of Nursing, University of Missouri at Kansas City, 1995.
54. Hart D. Assessing culture: pediatric nurses' beliefs and self-reported practices. *J Pediatr Nurs* 1999;14: 255–262.

55. Kotzer A, Coy J, LeClaire A. The effectiveness of a standardized educational program for children using patient-controlled analgesia. *J Soc Pediatr Nurs* 1998; 3:117–26.
56. Broome M, Huth M. Preparation of children for hospitalization, surgery and procedures. In: Craft-Rosenberg M, Denehy J, ed. *Nursing interventions for children and families*. Philadelphia: Saunders, 2000.
57. Yap JN. A critical review of pediatric preoperative preparation procedures: processes, outcomes, and future directions. *J Appl Devel Psychol* 1988;4:359–389.
58. Romsing J, Walther-Larsen J. Post-operative pain in children: a survey of parents expectations and perceptions of children's experiences. *Paediatr Anaesth* 1996; 3:215–218.
59. Broome M. Helping parents support their child in pain. *Pediatr Nurs* 2000;3:315–317.
60. Bauchner H, Vinci R, Waring C. Parental presence during procedures in an emergency room: results from 50 operations. *Pediatrics* 1991;4:544–548.
61. Bauchner H, Vinci R, Waring C. Pediatric procedures: do parents want to stay? *Pediatrics* 1989;84:907–909.
62. Broome M, Endsley R. Parent and child reactions to an immunization. *Pain* 1989;1:85–92.
63. Blount R, Landolf-Fritsche B, Powers S, et al. Differences between high and low coping children and between parent and staff behaviors during painful procedures. *J Pediatr Psychol* 1991;16:795–809.
64. Broome M, Lillis P, McGahee T, et al. The use of distraction and imagery with children during painful procedures. *Oncol Nurs Forum* 1992;19:499–502.
65. Broome M, Rehwaldt M, Fogg L. Relationships between cognitive-behavioral techniques, temperament, observed distress and pain reports in children and adolescents during lumbar puncture. *J Pediatr Nurs* 1998; 1:48–54.
66. Pederson C. Nonpharmacologic interventions to manage children's pain: immediate and short-term effects of a continuing education program. *J Contin Educ Nurs* 1996;3:131–140.
67. Shaw E, Routh D. Effect of mother presence on children's reactions to aversive procedures. *J Pediatr Psychol* 1982;7:33–42.
68. Jacobsen P, Manne S, Gorfinkle K, et al. Analysis of child and parent behavior during painful medical procedures. *Health Psychol* 1990;5:559–576.
69. Broome M, Endsley R. Maternal presence, childrearing practices and child response to an injection. *Res Nurs Health* 1989;12:229–235.
70. Doctor M. Parent participation during painful wound care procedures. *J Burn Care Rehabil* 1994;3:288–292.
71. Dahlquist L, Power T, Carlson L. Physician and parent behavior during invasive pediatric cancer procedures: relationships to child behavioral distress. *J Pediatr Psychol* 1995;4:477–490.
72. Naber S, Halstead L, Broome M, et al. Communication and control: parent, child and health professionals' interactions during painful procedures. *Issues Compr Pediatr Nurs* 1995;18:79–90.
73. O'Laughlin E, Ridley-Johnson R. Maternal presence during children's routine physical examinations: the effect of mother as observer in reducing children's distress. *Child Health Care* 1995;3:175–191.
74. Maikler V. Pharmacologic pain management in children: a review of intervention research. *J Pediatr Nurs* 1998;1:3–14.
75. Boughton K, Blower C, Chartrand C, et al. Impact of research and pediatric pain assessment and outcomes. *Pediatr Nurs* 1998;1:31–35.
76. McCaffery M, Ferrell B. Correcting misconceptions about pain assessment and use of opioid analgesics: educational strategies aimed at public concerns. *Nurs Outlook* 1991;4:184–190.
77. Romsing J. Assessment of nurses' judgement for analgesic requirements of postoperative children. *J Clinic Pharm Ther* 1996;3:159–163.
78. Weldon BC, Connor M, White PF. The role of concurrent opioid infusions and nurse-controlled analgesia. *Clin J Pain* 1993;9:26–33.
79. Mitchell P, Heinrich J, Moritz P, et al. Measurement into practice. *Med Care* 1997;11:124–130.
80. Ross PJ, Fochtman D. Conscious sedation: a quality management project. *J Pediatr Oncol Nurs* 1995;3: 115–121.
81. Lambert S. Distraction, imagery and hypnosis: techniques for management of children's pain. *J Child Fam Nurs* 1999;6:5–15.
82. Vessey J, Carlson K. Nonpharmacological interventions to use with children in pain. *Issues Compr Pediatr Nurs* 1996;19:169–182.
83. McCarthy AM, Cool V, Hanrahan K. Cognitive behavioral interventions for children during painful procedures: research challenges and program development. *J Pediatr Nurs* 1998;7:119–120.
84. Pederson C, Harbaugh BL. Nurses' use of nonpharmacologic techniques with hospitalized children. *Issues Compr Pediatr Nurs* 1995;2:91–109.
85. Marek K. Measuring the effectiveness of nursing care. *Outcomes Manage Nurs Pract*1998;1:8–11.
86. Wong S. Outcomes of nursing care: how do we know? *Clin Nurs Spec* 1998;12:147–151.
87. Vincent K. Nurses analgesic practices with hospitalized children. *J Child Fam Nurs* 2001;2:1–12.
88. Fanurik D, Koh J, Schmitz M. Distraction techniques combined with EMLA: effects on I.V. insertion pain and distress in children. *Child Health Care* 2000;2:87–101.
89. Frank NC, Blount RL, Smith AJ, et al. Parent and staff behavior, and previous medical experience and maternal anxiety as they relate to child distress and coping. *J Pediatr Psychol* 1995;20:277–289.
90. Macnab A, Thiessan P, McLeod E, et al. Parent assessment of family-centered care practices in a children's hospital. *Child Health Care* 2000;2:113–128.
91. McGrath P, Findley GA, Ritchie JA. *Pain, pain go away: helping children with pain*. Halifax, NS: Department of Psychology, 1994.
92. Kuttner L. *A child in pain: how to help, what to do*. Vancouver: Hartley & Marks, 1996.
93. Meyers T, Eichorn D, Guzzetta C, et al. Family presence during invasive procedures and resuscitation. *Am J Nurs* 2000;2:1–23.
94. Pederson C. Ways to feel comfortable: teaching aids to promote children's comfort. *Issues Compr Pediatr Nurs* 1994;17:37–46.
95. Campos R. Rocking and pacifiers; two comforting interventions for heelstick. *Nurs Res Health* 1994;11: 321–331.
96. Vessey JA, Carlson KL, McGill J. Use of distraction

during an acute painful experience. *Nurs Res* 1994;6: 369–372.

97. French GM, Painter EC, Coury DL. Blowing away shot pain: a technique for pain management during immunizations. *Pediatrics* 1994;93:384–388.
98. Broome M. *To tame the hurting thing: relaxation and imagery for children*. Birmingham: University of Alabama at Birmingham, 1994.
99. Carlson K. Selected resources on pediatric pain. *J Pediatr Nurs* 1998;1:64–66.
100. Johnson M, Maas M, Moorehead S. *Nursing outcomes classification*, 2nd ed. St. Louis: Mosby Year Book, 2000.
101. Gedaly-Duff V, Huff-Slankard J. Sleep as an indicator for pain relief in an infant: a case study. *J Pediatr Nurs* 1998;1:32–39.
102. Forward PS, Brown TL, McGrath PJ. Mothers' attitudes and behavior toward medicating children's pain. *Pain* 1996;67:469–474.
103. Weisz JR, McCabe MA, Dennig MD. Primary and secondary control among children undergoing medical procedures: adjustment as a function of coping style. *J Consult Clin Psychol* 1994;62:324–332.
104. Whaley LF, Wong DL. *Nursing care of infants and children*, 5th ed. St. Louis: Mosby Year Book, 1995.
105. Savedra MC, Holzemer WL, Tesler MD Assessment of postoperative pain in children using the Adolescent Pediatric Pain tool. *Nurs Res* 1993;42:50–63.
106. McGrath PA, deVerber LL, Hearn MT. Multidimensional pain assessment in children. In: Fields H, Dubner R, Cervero F, eds. *Advances in pain research and therapy*. New York: Raven, 1985:387–393.
107. Maikler V. Diaries as a data collection tool. *J Child Fam Nurs* 2000;1:65–69.

24

Physical Therapy Management of Pain in Children

Claire F. McCarthy, Alice M. Shea, and Penny Sullivan

Physical therapy intervention is an integral component in the management of a wide range of acute and chronic conditions involving pain. Physical therapists use the science and art of exercise and physical modalities to promote healing. The goal is to return all systems, including the pain transmission system, to optimal functioning.

Successful physical therapy management of pediatric and adolescent patients with pain ideally takes place in an environment of integrated care. Physical therapists participate as members of multidisciplinary groups or, ideally, with interdisciplinary teams to address the multifaceted issues involved in the treatment of pain. Whatever the setting, because each discipline serves to enhance the effectiveness of the others, communication among practitioners is essential. The pediatric physical therapist approaches pain management from a background of treating a wide variety of neuromuscular and musculoskeletal conditions involving acute and chronic pain from infancy through adolescence. Intervention by the physical therapist reflects this knowledge and experience.

This chapter highlights five areas of physical therapy management of pain: evaluation, program design (goals and treatment), strategies used in acute and chronic pain management, patient and parent education, and organization of physical therapy services for pain treatment.

EVALUATION

The initial physical therapy evaluation of a patient referred with a significant level of pain must be comprehensive. Observation, history taking including pain measurement and assessment, physical examination, and functional evaluation including performance of activities are equally important components. Selection of relevant components will relate to the presenting problem. Is it acute, chronic, or a combination of symptoms? Because of the special attention required by the child or adolescent in pain, the evaluation can be time-consuming. The short attention span of a younger child when combined with limited tolerance because of pain may necessitate dividing the evaluation into several short sessions. Table 24.1 illustrates an evaluation used for complex regional pain syndrome (CRPS).

Observation

Observations made by the therapist on initial contact with the child and/or family and those made throughout the evaluation process provide important information and insights for planning of management. Posture, movement, behavior, and interactions with people are readily observable. The type of assistive devices such as crutches, splints, or orthotics should be identified. The use and function of the devices are recorded. These observations serve to focus the evaluation.

History

The medical history illustrates the role of health issues and pain in the life of the child and family. A thorough review of the medical

TABLE 24.1. *Complex regional pain syndrome study physical therapy evaluation*

Evaluation	Measure
History of problem	Interview of patient and family
Assess patient knowledge of physical therapy	When problem recognized
Assess knowledge of approach to complex regional pain syndrome to be used	How long problem existed
	Impact on activities
	Assistive devices used, length of time
	Major restriction in activities
	Observation of family interaction
	Note who "gives" answers
	Listen to and for important facts
Pain assessment	
Intensity	Visual analog scale
Location	Patient identification
Affect	Visual analog scale
Descriptors	Patient idescriptors
Skin changes	
Color, temperature, dryness	Observation, patient report, palpation
Allodynia	
Degree/severity	Developed ordinal scale, built on tolerance to touch and time tolerated
Location, extent	Self-report
Clothes aversion	Goniometric assessment
Joint motion	Manual examination + isokinetic testing
Muscle strength and performance	Limb circumference
Limb atrophy	Rancho Los Amigos Observation Gait Analysis
Function	Time-distance tests
	Stair climbing

history, including illnesses, surgical procedures, hospitalizations, previous or current physical therapy intervention, psychotherapy, and previous pain treatment will have an impact on the design of the physical therapy regimen.

The history of the presenting condition includes its onset and any precipitating event, the recent course and components of management, if any, and projected outcomes. History should also include information on pain onset, location, intensity, duration, frequency, types of sensations, and the course of the pain experience. Other determinants in treatment planning include the knowledge of activities that relieve or aggravate the pain, the effectiveness of pain medications, and the impact that the pain is having on the child directly, as well as on the child's family, social life, school, and extracurricular activities. If cultural differences or concerns are present, attention to the child, family, and therapist interactions and responses can be invaluable. The specifics of previous physical therapy treatment for pain management, treatment outcome, and any intervention for pain control are important. If the child is young or unable to communicate, history from the parent(s) should include as much of the above information as possible. If assistive devices are used, information on the reason for use, length of time worn, satisfaction, and comfort level is important. During the time such information is being gathered, a rapport is being established between the patient and parent(s) and the therapist.

The extent to which the parents or child answer questions during the session may reflect the child's level of autonomy. It can also reflect the level of understanding of the problem. Encouraging children to answer questions themselves increases their sense of control, fosters a pattern of independence and accountability for future therapy sessions, and allows assessment of the child's level of understanding of the treatment process.

Pain Tests and Measurements

Pain is defined as an unpleasant sensory and emotional experience (1). Physical therapists, however, must attempt to objectively assess this subjective phenomenon not only as a component of current history but also as baseline data to design treatment programs and assess outcomes. The ability to proceed with the hands-on and movement analysis components of an evaluation can be affected. Both the quality and quantity of pain and the resultant effect on movement and function are used as guideposts throughout and contribute to clinical decisions (2). Quality addresses intensity, type, and consistency of pain; quantity addresses frequency, number of areas involved, and the extent of each area involved.

The developmental stage of the child influences the response to pain. According to Jean Piaget, the way a child perceives the world, thinks, reasons, and uses language is qualitatively different according to stages. These are described as sensorimotor (birth to 2 years), preoperational (2 to 7 years), concrete operations (7 to 12 years), and adolescent/adult (12 years and older) (3). For example, an infant or 6-month-old child may well become irritable or wince with a quick, rough, or cold touch, a loud sound or voice, or very bright lighting; a 2- or 3-year-old child may allow use of instruments after touching or feeling them. Time used to assess and prepare a child's environment can prevent a response of fear, irritation, or unwillingness to move from being misconstrued as caused by pain.

Physical therapists are becoming increasingly familiar with methods of rating and recording the level of pain sensation. These include self-report, behavioral, and physiologic methods. Recent inclusion of pain management standards by the Joint Commission on Accreditation of Healthcare Organizations (JCAHO) has focused additional attention on documentation in this area (4).

Self-report scales are considered the best indicators of a child's pain experience. Children as young as 4 years can point to a picture of the face on a scale that indicates the intensity of their pain (5); children by the age of 7 years can also use a visual analog scale or a numeric rating scale (6–8). Older children can also provide information about the characteristics of the pain sensation such as sharp, aching, stinging, or intermittent.

Assessment of the emotional aspects of pain is also important. Children 6 years of age and older should be given the opportunity to express the emotions of pain. Quantification of the emotional aspect of the pain experience can be done using the self-report scales (8). Few children have difficulty understanding the distinction between being "scared" and being "hurt."

Pediatric physical therapists are often involved in the care of children with developmental disabilities. Although research is being done in this area, no valid measurement tools currently exist (9). Careful observation of behavioral and physiologic changes combined with discussion with parents or caregivers is important to determine the best methods of communication. With some children, self-report may be possible with the use of communication boards or electronic devices, sign language, facial movements, and cues that are understood by families and caregivers.

Multidimensional scales and composite measures have been developed and should be considered by therapists for use with infants as well as children and adolescents with complex pain problems (10).

In interpreting findings, the therapist determines whether the pain is expected given the pathology. Anticipated pain can be addressed; unexpected or excessive pain is an alert to the therapist. Additional analysis may be necessary, and consultation with the referring physician is indicated. An example of such a situation is point tenderness over a specific location and unwillingness to accept pressure, as might occur in the malunion of a fracture. Pain, therefore, is always viewed in the context of the total clinical picture and not as an isolated entity. Clinical decisions are based on the therapist's judgment of the severity of the sensation and the level of distress the child is experiencing. These aspects must be differentiated in assessing the whole experience of pain because each requires a different approach.

During an initial evaluation and using appropriate measurement tools, therapists measure the level of pain and the accompanying emotion that the child is experiencing. The initial measurement is then used as a baseline for the scope of the painful problem and as a measure for judging improvement. When combined with history and observations, the information helps the therapist to make the remaining components of the evaluation as comfortable as possible and allows valid interpretation of test findings.

Physical Examination

Physical examination is always done with care so that the patient is as comfortable as possible to lessen fear and apprehension. The therapist continues to develop a positive and trusting relationship with the patient and parents. Both are actively engaged in the therapeutic process by discussing the purpose and rationale for the evaluation and getting assurance of their understanding. A brief description of each test procedure and any expectation of pain is given.

The therapist must be flexible in administering an evaluation and alter the sequence or techniques in response to the patient's tolerance. Initially, procedures performed with the patient in an upright position, such as sitting or standing, are less threatening than those performed with the patient supine. It is important to maximize the patient's feeling of control during each therapy session. Such consideration adds to the trust and comfort level.

Posture (11,12) and gait (13,14) are evaluated to establish current deviations and habitual patterns. Abnormal posture and walking patterns resulting from pain may often lead to stresses on other parts of the body. Muscle splinting and weight shifting away from the site of pain are frequently observed. Such compensatory actions may lead to the development of secondary problems and should be addressed (Fig. 24.1).

Soft tissue is examined by observation and palpation. The presence of tenderness or trigger points is noted. Skin changes such as discoloration, dryness, excessive sweating, scarring, shininess, hair growth or loss, and soft-tissue contractures are recorded. The patient's avoidance of clothing on a hypersensitive extremity is noted.

Palpation further identifies the areas affected and differentiates the type of touch that can be tolerated. The term *allodynia* refers to pain evoked by light touch of the skin. *Hyperalgesia* refers to disproportionately severe pain produced by stimuli that would normally require much higher stimulus intensities to evoke the same severity of pain. If allodynia is present, the extent of the area and any focal points are described. A nominal scale is being developed to describe the degree of hypersensitivity. Awareness of areas of hypersensitivity of a limb directs hand placement and positioning. Edema is quantified by a girth measurement; palpation reveals pitting characteristics. Temperature differences between limbs are felt by palpation and can be measured by a skin thermometer.

Strength and flexibility are measured using standardized manual muscle tests (11,15) and range of motion measurements (16,17). Involving children in the test procedures by having them demonstrate their arcs of motion and painful positions will engage them in the evaluative process and alleviate their fears. When the therapist does hands-on testing, measuring the uninvolved side teaches the child about what to expect, provides a comparison with the involved side, and helps to allay apprehensions.

Function is of prime importance. If assistive devices are used, a further check of fit, use, and appropriateness is necessary. Observation of gait and stair climbing with and without assistive devices is important. An-

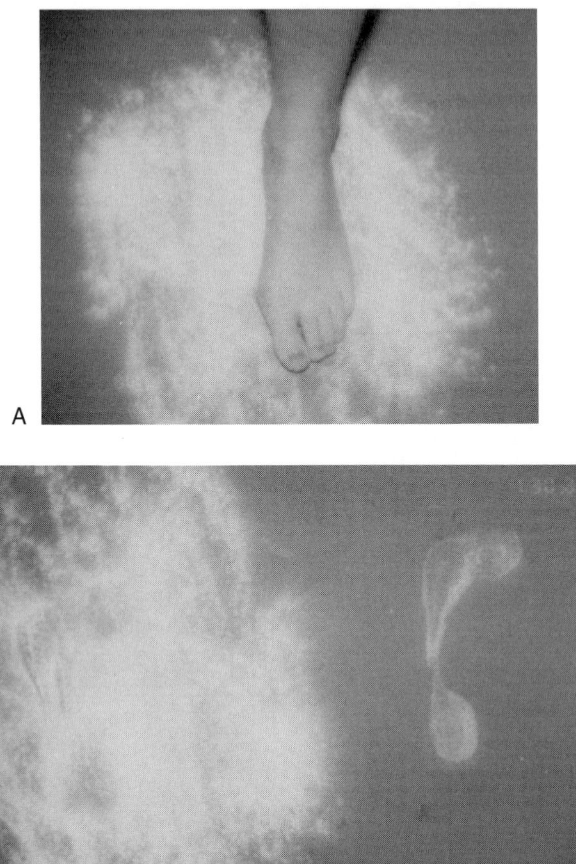

FIG. 24.1. This patient illustrates the use of powder footprints to encourage weight bearing through a painful extremity.

swers to questions about getting to and from school, managing books, and engaging in usual leisure time activities also illustrate the current level of function. Are tasks at home done in the usual way, modified, or assumed by parents or siblings? Are there changes in eating or sleeping habits? An analysis of body mechanics involved in daily activities may reveal other areas that need intervention. The use of standardized functional assessments can be helpful in documenting progress (18–20).

In summary, the measurement of pain and its effect on function sets baseline data, helps to design treatment regimes, and facilitates measuring progress at specified intervals. Additional pain information obtained throughout the evaluation leads to the selection of appropriate treatment techniques. Such pain information may modify the initial plan. The same measurement tools should be used for documenting baseline data as well as judging the effect of a specific intervention. Consistent use of a tool when comparing baseline and subsequent evaluation data is very important, particularly if more than one therapist is involved.

PROGRAM DESIGN

When designing a program for a young patient with pain, the pediatric physical therapist considers developmental, family, school, and social concerns. If present, awareness of cultural differences and their potential impact on the selected management strategy is very important. The child's age, cognitive abilities, emotional maturity, behavioral development, and level of independence all have an impact on the goals and selected intervention strategies. The plan focuses on four main areas: pain reduction, alleviation of impairments, managing functional activities, and patient and family education. Each area is dependent on the others. As gains are made in one area, improvements often occur in one of the other areas. Educating patients and parents from the beginning and including them in the selection of management strategies through every phase of treatment contributes to an optimal outcome and long-term control of pain. To prevent confusion or misunderstandings at any age, use and choice of language by the therapist should be age appropriate, simple, unambiguous, positive, and truthful.

Time is an important consideration when caring for children who have pain. Careful explanation of procedures and unfamiliar instruments is always beneficial and can contribute to positive outcomes. Parents need detailed explanations, particularly if there is a negative response to treatment. Taking time to alleviate the anxiety of a child and the parents is invaluable.

Goals

Goals for physical therapy intervention are based on the evaluative findings and the expected course of recovery from the pathology or injury. Acute pain that is expected to diminish quickly and naturally will require different goals, priorities, and treatment approaches than chronic pain that persists over time. In either case, an early focus on goals and plans engages the patient in the therapeutic process. Participation by the child or adolescent in setting interim and long-term objectives promotes understanding of treatment rationale and improves compliance with the program.

A correlative goal is effective communication among the child, parents, and the therapist. Optimal treatment choices can be made if a child communicates his or her needs and discusses the treatment program. In the very young child or one who cannot express his or her needs, discussion between parents and therapist and parental participation in treatment planning are essential.

Treatment

The individualized treatment program design is based on prioritized goals that reflect the acuity level or chronicity of the pain and the positive clinical findings. Appropriate treatment modes are then selected to create a program designed for optimal care. Initially, treatment is aimed at decreasing pain as quickly and completely as possible. As patients respond to the efforts to improve their comfort, the focus of therapy shifts to improvement in function. The positive findings of the evaluation are addressed, and treatment focuses on remediation of the underlying causes of pain and dysfunction. Many modalities and treatment strategies are used in the treatment of acute and chronic pain and pain producing pathology (Table 24.2). Therapeutic intervention is facilitated when combined with relaxation, deep breathing, imagery, and distraction techniques (Chapter 17). A brief presentation of some of the modalities that are used frequently follows.

Modalities

A modality can be beneficial either as a primary mode of treatment or an adjunct to enhance the effects of other interventions such as massage, therapeutic exercise, and joint mobilization. When selecting a modality, appropriateness for children and any contraindications related to a child's age should be considered.

Transcutaneous electrical nerve stimulation (TENS) is a safe, noninvasive, and highly effective modality for partially or completely blocking the pain sensation. The analgesic effect of TENS has been ascribed to the gate control theory of pain, which suggests that stimu-

TABLE 24.2. *Schematic of physical therapy approaches used in complex regional pain syndrome*

Impairment	Goal	Approach
Knowledge deficits Understanding of the problem, reason for PT intervention, expectations for results of PT	Increase knowledge and understanding of problem, improve understanding of PT rationale, goals, and interventions	Education and explanation throughout 6-wk period
Pain	Diminish pain	Transcutaneous electrical nerve stimulation, thermal modalities, progressive weight bearing
Hypersensitivity (allodynia)	Desensitization to touch and weight bearing	Progressive sensory input
Limited range of motion	Increase range of motion	Active exercise and active stretching, neuromuscular facilitation
Decreased limb strength	Improve muscle strength and performance	Exercises for strength and use of movement patterns, progressive gross motor skills
Decreased limb circulation	Improve capillary blood flow, diminish swelling, blunt reflex vasoconstriction	Progressive active exercise, water-based activity, massage, contrast baths
Gait deviations	Improve strength, balance, and coordination; diminish deviations	Progressive weight bearing, gait training
Functional limitations Dependence in activities of daily living	Increase independence, achieve acceptance of role in recovery and self-care	Strategize and set progressive objectives for achieving functional goals
Disability Decreased participation in normal life roles	Facilitate return to previous activities, e.g., school, social and physical activities	Strategize and set goals with patient, family, and team members

PT, physical therapy.
Data from Lee BH, Scharff L, Sethna NF, et al. Physical and cognitive-behavioral treatment for complex regional pain syndromes. *J Pediatr* 2002, *in press.*

lation of large-diameter cutaneous afferent nerve fibers can inhibit pain transmission to the spinal cord via small-diameter nociceptive afferents (21). Another explanation is that endorphins are produced, resulting in pain relief via descending pain-inhibitory pathways (22,23).

TENS is contraindicated in patients with cardiac pacemakers, over a pregnant uterus, carotid arteries, eyes, and while driving. Use with incompetent or confused patients is also not recommended.

TENS has traditionally been used with children who are cognitively mature enough to communicate. Children can be fearful of TENS, particularly when the word electrical is used. Successful use of TENS with children depends on the skill of the therapist and the teaching strategies used with the child and parents. A simple explanation of pain pathways helps the child and parents to understand the concept of pain control. With instruction and practice, children, some as young as 8 years of age, can become independent in the use of TENS, gain control over their pain, and learn to take responsibility for their treatment.

Based on the child's report of pain, the therapist selects the appropriate electrode placement site on the affected body part and determines the mode and the rate and width parameters. A suggested approach to introducing TENS to a child is placing the electrodes on an unaffected part or on the parent (24). To reduce apprehension during the initial trial, the child can be allowed to control the intensity. Duration in time and frequency of use are determined by the degree of relief of pain reported by the child.

Electrodes are most commonly placed around the painful region but can also be placed along peripheral nerve routes or cutaneous branches, at acupuncture, motor, and trigger points, or at spinal segments (25). The conventional mode and acupuncture-like mode are the two basic modes of stimulation. At the initial trial session, conventional TENS is the mode most frequently used. The stimulation produced is at the more comfortable sensory level. The parameters of high rate, low pulse width produce a buzzing or tingling sensation in the painful area. The sensation should be strong but not unpleasant; a muscle contraction does not occur. When the conventional mode is used, pain relief is experienced with the unit on and patients can wear the unit for several hours at a time. The nervous system can accommodate conventional mode stimulation, and children may find that they need to increase intensity to obtain relief. The rate and/or width parameter can also be adjusted with successful continuation of pain relief.

Acupuncture-like TENS uses parameters of low rate, high pulse width. The sensation is that of a heartbeat, with a muscle contraction visible in the myotomes of the painful area. Children who do best with this mode seem to have higher pain tolerance, can "bite the bullet" and tolerate a higher intensity. When the acupuncture-like TENS mode is used, stimulation is only for 1 to 2 hours because muscles can become fatigued by constant contraction. There is less likelihood of nervous system accommodation. Because one mechanism for pain relief using the acupuncture-like TENS mode is the release of endorphins, pain relief can continue after the unit is turned off.

After being fitted with TENS, the patient ideally wears it for an hour. The therapist then checks for skin tolerance, monitors effectiveness, and resets parameters, if necessary. TENS is a modality that should not be used alone but as part of a comprehensive treatment program with other interventions such as skilled physical therapy, biobehavioral intervention, and medications. TENS can be used during a physical therapy treatment session (Fig. 24.2). The unit can be worn outside, to school, and during normal activities. Follow-up with the therapist is done to monitor the use and effectiveness of the unit.

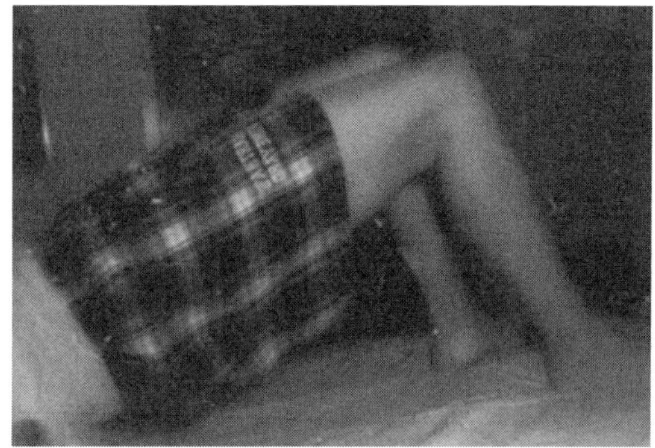

FIG. 24.2. Illustration of the use of transcutaneous electrical stimulation during an exercise session with a patient with complex regional pain syndrome of the left foot.

Written instructions, including illustrations of proper electrode placement, should always be given to the family. A diary should be given to the child to record changes in pain but, more important, to document improvement in function. This can be helpful if justification for use of the unit is required by insurance companies.

Ultrasound delivers thermal and nonthermal energy to subcutaneous tissues (e.g., muscle, tendon, bursa). Continuous ultrasonography acts by heating the tissues, whereas pulsed ultrasound provides nonthermal, acoustic streaming effects (26). Ultrasound is contraindicated in younger children in whom growth plates have not closed (27).

Electrical stimulation, using direct and alternating currents, causes change in muscle functioning and tissue homeostasis in a variety of ways. Muscle and nerve fibers are selectively stimulated depending on the type of waveform, amplitude, electrode pattern, and placement applied. Electrical stimulation is used to reduce pain, edema, and muscle spasm; it can also assist with muscle re-education. Combined electrical stimulation with ultrasonography delivers both types of stimulation simultaneously and may be most effective in decreasing pain (28).

Electromyogram biofeedback is used in the re-education of muscles in one of two ways: for relaxation of overactive or spastic muscles or for motor unit recruitment in a poorly contracting muscle. Children quickly learn the significance of the feedback (auditory and/or visual) and can be taught to use the modality independently at home. Temperature biofeedback may be used to increase circulation and facilitate an appropriate temperature response locally (29).

Iontophoresis is the introduction of topically applied, physiologically active ions into the epidermis and mucous membranes of the body by the use of continuous direct current, e.g., the use of a steroid such as dexamethasone over an inflamed tendon. The purpose of iontophoresis is to provide a local anesthetic, reduce edema, and reduce inflammation, and it is used in a variety of musculoskeletal inflammatory conditions (30).

Fluidotherapy, a heat modality, uses air-filtered solids as a medium for heat transfer. Active and passive range of motion can be performed while warming the involved extremity. Patients with a diagnosis that clinically presents with localized extremity pain, edema, decreased range of motion, and reduced circulation tolerate this modality well (31,32). It can be used as a method of desensitization on a limb with hypersensitivity, e.g., in CRPS. In addition, children enjoy this modality. Clinical experience has shown that some children at 2 years of age are developmentally ready for the use of this modality.

The application of *superficial cold or heat* is used in the presence of pain. Cold is recommended for use within 24 to 48 hours of injury to prevent swelling. Ice massage and cold packs are the frequently used two methods. Heat is generally used after the first 24 to 48 hours. Hot packs or moist heat are preferred.

Hydrotherapeutic techniques are especially soothing to painful conditions, including warm or tepid whirlpool for local relief or whole-body submersion. The action of the water increases cutaneous circulation, provides gentle tactile stimulation on all surfaces, and produces generalized muscle relaxation. Contrast baths are used to stimulate local circulation. Hydrotherapy is particularly useful for gaining function. The water provides buoyancy and decreases weight-bearing forces while being an enjoyable medium for the patient. Circulation and nutritional supply of joint surfaces and surrounding tissues are increased by active motion during emersion (33).

Exercise and Manual Techniques

Therapeutic exercise programs are based on evaluative findings and address specific impairments and loss of function. The selection and type of exercises used reflect the goals to be achieved and desired outcomes. Exercise can facilitate movement, strengthen muscle, improve muscle sequencing, improve postural awareness, correct gait deviations, improve local and systemic circulation, increase bone density, and improve endurance (34) (Fig. 24.3).

Manual techniques make the patient aware of specific areas of the body. Tissue manipulation, massage techniques, and trigger-point release are used to identify and treat soft-tis-

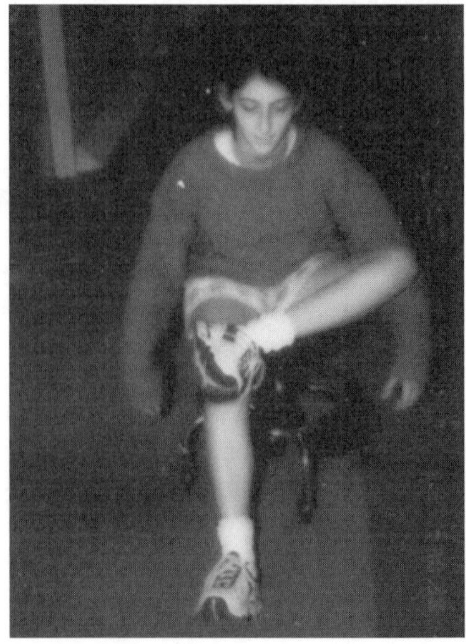

FIG. 24.3. This patient illustrates the propulsion of a stool with the involved limb to increase strength. The carpeted floor surface adds resistance.

sue dysfunction. The specific techniques used are too numerous to describe; however, all employ hands-on facilitation and inhibition of movement in conjunction with education to enable patients to better cope with and decrease their level of pain.

STRATEGIES IN ACUTE AND CHRONIC PAIN

Physical therapists participate in the treatment of both acute and chronic pain. This section uses the work of Jacobson and Mariano (35) to define these types of pain to describe treatment by the therapist.

> Pain that extends beyond the period of healing, in the absence of ongoing pathology, should be viewed as chronic pain. Pain of relatively short duration elicited by injury of body tissues and activation of nociceptive transducers at the site of local tissue damage should be viewed as acute pain. Pain, however, that extends over periods for which there is ongoing pathology might best be viewed as acute and chronic pain.

Acute Pain

Acute pain is expected to be of short duration, improve as healing progresses, and follow a reasonable timetable with a fairly predictable end point. Causes of acute pain are trauma, postoperative pain, and pain caused by conditions frequently seen by pediatric therapists (e.g., patellofemoral stress syndrome, Osgood–Schlatter disease). If pain and functional improvement are not observed within the expected time frame, a therapist should be proactive and contact the referring physician.

In the ambulatory setting, treatment strategies for conditions presenting with acute pain generally focus on relief of symptoms, resolution of impairments, and improvement of functional abilities. The goal is for the child to return to his/her baseline functional activity level.

With acute pain, an immediate and direct approach is most appropriate. Early intervention to reduce pain limits impairments and improves the level of function. Modalities previously described may be used. As pain decreases and function improves, the treatment regimen and home program are appropriately modified, and the child assumes more responsibility.

For children and adolescents, admission to an acute care facility is an anxiety-provoking experience. The hospital is new and bewildering and can be a frightening environment. Children may feel overwhelmed by the number of health professionals involved in their care and may react with apprehension each time they are approached. Adolescents may be more reluctant than children to express their concerns. Therapists in this setting need to be particularly sensitive to the presence of pain and an increased level of anxiety of both child and parents. Clear, concise, and age-appropriate explanations are important.

To maximize a child's cooperation, treatment times are coordinated with pain medication administration. Analgesics, when taken before the treatment, allow the patient to be more relaxed and compliant during the physical therapy program. In some situations, in which pain is a guidepost, medication may be delayed.

Postoperatively, parenteral infusion is the most frequently used method to administer opioids. Continuous infusions and/or nurse-controlled analgesia are used for children younger than 5 or 6 years of age. Children as young as 6 years of age can use a patient-controlled analgesia (PCA) pump that allows small boluses of opioid to be delivered immediately before or during a physical therapy session. Either nurse-controlled analgesia or PCA permits dosing in anticipation of a physical therapy session to provide supplemental analgesia for relief of movement-related pain Timing of these supplemental doses is especially useful for patients receiving pulmonary physical therapy after a thoracotomy or for patients with spinal fusions who begin ambulation in the first days postoperatively.

Pediatric therapists in acute care settings have become accustomed to treating children and adolescents who are receiving epidural delivery of opiates and local anesthetics. In these situations, knowledge of the motor and/or sensory effect of the specific procedure becomes very important to both maximize the positive effects on the therapeutic program and take proper precautions. For example, programs are initiated earlier, airway clearance is better tolerated and ambulation is possible. Precautions need to be taken to prevent dislodging of the catheter, assure safety of the patient in the presence of any motor or sensory loss, and protect the pump during ambulation. Communication and collaborative planning with pain service physicians can often be beneficial to coordinate decisions to increase or decrease epidural infusion rates before a physical therapy treatment session. For example, a patient with severe pain and contractures might benefit from an epidural bolus or increased infusion rate before physical therapy treatment. Conversely, a patient receiving a lumbar or low thoracic epidural infusion after abdominal surgery may require a reduced infusion rate if excessive motor blockade of the lower extremities has interfered with ambulation. Similar considerations apply when epidural infusions are used for patients with complex regional pain syndromes (see below and Chapter 34).

Chronic Pain

Pediatric physical therapists also see patients who experience pain in the absence of ongoing pathology or with a condition that is stable. Examples of these are headaches, back pain, neuropathic pain, CRPS, fibromyalgia, and chronic fatigue syndrome. Pain management is best approached from an interdisciplinary perspective, integrating pharmacologic, cognitive-behavioral, and physical therapeutic approaches preferably within the structure of a pain clinic (Chapter 27).

Many children with chronic pain function quite well. They do not allow their pain to be the guiding force in their lives and do not regard their pain as disabling. They receive appropriate intervention for treatable impairments, have learned physical and/or biobehavioral self-management techniques, and, although they may need to make some modifications, they lead fairly normal lives. There are some children, however, in whom pain becomes the primary focus of attention for both them and their family (36,37). School absenteeism or school avoidance can be high. Social interactions with friends are affected. Sleep patterns are poor, and family dynamics can be disrupted. Dependence on pain medications can occur. Fear–avoidance behavior results in severe restrictions of physical activity and increased deconditioning (38). Subjective reports of pain do not correlate with objective physical findings, and the child is more disabled than one would expect. These patients present a challenge to the treating therapist.

Wittink et al. (39) discuss the physical therapy management of adult patients with chronic pain using a modified functional restoration model. Their philosophy can be extrapolated to the child with chronic pain. The treatment is geared toward meaningful, functional goals that the child has identified, for example, "I want to return to school," "I want to be able to go to the mall with my friends." The child may need help in setting functional goals that are realistic. If he or she has not been attending school for some time, a short-term goal of returning for half days may be reasonable. The focus is taken away from pain and is placed on improvement in function, and disability is de-emphasized. Education about the pathophysiology of pain and its effect on function is a major component in the treatment approach. For instance, neuropathic pain (complex regional pain syndrome type I) is nonprotective pain. Although there is pain with attempts to use the joint, there is no worsening of an underlying process, and the use of the joint will not cause tissue injury. The latter information can be reassuring to patients and families and can have an impact on their perception of the problem. Treatable impairments are addressed by the therapist with a hands-on approach using any of the modalities previously described, but pain must be related to function and correlate with objective findings. Overmedicalization can be counterproductive in these patients. Self-management skills are emphasized that can be used at any time if a flare-up of acute symptoms occurs. A quota-based exercise program using a flow sheet can be used to monitor compliance with a home program and to help with pacing as activities increase (40). The flow sheet also serves as a motivating tool for the child. The patient and therapist agree on a quota for an exercise (duration and repetitions), and the patient records exactly what was performed. Exercises increase in intensity with the addition of aerobic conditioning. Exercise can improve mood, quality of sleep, self-esteem as well as activate endogenous pain-inhibiting systems.

Biobehavioral intervention is an integral component of the rehabilitation process. The child learns self-management skills through biofeedback, relaxation, training and other techniques. These help to modify pain behaviors and provide a means to cope with the pain. Adults with chronic pain can be expected to take primary responsibility for their pain management. With children, responsibility is a combined effort between the child and parents. Parents must embrace the same philosophy as the management team. Unintentionally, parents may compromise the efforts of the team by reinforcing pain behaviors based on personal beliefs or experiences with pain.

It has been suggested that persistent, painful pain conditions may produce irreversible changes in the structure and neurochemical function of the central nervous system and that these changes are encoded in the brain as pain memory (41). A pattern in the central nervous system is created, and the patient believes pain is present. This can make chronic pain resistant to traditional therapeutic interventions. Aggressive physical therapy, behavioral medicine, and pharmacologic interventions may retard the development of these changes in the function of the central nervous system and in pain memory. Perhaps increasing disability can be averted in the child, and return to full functional activities can be achieved.

Acute Chronic Pain

Physical therapists are frequently involved in treatment of conditions that present with acute and chronic pain, e.g., juvenile rheumatoid arthritis, hemophilia, cystic fibrosis. Ongoing pathology exists, with recurring episodes of acute, nociceptive pain. With an acute episode, emphasis is placed on alleviating the acute pain with strategies previously described. When the acute episode is resolved, the underlying pathology again becomes the focus. Because of underlying chronicity, both psychologic and social stressors can exist. Over time, these stressors can contribute to more emotional distress and additional limitations in functional abilities.

Children who experience both acute and chronic pain present a particular challenge to therapists. Acute events may not be anticipated and may have an effect on the ongoing pathology. Measurement of pain intensity over the course of each acute episode is important: continuing to measure the intensity level of the chronic pain and pain affect over time is essential. With children, treatment programs and management strategies need periodic and systematic comprehensive review.

PATIENT AND FAMILY EDUCATION

Functional goals are primarily addressed in the home program. The age and cognitive functioning of the child determine the degree to which monitoring, direct participation, or supervision is needed from the parent(s). Parents need to understand the importance of allowing children to take appropriate responsibility for their rehabilitation program. Sharing participation in the program is possible, but the goal is to have children take as much responsibility for their pain management and rehabilitation program as their cognitive and emotional development will allow.

Children or teenagers can learn to be cognizant of their pain while engaged in daily activities and, when appropriate, to use pain as an indicator for stopping an activity. Selected activities are carried out for short periods only, performed at a moderate pace in an easy, relaxed manner, and stopped before pain increases. The activity level is upgraded daily if there is no increase in pain. Some patients may need to build tolerance more gradually. The key is to develop a graduated regimen of slow increases in activity. If the pain worsens, the child waits until the pain level has returned to its minimal level. The child then starts again at a lower activity level or with a change in program. The goal is to gradually increase function without causing more pain.

Psychosocial elements need consideration and can heavily influence the patient's compliance. Activities are found that are motivating. Socialization may be incorporated into an activity, such as walking in the mall, playing ball, and swimming. An example of the importance of education is found in the treatment of sports-related injuries. The basic principles of pain management continue as the focus: the reduction of pain, restoration of physical function, management of the return to athletic or recreational activity, and the education of the child, family, and coach. The therapist's recognition of the influence of peer groups and coaches is particularly critical in selecting management strategies. Understanding the dynamics of the sport or activity involved, the associated environment and precipitating factors that led to dysfunction are important when problem solving and planning. Emphasis is placed on the athlete's participation in setting short-, interim-, and long-range objectives and accepting responsibility for achieving each objective in a timely fashion. The immediate goal of all concerned is the return to the athletic or recreational activity in preinjury condition as rapidly as possible. The long-range goal is the education of the young athlete, family members, or coaches in ways to prevent a recurrence or further injury.

Follow-up

Follow-up plans and strategies should begin either at the time of the initial evaluation in the ambulatory setting or at discharge from a facility. The diagnosis, acuity or chronicity of the pain, and the level of understanding demonstrated by the child and parents are important. In addition, a child's coping style, motivation, and level of cognitive development help to determine the type of program. Several visits may be needed before there is proficiency in carryover. Subsequent changes are made depending on the child's progress, understanding, and continued participation in goal setting and treatment planning, and overall compliance with the program.

ORGANIZATION OF PHYSICAL THERAPY SERVICES IN PAIN TREATMENT

The contribution of physical therapy to the pain management team is unique to each clinic and is determined by many factors. The practice philosophies and administrative organization of both the physical therapy department and the pain service will influence the scope and breadth of participation by the therapist(s). The role is further delineated by the patient population served within the facility, the needs of the team, and the resources of the physical therapy department.

Practice policies reflect the philosophy and structure of the physical therapy department. In some settings, the practice mode is to assign a primary therapist to each patient. The relationship that evolves between the therapist, patient, and family is an important one. If the relationship is positive, valuable information, important to clinical decisions, can be obtained. In addition, compliance with a long-range program can be anticipated. The therapist on the pain management team then acts as a liaison and a resource for the primary therapist. In other settings, the therapist on the team provides the care to all patients referred to the pain service.

The administrative organization of the pain service has an impact on physical therapy practice in the facility. Funding sources and need justification requirements will often dictate the service delivery system. The patient population seen by the pain service also has an impact on the nature and design of participation. Frequency of diagnoses, the age range of patients, and the volume of inpatient versus outpatient referrals are some of the relevant variables. The way that the needs are met is largely determined by the availability of physical therapy resources. The staffing complement and current level of the department, other patient care demands, and the competency level required by the pain management team must all be considered by the physical therapy department manager.

The administrative organization, practice policies, facility, and service delivery structures should be repeatedly reviewed and revised as needed. Health care delivery systems, governmental agencies, and regulatory agencies all have an impact on patient care issues. Pain management, implementation, documentation, and other components are a major aspect.

The physical therapist brings to a facility developing pain care standards, knowledge of the discipline, and its applicability to pain management, i.e., relevant practice modes, clinical approaches, and interventions. Active participation on committees, at team meetings, and at patient care conferences is essential.

Contributing to the understanding and management of pain in children and adolescents is of prime importance for health professionals. A recent prospective study of the effectiveness of physical therapy intervention with cognitive-behavioral treatment is described in Chapter 34 and recently submitted for publication (42). Because of limited information on the effectiveness of physical therapy management of pain in children, participation in research should be a major goal.

REFERENCES

1. Mersky H, ed. Classification of chronic pain: description of chronic pain syndrome and definition of pain terms. *Pain* 1986 [suppl 3]:S215–S221.
2. *Guide to Physical Therapy Practice*, 2nd ed. Alexandria, Virginia: American Physical Therapy Association, 2001.
3. Gruber HG, Jacques VJ. *The essential Piaget*. New York: Basic Books, 1977:447.
4. *2001 Comprehensive accreditation manual for hospitals*. Oakbrook Terrace, IL: Joint Commission Resources, Inc., 2001.
5. Wong D, Baker C. Pain in children: comparison of assessment scales. *Pediatr Neurosurg* 1998;14:9–17.
6. Abu-Saad H. Assessing children's responses to pain. *Pain* 1984:19:163–171.
7. Miller MD, Ferris DG. Measurement of subjective phenomenon in primary care research: the visual analogue scale. *Fam Pract Res J* 1993;13:15–24.
8. Jedlinsky BP, McCarthy CF, Michel TH. Validating pediatric pain measurement: sensory and affective components. *Pediatr Phys Ther* 1999;11:83–9
9. Breau CM, Camfield C, McGrath PJ, et al. Measuring pain accurately in children with cognitive impairments: refinement of a caregiver scale. *J Pediatr* 2001;138: 721–727.
10. Stevens B. Pain assessment in children: birth through adolescence. *Child Adolesc Psychiatr Clin North Am* 1997;6:725–743.
11. Kendall PF, McCreary ER, Provence PG. *Muscles-testing and function*, 3rd ed. Baltimore: Williams & Wilkins, 1993.
12. Sutherland DH, Biden EN, Wyatt MP, et al. In: *Clinics in developmental medicine #104-105: Developments of mature walking*. Oxford, UK: Blackwell Scientific Publications, 1988.
13. Gronley JK, Perry J. Gait analysis techniques: Rancho Los Amigos Hospital gait laboratory. *Phys Ther* 1984; 64:1831–1838.
14. Ranchos Los Amigos Medical Center. *Observation gait analysis*. Downey, CA: Los Amigos Research and Education Institute, Inc., 1996.
15. Hislop H, Montgomery J. *Danield and Worthingham's muscle testing*, 6th ed. Philadelphia: WB Saunders, 1995.
16. Norkin CC, White DJ, eds. *Measurement of joint motion: a guide to goniometry*, 2nd ed. Philadelphia: FA Davis, 1995.
17. Green WB, Hechman JD, eds. *The clinical measurement of joint motion*. Chicago: American Academy of Orthopedic Surgeons, 1994.
18. Beakley JM, Stratford PW, Lott SA, et al. The lower extremity functional scale (LEFS) scale development, measurement properties, and clinical application. *Phys Ther* 1999;79:371–378.
19. Jebsen RH, Taylor N, Trieschmann RB, et al. An objective and standardized test of hand function. *Arch Phys Med & Rehab* 1969;50:311–319.
20. Wall JC, Bell C, Campbell S, et al. The timed get-up-and-go test revisited: measurement of the component tasks. *J Rehabil Res Dev* 2000;37:109–113.
21. Melzack R, Wall PD. Pain mechanisms: a new theory. *Science* 1965;150:971–979.
22. Pomeranz B, Chiu D. Naloxone blockade of acupuncture analgesia: endorphin implicated. *Life Sci* 1976;19: 1757–1762.
23. Sjolund BH, Eriksson MBE. The influence of naloxone on analgesia produced by peripheral conditioning stimulation. *Brain Res* 1979;173:295–301.
24. Eland J. The use of TENS with children. In: Schechter N, Berde C, Yaster M, eds. *Pain in infants, children, and adolescents, volume 1*. Baltimore: Williams & Wilkins, 1993:331–339.
25. Mannheimer JS, Lampe GN. *Clinical transcutaneous electrical nerve stimulation*. Philadelphia: FA Davis, 1983.
26. McDiarmid T, Ziskin M, Michlovitz SL. Therapeutic ultrasound. In: Michlovitz SL, ed. *Thermal agents in rehabilitation, volume 3*. Philadelphia: FA Davis, 1996: 168–212.

27. Vaughn JL, Bender LF. Effects of ultrasound on growing bone. *Arch Phys Med Rehabil* 1959;40:158.
28. Snyder-Mackler L. electrical stimulation for tissue repair. In: Robinson AJ, Snyder-Mackler L, eds. *Clinical electrophysiology: electrotherapy and electrophysiologic testing*, 2nd ed. Baltimore: Williams & Wilkins, 1995:312–333.
29. Binder-Madleod SA. Electromyographic biofeedback to improve voluntary motor control. In: Robinson AJ, Snyder-Mackler L, eds. *Clinical electrophysiology: electrotherapy and electrophysiologic testing*, 2nd ed. Baltimore: Williams & Wilkins, 1995:433–449.
30. Ciccone CD. Iontophoresis. In: Robinson AJ, Snyder-Mackler L, eds. *Clinical electrophysiology: electrotherapy and electrophysiologic testing*, 2nd ed. Baltimore: Williams & Wilkins, 1995:335–358.
31. Rennis GA, Michlovitz SL. Biophysical principles of heating and superficial heating agents. In: Michlovitz SL, ed. *Thermal agents in rehabilitation*, 3rd ed. Philadelphia: FA Davis, 1996:127–138.
32. Henley EJ. Fluidotherapy: clinical applications and techniques. *Crit Care Med* 1991;3:151.
33. Walsh MT. Hydrotherapy: the use of water as a therapeutic agent. In: Michlovitz SL, ed. *Thermal agents in rehabilitation, volume 3*. Philadelphia: FA Davis, 1996: 139–168.
34. Sullivan PE, Markos PD. *Clinical decision making in therapeutic exercise*. Stamford: Appleton & Lange, 1995.
35. Jacobson L, Mariano AJ. General considerations of chronic pain. In: Loeser JD, Butler SH, Chapman CR, et al., eds. *Bonica's management of pain, volume 3*. Philadelphia: Lippincott Williams & Wilkins, 2001:241–254.
36. Cassidy JT. Progress in diagnosis and understanding chronic pain syndrome in children and adolescents. *Adolesc Med* 1998;9:101–114.
37. Bursch B, Walco GA, Zeltzer L. Clinical assessment and management of chronic pain and pain-associated disability syndrome. *J Dev Behav Pediatr* 1998;19:45–53.
38. Fordyce W, McMahon R, Rainwater G, et al. Pain complaint-exercise performance relationships in chronic pain. *Pain* 1981;10:311–321.
39. Wittink H, Michel TH, Cohen LJ, et al. Physical therapy management. In: Wittink H, Michel TH, eds. *Chronic pain management for physical therapists*. Boston: Butterworth-Heinemann, 1997:119–153.
40. Cohen LJ. Documentation. In: Wittink H, Michel TH, eds. *Chronic pain management for physical therapists*. Boston: Butterworth-Heinemann, 1997:197–207.
41. Sandkuhler J. Learning and memory in pain pathways. *Pain* 2000;88:113–118.
42. Lee BH, Scharff L, Sethna NF, et al. Physical therapy and cognitive-behavioral treatment for complex regional pain syndromes. *J Pediatr* 2002, *in press*.

25

Complementary and Alternative Medical Therapies in Pediatric Pain Treatment

Kathi J. Kemper and Paula Gardiner

As more and more Americans turn to complementary and alternative medical (CAM) therapies for themselves and their children, physicians are being asked various questions for which their formal training may not have prepared them:

- Do you think acupuncture might help my child's pain?
- I'd like to try massage to help relieve my child's discomfort; can you help me find a pediatric massage therapist?
- Are there any problems with using aromatherapy to comfort my child?
- My Canadian cousin recommended homeopathic remedies to address my child's overall constitution and help him be healthier in dealing with his pain. What do you think?

Physicians need not be expert in every form of therapy nor abandon evidence-based medicine to be able to help answer questions like these. However, we do need to be aware of the kinds of therapies that patients are using, how to talk with families to elicit a complete history of the different therapies they might be considering for their child, basic information about CAM practices and CAM providers, and where to turn for additional information. This chapter provides an overview of CAM in pediatric pain, acknowledging that this is a rapidly changing field. Closely related topics are covered in Chapters 17, 18 and 26 of this text.

DEFINITIONS

CAM refers to therapies that are not generally taught at American medical schools, not provided in hospitals, not reimbursed by third party payers, and not proven effective (1); however, because of rapid changes in practice and research, this definition is problematic. For example, more than half of American medical schools now offer courses on complementary and alternative therapies or holistic medicine (2). Many therapies formerly considered alternative, such as acupuncture and hypnosis, are now among the therapies offered in children's hospitals. Approximately 75% of pediatric pain treatment services in teaching hospitals in North America now provide one or more therapies (such as acupuncture) that were formerly considered alternative. As a result of both science and public pressure, increasing numbers of third party payers reimburse families for services once considered alternative.

The Cochrane collaboration has defined CAM in more anthropologic terms as "a broad domain of healing resources that encompasses all health systems, modalities and practices and their accompanying theories and beliefs, other than those intrinsic to the politically dominant health systems of a particular society or culture in a given historical period" (3). Implicit in this definition is the view that boundaries within CAM practices and between CAM and mainstream medicine are blurred and changing.

Other names for alternative medicine include folk, holistic, and integrative medicine. All have slightly different meanings. Folk medicine refers to therapies that families or group members provide as part of a family or cultural tradition. Examples include chicken soup for upper respiratory infections, cold foods for "hot" illnesses, and religious or ritual healing practices such as coining and sand painting (4,5). Culturally competent practice requires familiarity with a variety of folk beliefs and healing practices.

Holistic medicine refers to care of the whole patient—body, mind, emotions, spirit, and relationships—in the context of the patient's values, beliefs, culture, and community. Examples include screening for depression and alcohol use in family members (6), promoting housecleaning to reduce allergic symptoms, and promoting literacy in the pediatric clinic (7). Integrative medicine means integrating CAM into mainstream practice, based on scientific evidence of its safety and effectiveness (8). Pediatricians who incorporate chamomile, chicken soup, vaporizers, and other home remedies in their advice about treatments for common conditions such as colic and colds may be said to practice integrative medicine (9,10).

EPIDEMIOLOGY

The percentage of American adults using CAM increased from 34% in 1990 to 42% in 1997; out-of-pocket expenditures increased 45% during this same period (11–13). CAM use is common in adults with chronic or recurrent pain, such as low back pain and premenstrual pain.

In 1994, the percentage of general pediatric patients using CAM was approximately 11% (14); this percentage increased to approximately 20% in 1997 (15). The prevalence is substantially higher for children and families faced with chronic, recurrent, or fatal conditions (16,17). In families facing these conditions, the rates of CAM use range from 30% to more than 70% depending on age, acculturation, and access to services (18). Thus, these therapies may be used quite often by pediatric patients with chronic or recurrent pain.

PATIENTS'/FAMILIES' REASONS FOR USING COMPLEMENTARY AND ALTERNATIVE MEDICINE

Conventional therapies for children with severe, chronic pain are often thought to be aggressive and disempowering of the patient and family. Treatment complications are accepted by most families because they are optimistic that therapy will control the pain. However, as the treatments begin to exhibit side effects and families feel an increasing loss of control, many parents look toward complementary therapies to alleviate their child's distress. Even when conventional therapies are effective, some families turn to CAM to strengthen their child's immune system and prevent recurrences. If therapies are unsuccessful, parents begin searching for any therapy that might offer reasonable hope. Parents are particularly concerned with relief of suffering at the end of the child's life—a concern that may not be adequately met with current mainstream care (19).

We have been impressed with the amount of time and resources that parents at our institution invest to learn about and acquire complementary therapies. When we inquire about the use of CAM, bottles of vitamins, supplements, homeopathic remedies, and teas appear from pocketbooks and backpacks. The Internet, books, family members, and friends offer testimonials of cures. Often practitioners of several different healing traditions are consulted, and families purchase product-specific video tapes, audio tapes, herbs, remedies, dietary supplements, and devices.

For the most part, families seek therapies that are consistent with their values, worldview, and culture and seek care from therapists who respect them as individuals who offer them time and attention (20,21). Families value highly the care that they receive from compassionate, comprehensive physicians who provide individualized care (22). They seek additional information on healthy lifestyle choices, dietary supplements, and environmental therapies over which they may exert some control (23). They also seek care from CAM therapists who offer personal attention, hope, time, and therapies consistent with their values. Families who seek out CAM therapies rarely abandon mainstream care, but they may not feel comfortable discussing those therapies if they perceive the physician to be antagonistic or judgmental toward them. Conversely, they value the opinion of fair-minded, knowledgeable physicians about the safety and efficacy of the products in which they are interested.

TALKING WITH PATIENTS AND FAMILIES

Despite the increased use of CAM therapies by pediatric pain patients, families are not substantially more likely to discuss these therapies with their physician now than they were in 1990. Families fail to communicate about their use of CAM therapies for a variety of reasons (Table 25.1). The two primary reasons are failure to consider "natural" therapies medically relevant or of interest to a physician and fear of physician disapproval, leading either to censure, argument, abandonment, or embarrassment. Regardless of a family's reasons for reluctance, it is important for physicians to initiate discussions in a collaborative, systematic fashion.

Opening a discussion about therapeutic options is facilitated by a thorough understanding of the families' goals and values. Treatment goals tend to fall in one of five major areas:

TABLE 25.1. *Parents' reasons for nondisclosure of complementary and alternative medical therapy usage*

CAM considered "natural" or not medically relevant and therefore not worth mentioning
Perceived lack of physician interest
Fear of censure
Fear of being dissuaded from use (argument/conflict)
Fear of physician abandoning the child or family at a time of great need
Cultural practice, may be embarrassed

1. *Curing* the condition causing the pain,
2. *Reducing* or *managing* pain and related symptoms,
3. *Preventing* pain and related symptoms,
4. Generally *enhancing* well-being and resilience or reducing toxins and stress,
5. *Promoting* harmony, cultural solidarity, and/or a sense of peace.

The first three goals are familiar to and shared by most physicians. The fourth goal, enhancing well-being and resilience, is frequently emphasized by common sense cultural precepts (e.g., getting a good night's sleep and eating well to build up one's strength) and by many health care providers (e.g., naturopaths, acupuncturists, chiropractors, massage therapists) who promote their services, not on the basis that they are curative, but that they help the body's natural healing systems to work more efficiently. Detoxification is a popular underlying theme in many alternative therapies, although it is an outmoded concept in scientific medicine. The fifth goal is difficult to define precisely but is often an implicit part of many spiritual healing approaches; another aspect of this factor is the drive to try anything that sounds promising to ease later guilt: "if only we had tried...our child would not be suffering today."

In addition to ascertaining the goals of treatment, important questions to assess before offering a medical opinion about a particular therapy include the name of the therapy, who recommended it to the family, the family's current sources of information about the therapy, their baseline opinion about and experience with it, and their interest in learning more or pursuing this therapy while under the primary care of the medical team (Table 25.2). For example, they may not be as interested in the scientifically proven efficacy as they are in the potential side effects of a particular therapy. Exploring the family's sense of expected end points of therapy and the timeline for achieving their goals can aid in developing realistic expectations and contingency plans.

Having a ready supply of patient information materials about the more commonly used

TABLE 25.2. *Baseline questions to address with families about specific therapies*

Questions	Example
Name of therapy	Acupuncture
Recommended by	Family physician
Information sources	Physician, Internet, magazines, family
Purpose of therapy	Reduce pain
Baseline opinion	Eager to try it but would like an alternative to needles
Experience	Patient's father had acupuncture treatment for tennis elbow with good relief
Desire for therapy	Moderate-to-strong interest

therapies and therapists is invaluable in addressing common concerns. The Center for Families at Boston Children's Hospital, the Blum Resource Center at the Dana Farber Cancer Institute, and the National Institutes of Health's National Center for Complementary and Alternative Medicine have developed patient information materials regarding acupuncture, chi kung, chiropractic, homeopathy, massage, meditation, music and sound therapy, naturopathy, Reiki, the relaxation response, Therapeutic Touch, and yoga. The National Center for Complementary and Alternative Medicine website is http://nccam.nih.gov/nccam/fcp/factsheets/; Children's Hospital and Dana Farber Cancer Institute materials are available on the institutional internal web pages for easy access by staff and will soon be available on external web pages as well. In addition, the Center for Holistic Pediatric Education and Research in conjunction with the Longwood Herbal Task Force has developed patient information sheets and clinician summary information on the most commonly used herbs and dietary supplements (http://www.mcp.edu/herbal/).

No matter how well prepared, physicians need to anticipate the inevitable fact that patients will inquire about unfamiliar therapies and therapists. For these instances, it is helpful to collaborate with medical center librarians, pharmacists, and nutritionists to develop a list of reliable references. There may be hidden resources within the institution such as nurses or pharmacists who are also homeopathic practitioners or physical therapists who also practice massage, Reiki or Therapeutic Touch. We have compiled a brief list of general books and websites devoted to evidence-based information on complementary therapies (see the Appendix at the end of the chapter). Families have far more respect for a physician whose response to a question about an alternative therapy is "I don't know, but I'll do my best to find out to help your child," than to a physician who ignores, disparages, or dismisses their concerns.

By better understanding the patient and family viewpoints, experiences, and expectations and by anticipating common questions and informational needs about specific treatments, the physician can offer better advice in a focused, efficient manner. Even after taking a complete history about a particular therapeutic option raised by a family, it is wise to step back and ask in a systematic fashion about all the other therapies that the family may have considered before rushing in to offer advice. Frequently, we have found that the initial question raised by the family (e.g., is massage safe for a child with a brain tumor?) is the family's way of testing the waters of physician communication and empathy before raising questions about more challenging or sensitive issues.

THERAPIES AND THERAPISTS

Just as it is essential when diagnosing a perplexing symptom to have a systematic approach to differential diagnosis (e.g., congenital, autoimmune, toxin, neoplastic, infectious, trauma, psychosocial) and in taking care of a critically ill patient to use an organ-system approach to evaluating problems, it is essential when considering therapies to have a systematic approach to considering the potential risks and benefits of different therapies. Although it is tempting to focus solely on the first issue raised by parents, it is prudent to assess thoroughly all the different kinds of therapies that the family may be considering before responding fully to the presenting question.

We have found it useful to consider potential therapies in four major categories: (a) biochemical, (b) lifestyle, (c) biomechanical, and (d) bioenergetic. Each of these major categories has several subcategories, some of which may be considered mainstream and others of which may be considered complementary, depending on cultural circumstances and definitions (Table 25.3). For example, within the general category of biochemical therapies fall medications (both prescription and nonprescription medications), herbs, vitamins, and other dietary supplements.

Biochemical Therapies

Herbs, vitamins, minerals, and other dietary supplements are increasingly used to treat specific conditions and to promote general health. This may be less true for problems such as chronic pain than for other serious medical conditions, but we have still found that questions for which we are most often consulted have to do with the use of herbs and other dietary supplements. Physicians are well aware of the detrimental effects of combining some nutritional supplements with mainstream medications (e.g., folate with methotrexate therapy) but may be less familiar with the range of other supplements in which parents express interest. One factor complicating responsible care in this area is the rapid shift in popularity; one year, it is laetrile, another year it is Echinacea or blue green algae and within another year, it may be Japanese medicinal mushrooms accompanied by intense marketing efforts.

TABLE 25.3. *Systematic integrative therapeutic history*

A. Biochemical therapies
  1. Medications
    a. Prescription (e.g., birth control pills)
    b. Nonprescription (e.g., acetaminophen)
  2. Vitamins and minerals
  3. Herbs and other dietary supplements
    a. Herbs, e.g., willow bark, devil's claw
    b. Amino acids, e.g., glutamine
    c. Animal products and glandulars, fish oil
    d. Hormones, e.g., melatonin, DHEA
    e. Others, e.g., coenzyme Q_{10}

B. Lifestyle
  1. Diet, e.g., vegetarian, macrobiotic
  2. Exercise/rest
  3. Environment
    a. Light/dark/colors
    b. Sound/music/silence
    c. Aromatherapy
    d. Heat/cold
    e. Magnets/vibration/crystals

C. Biomechanical
  1. Massage or bodywork
  2. Spinal adjustment: chiropractic, osteopathic adjustment, craniosacral work
  3. Surgery and radiation therapy

D. Bioenergetic
  1. Acupuncture/acupressure
  2. Healing touch/Reiki/Therapeutic Touch
  3. Prayer/meditation/other spiritual practices
  4. Homeopathy

Because of the rapid shifts in the popularity of different dietary supplements, it is important for physicians to have reliable sources of information to address patient questions in this area. The tables at the end of the chapter describe list of the sources on which we depend for reliable information. Based on extensive, systematic literature reviews, we have prepared scientific monographs, clinician summary sheets, and patient handouts on some of the most commonly used supplements and provided linkages to other evidence-based sources of information (http://www.mcp.edu/herbal/). Hospital pharmacists and nutritionists and regional poison control center toxicologists are also very helpful sources of information.

Dietary Supplements Used to Treat Pain: White Willow Bark and Devil's Claw

Historically, many modern pain medications have been derived from herbal remedies. Willow bark contains salicylate compounds (which are actually more abundant in other plants such as wintergreen), which formed the backbone for aspirin. Poppy seeds provided opium and its many modern derivatives; chili peppers contain capsaicin, a potent topical counterirritant and analgesic. Devil's claw root is a South African pain remedy that has become popular as a European treatment for the pain of arthritis, headache, backache, and menstrual pain; although many of these herbal remedies have proven more effective than placebo in treating pain, they tend to be less potent than modern pharmacologic therapies, and most patients with severe pain who try them quickly return to mainstream medications. Herb–drug interactions with these compounds have not been fully described.

Several herbal remedies have mild to moderate anti-inflammatory effects. One of the most commonly used of these is chamomile. Patients and families are often happy to try chamomile tea as a mouthwash for mild oral mucositis because it is familiar and nontoxic and offers families a means of self-help. Licorice root is a moderately potent anti-inflammatory used both orally and topically. Licorice root works by inhibiting cortisol metabolism; patients taking steroid medications who begin using licorice root should be monitored closely for potential steroid side effects.

Although physicians unaccustomed to using herbs may suggest that patients discontinue their use during hospitalizations or intensive medical regimens, there are actually few studies documenting adverse herb–drug interactions, but the potential certainly exists for specific herb–drug adverse events. Some herbal supplements, such as ginkgo and garlic, may potentiate anticoagulant medications; patients using these herbs should be monitored closely. Other herbs that may potentiate platelet aggregation inhibitors include bromelain, Chinese skullcap, garlic, papain, and turmeric. Coumarin is found in several common herbs: horse chestnut bark, sweet clover, sweet vernal grass leaves, and tonka bean seeds (24). All patients who are taking antidepressant medications for pain should be warned against taking St. John's wort concurrently due to potentially serious interactions; St. John's wort may also substantially reduce serum levels of other medications such as protease inhibitors and digoxin. Patients who have received prescriptions for anxiolytic or sedative medications should be advised *not* to mix these medications with herbal sedatives such as valerian and kava kava to minimize potential additive effects.

All patients who choose to take herbs and other dietary supplements should be informed about the relative lack of federal regulation regarding the purity and potency of dietary supplements. These products are not regulated the same way that medications are. Manufacturers are allowed to make broad "structure/function" claims without testing for efficacy. The burden is on the U.S. Food and Drug Administration to establish toxicity *after* a product is on the market; manufacturers are not required to prove safety before selling products, even those products marketed to children. Label claims are no guarantee of the purity of the product contained in the package. *Consumer Reports* and other watch dog organizations have documented tenfold variations in the strength of products with the same labeling, and as many as 30% of imports from developing countries have been contaminated with pharmaceuticals, heavy metals, and other potentially serious compounds. We advise patients not to take a product unless they have a good reason to trust the manufacturer or if they themselves feel they can accurately determine the contents, e.g., ginger root for nausea or chamomile flowers as anti-inflammatory.

Lifestyle: Diet, Exercise, Environment, and Mind–Body Therapies

Diet

Because diet is something over which families have some control, it is one of the lifestyle therapies of greatest interest. Physicians typically consider diet in terms of caloric needs. Families frequently turn to other health care professionals, including naturopathic doctors, chiropractors, and acupuncturists about specific diets, and may consult with lay advisors as well. Although several specific diets have been recommended to families of children with cancer and attention deficit hyperactivity disorder, no clear dietary recommendations have emerged regarding specific diets for pediatric pain. Severe dietary restrictions run the risk of caloric deprivation and reduced quality of life. For example, the restrictive forms of macrobiotic diets have been associated with cases of scurvy, anemia, and hypoproteinemia (25).

Exercise

Although exercise is an important part of a healthy child's life, physical activity in children with pain may be quite limited. For many children who had been active in individual and team sports, there may be a sense of loss as their previous capabilities decline and their relationships with team mates are redefined. Several studies have documented an association between physical activity/exercise and improved psychologic outcomes, including reduced measures of depression and anxiety (26–29). Although intense exercise temporarily lowers natural killer cell activity, regular moderate physical exercise is associated epidemiologically with enhanced immune function (30–33). This is a ripe area for additional research.

Recently, there has been a growing interest in Eastern meditative exercises such as yoga, tai chi, and chi kung (qi gong) and their potential therapeutic influences on chronic illnesses such as asthma and cancer (34,35). Because these exercises can be done slowly and noncompetitively and can be practiced in a group or individually at home, they may be useful for children in pain. Theoretically, they have a lower risk of injuries than contact sports, running, weight lifting, or other intense exercises or sports.

Adequate rest is also vitally important for children with pain; "sleep is not a biological luxury" (36). Pain can interfere with sleep, and yet insufficient sleep appears to contribute to both pain and suffering. Chronic sleep disruption may be an important contributor to several chronic pain syndromes such as fibromyalgia. Much research remains to be done to elucidate the optimal strategies for enhancing healthy, restorative sleep in pediatric pain patients.

Environment

Patients experience a broad range of environmental influences as helpful or stressful. Pediatricians routinely discuss environmental recommendations such as light (phototherapy for jaundice), sound (white noise and vibration for colic, music to reduce stress), and temperature (cold to minimize pruritus). Skin-to-skin contact is a common strategy in the postpartum period to enhance mother–infant bonding. It also appears to have potent analgesic effects (37).

Families may also be interested in a variety of other environmental strategies to help the child feel more comfortable. Most of these approaches rely on common sense and attention to individual preferences. Bright or dim lights; bright, pastel, or neutral colors; photographs and other visual art; sounds and music; television and video games; books and homework; hot and cold packs; favorite pillows; and other objects can all contribute to comfort and decreased anxiety (when they fit with the child's perceived needs) or stress (when there is poor fit with the child's needs) (38,39). There are data supporting the use of music therapy in both adult and pediatric hospitalized patients (40–43). Aromatherapy, either alone or in combination with therapeutic massage, can also be helpful in reducing pain and anxiety (44). Various forms of electromagnetic stimulation ranging from transcutaneous electrical nerve stimulation devices to kitchen magnets are under scrutiny as ultramodern pain treatments (39,45,46). These therapies entail few risks and modest costs.

Mind–Body

Mind–body therapies encompass a broad range of practices including individual psychotherapy, group therapy, art and expressive therapies, support groups, and personal practices such as meditation. These therapies are discussed in other chapters 17 and 18.

Biomechanical: Massage and Spinal Adjustments

Massage

There are hundreds of types of bodywork and massage, but the four major categories practiced in the United States are Swedish massage (long, gliding strokes, kneading, and stroking), deep tissue massage (e.g., Rolfing and Hellerwork), pressure point techniques (e.g., shiatsu and acupressure), and movement integration (e.g., Feldenkrais and Alexander techniques). Nearly every cultural group in the world has a historic tradition of massage therapy. However, most professional massage schools in the United States provide little training in pediatrics, and most massage therapists rarely treat children.

Therapeutic massage can also be provided by physicians, nurses, and physical therapists as well as by parents and other family members. Massage can be provided alone or in conjunction with guided imagery, music therapy, aromatherapy, or healing touch.

Several scientific studies have documented the benefits of massage for infants, children, and adolescents with diverse health conditions including pain (47–56). Massage helps to improve circulation, loosens tight joints, decrease levels of stress hormones, enhance endogenous levels of serotonin, promote sleep, and enhance an overall sense of relaxation and well-being (51,52). Massage provides tangible reassurance that the patient is cared for, enhancing self-esteem and a sense of psychologic and emotional support (57).

Massage is probably one of the most underused therapies in pediatrics. It has few contraindications; common sense precludes the use of vigorous massage over a surgical wound, skin infections, abrasions, or burns. Although time intensive, massage can be provided inexpensively if parents or other family members are trained to do it. We have found it one of the most helpful adjunctive treatments for patients with chronic pain, particularly because it empowers the family to take an active role in helping to reduce a child's symptoms.

Spinal/Cranial Adjustment: Chiropractic

Chiropractic is the leading CAM therapy offered by licensed professionals in the United States. Chiropractors are licensed in all 50 states, and most major insurance carriers cover professional chiropractic care (58). Children and adolescents typically account for 10% to 20% of all visits to chiropractors. Nearly all chiropractic schools now offer courses in pediatric care. Although many chiropractors claim to treat otitis media, asthma, allergies, infantile colic, enuresis, and other common childhood health problems, most restrict its use to treating musculoskeletal problems.

There are no randomized, controlled trials demonstrating chiropractic's effectiveness in preventing or treating mild or serious pediatric disorders and none specifically evaluating its effectiveness in treating any particular kind of childhood pain. Conversely, acute significant adverse effects from chiropractic adjustments are very rare, and the rate of malpractice claims against chiropractors is much lower than the rate of suits against medical doctors (59). We have heard testimonials from several patients that chiropractic or osteopathic adjustment was the most helpful therapy that they had tried in treating chronic headaches and chronic back, shoulder, or joint pain. Research is needed to better understand the use of chiropractic services by pediatric patients with pain, their satisfaction with care, and the cost-effectiveness of chiropractic in treating pain.

Bioenergetic

Acupuncture

Acupuncture is one component of traditional Chinese medicine (60). It is based on the theory of a vital energy [chi (qi)] that circulates through the body in 12 channels or meridians. When the flow of chi is blocked or disrupted, disease occurs; when the flow is balanced, harmonized, and restored, the patient experiences health. The flow of chi can be affected by stimulating specific points along the energy meridians. Approximately 80% of licensed acupuncturists also recommend dietary changes, herbs and other supplements, and changes in lifestyle, exercise, rest, and relationships.

Despite its exotic nature and its reliance on a different set of assumptions than mainstream medicine, acupuncture is frequently recommended by physicians and requested by patients, particularly for symptomatic treatment of pain and other symptoms such as nausea and breathlessness (61–69), the National Institutes of Health Consensus conference on acupuncture concluded that acupuncture is effective in treating several kinds of pain and nausea in adults (70–73).

For children, nonneedle techniques, such as "sea bands" for nausea, can be used to minimize the risks and fears associated with needles (74). Among major teaching hospitals with a pediatric pain treatment service, nearly one-third offer acupuncture therapy to treat chronic pain in children (75). Despite initial misgivings, most pediatric patients readily accept acupuncture therapy after an age-appropriate introduction to it and an initial treatment (76).

Side effects from acupuncture treatment, such as infections, broken or retained needles, pneumothorax, and cardiac tamponade, are quite rare (77,78). Physicians should be aware that acupuncture therapists may also recommend herbal remedies and dietary changes and should discuss the appropriateness and risks of these therapies specifically with patients, families, and the consulting acupuncturist directly.

Healing Touch/Reiki/Therapeutic Touch

Healing Touch, Therapeutic Touch, and Reiki are three different kinds of bioenergetic therapy in which the healer transmits a spiritual or invisible healing energy through their hands to help patients. They are nonreligious forms of "laying on of hands" healing.

Although these kinds of energy healing techniques seem far-fetched to many physicians, they can be profoundly meaningful to children and families. In fact, several families of children for whom we have cared in the intensive care unit have reported that they felt that these therapies were at least as helpful as some of the most potent medical and surgical therapies provided to their children.

Therapeutic Touch was invented in the 1970s by Dolores Krieger, a nursing professor at New York University, and Dora Kunz, a clairvoyant healer, based on their observations on numerous religious healers. Therapeutic Touch is taught in nursing schools across the United States, and formal policies and procedures for performing Therapeutic Touch are part of nursing practice in many children's hospitals. There are no national certifying examinations, and no states separately license Therapeutic Touch practitioners.

Numerous studies in adult, adolescent, and pediatric populations support the use of Therapeutic Touch to reduce pain and anxiety and to promote relaxation and a sense of well-being (79–84). Side effects are rare. Costs vary depending on whether the practice is provided as part of routine nursing care or by a parent or other family member.

Reiki is a similar practice that grew out of a Japanese tradition (85,86). Reiki practitioners are trained by a Reiki master through a workshop and an "empowerment" or "attunement." In some cases, Reiki healers do long-distance healing in which the patient is visualized and energy is sent through intention rather than being transmitted by direct physical contact. Few studies have specifically evaluated the effectiveness of Reiki in treating pain (87,88); conversely, no side effects have been reported either.

Prayer

As physicians know, every serious diagnosis presents a potential spiritual crisis for a child and the family. Our experience and numerous studies suggests that families are eager to discuss the impact of their diagnosis or condition on their spiritual or religious beliefs and often rely on these beliefs as an important coping strategy (89–92). Most patients and physicians believe that spiritual well-being is an important component of overall health and strongly linked to functional status (93–95); yet many physicians feel poorly prepared to address families' questions and concerns in this area.

When used as an adjunctive therapy, intercessory prayer on behalf of patients is low in cost and free of side effects. Scientific studies suggest that it may actually offer tangible health benefits (96–99). Regardless of its impact on disease or symptom management, it often helps families feel that they are doing everything they can to help the child, reinforces the family's sense of culture and meaning, and promotes a sense of peace and harmony.

Homeopathy

Homeopathic remedies are widely available in the United States (100,101). Homeopathy is a nearly 200-year-old European system of medical treatment. It is based on two principles: (a) the Law of Similars or "like cures like" and (b) the Law of Dilutions. The Law of Similars means that a remedy that would cause a symptom in a healthy person is used to treat the same symptom in a sick person. For example, a homeopathic remedy made from coffee might be used to treat a child suffering from insomnia. Although such remedies raise immediate concerns about safety, serious side effects from homeopathic treatment are incredibly rare owing to the second principle of homeopathic treatment, the Law of Dilutions, which says that the more the remedy is diluted, the more powerful it becomes. Homeopathic practitioners believe that these very dilute remedies contain an energy or information that is used by the patient to heal their symptoms.

Although 20% to 30% of a homeopath's patient load is pediatric and adolescent patients, few studies have evaluated the effectiveness of homeopathy in treating pediatric pain (56,102). A recent review suggested that the evidence was insufficient to recommend homeopathy as a prophylactic therapy for migraine headaches, but a more recent randomized, controlled trial suggested some benefit (103,104). These remedies are extremely safe and are rarely contraindicated in patients who can tolerate oral preparations. Therefore, we typically support families in their experimental use of homeopathic remedies; our willingness to support their choice typically results in greater acceptance of and enthusiasm for recommended medical regimens.

SUMMARY

The use of CAM in pediatric pain patients is common and increasing. Physicians need to be aware of the most common types of therapies, families' reasons and goals in using them, and the resources available within their institutions and available through articles, books, and the Internet to provide truly comprehensive and compassionate multidisciplinary care. Resources are listed below in the Appendix.

APPENDIX

Books

Dillard, J. Alternative medicine for dummies. New York: Hungry Minds, Inc., 1998

Jonas WB, Levin JS. *Essentials of complementary and alternative medicine.* New York: Lippincott Williams & Wilkins, 1999

Kemper KJ. *The holistic pediatrician.* New York: Harper Collins, 1996, 2002

Sierpina V. *Integrative healthcare: complementary and alternative therapies for the whole person* Philadelphia: F.A. Davis, Co., 2001

Periodicals

Nutrition Action Newsletter (Center for Science in the Public Interest)

Prescriber's Letter

HerbalGram

Websites

Center for Holistic Pediatric Education and Research: *http://www.holistickids.org*

Longwood Herbal Task Force: *http://www.mcp.edu/herbal/*

NIH Center for Alternative Medicine: *http://nccam.nih.gov*

Rosenthal Center for Complementary and Alternative Medicine: *http://cpmcnet.columbia.edu/dept/rosenthal/*

Comprehensive Natural Products Database (commercial): *www.naturaldatabase.com*

ConsumerLabs (independent testing of herbal products): *http://www.consumerlabs.com*

Recent articles

General overviews

Kemper KJ. Integrative medicine: talking with families about complementary, alternative and mainstream medical therapies in acute care settings. *Emerg Office Pediatr* 2000;13:45–49

Kemper KJ. Integrative medicine: does it work? *Arch Dis Child* 2001;84:6–9

Kemper KJ, Wornham WL. Consultations for holistic pediatric services for inpatients and outpatient oncology patients at a Children's Hospital. *Arch Pediatr Adolesc Med* 2001;155:449–454

Specific therapies

Lee A, Highfield ES, Berde CB, et al. Acupuncturists: practice characteristics and pediatric care. *Western J Med* 1999;171:153–157

Gardiner P, Kemper KJ. Peripheral brain: herbs in pediatric and adolescent medicine. *Pediatr Rev* 2000;21:44–57

Lee A, Kemper KJ. Homeopathy and naturopathy: practice characteristics and pediatric care. *Arch Pediatr Adolesc Med* 2000;154:75–80

Lee A, Li DH, Berde CB, et al. Practice characteristics of chiropractors who treat children. *Arch Pediatr Adolesc Med* 2000;154:401–407

Kemper KJ, Sarah R, Silver-Highfield E, et al. On pins and needles: pediatric pain patients' experience with acupuncture. *Pediatrics* 2000;105:941–947

REFERENCES

1. Eisenberg DM, Kessler RC, Foster C, et al. Unconventional medicine in the United States. Prevalence, costs, and patterns of use. *N Engl J Med* 1993;328:246–252.
2. Wetzel MS, Eisenberg DM, Kaptchuk TJ. Courses involving complementary and alternative medicine at US medical schools. *JAMA* 1998;280:784–787.
3. Zollman C, Vickers A. What is complementary medicine? *BMJ* 1999;319:693–696.
4. Pachter LM. Culture and clinical care. Folk illness beliefs and behaviors and their implications for health care delivery. *JAMA* 1994;271:690–694.
5. Pachter L. Practicing culturally sensitive pediatrics. *Contemp Pediatr* 1997;Sept:139–154.
6. Kemper KJ, Osborn LM, Hansen DF, et al. Family psychosocial screening: should we focus on high-risk settings? *J Dev Behav Pediatr* 1994;15:336–341.
7. Needlman R, Fried LE, Morley DS, et al. Clinic-based intervention to promote literacy. A pilot study. *Am J Dis Child* 1991;145:881–884.
8. Kemper KJ, Cassileth B, Ferris T. Holistic pediatrics: a research agenda. *Pediatrics* 1999;103:902–909.
9. Kemper KJ. Separation or synthesis: a holistic approach to therapeutics. *Pediatr Rev* 1996;17:279–283.
10. Kemper KJ. *The holistic pediatrician: a parent's comprehensive guide to safe and effective therapies for the 25 most common childhood ailments.* New York: Harper Perennial, 1996:408.
11. Eisenberg DM, Davis RB, Ettner SL, et al. Trends in alternative medicine use in the United States, 1990–1997: results of a follow-up national survey. *JAMA* 1998;280:1569–1575.
12. Elder NC, Gillcrist A, Minz R. Use of alternative health care by family practice patients. *Arch Fam Med* 1997;6:181–184.
13. Cassileth BR, Lusk EJ, Guerry D, et al. Survival and quality of life among patients receiving unproven as compared with conventional cancer therapy. *N Engl J Med* 1991;324:1180–1185.
14. Spigelblatt L, Laine-Ammara G, Ples B, et al. The use of alternative medical care by children. *Pediatrics* 1994;94:811–814.
15. Ottolini M, Hamburger E, Loprieto J, et al. Alternative Medicine Use Among Children in the Washington, DC Area, Pediatric Academic Societies, San Francisco, May 4, 1999.
16. Grootenhuis MA, deGraaf-Nijkerk JH, Wel Mvd. Use of alternative treatment in pediatric oncology. *Cancer Nurs* 1998;21:282–288.
17. Stern RC, Canda ER, Doershuk CF. Use of nonmedical treatment by cystic fibrosis patients. *J Adolesc Health* 1992;13:612–615.
18. Breuner CC, Barry PJ, Kemper KJ. Alternative medicine use by homeless youth. *Arch Pediatr Adolesc Med* 1998;152:1071–1075.
19. Wolfe J, Grier HE, Klar N, et al. Symptoms and suffering at the end of life in children with cancer. *N Engl J Med* 2000;342:326–333.
20. Astin JA.Why patients use alternative medicine: results of a national study. *JAMA* 1998; 279:1548–1553.
21. Neuberger J. Primary care: core values. Patients' priorities. *BMJ* 1998;317:260–262.
22. Maizes V, Caspi O. The principles and challenges of integrative medicine. *West J Med* 1999;171:148–149.
23. Kaptchuk TJ, Eisenberg DM. The persuasive appeal of alternative medicine. *Ann Intern Med* 1998;129: 1061–1065.
24. Brinker FJ. *Herb contraindications and drug interactions: with appendices addressing specific conditions and medicines.* Sandy, OR: Eclectic Institute, 1997:146.
25. Anonymous. Macrobiotic diets for the treatment of cancer. *CA Cancer J Clin* 1989;39:248–251.
26. Keats MR, Courneya KS, Danielsen S, et al. Leisure-time physical activity and psychosocial well-being in adolescents after cancer diagnosis. *J Pediatr Oncol Nurs* 1999;16:180–188.
27. DiLorenzo TM, Bargman EP, Stucky-Ropp R, et al. Long-term effects of aerobic exercise on psychological outcomes. *Prev Med* 1999;28:75–85.
28. Martinsen EW. Physical activity and depression: clinical experience. *Acta Psychiatr Scand Suppl* 1994;377: 23–27.
29. Brown SW, Welsh MC, Labbe EE, et al. Aerobic exercise in the psychological treatment of adolescents. *Percept Mot Skills* 1992;74:555–560.
30. Shephard RJ, Shek PN. Effects of exercise and training on natural killer cell counts and cytolytic activity: a meta-analysis. *Sports Med* 1999;28:177–195.
31. Peters C, Lotzerich H, Niemeier B, et al. Influence of a moderate exercise training on natural killer cytotoxicity and personality traits in cancer patients. *Anticancer Res* 1994;14:1033–1036.
32. Woods JA, Davis JM, Smith JA, et al. Exercise and cellular innate immune function. *Med Sci Sports Exerc* 1999;31:57–66.
33. Kiningham RB. Physical activity and the primary prevention of cancer. *Prim Care* 1998;25:515–536.
34. Kemper K, Lester M. Alternative asthma therapies: an evidence based review. *Contemp Pediatr* 1999;16: 162–195.
35. Cassileth BR. Complementary therapies: overview and state of the art. *Cancer Nurs* 1999;22:85–90.
36. Lewin D, Dahl R. Importance of sleep in the management of pediatric pain. *Dev Behav Pediatr* 1999;20: 244–252.
37. Gray L, Watt L, Blass E. Skin-skin contact is analgesic in healthy newborns. *Pediatrics* 2000;105:e14.
38. Field T, Martinez A, Nawrocki T, et al. Music shifts frontal EEG in depressed adolescents. *Adolescence* 1998;33:109–116.
39. Weintraub M. Chronic submaximal magnetic stimulation in peripheral neuropathy: is there a beneficial therapeutic relationship. *AJMN* 1998;8:12–16.
40. Weber S, Nuessler V, Wilmanns W. A pilot study on the influence of receptive music listening on cancer patients during chemotherapy. *Int J Arts Med* 1997;5: 27–35.
41. Bellamy M, Willard P. Music therapy: an integral com-

ponent of the oncology experience. *Int J Arts Med* 1993;7:14–49.
42. Chlan L. Effectiveness of a music therapy intervention on relaxation and anxiety for patients receiving ventilatory assistance. *Heart Lung* 1998;27:169–176.
43. Coleman J, Pratt R, Stoddard R, et al. The effects of male and female singing and speaking voices on selected physiological and behavioral measures of premature infants in the intensive care unit. *Int J Arts Med* 1997;5:4–11.
44. Wilkinson S, Aldridge J, Salmon I, et al. An evaluation of aromatherapy massage in palliative care. *Palliat Med* 1999;13:409–417.
45. Brown CS, Parker N, Ling F, et al. Effect of magnets on chronic pelvic pain. *Obstet Gynecol* 2000;95:529.
46. Collacott EA, Zimmerman JT, White DW, et al. Bipolar permanent magnets for the treatment of chronic low back pain: a pilot study. *JAMA* 2000;283:1322–1325.
47. Field T. Supplemental stimulation of preterm neonates. *Early Hum Dev* 1980;4:301–314.
48. Field T, Morrow C, Valdeon C, et al. Massage reduces anxiety in child and adolescent psychiatric patients. *J Am Acad Child Adolesc Psychiatry* 1992;31:125–131.
49. Field T, Ironson G, Scafidi F, et al. Massage therapy reduces anxiety and enhances EEG pattern of alertness and math computations. *Int J Neurosci* 1996;86: 197–205.
50. Hernandez-Reif M, Field T, Krasnegor J, et al. Children with cystic fibrosis benefit from massage therapy. *J Pediatr Psychol* 1999;24:175–181.
51. Field T, Hernandez-Reif M, Seligman S, et al. Juvenile rheumatoid arthritis: benefits from massage therapy. *J Pediatr Psychol* 1997;22:607–617.
52. Field T, Peck M, Krugman S, et al. Burn injuries benefit from massage therapy. *J Burn Care Rehabil* 1998; 19:241–244.
53. Ferrell-Torry AT, Glick OJ. The use of therapeutic massage as a nursing intervention to modify anxiety and the perception of cancer pain. *Cancer Nurs* 1993; 16:93–101.
54. King CR. Nonpharmacologic management of chemotherapy-induced nausea and vomiting. *Oncol Nurs Forum* 1997;24:41–48.
55. Lawvere S, Moscato B, Donahue R, et al. The effect of massage therapy on self-reported anxiety, depressive mood and pain in ovarian cancer patients: initial findings. *Am J Epidemiol* 1999;149:530.
56. Lee AC, Kemper KJ. Homeopathy and naturopathy: practice characteristics and pediatric care. *Arch Pediatr Adolesc Med* 2000;154:75–80.
57. Bredin M. Mastectomy, body image and therapeutic massage: a qualitative study of women's experience. *J Adv Nurs* 1999;29:1113–1120.
58. Kaptchuk TJ, Eisenberg DM. Chiropractic: origins, controversies and contributions. *Arch Intern Med* 1998;158:2215–2224.
59. Studdert DM, Eisenberg D, Miller F, et al. Medical malpractice implications of alternative medicine. *JAMA* 1998;280:1610–1615.
60. Vickers A, Zollman C. ABC of complementary medicine. Acupuncture. *BMJ* 1999;319:973–976.
61. Zaza C, Sellick SM, Willan A, et al. Health care professionals' familiarity with non-pharmacological strategies for managing cancer pain. *Psychooncology* 1999;8:99–111.
62. Kemper KJ, Vincent EC, Scardapane JN. Teaching an integrated approach to complementary, alternative, and mainstream therapies for children: a curriculum evaluation. *J Altern Complement Med* 1999;5:261–268.
63. Coss RA, McGrath P, Caggiano V. Alternative care. Patient choices for adjunct therapies within a cancer center. *Cancer Pract* 1998;6:176–181.
64. Verhoef MJ, Sutherland LR. Alternative medicine and general practitioners. Opinions and behaviour. *Can Fam Phys* 1995;41:1005–1011.
65. Sjogren P, Banning AM, Jensen NH, et al. Management of cancer pain in Denmark: a nationwide questionnaire survey. *Pain* 1996;64:519–525.
66. Helms J. An overview of medical acupuncture. *Altern Ther Helath Med* 1998;4:35–45.
67. Pearl D, Schrollinger E. Acupuncture: its use in medicine. *West J Med* 1999;171:176–180.
68. Zhou J, Li Z, Jin P. A clinical study on acupuncture for prevention and treatment of toxic side-effects during radiotherapy and chemotherapy. *J Tradit Chin Med* 1999;19:16–21.
69. Dundee JW, Yang J. Prolongation of the antiemetic action of P6 acupuncture by acupressure in patients having cancer chemotherapy. *J R Soc Med* 1990;83: 360–362.
70. Acupuncture NCDPO. NIH Consensus Conference. Acupuncture. *JAMA* 1998;280:1518–1524.
71. He JP, Friedrich M, Ertan AK, et al. Pain-relief and movement improvement by acupuncture after ablation and axillary lymphadenectomy in patients with mammary cancer. *Clin Exp Obstet Gynecol* 1999;26:81–84.
72. Ahmed HE, Craig WF, White PF, et al. Percutaneous electrical nerve stimulation (PENS): a complementary therapy for the management of pain secondary to bony metastasis. *Clin J Pain* 1998;14:320–323.
73. Alkaissi A, Stalnert M, Kalman S. Effect and placebo effect of acupressure (P6) on nausea and vomiting after outpatient gynaecological surgery. *Acta Anaesthesiol Scand* 1999;43:270–274.
74. Dundee JW, Yang J, McMillan C. Non-invasive stimulation of the P6 (Neiguan) antiemetic acupuncture point in cancer chemotherapy. *J R Soc Med* 1991;84:210–212.
75. Lee AC, Highfield ES, Berde CB, et al. Survey of acupuncturists: practice characteristics and pediatric care. *West J Med* 1999;171:153–157.
76. Kemper K, Sarah R, Silver-Highfield E, et al. On pins and needles: pediatric pain patients' experience with acupuncture. *Pediatrics* 2000;105:941–947.
77. Ernst E, White AR. Indwelling needles carry greater risks than acupuncture techniques. *BMJ* 1999;318:536.
78. Ernst E, White A. Life-threatening adverse reactions after acupuncture? A systematic review. *Pain* 1997;71: 123–126.
79. Hughes PP, Meize-Grochowski R, Harris CN. Therapeutic touch with adolescent psychiatric patients. *J Holist Nurs* 1996;14:6–23.
80. Turner JG, Clark AJ, Gauthier DK, et al. The effect of therapeutic touch on pain and anxiety in burn patients. *J Adv Nurs* 1998;28:10–20.
81. Peck SD. The efficacy of therapeutic touch for improving functional ability in elders with degenerative arthritis. *Nurs Sci Q* 1998;11:123–132.
82. Giasson M, Bouchard L. Effect of therapeutic touch on the well-being of persons with terminal cancer. *J Holist Nurs* 1998;16:383–398.

83. Gordon A, Merenstein JH, D'Amico F, et al. The effects of therapeutic touch on patients with osteoarthritis of the knee. *J Fam Pract* 1998;47:271–277.
84. Ireland M. Therapeutic touch with HIV-infected children: a pilot study. *J Assoc Nurses AIDS Care* 1998;9: 68–77.
85. Kelner M, Wellman B. Who seeks alternative health care? A profile of the users of five modes of treatment. *J Altern Complement Med* 1997;3:127–140.
86. Muller B, Gunther H. *A complete nook of Reiki healing*. Mendocino, CA: LifeRhythm, 1995.
87. Sawyer J. The first Reiki practitioner in our OR. *AORN J* 1998;67:674–677.
88. Olson K, Hanson J. Using Reiki to manage pain: a preliminary report. *Cancer Prev Control* 1997;1:108–113.
89. King DE, Bushwick B. Beliefs and attitudes of hospital inpatients about faith healing and prayer. *J Fam Pract* 1994;39:349–352.
90. Ehman JW, Ott BB, Short TH, et al. Do patients want physicians to inquire about their spiritual or religious beliefs if they become gravely ill? *Arch Intern Med* 1999;159:1803–1806.
91. Rosner F. Can an amulet cure leukemia? *JAMA* 1999; 282:307.
92. Daaleman TP, Nease DE Jr. Patient attitudes regarding physician inquiry into spiritual and religious issues. *J Fam Pract* 1994;39:564–568.
93. Ellis MR, Vinson DC, Ewigrnan B. Addressing spiritual concerns of patients: family physicians' attitudes and practices. *J Fam Pract* 1999;48:105–109.
94. Fernsler JI, Klemm P, Miller MA. Spiritual well-being and demands of illness in people with colorectal cancer. *Cancer Nurs* 1999;22:134–140.
95. Matthews DA, McCullough ME, Larson DB, et al. Religious commitment and health status: a review of the research and implications for family medicine. *Arch Fam Med* 1998;7:118–124.
96. Byrd RC. Positive therapeutic effects of intercessory prayer in a coronary care unit population. *South Med J* 1988;81:826–829.
97. Harris WS, Gowda M, Kolb JW, et al. A randomized, controlled trial of the effects of remote, intercessory prayer on outcomes in patients admitted to the coronary care unit. *Arch Intern Med* 1999;159:2273–2278.
98. Sicher F, Targ E, Moore D 2nd, et al. A randomized double-blind study of the effect of distant healing in a population with advanced AIDS. Report of a small scale study. *West J Med* 1998;169:356–363.
99. Collipp P. The efficacy of prayer: a triple blind study. *Med Times* 1969;97:201–204.
100. Ullman D. Homeopathy and managed care: manageable or unmanageable. *J Altern Complement Med* 1999;5:65–73.
101. Berman BM, Singh BK, Lao L, et al. Physicians' attitudes toward complementary or alternative medicine: a regional survey. *J Am Board Fam Pract* 1995;8: 361–366.
102. Friese KH, Kruse S, Ludtkc P, et al. The homeopathic treatment of otitis media in children—comparisons with conventional therapy. *Int J Clin Pharmacol Ther* 1997;35:296–301.
103. Ernst E. Homeopathic prophylaxis of headaches and migraine? A systematic review. *J Pain Symptom Manage* 1999;18:353–357.
104. Straumsheim P, Borchgrevink C, Mowinckel P, et al. Homeopathic treatment of migraine: a double blind, placebo controlled trial of 68 patients. *Br Homeopath J* 2000;89:4–7.

26
Acupuncture

Yuan-Chi Lin

Acupuncture is one of the treatment modalities within comprehensive traditional Chinese medicine (TCM) developed for more than three millennia. Acupuncture is used in the treatment of many medical conditions; pain is one of the most frequent indications for its use.

The word acupuncture is derived from the Latin words *acus*, "needle," and *punctura*, "a pricking." Acupuncture treatment is performed by inserting special needles into the skin at specific sites, known as acupuncture points, for a desired therapeutic effect. The original terminology of acupuncture in Chinese is *jin jiao*, which consists of the practice of acupuncture and moxibustion. Moxibustion, burning of moxa (Artemisia vulgaris) over the acupuncture points, can be also used for the treatment of various illnesses.

Needles of flint, bamboo, and bone from the Neolithic period suggest that acupuncture existed long before the discovery of metal. The *Yellow Emperor's Classic of Internal Medicine* from the fourth century B.C. described the practice of puncturing the body for pain relief. Acupuncture as a therapeutic intervention is now widely practiced in the United States.

Promising results support the efficacy of acupuncture in adult postoperative and chemotherapy-related nausea and vomiting and postoperative dental pain. Acupuncture may be useful as an adjunct treatment, an acceptable alternative, or included in a comprehensive management program for other conditions such as addiction, stroke rehabilitation, headache, menstrual cramps, tennis elbow, fibromyalgia, myofascial pain, osteoarthritis, low back pain, carpal tunnel syndrome, and asthma (1). A recent study revealed that use of alternative therapy is not limited to children with a life-threatening illness but is commonly used for those children with routine medical problems (2). Acupuncture is one of the alternative therapies frequently used in children (3).

This chapter provides a practical and theoretic understanding of acupuncture from both traditional Chinese and Western biomedical perspectives. This chapter does not intend to provide specific instructions on the techniques of acupuncture. The literature on the use of acupuncture is reviewed, with particular focus on children and adolescents. The training and licensing requirements for acupuncturists and the insurance coverage and potential risks of acupuncture are addressed.

MECHANISM OF ACUPUNCTURE

Traditional Chinese Medicine Perspective

Within TCM, sharp distinctions are not made between the physical, psychologic, and synthetic. This is in contrast to Western biomedical science, which tends to be reductionistic in its attempts to trace a linear cause-and-effect chain of events to a single identifiable cause. In the TCM framework, illness is understood as an overall pattern of multiple physical, psychologic, and environmental factors.

The concepts of yin and yang and the five elements are contrived by the ancient Chinese as one of the methods of defining and explaining the nature phenomena and the theory of acupuncture. The theoretic basis of TCM stems from a system of metaphysics that focuses on a balance between two opposing forces: yin and yang. Yin and yang are nature phenomena that also exist in the body. Yin is present in the qualities of cold, rest, passivity, dark, inward, decrease, and female. Yang is associated with hot, activity, activity, light, outward, increase, and male. Health requires a balance of yin and yang within a given person. Disease is characterized by a disharmony or lack of balance between yin and yang. Within the body, the balance of yin and yang is manifest in the flow of *qi* (pronounced "chee").

The theory of five elements based on the notion that all phenomena in the universe are the products of the evolution of five qualities: wood → fire → earth → metal → water → wood. In TCM, the five elements theory corresponds with normal physiology, influences the pathologic changes, and affects ailment management.

Qi is not easily translatable or definable because a clear distinction between matter and energy is not made in Chinese metaphysics. *Qi* flows through a complex system of meridians throughout the body, maintaining life and health. The meridians are not defined by physical structures such as blood or lymphatic vessels, but by their function. The body is viewed as a dynamic system of organs connected by the flow of *qi* within the meridians.

Illness results from the improper flow of *qi* through the meridians. The proper flow of *qi* may be restored by the insertion of several very fine needles at a properly determined combination of the 365 classic acupuncture points along the meridians. The classic diagram of the spleen meridian is shown is Figure 26.1. Manual twirling of the needles produces a sore, heavy, or numb sensation known as *de qi* ("obtaining *qi*"). Practitioners of TCM observed that stimulating specific acupuncture points resulted in predictable responses in patients with a given pattern of signs and symptoms. The great treatises of TCM such as the *Huang Ti Nei Ching* (*Yellow Emperor's Treatise on Internal Medicine*) guide the practitioner to select the correct points for a particular condition. Several treatments may be required over the course of weeks or months.

Practitioners of acupuncture routinely require a detailed medical history and information on current illness in pursuing the diagnosis. In addition, attention is focused on the character of the pulse and the appearance of the tongue. The goal of the history and physical examination is to assess the balance of yin and yang. The aim of therapy is to restore deficiencies or correct excesses in *qi* and thus restore health.

TCM has evolved over the past 3,000 years and continues to be used today in China and in Asian communities around the world. The theory and practice of TCM differ dramatically from those of Western medicine, making TCM not easy to understand and accept. The utility and validity of TCM lie in its demonstrated effectiveness. Similarly, the lack of understanding of the biologic mechanism of modern inhaled anesthetics does not prevent their use in practice. However, as with any new therapy, properly conducted laboratory

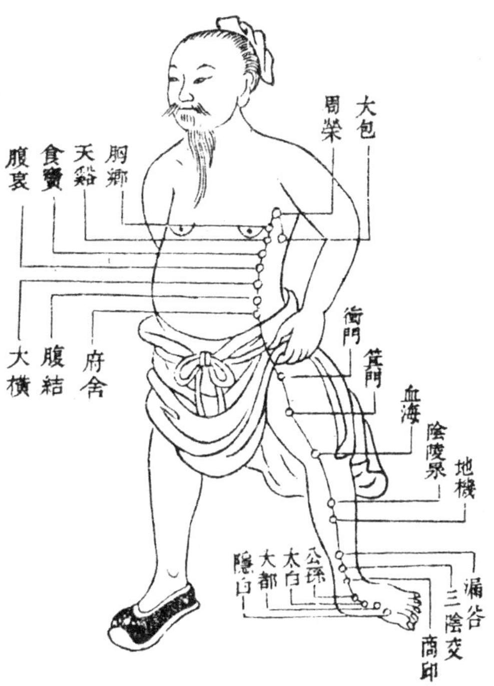

FIG. 26.1. The classic diagram of the spleen meridian.

and clinical studies are necessary to establish the safety and effectiveness of acupuncture.

Western Biomedical Perspective

Interest in acupuncture developed in the West in the 1970s. Stories of the use of acupuncture for anesthesia during major surgery in China appeared in the Western press. This popular interest soon led to scientific efforts to test the clinical effectiveness and elucidate the underlying physiologic mechanism of acupuncture for analgesia. In the West, basic scientific and clinical research has focused on the use of acupuncture for analgesia. Scientific research has not historically been part of TCM, which has been derived empirically through many years of experience.

Basic Research

Basic scientific research has focused on understanding acupuncture from a neurobiologic perspective. One theory proposes that acupuncture inhibits the transmission of pain according to the gate control theory put forth by Wall and Melzack in 1965 (4). In this model, acupuncture may act by stimulating sensory Aβ fibers, directly inhibiting the spinal transmission of pain by smaller Aδ and C fibers (5).

The subject of most basic research has been the relationship between acupuncture and the production of endogenous opioid peptides, such as the endorphins and enkephalins, and stimulation of the endogenous descending inhibitory pathways. In human studies, analysis of cerebrospinal fluid after acupuncture treatment showed elevated levels of serotonin, endorphins, and enkephalins (6). Although the mechanism of acupuncture analgesia is not entirely clear, a growing body of scientific knowledge indicates, "the essence of acupuncture analgesia is mainly the activation of the endogenous antinociceptive system to modulate pain transmission and pain response" (7). Low (2 Hz) and high (100 Hz) frequency of electrical acupuncture selectively induces the release of enkephalins and dynorphins in both experimental animals and humans (8).

An early human study by Mayer et al. (9) indicated that acupuncture analgesia might be reversed by naloxone. Similar findings were reported in animal studies. A subsequent human study by Chapman et al. (10) failed to show evidence of naloxone reversal of analgesia. It was postulated that the increased cerebrospinal fluid and plasma levels of opioids might be the result of stress induced by the experimental situation rather than the acupuncture treatment.

Pomeranz and Stux (11) offered a comprehensive theory that proposes that acupuncture activates small myelinated nerve fibers in the muscle, sending impulses to the spinal cord that then activate centers in the spinal cord, midbrain, and pituitary–hypothalamus to produce analgesia. The spinal cord may use enkephalin and dynorphin to block incoming pain signals. In the midbrain, enkephalin may activate the raphe descending system, which inhibits pain transmission at the level of the spinal cord with the monoamines serotonin and epinephrine. The pituitary–hypothalamus may act to release β endorphin into the blood and cerebrospinal fluid to produce analgesia at a distance. He (7) postulated a similar mechanism, emphasizing the importance of the periaqueductal gray in initiating descending as well as ascending pain inhibitory pathways.

Functional magnetic resonance is used to investigate the effect of acupuncture in normal subjects to provide the foundation for understanding the mechanism of acupuncture. Correlations between the BL 62 acupuncture point with the visual cortex was investigated (12). Acupuncture needle manipulation on the LI 4 (Hegu) point modulates the activity of the limbic system and subcortical structure revealed in functional magnetic resonance imaging.

Clinical Research

Clinical research has largely consisted of uncontrolled trials of acupuncture for the treatment of chronic pain in adults. Although beneficial results have been frequently demonstrated, the flawed design of many studies limits the value of the results.

Several difficulties are inherent in designing valid blinded, randomized, controlled trials of acupuncture (13,14). First, the studies can be best when single blinded because a trained acupuncturist must do all the needling. Second, difficulties arise in determining an appropriate placebo for the control group. Various studies have used "sham" acupuncture sites (needles placed at incorrect sites), other devices (such as a nonfunctional transcutaneous electrical nerve stimulation unit), or no treatment at all. This factor is important because as many as 30% of subjects may respond positively to some placebos. Third, acupuncture analgesia may require multiple treatment sessions over an extended period of time to demonstrate treatment effectiveness. Extended follow-up would be required to demonstrate the statistical significance only produced by studying large numbers of patients.

Richardson and Vincent (15) reviewed 27 controlled studies of acupuncture for treating acute and chronic pain as well as several large, uncontrolled studies. Fifty percent to 80% of patients showed short-term benefit from acupuncture. Lack of follow-up data made assessment of long-term effectiveness difficult. In a meta-analysis of 14 randomized, controlled trials of acupuncture for chronic pain in adults, Patel et al. (16) found that, although few of the individual trials demonstrated statistically significant benefit from acupuncture, the pooled results for several subgroups attained statistical significance of the benefit of acupuncture. The results of studies examining the use of acupuncture for other medical conditions are less clear (17).

CLINICAL USE OF ACUPUNCTURE PAIN MANAGEMENT IN CHILDREN AND ADOLESCENTS

Most clinical trials of acupuncture have involved adult patients. At present, very few studies have been addressed the problems particular to children and adolescents.

Acute Pain

Acute pain is common in children and adolescents. Accidents and injuries are leading causes of morbidity in this age group. For severe acute, subacute, or recurrent acute pain, lasting hours or days, acupuncture may be of benefit.

Gunsberger (18) reported the use of acupuncture for treating sore throat symptoms. Of 100 patients treated at one acupuncture point, 93 reported immediate relief of pain and 85 reported relief 2 to 3 hours after treatment. However, the study design is flawed. Patients who refused treatment were used as the control group; patients who chose to participate were therefore not part of a random sample.

Acupuncture may be more useful in predictable situations involving acute pain, such as dental procedures and postoperative pain, or in medical conditions with recurrent episodes of acute pain, such as sickle cell crisis and recurrent abdominal pain. Although effective treatment is available in many cases (i.e., local anesthetics for dental procedures, opioids for severe postoperative pain), side effects such as respiratory depression may be seen. Taub and colleagues (19) used acupuncture for the treatment of dental pain in a single-blind, randomized, controlled trial in 39 adult patients undergoing dental restoration for caries. Patients were randomized to real (experimental group) or sham (control group) acupuncture. Seventy percent of the experimental group reported good or excellent pain reduction; 53% of the control group reported good or excellent pain reduction. The results for the two groups showed no statistical significance. Systematic review showed that acupuncture is effective in relieving dental pain (20).

Co (21) reported effective treatment of sickle cell crisis pain. This study included ten adult patients experiencing 16 crises involving roughly symmetric bilateral extremity pain. Patients served as their own controls: real acupuncture points were used on one side and sham points on the other. By patient self-assessment, favorable responses were seen in

15 of the 16 treatments: seven responses at the genuine acupuncture points, two responses at the sham sites, and six responses at both sites. It is not clear whether coanalgesics were also used. The effect may not be related to needling of a prescribed point. However, the number of subjects was very small, making it difficult to assess the difference between real and sham acupuncture.

Facco et al. (22) compared the use of acupuncture and pentazocine for the treatment of postoperative pain (hysterectomy). Thirty-four adult women chose to receive either acupuncture or 30 mg pentazocine after undergoing laparotomy. The treatments did not differ in their analgesic effects. Interestingly, the study demonstrated that the acupuncture patients' postoperative vital capacity exceeded their preoperative vital capacity; the preoperative values of pentazocine group did not change.

The studies cited here all suggest that acupuncture is beneficial in the treatment of acute pain. However, it is important to note that, on close examination, each of them has methodologic flaws that limit the value of the results. Further studies are required to demonstrate the benefit of acupuncture in children and adolescents with acute pain.

Chronic Pain

Chronic pain, especially low back pain, is less prevalent among children than adults. Acupuncture was shown to be superior to various control interventions for low back pain treatment (23). However, chronic painful conditions such as reflex sympathetic dystrophy or migraine headaches are not rare in children and adolescents. Existing treatments may lack effectiveness or have unacceptable side effects. In these settings, acupuncture may serve as a valuable therapy or adjunct treatment.

Reports have appeared about the benefits of traditional acupuncture therapy and auricular therapy the in treating reflex sympathetic dystrophy (24,25). However, each of these reports involves only one to five patients in uncontrolled studies. In addition, the intermittent natural history of pain in reflex sympathetic dystrophy makes reassessment of treatment effect difficult.

Acupuncture therapy for migraine headaches has also been reported to be effective in several adult studies (26,27). Acupuncture may be useful for the treatment of chronic myofascial pain. In an uncontrolled study, Lewit (28) reported immediate relief in 87% of cases and long-term benefit in at least 92 of 288 cases. Melzack and colleagues (29) reported a 71% correlation between acupuncture points and trigger points used in the treatment of myofascial pain.

In a perspective, randomized, placebo-controlled trial, Helms (30) demonstrated a significant benefit from acupuncture in the treatment of primary dysmenorrhea. Forty-three subjects were divided into four groups: real acupuncture, sham acupuncture, no treatment, and a visitation group (i.e., visited physician as frequently as treatment groups but received no treatment). A larger proportion of subjects in the real acupuncture group showed improvement than in the other groups; analgesic usage was reduced by 41% in the acupuncture group. However, the small number of subjects and lack of blinding remain problematic.

The lack of literature on the use of acupuncture for treating chronic pain in children makes it difficult to reach any firm conclusions. As mentioned above, 50% to 70% of adults with chronic pain received at least short-term benefit from acupuncture therapy. However, the underlying causes of chronic pain differ between children and adults. Although the effectiveness of acupuncture analgesia is unclear, acupuncture appears to be quite safe. It may serve as a useful adjunct to existing therapies. In the case of chronic pain, a multidisciplinary approach is often helpful, and an acupuncturist may be a valuable in the team approach.

Acupuncture Therapy for Other Medical Conditions

In TCM, acupuncture is used for treating many conditions other than acute or chronic pain. In the West, acupuncture has treated smoking cessation, alcoholism, and opioid addiction (31,32), conditions more common in adults than children. Acupuncture has also been studied for the treatment of asthma and obesity and the prophylaxis of chemotherapy-induced sickness, all of which may be pertinent to children and adolescents.

Fung and colleagues (33) studied the effects of real and sham acupuncture on exercise-induced asthma in a prospective, randomized, single-blind study of 19 children. Treatment was given to known asthmatics 20 minutes before treadmill exercise. Although basal bronchomotor tone was not altered, both real and sham acupuncture attenuated bronchoconstriction after exercise. The mean maximal percentage decreases in forced expiratory volume in 1 second, forced vital capacity, and peak expiratory flow rate were 44%, 33.3%, and 49.5%, respectively, with no treatment; 23.8%, 15.8%, and 25.9%, respectively, after real acupuncture; and 32.6%, 26.1%, and 34.3%, respectively, after sham acupuncture. Several adult studies have also reported mixed results from acupuncture in the treatment of asthma (34–37).

In a well-designed, randomized, placebo-controlled crossover study, Dundee et al. (38) demonstrated that acupuncture might serve as an effective antiemetic for patients undergoing cancer chemotherapy. The study involved 130 adult patients with a history of distressing sickness with chemotherapy treatments. With acupuncture, sickness was absent or reduced in 97% of the patients. This study is of note because tolerable doses of available antiemetics are often ineffective. Although only adult patients were included, the toxicity of drug protocols is similar to those used for children and adolescents. Systematic review of 33 randomized controlled trials has shown that acupuncture is more effective than placebo in postoperative nausea and vomiting and chemotherapy-induced nausea and vomiting (39).

Clinical trials of acupuncture therapy for many other medical conditions have been carried out. Many trials have the methodologic flaws mentioned previously, making it difficult to reach any clear scientific conclusions for many indications. As Vincent and Richardson (13) point out: "Even if there are currently no clear indications for or against the use of acupuncture in a particular disorder an individual patient who finds the method and philosophy sympathetic might derive considerable benefit from it."

PRACTICAL GUIDE

Various acupuncture needles are available. Most needles used in clinical practice are made of stainless steel, although needles of other metals such as gold are available. Both disposable and reusable needles are available. Reusable needles must be sterilized by appropriate autoclave techniques between uses. Needles vary from 0.5 to 5 in. in length and from 26 to 36 gauge in diameter. A steel or plastic insertion tube can be a guide for the placement of the needle. The needle is tapped through the epidermis while the tube is in place. Deeper insertion is achieved by manipulation of the needle after the tube is removed (Fig. 26.2).

After insertion, stimulation of the acupuncture may be achieved manually or by use of electroacupuncture. Each acupuncture point has a prescribed depth of insertion. Manual techniques may involve the lifting and thrusting of the needle or twisting and twirling of the needle. Electroacupuncture achieves a similar effect by attaching low-voltage elec-

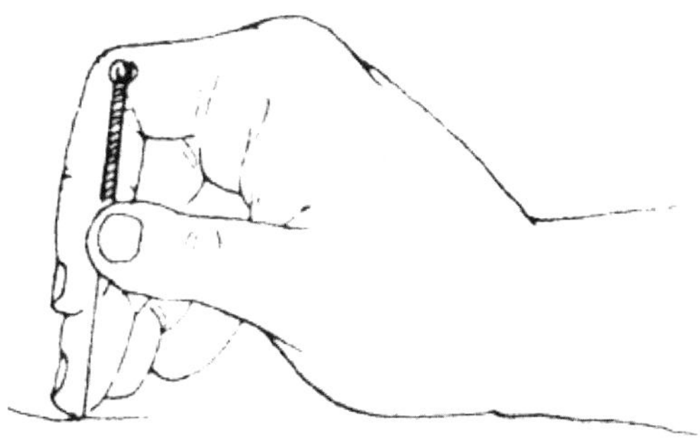

FIG. 26.2. Manual insertion of an acupuncture needle.

trodes to the needles. The intensity, pulse width, and duration may be varied, much in the same way as in transcutaneous electrical nerve stimulation.

Relatively little pain results in the insertion of the needles. Most acupuncturists are quite skilled in the painless insertion of needles. In my experience, most children can accept acupuncture treatment well (40). Acupuncture is extremely safe. Occasionally, a patient may have some bruising at an acupuncture site. The principal risk is infection from use of improperly sterilized needles. Cases of hepatitis B (41), human immunodeficiency virus infection (42), and fatality (43) have been reported. This can be avoided by using disposable sterile acupuncture needles and by proper insertion of the needles.

Licensing of the practice of acupuncture is determined by each state. The National Commission for the Certification of Acupuncturists has established standards for training and certification of knowledge and proficiency. Most states use the National Commission for the Certification of Acupuncturists examination process to license acupuncturists. Some states require acupuncturists to be supervised by licensed physicians. This includes confirming the diagnosis of the patient before treatment. Some states allow licensed acupuncturists to practice independently. There are an estimated 14,000 licensed acupuncturists in the United States. Most acupuncturists receive 2 to 3 years of academic training including supervised clinical experience in the treatment of a variety of medical disorders. Most of the training programs include some pediatric training, and most standard acupuncture textbooks contain instruction on the treatment of children (44).

Most states allow physicians to practice acupuncture after proper training. A minimum of 300 hours of formal training is necessary. The American Academy of Medical Acupuncture is one of the largest physician–acupuncturist associations. The American Board of Medical Acupuncture has developed a comprehensive board certification process for physician acupuncturists. It is estimated that there are 3,000 trained physician acupuncturists in the United States. A recent survey revealed that more than 30% of the major pediatric academic pain centers offer acupuncture for the treatment of pediatric pain. Physician–acupuncturists perform most of the acupuncture therapy for pediatric patients (45).

More health maintenance organizations are now covering the cost of acupuncture treatment. Some workmen's compensation insurance and personal injury insurance policies also cover acupuncture treatment.

CONCLUSION

Acupuncture can be integrated to the standard pediatric pain management program. The referring physician should provide the patient, or the parents in the case of the pediatric patients, with some understanding of how the theoretic orientation of the acupuncturist differs from that of Western medical issues such as the use of needles. Sterilization should be discussed. Patients may be somewhat skeptical initially, but a reassuring and confident attitude of the physician is very helpful for the acupuncturist and beneficial for the patient.

Clinical experience suggests that acupuncture may offer relief to children and adolescents in pain or with other medical conditions. Within TCM, acupuncture has been used for a wide range of illnesses for more than three millennia. From a Western biomedical perspective, the underlying neurobiologic mechanism of acupuncture analgesia is becoming apparent. However, the lack of randomized, controlled clinical studies in children makes it difficult to form any definitive conclusions about clinical use at present.

The value of any new therapy depends on its relative safety and effectiveness in light of other available treatments and the seriousness of the condition being treated. The ideal treatment is one that is both highly effective and safe. In some cases (e.g., acute pain), effective treatment is currently available (e.g., opioid analgesia), but serious adverse effects may result (e.g., respiratory depression, addiction). In other cases, a highly effective treatment is not available or known treatments may not work for some patients (e.g., chronic pain, smoking cessation, obesity).

The philosophy, theory, and practice of TCM and those of Western biomedical science differ markedly. The differences make it difficult for Western-trained health care providers to understand and accept acupuncture. Although differing worldviews are probably irreconcilable, the underlying laws of nature, however, are universal. If acupuncture is a valid method of treatment, continued research, both basic and clinical, may further clarify acupuncture's underlying mechanism and clinical effectiveness, allowing it to be rationally incorporated into Western medical practice.

REFERENCES

1. NIH Consensus Conference. Acupuncture. *JAMA* 1998; 280:1518–1524.
2. Friedman T, Slayton W, Allen L, et al. Use of alternative therapies for children with cancer. *Pediatrics* 1997; 100:e1.
3. Spigelblatt L, Laine-Ammara G, Pless B, et al. The use of alternative medicine by children. *Pediatrics* 1994;94: 811–814.
4. Melzack R, Wall PD. Pain mechanism: a new theory. *Science* 1965;150:971–979.
5. Lewith GT, Kenyon JN. Physiological and psychological explanations for the mechanism of acupuncture as a treatment for chronic pain. *Soc Sci Med* 1984;19: 1367–1378.
6. Sjolund B, Terenius L, Eriksson M. Increased cerebrospinal fluid levels of endorphins after electro-acupuncture. *Acta Physiol Scand* 1977;100:382–384.
7. He L. Involvement of endogenous opioid peptides in acupuncture analgesia. *Pain* 1987;31:99–121.
8. Ulett G, Han S, Han J. Electroacupuncture: mechanisms and clinical application. *Biol Psychiatry* 1998; 44:129–138.
9. Mayer D, Price D, Raffii A. Antagonism of acupuncture analgesia in man by the narcotic antagonist naloxone. *Brain Res* 1977;121:368–372.
10. Chapman CR, Benedetti C, Colpitts YH, et al. Naloxone fails to reverse pain thresholds elevated by acupuncture: acupuncture analgesia reconsidered. *Pain* 1983;16:13–31.
11. Pomeranz B, Stux G. *The scientific basis of acupuncture*. Berlin: Springer-Verlag, 1987:6–72.
12. Cho Z, Chung S, Jones J, et al. Findings of the correlation between acupoints and corresponding brain cortical using functional MRI. *Proc Natl Acad Sci U S A* 1998;95:2670–2673.
13. Vincent CA, Richardson PH. The evaluation of therapeutic acupuncture: concepts and methods. *Pain* 1986; 24:1–13.
14. Lewith GT, Machin D. On the evaluation of the clinical effects of acupuncture. *Pain* 1983;16:111–127.
15. Richardson P, Vincent C. Acupuncture for treatment of pain. *Pain* 1986;24:15–40.
16. Patel M, Gutzwiller F, Paccaud F, et al. A meta-analysis of acupuncture for chronic pain. *Int J Epidemiol* 1989; 18:900–906.
17. Vincent CA, Richardson PH. Acupuncture for some common disorders: a review of evaluative research. *J R Coll Gen Pract* 1987;37:77–81.
18. Gunsberger M. Acupuncture in the treatment of sore throat symptomatology. *Am J Chin Med* 1973;1:337–340.
19. Taub H, Beard, MC, Eisenberg L, et al. Studies of acupuncture for operative dentistry. *J Am Dent Assoc* 1977;99:555–561.
20. Ernst E, Pittler M. The effectiveness of acupuncture in treating dental pain. *Br Dent J* 1998;184:443–447.
21. Co L. Acupuncture: an evaluation in the painful crises of sickle-cell anemia. *Pain* 1979;7:181–185.
22. Facco E, Manani G, Angel A, et al. Comparison study between acupuncture and pentazocine analgesic and respiratory post-operative effects. *Am J Chin Med* 1981; 9:225–235.
23. Ernest E, White A. Acupuncture for back pain. *Arch Intern Med* 1998;158:2235–2241.
24. Leo K. Use of electrical stimulation at acupuncture points for the treatment of reflex sympathetic dystrophy in a child: a case report. *Phys Ther* 1983;63:957–959.
25. Spoerel W, Varkey, M, Leung CY. Acupuncture in chronic pain. *Am J Chin Med* 1976;4:267–279.
26. Dowson D, Lewith GT, Machin D. The effects of acupuncture versus placebo in the treatment of headache. *Pain* 1985;21:35–42.
27. Loh L, Nathan PW, Schott GD, et al. Acupuncture versus medical treatment for migraine and muscle tension headaches. *J Neurol Neurosurg Psychiatry* 1984;47: 333–337.
28. Lewit K. The needle effect in the relief of myofascial pain. *Pain* 1979;3:83–90.
29. Melzack T, Stillwell DM, Fox EJ. Trigger points and acupuncture points for pain: correlations and implications. *Pain* 1977;3:3–23.
30. Helms J. Acupuncture for the management of primary dysmenorrhea. *Obstet Gynecol* 1987;69:51–56.
31. Clavel F, Benhamou S, Company-Huertas A, et al. Helping people to stop smoking: randomised comparison of groups being treated with acupuncture and nicotine gum with control groups. *BMJ* 1985;291: 1538–1539.
32. Smith M, Khan I. An acupuncture programme for the treatment of drug-addicted persons. *Bull Narc* 1988;40: 35–41.
33. Fung K, Chow OKW, So SY. Attenuation of exercise-induced asthma by acupuncture. *Lancet* 1986;27: 1419–1421.
34. Tandon M, Soh PF. Comparison of real and placebo acupuncture in histamine-induced asthma: a double-blind crossover study. *Chest* 1989;96:102–105.
35. Tashkin D, Kroening RJ, Bresler DE, et al. A controlled trial of real and stimulated acupuncture in the management of chronic asthma. *J Allerg Clin Immunol* 1985; 76:6855–864.
36. Jobst K, McPherson K, Brown V, et al. Controlled trial of acupuncture for disabling breathlessness. *Lancet* 1986;27:1416–1418.
37. Tashkin D, Bresler DE, Kroenin RJ, et al. Comparison of real and simulated acupuncture and isoproterenol in methacholine-induced asthma. *Ann Allergy* 1977;39: 379–387.

38. Dundee J, Ghaly R, Fitzpatrick K, et al. Acupuncture prophylaxis of cancer chemotherapy-induced sickness. *J R Soc Med* 1989;82:268–271.
39. Vickers A. Can acupuncture have specific effects on health? A systemic review of acupuncture antiemetic trials. *J R Soc Med* 1996;89:303–311.
40. Lin Y. Acupuncture as an adjunctive treatment for chronic pain in children: patients' perspective. *Anesth Analg* 2001;92:262.
41. Kent G, Brondum J, Keenlyside RA, et al. A large outbreak of acupuncture-associated hepatitis B. *Am J Epidemiol* 1988;127:591–598.
42. Vittecoq D, Mettetal JF, Rouzioux C, et al. Acute HIV infection after acupuncture treatments. *N Engl J Med* 1989;320:250–251.
43 Ernst E, White A. Life-threatening adverse reactions after acupuncture? A systemic review. *Pain* 1997;71: 123–126.
44. Lee AC, Highfield ES, Berde CB, et al. Survey of acupuncturists: practice characteristics and pediatric care. *West J Med* 1999;171:153–157.
45. Lin Y, Lee A, Kemper K, et al. Integrating complementary and alternative medicine in pediatric pain management. *Anesthesiology* 1999;91:939.

27

Multidisciplinary Programs for Management of Acute and Chronic Pain in Children

Charles B. Berde and Jean Solodiuk

Management of acute or chronic pain in infants and children is a shared task among diverse clinicians. Programs for pain management can take a variety of forms, depending on the type and number of patients treated, resources and economic limitations, and availability of staff in different disciplines. There is no one form of organization that is right for all hospitals. In this chapter, we summarize some of the considerations relevant to the organization of acute and chronic pain management services for children.

In the past 3 years in the United States, the Joint Commission on Accreditation of Health Care Organizations has mandated a very explicit set of new standards for systematic approaches to pain and symptom management in hospitals and clinics. With the considerable leverage that the Joint Commission on Accreditation of Health Care Organizations has over hospitals, the result has been an enormous effort by hospitals to comply with these standards.

ACUTE PAIN MANAGEMENT PROGRAMS

Programmatic approaches to acute pain management may range from a formal acute pain service (1–3) to a model of care by individual primary services, with a set of hospital-wide practice standards for pain assessment and analgesic prescribing. Regardless of the details of how an acute pain management program is organized, in our view, there are some desirable features, which are listed in Table 27.1.

Advantages and disadvantages of acute pain service versus primary service models for acute pain care are listed in Tables 27.2 and 27.3.

It is possible to implement "hybrid" models that combine features of both models listed in Tables 27.2 and 27.3 or to employ both models in parallel for different patient subgroups.

SYSTEMATIC PAIN ASSESSMENT

Systematic pain assessment and measurement are a crucial aspect of pain management practice. One way of implementing the Joint Commission on Accreditation of Health Care Organizations standard RI 1.2.8 ("patients have the right to appropriate assessment and management of pain") is to regard pain measurement as the fifth vital sign. Formal pain intensity scoring is to be conducted and recorded for hospitalized patients at regular intervals, as is done routinely for heart rate, blood pressure, respiratory rate, and temperature. Scales are chosen based on patients' age and cognitive status, as described in detail in Chapters 7 and 8. Commonly, a visual analog scale or verbal analog scale is used for older children and adolescents, a faces scale or color analog scale (4,5) is used for children ages 4 to 8 years of age, and behavioral scales are used for infants, toddlers, and children with developmental disabilities. The FLACC (*f*acial expression, *l*eg movement, *a*ctivity, *c*ry, and *c*onsolability) scale (6) is used for most nonverbal children, infants, and toddlers, and the Premature Infant Pain Profile scale (7) is used predominantly in the newborn intensive care unit.

TABLE 27.1. *Desirable features of acute pain management programs*

1. Multidisciplinary commitment to pain prevention and prompt relief of pain and other symptoms
2. Guidelines/protocols/standards for:
   a. Documentation of pain history including child's word for pain and typical pain behaviors
   b. Systematic assessment and documentation of pain and other symptoms
   c. Pharmacologic and cognitive-behavioral management of pain and other symptoms
   d. Strategies to prevent pain and other symptoms whenever possible
   e. Management of side effects
   f. Monitoring of pain, vital signs, and level of consciousness
   g. Use of all specialized techniques available in the hospital such as intravenous patient-controlled analgesia, epidural infusions, PCEA, spinal infusions, plexus infusions, implantable baclofen pumps
3. Consensus regarding assignment of responsibilities and oversight
4. Tracking of outcomes and a quality improvement program
5. Education program for clinicians
6. Education program for parents and children
7. Multidisciplinary commitment to patient/parent involvement in pain assessment and management

PCEA, patient-controlled epidural analgesia.

EDUCATION PROGRAMS FOR CLINICIANS, PATIENTS, AND PARENTS

It is ideal for hospitals to develop standardized pain education programs for all clinicians, with formal pre- and post-assessments of clinicians' knowledge and beliefs. At Boston Children's Hospital, an illustrated information packet on pain is given routinely to parents and patients; it is printed through the Center for Families at Children's Hospital. Various print and web-based resources are now available. We especially recommend the materials available at http://pedspain.nursing.uiowa.edu and http://is.dal.ca/>pedpain/pedpain.html.

SYSTEMIC OPIOID ADMINISTRATION

Systemic opioids are a central part of any approach to acute pain management, even with the "opioid-sparing" strategy espoused by Kehlet et al. (8). As with the choice of care delivery model, there is no single "right

TABLE 27.2. *Acute pain service model*

A. Characteristics
   1. A group of physicians and nurses (and/or other clinicians, including pharmacists) takes hospital-wide responsibility for development of standards for pain assessment and management and provides hands-on, 24-hour, 7 days per week care of pain and symptom management for a large cohort of patients.
   2. These nurses and physicians have pain and symptom management as their primary daily task, not just as an afterthought.
B. Advantages
   1. Pain management is handled by clinicians with expertise and a commitment to do it well. As they develop experience, they become expert at identifying and solving the problems commonly faced by hospitalized patients with acute pain.
   2. Pain management becomes the clear responsibility of clinicians who are identified to the entire hospital.
   3. Outcomes can be tracked, and quality can be improved by learning from experience.
   4. There is some evidence (3) that pain and symptoms are treated more promptly in this model.
C. Disadvantages
   1. With shifting of responsibility to the acute pain service, primary service clinicians, including their residents and fellows, may become less skilled at pain management.
   2. Pain service clinicians may at times be less aware of some medical and surgical conditions that influence responses to analgesics and other medications. It is necessary for pain service clinicians to be very attentive to the types of medical and surgical problems that require intervention by the primary service clinicians.
   3. There are costs associated with funding positions for pain service physicians, nurses, and clinical nurse specialists. In the current medical economic climate, it may be difficult to find funding for these positions or to generate sufficient billing and collections to support these positions based on clinical revenue.

TABLE 27.3. *Primary service/hospital practice standards model*

A. Characteristics
   1. Pain management is implemented by primary services, either through resident or attending physicians.
   2. A multidisciplinary committee sets standards for analgesic prescribing and pain assessment.
   3. Education programs are developed and implemented for physicians, nurses, pharmacists, and other clinicians.

B. Advantages
   1. If ideally implemented, a wide group of primary service clinicians (e.g., surgeons, pediatricians, pediatric subspecialists) will develop expertise in pain assessment and management. This may carry over to other practice settings in the future.
   2. In most cases, primary service clinicians know the spectrum of their patients' medical and surgical issues and can evaluate pain and other symptoms in the context of the patient's overall condition.
   3. Costs of operations are lower than with an acute pain service.

C. Disadvantages
   1. Unless implemented in an optimal manner, there is a risk that pain management will be no one's responsibility or will fall to the most junior clinicians who may be preoccupied with other aspects of care, leading to suboptimal management.
   2. In the busy world of modern-day medicine, it may be overly optimistic to think that physicians' practices can be changed to a uniformly high standard simply by education and guidelines. Undertreatment of pain has been widespread, and there is a considerable potential for "backsliding" to a lower standard of care.
   3. If primary service physicians, especially residents, are occupied with other tasks, such as assessing or admitting other patients or assisting in the operating room, then delays in pain treatment become more likely.
   4. A clinician who continues to provide mediocre, but not overtly dangerous, pain treatment may receive little feedback to improve care.

way" to administer opioids; choice of routes, schedules, infusions, bolus options, and so on depends in part on local resource availability.

Intermittent Intravenous Opioid Dosing

In our institution, there is a general practice of administering opioids via an "intravenous push," primarily in higher acuity locations, such as the postanesthetic care unit and intensive care units. For most other intermittent dosing in lower acuity locations, intermittent intravenous doses are administered over 20 minutes, either via a syringe pump or dilution into a burette of maintenance intravenous fluid, with the infusion rate controlled by a volumetric pump.

With intermittent dosing, it is essential that clinicians appreciate the importance of repeated patient observation, both during the infusion and after its conclusion. The peak respiratory depressant effect of intravenous morphine is commonly stated as occurring 15 to 20 minutes after dosing, with rapid reduction in respiratory depressant effect thereafter. A review of published and unpublished cases of respiratory depression indicates that this view is an oversimplification. Respiratory depression is state dependent; it is exacerbated by sleep. Thus, a not uncommon scenario in critical incidents is as follows. A patient is alert and in pain, he or she receives a morphine dose; 20 minutes later, he or she is more comfortable and calm, 10 minutes later, he or she falls asleep; 20 minutes later, an episode of hypoventilation or airway obstruction occurs.

Patient-, Nurse-, and Parent-Controlled Analgesia

Patient-controlled analgesia (PCA) has been used widely for children since the late 1980s, and there is now a considerable literature on clinical outcomes (9–16). In general, PCA provides good analgesia, high satisfaction among patients, parents, and caregivers, and a very good safety record, both in tertiary centers and in a wide range of tertiary or community hospital settings worldwide (17).

Most pediatric centers in the United States permit PCA for children approximately 6 years of age and older. Although there are case reports suggesting that children as young as 3 or 4 years can use PCA, our view is that there is a high failure rate when children 3 to 5 years of age with acute pain use PCA. In most cases, this involves an inability of the child to understand a causal connection between pushing the button and obtaining relief. We have observed that children ages 3 to 5 years who have used PCA successfully are children with severe and long-standing pain such as cancer pain with attentive parents who are able to recognize their child's pain behaviors and gently guide their child in using PCA appropriately (Table 27.4).

Choice among agents for PCA is governed largely by custom, convenience, and an individual patient's history of effectiveness or side effects. Comparative studies support the use of morphine as an initial choice for most patients, both in the postoperative setting and after bone marrow transplantation (18,19).

Nurse-controlled analgesia appears to be a very convenient and safe method for titrating opioid dosing for infants and younger children or for children with developmental disabilities.

Parent-controlled analgesia has generated some controversy. In home palliative care, it is a well-established method for permitting dose titration and escalation and for adjusting dosing for breakthrough pain. The controversy mainly concerns parents pushing the PCA button for opioid-naïve children after surgery. Those who favor its use point out that parents know their child well and are in an ideal position to assess his or her pain. They note that on a busy ward, there may be delays in treatment if a nurse is not available to respond to a call from the parent. In some cases, parents may accompany the child through multiple hospitalizations and may become quite experienced and sophisticated in their knowledge of medical issues.

TABLE 27.4. *Making patient-controlled analgesia work*

1. Choose patients wisely
2. Develop a system for education of physicians, nurses, parents, and patients
3. Assess pain and side effects
4. Individualize dosing parameters according to medical and psychologic factors
5. Use a proactive program for side effect management

A counterargument is as follows. The inherent safety of PCA is that when the patient begins to become narcotized, he or she falls asleep, dosing stops, and plasma and brain concentrations return to a more acceptable range. If another individual pushes the button for a somnolent patient, then hypoventilation may ensue. Parents may vary widely in their understanding of how pain is assessed postoperatively or whether there is impending overnarcotization. There have been numerous cases brought to our attention by risk management departments in other hospitals that involved respiratory or cardiac arrests, and in at least two cases, death owing to parents pushing the PCA button. Among these cases, the following features were common:

1. patient risk factors, including airway narrowing, respiratory disease, or motor impairment;
2. no protocol for parent education;
3. no protocol for frequent or continuous patient observation or monitoring;
4. adverse events occurred in the middle of the night or very early morning hours.

A recent case series by Monitto et al. (20) from Johns Hopkins Hospital showed generally good effectiveness and safety in a series of patients who received either nurse- or parent-controlled analgesia. It is important to note that hypoventilation requiring naloxone occurred in a few cases and this series was accumulated in a hospital with extensive experience in pediatric PCA use. In a hospital with less experienced staff and with a less vigilant system of observation, these hypoventilation episodes could have resulted in much less favorable outcomes.

Based on these concerns, our current practice is to make widespread use of nurse-controlled analgesia but to restrict parent-controlled analgesia to parents of children who are in palliative care or for a small subset of children who are chronically receiving parenteral opioids at home. Further large-scale outcome studies in this area are needed.

In the United States, pediatric hospitals commonly use programmable pumps that permit selection of parameters including a loading dose, bolus dose, lock-out interval, continuous (basal) rate, and 1- or 4-hour maximal dose. Not all PCA pumps are adaptable for use with children (Table 27.5). Some these pumps are quite bulky and are routinely mounted on an intravenous pole. Others are more portable, which makes them attractive for home care or palliative care. In other parts of the world, there is more widespread use of simple, inexpensive hydraulic devices, such as the Edmonton infuser.

The inclusion of basal infusions with PCA is another controversial area. The theoretic advantage of including a basal infusion is that one maintains a degree of analgesic effect at all times but especially during nighttime sleep (Fig. 27.1A), so that the patient does not awaken frequently in pain and find him- or herself unable to "catch up" owing to the restricted dosing permitted by the PCA boluses (Fig. 27.1C).

Those opposed to basal infusions cite both safety concerns and a potential reduction in side effects as reasons to avoid them. They note that with a basal infusion, a patient who has dosed him- or herself to the point of impending narcosis will continue to receive opioid while asleep, increasing the chance of dangerous hypoventilation (Fig. 27.1B). In addition, for patients whose analgesic requirements are less than anticipated, a basal infusion will increase their overall opioid consumption and thereby increase the chance for opioid-induced side effects.

Available studies on this issue have drawn mixed conclusions for reasons outlined below. In our first controlled study of pediatric PCA, patients were randomized to receive morphine delivered via either (a) PCA alone, (b) PCA plus basal infusion, or (c) nurse-administered intermittent injections. In this study, pain scores were lower and patient satisfaction scores were higher in the PCA plus basal infusion group compared with the PCA alone group. There were no group differences in either total opioid use or opioid-related side effects. McNeely and Trentadue (21) compared PCA with PCA plus basal infusion and reported a higher frequency of brief episodes of desaturation during sleep in the PCA plus basal infusion group, although none of these episodes produced clinically apparent adverse consequences. Subsequently, Doyle et al. (13,14) attempted a more systematic examination of basal infusions in pediatric PCA. They concluded that a very low basal rate, approximately 4 μg/kg per hour (0.004 mg/kg per hour), was optimal for a basal morphine infusion rate along with PCA. Although these studies were carefully conducted, their relevance is limited somewhat by the fact that a high percentage of these patients had comparatively minor operations such as appendectomies. These patients typically receive much lower opioid dosing than those undergoing major procedures such as scoliosis repairs and other major orthopedic procedures, thoracotomies, and major abdominal and pelvic surgeries.

Our position in this controversy is that "it depends on the individual case." Psychologic factors also influence choice of PCA parameters

TABLE 27.5. *Desirable features of patient-controlled analgesia pumps for pediatric use*

1. Accuracy of infusion at low volumes
2. Intuitive programming to minimize amount of information that users must remember to operate device
   a. Controls logically grouped and clearly labeled
   b. Clear language in wording of display
   c. Simple error recovery
3. No default settings so that clinicians must consciously program settings, especially for concentration
4. Review of programming mandatory before starting the pump
5. Tamper proof
6. Flexibility in dosing
7. Portability for ease of transporting patient to physical therapy and to the playroom
8. Disposables (bags, syringes, tubing) convenient and reasonable in cost

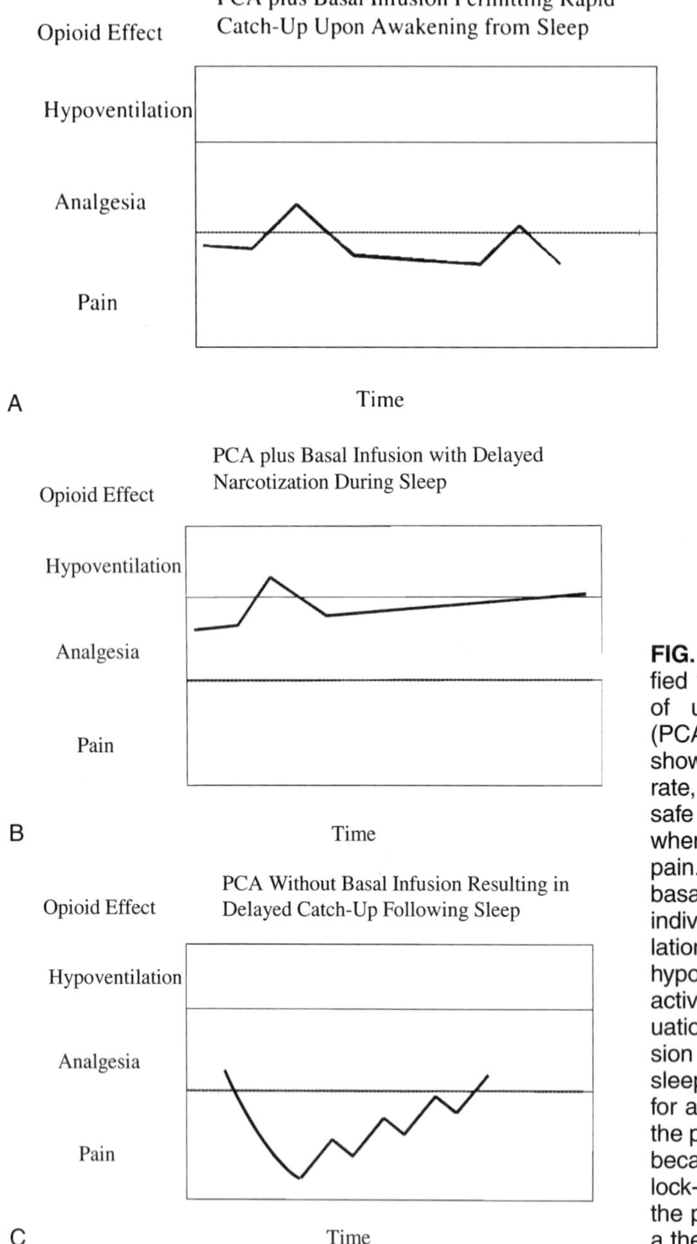

FIG. 27.1. The diagrams depict a simplified view of the different consequences of using patient-controlled analgesia (PCA) with or without a basal infusion. **A** shows how, with an ideal basal infusion rate, PCA plus basal infusion can permit safe dosing along with rapid "catch up" when patients awaken from sleep with pain. **B** shows a situation in which the basal rate is comparatively high for this individual patient, so that drug accumulation during sleep can result in delayed hypoventilation even without the patient activating the PCA button. **C** shows a situation using PCA without a basal infusion in which the patient awakens from sleep without having pushed the button for an extended period of time, in which the process of "catching up" is prolonged because multiple doses and multiple lock-out intervals are required to return the plasma/brain opioid concentration to a therapeutic range.

(22). In Table 27.6, we list factors that would argue for or against inclusion of a basal infusion.

In practice, basal infusions are used in our hospital for almost all oncology patients, almost all patients with sickle cell disease having vaso-occlusive pain episodes (23), and almost all scoliosis patients for the first postoperative night. If an opioid-naïve postoperative patient requires a basal infusion on a regular ward, then we would be inclined to use electronic monitoring (see section on monitoring).

Conversion To Oral Opioids

A major issue for postoperative pain treatment is to identify ways to ensure the success

TABLE 27.6. *Factors that influence inclusion of a basal infusion with patient-controlled analgesia*

A. Factors that bias toward inclusion of a basal infusion
  1. Long-standing opioid use
  2. Chronic illnesses, e.g., cancer and sickle cell disease
  3. High pain severity
  4. Very extensive surgery, especially for the first postoperative night
  5. A history of inadequate analgesia with previous parameter choices
  6. Depressed mood, anxiety disorders, or other emotional factors that would decrease the patient's patience or ability to cope with delays in attaining relief

B. Factors that bias against inclusion of a basal infusion
  1. Significant airway, neurologic, or respiratory compromise
  2. Relatively mild pain
  3. No previous exposure to opioids
  4. Surgery that could result in bleeding into the airway, e.g., maxillofacial procedures, alveolar bone grafting, pharyngeal flaps
  5. Not very extensive surgery
  6. More than 1 to 2 days postoperatively
  7. A history of somnolence or hypoventilation with previous opioid administration

of conversion to oral opioid administration after discontinuation of parenteral or neuraxial analgesic administration. In many cases, this is a principal determinant of a child's readiness for hospital discharge.

One common problem in conversion to oral opioids is administration of insufficient doses to account for the low oral-to-parenteral relative potency of most opioids. For example, if one converts from intravenous morphine to oral morphine, then a threefold increase in the daily morphine dose is generally recommended.

Codeine is commonly used as a first-line oral opioid. Codeine has the advantage of ready availability; in many locations, it is the only oral opioid that can be prescribed by telephone order to local pharmacies (generally in combination with acetaminophen). Codeine nevertheless has two major disadvantages as a first-line oral analgesic.

1. In standard doses (0.5 to 1 mg/kg), codeine is a remarkably weak analgesic. For example, in systematic reviews in adults, 30 to 45 mg codeine orally provides less consistent analgesia in several models than 600 mg ibuprofen. Although the analgesia of codeine may be increased by further dose escalation, a limited literature from the 1960s suggests that escalation to 2 mg/kg produces an unacceptably high incidence of side effects. This common belief is based on only limited data and deserves further study.

2. Codeine is essentially a prodrug of morphine with little intrinsic analgesia by itself; it is activated by hepatic O-demethylation to convert it to morphine. Between 4% and 12% of subjects lack the enzyme that converts codeine to morphine; for these subjects, codeine is essentially inert as an analgesic (24).

For these two reasons, we encourage more routine first-line use of "stronger" oral opioids, particularly after significantly painful surgeries.

EPIDURAL ANALGESIA

Epidural analgesia can provide optimal relief of pain and can improve postoperative outcome, particularly if it used in combination with a postoperative rehabilitation program that emphasizes early mobilization, oral nutrition, and early return to normal activities (25,26). Detailed discussion of techniques of placement and pharmacology of epidural local anesthetics, opioids, and adjuvants is provided in other chapters (Chapters 14, 20, and 22). Here we concentrate more on "how to make it work."

Epidural analgesia is labor intensive and requires a high degree of physician and nursing expertise and attention. Hospitals that treat children only infrequently, in our view, should concentrate first on establishing uniform standards for pain assessment and treatment and optimal delivery of opioids and treatment of their side effects. Conversely, in our view, providing epidural analgesia should become the standard of care for most major tertiary pediatric centers in developed countries.

Tables 27.7, 27.8, and 27.9 list some of our opinions about how to make epidural analgesia work optimally.

TABLE 27.7. *Making epidural analgesia work*

1. Select patients properly. Selection of patients for epidural analgesia should involve a consideration of the patient's medical and psychosocial condition, the type of surgery or other sources of pain, and technical factors that will have an impact on the success of placement.
2. Prove that all catheters are properly placed.
   a. Because most pediatric epidural catheters are placed under sedation or general anesthesia, anesthesiologists must use more indirect methods to confirm proper location.
   b. Radiographic methods (fluoroscopy, contrast epidurography, use of radio-opaque catheters) can provide extremely reliable confirmation in selected cases, but they incur additional expense, time, and radiation exposure. We use them routinely for high-risk situations, including patients undergoing lung transplantation or patients receiving long-term epidural catheters for palliative care or for treatment of complex regional pain syndrome.
   c. The recently developed method of electrical stimulation guidance by Tsui et al.[1] is a noteworthy advance. This method is quick, inexpensive, and reliable.
   d. Use a chloroprocaine test for patients in the postanesthetic care unit or on the wards to reconfirm positioning (Table 27.8) if there is any doubt.
3. Use optimal choice of epidural infusions (Table 27.9).
   a. Local anesthetics are effective only if applied at or near the dermatomal level of the surgery.
   b. Local anesthetics are frequently inadequate as the sole agent in epidural infusions. We routinely recommend combining local anesthetics with either opioids or clonidine.
   c. If low-lying catheter tips are used for upper abdominal or thoracic surgery, consider the use of hydrophilic opioids, especially hydromorphone.
4. Fix inadequate infusions rapidly, not slowly.
   a. If a patient in a postoperative unit develops significant pain while receiving an epidural infusion, it is an inadequate response to simply increase the infusion rate by 15% to 25%. If no bolus is given, it is highly probable that it will take 3 to 4 hours to reach a new steady state. This results in an unacceptably long period of insufficient pain relief.
   b. Alternatives for rapid correction include (details in Tables 27.8 and 27.9):
      i. A chloroprocaine bolus,
      ii. 1 to 2 hours of the existing infusion as a bolus over 10 to 20 minutes,
      iii. A bolus of epidural hydromorphone,
      iv. Use of epidural local anesthetic + clonidine, with nurse-administered intermittent intravenous opioid dosing for rescue,
      v. After rapid correction per options i to iv above, the maintenance rate is increased by approximately 25%.

[1]Data from Tsui BC, Seal R, Koller J, et al. Thoracic epidural analgesia via the caudal approach in pediatric patients undergoing fundoplication using nerve stimulation guidance. *Anesth Analg* 2001;93:1152–1155.

TABLE 27.8. *Chloroprocaine test for epidural catheter tip location*

Indication: For a patient postoperatively who had inadequate analgesia and incomplete confirmation of epidural catheter tip positioning. The presumption is that the catheter has previously been test-dosed and that the patient has subsequently received a loading dose of an amino amide local anesthetic, e.g., lidocaine or bupivacaine, with or without a subsequent infusion. The presumption is that the catheter cannot be intrathecal, otherwise there would already be clear evidence of conduction blockade. The rationale for using chloroprocaine, an amino ester, is that in this circumstance, a repeat loading dose of an amino amide would result in "staircasing" of plasma drug concentration, increasing the risk of systemic local anesthetic toxicity, including seizures and arrhythmias. Because chloroprocaine is metabolized extremely rapidly by plasma esterases ($t_{½}$ β <1 minute even in former preterm infants), one can give repeat loading doses with much less risk of drug accumulation.

Monitoring and equipment: As with any major conduction blockade, there should be ready availability of a blood pressure cuff, an electrocardiogram machine, an oxygen source, a bag and mask, and resuscitative medications, including a vasopressor such as ephedrine and an anticonvulsant such as midazolam and thiopental. Continuous assessment of heart rate is desirable during any bolus dosing for major conduction blockade.

Dosing: Chloroprocaine (3% solution) is used to provide objective signs of sensory and motor blockade. Dosing is administered in four increments over 4 minutes according to age:

Age	Incremental dose (mL/kg)	Total dose (mL/kg)
0–2 yr	0.2	0.8
3–8 yr	0.15	0.6
>9 yr	0.1 (to a max of 4 mL)	0.4 (to a max of 16 mL)

Findings and interpretation:

a. No signs of lower extremity sensory or motor block and no change in heart rate or blood pressure → catheter tip is probably not in the epidural space.
b. Bilateral partial or complete sensory and motor block of the lower extremities with or without change reductions in blood pressure or heart rate → catheter tip is probably in a lumbar or sacral epidural position.
c. Minimal sensory or motor block in the legs, but clear reductions in heart rate and blood pressure and clear evidence of analgesia; may show signs of abdominal muscle motor blockade → catheter tip is probably in a thoracic epidural position.
d. Unilateral partial sensory or motor blockade → catheter tip may have passed through an intervertebral foramen.

TABLE 27.9. *Examples of interventions to improve epidural analgesia once the catheter tip location is presumptively determined (modify according to clinical indications; use hydromorphone with extreme caution in infants younger than 3 months of age)*

a. If the catheter tip is not epidural, abandon the technique and begin systemic analgesia. In unusual cases, there may be an indication for replacement of the epidural catheter.
b. If the catheter tip is lumbosacral and the surgical site is thoracic, upper abdominal, or mid-abdominal, consider the addition to the preexisting epidural local anesthetic infusion of a hydrophilic opioid, e.g., hydromorphone. A conservative initial hydromorphone bolus dose would be approximately 6 μg/kg, followed by infusion of 0.5 to 2 μg/kg/hr. For example, if the infusion contains 0.1% bupivacaine with 10 μg/mL hydromorphone, then 0.2 mL/kg/hr gives a hydromorphone dosing of 2 μg/kg/hr.
c. If the catheter tip is thoracic and the surgical site is thoracic, upper abdominal, or mid-abdominal, consider the addition to the preexisting epidural local anesthetic infusion of one or the other (not both) of the following two options:
   i. An initial hydromorphone bolus dose of approximately 4 μg/kg, followed by hydromorphone added to the preexisting epidural infusion to yield a dose of 0.5 to 1.5 μg/kg/hr.
   ii. Addition of 2 μg/mL fentanyl + 0.4 μg/kg clonidine to the preexisting epidural infusion to infuse at approximately 0.3 mL/kg/hr. This would yield 0.6 μg/kg/hr fentanyl and 0.12 μg/kg/hr clonidine.
d. If the catheter tip is lumbosacral and the surgical site is lumbosacral or lower abdominal, consider the addition to the epidural local anesthetic infusion of one or the other (not both) of the following:
   i. 2 μg/mL fentanyl + 0.4 μg/mL clonidine per option c.
   ii. Hydromorphone, at bolus doses or infusion rates starting at approximate 50% to 70% of those described in options b and c.
e. If the catheter tip is in the appropriate dermatomal level for surgery, another option is to infuse local anesthetic + clonidine via the epidural, plus intravenous opioids as needed. This permits convenient rescue analgesia while avoiding the complications and risks associated with the combined use of systemic and epidural opioids.
f. Along with any of interventions b through e, consider the addition of a systemic nonsteroidal anti-inflammatory drug or cyclooxygenase 2 inhibitor. This will rarely be sufficient by itself but may make interventions b through e more effective.

MONITORING FOR RESPIRATORY DEPRESSION

There is wide variation in standards for patient observation and electronic monitoring for patients receiving systemic or epidural opioids and local anesthetics. Most practices (including our own) are not evidence based. Our opinions are the following.

1. No electronic system can substitute for skilled patient observation and assessment. Level of consciousness is a very useful guide to opioid effect; we recommend assessment of this every 4 hours.
2. Electronic monitors that do not ring throughout a ward and at the nurses' station give a false sense of security.
3. An excessive frequency of false alarms can make clinicians ignore them or shut off monitors.
4. A form of electronic monitoring that may detect a physiologically ideal parameter, such as end-tidal or transcutaneous P_{CO_2}, may become impractical in daily use if it generates too many false-positive alarms or has too many false-negative failures, for example, owing to partial dislodgement.

At Children's Hospital in Boston, every bed space in the entire hospital has the potential for two-channel electronic monitoring with alarms that ring throughout the hallways and at the nurses' station. There is very ready availability of monitors that detect heart rate and chest wall impedance for apnea monitoring. The low and high heart rate and respiratory rate alarm parameters can be individualized according to patient age and physiologic status. In addition, one of these two channels can be used for pulse oximetry for approximately 15 to 20 patients each day who are not in the intensive care unit or pediatric acute care unit.

IMMEDIATE RESPONSE SYSTEMS

Regardless of the model for acute pain care used, there is a need for immediate response to critical incidents. Depending on the type of hospital setting, this may involve a pediatric anesthesiologist, a pediatric intensivist, a house physician, a pediatric senior resident, or a variety of other clinicians. At a minimum, this clinician should be expert at pediatric airway management and should have extensive experience with assessment and management of pain and effects of analgesics.

PHARMACY SERVICES

Pharmacists play a number of roles in acute pain services. They are responsible for drug dispensing, formulation of infusions, prevention of drug-dosing errors, identifying potential drug interactions, and identifying other patient-specific factors that may modify responses to analgesics. It is essential that they be integrally involved in acute pain services, at the stage of protocol development, in the consideration of introduction of new analgesics or forms of analgesic delivery, and for ongoing aspects of patient care.

INFORMATION MANAGEMENT

An acute pain service requires transfer of clinical information among clinicians. It is ideal to have an information management program that combines some of the following features:

1. generation of a readable sign-out list that posts patients' names, ages, weights, diagnoses, locations, and types of analgesic treatments being administered;
2. maintenance of a relational database to track outcomes, complications, sentinel events, and clinical volume;
3. generation of bills based on menu-driven coding of diagnoses and procedures;
4. clinical note writing for the medical record according to standards expected by the Health Care Financing Administration.

Over a 10-year period, our acute pain service has used a program known as PTS written as an Oracle database to be compatible with our hospital's computer network. This program accomplished goals 1 through 3, although data entry was somewhat cumbersome. Recently, we developed modules to add goal 4 to make a more intuitive, point-and-click–based interface and to have a hand-held pocket PC interface. This system is undergoing testing at present.

CODING AND BILLING, ECONOMICS, AND STAFFING MODELS

The predominant operating costs of an acute pain service are personnel costs for the time spent by physicians, nurses, and pharmacists. Many pediatric centers try to offset physician costs by having staff physicians, generally anesthesiologists, spend a portion of their day making rounds on the acute pain service and a portion of their day covering sedation services, the pediatric acute care unit, or other locations. Similarly, in some centers, a clinical nurse specialist or nurse practitioner will multitask coverage of other locations in the hospital. The decisions regarding staffing depend in part on local patient volume and staff availability. Even in situations in which attending physicians cover an acute pain service along with other clinical roles, we believe that it should be the standard of care for the attending physician to check on all patients at least once daily.

It is unlikely that an acute pain service in the current medical climate can generate any significant profit. The major aims should be to provide optimal clinical service while minimizing economic loss or subsidizing the service from other activities. Proper choice of current procedural terminology codes may improve billing and collection. Collection depends on local payer mix and on negotiated rates with insurance companies and managed care organizations. We have frequently taken the position that provision of postoperative pain care for children is a specialized area of expertise that is not necessarily found among residents from other services who may rotate from adult hospitals.

CHRONIC PAIN MANAGEMENT PROGRAMS

Although many individual pediatric subspecialists care for children with chronic pain, numerous pediatric tertiary centers worldwide have developed multidisciplinary clinics for pediatric chronic pain management, modeled in many respects after the example of adult pain clinics espoused by McQuay et al. (27).

Physicians from a range of subspecialties may be involved in pediatric chronic pain management; at centers around the world, developmental pediatricians, neurologists, anesthesiologists, oncologists, rheumatologists, physiatrists, and psychiatrists have all served in this role. Again, no single model can be applied in all settings (Table 27.10).

In our view, it is optimal to have a clinic structure in which patients meet with a physician, a psychologist (or other mental health professional), and a physical therapist for a comprehensive evaluation on their first visit to the clinic. In our clinic, each of these three clinicians meets with the patient and family for 1 hour, then there is a team conference, and then there is a group session for presentation of a treatment plan to the patient and family. Although this approach is extremely time-consuming (typically only three new patients are seen in a clinic day), it helps to ensure a comprehensive approach. In other clinics, there is a combined interview for 1 to 2 hours with all three clinicians meeting with the family and patient. There are advantages and disadvantages of each approach.

TABLE 27.10. *Essential aspects of chronic pain management programs*

1. Clinicians from several disciplines; often this will include physicians, nurses, psychologists, and physical therapists.
2. Protected time for clinicians to permit adequate attention to these complex patients.
3. Clinic space with examination rooms, interview rooms, and a waiting area.
4. Sufficient administrative support staff to manage telephone calls, scheduling, insurance authorization, and related business aspects.
5. Office space equipped with sufficient computer resources, space for patient files, and so on.
6. Institutional commitment to support the program even if it does not generate much income.

There is an enormous volume of telephone calls required for the proper care of these patients. In our clinic, each weekday, a senior staff nurse manages patient callbacks, refills prescriptions, titrates medications based on efficacy and side effects, and keeps all clinicians informed about patients' progress. We have developed a relational database program known as Axon–Hillock that facilitates group task management and automated e-mail notification for involved clinicians. As with much of the medical software, the utility of such a program is dependent in part on how it interfaces with the rest of the local hospital's information infrastructure.

PSYCHOLOGIC ASSESSMENT, PSYCHOTHERAPY, AND COGNITIVE-BEHAVIORAL TREATMENT

It is a common misconception that the primary purpose of psychologists' involvement in pain clinics is to discover and/or diagnose "psychopathology" (28). A considerable percentage of patients does exhibit anxiety, exaggerated worry (29), depressed mood, and posttraumatic stress disorders; psychologic diagnoses and learning difficulties are frequently identified for the first time during their initial pain clinic visit. Nevertheless, effective psychologic interventions for children with chronic pain are not limited to those with "*DSM* diagnoses." Cognitive-behavioral treatments have a robust track record of effectiveness in a wide spectrum of chronic pain conditions (30). These issues are discussed in much greater detail in other chapters. Local factors may have a great affect on how psychologic interventions are delivered. Group treatment, individual treatment in the clinic, and treatment models that emphasize self-directed interventions (31) may all be appropriate in some settings. We maintain the view that psychologic assessment should be an integral part of the first visits for the overwhelming majority of children attending chronic pain clinics.

PATIENT AND FAMILY EDUCATION AND ATTITUDINAL CHANGE

A major task during the meeting with patients and families at the end of their first clinic day is to provide education and a different viewpoint on chronic pain, impairment, and disability. It is essential to understand patients' and parents views' of the nature of pain (32,33) and appropriate responses to pain. A common, frequently mistaken, belief in some families is that the child should refrain from many normal activities, including school attendance, until "the answer is found and the problem is fixed." Parents and patients are encouraged to diminish catastrophizing (34) and to promote more adaptive and positive coping styles (35–37).

MEDICATION PRESCRIBING FOR CHRONIC PAIN

Medical therapies for many forms of chronic pain, including neuropathic pain and migraine, require patience in dose titration and in longitudinal assessment of effectiveness and side effects. Detailed discussions of the pharmacology of these agents are provided in other chapters. The emphasis here is on the process of dose titration and assessment. In our clinic, it has been useful to give patients printed information sheets for the common types of medications and to employ weekly telephone calls with our clinic nurses, particularly in the initial dose titration phase. Our clinic task management program, Axon–Hillock (see previous section), has been invaluable in tracking prescription refills, symptoms, side effects, and analgesic responses. The framework for medication prescribing varies greatly in different clinics with different resources. Telephone messages through administrative support staff, direct paging of clinicians, voice mail, or other forms of messaging are commonly used methods for patients communicating with clinicians about medication adjustments.

CHRONIC OPIOID THERAPY

Among the patients in our chronic pain clinic, only a very small percentage receives opioids on a long-term basis. Some these patients have diseases with the potential for a short life expectancy, such as cancer or some neurodegenerative disorders, a few have severe skeletal conditions with no immediate surgical options, and others have long-standing neuropathic pain owing to injuries to the peripheral or central nervous system. For patients who are not clearly in a palliative treatment mode, we require an opioid-prescribing contract between the patient, their family, and our clinic providers (Table 27.11).

A recent review of our database listed 21 patients not in palliative care who were receiving opioids on a long-term basis. This represents less than 4% of a cohort of approximately 550 patients who are regarded as in active, ongoing treatment at any given time, including approximately 350 new patients evaluated annually for multidisciplinary chronic pain care. An additional 25 to 40 clinic patients annually are prescribed opioids on a short-term basis, e.g., for 1 to 2 months, while other therapies are being implemented. A major feature of the Axon–Hillock database is that it permits close tracking of opioid prescribing and helps to detect deviations from expected medication requirements. The risk–benefit issues of long-term use of opioids for children with chronic pain need to be determined; this is a subject that merits broad-based prospective longitudinal study (38).

FISCAL ISSUES

Care of children and adolescents with chronic pain is labor- and time intensive. As with acute pain management programs, it is unlikely that these programs will be profitable in the current medical climate in most countries. Anesthesia-based chronic pain clinics for adults generate considerable revenue from nerve-blocking procedures. The situation for children differs greatly from the adult models in this regard because neural blockade is less commonly indicated for most pediatric chronic pain conditions and because children typically require either conscious sedation or general anesthesia for procedures, which necessitates

TABLE 27.11. *Pain treatment service chronic opioid pain medication agreement*

The following agreement relates to my/my child's use of opioid pain medications prescribed for chronic pain by a physician at the Pain Treatment Service, Children's Hospital, Boston. I recognize that specific policies regarding the use of opioids and related controlled substances are followed by the staff of the Pain Treatment Service. I will be provided with the controlled substances while actively participating in this program only if I adhere to the following regulations:

1. I will use the substances only within the parameters given by the Pain Treatment Service physician.
2. I will not receive replacements for lost or stolen medications.
3. I will receive controlled substances only from the Children's Hospital Pain Treatment Service staff. My violation of this will result in a discontinuation of treatment.
4. I will not expect to receive additional medication before my/my child's next scheduled refill, even if my prescription runs out.
5. I will accept generic brands of my prescription medication.
6. If it appears to the physician that my/my child's daily functioning and quality of life are not benefiting from treatment with the controlled substances, I will gradually taper my/my child's medication as prescribed by the physician. I will not hold any member of the Pain Treatment Service liable for problems caused by discontinuance of controlled substances, provided that I receive 30 days' notice of termination.
7. I agree to submit to urine and blood screening to detect the use of nonprescription medications at any time.
8. I recognize that my/my child's chronic pain represents a complex problem that may benefit from physical therapy, psychotherapy, and behavioral medicine strategies. I also recognize that my participation in the management of my/my child's pain is extremely important. I agree to actively participate in all aspects of the pain management program to maximize the likelihood that my/my child's level of functioning will increase and my/my child's ability to cope with my/my child's condition will improve.

Patient signature	Date
Physician signature	Date
Family member signature	Date

performing these procedures in a procedure room or anesthetizing location rather than in a typical clinic setting. Nevertheless, attention to proper diagnostic and procedure codes can help to improve revenue in clinics in the United States and other countries in which reimbursement is based on the number and complexity of clinic visits. Clinicians involved in pediatric chronic pain management often dedicate a portion of their time to the pain clinic, while continuing part-time practice in another clinical setting that provides better reimbursement. Grant support, private donations, or institutional support is generally necessary to make pediatric chronic pain programs fiscally viable.

LONG-DISTANCE TREATMENT

Because relatively few pediatric chronic pain programs are available, it is inevitable that a considerable percentage of children and their families seeking treatment for chronic pain live at some distance from the clinic in a tertiary pediatric center. It is often helpful to conduct a detailed review of patient records and a telephone interview with the family before the first long-distance visit so that there can be some preliminary expectations regarding goals of treatment, duration of a possible hospital stay, and so on. Conversely, clinicians should be careful in making firm promises about a course of treatment before the in-person evaluation because "things are not always what they seem" from a telephone discussion. If an ongoing treatment relationship is formed, it is often ideal to establish a collaborative treatment plan between clinicians at the pain clinic and clinicians in the patient's local area. Prospective study of a model of long-distance treatment is in progress (P. J. McGrath, personal communication, 2002).

INPATIENT TREATMENT OF CHILDREN AND ADOLESCENTS WITH CHRONIC PAIN

Most children with chronic pain can be treated on an outpatient basis, and it is desirable to do so that they can maintain ongoing involvement in school and family life. In a small subgroup of cases, there is a need for short- or longer term inpatient treatment.

Short-term hospitalization is commonly used when there is a need for adjustment of medications in a medically complex patient for whom outpatient titration may involve some risk. For example, initial trial bolus dosing of intrathecal baclofen may be performed with an overnight hospitalization for a patient with spasticity of supraspinal origin. A second common indication for short-term hospitalization is for a patient with severe extremity pain with long-standing immobility or joint contractures, e.g., more severe cases of complex regional pain syndromes, for whom intensive physical therapy may be facilitated by continuous epidural analgesia or continuous plexus blockade for a period of 5 to 10 days. In both situations, children are admitted to a regular medical-surgical inpatient unit. When feasible, we prefer to admit them to a particular unit in which the nurses have very extensive and regular experience with children with chronic pain and disability.

In contrast, there is a subgroup of children and adolescents with chronic pain and long-standing disability (39) who require more prolonged hospitalization to permit an intensive program of physical and psychologic rehabilitation. Several types of hospital settings can be used for this situation, with attendant advantages and disadvantages: an acute care medical/surgical ward, a rehabilitation unit, an open medical/psychiatric unit, and a locked psychiatric unit. In the United States at present, and probably in many other countries, these patients frequently present a dilemma in terms of where to find optimal treatment. There is a profound shortage of inpatient beds for psychiatric/psychologic treatment, and most inpatient psychiatric settings consist of locked units for short-term treatment of children who are acutely depressed, acutely psychotic, or dangerous to themselves or others.

Many children and adolescents with chronic pain and disability refractory to outpatient treatment would benefit from an inpatient milieu that includes intensive psychiatric/psychologic services, intensive physical rehabilitation, intensive academic rehabilitation (i.e., tutoring), and some medical interventions. These patients are almost never psychotic, are only very rarely dangerous to themselves or others, and in most cases, they have excellent cognitive development and communication skills. In a small percentage of cases, a child's depressed mood or agitation is appropriately managed in a typical inpatient pediatric psychiatric unit. However, a typical locked pediatric psychiatric ward, as currently established in the United States, may be suboptimal for treatment for many other of these children and adolescents, despite the severity of their physical and psychologic impairments because the milieu is too oriented toward acute psychiatric care of children who are more severely mentally ill.

Pediatric inpatient rehabilitation units often have a mix of children with major disabilities, including hypoxic-ischemic brain injury, spinal cord injury, congenital neurologic disorders, and chronic respiratory failure. The orientation toward physical rehabilitation and stepwise return to normal functioning may be ideal for many children with chronic pain. What is often a challenge in pediatric rehabilitation units is to provide sufficient staffing with psychiatrists, psychologists, and other mental health clinicians as well as skilled tutors who are specifically experienced in the needs of children with chronic pain and pain-related disability.

Adult inpatient pain units are more widely available, often in conjunction with adult rehabilitation services. Although these units have an orientation toward reducing pain-related disability and an expertise in pharmacotherapy and physical therapy, they are generally an ideal therapeutic milieu for children and adolescents.

Several alternative models for inpatient treatment and day treatment are currently under discussion. It will be important to begin a prospective examination of the effectiveness of these treatment settings.

CONCLUSIONS

Multidisciplinary programs for acute and chronic pain management are evolving along several types of models worldwide. Prospective and, in many cases, multicenter clinical trials are needed to examine advantages and disadvantages of different treatment models.

REFERENCES

1. Ready LB, Oden R, Chadwick HS, et al. Development of an anesthesiology-based postoperative pain management service. *Anesthesiology* 1988;68:100–106.
2. Berde C, Sethna N, Levin L, et al. Regional analgesia on pediatric medical and surgical wards. *Intensive Care Med* 1989;15:S40–S43.
3. Miaskowski C, Crews J, Ready LB, et al. Anesthesia-based pain services improve the quality of postoperative pain management. *Pain* 1999;80:23–29.
4. Grossi E, Borghi C, Cerchiari EL, et al. Analogue chromatic continuous scale (ACCS): a new method for pain assessment. *Clin Exp Rheumatol* 1983;1:337–340.
5. McGrath P, Seifert C, Speechley K, et al. A new analogue scale for assessing children's pain: an initial validation study. *Pain* 1996;64:435–443.
6. Merkel SI, Voepel-Lewis T, Shayevitz JR, et al. The FLACC: a behavioral scale for scoring postoperative pain in young children. *Pediatr Nurs* 1997;23:293–297.
7. Stevens B, Johnston C, Petryshen P, et al. Premature Infant Pain Profile: development and initial validation. *Clin J Pain* 1996;12:13–22.
8. Kehlet H, Rung GW, Callesen T. Postoperative opioid analgesia: time for a reconsideration? *J Clin Anesth* 1996;8:441–445.
9. Gaukroger PB, Tomkins DP, van der Walt JH. Patient-controlled analgesia as postoperative pain treatment for children. *J Pediatr Nurs* 1989;4:162–171.
10. Berde CB, Lehn BM, Yee JD, et al. Patient-controlled analgesia in children and adolescents: a randomized, prospective comparison with intramuscular administration of morphine for postoperative analgesia. *J Pediatr* 1991;118:460–466.
11. Mackie AM, Coda BC, Hill HF. Adolescents use patient-controlled analgesia effectively for relief from prolonged oropharyngeal mucositis pain. *Pain* 1991;46: 265–269.
12. Doyle E, Mottart KJ, Marshall C, et al. Comparison of different bolus doses of morphine for patient-controlled analgesia in children. *Br J Anaesth* 1994;72:160–163.
13. Doyle E, Harper I, Morton NS. Patient-controlled analgesia with low dose background infusions after lower abdominal surgery in children. *Br J Anaesth* 1993;71: 818–822.
14. Doyle E, Robinson D, Morton NS. Comparison of patient-controlled analgesia with and without a background infusion after lower abdominal surgery in children. *Br J Anaesth* 1993; 71:670–673.
15. Bray RJ, Woodhams AM, Vallis CJ, et al. Morphine consumption and respiratory depression in children receiving postoperative analgesia from continuous morphine infusion or patient controlled analgesia. *Paediatr Anaesth* 1996;6:129–134.
16. Collins JJ, Geake J, Grier HE, et al. Patient-controlled analgesia for mucositis pain in children: a three- period crossover study comparing morphine and hydromorphone. *J Pediatr* 1996;129:722–728.
17. Veyckemans F. Patient-controlled analgesia. Its South African debut in a provincial hospital. *S Afr Med J* 1992;81:74–76.
18. Coda BA, O'Sullivan B, Donaldson G, et al. Comparative efficacy of patient-controlled administration of morphine, hydromorphone, or sufentanil for the treatment of oral mucositis pain after bone marrow transplantation. *Pain* 1997;72:333–346.
19. Dunbar PJ, Chapman CR, Buckley FP, et al. Clinical analgesic equivalence for morphine and hydromorphone with prolonged PCA. *Pain* 1996;68:265–270.
20. Monitto CL, Greenberg RS, Kost-Byerly S, et al. The safety and efficacy of parent-/nurse-controlled analgesia in patients less than six years of age. *Anesth Analg* 2000;91:573–579.
21. McNeely JK, Trentadue NC. Comparison of patient-controlled analgesia with and without nighttime morphine infusion following lower extremity surgery in children. *J Pain Symptom Manage* 1997;13:268–273.
22. Wermeling DP, Greene SA, Boucher BA, et al. Patient controlled analgesia: the relation of psychological factors to pain and analgesic use in adolescents with postoperative pain. *Clin J Pain* 1992;8:215–221.
23. Shapiro BS, Cohen DE, Howe CJ. Patient-controlled analgesia for sickle-cell-related pain. *J Pain Symptom Manage* 1993;8:22–28.
24. Caraco Y, Sheller J, Wood AJ. Pharmacogenetic determination of the effects of codeine and prediction of drug interactions. *J Pharmacol Exp Ther* 1996;278:1165–1174.
25. Moiniche S, Bulow S, Hesselfeldt P, et al. Convalescence and hospital stay after colonic surgery with balanced analgesia, early oral feeding, and enforced mobilisation. *Eur J Surg* 1995;161:283–288.
26. Kehlet H. Acute pain control and accelerated postoperative surgical recovery. *Surg Clin North Am* 1999;79: 431–443.
27. McQuay HJ, Moore RA, Eccleston C, et al. Systematic review of outpatient services for chronic pain control. *Health Technol Assess* 1997;1:i–iv, 1–135.
28. Eccleston C. Role of psychology in pain management. *Br J Anaesth* 2001;87:144–152.
29. Eccleston C, Crombez G, Aldrich S, et al. Worry and chronic pain patients: a description and analysis of individual differences. *Eur J Pain* 2001;5:309–318.
30. Morley S, Eccleston C, Williams A. Systematic review and meta-analysis of randomized controlled trials of cognitive behaviour therapy and behaviour therapy for chronic pain in adults, excluding headache. *Pain* 1999; 80:1–13.
31. Richardson GM, McGrath PJ. Cognitive-behavioral therapy for migraine headaches: a minimal-therapist-contact approach versus a clinic-based approach. *Headache* 1989;29:352–357.
32. Aldrich S, Eccleston C. Making sense of everyday pain. *Soc Sci Med* 2000;50:1631–1641.
33. Eccleston C, Williams AC, Rogers WS. Patients' and professionals' understandings of the causes of chronic pain: blame, responsibility and identity protection. *Soc Sci Med* 1997;45:699–709.

34. Crombez G, Eccleston C, Baeyens F, et al. When somatic information threatens, catastrophic thinking enhances attentional interference. *Pain* 1998;75:187–198.
35. Scharff L, Turk DC, Marcus DA. Psychosocial and behavioral characteristics in chronic headache patients: support for a continuum and dual-diagnostic approach. *Cephalalgia* 1995;15:216–223.
36. Schanberg LE, Lefebvre JC, Keefe FJ, et al. Pain coping and the pain experience in children with juvenile chronic arthritis. *Pain* 1997;73:181–189.
37. Gil KM, Carson JW, Sedway JA, et al. Follow-up of coping skills training in adults with sickle cell disease: analysis of daily pain and coping practice diaries. *Health Psychol* 2000;19:85–90.
38. McQuay H. Opioids in chronic non-malignant pain. *BMJ* 2001;322:1134–1135.
39. Bursch B, Walco GA, Zeltzer L. Clinical assessment and management of chronic pain and pain-associated disability syndrome. *J Dev Behav Pediatr* 1998;19: 45–53.

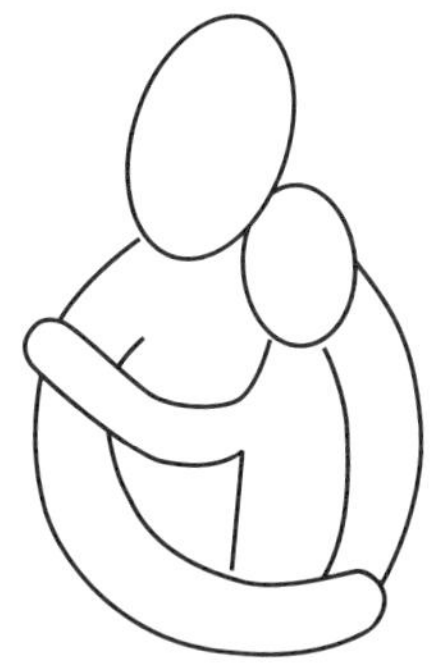

PART III

Specific Pain Problems

28

Management of Pain in Sickle Cell Disease

Carlton Dampier and Barbara S. Shapiro

OVERVIEW

Importance

Sickle cell disease is an inherited disorder that affects ethnic groups originating from areas in which malaria was endemic, such as Africa, the Mediterranean basin, and India. The gene frequency is highest in African populations and second highest in Americans of African ancestry. The disease is a significant problem in both Africa and the United States; approximately one in 500 African Americans has sickle cell disease (1,2).

The painful episode is the most common problem affecting children, adolescents, and adults with sickle hemoglobinopathies and is the most frequent cause for emergency department (ED) visits and hospital admissions (3–5). Sickle cell disease–related pain, often called "crisis" pain, is a discrete occurrence of pain, followed by a return to the usual baseline. The pain significantly undermines normal activities because patients are often unable to attend school or work (6).

Pathophysiology

Sickle cell disease results from an inherited and stable alteration in the genetic locus that codes for the β-globin subunit of the hemoglobin molecule. If only one of the genes at this locus is affected, the patient has the sickle cell trait, which is benign. Modification of both genes at this locus (i.e., on both chromosomes) is necessary to produce sickle cell disease. Sickle hemoglobinopathies vary in type depending on the precise nature of the genetic alteration on each chromosome. Homozygous sickle cell disease, in which the β-globin gene on each chromosome contains the classic sickle mutation, is the prototype. However, one of the β-globin genes may contain a different mutation, such as β-thalassemia or hemoglobin C, producing entities such as sickle β-thalassemia or SC disease. The subgroups predictably vary in hemolytic severity, but there is a great deal of overlap in the severity or frequency of sickle complications (2,7).

When deoxygenated, the altered hemoglobin, unlike the normal molecule, readily forms polymers that distort the red blood cells, producing the pathognomonic sickled cells. These cells are inflexible, adhere to endothelium, and have a prolonged transit time in capillary and postcapillary beds. At times, a large number of sickle red blood cells aggregates and occludes local flow. Usually the occlusion is temporary, and the tissues distal to the occlusion are protected by collateral flow. However, if the collateral vessels also are occluded by an acceleration of the sickling process, ischemia, infarction, and then tissue necrosis result (8). The process becomes evident as a painful episode when the affected area contains either nociceptors or nerves and is large enough for the effect to be perceived as pain.

Natural History of the Disease

Although pain is the most frequent problem experienced by people with sickle cell disease, it is far from the only complication. Infection is the most common cause of death in the pediatric age group, especially in children younger than 3 years of age. The advent of neonatal screening, with the early institution of penicillin prophylaxis, has dramatically decreased early mortality (9). Other life-threatening pediatric events include stroke, splenic sequestration, and acute chest syndrome (7). Some effects of the disease that are more typical of adolescents and young adults, such as aseptic necrosis of the hips and shoulders and compression fractures of the vertebrae, can produce severe chronic pain (10).

Despite the fact that the complications of sickle cell disease can be life threatening, with the institution of prophylactic antibiotics and appropriate supportive therapy, the average patient with sickle cell disease can expect to live until at least middle age. Thus, in treating the pain of children and young adults, we must consider the long-term effects of any intervention on development, function, and quality of life over a considerable future lifespan.

Natural History of the Pain

The hallmark of sickle cell disease pain is its extreme variability and unpredictability in timing, location, and intensity. Although patients often follow their own patterns, the unpredictability can be the bane of the patient's existence. In adult individuals, a large series reported an association between the frequency of painful episodes and increased mortality (11).

Duration

Painful episodes severe enough to require hospitalization typically last 3 to 7 days, whereas episodes managed at home may be as short as a few hours or as long as several weeks (12,13). In general, painful episodes in children are shorter than those in adults. Unfortunately for some severely affected adolescents and adults, their normal baseline can be daily pain, with intermittent acute exacerbations of more severe pain.

The pain may begin and end suddenly or gradually. Some patients report waking at night or in the morning with severe pain, whereas others have no temporal pattern. Many experience a prodrome, which may consist of fatigue, increased jaundice, or just a feeling of "not being right" (14). Generally, the episode intensity rises, plateaus, and then falls, but the pattern may be erratic (15).

Severity

The episode can vary in pain severity from mild to extremely intense (12,13,16). Episodes typically managed at home are of mild to moderate severity, but some patients even choose to manage severe pain at home, particularly if they have access to potent oral opioids (13). The magnitude of the pain is powerfully depicted in African tribal names for sickle cell disease. *Nuidudui* (Ewe) translates as "body chewing," *hemkom* (Adangme) means "body biting," and *adep* (Banyangi) means "beaten up." Some tribal names, such as *chwechweechwe* (Ga) and *nwiiwii* (Fante), onomatopoeically communicate the severity (17). Patients who have experienced surgical procedures rate their sickle cell disease pain as often more severe than their postoperative pain (16).

Character

The pain is usually nociceptive. Neuropathic pain syndromes occur but are unusual in childhood. Children typically use descriptors such as "deep," "aching," and "tiring" (18). Some patients report a strong affective character to their pain using such descriptors as "unbearable" or "intolerable" (19). The quality of the pain is often consistent from episode to episode.

Developmental Aspects

Painful episodes can occur as early as 6 to 9 months of age, in part as a consequence of the gradual loss of the protective effects of the large amounts of fetal hemoglobin present at birth (20). Dactylitis, which is pain and swelling of the hands and feet, occurs mostly in children younger than 3 years of age. However, some patients do not experience pain until adolescence or young adulthood. In general, when pain occurs frequently during childhood, it continues at the same or increased frequency and intensity during adolescence and young adulthood (11,21).

Region

Pain occurs in any part of the body that contains nociceptors or peripheral nerves and involves single or multiple body parts. Both flat bones and long bones are involved, as well as adjacent soft tissues or joint fluid. In some cases, the pain locations may be symmetric on both sides of the body. Periarticular pain may be more frequent in older adolescent and adult patients who have lost their metaphyseal circulation. The pain locations may migrate during early phases of an episode. Although most patients can accurately describe their pain locations, some patients describe pain episodes involving the entire body (22).

Diagnosis

Pain in patients with sickle cell disease may be a manifestation of vaso-occlusion or may be a symptom of another process, such as infection. Although vaso-occlusive pain occurs in the head, chest, abdomen, and limbs, the differential diagnosis must include stroke and intracranial hemorrhage, pneumonia and acute chest syndrome, cholecystitis, pelvic inflammatory disease, appendicitis and other abdominal events, osteomyelitis, trauma, and avascular necrosis (7,10). Assessment includes a thorough history, physical examination, and appropriate laboratory studies to identify these disease processes. Fever can be associated with uncomplicated painful episodes or infection. Fever should not be dismissed lightly because infections can be rapidly life threatening in patients with sickle cell disease and may precipitate what feels to the patient like a typical painful episode. Patients, including young children, can often tell the difference between their typical "crisis" pain and other processes; a patient's admonition that this pain is different should be taken seriously (2). Other pain syndromes that are common in children and adolescents (such as migraine headaches, recurrent abdominal pain, and somatization disorder) can also occur in patients with sickle hemoglobinopathies (10).

Investigators have searched for an "objective" marker for vaso-occlusive pain (10,23, 24). However, no parameter, including vital signs, physical examination, radiologic studies, hemoglobin, bilirubin, erythrocyte sedimentation rate, C-reactive protein, or the number of irreversibly sickled cells is both sensitive and specific. Considering the multifactorial nature of pain and the poorly understood mechanisms of vaso-occlusive pain (25, 26), it is not surprising that no such marker has emerged.

Temporal Factors

The frequency of the episodes varies greatly among patients. Approximately 30% of people with this illness never or rarely have pain in any given year, 50% have a few episodes yearly, and the remaining 20% experience frequent and severe pain (11,27). Patients who are severely affected may have pain on most days, and those who come to the hospital for pain management may be admitted as often as several times each month. In many programs, a large percentage of the admissions for sickle cell disease–related pain involves a minority of their patients (27). The frequency and regularity of painful episodes vary over time in individual patients. For example, several months punctuated by frequent severe episodes may be followed by a long pain-free interlude (12,13,28).

Precipitating Factors

Painful episodes may be precipitated by infection, hypoxemia, dehydration, acidosis, fatigue, strenuous exercise, exposure to cold (including swimming in cool water), stress, menses, or pregnancy (2,10,29,30). A relationship to sleep apnea has been proposed but remains controversial (31,32). However, most painful episodes have no identifiable precipitant, and factors that result in pain in one patient may not affect another. Data about the influence of weather and seasonal factors are conflicting (21,33–36). Many patients report increased frequency of pain in some seasons. Known precipitating factors occur in all climates and are influenced by behavior. Exposure to cold in the winter and dehydration from heat in the summer can result in pain. Knowing this, a patient may take care to dress warmly in the winter but forget to bring a sweater to air-conditioned buildings in the summer. Similarly, depending on personal interests and anxieties, some children may play sports in the summer to the point of fatigue and dehydration or become stressed and tired after school begins in the fall. The clinical observation of seasonal variation in some patients is unlikely to be demonstrated in studies that do not take into account the multitude of precipitants and behaviors.

Disease Severity

Factors that modulate pain frequency of both severe hospitalized episodes or milder outpatient episodes include the quantity and cellular distribution of fetal hemoglobin, the baseline hematocrit, and gender (7,37–39). However, patients who are similar in these respects can still differ in the severity of the pain. There is some evidence linking genetically controlled endothelial, microvascular, and serum factors to the expression of the disease (8,39–42). Factors associated with increased frequency of pain sometimes parallel those of acute chest syndrome and bone infarcts (43) but not necessarily other manifestations of the disease, such as stroke or aseptic necrosis (10,44). Although genetic and physiologic influences modulate the disease severity, the psychosocial context and the patient's coping strategies have a powerful effect on the evolution of the illness (45). Thus, the biologic, psychologic, and social spheres cannot, in the final analysis, be separated.

Acute and Chronic Pain in Sickle Cell Disease

The definitions of acute and chronic pain are controversial. Rigid temporal distinctions (i.e., pain that lasts for more than 3 months is chronic) are arbitrary at best, misleading at worst, and difficult to apply to recurrent pain syndromes. Additionally, the effects of time may vary with developmental stage and age. A period of time perceived by an adult as short (e.g., 1 week) may be perceived by a young child as endless. Especially for recurrent pain, and for pain affecting children and adolescents, the definitions of acute and chronic rest on the individual's perception of the pain and the effect of the pain on mood, expectations, function, and social interactions (Fig. 28.1).

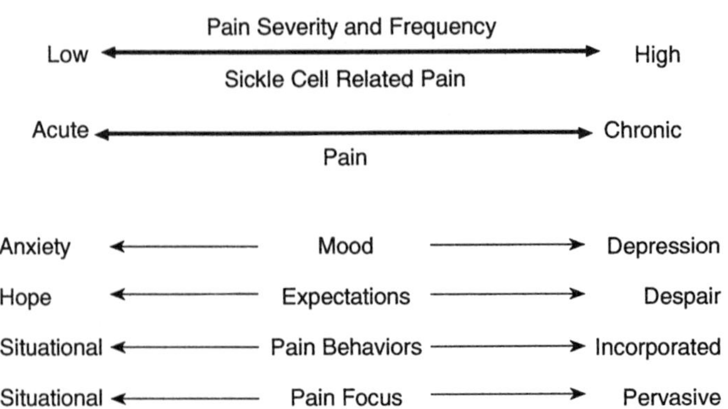

FIG. 28.1. A model for acute and chronic pain.

Sickle cell disease pain forms a continuum from acute to chronic. Some patients have only occasional episodes of pain. This pain is unlikely to interfere with hopes and dreams or to become a major focus of the child's life and is optimally treated with approaches used for acute pain syndromes, such as postoperative pain. As the pain becomes more frequent and severe, it can be incorporated into everyday life. At the worst, a cycle of depression, splintered relationships, and worsening pain develops. Frequent sickle cell disease–related pain is a model for chronic intractable pain associated with nonmalignant disease; as such, pain is lifelong, and there is no cure for the disease or the pain. Pain management in such patients should follow the principles of chronic pain management, integrating pharmacologic, cognitive-behavioral and psychologic, and physical approaches within a supportive framework. The success of such an approach is optimized by the development of a therapeutic alliance between the patient (and the family) and the health care team.

Home Versus Hospital Management

Health care professionals tend to identify ED and inpatient admissions as the marker for severe painful episodes. Admissions have been used as outcome criteria to examine the efficacy of various interventions, and, in many centers, to identify patients who require alternative approaches for pain management. However, painful episodes managed at home and not at the hospital may not come to the attention of health caretakers. One study documented 90% of episodes in childhood and 60% of episodes in adults were managed at home if families had access to appropriate analgesics in a supportive environment (12, 13). Some patients manage very severe pain at home if they are not vomiting or otherwise ill (6,13,16). Coming to the hospital for pain management is a learned behavior, influenced by variables such as past experiences, social supports, coping skills and style, instruction in home management, and health beliefs. The need for inpatient management is determined more by the patient's previous encounters with the medical system and by both the patient's and physician's beliefs about the proper use of such resources than by standard measures of pain intensity (46). Alternatively, some patients and their families may find the acute care or hospital experience so aversive or distressing that they will attempt to manage pain or other complications at home even when not medically appropriate.

Although the ability to manage pain at home is often correlated with effective coping skills and social supports (27), a decrease in hospital admissions may not necessarily be related to improvement in function. Pain that is managed at home can be as disruptive of activities of daily living, such as school attendance and social encounters, as pain that is managed in the hospital (6). Similarly, although home management is generally less disruptive to family life, some patients may encounter extreme difficulties. For example, if no adult is at home to help the patient, even moderate pain can be difficult to manage.

Health care professionals must view painful episodes from the patient's perspective of pain and function as a continuum in ongoing daily life rather than just from their perspective of the hospital encounter. If the goal of treatment is to decrease medical costs or usage, it is reasonable to use the number of admissions as a measure of success. However, if the goal is to improve function, factors such as school attendance and psychosocial status must be assessed.

ISSUES AFFECTING PATIENTS WITH SICKLE CELL DISEASE PAIN

Illness does not exist within a societal vacuum. Cultural mores and values influence the manner in which an illness and patients with that illness are treated medically. The attitudes and interactions of health care professionals around an illness are as profound for the patients as the family constellation is for a child. If we are to provide culturally competent treatment for sickle cell disease pain, we must view the illness within its context.

Racial and Socioeconomic Factors

Although rarely addressed in the literature, it is striking that in the English-speaking countries, most of the patients are black and most of the health care professionals are white. This racial difference between patients and caretakers is often accompanied by large socioeconomic disparities and by differences in culturally determined beliefs about health and pain. Communication among races, cultures, and socioeconomic groups has historically been fraught with problems. It is inevitable that preexisting attitudes and tensions will affect the very human interactions that occur around the care of a patient. Pain, intrinsically, is subjective and to be treated, its presence must be communicated; pain cannot be palpated, weighed, or measured. Trust and a common language are necessary for effective communication.

Poverty affects access to the health care system. Outpatient visits may be difficult for a single mother with several small children who is dependent on public transportation. Services for psychologic approaches to pain often are not available in facilities treating patients with sickle cell disease, and the families may be unable to afford private services. Inner-city pharmacies may not provide the potent opioid analgesics many patients need to manage their severe pain (47). Patients with little education are disadvantaged when bargaining with bureaucracies. Family structure and integrity can be undermined by poverty, and there may be little energy for caring for a child with frequent painful episodes. The effect of the illness and the pain on function and future opportunities is also influenced by socioeconomic characteristics. Welfare reform has sent many single parents out to work, and they are not available to care for a child at home with frequent pain.

Children and adolescents with frequent pain are absent from school on a significant number of school days (6). Many patients attend large, understaffed city schools, which are ill equipped to help these students maintain their academic standing in the face of frequent absences. Some children may also have significant cognitive difficulties as a result of silent infarcts (48).

Context of Care

Most patients with sickle cell disease receive medical care in large academic centers where state-of-the-art medical technology is available. Many such centers employ a rotating system of medical care, with a different attending physician, fellow, and resident on service every month. Unless one physician assumes the primary responsibility for the patient, both in and out of the hospital, continuity of care is lacking, and the pain may be treated in a different manner during each admission. This adds unpredictability of treatment to the unpredictability of the pain, and weakens adherence to long-term goals of pain management.

The separation of care of patients with sickle cell disease (and other chronic illnesses) into pediatric and adult facilities poses problems in transition. The philosophies and goals of pain management may differ, and patients usually change from pediatric to adult care facilities during the tumultuous years of late adolescence, when pain may be a severe problem. Even some older adolescent patients may not have learned to manage their own health care, making such a transition even more problematic. A more effective transition approach is to promote disease self-care as a developmental task to be achieved with increasing success and complexity as the child becomes an adolescent and then a young adult.

Nature of the Pain and Effect on Psychosocial Function

The pain in sickle cell disease is intermittent, unpredictable, often severe, and usually unavoidable. Pain of this type erodes the patient's perception of control over life events and is reminiscent of the learned helplessness seen in experimental subjects, who, when exposed to repetitive, unavoidable, and unpredictable noxious stimuli, eventually cease attempting to avoid the stimulus (49). One can speculate that the nature of the pain may interact with personal characteristics of explanatory style and temperament, predisposing some patients to depression and passivity (50). It is during childhood and adolescence that the development of independence and a positive body image are central issues, and patients may be exceptionally vulnerable to the effects of unavoidable pain. Passivity and negative thinking are correlated with increased pain severity (46), and when these attributes are pervasive, psychologic and home care approaches to pain management may be difficult to implement.

The effects of pain on psychosocial status have not been defined. Studies of psychosocial status in children show no differences between patients with sickle cell disease and controls matched for race and socioeconomic level (51,52). There is some evidence that psychosocial problems first appear in adolescence, particularly in males (53–55). Adults with sickle cell disease have significant psychopathology and social dysfunction compared with adults with diabetes matched for disease severity, race, and socioeconomic status (56,57). To date, patients with frequent and severe pain have not been compared with patients with little or no pain. Despite the apparent absence of psychosocial problems in children with sickle cell disease, the general undermining of mood and social interactions by chronic pain suggests that it is reasonable to provide intervention early in childhood and adolescence to minimize later consequences.

Societal Issues

Drug abuse is a major and visible problem in our society. Concerns about this issue affect health care professionals, patients, and families alike, and fears about abuse likely hinder the appropriate use of opioids in pain management. The incidence of addiction in adults with sickle cell disease has varied from 0% to 11% in three surveys done in different cities (27,58,59). In the two surveys showing addiction in sickle cell disease, the factors leading to addiction were not explored (27,59). However, the perception of many health care providers is that patients in pain, and patients with sickle cell disease in particular, have a higher incidence of opioid dependence than the general population (60,61). Chance alone dictates that the incidence of addiction in patients with any disease would parallel the baseline rate of addiction in an equivalent healthy population, unless the disease itself affects risk. It is clear that most patients with sickle cell disease are not addicted, even though opioids may be used on a lifelong basis for pain control. This is consistent with the finding that the use of opioids in patients with other pain syndromes does not lead to addiction (62). Therefore, there is no reason to withhold adequate analgesia. Families are often concerned about the possibility of addiction; education about the appropriate use of opioids for pain should be introduced at an early age.

We live in an age of societal adulation of technologic and mechanical wizardry. The fabric of medical practice inevitably reflects this outlook. The biomedical approach has resulted in enormous strides in our understanding of the pathophysiology of sickle cell disease. However, all aspects of that person shape the individual's response to this pathophysiologic mechanism. The current biomedical model of this disease is necessary, but not sufficient, as a basis for the management of patients with their chronic illness and chronic pain. A biopsychosocial model is more appropriate.

Lack of Visibility in the Hematology Community

Clinical descriptions and studies of pain in patients with sickle cell disease have been sparse. *Pain,* the journal of the International Association for the Study of Pain, contained no articles on sickle cell disease pain from January 1981 to December 1990, and only two from January 1991 to July 2000. The schema developed by the International Association for the Study of Pain for coding chronic pain diagnoses contains no reference to sickle cell disease pain. Two major textbooks about pain contain only brief descriptions of sickle cell disease (63,64). Similarly, *Blood*, the journal of the American Society of Hematology, has published only one clinical treatment study of sickle cell disease pain from January 1981 to December 1990 (65), and five from January 1991 to July 2000.

In contrast, sickle cell disease pain treatment is beginning to receive recognition within the pain community. The American Pain Society published a monograph in 1999 describing clinical practice guidelines for the management of acute and chronic pain in sickle cell disease (66). A treatment algorithm for EDs has been developed based on these guidelines. The International Association for the Study of Pain has also recently published a monograph on clinical aspects of sickle cell disease pain (10).

Health care professionals concerned about pain management have made major changes in the management of cancer pain over the past 10 to 15 years. These changes were accomplished via collaboration with oncologists, formation of cancer pain services, education of health care professionals and families, and the organization of cancer pain initiatives. Similar efforts are necessary to improve the management of pain in patients with sickle cell disease.

Problems with Research

The treatment of painful episodes in sickle cell disease is essentially the same now as it was 20 to 25 years ago (10,67). Although there is increasing research on the natural history of the pain, few clinical trials to develop more effective ways to treat the pain have been conducted. The wide variability among and within patients is a problem in designing clinical studies because large numbers of subjects and long follow-up periods are required for meaningful analysis. Adherence to study protocols may be viewed by potential investigators as problematic in patients in lower socioeconomic groups, although this has not been substantiated (6,12,13,68). Collaboration among hematologists and pain specialists is essential for successful research.

TREATMENT

General Principles

Various treatments are available for vaso-occlusive pain. Although pharmacologic intervention is the mainstay of therapy for the acute episode, it must be embedded within an individualized and integrated multidisciplinary framework for patients with frequent and severe pain (27,46). When treating children and adolescents, the multidisciplinary approach is tailored to the developmental level of the child (Table 28.1).

Sickle cell disease produces the only common pain syndrome in which opioids are considered the major therapy and are started in early childhood and continued throughout adult life. The issues and implications of lifelong opioid treatment are not known. Treating patients with frequent courses of opioids without also providing adjunctive methods of pain control, close support, and therapeutic supervision is irresponsible. The goal of treatment of the acute episode is not to take all the pain away, which is usually impossible, but to make the pain tolerable to the patient until the episode resolves. One works with the patient to de-emphasize the crisis nature of the pain, so that the pain fits more smoothly into daily life. For this reason, many health care professionals do not use the word crisis to describe the pain, as the word itself reinforces the connotation of catastrophe.

Current analgesic agents, even when used aggressively in a manner similar to the treatment of cancer pain, can be inadequate in controlling some of the most severe painful episodes. This can be a source of enormous frustration for patients, physicians, and nurses. Unfortunately, the helplessness and frustration felt by the health care professionals may be channeled into blaming the patient for not responding to the physician's

TABLE 28.1. *Integrated cognitive-behavioral-pharmacologic approach*

A. Age 6 months to 4 years
   1. Infusion with rescue doses or around the clock doses
   2. Stepwise pharmacologic approach at home
      a. Acetaminophen
      b. Mild opioid
   3. Education of parents
B. Age 4 to 7 years
   1. Continue the same pharmacologic approach
   2. Introduce cognitive-behavioral methods
   3. Education focused on parent and child
C. Age 7 to 12 years
   1. Introduce flexible dosing schedule or patient-controlled analgesia; discuss during outpatient visit
   2. Continue stepwise pharmacologic approach at home; can introduce strong opioid by mouth when necessary, if family is able to manage severe pain at home
   3. Emphasize continuity of care
   4. Refine cognitive-behavioral intervention
   5. Educate emphasizing more child responsibility
   6. Identify school problems, intervene with schools, neuropsychologic testing when necessary
   7. Family therapy when necessary
D. Age 12 to 17 years
   1. Identify high-risk behavior early (137,138; K. Covelman and M. Russel, unpublished, 1980)
      a. Increasing medication use
      b. School failure
      c. Increasing number of hospitalizations
      d. Adversarial relationship with health caretakers
   2. Emphasize appropriate pharmacologic management at home
   3. Consistent pharmacologic approach when hospitalized
   4. Cognitive-behavioral intervention
   5. Treat depression
   6. Train nurses and other staff in positive reinforcement of appropriate behavior and limit setting
   7. Introduce contracts when necessary; involve family
   8. Family therapy when necessary
   9. Education focused toward self-regulation and responsibility
   10. Prepare for transfer to adult program
   11. Employment and career counseling

best efforts. Similarly, nurses may blame physicians and vice versa. Open discussions with patients, families, and medical and nursing caretakers about the limitations of treatment are necessary to avoid the tendency to blame others.

Assessment

The assessment of vaso-occlusive pain is similar to assessment in other pain syndromes. Self-report is primary. Simple, easily used, and understood tools are most useful in acute care settings to guide medication dosing. Verbal self-report scales and categoric scales are typical examples. For children, these categoric scales may include faces either as pictures or cartoons to facilitate comprehension (69). More detailed multidimensional scales may be most helpful in the outpatient setting as part of yearly comprehensive pain assessments (19,70). Unfortunately, there are no currently validated assessment tools for the many preverbal young children with sickle cell disease pain.

Observation of behavior helps caregivers understand the patient's coping style and skills and the need for adjunctive techniques. Patients who have had frequent painful episodes behave in a manner learned from previous experiences. For example, the adolescent who has received medication on an as-needed basis for years may perceive that medication is given only if behavior indicates severe pain. The patient may lie quietly in bed when alone and then begin to writhe and moan when a caretaker enters the room. Such behavior does not indicate that the pain is not severe but merely reflects the individual's response to environmental contingencies.

Assessment includes an evaluation of the pain and the psychosocial context. During an acute episode, the assessment should focus on the pain to determine immediate treatment. When the patient becomes more comfortable, a complete evaluation can be performed. Patients can be depressed or anxious during an acute episode, and it can be difficult to discern whether changes in mood or affect are primary or secondary. If concerns about mood or function emerge, the evaluation should be continued after resolution of the pain.

Assessment during pain-free interludes includes evaluation of the patient's and family's understanding of the pain, its effects and management, the reaction of the family, performance in school and other activities of daily living, social interactions, coping skills and style, mood and self-esteem, and interactions with the health care system. Family assessment is essential and should include all key family members because relatives may have divergent attitudes toward the pain. The disbelief of pain that often plagues patients with sickle cell disease when they interact with health care professionals may be encountered within the family. Conversely, parents may be overprotective and oversolicitous, undermining coping skills and normal development. Conflicts at home may be reenacted within the hospital. For example, a child with one oversolicitous parent and one parent who believes the child is malingering can develop exacerbated pain behaviors. When this behavior occurs in the hospital, the staff may become split, with some defending and others dismissing the pain. Such situations cannot be remedied unless the home and hospital contexts are carefully examined. The process of assessment can be therapeutic as well as evaluative.

When there is an adversarial relationship between the patient and the health caretakers, a careful and compassionate assessment can promote trust. The assessment can be performed in a manner that enhances functional coping rather than behaviors focusing on pain. It is difficult to remain calm in the presence of a patient behaving in a manner consistent with severe pain, but an oversolicitous or alarmed reaction adds to the patient's perception of crisis and catastrophe. While the patient describes the pain, the physician or nurse should look directly at the patient rather than at the body part. Pain can be acknowledged while praising appropriate attempts at activity and self-care. Evaluation of provocative and palliative factors can clarify for the patient possible avenues for pain control. For example, many patients use distraction effectively but do not consciously appreciate their abilities. Having patients scale the intensity of the pain helps them to perceive pain as variable, with a certain degree of pain being tolerable, rather than as an all-or-none phenomenon. Finally, a patient-centered assessment underlines that the pain belongs to the patient and provides the foundation for encouraging self-care and responsibility.

Pharmacologic Agents

The stepwise approach recommended by the World Health Organization for the management of cancer pain (66,71) is applicable to the management of sickle cell disease pain. A nonsteroidal anti-inflammatory drug (NSAID) or acetaminophen is used as needed for mild pain. For moderate pain, the NSAID or acetaminophen is taken around the clock, and a mild opioid, such as codeine or oxycodone, is added, first as needed and then around the clock. A strong opioid is used with acetaminophen or the NSAID for severe pain.

When parenteral administration is necessary, the intravenous route should be used. Intramuscular injections are painful and frightening, especially for children, and when used repetitively produce fibrosis and sterile abscesses (10). The subcutaneous route can be used for some opioids if intravenous access is not reliable and the patient is not dehydrated or requires other parenteral medications.

Patients with frequent episodes of pain usually develop preferences for particular drugs. In general, requests should be honored as the patient has often made a personal judgment of analgesia versus adverse effect profiles. Problems emerge as the state of the art of pain management advances. For example, many sickle cell disease treatment centers are now using morphine in preference to meperidine, and patients who have been treated with meperidine for years may view this change with trepidation. Similarly, the use of oral opioids equianalgesic to previously used parenteral opioids may be seen as a dismissal of the severity of the pain. No matter how positively the new agent or route is presented, the degree of pain relief may be inferior. This is in accord with the demonstrated power of learned expectation in determining the degree of pain relief (72). Unless medical considerations dictate an immediate change, it is preferable to discuss proposed medication modifications with the patient before admission. Abrupt changes when pain is acute decrease trust and undermine the efficacy of therapy. One could also develop with the patient a stepwise approach to change, accomplished over several admissions.

Nonsteroidal Anti-inflammatory Drugs and Acetaminophen

These agents have been extensively studied in the treatment of other pain syndromes and have proven efficacy in the management of mild to moderate pain (73). Their role in the management of severe vaso-occlusive pain is not clear (74). The action of NSAIDs on prostaglandin synthesis may be salutary in somatic pain, especially that involving bony infarction. Parenteral NSAIDs are available (75,76), but studies have shown variable efficacy against severe sickle cell disease pain (77,78). The physician must closely supervise use of NSAIDs and acetaminophen, especially at home, because patients may exceed maximal safe doses in an effort to avoid the use of opioids or hospitalization.

NSAIDs and acetaminophen can produce analgesic nephropathy, especially when used frequently (79). Many patients with sickle cell disease use NSAIDs or acetaminophen almost daily for years, starting in childhood or adolescence. Renal pathology, sometimes developing into nephropathy and renal failure, is a well-described complication of sickle cell disease (2,7,80). Until data are available about the role of NSAIDs and acetaminophen in the nephropathy of sickle cell disease, the chronic use of these agents should not be regarded as benign. Regular testing of renal function is necessary, and medication should be discontinued if there is any deterioration.

Opioids

As in cancer pain, oral opioids should be used whenever possible. Strong oral opioids, used in appropriate doses, are equianalgesic to parenterally administered agents (81). Parenteral administration is necessary if the patient is vomiting or otherwise unable to take oral medication or hydration or if the pain is severe, requiring rapid management. The unnecessary use of parenteral agents reinforces the sense of "crisis," and repetitive use of the intravenous route can cause future difficulty in obtaining intravenous access. However, the ability to use oral opioids does not always indicate that the pain should be managed at home. Large doses of oral opioids used acutely require frequent monitoring of vital signs. Severe painful episodes can evolve rapidly into life-threatening events. Last, some patients live in areas where their supply of analgesics may be stolen.

Oral codeine or oxycodone is indicated for mild to moderate pain. They can be used as a single agent or conjunction with an NSAID or acetaminophen. The single agent facilitates titration, but the combined preparations may be simpler for home administration. Patients who cannot tolerate codeine or oxycodone may be able to use equianalgesic doses of morphine or hydromorphone. Morphine, used orally or parenterally, is the preferred drug for the management of severe sickle cell disease pain (82,83). Sustained-release oral morphine preparations also provide effective analgesia (84) but require titration and have a slower onset of action. If oral analgesia is initiated when the pain is resolving or the patient has a history of short-lived episodes, the pain may be better managed with an immediate-release preparation that can be rapidly and easily titrated. Hydromorphone is useful for patients who cannot tolerate morphine. Oral methadone can be difficult to titrate because of its long half-life and can cause substantial sedation. However, it is gaining popularity among some physicians as a valuable agent for chronic sickle cell disease pain.

Historically, meperidine has been widely used in the management of sickle cell disease pain. However, there are problems associated with its use. Meperidine has a long-acting metabolite, normeperidine, which is not analgesic and can cause hallucinations and seizures (85–87). Renal vaso-occlusion produces renal tubular acidosis (88), and normeperidine is excreted even more slowly in alkaline urine (85). Significant dysphoria has been reported in patients with cancer who receive meperidine for more than 24 hours (89). The serum levels of meperidine are lower in patients with sickle cell disease than in other patients given equal doses, and they are below the levels needed for adequate analgesia (90). These issues are responsible for the recommendation of morphine as a first-line agent (66,91).

Agonist–antagonist preparations have not been well studied in sickle cell disease pain (92,93). They are useful for situations in which increases in intrabiliary pressure or spasm of the sphincter of Oddi are problematic (e.g., pancreatitis, cholelithiasis) or when intestinal motility is a significant problem (94–96). However, increased doses beyond a certain maximum do not produce increased analgesia (analgesic ceiling) (97), and although there is a similar limit to respiratory depression, this limit generally does not occur until the dose is close to the analgesic ceiling (98). Activation of the μ receptor can produce psychotomimetic effects, although the frequency of occurrence varies with the agent (99,100). It is possible that some agonist–antagonist preparations (such as buprenorphine) may produce adequate analgesia with fewer side effects such as respiratory depression, nausea, vomiting, and pruritus (93,99,100). Data regarding efficacy and side effects are needed before accepting their potential as effective agents in patients with sickle cell disease pain.

Various schedules are possible using permutations of oral and parenteral administration (Table 28.2). These schedules should be tailored to individual needs and preferences. Intravenous infusions with intermittent rescue doses are probably safer than using higher dose infusions without rescues. Administration as needed should be avoided, except when the pain is truly intermittent and unpredictable. Patients older than the age of 6 or 7 years can have the option of refusing an offered dose if it is not necessary or of choosing between a larger or smaller dose.

Patient-controlled analgesia (PCA) provides safe and effective analgesia for children and adolescents with postoperative pain (101). It has been used for sickle cell disease–related pain (102–105), where it has theoretic pharmacologic and psychologic advantages. PCA encourages self-regulation and responsibility and reinforces the ownership of the pain by the patient. Additionally, because the intensity of the pain may wax and wane rapidly, patient-controlled dosing can provide rapid and safe titration of analgesia to the level of the pain. It is difficult to adjust regularly scheduled doses or infusions in such a timely manner in most hospital settings. PCA may also have a role in the ED management of pain.

TABLE 28.2. *Methods for administering opioid analgesia in the hospital*

1. Intermittent i.v. doses around the clock
2. i.v. infusion
3. i.v. infusion with intermittent i.v. doses
4. Sustained-release or immediate-acting agents given orally around the clock, with intermittent i.v. doses
5. PCA with or without basal infusion
6. Sustained-release or immediate-acting agents given orally around the clock, with PCA without basal infusion

i.v., intravenous; PCA, patient-controlled analgesia.

The dosing parameters for PCA often need to be different in sickle cell disease pain than in postoperative or cancer pain. A larger, patient-controlled dose is often necessary for rapid titration in opioid-tolerant patients, without the frustration of triggering the device many times each hour. For example, four allowed doses per hour of 2 mg each are preferable to eight allowed doses of 1 mg each. The lock-out interval should be short (6 to 10 minutes). It is particularly important to avoid frustration when introducing PCA to a patient who has been accustomed to large intermittent doses. Low-dose basal infusions prevent inadvertent excessive sedation if the pain should resolve rapidly (105). Higher dose basal infusions may be needed in some patients, particularly at night to allow adequate analgesia during sleep without the need for frequent patient-controlled doses.

The opioid dose may need to be very large in severe pain episodes, both because of the intense pain and because some patients with severe pain may also be opioid tolerant. An infusion rate of 40 mg per hour in an adult has been reported (100), and our experience thus far with PCA has been that the actual delivered dose for severe pain can be as high as 0.4 mg/kg per hour, with an average of 0.1 mg/kg per hour (106). A series of nonopioid-tolerant adult patients at a large medical center treated with morphine PCA used hourly continuous infusion rates ranging from 0.026 to 0.02 mg/kg and demand doses ranging from 0.06 to 0.03 mg/kg (105). Such doses are higher than those needed for postoperative pain and are far lower than those often needed for the management of severe cancer pain.

The difficulties and dangers of such large doses of opioids are very different in sickle cell disease than in cancer pain. Patients with acute severe episodes interspersed with pain-free intervals, during which no opioids are required, may be tolerant of opioids to a greater or lesser extent, and the degree of tolerance is not as predictable as in cancer pain. If there is even mild depression of respiration, atelectasis may occur, and hypoxemia may increase intravascular sickling. However, to date, there are no reliable data on the association between opioid therapy and the development of pulmonary insufficiency or hypoxemia in patients with sickle cell disease.

Adequate analgesia is necessary, however, and the potential hazards of opioid therapy are balanced by the risks of inadequate respiratory excursion and atelectasis from splinting of the chest wall because of pain (107). There is some evidence that patients who develop acute chest syndrome do so because of infection, fat embolism from marrow infarction, overhydration, inactivity, and continued recumbency rather than as a direct result of opioid therapy (107–109). The opioid dose should be carefully and frequently titrated according to the extent of analgesia and sedation. Pulse oximetry may be useful in determining the need for supplemental oxygen administration but may overestimate the degree of hypoxemia. Ambulation, frequent position changes, and the regular use of incentive spirometry (110) should be encouraged.

Adjuvants

There have been no published studies of the use of medications such as tricyclic antidepressants and stimulants in sickle cell disease pain. Without data on efficacy and risks, suggestions for clinical use must be extrapolated from studies in other pain syndromes. The use of tricyclic antidepressants during an acute episode is unlikely to add analgesia before the episode resolves (111,112), and it may increase sedation, ileus, and other side effects. However, these agents may be useful when given on a daily basis to patients with frequent severe episodes or chronic daily pain. Sleep is often a problem for patients during an acute episode. Low doses of tricyclic antidepressants given at bedtime produce a soporific effect, which is useful in other pain syndromes. However, until more is known about the effect of opioids on oxygen saturation and blood pH in patients with sickle cell disease, especially during sleep, the routine use of tricyclic antidepressants and hypnotics for sleep when opioids are also being administered cannot be recommended unless the patient is closely monitored.

Stimulants augment opioid analgesia without causing further sedation or respiratory depression (113–115). However, to consistently avoid respiratory depression, they have to be given around the clock, which would disrupt sleep. Because the pain usually is time limited in sickle cell disease, it is unnecessary to use stimulants to improve the quality of awake time, as one does with patients with cancer. Parents may view these agents with concern, as drugs of abuse. Without further investigation of efficacy and risks (116), stimulants cannot be recommended for routine use. They may be helpful in special circumstances, such as for patients with acute chest syndrome, when opioid analgesia is inadequate or is adding to respiratory problems.

Similarly, there is no published information on the use of antiepileptic medications, such as carbamazepine or gabapentin, for chronic sickle cell disease pain. Although these medications have documented efficacy in neuropathic pain, there is little clinical evidence that sickle cell disease pain typically has neuropathic features.

Anxiolytics, such as the benzodiazepines, add no analgesia and potentiate sedation and respiratory depression. Anxiety is usually secondary to pain, but not always. Benzodiazepines are recommended only when anxiety is a primary component of distress. Hydroxyzine is commonly used as an adjuvant to analgesia. However, large doses are required for the analgesic effects (73) and increase sedation. Hydroxyzine is recommended only for pruritus.

Epidural Analgesia

In recent years, epidural analgesia has been used with increasing frequency in a variety of pain syndromes (117) and has been used for patients with sickle cell disease (118,119). Although the epidural administration of opioids or mixtures of opioids and local anesthetics would be likely to produce excellent analgesia, the repetitive nature of the pain must be considered when contemplating use for sickle cell disease–related pain. It is not clear how often an epidural catheter can be inserted during a patient's lifetime without producing local fibrosis or other complications. Additionally, the use of epidural analgesia may reinforce the crisis nature of the painful episode and undermine the patient's role in managing the pain. Until further data are available, the use of epidural catheters should be restricted to painful episodes that are truly out of the ordinary for that patient, in which the use of systemic opioids may give inadequate pain relief while causing serious adverse effects.

Other Pharmacologic Approaches

There have been many studies of agents that inhibit hemoglobin gelation or act on membranes to reduce sickling (65,120). For the most part, these drugs have thus far been ineffective *in vivo* or too toxic for use. Aspirin has been shown ineffective when used as prophylaxis for vaso-occlusive pain (121). However, a chemotherapeutic agent, hydroxyurea, has been shown in a large, randomized clinical trial to increase the concentration of fetal hemoglobin and decrease the frequency of painful episodes and acute chest syndromes (122). It is now approved by the U.S. Food and Drug Administration for this indication in adult patients.

Intravenous high-dose steroids have been demonstrated in a randomized, controlled trial to reduce the duration of hospitalization for sickle cell disease pain (123). Whether this represented a primary analgesic effect or an anti-inflammatory effect is unclear. Concern has been raised about the potential adverse effects of repeated doses of steroids on the immune system for patients with frequent pain as well as the potential increased risk for avascular necrosis. Patients who received steroids also had an increased number of rebound pain episodes after therapy was discontinued. Future studies are necessary to determine whether newer potent anti-inflammatory agents will have similar beneficial or adverse effects.

Nonpharmacologic Medical Approaches

Hydration has traditionally been used to treat vaso-occlusive pain, even though there are no controlled studies confirming its efficacy (7,10). However, hydration is necessary to replenish the isosthenuric losses of sickle cell disease–related kidney damage. Fluid intake should be calculated to supply 1.25 to 1.5 times the calculated fluid maintenance. Intravenous hydration exceeding these rates may produce pulmonary edema (109) and may need to be reduced in the presence of pulmonary parenchymal damage during acute chest syndromes.

The use of supplemental oxygen during sickle pain remains a frequent practice at many hospitals and EDs. However, a randomized clinical trial of supplemental oxygen during acute painful episodes demonstrated no clinical benefit (124). Certainly, it is indicated in the presence of hypoxemia. Supplemental oxygen administered continuously to a patient who is not hypoxic decreases the production of erythropoietin (125) and contributes to increased transfusion requirements.

Regular red blood cell transfusions, given every 3 to 4 weeks, can be used to reduce the frequency of vaso-occlusive pain (126). Transfusion carries many risks for all recipients, and patients with sickle cell disease have a high incidence of alloimmunization (126,127). Severe alloimmunization may render subsequent transfusions for life-threatening events difficult, if not impossible. Therefore, transfusions should not be used without strong indications (7). During an acute event, they should be given only for life-threatening problems, such as severe anemia or progressive acute chest syndrome, and not to hasten resolution of the pain. Patients with very frequent and severe painful events, whose function is severely impaired by the pain, may benefit from prophylactic transfusions (2,7,126). Some patients continue to have painful episodes even after the initiation of such therapy. It is unclear whether this is secondary to physiologic changes from the previous vaso-occlusive events or from psychosocial factors that maintain the pain, or both.

Psychologic and Cognitive-Behavioral Methods

As with pharmacologic interventions, psychologic and cognitive-behavioral interventions should be individualized to age, needs, and coping style. It is best to introduce these techniques when pain first becomes an issue rather than waiting until the patient is identified as a "problem" by medical and nursing staff. By this time, adversarial relationships and unhelpful coping skills have often become entrenched, rendering such intervention much more difficult. It is vital that the physician work on an ongoing basis with the mental health professional to introduce, explain, and strongly endorse these techniques because otherwise the patient and family may perceive these approaches as "second class" or punitive. The family should be included in the intervention because the coping styles of children are often similar to those of their parents (128).

Hypnosis and biofeedback have been used for patients with sickle cell disease (129–132). Studies have not included appropriate controls, so it is unclear whether improvements resulted from active intervention or from nonspecific effects. However, these techniques are easily taught and free of side effects and may enhance coping skills. Pending further investigation, these approaches should be available for patients with frequent painful episodes. Ideally, they should be introduced when the patient is relatively free of pain, but their use can be quite effective even when initiated at other times.

Education of the patient and family about pain and its management should be ongoing. Children and parents can be taught to use a pain scale. Individualized treatment plans for home management can be worked out with the family and posted in a prominent position in the house (Fig. 28.2). Children and parents can keep home records of pain and medication used. Such diaries can be helpful to the medical professional in adjusting pain management and can make the patient and the family part of the treatment team (133). Fi-

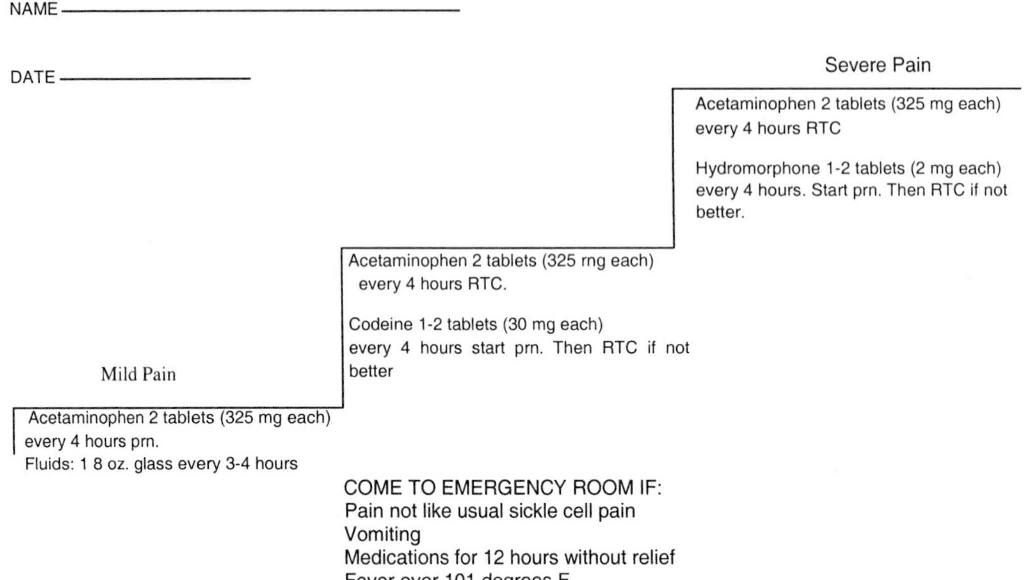

NAME
DATE
Severe Pain
Acetaminophen 2 tablets (325 mg each) every 4 hours RTC
Hydromorphone 1-2 tablets (2 mg each) every 4 hours. Start prn. Then RTC if not better.
Acetaminophen 2 tablets (325 rng each) every 4 hours RTC.
Codeine 1-2 tablets (30 mg each) every 4 hours start prn. Then RTC if not better
Mild Pain
Acetaminophen 2 tablets (325 mg each) every 4 hours prn.
Fluids: 1 8 oz. glass every 3-4 hours
COME TO EMERGENCY ROOM IF:
Pain not like usual sickle cell pain
Vomiting
Medications for 12 hours without relief
Fever over 101 degrees F.

FIG. 28.2. Stepwise guide for home management of pain.

nally, the health care system, especially in a tertiary care center, can be a perpetual source of frustration and confusion for many patients and families. Education can help families understand the structure and how they can effectively advocate for themselves and their child.

Education of medical and nursing staff about sickle cell disease pain is necessary to provide competent treatment, to prevent the development of adversarial relationships, and to provide continuity of care. A single educational session is inadequate; the process must be ongoing, and the frustrations of the health caretakers should be taken as seriously as the frustrations of the patients.

Psychotherapy for the child and family is necessary when there is ongoing or significant dysfunction. Even when regular involvement of a mental health professional is not required, the sickle cell disease physician and nurse should provide supportive counseling. The potential for secondary gain exists for patients with any chronic problem (134), even in the most functional of families (although secondary gain should not be regarded as an indication that pain is not present). Parents need help in deciding appropriate limits and responsibilities, especially when the child has pain. Support groups for families and patients can be very helpful (27); a mixed group of adolescents and adults may help smooth the transition to care in an adult facility.

Contracts are written agreements involving the patient, family, and health caretakers, in which the responsibilities of all are defined in variable detail (135). The process of working out a contract is usually more therapeutic than the actual document because it involves the patient and family in an active therapeutic alliance. Contracts can be helpful for some adolescents with frequent admissions to the hospital for pain (136–139; K. Covelman and M. Russel, unpublished, 1980). The terms of the contract vary according to the situation but may include criteria for admission, the dose and schedule for medication, expectations for self-care, and weaning. They may be quite extensive or very brief. If the contract is to be effective, the terms cannot be changed, except by mutual agreement of all involved in drawing up the document, and the pain must be managed in a pharmacologically sound manner (Fig. 28.3). In some cases in which staff and patient conflict is significant, these contracts must also address staff as well as patient responsibilities to avoid being punitive.

Children and adolescents with frequent and severe pain may miss a significant amount of school (as much as 1 of every 5 days) (6). Unfortunately, many states require home tutoring only for absence from school for 2 successive weeks (140). Children with sickle cell disease pain usually miss only 3 or 4 days in a row, but this can occur at frequent intervals throughout the year (6). With such frequent absences, the patient may get behind in school, often to the extent of repeating a grade, and develop a fear and avoidance of returning to school. Interactions with peers are affected, and coping skills are eroded. These factors maintain and intensify any pain. Health care professionals can help by providing personnel at the school with information about sickle cell disease and painful episodes and by acting as advocates for changes in public policy.

Physical Methods

Heating packs and hot baths are helpful for many patients. Cold generally worsens the pain, although an occasional patient benefits from limited application to an extremity. Light massage is intolerable to some people and helpful for others. Transcutaneous electrical nerve stimulation may decrease the intensity of the pain, although the one study of this treatment for acute sickle cell disease pain showed that it did not decrease the length of hospital stay (141). There have been no published studies of its use in chronic pain states of sickle cell disease. Fluidotherapy has been shown to be helpful (142) but is usually not readily accessible. Extremities can be splinted or braced to prevent painful motion and to facilitate ambulation. Although rest is necessary, simple exercises help maintain strength and flexibility, especially during a protracted episode of pain.

Other Interventions

Support systems in the family and community are vital. Many patients and families cite religion as a powerful source of support in coping with the pain. Contact with clergy by health caretakers may be helpful. Some cultural groups use folk remedies for the pain. As long as no dangerous methods are used, these can be incorporated into the care plan. It is important for healthcare professionals to realize that religion, family, and the community provide more powerful methods for pain control and coping for many families than the treatments offered by a medical center.

OUTPATIENT MANAGEMENT OF PAIN

Education is the foundation for successful home management of pain. A stepwise approach to pain management should be specific and readily understandable, with doses defined in number of tablets as well as in milligrams and with the amount of fluid necessary for adequate hydration defined as the number of glasses of a particular size necessary in 24 hours. Cognitive behavioral techniques can be included on the stepwise guide. As appropriate, patients and families should also be instructed in the use of around-the-clock analgesic schedules for persistent pain, use of appropriate analgesic combinations for refractory pain, and the use of long-acting medications for chronic pain. Avoidance of precipitating factors should be discussed with awareness of normal development because strict avoidance may severely restrict daily activities (138,139). Families and patients should know when to come to the hospital or clinic for acute care.

Various oral analgesics, including potent opioids, can be used safely at home with proper education and supervision. Adolescents should discuss medication usage with

CONTRACT

Patient:
Date:

Management Guidelines for James/Lisa's Admissions for Sickle Cell Pain

The goal of this contract is to develop a plan to manage James/Lisa's pain both pharmacologically and behaviorally so that he/she can return to normal daily activity as soon as possible. The plan is comprised of four levels of intervention. If James/Lisa is meeting the staff's and his/her parent's expectations he/she should be given access to Nintendo, game room, videos, supper club, etc. If he/she is unable to engage in expected activity, he/she should not be given special access. The length of time James/Lisa should remain on each level will be negotiated between him/her and the physician and nursing staff. Recommended time frames are offered.

Level 1 (1-3 days)
This represents the initial stage of hospitalization. This is when pharmacologic treatment will need to be most aggressive and activity will be limited

Medication:
PCA with morphine
If he/she is not vomiting, acetaminophen with codeine orally A TC will be substituted for the basal infusion on the PCA.

Activity:
1. James/Lisa should change positions in bed at least every four hours.
2. Encourage personal hygiene care.
3. James/Lisa should do relaxation and respiratory exercises every 4 hours during day and evening shifts.

IF JAMES/LISA FEELS UP TO GETTING OUT OF BED, SUPPORT HIM/HER FOR DOING SO. Please encourage him/her to meet these criteria but try not to give him/her a great deal of attention for refusing to comply. Rather, focus on the positives he/she has access to if he/she complies. If James/Lisa is able to sit up and watch TV, he/she should be permitted to do so.

Level 2 (1-2 days)
The focus of this level is on increasing mobility and activity while maintaining a medication regimen equivalent to level 1.

Medication:
Stop basal infusion on PCA, if being used.
Start acetaminophen and codeine around-the-clock, if not being used.

Activity:
The importance of mobility should be underscored to James/Lisa while continuing to acknowledge his/her pain. Continue to reinforce (e.g., verbal praise and social attention) efforts to engage in activities. Again, gradually increase the demand to help in his/her own care.

1. James/Lisa should get out of bed at least once a shift (e.g., sit in a chair) for a minimum of 30 minutes. If he/she would like to be out longer, encourage him/her to do so.
2. James/Lisa should do his/her relaxation and respiratory exercises every 4 hours during day and evening
3. Nursing and James/Lisa should negotiate the daily schedule or responsibilities (e.g., getting up out of bed). The more structured James/Lisa's day is the easier the transition to home and school will be.

Level 3 (1-2 days)
The focus here is on increasing function on the unit while decreasing pain medications.

Medication:
Acetaminophen with either codeine or oral morphine around-the-clock. Stop PCA.

Activity
1. Encourage personal hygiene to be conducted away from the bed area.

2. James/Lisa should get out of bed and walk at least once a shift for as long as possible. This is a great opportunity to let him/her know that you are pleased he/she is up even though he/she has pain. Encourage attendance at supper club and movies on the unit. etc.
3. James/Lisa should continue to do relaxation and respiratory exercises every 4 hours during day and evening shifts.
4. Nursing and James/Lisa should negotiate daily schedule of responsibilities.

Level 4 (1 day)
Prepare for discharge!

Medication:
Decrease dose if possible.

Activity:
1. Encourage as much independence and activity as possible.
2. Discuss plan for school return and home management of pain.

James/Lisa has agreed to the above contract and in doing so is working to decrease the number and length of hospital stays to manage his/her pain. His/her parent is also in support of the plan. In addition to agreeing with the above contract, James/Lisa agrees to try to manage his/her pain as an outpatient by taking pain medication by mouth and doing relaxation exercises right at the start of the pain.

Signed: ______________________________
James/Lisa

____
Parent

____
Physician

____
Nurse

____
Mental Health Professional

FIG. 28.3. Example of a contract. Management guidelines for James's/Lisa's admissions for sickle cell pain. (Developed by Kenneth Covelman, The Child Guidance Center, Philadelphia, PA, and Mary Osborne, Ph.D., Children's Seashore House, Philadelphia, PA.)

their parents during their steady-state periods, so that misunderstandings do not arise during periods of pain. The method for obtaining telephone contact with medical caretakers must be defined and easily accessible. Once a successful medication regimen is developed, it should be kept consistent unless circumstances change. A record should be kept of the number of prescriptions issued and the dates. An increase of medication use may signify a physiologic change (increase in weight) or the need for adjunctive pain management techniques. Physicians who are not directly involved in the continuing care of a patient should notify the sickle cell disease physician when writing analgesic prescriptions.

MANAGEMENT IN THE EMERGENCY DEPARTMENT

The ED is the interface between family-centered home management and hospital-centered management of sickle cell disease–related pain. It is helpful to maintain a card file, notebook, or some other data source in the ED on frequently seen patients that contains information about diagnosis, previous complications, and suggested pain management and contracts. The physician responsible for sickle cell disease problems should be contacted as soon as possible.

The initial history should include questions about home management, past management of pain and what has worked, the presence of nausea and vomiting, the intensity and nature of the pain, the approximate amount of opioids during the previous day and week, and the usual pattern for vaso-occlusive episodes. The patient who is vomiting or who has failed consistent and adequate home pain management is likely to require admission, whereas the patient who has not used any medication may respond well to a mild opioid with acetaminophen or an NSAID. Many patients have short episodes of severe pain, requiring intravenous hydration and analgesia. A holding area in the ED where such therapy can be provided for 12 to 24 hours may decrease the number of inpatient admissions (143). Patients frequently are quite knowledgeable about the drugs and doses that have worked for them in the past. Requests for specific drugs and doses should not be interpreted as necessarily signifying drug-seeking or manipulative behavior.

Pharmacologic management of painful episodes in the ED proceeds in four stages. First, the starting opioid dose and route are determined. Second, the degree of analgesia and sedation is determined after the initial dose, and subsequent smaller doses are given every 15 to 30 minutes until the pain is tolerable or until side effects are intolerable, in which case, these adverse effects may also require pharmacologic management. Third, a decision about disposition is made. Fourth, analgesia is maintained until the patient is either admitted or sent home to resume home management (Fig. 28.4).

The initial opioid dose is based on the home use of opioids, estimated degree of opioid tolerance, and adequacy of home management. If opioids have been used consistently and without success at home, a reasonable starting dose would offer at least two times the analgesia given at home. For example, if a patient has been using 60 mg codeine, 20 mg oral morphine (4 to 5 mg intravenous morphine) will approximately double the analgesia. If the patient is in severe pain or is opioid tolerant, it is reasonable to provide three times or more the analgesia given at home.

If opioids have not been used at home, the patient with severe pain should be given the usual starting dose (Table 28.3), even if higher doses have been required in the past. The patient who has been using large doses of strong opioids at home may be given approximately 1.5 times the traditional starting dose. He or she may actually require three to four times this amount, but this should not be given in a single dose; rather, it can be given by dose titration every 15 to 30 minutes. The physician must remember that cross-tolerance among opioids may be incomplete. Thus, the patient maintained on oral morphine at home may not tolerate an equi-analgesic dose of hydromorphone.

Analgesia and sedation should be assessed at the time of peak effect (approximately 30 to 45 minutes for oral opioids and 10 to 15 minutes for intravenous opioids). Frequent

TABLE 28.3. *Severe pain: recommended starting doses*

		Body weight	
Drug	Route	>50 kg (mg)	<50 kg (mg/kg)
Morphine	i.v.	5–10	0.1
	p.o.	15–30	0.3
Hydromorphone	i.v.	1–1.5	0.015
	p.o.	4–8	0.08

i.v., intravenous; p.o., orally.

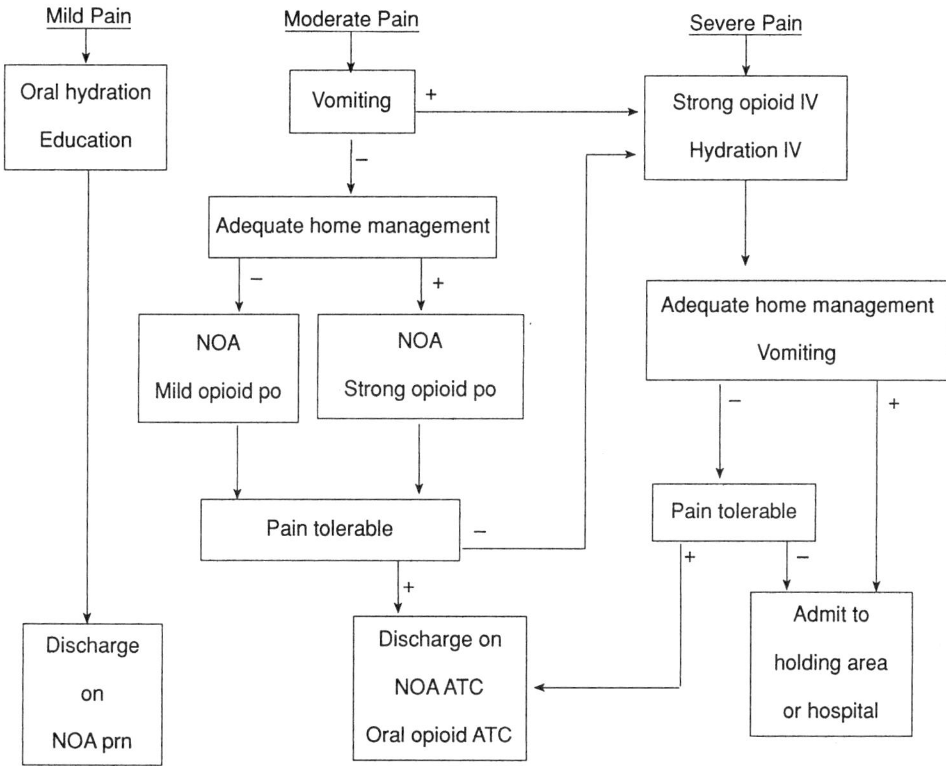

FIG. 28.4. Management of painful episodes in the emergency department. PCA, patient-controlled analgesia. *NOA*, nonopioid analgesic; *ATC*, around the clock.

small doses can be given every 15 to 30 minutes by the intravenous route, and the oral dose can be supplemented after approximately 45 minutes to 1 hour if adequate analgesia is not achieved with the first dose (Table 28.4). The physician experienced in the use of opioids may choose to use higher doses than those recommended here for opioid-tolerant patients.

Patients are often deprived of sleep, and adequate analgesia results in sleep. The respiratory rate may decline to normal, if it has been elevated as a result of the pain. Careful titration of analgesia rarely results in significant respiratory depression. However, the patient should be closely monitored. If naloxone is necessary, small amounts should be used (e.g., a starting dose of 1 to 2 mg/kg, with the dose doubled every few minutes until the respiratory rate returns to normal). Large doses of naloxone can produce withdrawal symptoms in the opioid-dependent patient and make subsequent analgesia difficult until the drug is excreted.

Because people vary in their ability to manage pain at home and because pain is not comparable from one patient to another, determination of the need for admission must be made in consultation with the family. A pain intensity score is useful only for following the course of the vaso-occlusive episode because some patients may be able to manage severe pain at home.

Patients may remain in the ED for at least several hours. Once adequate analgesia is achieved, it must be maintained. The pain may return in less than 1 hour or not for several hours, depending on the severity of the pain and the pharmacokinetics of the drug administered. When the pain returns, the patient

TABLE 28.4. *Guide to intravenous dose titration*[a]

Sedation	No analgesia	Partial analgesia	Adequate analgesia
None	Repeat half to full dose	Repeat quarter to half dose	Observe duration of analgesia
Moderate	Repeat half dose	Repeat quarter dose	Observe duration of analgesia
Profound	Reassess patient Monitor Maximize nonopioid intervention dose	Monitor patient Maximize nonopioid intervention doses Decrease subsequent doses	Monitor patient Decrease subsequent doses

[a]Analgesia and sedation are assessed 15 to 30 minutes after the initial intravenous dose.

should receive another dose of opioid (Fig. 28.5). The time of return should be noted on the chart. If the patient is admitted to the hospital, an extra opioid dose may help to maintain pain control during transport to the inpatient unit.

INPATIENT MANAGEMENT

The stages of inpatient management are (a) assessment of the patient and the pain, (b) determination of the method of management, (c) dose titration if not done in the ED, (d) maintenance of analgesia, (e) weaning, and (f) discharge. Determination of the method of management should be based on the considerations outlined in the section on pharmacologic management. Early contact with the primary caretaker is important. Unless there are problems, the method of management started on admission should be continued throughout the hospital stay, so the patient will not have to adjust to multiple changes in management. Pain often increases at night, precipitating requests for changes in the management. If this is a pattern, it is helpful to discuss this possibility with the patient and health care staff and decide on a plan because physicians present

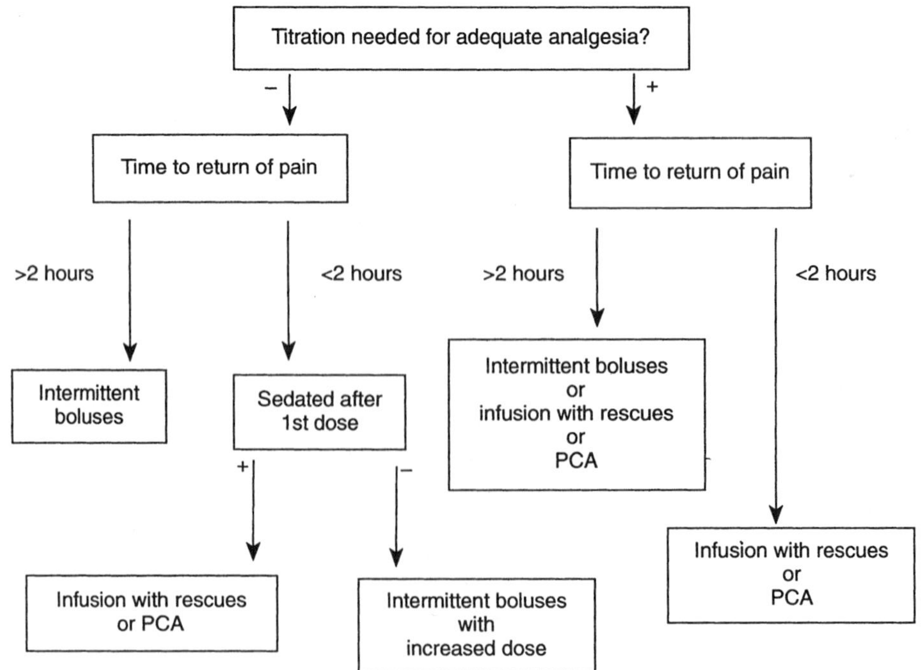

FIG. 28.5. Maintenance of analgesia. *PCA*, patient-controlled analgesia.

during the nighttime hours may not know the patient.

Weaning can be a source of discord between the caretakers and the patient, especially if the patient perceives the weaning as precipitous or coerced. The method of weaning should be discussed in advance with the patient. In general, weaning should proceed slowly to prevent the need to backtrack. While the pain continues, the dose of the medication should be decreased, but the interval should not be lengthened because this increases anxiety and the likelihood of breakthrough pain. The method and rate of weaning are as variable as the patients. Patients with slowly resolving pain may need a decrease of approximately 10% to 25% per day. Other patients may experience total resolution of the pain within a very short interval and can be abruptly tapered. Therefore, no formula for weaning can be applied to all patients.

For example, if the patient is receiving intravenous medication, the first step for weaning may be the introduction of oral opioid analgesia at an equianalgesic dose given around the clock. Smaller intravenous doses can then be offered as rescues. If high doses of parenteral opioids are being used, it may be better to wean to approximately half the original dose and then to substitute the oral opioid. Weaning from PCA can be accomplished very smoothly. If a basal infusion is being used, this can be stopped, with substitution of a sustained-release oral opioid given around the clock. Most patients will stop using the patient-controlled dose spontaneously which can be replaced with a short-acting opioid (105).

MANAGEMENT OF THE HIGH-RISK PATIENT

Patients with very frequent and severe pain are at high risk of psychosocial dysfunction (138,139; K. Covelman and M. Russel, unpublished, 1980). The dysfunction often becomes evident during adolescence. Because a critical element of this developmental phase is the assertion of autonomy and independence, which is especially difficult in light of the chronic dependence on medical caretakers, the issues of chronic pain become intertwined with developmental and emotional issues. This is when an adversarial relationship between the patient and the health care system often develops (138,139).

Ideally, multidisciplinary intervention is instituted when the pain becomes frequent and severe, when family issues are identified, and when difficulties in school are encountered. However, our care system is not ideal, and there may be no intervention until the relationship between the patient and the health care system reaches a crisis.

Management includes the development of a contract and the provision of cognitive-behavioral coping skills training and psychotherapy. Depression may be present and should be treated. Strict continuity of care, sound pharmacologic management of the pain with long-acting analgesics, and inclusion of the family in treatment are vital (138, 139,144; K. Covelman and M. Russel, unpublished, 1980).

High-risk patients often have problems maintaining outpatient appointments. A pattern develops in which the patient is discharged from the hospital with plans for psychosocial follow-up as an outpatient, even though historically the family does not show up for these appointments. Medical and nursing professionals, frustrated in their attempts to provide care and focus on the inpatient problems, discharge the patient as soon as possible. The patient and family, also frustrated by the problems in the hospital, agree to the follow-up appointments but privately see no reason to commit to a therapeutic alliance (Fig. 28.6). A common coping mechanism for recurrent pain is to operate in a crisis mode, and the resolution of the pain is accompanied by resumption of normal life, with a denial of future problems. This is adaptive when pain is infrequent but is maladaptive when pain is frequent.

Difficulties with follow-up need to be faced squarely, without the illusion that immediate changes can be accomplished. It

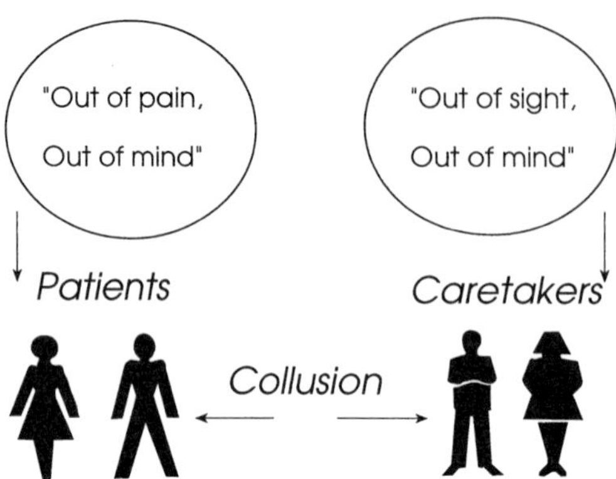

FIG. 28.6. Collusion between patient and health care professional.

takes time and work to build trust. If health caretakers recognize that a patient has historically experienced difficulty, for whatever reason, in keeping outpatient appointments, the hospital can be used as a forum for intervention. Once the pain has eased, work can begin to establish a contract for the next admission and to teach coping skills. Even if the family is unable to visit the patient during the admission, someone from the family must be present on the day of discharge. Thus, the day of discharge can be extended and can be used to assess at least part of the family and to provide education and participation in the contract. Subsequent admissions are used to build on this foundation. During this process, the factors impeding outpatient visits can be explored and assistance rendered. This approach requires commitment and flexibility on the part of the health care professionals.

Health care professionals often experience considerable difficulty dealing with adolescents who are known or suspected to be substance abusers. Although there is little information in this area, suggestions can be made for managing adolescents with severe sickle cell disease pain who are also substance abusers. These patients can be treated like the high-risk patient who is not a substance abuser. Contracts are particularly useful, and health care professionals should be very clear and consistent with themselves and the patient and family about expectations, limits, and concerns. Additionally, the following recommendations are offered:

1. Optimize the use of nonopioid analgesics and cognitive-behavioral skills.
2. Use opioids in adequate doses to control the pain. Patients who abuse substances may be tolerant and may require very high doses.
3. Do not use analgesia on an as-needed basis under any circumstances because this encourages drug-seeking behavior. Provide medication within a structured predictable framework.
4. Distinguish between a history of drug abuse and current abuse because the concerns may be different (49).
5. Discuss the issue honestly, but kindly, with the patient. It is inappropriate for the chart to contain remarks about drug-seeking behaviors that have not been discussed with the patient.
6. Provide previously agreed on amounts of opioids for outpatient management.
7. Emphasize oral rather than intravenous opioids. Sustained-release or long-acting opioids may be particularly useful.

DIRECTIONS FOR THE FUTURE

Much clinical and research work is needed to better understand and treat vaso-occlusive pain. The effects of the pain on function, mood, and development have not been well delineated. Pain assessment techniques for preverbal or cognitively impaired individuals need to be validated. We need improved knowledge of the pharmacokinetics of analgesic agents in this population and dose schedules for PCA. We need careful studies of the efficacy of adjuvant drugs. Many investigators are now exploring cognitive-behavioral approaches to pain control. Psychotherapy, although described in other chronic problems, has not been well studied in patients with sickle cell disease. The early identification and management of the high-risk patient are of great importance. Management of pain in the adolescent or adult who abuses substances is a controversial and largely unexplored area.

Socioeconomic, racial, and cultural differences between patients and the caretakers pose problems in clinical management and in the design of clinical studies. We must explore attitudes and examine methods for improving communication, if the management of pain is to show a meaningful rather than a cosmetic improvement. Finally, advocacy for children and adolescents with sickle cell disease and other chronic problems is necessary to change public policy regarding education and funding for health care and research.

REFERENCES

1. Ohene-Frempong K. Sickle cell disease in the United States of America and Africa. *Blood* 1999[Suppl 1]: 64–72.
2. Serjeant GR. *Sickle cell disease.* Oxford: Oxford University Press, 1985.
3. Brozovic M, Anionwu E. Sickle cell disease in Britain. *J Clin Pathol* 1984;37:1321–1326.
4. Brozovic M, Davies S, Brownell A. Acute admissions of patients with sickle cell disease who live in Britain. *BMJ* 1987;294:1206–1208.
5. Tetrault SM, Scott RB. Five year retrospective study on hospitalization and treatment of sickle cell anemia patients. In: *Proceedings of the First National Symposium on Sickle Cell Disease.* Bethesda, MD, 1974.
6. Shapiro B, Dinges D, Beningo L, et al. Home management of sickle cell-related pain in children and adolescents: natural history and impact on school attendance *Pain* 1995;1:139–144.
7. Embry SH, Hebbel RP, Mohandas N, et al. eds. *Sickle cell disease: basic principles and clinical practice.* Philadelphia: Lippincott–Raven, 1994.
8. Ballas SK. Sickle cell pain. In: *Progress in pain research and management, volume 11.* Seattle: IASP Press, 1998.
9. Gaston MH, Verter JI, Woods G, et al. Prophylaxis with oral penicillin in children with sickle cell anemia: a randomized trial. *N Engl J Med* 1986;314:1593–1599.
10. Nagel RL, Fabry ME, Billett HH, et al. Sickle cell painful crisis: a multifactorial event. *Prog Clin Biol Res* 1987;240:361–380.
11. Platt OS, Thorington BD, Brambilla DJ, et al. Pain in sickle cell disease: rates and risk factors. *N Engl J Med* 1991;325:11–16.
12. Westerman MP, Bailey K, Freels S, et al. Assessment of painful episode frequency in sickle cell disease. *Am J Hematol* 1997;54:183–188.
13. Dampier C, Reber D, Bauer NK. Characteristics of out-patient painful episodes in pediatric patients with sickle cell disease. Presented at the 8th World Congress on Pain, August 1996.
14. Murray N, May A. Painful crises in sickle cell disease-patients' perspectives. *BMJ* 1988;297:452–454.
15. Beyer JE, Simmons LE, Woods GM, et al. A chronology of pain and comfort in children with sickle cell disease. *Arch Pediatr Adolesc Med* 1999;153:913–920.
16. Conner-Warren RL. Pain intensity and home pain management of children with sickle cell disease. *Issues Compr Pediatr Nurs* 1996;19:183–195.
17. Konotey-Ahulu FID. The sickle cell diseases. *Arch Intern Med* 1974;133:611–619.
18. Walco GA, Dampier CD, Djordjevic D. Pain assessment in children and adolescents with sickle cell disease. Presented at the Sixteenth Annual Postgraduate Conference on Sickle Cell Disease in the Next Decade: innovative therapeutic approaches. Washington, DC, 1987(abst).
19. Walco GA, Dampier CD. Pain in children and adolescents with sickle cell disease: a descriptive study. *J Pediatr Psychol* 1990;15:643–658.
20. Stevens MCG, Padwick M, Serjeant GR. Observations on the natural history of dactylitis in homozygous sickle cell disease. *Clin Pediatr* 1981;20:311–317.
21. Baum KF, Dunn DT, Maude GH, et al. The painful crisis of homozygous sickle cell disease. *Arch Intern Med* 1987;147:1231–1234.
22. Gil KM, Phillips G, Abrams MR, et al. Pain drawings and sickle cell disease pain. *Clin J Pain* 1990;6: 105–109.
23. Lawrence C, Fabry MR. Objective indices of sickle cell painful crisis: decrease in RDW and percent dense cells and increase in ESR and fibrinogen. *Prog Clin Biol Res* 1987;240:329–336.
24. Mankad YN, Williams P, Harpen M, et al. Magnetic resonance imaging, percentage of dense cells and serum prostanoids as tools for objective assessment of pain crisis: a preliminary report. *Prog Clin Biol Res* 1987;240:337–350.
25. Charache S, Zohoun I. Pathogenesis of painful sickle cell crisis. *Prog Clin Biol Res* 1987;240:265–275.
26. Steinberg MH. Determinants of vaso-occlusive severity in sickle cell disease. *Prog Clin Biol Res* 1987;240: 413–428.
27. Vichinsky EP, Johnson R, Lubin BH. Multidisciplinary approach to pain management in sickle cell disease. *Am J Pediatr Hematol Oncol* 1982;4:328–333.
28. Diggs LW, Flowers E. Sickle cell anemia in the home environment. *Clin Pediatr* 1971;10:697–700.
29. Rather SJ, Athanasian EA. Water sports and sickle cell anemia. *Ann Intern Med* 1986;105:971.
30. Samuels-Reid J, Scott RB. Painful crises and menstruation in sickle cell disease. *South Med J* 1985;78: 384–385.
31. Castele R, Strohl K, Chester C, et al. Oxygen saturation with sleep in patients with sickle cell disease. *Arch Intern Med* 1986;146:722–725.
32. Scharf M, Lobel J, Caldwell E, et al. Nocturnal oxygen desaturation in patients with sickle cell anemia. *JAMA* 1983;249:1753–1755.
33. Addae S. Mechanism for the high incidence of sickle cell crisis in the tropical cool season. *Lancet* 1971;2: 1256.
34. Redwood AM, Williams EM, Desai P, et al. Climate and painful crisis of sickle cell disease in Jamaica. *BMJ* 1976;1:66–68.
35. Seeler RA. Non-seasonality of sickle cell crisis. *Lancet* 1973;2:743.
36. Slovis C, Tailey J, Pitts R. Non relationship of clima-

tologic factors and painful sickle cell anemia crisis. *J Chronic Dis* 1986;39:121–126.
37. Schechter AN, Bunn HF. What determines severity in sickle-cell disease? [Editorial]. *N Engl J Med* 1982; 306:295–297.
38. Dover GI, Charache S. The effect on increased fetal hemoglobin production on the frequency of vaso-occlusive crisis in sickle cell disease. *Prog Clin Biol Res* 1987;240:277–285.
39. Dampier C, Brodecki D, Bauer NK. Characteristics of out-patient painful episodes in pediatric patients with sickle cell disease—predictors of episode frequency. Presented at the 18th Annual Scientific Meeting of the American Pain Society, October 1999.
40. Ballas SK, Lamer J, Smith ED. Rheological properties of sickle erythrocytes in the steady state predict the frequency and severity of the sickle cell painful crisis. *Blood* 1987;70:558a.
41. Chien S. Rheology of sickle cells and microcirculation. *N Engl J Med* 1987;311:1567–1569.
42. Hebbel RP, Moldow CF, Steinberg MH. Modulation of erythrocyte-endothelial interactions and the vaso-occlusive severity of sickling disorders. *Blood* 1981;58: 947–952.
43. Milner PF, Kraus AP, Sebes JI, et al. Sickle cell disease as a cause of osteonecrosis of the femoral head. *N Engl J Med* 1991;325:1476–1481.
44. Ohene-Frempong K, Weiner SJ, Sleeper LA, et al. Cerebrovascular accidents in sickle cell disease: rates and risk factors. *Blood* 1998;91:288–294.
45. Gil KM, Abrams MR, Phillips G, et al. Sickle cell disease pain: relation of coping strategies to adjustment. *J Consult Clin Psychol* 1989;57:1–7.
46. Maxwell K, Streetly A, Bevan D. Experiences of hospital care and treatment seeking for pain from sickle cell disease: qualitative study. *BMJ* 1999;318:1585–1590.
47. Morrison RS, Wallenstein S, Natale DK, et al. 'We don't carry that'—failure of pharmacies in predominantly nonwhite neighborhoods to stock opioid analgesics. *N Engl J Med* 2000;342:1023–1026.
48. Schatz J, Brown RT, Pascual JM, et al. Poor school and cognitive functioning with silent cerebral infarcts and sickle cell disease. *Neurology* 2001;56:1109–1111.
49. Maier SF, Seligman MEP. Learned helplessness: theory and evidence. *J Exp Psychol* 1976;105:346.
50. Nolen-Hoeksema S, Girgus JS, Seligman MEP. Learned helplessness in children: a longitudinal study of depression, achievement, and explanatory style. *J Pers Soc Psychol* 1986;51:1–8.
51. Kumar S, Powars D, Allen J, et al. Anxiety, self-concept, and personal and social adjustments in children with sickle cell anemia. *Pediatrics* 1976;8:859–863.
52. Lemanek LK, Moure SL, Gresham FM, et al. Psychological adjustment of children with sickle cell anemia. *J Pediatr Psychol* 1986;11:397–409.
53. Hertig AL, White LS. Psychosocial adjustment in children and adolescents with sickle cell disease. *J Pediatr Psychol* 1986;11:411–427.
54. Morgan SA, Jackson J. Psychological and social concomitants of sickle cell anemia in adolescents. *J Pediatr Psychol* 1986;11:429–440.
55. Whitworth E, Abrams M, Martin A, et al. Self esteem of sickle cell patients: a developmental perspective. Presented at the Sixteenth Annual Postgraduate Conference on Sickle Cell Disease in the Next Decade: Innovative Therapeutic Approaches. Washington, DC, 1987(abst).
56. Damlouji NF, Georgopoulos A, Kevess-Cohen R, et al. Social disability and psychiatric morbidity in sickle cell anemia and diabetes patients. *Psychosomatics* 1982;23:925–931.
57. Leavell SR, Ford CY. Psychopathology in patients with sickle cell disease. *Psychosomatics* 1983;24:23–37.
58. Brozovic M, Davies S, Yardumian A, et al. Pain relief in sickle cell crisis [Letter]. *Lancet* 1986;2:624–625.
59. Payne R. American Pain Society Workshop on the Management of Sickle Cell Pain. St. Louis, 1990.
60. Waldrop RD, Mandry C. Health professional perceptions of opioid dependence among patients with pain. *Am J Emerg Med* 1995;13:529–531.
61. Shapiro BS, Benjamin LJ, Payne R, et al. Sickle cell-related pain: perceptions of medical practitioners. *J Pain Symptom Manage* 1997;14:168–174.
62. Porter J, Jick H. Addiction rare in patients treated with narcotics. *N Engl J Med* 1980;302:123.
63. Bonica JJ. *The management of pain*, 2nd ed. Philadelphia: Lea & Febiger, 1990.
64. Wall PD, Melzack R, eds. *Textbook of pain*, 2nd ed. New York: Churchill-Livingstone, 1989.
65. Benjamin LJ, Berkowitz LR, Orringer E, et al. A collaborative, double blind randomized study of cetiedil citrate in sickle cell crisis. *Blood* 1986;67:1442–1447.
66. Benjamin LJ, Dampier CD, Jacox A, et al. *Guidelines for the management of acute and chronic pain in sickle cell disease. APS Clinical Practice Guideline Series, no. 1.* Glenview, IL: American Pain Society, 1999.
67. Desforges JF, Wang M. Sickle cell anemia. *Med Clin North Am* 1966;50:1519–1529.
68. Buchanan GR, Siegel JD, Smith SJ, et al. Oral penicillin prophylaxis in children with impaired splenic function: a study of compliance. *Pediatrics* 1982;70: 926–930.
69. Schechter NL, Berde CB, Yaster M. *Pain in infants, children, and adolescents*. Baltimore: Williams & Wilkins, 1993.
70. McGrath PA, ed. *Pain in children: nature, assessment, treatment*. New York: Guilford Press, 1990.
71. World Health Organization. *Cancer pain relief*. Geneva: Office of Publications, 1986.
72. Voudouris N, Peck CL, Coleman G. The role of conditioning and verbal expectancy in the placebo response. *Pain* 1990;43:121–128.
73. Beaver WT. Combination analgesics. *Am J Med* 1984; 15:38–53.
74. Perlin E, Castro O, Finke H, et al. The value of diflunisal (Dolobid) in the treatment of painful sickle cell crisis. *Blood* 1986;68:S64a.
75. Pandit UA, Kothary SP, Pandit SK. Intravenous dezocine for postoperative pain: a double-blind, placebo-controlled comparison with morphine. *J Clin Pharmacol* 1986;26:275–280.
76. Ketorolac tromethamine. *Med Lett Drugs Ther* 1990; 32:79–82.
77. Hardwick WE, Givens TG, Monroe KW, et al. Effect of ketorolac in pediatric sickle cell vaso-occlusive pain crisis. *Pediatr Emerg Care* 1999;15:179–182.
78. Perlin E, Finke H, Castro O, et al. Enhancement of pain control with ketorolac tromethamine in patients with sickle cell vaso-occlusive crisis. *Am J Hematol* 1994;46:43–47.

79. Dubach UC, Rosner B, Sturmer T. An epidemiologic study of abuse of analgesic drugs: effects of phenacetin and salicylate on mortality and cardiovascular morbidity (1968 to 1987). *N Engl J Med* 1991; 324:155–160.
80. Matustik MC, Carpentieri U, Corn C, et al. Hyperreninemia and hyperaldosteronism in sickle cell anemia. *Pediatrics* 1979;95:206–209.
81. Twycross RG, McQuay HJ. Opioids. In: Wall PD, Melzack R, eds. *Textbook of pain*, 2nd ed. Edinburgh: Churchill-Livingstone, 1989.
82. Freidman EW, Webber AB, Osborne HH, et al. Oral analgesia for treatment of painful crisis in sickle cell anemia. *Ann Emerg Med* 1986;15:787–791.
83. Jacobson SJ, Kopecky EA, Joshi P, et al. Randomized trial of oral morphine for painful episodes of sickle cell disease in children. *Lancet* 1997;350:1358–1361.
84. Brookoff D, Polomano R, Callans D. Management of sickle cell pain with controlled release morphine. American Pain Society Annual Meeting, Phoenix, AZ, 1989.
85. Mather LE, Meffin PJ. Clinical pharmacokinetics of pethidine. *Clin Pharmacokinet* 1978;3:352–368.
86. Szeto H, Inturrisi CE, Houde R, et al. Accumulation of normeperidine, an active metabolite of meperidine, in patients with renal failure or cancer. *Ann Intern Med* 1977;86:738–741.
87. Tang R, Shimomura S, Rotblatt M. Meperidine-induced seizures in sickle cell patients. *Hosp Formul* 1980;76:764–772.
88. Oster JR, Lespier LE, Lee SM, et al. Renal acidification in sickle cell disease. *J Lab Clin Med* 1976;88: 389–401.
89. Kaiko R, Foley K, Grabinski P, et al. Central nervous system excitatory effects of meperidine in cancer patients. *Ann Neurol* 1983;13:180–185.
90. Abbuhl S, Jacobson S, Murphy J, et al. Serum concentration of meperidine in patients with sickle cell crisis. *Ann Emerg Med* 1986;15:433–438.
91. Howland MA, Goldfrank L, Paris P, et al. Meperidine usage in patients with sickle cell crisis [Letter]. *Ann Emerg Med* 1986;15:180–182.
92. Woods GM, Parson PM, Strickland DK. Efficacy of nalbuphine as a parenteral analgesic for the treatment of painful episodes in children with sickle cell disease. *J Assoc Acad Minor Phys* 1990;1:90–92.
93. Gonzalez ER, Ornato JP, Ware D, et al. Comparison of intramuscular analgesic activity of butorphanol and morphine in patients with sickle cell disease. *Ann Emerg Med* 1988;17:788–791.
94. McCammon RI, Stoelting RK, Madura JA. Effects of butorphanol, nalbuphine, and fentanyl on intrabiliary tract dynamics. *Anesth Analg* 1984;63:139–142.
95. Gawrisch E, Cheng E. Buprenorphine sedation of intensive care patients and ileus reversal. *Crit Care Med* 1990;18:1034–1036.
96. Yukioka H, Rosen M, Evans KT, et al. Gastric emptying and small bowel transit times in volunteers after intravenous morphine and nalbuphine. *Anaesthesia* 1987;42:704–710.
97. Flacke JW. Antagonism of opioid analgesics with nalbuphine and naloxone. *Semin Anesth* 1988;7:178–191.
98. Roinagnoli A, Keats AS. Ceiling effect for respiratory depression by nalbuphine. *Clin Pharmacol Ther* 1980; 27:478–485.
99. Errick JK, Heel RC. Nalbuphine: a preliminary review of its pharmacological properties and therapeutic efficacy. *Drugs* 1983;26:191–211.
100. McQuay HJ, Moore RA, Bullingham RES. Buprenorphine kinetics. *Adv Pain Res Ther* 1986;8:271–278.
101. Berde CB, Lehn B, Yee J, et al. Patient-controlled analgesia in children and adolescents: a randomized perspective comparison of intramuscular administration of morphine for post-operative analgesia. *J Pediatr* 1991;118:460–466.
102. Batenhorst RL, Maurer HS, Bertch KA, et al. Patient controlled analgesia in uncomplicated sickle cell pain crisis. *Blood* 1987;70:S58a.
103. Schechter NL, Berrian FB, Katz SM. The use of patient-controlled analgesia in adolescents with sickle cell pain crisis: a preliminary report. *J Pain Symptom Manage* 1988;3:109–113.
104. Holbrook CT. Patient-controlled analgesia pain management for children with sickle cell disease. *J Assoc Acad Minor Phys* 1990;1:93–96.
105. Glasson JC, Ginsberg B. Individualized PCA dosing recommendations for sickle cell crisis pain. Presented at the annual meeting of the American Pain Society, San Diego, CA, 1999(abst).
106. Shapiro B, Cohen D, Howe C. Use of patient-controlled analgesia for patients with sickle cell disease. Presented at The Second International Symposium on Pediatric Pain. Montreal, Canada, 1991(abst).
107. Rucknagel DL, Kalinyak KA, Gelfan MJ. Rib infarcts and acute chest syndrome in sickle cell diseases. *Lancet* 1991;337:831–833.
108. Sprinkle RH, Cole T, Smith SL, et al. Acute chest syndrome in pediatric patients with sickle cell disease: a retrospective analysis of 100 hospitalized patients. *Am J Pediatr Hematol Oncol* 1986;8:105–110.
109. Haynes L, Allison RC. Pulmonary edema: complication in the management of sickle cell pain crisis. *Am J Med* 1986;80:833–840.
110. Bellet PS, Kalinyak KA, Shukla R, et al. Incentive spirometry to prevent pulmonary complications in sickle cell disease. *N Engl J Med* 1995;333:699–703.
111. Feinmann C. Pain relief by antidepressants: possible modes of action. *Pain* 1985;23:1–8.
112. Sharav Y, Singer E, Schmidt E, et al. The analgesic effect of amitriptyline on chronic facial pain. *Pain* 1987; 31:199–209.
113. Bruera E, Chadwick S, Brenneis C. Methylphenidate associated with narcotics for the treatment of cancer pain. *Cancer Treat Rep* 1987;71:120–127.
114. Forrest WH, Brown BW, Brown CR, et al. Dextroamphetamine with morphine for treatment of postoperative pain. *N Engl J Med* 1977;296:712–715.
115. Laska EM, Sunshine A, Mueller F, et al. Caffeine as an analgesic adjuvant. *JAMA* 1984;251:1711–1718.
116. Gawin FH, Ellinwood EH. Cocaine and other stimulants. *N Engl J Med* 1988;318:1173–1182.
117. McIlvaine WB. Spinal opioids for the pediatric patient. *J Pain Symptom Manage* 1990;5:183–190.
118. Finer P, Blair L, Rowe P. Epidural analgesia in the management of labor pain and sickle cell crisis: a case report. *Anaesthesiology* 1988;68:799–800.
119. Yaster M, Tobin JR, Billet C, et al. Epidural analgesia in the management of severe vaso-occlusive sickle cell crisis. *Pediatrics* 1994;93:310–315.
120. Aluoch JR. The treatment of sickle cell disease. A his-

torical and chronological literature review of the therapies applied since 1910. *Trop Geogr Med* 1984;36: S1–26.
121. Greenberg J, Ohene-Frempong K, Halus L, et al. Trial low doses of aspirin as prophylaxis in sickle cell disease. *J Pediatr* 1983;102:781–784.
122. Charache S, Terrin ML, Moore RD, et al. Effect of hydroxyurea on the frequency of painful crises in sickle cell anemia. *N Engl J Med* 1995;332:1317–1322.
123. Griffin TC, McIntire D, Buchanan GR. High-dose intravenous methylprednisolone therapy for pain in children and adolescents with sickle cell disease. *N Engl J Med* 1994;330:733–737.
124. Robieux IC, Kellner JD, Coppes MJ, et al Analgesia in children with sickle cell crisis: comparison of intermittent opioids vs continuous intravenous infusion of morphine and placebo-controlled study of oxygen inhalation. *Pediatr Hematol Oncol* 1992;9:317–326.
125. Embury SH, Garcia JF, Mohandas N, et al. Effects of oxygen inhalation on endogenous erythropoietin kinetics, erythropoiesis, and properties of blood cells in sickle cell anemia. *N Engl J Med* 1984;311: 291–295.
126. Styles LA, Vichinsky EP. Effects of a long-term transfusion regimen on sickle cell-related illness. *J Pediatr* 1994;125:909–911.
127. Vichinsky E, Earles A, Johnson R, et al. Alloimmunization in sickle cell anemia and transfusion of racially unmatched blood. *N Engl J Med* 1990;322: 1617–1621.
128. Gil KM, Williams DA, Thompson RJ, et al. Sickle cell disease in children and adolescents: the relation of child and parent pain coping strategies to adjustment. *J Pediatr Psychol* 1991;16:643–663.
129. Zeltzer L, Dash J, Holland JP. Hypnotically induced pain control in sickle cell anemia. *Pediatrics* 1979;64: 533–536.
130. Cozzi J, Tryon WW, Sedlacek K. The effectiveness of biofeedback-assisted relaxation in modifying sickle cell crises. *Biofeedback Self Regul* 1987;12:51–61.
131. Thomas JE, Koshy M, Patterson L, et al. Management of pain in sickle cell disease using biofeedback therapy: a preliminary study. *Biofeedback Self Regul* 1984; 9:413–420.
132. Dinges DF, Whitehouse WG, Orne EC, et al. Self-hypnosis training as an adjustive treatment in the management of pain associated with sickle cell disease. *Int J Clin Exp Hypnosis* 1997;45:417–432.
133. Cherry GO. Protocol for comprehensive management of patients with sickle cell disease. NC Department of Human Resources, Division of Health Services, 1983.
134. Krener P, Adelman A. Parent salvage and parent sabotage in the care of chronically ill children. *Am J Dis Child* 1988;142:945–951.
135. Turk DC, Meichenbaum D, Genest M. *Pain and behavioral medicine*. New York: Guilford Press, 1983.
136. Powers R. Management protocol for sickle cell disease patients with acute pain: impact on emergency department and narcotic use. *Am J Emerg Med* 1986;4: 267–268.
137. Burghardt-Fitzgerald DC. Pain-behavior contracts: effective management of the adolescent in sickle-cell crisis. *J Pediatr Nurs* 1989;4:320–324.
138. Covelman K. Psychosomatic aspects of sickle cell disease: an open systems model. Presented at the Annual Conference of the National Council on Family Relations. Washington, DC, 1982.
139. Covelman K. Adaptation of a family therapy model for sickle cell crisis: Significance of patient population and symptom characteristics. Presented at the American Orthopsychiatric Association. Chicago, IL, 1986.
140. Hobbs N, Perrin J, Ireys H. *Chronically ill children and their families*. San Francisco: Jossey-Bass, 1985.
141. Wang WC, George SL, Wilimas JA. Transcutaneous electrical nerve stimulation (TENS) treatment of sickle cell painful crises. *Acta Haematol* 1990;80:90–102.
142. Alcorn R, Bowser B, Henley EJ, et al. Fluidotherapy and exercise in the management of sickle cell anemia. *Phys Ther* 1984;64:1520–1522.
143. Benjamin LJ, Swinson GI, Nagel RL. Sickle cell anemia day hospital: an approach for the management of uncomplicated painful crises. *Blood* 2000;95: 1130–1136.
144. Hall H, Chiarucci K, Lawson MK, et al. Management approaches for sickle cell anemia patients experiencing recurrent vaso-occlusive pain. Presented at Sixteenth Annual Meeting of the National Sickle Cell Disease Program. Mobile, AL, 1991(abst).

29

Management of Pain in Childhood Cancer

John J. Collins and Steven J. Weisman

The recognition and treatment of cancer pain for both children and adults have helped to facilitate the development of pain treatment services dedicated to the management of both malignant and nonmalignant pain. Ever since the first consensus conference meetings that led to the publication of the World Health Organization's monograph, *Cancer Pain Relief*, in 1990, treatment programs for the relief of cancer pain have expanded (1). In fact, the first published guidelines for the treatment of cancer pain in children were published in 1990, after a retreat in rural Connecticut attended by international experts in pediatric pain relief (2–4). Since that time, several other guidelines and monographs have been released that provide a very useful framework for the treatment of pain in children with cancer (5,6).

Over the past 40 years, treatment of childhood cancer has advanced beyond almost anyone's wildest imagination. In these first years of the new millennium, we can expect more than 75% of all children diagnosed with a malignancy to achieve long-term survival and cure (Fig. 29.1). In fact, the overall mortality rate in children owing to cancer has fallen from 5.4 per 100,000 population to 2.8 per 100,000 between 1975 and 1998 (7) (Fig. 29.2). These facts, coupled with a relatively stable rate of diagnosed malignant cases (12.8 per 100,000 in 1975 versus 16.1 per 100,000 in 1998), might lead one to imagine less need for pain management in these children (7) (Fig. 29.3). Unfortunately, this is not the case. The revolution and evolution of these highly successful treatment regimens have taken place only because of the significant burden of very aggressive treatment programs for our patients.

Such programs now include aggressive forms of medical, surgical, and radiotherapeutic regimens that challenge our abilities to care for these children. Patients experience prolonged periods of malaise and painful mucositis from aggressive multidrug cancer treatment protocols. Many of these regimens include total body or extended-field radiation therapy as well. Orthopedic surgeons have developed major limb-sparing procedures that involve limb or even quadrant reconstruction with attendant tissue damage or direct nerve injury or neurapraxia. These intensive, at times invasive, therapies mandate more aggressive and often more prolonged courses of analgesic management. The complexity of the pain problems also mandate a broad understanding of the pathophysiology of the pain states, so that targeted analgesic regimens can be employed.

Finally, in the minority of children who fail the improved antitumor therapies, there is a need for coordinated end-of-life supportive care that includes aggressive pain management. This topic remains beyond the scope of this chapter and is presented in Chapter 30 of this book

CANCER PAIN IN CHILDREN: THE EXTENT OF THE PROBLEM

Pain is a common symptom experienced by children with cancer. In acknowledgment of the prevalence of this symptom and the importance of adequate management, the World Health Organization produced a document with the expectation that the principles of pain management and palliative care would

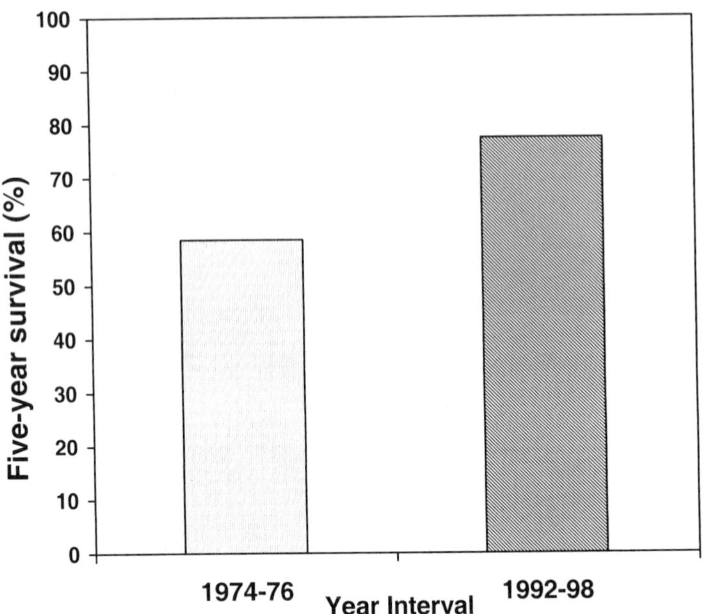

FIG. 29.1. Five-year survival rate in children with cancer.

be applicable to all children with cancer, irrespective of geographic location (8).

Information was acquired about symptom characteristics from a heterogeneous population of children with cancer 10 to 18 years of age at Memorial Sloan-Kettering Cancer Center in New York (9). Children were asked about their symptoms during the preceding week. Pain was the most prevalent symptom in the inpatient group (84.4%) and was rated as moderate to severe by 86.8% and highly distressing ("quite a bit to very much") by 52.8% of these children. Pain was experienced by 35.1% of the outpatient group, of

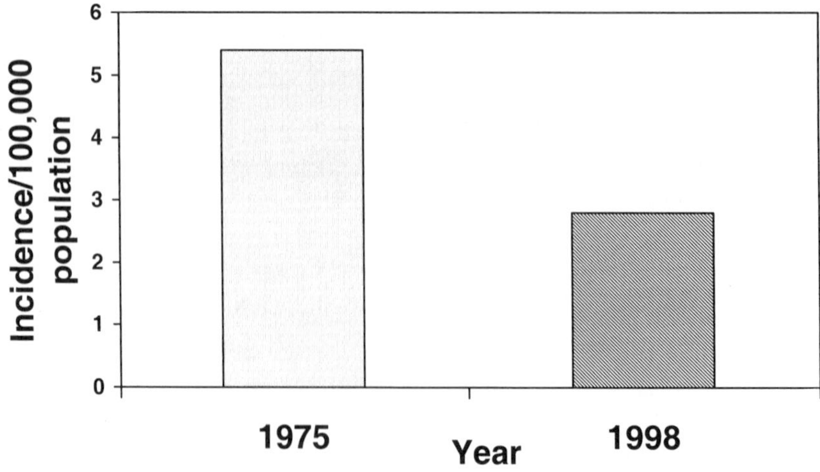

FIG. 29.2. Mortality rate of children with cancer. Birth through 18 years of age. Data are reported as incidence per 100,000 population (7). In 1975, the overall mortality rate owing to cancer for children was 5.4 per 100,000. In 1998, the reported rate was 2.8 per 100,000.

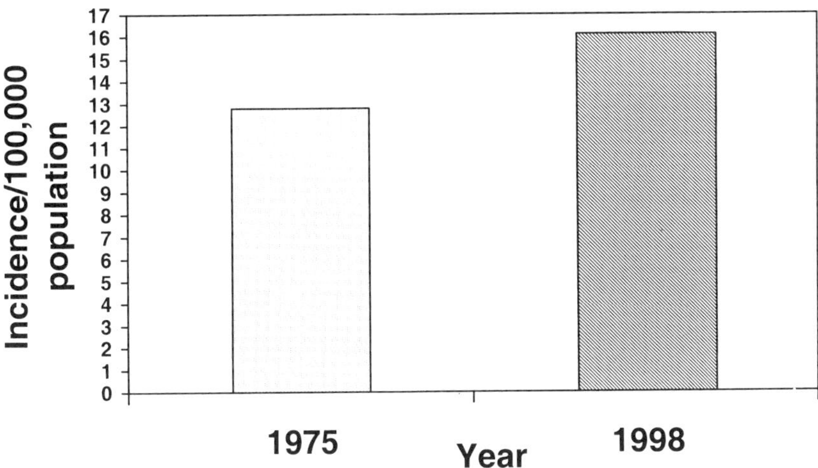

FIG. 29.3. Cancer incidence in children. Birth through 18 years of age. Data are reported as incidence per 100,000 population (7). In 1975, the overall incidence of cancer in all sites and in all races was 12.8 per 100,000. In 1998, the reported rate was 16.1 per 100,000.

whom 75% rated it as being moderate to severe and 26.3% rated distress as "quite a bit to very much" (9).

A cohort of 149 British and Australian children with cancer aged 7 to 12 was surveyed about their experience of symptoms during the preceding 48 hours (J. J. Collins, unpublished data). Approximately one-third had experienced pain in the previous 48 hours. More than half of this group had pain severity in the medium to severe range, and one-third were highly distressed by their experience (J. J. Collins, unpublished data). Pain is one of many symptoms experienced by children with cancer. Pain assessment must be considered in light of highly symptomatic children with complex disease processes.

A study of children with cancer at the National Cancer Institute found that 62% presented to their practitioner with a complaint of pain before their cancer diagnosis (10). Pain had been present for a median of 74 days before anticancer treatment was begun. The duration of pain experienced was not related to the extent of disease at diagnosis. After the initiation of anticancer therapy, most children had resolution of their pain, with the rare patient requiring long-term opioid therapy. Children with hematologic malignancy had a shorter duration of pain than children with solid tumors (10).

There is little information about the epidemiology of pain related to pediatric brain or spinal cord tumors. Children with brain tumors commonly present with either abnormal neurologic signs or symptoms of raised intracranial pressure (11). Most children with spinal cord tumors present with a complaint of pain (12). Back pain is more common than abnormal neurologic signs as a sign of spinal cord compression in children (13). Spinal cord compression owing to metastatic disease is more likely to occur late in a child's illness (13).

As cancer treatment protocols evolve for each patient, treatment-related, rather than tumor-related, causes of pain predominate (14, 15). Causes of treatment-related pain include postoperative pain, mucositis, phantom limb pain, infection, antineoplastic therapy–related pain, and procedure-related pain (e.g., bone marrow aspiration, needle puncture, lumbar puncture, removal of central venous line). Ljungman et al. (16) recently surveyed a group of Swedish children to describe the sources of pain in children being treated for cancer. This survey demonstrates again that the greatest sources of pain in children with cancer are from treatment and procedures.

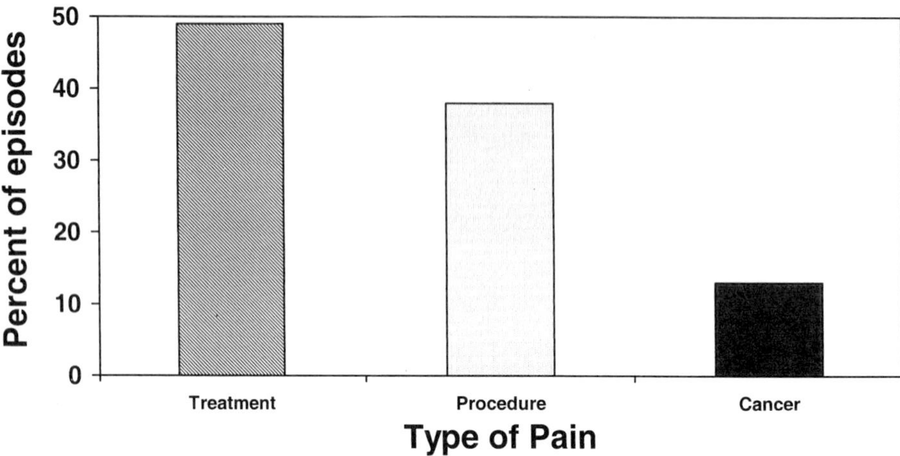

FIG. 29.4. Origin of pain in children with cancer. Breakdown of the causes of cancer pain in a group of 55 Swedish children who were given a structured interview. Results are reported as the percentage of the total episodes of pain (16).

At relapse or when tumors become resistant to treatment, tumor-related pain frequently occurs. Palliative chemotherapy and radiation may be used as modalities of pain control in terminal pediatric malignancy, depending on tumor type and sensitivity. Intractable pain in terminal pediatric malignancy occurs more commonly in patients with solid tumors metastatic to the central or peripheral nervous system (17).

Various nonmalignant chronic pain conditions have been encountered in young adult survivors of childhood cancer as a direct consequence of cancer and/or its treatment (18). The causes of these conditions include complex regional pain syndrome (CRPS) type II (causalgia) of the lower extremity, phantom limb pain, avascular necrosis, mechanical pain owing to failure of bony union after tumor resection, and rarely postherpetic neuralgia. Some patients require opioid therapy for the management of nonmalignant pain (18) (Fig. 29.4).

TUMOR-RELATED CAUSES OF PEDIATRIC CANCER PAIN

A number of children continue to have pain related to tumor despite the initial response of their pain to treatment. Miser et al. (14) found that one-third of the pain experienced by inpatients and approximately 20% of pain experienced by outpatients was owing to tumor.

Tumor-related pain commonly results in somatic, visceral, and neuropathic pain (Table 29.1). Somatic pain is usually well localized and frequently described as "aching" or "gnawing." Examples of somatic pain include pain associated with either primary or metastatic bone disease or postsurgical incisional pain. Visceral pain results from the infiltration, compression, distention, or stretching of thoracic and abdominal viscera by primary or metastatic tumor. This pain is poorly localized, is often described as "deep," "squeezing," and "pressure," and may be associated with nausea, vomiting, and diaphoresis, particularly when acute. An example of visceral pain includes pain associated with tumor of the liver, either primary (e.g., hepatoblastoma) or metastatic (e.g., neuroblastoma). Neuropathic pain most commonly results

TABLE 29.1. *Disease-related pain*

Bone pain (metastatic, leukemia)
Somatic pain (osteosarcoma, rhabdomyosarcoma)
Visceral pain (hepatocellular carcinoma)
Neuropathic pain (neuroblastoma/Ewing sarcoma of the spine)

from tumor compression or infiltration of peripheral nerves or the spinal cord. The clinical features of pain resulting from neural injury include dysesthesias with a burning and/or electrical quality, paroxysmal brief shooting or stabbing qualities, allodynia or pain that is induced by stimuli that are not normally painful (e.g., light touch of the skin), or pain that may be felt in the region of a sensory deficit (19).

Disease-related pain is best treated early on by administration of suitable analgesics. After antitumor therapy is initiated, it is common for disease-related pain to resolve quite expeditiously (10). For example, although most children with acute leukemia present with diffuse bone pain, within just a few days of initiating antileukemic therapy, all pain resolves.

TREATMENT-RELATED CAUSES OF PEDIATRIC CANCER PAIN

Treatment-related causes of pediatric cancer pain are outlined below and in Table 29.2.

Mucositis

The optimal management of pain related to radiation- and chemotherapy-induced mucositis is not established. A survey of U.S. hospitals indicated that there was wide variation in the management of oral mucositis in the adult population and no consistent approach to pain management despite National Institutes of Health guidelines (20,21). Initial therapy for treating mucositis includes single agents (saline, opioids, sodium bicarbonate, hydrogen peroxide, sucralfate suspension, clotrimazole, nystatin, viscous lidocaine, amphotericin B, dyclonine) or mouthwash mixtures often using combinations of single agents. Second- and third-line regimens for the management of mucositis are common and include opioids; however, there was no consistent pattern (20). A recent evaluation of three mouthwash regimens in adults (salt and soda, chlorhexidine, and lidocaine/diphenhydramine/antacid) showed no differences in time to resolution of mucositis symptoms (22).

TABLE 29.2. *Treatment-related pain*

Chemotherapy: mucositis, extravasation, neuropathy
Radiation therapy: mucositis, local tissue damage
Postoperative: phantom limb
Immune: graft-versus-host disease, infection
Postoperative

TABLE 29.3. *Mucositis mouthwash*

1 part viscous lidocaine (2%)
1 part diphenhydramine elixir
2 parts antacid suspension (Maalox or Mylanta)
1–2 parts water
Optional: flavoring of choice (vanilla)

The mucositis after conditioning for bone marrow transplantation is often intense and prolonged. Mucositis pain in transplant patients is typically continuous, with exacerbation during mouth care and on swallowing and awakening. The pain often precludes talking, eating, and, on occasions, swallowing (23). For patients with severe mucositis, our practice is to use parenteral opioids, primarily administered as a continuous infusion or by patient-controlled analgesia (PCA). Data are emerging regarding the safety and efficacy of PCA for mucositis pain after bone marrow transplantation in children (24).

The use of various mouthwash mixtures may be helpful to children with mucositis (25). It is important to be sure that the child is able to swish and spit the mixtures that contain absorbable active agents such as lidocaine or diphenhydramine (26) (Table 29.3). Capsaicin has been used as a counterstimulant to alleviate the pain of mucositis (27,28). In the report by Berger et al. (27), a formula for capsaicin-laced caramel lozenges is described.

Graft Versus Host Disease

Acute graft versus host disease may be associated with severe abdominal pain. This is not an uncommon cause of pain after allogeneic bone marrow transplantation and frequently requires the administration of opioids (24).

Phantom Limb Pain

Phantom sensations and phantom limb pain are common in children after an amputation. Unlike adults, this pain in children tends to decrease with time (29). Preoperative pain in the diseased extremity may be a predictor of subsequent phantom pain (29). In adults, preoperative regional anesthesia may be effective in preventing phantom limb pain (30). Gabapentin has proven to be quite useful in treating this type of pain (31–33).

Infection

Infection is common in children with cancer and often is associated with pain. Common locations of pain owing to infection in the immunocompromised child include perioral, perirectal, abdominal, and skin infection. Severe abdominal pain can be owing to typhlitis (infection of the cecum) in the immunocompromised, neutropenic patient (34–37). Resolution of pain is usually associated with treatment and resolution of the infection. It is common for acute herpes zoster to be associated with pain (38–40). Fortunately, it is uncommon for zoster infection to be associated with postherpetic neuralgia in children. In adults, treatment for postherpetic neuralgia includes tricyclic antidepressants, topical, regional, and systemic local anesthetics, and opioids.

Antineoplastic Therapy–Related Pain

Peripheral venous injection of some chemotherapeutic agents (e.g., leucovorin, thiotepa) may be associated with local pain at the time of injection. Thrombophlebitis occasionally develops after the injection of chemotherapy into a peripheral vein (41–43). Intrathecal chemotherapy has been associated with arachnoiditis and meningeal irritation syndrome (headache, nuchal rigidity, fever, nausea, vomiting) (44–46).

Extravasation of antineoplastic agents has become much less common because of the increased use of central venous lines and peripherally inserted central catheters. Vesicants, when extravasated, produce local necrosis, whereas irritants produce burning or inflammation without necrosis. For many years, vincristine, anthracyclines (doxorubicin or daunorubicin), and actinomycin D have been used extensively to treat childhood cancer. These agents cause severe local reaction with tissue necrosis when extravasated and should be managed immediately with one of several antidote techniques (47–49). Extravasation of sclerosing chemotherapeutic agents has even been described in damaged intrathoracic catheters (50). Severe local tissue necrosis with possible local nerve injury may require multimodal pain management including opioids and antineuropathic therapy.

Administration of vincristine can commonly cause a peripheral neuropathy that is associated with pain (51). Radiation to the spine or areas involving peripheral nerves may contribute to worsening of this peripheral neuropathy. Treatment is usually successful by reducing or eliminating the vincristine or by administration of a tricyclic antidepressant or gabapentin (52,53). A long-term pain management problem may be associated with painful vincristine neuropathy. Although this is uncommon in childhood and is usually a self-limiting condition, it may cause severe pain requiring treatment with opioids and adjuvant analgesics.

As new antineoplastic agents become available for the treatment of childhood cancer, the practitioner must be aware of the possibility of new pain syndromes arising. The monoclonal antibody 3F8 is a novel antiganglioside agent for the treatment of stage 4 neuroblastoma. The infusion of this agent has been associated with severe abdominal and limb pain in children despite opioid premedication (54).

Even otherwise salutary therapies used in the supportive care of patients with cancer may cause painful syndromes. For example, granulocyte colony–stimulating factor and granulocyte-monocyte–stimulating factor have been associated with significant bone pain (55–57). The predominant side effect associated with administration of granulocyte colony–stimulating factor in adults is medullary bone pain, and this effect is dose related (58). It is most often observed shortly after administration of granulocyte colony–stimulating factor and again just before the onset of neutrophil recovery. The pain associated with granulocyte colony–stimulating factor usually responds to nonopioid analgesics.

Postoperative Pain

The management of postoperative pain in the child with cancer is similar to the management in patients without malignancy, and this has been reviewed elsewhere in this volume. Patients who have been receiving preoperative opioids should have their daily dose of opioids calculated, and this dose used as a baseline to which additional opioids are added for the purposes of postoperative pain control. If this principle is ignored in postoperative care, there will be dramatic undermedication in opioid-dependent oncology patients.

Procedure-Related Pain

In 1987, Miser et al. (14) first reported the observation that much of the pain of childhood cancer was related to invasive procedures. In 1999 and 2000, when Ljungman et al. (16,59) readdressed this issue, they found that the relative proportion of pain owing to procedures had actually risen to almost 40% of all pain episodes in children with cancer. Survivors of childhood cancer vividly recall the difficulties in experiencing repeated painful procedures (60). There is no clear evidence to confirm the importance of aggressive management of painful procedures in children with cancer. However, there is some contextual support for the notion that it is important to proactively manage painful procedures in children who can be expected to have many such procedures in the course of their treatment (61). In this brief follow-up study of children undergoing bone marrow aspirations and/or lumbar puncture, the authors demonstrated that in children who received placebos for their first painful procedure, pain scores did not decrease even when otherwise adequate analgesia was provided in the future.

TABLE 29.4. *Procedure-related pain*

Needles: intravenous lines, port access, phlebotomy
Bone marrow aspiration/biopsy
Lumbar puncture
Central line removal
Diagnostic procedures

Procedure-related causes of pain in children with cancer are outlined below and in Table 29.4.

Needle Puncture

Needle procedures are a major source of distress for children (62). Needle puncture is required for obtaining blood specimens, administration of intravenous or intramuscular chemotherapy (e.g., methotrexate or L-asparaginase), or access to implanted intravenous access devices.

Children need adequate preparation before their first needle puncture to minimize fear and anxiety. This preparation starts with the practitioner working with a child's parents to obtain insight into the child's coping style, to explain to them the nature of the procedure, and to enlist their support (63). An age-appropriate explanation to the child should follow with consideration of that particular child's previous experience of painful procedures and coping style (64).

Various topical treatments have been used to provide analgesia for needle procedures. Skin cooling with either ice or fluorocarbon coolant sprays has been used with some success (65). The eutectic mixture of local anesthetics [lidocaine-prilocaine cream (EMLA)] has become a useful method of topical anesthesia (66,67). The depth of penetration of this anesthesia increases in proportion to the duration of the application of the lidocaine-prilocaine cream (68). Lidocaine-prilocaine cream has proved safe, with low plasma local anesthetic concentrations and a negligible risk of methemoglobinemia (69–73). Lidocaine-prilocaine cream provides no analgesia for structures deep to the dermis but can make subsequent deeper infiltration with local anesthetic less painful. Both skin cooling and lidocaine-prilocaine cream may produce vasoconstriction, which may make venous cannulation more difficult in some patients. Preliminary studies of topical amethocaine (tetracaine) for cutaneous analgesia before venous cannulation, subcutaneous port access, and neonatal skin prick has demonstrated promising safety and efficacy data (74–80).

Lumbar Puncture

The pain related to lumbar puncture is mainly related to the skin puncture by the spinal needle and the inadvertent encounter with the periosteum in one of the bony vertebral structures. Although the dura is a pain-sensitive structure, it is uncommon for patients to experience pain as the dura is punctured or as intrathecal medication is instilled. Lidocaine-prilocaine cream or other topical local anesthetics may be useful when applied before the administration of local anesthesia (81). The main distress of lumbar puncture for children is often related to the required body position and the necessity to remain still until the procedure is complete. It is therefore essential that the personnel performing this procedure in children be highly skilled and quite familiar with normal anatomy so that the child does not experience inordinate discomfort from "probing" for the subarachnoid space. Some children are unable to comply with these requirements, and they should be offered conscious sedation or general anesthesia.

Lumbar puncture may produce a sustained cerebrospinal fluid leak, leading to low intracranial pressure. The epidemiology of postdural puncture headache in children with cancer is not known (45,46,82,83). Although it is presumed to be owing to the same physiology of low cerebral spinal fluid pressure owing to a leak at the puncture site, the contributory role of various intrathecal medications remains undefined (82,83). The treatment of postdural puncture headache is generally with simple analgesics, caffeine, and adequate hydration and placing the patient in the supine position. In refractory cases, an epidural blood patch (i.e., the injection of autologous blood in the epidural space) may be required (84–86). It is also easily prevented by the use of noncutting, pencil-point spinal needles (e.g., Sprotte, Whitacre) of the smallest caliber (24 to 29 gauge) that can be used to both sample cerebral spinal fluid and inject intrathecal medications (87–89).

Bone Marrow Aspiration/Biopsy

The almost universal distress of children having bone marrow aspiration has been previously documented (90,91). The pain related to bone marrow aspiration is related to the insertion of a large needle into the posterior iliac space and to the unpleasant sensation experienced at the time of marrow aspiration. The latter pain is not alleviated by the administration of local anesthetic. Cognitive-behavioral therapy (e.g., guided imagery, relaxation, hypnosis), conscious sedation, and general anesthesia have been shown to be effective modalities for the control of pain and distress (92–101). Every center caring for children with cancer should develop suitable algorithms in their institution to facilitate good pain management for children undergoing bone marrow aspiration or biopsy. No particular method can be advocated as absolutely superior; however, the choice should be based on the age of the patient, patient preference, previous painful experiences, temperament, and availability of supportive services. Options should be tailored to individual needs (102).

Removal of Central Venous Lines

The increasing use of tunneled central venous lines in children with cancer has created the need for sedation or brief general anesthesia for the removal of central venous lines.

Other Invasive Diagnostic Procedures

Children with malignancies frequently require diagnostic evaluation of new lesions, infectious or malignant. These are now commonly performed in radiology suites where needle-guided sampling is performed using procedural sedation or general anesthesia. When children are sent for these potentially painful procedures, it is important to ensure that a suitable pain management plan is established.

NONTREATMENT AND NONTUMOR CAUSES OF PAIN IN CHILDREN WITH CANCER

The pediatric oncology patient is just as prone to causes of pain unrelated to either the tumor or its treatment as the general pediatric population. Potential causes related to the tumor or its treatment must be excluded. Acute appendicitis in children with cancer may present a diagnostic dilemma and is associated with a high diagnostic error rate (103).

Chronic Pain in Survivors of Childhood Cancer

Practitioners must be alert to the potential for chronic pain management problems to arise as a consequence of treatment. There is little literature about chronic pain as a consequence of treatment in children with cancer (104,105). Various problems have been encountered in long-term survivors of childhood cancer including chronic abdominal pain of uncertain origin, complex regional pain syndrome type I of the lower extremity, phantom limb pain, chronic lower extremity pain owing to a mechanical problem with an internal prosthesis, avascular necrosis of multiple joints, neuralgia and mechanical pain owing to failure of bony union after tumor resection, and postherpetic neuralgia. Patients may develop scoliosis and then musculoskeletal pain as a result of therapy in the chest such as rib resections or radiation therapy. Some patients require chronic opioids or long-term adjuvant therapy for neuropathic pain syndromes.

Nonpharmacologic Approaches to Pain Management in Children with Cancer

The techniques employed for nonpharmacologic methods of pain control in children include physical (e.g., physical therapy, massage, heat and cold stimulation, electrical nerve stimulation, acupuncture), behavioral (e.g., exercise, relaxation, biofeedback, modeling, desensitization, art and play therapy), and cognitive (e.g., distraction, attention, imagery, thought stopping, hypnosis, music therapy, psychotherapy). Selection of an appropriate method is determined by whether the intervention is focused on modifying an individual's sensory perception, behaviors, or thoughts and coping abilities (106).

In the context of childhood cancer, cognitive-behavioral techniques are most commonly used to decrease distress and enhance a child's ability to cope with medical procedures (107–110). These techniques have also been popularized as adjuvant therapy for the treatment of nausea and vomiting during administration of chemotherapy (111–114). During nonpainful procedures, such as radiotherapy, children can be assisted by hypnotic techniques (115). There also appears to be a role for incorporating cognitive-behavioral techniques into the end-of-life care plan for children with cancer (116–118).

Cognitive-behavioral approaches have the advantage that learning them for one situation may generalize to their use in another situation. A child who learns relaxation training and guided imagery to manage needle procedures may then apply this method to managing headache, dyspnea, nausea, or other symptoms. In a recent film by Dr. Leora Kuttner, several survivors of childhood cancer recount the importance and utility of learning cognitive-behavioral methods (119). Several of them commented on how they incorporated these skills as lifelong tools to cope with stress, illness, and childbearing.

The decision to use a psychologic or pharmacologic approach or both for pain procedures depends on the nature of the procedure and skill of the practitioner, an understanding of the child and family, and the expectations of pain and anxiety for that child undergoing that procedure. The choice of which nonpharmacologic method to use is based on factors such as the child's age, behavioral factors, coping ability, fear and anxiety, and the type of pain experienced in the past.

The preparation of a child undergoing a painful procedure involves providing a description of the steps of a given procedure and the sensations experienced. This is perhaps the most common intervention for children about to undergo invasive medical procedures. The rationale for this intervention is that unexpected stress is more anxiety provoking and more difficult to cope with than anticipated or predictable stress (64,120). It is helpful to perform the procedure in a quiet, calm environment conducive to reducing stress and anxiety and in a location separate from the child's room.

The effectiveness of hypnosis in the reduction of pain and anxiety during bone marrow aspiration and lumbar puncture in children has been confirmed by several reports (107–109,121). Similarly, the role of distraction techniques in reducing children's distress during procedures has been examined by several investigators and shown to be effective. One study demonstrated distraction to be less effective for younger children (122). Another study enlisted the support of parents and showed a reduction in the children's behavioral distress and lowering of the parents' anxiety (123). Several investigators have examined and shown the effectiveness of cognitive-behavioral interventions that have included preparatory information, relaxation, imagery, positive coping statements, modeling, and behavioral rehearsal (124,125).

PHARMACOTHERAPY FOR THE MANAGEMENT OF CANCER PAIN IN CHILDREN

Analgesic Studies in Children with Cancer

Improvement in pediatric pain management will depend in part on advances in analgesic therapeutics. The few analgesic studies that have been performed in children with cancer generally had few subjects and few were controlled (126). There have been no controlled clinical trials of adjuvant analgesics in pediatrics. Although the pharmacokinetic and major pharmacodynamic properties of most opioids have been studied in pediatrics, little information is available about oral bioavailability and potency ratios.

Analgesics

The prescription of analgesics for children with cancer pain is based on the World Health Organization analgesic ladder. The prescription of analgesics should be according to pain severity, ranging from acetaminophen and nonsteroidal anti-inflammatory drugs for mild pain (step 1 of the ladder) to mild opioids with or without step 1 drugs (step 2) and finally to opioids for moderate and severe pain (step 3). The choice of analgesic is individualized to achieve an optimal balance between analgesia and side effects. In patients with known recognized severe pain problems, it is not necessary to slowly advance up this so-called analgesic ladder. Initiation of therapy with a parenteral opioid may very well be the initial intervention.

Nonopioid Analgesics

Acetaminophen inhibits prostaglandin synthesis primarily in the central nervous system. It is one of the most commonly used nonopioid analgesics in children and does not have the side effects of gastritis and inhibition of platelet function found with aspirin and other older nonsteroidal anti-inflammatory drugs. Although acetaminophen has a potential for hepatic and renal injury, this is uncommon in therapeutic doses (127). Acetaminophen does not have an association with Reye syndrome (128–132).

The antipyretic action of acetaminophen may be contraindicated in neutropenic patients in whom it is important to monitor fever. Oral dosing of 15 mg/kg every 4 hours is recommended, with a maximal daily dose of 90 mg/kg in children and 60 mg/kg in infants and neonates. There are no data on the safety of chronic administration of acetaminophen in infants and children.

In selected children with adequate platelet number and function, nonsteroidal anti-inflammatory drugs may be helpful analgesics, both alone and in combination with opioids. However, aspirin and, nonsteroidal anti-inflammatory drugs are often contraindicated in pediatric oncology patients at risk of bleeding owing to thrombocytopenia. Choline magnesium trisalicylate (Trilisate) has been recommended because of adult reports of minimal effects on platelet function *in vitro* and experimental studies showing minimal gastric irritation in rats in contrast to aspirin (133). Such data should be viewed with caution because they do not include medically ill patients with thrombocytopenia or other morbidities. There are no data on the safety, efficacy, and tolerability of new cyclooxygenase-2 inhibitors (celecoxib, refecoxib, and valdecoxib) in children with cancer, although these new agents do not inhibit platelet function and have markedly reduced gastrointestinal side effects (134,135).

Opioid Analgesics

Codeine is a phenanthrene alkaloid derived from morphine and is generally prescribed for moderate pain. Codeine is commonly administered orally in children and often in combination with acetaminophen. Codeine is often administered in pediatrics in oral doses of 0.5 to 1 mg/kg every 4 hours for children older than 6 months of age.

Oxycodone is a semisynthetic opioid and is used for moderate to severe pain. Oxycodone is available as a long-acting preparation and as an oral preparation in combination with acetaminophen or ibuprofen. The long-acting preparation (OxyContin) has a more rapid onset of clinical analgesia than long-acting morphine, but it is formulated in a pill that must be swallowed intact (136,137). Oxycodone has a higher clearance value and a shorter elimination half-life in children 2 to 20 years of age than adults (138–140).

Morphine is perhaps the most widely used opioid for moderate to severe cancer pain in children. It can be employed via the oral, intravenous, subcutaneous, epidural, and intrathecal routes. The major hepatic metabolite of morphine (morphine-6-glucuronide) produces analgesia and side effects comparable with those of morphine with long-term dosing (141,142). Morphine-6-glucuronide may accumulate and result in opioid side effects in patients with renal insufficiency.

Morphine clearance is delayed in the first 1 to 3 months of life. The half-life of morphine changes from 10 to 20 hours in preterm infants to 1 to 2 hours in young children (143–145). Starting doses in very young infants should be reduced by approximately 25% to 50% on a per kilogram basis relative to the dosing recommended for older children. During the neonatal period for term infants, the volume of distribution is linearly related to age and body surface area (143,146,147). A recent study suggested that when given an equivalent dose for weight, younger children are likely to have significantly lower plasma morphine and metabolite concentrations (148). Nonetheless, young infants may be more prone to the respiratory depressive effects of opioids, and caution should be exercised in choosing a dose. A starting dose for oral morphine of 0.2 to 0.3 mg/kg per dose is recommended for children with pain unrelieved by mild or moderate strength analgesics (148).

Oral morphine has a significant first-pass metabolism in the liver. An oral-to-parenteral potency ratio of approximately 3:1 is commonly employed during long-term administration (149). Typical starting intravenous morphine infusion rates are 0.02 to 0.03 mg/kg per hour after the first 4 months of life and 0.015 mg/kg per hour in younger infants. Sustained-release oral tablets of morphine (MS Contin) are available for use and are usually administered at twice-daily intervals. Dosing at 8-hour intervals may be appropriate in children (148). Crushing sustained-released tablets produces immediate release of morphine and is not recommended. Sustained-release capsules (Kadian) with time-released pellets are also available (150). These have the advantage of being able to be mixed with semisolids for administration to children who cannot swallow pills.

Hydromorphone is an alternative opioid when dose-limiting side effects of morphine develop. In addition, hydromorphone appears to be safe to use in patients with impaired renal function. Hydromorphone is available for oral, intravenous, subcutaneous, epidural, and intrathecal administration. It has been reported as an effective analgesic agent in several studies of children with cancer (24,151, 152). A double-blind, randomized, crossover comparison of morphine to hydromorphone using PCA in children and adolescents with mucositis after bone marrow transplantation showed that hydromorphone was well tolerated and had a potency ratio of approximately 6:1 relative to morphine in this setting (153). Adult studies indicate that intravenous hydromorphone is five to eight times as potent as morphine (154). Hydromorphone is convenient for subcutaneous infusion because of its high potency and aqueous solubility. Little is known about the pharmacokinetics of hydromorphone in infants and children.

Fentanyl is a synthetic opioid approximately 50 to 100 times more potent than morphine during single intravenous administration (155–157). Fentanyl is highly lipid soluble and has a very rapid onset of action after intravenous administration. Fentanyl is eliminated almost entirely by hepatic metabolism. The half-life of fentanyl is prolonged in preterm infants undergoing cardiac surgery (158), but values comparable with those of adults are reached within the first months of life (156,159–162). The clearance of fentanyl is higher in infants and young children than in adults (162).

The duration of action of fentanyl after single intravenous bolus administration is shorter than that for morphine. This feature makes fentanyl useful for procedures in which rapid onset and short duration are important. Fentanyl may be used as an alternative opioid for patients with dose-limiting side effects with morphine (163–165). Rapid administration of high doses of intravenous fentanyl may result in chest wall rigidity and severe ventilatory difficulty (166–169).

The use of oral transmucosal fentanyl for sedation/analgesia during bone marrow biopsy/aspiration and lumbar puncture in children with cancer has been described (170). The frequency of vomiting seen in this study may limit the usefulness of this technique. In a small study using a clinical protocol, the utility, feasibility, and tolerability of transdermal fentanyl were demonstrated in children with cancer pain (171). The mean clearance and volume of distribution of transdermal fentanyl were the same for both adults and children, but the variability was higher for adults (171). A larger study is required to confirm these findings.

Meperidine is a short half-life synthetic opioid and has been used for procedural and postoperative pain in children. Neonates have a slower elimination of meperidine than children and young infants (172–175). Normeperidine, a metabolite of meperidine, can cause central nervous system excitatory effects including tremors and convulsions (176–179). This can occur particularly in patients with renal impairment. Meperidine is not generally recommended for children with chronic pain requiring opioids. Meperidine in low doses (0.25 to 0.5 mg/kg intravenously) is used for the prophylaxis and treatment of rigors after the infusion of amphotericin (180–182) or after administration of general anesthesia (183–185).

Methadone is a synthetic opioid that has a long and variable half-life in children. The oral-to-parenteral potency ratio is approximately 2:1. In children receiving postoperative analgesia, methadone produced equivalent but more prolonged analgesia than morphine (186,187). Because of its prolonged half-life, methadone has a risk of delayed sedation and overdose occurring several days after initiating treatment.

Frequent patient assessment is the key to the safe and effective use of methadone. If a patient becomes oversedated, it is recommended that the drug be held and the patient be observed until alertness has improved. Although as-needed dosing is discouraged for most patients with cancer pain, some clinicians find this approach a useful way to establish a dosing schedule for methadone (186). Methadone remains a long-acting agent when administered either as an elixir or as crushed tablets.

ROUTES AND METHODS OF ANALGESIC ADMINISTRATION

Analgesics should be administered to children by the simplest, safest, most effective, and least painful route. The oral route of administration of analgesics is therefore the first choice for most patients. Oral dosing is generally predictable and inexpensive and does not require invasive procedures or technologies. The intramuscular administration of an opioid is painful and may lead to the underreporting of pain. This route of administration does not permit easy dose titration or infusion and should be avoided. Rectal administration is discouraged in children with cancer because of concern regarding infection, the variability of rectal absorption of drugs, and the undesirability of this delivery route (81).

Intravenous administration of opioids has the advantage of rapid onset of analgesia, easier opioid dose titration, bioavailability, and continuous effect when infusions are used. The subcutaneous route is an alternative route of administration for children with poor intravenous access (188). Subcutaneous infusion rates generally do not exceed 1 to 3 mL per hour (189). A small catheter or butterfly needle (25 to 27 gauge) may be placed under the skin of the thorax, abdomen, or thigh. Subcutaneous infusion sites are changed approximately every 3 to 7 days.

PCA has been used for the management of prolonged oropharyngeal mucositis pain after bone marrow transplantation in children and adolescents (23,24,153). PCA is a method of opioid administration that permits the patient to self-administer a small bolus dose of opioid within set time limits. In postoperative use, PCA is widely used by children 6 to 7 years of age and older (190–193).

PCA allows appropriate children to have control over their analgesia and to choose a balance between the benefits of analgesia versus the side effects of opioids. In patients with severe mucositis, for example, opioid dosing can be timed with routine mouth care and other causes of incidental mouth pain. A controlled comparison of staff-controlled continuous infusion of morphine and PCA in adolescents with severe oropharyngeal mucositis found that the PCA group had equivalent analgesia but less sedation and less difficulty concentrating (23).

Opioid Dose Schedules

Unless painful episodes are truly incidental and unpredictable, analgesics should generally be administered at regular times to provide continuous pain relief. Should breakthrough pain occur, as-needed doses of opioid are incorporated into the analgesic regimen to allow a patient to have additional analgesia. Rescue doses of opioid may be calculated as approximately 5% to 10% of the total daily opioid requirement and may be administered every hour (149).

Opioid dose escalation may be required after opioid administration begins and periodically thereafter. The size of an opioid dose increment may be calculated as follows:

1. If greater than approximately six rescue doses of opioid are given in a 24-hour period, then the total daily opioid dose should be increased by the total of opioid given as rescue medication. For example, the hourly average of the total daily rescue opioid should be added to the baseline opioid infusion. An alternative to this method would be to increase the baseline infusion by 50% (149).
2. Rescue doses are kept as a proportion of the baseline opioid dose. This dose can be 5% to 10% of the total daily dose (149). An alternative to this method could be between 50% to 200% of the hourly basal infusion rate (149).

Opioid Switching

The indication for an opioid switch to an alternative opioid is dose-limiting side effects. In other words, the dose of opioid required to achieve adequate analgesia is limited by opioid side effects experienced by an individual.

These usually include pruritus, nausea/vomiting, and sedation/dysphoria. A favorable change in analgesia to side effect profile will be experienced if there is less cross-tolerance at the opioid receptors mediating analgesia than at those mediating adverse effects (194).

After long-term opioid dosing of short-acting opioids, equivalent analgesia may be attained with a dose of a second opioid that is approximately 50% lower than that calculated from an equianalgesic table (194). In contrast to short half-life opioids, the doses of methadone required for equivalent analgesia after switching may be 10% to 20% of the equianalgesic dose of the previously used short half-life opioid. A protocol for methadone dose conversion and titration has been reported (195).

Opioid Side Effects

Children do not necessarily report opioid side effects voluntarily (e.g., constipation, pruritus, unpleasant dreams) and should be asked specifically about these problems. An assessment of opioid side effects should be included in an assessment of analgesic effectiveness. All opioids can potentially cause the same constellation of side effects. If side effects limit opioid dose escalation, then consideration should be given to an opioid switch. Tolerance to some opioid side effects (e.g., sedation, nausea/vomiting, pruritus) often develops within the first week of starting these drugs. Children do not develop tolerance to constipation, and concurrent treatment with laxatives should be considered.

Adjuvant Analgesics in Children with Cancer

Adjuvant analgesics are a heterogeneous group of medications that have a primary indication other than pain management but are analgesic in some painful conditions (196). Commonly, these drugs are prescribed in conjunction with primary analgesics. Classes of adjuvant agents include antidepressants, anticonvulsants, neuroleptics, psychostimulants, antihistamines, corticosteroids, and centrally acting skeletal muscle relaxants.

Antidepressants

Tricyclic antidepressants have been used for a variety of pain conditions in adults including cancer pain (197). A recent review of the published data on the efficacy of a variety of adjuvant drugs used in the treatment of neuropathic pain showed that the tricyclic antidepressants required the fewest patients to treat for positive effects (198). Data from adult studies have guided the use of antidepressants as adjuvant analgesics in pediatrics (199–201). Baseline hematology and biochemistry tests and an electrocardiogram to exclude Wolff–Parkinson–White syndrome or other cardiac conduction defects have been recommended before starting treatment with tricyclic antidepressants (202). An electrocardiogram is recommended periodically during long-term use or if standard milligram per kilogram doses are exceeded (203–205).

Psychostimulants

The use of dextroamphetamine and methylphenidate was reported in a survey of 11 children receiving opioids for a variety of painful conditions including cancer pain (206). Somnolence was reduced in these patients without significant adverse side effects. Dextroamphetamine potentiates opioid analgesia in postoperative adult patients, and methylphenidate counteracts opioid-induced sedation and cognitive dysfunction in patients with advance-stage cancer (207–209). The potential side effects of methylphenidate include anorexia, insomnia, and dysphoria.

Corticosteroids

Corticosteroids may have a role in bone pain owing to metastatic bone disease (210–212) and cerebral edema owing to either primary or metastatic tumor (213–217) and epidural spinal cord compression (13,217,

218). Dexamethasone tends to be the most frequently used corticosteroid because of its high potency, duration of action, and minimal mineralocorticoid effect.

Corticosteroids may produce analgesia by a variety of mechanisms including anti-inflammatory effects, reduction of tumor edema, and potentially by a reduction of spontaneous discharge in injured nerves (219).

Anticonvulsants

The mechanism of action of anticonvulsants in controlling lancinating pain is not understood but is probably related to reducing paroxysmal discharges of neurons (220,221). Standard anticonvulsants may be problematic in children with cancer because of their potential adverse effects on the hematologic profile. Nonetheless, several of them have been shown to have efficacy in relieving neuropathic pain. Carbamazepine, phenytoin, and valproic acid have been the mainstay anticonvulsants for neuropathic pain for some time (221–225). Gabapentin, which is well tolerated, appears to be useful for the treatment of neuropathic pain (226–228). Gabapentin does not appear to have significant effects on hematopoiesis and, therefore, may be the drug of choice in children with cancer and neuropathic pain (229–231). It has been used successfully in the treatment of phantom limb pain in children and adolescents (31). The newer anticonvulsants oxcarbazepine, lamotrigine, and topiramate have not been evaluated for treatment of neuropathic pain in children (221,232,233).

Radionuclides

Radionuclide therapy for painful osseous metastases has been reported in the adult literature (90). Bone-seeking radionuclides used include strontium 89, phosphorus 32, iodine 131, and tin 117m (234–237). ^{131}I-iodine-meta-iodobenzylguanidine has been studied in children with disseminated and painful metastatic bone disease owing to neuroblastoma (236,238–240). The side effects of ^{131}I-iodine-meta-iodobenzylguanidine were thrombocytopenia and cystitis.

Neuroleptics

Some authors suggest that some of the neuroleptic drugs can be used in the treatment of cancer pain (241–243). Although for many years, these drugs were thought to be coanalgesics with the opioids, there is little direct proof of this concept. This class of drug does have profound sedating properties, which probably explain the perception of coanalgesia (244).

Methotrimeprazine, a phenothiazine, appears to have analgesic properties in adult cancer pain (245). It should not be used as a substitute for opioid analgesia, even though there are reports of its analgesic efficacy (241,246–248). The mechanism by which methotrimeprazine produces analgesia and its role as an adjuvant analgesic agent in children with cancer pain is unclear. Methotrimeprazine may be useful as an adjuvant in patients with disseminated cancer who experience pain associated with anxiety, restlessness, or nausea (245,248,249).

CONCLUSION

Pain is a common symptom in children with cancer and is most commonly related to treatment. The World Health Organization created a set of guidelines for the universal application of the principles of pain management and palliative care for all children with cancer. Intractable cancer pain is rare in children and is most common in children with a solid tumor metastatic to spinal nerve roots, spinal cord, or larger peripheral nerves. The approach to cancer pain management should involve a multidisciplinary approach and employ both pharmacologic agents and nonpharmacologic methods of pain control.

REFERENCES

1. World Health Organization. Cancer pain relief and palliative care. Report of a WHO Expert Committee. *WHO Tech Rep Ser* 1990;804:1–75.
2. Berde C, Ablin A, Glazer J, et al. Report of the Sub-

committee on Disease-Related Pain in Childhood Cancer. *Pediatrics* 1990;86:818–825.
3. Zeltzer LK, Altman A, Cohen D, et al. Report of the Subcommittee on the Management of Pain Associated with Procedures in Children with Cancer. *Pediatrics* 1990;86[Suppl 5]:826–831.
4. McGrath PJ, Beyer J, Cleeland C, et al. Report of the Subcommittee on Assessment and Methodologic Issues in the Management of Pain in Childhood Cancer. *Pediatrics* 1990;86:814–817.
5. World Health Organization. *Cancer pain relief: with a guide to opioid availability*, 2nd ed. Geneva: World Health Organization, 1996.
6. Benedetti C, Brock C, Cleeland C, et al. NCCN practice guidelines for cancer pain. *Oncology (Huntingt)* 2000;14:135–150.
7. Ries LAG, Eisner MP, Kosary CL, et al., eds. *SEER Cancer Statistics Review, 1973–1998*. Bethesda, MD: National Cancer Institute, 2001.
8. World Health Organization. *Cancer pain relief and palliative care in children*. Geneva: World Health Organization, 1998.
9. Collins JJ, Byrnes ME, Dunkel IJ, et al. The measurement of symptoms in children with cancer. *J Pain Symptom Manage* 2000;19:363–377.
10. Miser AW, McCalla J, Dothage JA, et al. Pain as a presenting symptom in children and young adults with newly diagnosed malignancy. *Pain* 1987;29:85–90.
11. Heideman R, Packer R, Albright L, et al. *Tumors of the central nervous system*, 3rd ed. Philadelphia: Lippincott–Raven, 1997.
12. Hahn Y, McClone D. Pain in children with spinal cord tumors. *Child Brain* 1984;11:36–46.
13. Lewis DW, Packer RJ, Raney B, et al. Incidence, presentation, and outcome of spinal cord disease in children with systemic cancer. *Pediatrics* 1986;78:438–443.
14. Miser A, Dothage J, Wesley R, et al. The prevalence of pain in a pediatric and young adult cancer population. *Pain* 1987;29:73–83.
15. Elliott S, Miser A, Dose A, et al. Epidemiologic features of pain in pediatric cancer patients: a co-operative community-based study. *Clin J Pain* 1991;7: 263–268.
16. Ljungman G, Gordh T, Sorensen S, et al. Pain in paediatric oncology: interviews with children, adolescents and their parents. *Acta Paediatr* 1999;88:623–630.
17. Collins JJ, Grier HE, Kinney HC, et al. Control of severe pain in children with terminal malignancy. *J Pediatr* 1995;126:653–657.
18. Collins JJ, Berde CB. Management of pain in children. In: Pizzo PA, Poplack DG, eds. *Principles and practice of pediatric oncology*, 3rd ed. Philadelphia: Lippincott–Raven, 1997:1183–1199.
19. Loeser JD, Bonica JJ. *Bonica's management of pain*, 3rd ed. Philadelphia: Lippincott Williams & Wilkins, 2001.
20. Mueller BA, Millheim ET, Farrington EA, et al. Mucositis management practices for hospitalized patients: national survey results. *J Pain Symptom Manage* 1995; 10:510–520.
21. National Institutes of Health. *National Institutes of Health Consensus Development Conference Statement: oral complications of cancer therapies: diagnosis, prevention, and treatment*. Bethesda, MD; National Institutes of Health, 1989.
22. Dodd MJ, Dibble SL, Miaskowski C, et al. Randomized clinical trial of the effectiveness of 3 commonly used mouthwashes to treat chemotherapy-induced mucositis. *Oral Surg Oral Med Oral Pathol Oral Radiol Endod* 2000;90:39–47.
23. Mackie AM, Coda BC, Hill HF. Adolescents use patient-controlled analgesia effectively for relief from prolonged oropharyngeal mucositis pain. *Pain* 1991; 46:265–269.
24. Dunbar PJ, Buckley P, Gavrin JR, et al. Use of patient-controlled analgesia for pain control for children receiving bone marrow transplant. *J Pain Symptom Manage* 1995;10:604–611.
25. Kennedy L, Diamond J. Assessment and management of chemotherapy-induced mucositis in children. *J Pediatr Oncol Nurs* 1997;14:164–174, quiz 75–77.
26. Elad S, Cohen G, Zylber-Katz E, et al. Systemic absorption of lidocaine after topical application for the treatment of oral mucositis in bone marrow transplantation patients. *J Oral Pathol Med* 1999;28:170–172.
27. Berger A, Henderson M, Nadoolman W, et al. Oral capsaicin provides temporary relief for oral mucositis pain secondary to chemotherapy/radiation therapy. *J Pain Symptom Manage* 1995;10:243–248.
28. Hautkappe M, Roizen MF, Toledano A, et al. Review of the effectiveness of capsaicin for painful cutaneous disorders and neural dysfunction. *Clin J Pain* 1998;14: 97–106.
29. Krane EJ, Heller LB. The prevalence of phantom sensation and pain in pediatric amputees. *J Pain Symptom Manage* 1995;10:21–29.
30. Bach S, Noreng M, Tjellden N. Phantom limb pain in amputees during the first twelve months following limb amputation after preoperative lumbar epidural blockade. *Pain* 1988;33:297–301.
31. Rusy LM, Troshynski TJ, Weisman SJ. Gabapentin in phantom limb pain management in children and young adults: report of seven cases. *J Pain Symptom Manage* 2001;21:78–82.
32. Dangel T. Chronic pain management in children. Part I: cancer and phantom pain. *Paediatr Anaesth* 1998;8: 5–10.
33. Rosenberg JM, Harrell C, Ristic H, et al. The effect of gabapentin on neuropathic pain. *Clin J Pain* 1997;13: 251–255.
34. Schwartz IS. Typhlitis. *N Y State J Med* 1989;89:426.
35. Hiruki T, Fernandes B, Ramsay J, et al. Acute typhlitis in an immunocompromised host. Report of an unusual case and review of the literature. *Dig Dis Sci* 1992;37: 1292–1296.
36. Moir DH, Bale PM. Necropsy findings in childhood leukaemia, emphasizing neutropenic enterocolitis and cerebral calcification. *Pathology* 1976;8:247–258.
37. Alexander JE, Williamson SL, Seibert JJ, et al. The ultrasonographic diagnosis of typhlitis (neutropenic colitis). *Pediatr Radiol* 1988;18:200–204.
38. Portenoy RK, Duma C, Foley KM. Acute herpetic and postherpetic neuralgia: clinical review and current management. *Ann Neurol* 1986;20:651–664.
39. King RB. Concerning the management of pain associated with herpes zoster and of postherpetic neuralgia. *Pain* 1988;33:73–78.
40. Koc Y, Miller KB, Schenkein DP, et al. Varicella zoster virus infections following allogeneic bone marrow transplantation: frequency, risk factors, and clinical

outcome. *Biol Blood Marrow Transplant* 2000;6:44–49.
41. Nguyen LT, Laberge JM, Guttman FM, et al. Spontaneous deep vein thrombosis in childhood and adolescence. *J Pediatr Surg* 1986;21:640–643.
42. Rickles FR, Levine MN. Venous thromboembolism in malignancy and malignancy in venous thromboembolism. *Haemostasis* 1998;28[Suppl 3]:43–49.
43. Booth BW, Weiss RB. Venous thrombosis during adjuvant chemotherapy. *N Engl J Med* 1981;305:170.
44. D'Angio GJ. Early and delayed complications of therapy. *Cancer* 1983;51[Suppl 12]:2515–2518.
45. Geiser CF, Bishop Y, Jaffe N, et al. Adverse effects of intrathecal methotrexate in children with acute leukemia in remission. *Blood* 1975;45:189–195.
46. Steinherz P, Jereb B, Galicich J. Therapy of CNS leukemia with intraventricular chemotherapy and low-dose neuraxis radiotherapy. *J Clin Oncol* 1985;3:1217–1226.
47. Buchanan GR, Buchsbaum HJ, O'Banion K, et al. Extravasation of dactinomycin, vincristine, and cisplatin: studies in an animal model. *Med Pediatr Oncol* 1985;13:375–380.
48. Kassner E. Evaluation and treatment of chemotherapy extravasation injuries. *J Pediatr Oncol Nurs* 2000;17:135–148.
49. Dorr RT. Antidotes to vesicant chemotherapy extravasations. *Blood Rev* 1990;4:41–60.
50. Watterson J, Heisel M, Cich JA, et al. Intrathoracic extravasation of sclerosing agents associated with central venous catheters. *Am J Pediatr Hematol Oncol* 1988;10:249–251.
51. Allen JC. The effects of cancer therapy on the nervous system. *J Pediatr* 1978;93:903–909.
52. Heiligenstein E, Steif BL. Tricyclics for pain. *J Am Acad Child Adolesc Psychiatry* 1989;28:804–805.
53. Uhm JH, Yung WK. Neurologic complications of cancer therapy. *Curr Treat Options Neurol* 1999;1:428–437.
54. Cheung NK, Lazarus H, Miraldi FD, et al. Ganglioside GD2 specific monoclonal antibody 3F8: a phase I study in patients with neuroblastoma and malignant melanoma. *J Clin Oncol* 1987;5:1430–1440.
55. Fischmeister G, Kurz M, Haas OA, et al. G-CSF versus GM-CSF for stimulation of peripheral blood progenitor cells (PBPC) and leukocytes in healthy volunteers: comparison of efficacy and tolerability. *Ann Hematol* 1999;78:117–123.
56. Milkovich G, Moleski RJ, Reitan JF, et al. Comparative safety of filgrastim versus sargramostim in patients receiving myelosuppressive chemotherapy. *Pharmacotherapy* 2000;20:1432–1440.
57. Ayan I, Kebudi R, Dogan S, et al. Granulocyte colony-stimulating factor in neutropenic, pediatric solid tumor patients following chemotherapy. *Pediatr Hematol Oncol* 1996;13:417–424.
58. American Society of Clinical Oncology. Recommendations for the use of hematopoietic colony-stimulating factors: evidence-based, clinical practice guidelines. *J Clin Oncol* 1994;12:2471–2508.
59. Ljungman G, Gordh T, Sorensen S, et al. Pain variations during cancer treatment in children: a descriptive survey. *Pediatr Hematol Oncol* 2000;17:211–221.
60. Fowler-Kerry S. Adolescent oncology survivors' recollection of pain. In: Tyler D, Krane E, eds. *Advances in pain research and therapy: pediatric pain*. New York: Raven Press, 1990:365–371.
61. Weisman SJ, Bernstein B, Schechter NL. Consequences of inadequate analgesia during painful procedures in children. *Arch Pediatr Adolesc Med* 1998;152:147–149.
62. Rice LJ. Needle phobia: an anesthesiologist's perspective. *J Pediatr* 1993;122:S9–S13.
63. Schechter NL, Bernstein BA, Beck A, et al. Individual differences in children's response to pain: Role of temperament and parental characteristics. *Pediatrics* 1991;87:171–177.
64. Zeltzer LK, Jay SM, Fisher DM. The management of pain associated with pediatric procedures. *Pediatr Clin North Am* 1989;36:941–964.
65. Cohen Reis E, Holubkov R. Vapocoolant spray is equally effective as EMLA cream in reducing immunization pain in school-aged children. *Pediatrics* 1997;100:E5.
66. Halperin DL, Koren G, Attias D, et al. Topical skin anesthesia for venous, subcutaneous drug reservoir and lumbar punctures in children. *Pediatrics* 1989;84:281–284.
67. Miser AW, Goh S, Dose AM, et al. Trial of a topically administered local anesthetic (EMLA cream) for pain relief during central venous port access in children with cancer. *J Pain Symptom Manage* 1994;9:259–264.
68. Bjerring P, Arendt-Nielsen L. Depth and duration of skin analgesia to needle insertion after topical application of EMLA cream. *Br J Anaesth* 1993;64:173–177.
69. Essink-Tjebbes CM, Hekster YA, Liem KD, et al. Topical use of local anesthetics in neonates. *Pharm World Sci* 1999;21:173–176.
70. Hopkins CS, Buckley CJ, Bush GH. Pain-free injection in infants. Use of a lignocaine-prilocaine cream to prevent pain at intravenous induction of general anaesthesia in 1–5-year-old children. *Anaesthesia* 1988;43:198–201.
71. Law RMT, Halpern S, Martins RF, et al. Measurement of methemoglobin after EMLA analgesia in newborn circumcision. *Biol Neonate* 1996;70:213–217.
72. Taddio A, Shennaan A, Stevens B, et al. Safety of lidocaine-prilocaine (EMLA) in neonates > 30 weeks gestation. In: *8th World Congress on Pain. Vancouver, British Columbia, Canada*. Seattle: IASP Press, 1996:182.
73. Taddio A, Shennan AT, Stevens B, et al. Safety of lidocaine-prilocaine cream in the treatment of preterm neonates. *J Pediatr* 1995;127:1002–1005.
74. Lawson RA, Smart NG, Gudgeon, AC, et al. Evaluation of an amethocaine gel preparation for percutaneous analgesia before venous cannulation in children. *Br J Anaesth* 1995;75:282–285.
75. van Kan HJ, Egberts AC, Rijnvos WP, et al. Tetracaine versus lidocaine-prilocaine for preventing venipuncture-induced pain in children. *Am J Health Syst Pharm* 1997;54:388–392.
76. Doyle E, Freeman J, Im NT, et al. An evaluation of a new self-adhesive patch preparation of amethocaine for topical anaesthesia prior to venous cannulation in children. *Anaesthesia* 1993;48:1050–1052.
77. Jain A, Rutter N. Local anaesthetic effect of topical amethocaine gel in neonates: randomised controlled trial. *Arch Dis Child Fetal Neonatal Ed* 2000;82:F42–F45.

78. Browne J, Awad I, Plant R, et al. Topical amethocaine (Ametop) is superior to EMLA for intravenous cannulation. Eutectic mixture of local anesthetics. *Can J Anaesth* 1999;46:1014–1018.
79. Bishai R, Taddio A, Bar-Oz B, et al. Relative efficacy of amethocaine gel and lidocaine-prilocaine cream for Port-a-Cath puncture in children. *Pediatrics* 1999;104: E31.
80. O'Connor B, Tomlinson AA. Evaluation of the efficacy and safety of amethocaine gel applied topically before venous cannulation in adults. *Br J Anaesth* 1995;74:706–708.
81. Kapelushnik J, Koren G, Solh H, et al. Evaluating the efficacy of EMLA in alleviating pain associated with lumbar puncture; comparison of open and double-blinded protocols in children. *Pain* 1990;42:31–34.
82. Burt N, Dorman BH, Reeves ST, et al. Postdural puncture headache in paediatric oncology patients. *Can J Anaesth* 1998;45:741–745.
83. Wee LH, Lam F, Cranston AJ. The incidence of post dural puncture headache in children. *Anaesthesia* 1996;51:1164–1166.
84. Seebacher J, Ribeiro V, LeGuillou JL, et al. Epidural blood patch in the treatment of post dural puncture headache: a double blind study. *Headache* 1989;29: 630–632.
85. Safa-Tisseront V, Thormann F, Malassine P, et al. Effectiveness of epidural blood patch in the management of post-dural puncture headache. *Anesthesiology* 2001; 95:334–339.
86. Flaatten H, Felthaus J, Kuwelker M, et al. Postural post-dural puncture headache. A prospective randomised study and a meta-analysis comparing two different 0.40 mm O.D. (27 g) spinal needles. *Acta Anaesthesiol Scand* 2000;44:643–647.
87. Dittmann M, Schaefer HG, Renkl F, et al. Spinal anaesthesia with 29 gauge Quincke point needles and post dural puncture headache in 2,378 patients. *Acta Anaesthesiol Scand* 1994;38:691–693.
88. Campbell DC, Douglas MJ, Pavy TJ, et al. Comparison of the 25-gauge Whitacre with the 24-gauge Sprotte spinal needle for elective caesarean section: cost implications. *Can J Anaesth* 1993;40:1131–1135.
89. Dahl JB, Schultz P, Anker-Moller E, et al. Spinal anaesthesia in young patients using a 29-gauge needle: technical considerations and an evaluation of postoperative complaints compared with general anaesthesia. *Br J Anaesth* 1990;64:178–182.
90. Jay S, Ozolins M, Elliott C, et al. Assessment of children's distress during painful medical procedures. *Health Psychol* 1983;2:133–147.
91. Katz ER, Kellerman J, Siegel SE. Behavioral distress in children with cancer undergoing medical procedures: developmental considerations. *J Consult Clin Psychol* 1980;48:356–365.
92. Tobias JD, Phipps S, Smith B, et al. Oral ketamine premedication to alleviate the distress of invasive procedures in pediatric oncology patients. *Pediatrics* 1992; 90:537–541.
93. Theroux MC, West DW, Corddry DH, et al. Efficacy of intranasal midazolam in facilitating suturing of lacerations in preschool children in the emergency department. *Pediatrics* 1993;91:624–627.
94. Sievers TD, Yee JD, Foley ME, et al. Midazolam for conscious sedation during pediatric oncology procedures: safety and recovery parameters. *Pediatrics* 1991;88:1172–1179.
95. Hennes HM, Wagner V, Bonadio WA, et al. The effect of oral midazolam on anxiety of preschool children during laceration repair. *Ann Emerg Med* 1990;19: 1006–1009.
96. Green SM, Nakamura R, Johnson NE. Ketamine sedation for pediatric procedures: Part 1, A prospective series. *Ann Emerg Med* 1990;19:1024–1032.
97. Gamis AS, Knapp JF, Glenski JA. Nitrous oxide analgesia in a pediatric emergency department. *Ann Emerg Med* 1989;18:177–181.
98. Annequin D, Carbajal R, Chauvin P, et al. Fixed 50% nitrous oxide oxygen mixture for painful procedures: a French survey. *Pediatrics* 2000;105:E47.
99. Friedman AG, Mulhern RK, Fairclough D, et al. Midazolam premedication for pediatric bone marrow aspiration and lumbar puncture. *Med Pediatr Oncol* 1991; 19:499–504.
100. Jay SM, Elliott CH, Katz E, et al. Cognitive-behavioral and pharmacologic interventions for children's distress during painful medical procedures. *J Consult Clin Psychol* 1987;55:860–865.
101. Jay S, Elliott CH, Fitzgibbons I, et al. A comparative study of cognitive behavior therapy versus general anesthesia for painful medical procedures in children. *Pain* 1995;62:3–9.
102. Berde C. Pediatric oncology procedures: to sleep or perchance to dream? *Pain* 1995;62:1–2.
103. Angel CA, Rao BN, Wrenn E Jr, et al. Acute appendicitis in children with leukemia and other malignancies: still a diagnostic dilemma. *J Pediatr Surg* 1992; 27:476–479.
104. Crom DB, Chathaway DK, Tolley EA, et al. Health status and health-related quality of life in long-term adult survivors of pediatric solid tumors. *Int J Cancer Suppl* 1999;12:25–31.
105. Barr RD, Furlong W, Dawson S, et al. An assessment of global health status in survivors of acute lymphoblastic leukemia in childhood. *Am J Pediatr Hematol Oncol* 1993;15:284–290.
106. McGrath PA. Intervention and management. In: Bush JP, Harkins SW, eds. *Children in pain: clinical and research issues from a developmental perspective*. New York: Springer-Verlag, 1991:476.
107. Zeltzer L, Lebaron S. Hypnosis and nonhypnotic techniques for reduction of pain and anxiety during painful procedures in children and adolescents with cancer. *J Pediatr* 1982;101:1032–1035.
108. Kellerman J, Zeltzer L, Ellenberg L, et al. Adolescents with cancer. Hypnosis for the reduction of the acute pain and anxiety associated with medical procedures. *J Adolesc Health Care* 1983;4:85–90.
109. Katz ER, Kellerman J, Ellenberg L. Hypnosis in the reduction of acute pain and distress in children with cancer. *J Pediatr Psychol* 1987;12:379–394.
110. Liossi C, Hatira P. Clinical hypnosis versus cognitive behavioral training for pain management with pediatric cancer patients undergoing bone marrow aspirations. *Int J Clin Exp Hypn* 1999;47:104–116.
111. Zeltzer L, Kellerman J, Ellenberg L, et al. Hypnosis for reduction of vomiting associated with chemotherapy and disease in adolescents with cancer. *J Adolesc Health Care* 1983;4:77–84.
112. Hockenberry MJ, Cotanch PH. Hypnosis as adjuvant

antiemetic therapy in childhood cancer. *Nurs Clin North Am* 1985;20:105–107.
113. Morrow GR, Hickok JT. Behavioral treatment of chemotherapy-induced nausea and vomiting. *Oncology (Huntingt)* 1993;7:83–89, discussion 93–94, 97.
114. Jacknow DS, Tschann JM, Link MP, et al. Hypnosis in the prevention of chemotherapy-related nausea and vomiting in children: a prospective study. *J Dev Behav Pediatr* 1994;15:258–264.
115. Bertoni F, Bonardi A, Magno L, et al. Hypnosis instead of general anaesthesia in paediatric radiotherapy: report of three cases. *Radiother Oncol* 1999;52:185–190.
116. Harper GW. A developmentally sensitive approach to clinical hypnosis for chronically and terminally ill adolescents. *Am J Clin Hypn* 1999;42:50–60.
117. Stevens MM, Dalla Pozza L, Cavalletto B, et al. Pain and symptom control in paediatric palliative care. *Cancer Surv* 1994;21:211–231.
118. Pettitt GA. Adjunctive trance and family therapy for terminal cancer. *N Z Med J* 1979;89:18–21.
119. Kuttner L. No fears, no tears: children with cancer coping with pain. In: Tyler DC, Krane EJ, eds. *Advances in pain research and therapy. vol. 15: pediatric pain.* New York: Raven Press, 1990:391–392.
120. Siegel LJ, Smith KE. Children's strategies for coping with pain. *Pediatrician* 1989;16:110–118.
121. Hilgard JR, LeBaron S. Relief of anxiety and pain in children and adolescents with cancer: quantitative measures and clinical observations. *Int J Clin Exp Hypn* 1982;30:417–442.
122. Kuttner L, Bowman M, Teasdale M. Psychological treatment of distress, pain, and anxiety for young children with cancer. *J Dev Behav Pediatr* 1988;9:374–381.
123. Manne SL, Redd WH, Jacobsen PB, et al. Behavioral intervention to reduce child and parent distress during venipuncture. *J Consult Clin Psychol* 1990;58:565–572.
124. McGrath PA, De Veber LL. The management of acute pain evoked by medical procedures in children with cancer. *J Pain Symptom Manage* 1986;1:145–150.
125. Jay SM, Elliott CH, Ozolins M, et al. Behavioral management of children's distress during painful medical procedures. *Behav Res Ther* 1985;23:513–520.
126. Collins JJ. Pharmacologic management of pediatric cancer pain. In: Portenoy RK, Bruera E, eds. *Topics in palliative care.* New York: Oxford University Press, 1998:7–28.
127. Sandler DP, Smith JC, Weinberg CR, et al. Analgesic use and chronic renal disease. *N Engl J Med* 1989;320: 1238–1243.
128. Hurwitz ES, Barrett MJ, Bregman D, et al. Public Health Service study on Reye's syndrome and medications. Report of the pilot phase. *N Engl J Med* 1985; 313:849–857.
129. Rumack BH, Peterson RG. Acetaminophen overdose: incidence, diagnosis, and management in 416 patients. *Pediatrics* 1978;62[Suppl]:898–903.
130. Halpin TJ, Holtzhauer FJ, Campbell RJ, et al. Reye's syndrome and medication use. *JAMA* 1982;248: 687–691.
131. Banco L. Use of aspirin and Reye's syndrome. *Am J Dis Child* 1987;141:240–241.
132. Lesko SM, Mitchell AA. The safety of acetaminophen and ibuprofen among children younger than two years old. *Pediatrics* 1999;104:E39.
133. Stuart JJ, Pisko EJ. Choline magnesium trisalicylate does not impair platelet aggregation. *Pharmatherapeutica* 1981;2:547–551.
134. Goldstein JL, Silverstein FE, Agrawal NM, et al. Reduced risk of upper gastrointestinal ulcer complications with celecoxib, a novel COX-2 inhibitor. *Am J Gastroenterol* 2000;95:1681–1690.
135. Leese PT, Hubbard RC, Karim A, et al. Effects of celecoxib, a novel cyclooxygenase-2 inhibitor, on platelet function in healthy adults: a randomized, controlled trial. *J Clin Pharmacol* 2000;40:124–132.
136. Mandema JW, Kaiko RF, Oshlack B, et al. Characterization and validation of a pharmacokinetic model for controlled-release oxycodone. *Br J Clin Pharmacol* 1996;42:747–756.
137. Benziger DP, Miotto J, Grandy RP, et al. A pharmacokinetic/pharmacodynamic study of controlled-release oxycodone. *J Pain Symptom Manage* 1997;13:75–82.
138. Olkkola KT, Hamunen K, Seppala T, et al. Pharmacokinetics and ventilatory effects of intravenous oxycodone in postoperative children. *Br J Clin Pharmacol* 1994;38:71–76.
139. Kalso E. Pharmacokinetics and ventilatory effects of intravenous oxycodone in postoperative children. *Br J Clin Pharmacol* 1995;39:214–215.
140. Poyhia R, Vainio A, Kalso E. A review of oxycodone's clinical pharmacokinetics and pharmacodynamics. *J Pain Symptom Manage* 1993;8:63–67.
141. Smith MT. Neuroexcitatory effects of morphine and hydromorphone: evidence implicating the 3-glucuronide metabolites. *Clin Exp Pharmacol Physiol* 2000;27:524–528.
142. Wright AW, Watt JA, Kennedy M, et al. Quantitation of morphine, morphine-3-glucuronide, and morphine-6-glucuronide in plasma and cerebrospinal fluid using solid-phase extraction and high-performance liquid chromatography with electrochemical detection [published erratum appears in *Ther Drug Monit* 1998; 20:218]. *Ther Drug Monit* 1994;16:200-208.
143. Bhat R, Chari G, Gulati A, et al. Pharmacokinetics of a single dose of morphine in preterm infants during the first week of life. *J Pediatr* 1990;117:477–481.
144. Lynn AM, Nespeca MK, Opheim KE, et al. Respiratory effects of intravenous morphine infusions in neonates, infants, and children after cardiac surgery. *Anesth Analg* 1993;77:695–701.
145. Olkkola KT, Maunuksela EL, Korpela R, et al. Kinetics and dynamics of postoperative intravenous morphine in children. *Clin Pharmacol Ther* 1988;44: 128–136.
146. Pokela ML, Olkkola KT, Seppala T, et al. Age-related morphine kinetics in infants. *Dev Pharmacol Ther* 1993;20:26–34.
147. McRorie TI, Lynn AM, Nespeca MK, et al. The maturation of morphine clearance and metabolism. *Am J Dis Child* 1992;146:972–976.
148. Hunt A, Joel S, Dick G, et al. Population pharmacokinetics of oral morphine and its glucuronides in children receiving morphine as immediate-release liquid or sustained-release tablets for cancer pain. *J Pediatr* 1999;135:47–55.
149. Cherny NI, Foley KM. Nonopioid and opioid analgesic pharmacotherapy of cancer pain. *Hematol Oncol Clin North Am* 1996;10:79–102.
150. Broomhead A, Kerr R, Tester W, et al. Comparison of a once-a-day sustained-release morphine formulation

with standard oral morphine treatment for cancer pain. *J Pain Symptom Manage* 1997;14:63–73.
151. Babul N, Darke AC, Hain R. Hydromorphone and metabolite pharmacokinetics in children. *J Pain Symptom Manage* 1995;10:335–337.
152. Weisman SJ, Wishnie E. Postoperative hydromorphone epidural analgesia in children. In: *8th World Congress on Pain. Vancouver, British Columbia, Canada* . Seattle: IASP Press, 1996:301.
153. Collins JJ, Geake J, Grier HE, et al. Patient-controlled analgesia for mucositis pain in children: a three-period crossover study comparing morphine and hydromorphone. *J Pediatr* 1996;129:722–728.
154. Lawlor P, Turner K, Hanson J, et al. Dose ratio between morphine and hydromorphone in patients with cancer pain: a retrospective study. *Pain* 1997;72:79–85.
155. Gourlay GK, Kowalski SR, Plummer JL, et al. Fentanyl blood concentration-analgesic response relationship in the treatment of post-operative pain. *Anesth Analg* 1988;67:329–337.
156. Singleton MA, Rosen JI, Fisher DM. Plasma concentrations of fentanyl in infants, children, and adults. *Can J Anaesth* 1987;34:152–155.
157. Koren G, Maurice L. Pediatric uses of opioids. *Pediatr Clin North Am* 1989;36:1141–1156.
158. Collins C, Koren G, Crean P, et al. Fentanyl pharmacokinetics and hemodynamic effects in preterm infants during ligation of patent ductus arteriosus. *Anesth Analg* 1985;64:1078–1080.
159. Hertzka RE, Gauntlett IS, Fisher DM, et al. Fentanyl-induced ventilatory depression: effects of age. *Anesthesiology* 1989;70:213–218.
160. Koren G, Goresky G, Crean P, et al. Pediatric fentanyl dosing based on pharmacokinetics during cardiac surgery. *Anesth Analg* 1984;63:577–582.
161. Koren G, Goresky G, Crean P, et al. Unexpected alterations in fentanyl pharmacokinetics in children undergoing cardiac surgery: age related or disease related? *Dev Pharmacol Ther* 1986;9:183–191.
162. Gauntlett IS, Fisher DM, Hertzka RE, et al. Pharmacokinetics of fentanyl in neonatal humans and lambs: effects of age. *Anesthesiology* 1988;69:683–687.
163. Cherny NJ, Chang V, Frager G, et al. Opioid pharmacotherapy in the management of cancer pain: a survey of strategies used by pain physicians for the selection of analgesic drugs and routes of administration. *Cancer* 1995;76:1283–1293.
164. Warner MA, Hosking MP, Gray JR, et al. Narcotic-induced histamine release: a comparison of morphine, oxymorphone, and fentanyl infusions. *J Cardiothorac Vasc Anesth* 1991;5:481–484.
165. Goodarzi M. Comparison of epidural morphine, hydromorphone and fentanyl for postoperative pain control in children undergoing orthopaedic surgery. *Paediatr Anaesth* 1999;9:419–422.
166. Irazuzta J, Pascucci R, Perlman N, et al. Effects of fentanyl administration on respiratory system compliance in infants. *Crit Care Med* 1993;21:1001–1004.
167. Wells S, Williamson M, Hooker D. Fentanyl-induced chest wall rigidity in a neonate: a case report. *Heart Lung* 1994;23:196–198.
168. Muller P, Vogtmann C. Three cases with different presentation of fentanyl-induced muscle rigidity—a rare problem in intensive care of neonates. *Am J Perinatol* 2000;17:23–26.
169. Vaughn RL, Bennett CR. Fentanyl chest wall rigidity syndrome—a case report. *Anesth Prog* 1981;28:50–51.
170. Schechter NL, Weisman SJ, Rosenblum M, et al. The use of oral transmucosal fentanyl citrate for painful procedures in children. *Pediatrics* 1995;95:335–339.
171. Collins JJ, Dunkel IJ, Gupta SK, et al. Transdermal fentanyl in children with cancer pain: feasibility, tolerability, and pharmacokinetic correlates. *J Pediatr* 1999;134:319–323.
172. Hamunen K, Maunuksela EL, Seppala T, et al. Pharmacokinetics of i.v. and rectal pethidine in children undergoing ophthalmic surgery. *Br J Anaesth* 1993;71:823–826.
173. Hamunen K. Ventilatory effects of morphine, pethidine and methadone in children. *Br J Anaesth* 1993;70:414–418.
174. Koska AJ 3rd, Kramer WG, Romagnoli A, et al. Pharmacokinetics of high-dose meperidine in surgical patients. *Anesth Analg* 1981;60:8–11.
175. Pokela ML, Olkkola KT, Koivisto M, et al. Pharmacokinetics and pharmacodynamics of intravenous meperidine in neonates and infants. *Clin Pharmacol Ther* 1992;52:342–349.
176. Kussman BD, Sethna NF. Pethidine-associated seizure in a healthy adolescent receiving pethidine for postoperative pain control. *Paediatr Anaesth* 1998;8:349–352.
177. Pryle BJ, Grech H, Stoddart PA, et al. Toxicity of norpethidine in sickle cell crisis. *BMJ* 1992;304:1478–1479.
178. Kaiko RF, Foley KM, Grabinski PY, et al. Central nervous system excitatory effects of meperidine in cancer patients. *Ann Neurol* 1983;13:180–185.
179. Kyff JV, Rice TL. Meperidine-associated seizures in a child. *Clin Pharm* 1990;9:337–338.
180. Burks LC, Aisner J, Fortner CL, et al. Meperidine for the treatment of shaking chills and fever. *Arch Intern Med* 1980;140:483–484.
181. Oldfield EC 3rd. Meperidine for prevention of amphotericin B-induced chills. *Clin Pharm* 1990;9:251–252.
182. Holtzclaw BJ. Control of febrile shivering during amphotericin B therapy. *Oncol Nurs Forum* 1990;17:521–524.
183. Pauca AL, Savage RT, Simpson S, et al. Effect of pethidine, fentanyl and morphine on post-operative shivering in man. *Acta Anaesthesiol Scand* 1984;28:138–143.
184. Wang JJ, Ho ST, Lee SC, et al. A comparison among nalbuphine, meperidine, and placebo for treating postanesthetic shivering. *Anesth Analg* 1999;88:686–689.
185. Schwarzkopf KR, Hoff H, Hartmann M, et al. A comparison between meperidine, clonidine and urapidil in the treatment of postanesthetic shivering. *Anesth Analg* 2001;92:257–260.
186. Berde CB, Beyer JE, Bournaki MC, et al. Comparison of morphine and methadone for prevention of postoperative pain in 3- to 7-year-old children. *J Pediatr* 1991;119:136–141.
187. Yaster M, Deshpande JK, Maxwell LG. The pharmacologic management of pain in children. *Compr Ther* 1989;15:14–26.
188. Miser AW, Davis DM, Hughes CS, et al. Continuous subcutaneous infusion of morphine in children with cancer. *Am J Dis Child* 1983;137:383–385.

189. Bruera E, Brenneis C, Michaud M, et al. Use of the subcutaneous route for the administration of narcotics in patients with cancer pain. *Cancer* 1988;62: 407–411.
190. Berde CB, Lehn BM, Yee JD, et al. Patient-controlled analgesia in children and adolescents: a randomized, prospective comparison with intramuscular administration of morphine for postoperative analgesia. *J Pediatr* 1991;118:460–466.
191. Gureno MA, Reisinger CL. Patient controlled analgesia for the young pediatric patient. *Pediatr Nurs* 1991; 17:251–254.
192. Till H, Lochbuhler H, Kellnar S, et al. Patient controlled analgesia (PCA) in paediatric surgery: a prospective study following laparoscopic and open appendicectomy. *Paediatr Anaesth* 1996;6:29–32.
193. Tobias JD, Baker DK. Patient-controlled analgesia with fentanyl in children. *Clin Pediatr (Phila)* 1992; 31:177–179.
194. Portenoy RK. Opioid tolerance and responsiveness: Research findings and clinical observations. In: Gebhart GF, Hammond DL, Jensen TS, eds. *Proceedings of the 7th World Congress on Pain*. Seattle: IASP Press, 1994:615–619.
195. Inturrisi CE, Portenoy RK, Max MB, et al. Pharmacokinetic-pharmacodynamic relationships of methadone infusions in patients with cancer pain. *Clin Pharmacol Ther* 1990;47:565–577.
196. Portenoy RK. Adjuvant analgesics in pain management. In: Doyle D, Hanks GWC, MacDonald N, eds. *Oxford textbook of palliative medicine*. Oxford/New York: Oxford University Press, 1993:187–203.
197. Magni G. The use of antidepressants in the treatment of chronic pain. A review of the current evidence. *Drugs* 1991;42:730–748.
198. Sindrup SH, Jensen TS. Efficacy of pharmacological treatments of neuropathic pain: an update and effect related to mechanism of drug action. *Pain* 1999;83: 389–400.
199. Magni G, Conlon P, Arsie D. Tricyclic antidepressants in the treatment of cancer pain: a review. *Pharmacopsychiatry* 1987;20:160–164.
200. McQuay HJ, Tramer M, Nye BA, et al. A systematic review of antidepressants in neuropathic pain. *Pain* 1996;68:217–227.
201. Galer BS. Neuropathic pain of peripheral origin: advances in pharmacologic treatment. *Neurology* 1995; 45[Suppl 9]:S17–S25, discussion S35–S36.
202. Watson CPN. Antidepressant drugs as adjuvant analgesics. *J Pain Symptom Manage* 1994;9:392–405.
203. Biederman J, Baldessarini RJ, Wright V, et al. A double-blind placebo controlled study of desipramine in the treatment ADD: II. Serum drug levels and cardiovascular findings. *J Am Acad Child Adolesc Psychiatry* 1989;28:903–911.
204. Wilens TE, Biederman J, Baldessarini RJ, et al. Electrocardiographic effects of desipramine and 2-hydroxydesipramine in children, adolescents, and adults treated with desipramine. *J Am Acad Child Adolesc Psychiatry* 1993;32:798–804.
205. Wilens TE, Biederman J, Baldessarini RJ, et al. Cardiovascular effects of therapeutic doses of tricyclic antidepressants in children and adolescents. *J Am Acad Child Adolesc Psychiatry* 1996;35:1491–1501.
206. Yee JD, Berde CB. Dextroamphetamine or methylphenidate as adjuvants to opioid analgesia for adolescents with cancer. *J Pain Symptom Manage* 1994;9: 122–125.
207. Forrest WH Jr, Brown BW Jr, Brown CR, et al. Dextroamphetamine with morphine for the treatment of postoperative pain. *N Engl J Med* 1977;296:712–715.
208. Bruera E, Fainsinger R, MacEachern T, et al. The use of methylphenidate in patients with incident cancer pain receiving regular opiates. A preliminary report. *Pain* 1992;50:75–77.
209. Bruera E, Miller MJ, Macmillan K, et al. Neuropsychological effects of methylphenidate in patients receiving a continuous infusion of narcotics for cancer pain. *Pain* 1992;48:163–166.
210. Thomsen CB, Crawford ME, Sjogren P. [Malignant bone pain]. *Ugeskr Laeger* 1997;159:2364–2369.
211. Tannock I, Gospodarowicz M, Meakin W, et al. Treatment of metastatic prostatic cancer with low-dose prednisone: evaluation of pain and quality of life as pragmatic indices of response. *J Clin Oncol* 1989;7: 590–597.
212. Hanks GW. The pharmacological treatment of bone pain. *Cancer Surv* 1988;7:87–101.
213. Gutin PH. Corticosteroid therapy in patients with cerebral tumors: benefits, mechanisms, problems, practicalities. *Semin Oncol* 1975;2:49–56.
214. Weinstein JD, Toy FJ, Jaffe ME, et al. The effect of dexamethasone on brain edema in patients with metastatic brain tumors. *Neurology* 1973;23:121–129.
215. Lieberman A, LeBrun Y, Glass P, et al. Use of high dose corticosteroids in patients with inoperable brain tumours. *J Neurol Neurosurg Psychiatry* 1977;40: 678–682.
216. Black P. Brain metastasis: current status and recommended guidelines for management. *Neurosurgery* 1979;5:617–631.
217. Koehler PJ. Use of corticosteroids in neuro-oncology. *Anticancer Drugs* 1995;6:19–33.
218. Greenberg HS, Kim JH, Posner JB. Epidural spinal cord compression from metastatic tumor: results with a new treatment protocol. *Ann Neurol* 1980;8:361–366.
219. Watanabe S, Bruera E. Corticosteroids as adjuvant analgesics. *J Pain Symptom Manage* 1994;9:442–445.
220. Tremont-Lukats IW, Megeff C, Backonja MM. Anticonvulsants for neuropathic pain syndromes: mechanisms of action and place in therapy. *Drugs* 2000;60:1029–1052.
221. Backonja MM. Anticonvulsants (antineuropathics) for neuropathic pain syndromes. *Clin J Pain* 2000;16 [Suppl]:S67–S72.
222. Rush AM, Elliott JR. Phenytoin and carbamazepine: differential inhibition of sodium currents in small cells from adult rat dorsal root ganglia. *Neurosci Lett* 1997; 226:95–98.
223. Harke H, Gretenkort P, Ladleif HU, et al. The response of neuropathic pain and pain in complex regional pain syndrome I to carbamazepine and sustained-release morphine in patients pretreated with spinal cord stimulation: a double-blinded randomized study. *Anesth Analg* 2001;92:488–495.
224. Loscher W. Valproate: a reappraisal of its pharmacodynamic properties and mechanisms of action. *Prog Neurobiol* 1999;58:31–59.
225. Hardy JR, Rees EA, Gwilliam B, et al. A phase II study to establish the efficacy and toxicity of sodium

valproate in patients with cancer-related neuropathic pain. *J Pain Symptom Manage* 2001;21:204–209.

226. Pan HL, Eisenach JC, Chen SR. Gabapentin suppresses ectopic nerve discharges and reverses allodynia in neuropathic rats. *J Pharmacol Exp Ther* 1999; 288:1026–1030.
227. Attal N, Brasseur L, Parker F, et al. Effects of gabapentin on the different components of peripheral and central neuropathic pain syndromes: a pilot study. *Eur Neurol* 1998;40:191–200.
228. Chapman V, Suzuki R, Chamarette HL, et al. Effects of systemic carbamazepine and gabapentin on spinal neuronal responses in spinal nerve ligated rats. *Pain* 1998;75:261–272.
229. Khurana DS, Riviello J, Helmers S, et al. Efficacy of gabapentin therapy in children with refractory partial seizures. *J Pediatr* 1996;128:829–833.
230. Marson AG, Kadir ZA, Hutton JL, et al. The new antiepileptic drugs: a systematic review of their efficacy and tolerability. *Epilepsia* 1997;38:859–880.
231. Morris GL 3rd. Efficacy and tolerability of gabapentin in clinical practice. *Clin Ther* 1995;17:891–900.
232. Ichikawa K, Koyama N, Kiguchi S, et al. Inhibitory effect of oxcarbazepine on high-frequency firing in peripheral nerve fibers. *Eur J Pharmacol* 2001;420: 119–122.
233. Curry WJ, Kulling DL. Newer antiepileptic drugs: gabapentin, lamotrigine, felbamate, topiramate and fosphenytoin. *Am Fam Physician* 1998;57:513–520.
234. Srivastava SC, Atkins HL, Krishnamurthy GT, et al. Treatment of metastatic bone pain with tin-117m Stannic diethylenetriaminepentaacetic acid: a phase I/II clinical study. *Clin Cancer Res* 1998;4:61–68.
235. Silberstein EB, Williams C. Strontium-89 therapy for the pain of osseous metastases. *J Nucl Med* 1985;26: 345–348.
236. Westlin JE, Letocha H, Jakobson A, et al. Rapid, reproducible pain relief with [131I]iodine-metaiodobenzylguanidine in a boy with disseminated neuroblastoma. *Pain* 1995;60:111–114.
237. Silberstein EB. The treatment of painful osseous metastases with phosphorus-32-labeled phosphates. *Semin Oncol* 1993;20[Suppl 2]:10–21.
238. Voute PA, Hoefnagel CA, de Kraker J. 131I-metaiodobenzylguanidine in diagnosis and treatment of neuroblastoma. *Bull Cancer* 1988;75:107–111.
239. Cheung NK, Kushner BH, LaQuaglia M, et al. N7: a novel multi-modality therapy of high risk neuroblastoma (NB) in children diagnosed over 1 year of age. *Med Pediatr Oncol* 2001;36:227–230.
240. Treuner J, Klingebiel T, Bruchelt G, et al. Treatment of neuroblastoma with metaiodobenzylguanidine: results and side effects. *Med Pediatr Oncol* 1987;15:199–202.
241. Rogers AG. The use of methotrimeprazine (Levoprome) in a patient sensitive to opioids and possible bowel shutdown. *J Pain Symptom Manage* 1989;4: 44–45.
242. Patt RB, Proper G, Reddy S. The neuroleptics as adjuvant analgesics. *J Pain Symptom Manage* 1994;9: 446–453.
243. Breitbart W. Psychotropic adjuvant analgesics for pain in cancer and AIDS. *Psychooncology* 1998;7: 333–445.
244. Richter PA, Burk MP. The potentiation of narcotic analgesics with phenothiazines. *J Foot Surg* 1992;31: 378–380.
245. Beaver WT, Wallenstein SL, Houde RW, et al. A comparison of the analgesic effects of methotrimeprazine and morphine in patients with cancer. *Clin Pharmacol Ther* 1966;7:436–446.
246. Methotrimeprazine (Levoprome)—a potent analgesic. *Med Lett Drugs Ther* 1967;9:49–50.
247. Stirman JA. A comparison of methotrimeprazine and meperidine as analgesic agents. *Anesth Analg* 1967;46: 176–180.
248. Oliver DJ. The use of methotrimeprazine in terminal care. *Br J Clin Pract* 1985;39:339–340.
249. Storey P, Hill HH Jr, St. Louis RH, et al. Subcutaneous infusions for control of cancer symptoms. *J Pain Symptom Manage* 1990;5:33–41.

30

Pain and Palliative Care

Ann Goldman, Gerri Frager, and Maureen Pomietto

The theme of this chapter is pain management in children for whom the focus of care is palliative. Because one of the fundamental precepts of palliative care is its integrated and holistic approach to the child and family, we particularly chose to consider pain within the broader picture of palliative care. We emphasize the importance of addressing pain assessment and management in the context of all the child's symptoms and the child's and family's psychosocial and spiritual needs, especially toward the end stages of the child's life.

WHAT IS PALLIATIVE CARE?

Palliative care developed initially in response to the unmet emotional, physical, psychologic, and spiritual needs of adults dying of cancer, and concern for all these aspects of care is essential to its philosophy. Hospice is sometimes more narrowly defined as care within this framework, provided within freestanding buildings or home-care programs. In many parts of the world, palliative care and hospice are synonymous.

In pediatrics, a broader and more appropriate approach that is now evolving is one that recognizes that the benefits of palliative care are applicable to and should be available for any child and family living with a life-threatening illness. The optimal time to introduce the concept of palliative care is early on, when the child is first diagnosed with a significant life-threatening illness that may, or is likely to, end in premature death. As in the traditional models of palliative care, support is provided not only for the sick child but also the wider circle of those affected by the illness: his or her family and peers. Such care should be provided by a team with multidisciplinary skills and one that can offer continuity. Often this is best ensured by ongoing involvement by a core of local health care professionals with pediatric skills who know the child and family well, who liaise with and are supported by health care professionals with experience in the specialized aspects of palliative care.

Experience, sensitivity, and confidence are needed in the assessment and management of these children and families, particularly in evaluating the complex interplay that occurs between psychosocial, spiritual, and physical factors over the course of the illness. Some of the specific skills needed include the ability to assess pain in the young, nonverbal, and cognitively impaired child; familiarity and experience with the range of pain management techniques available; awareness of children's understanding of illness and death; the ability and confidence to communicate with seriously ill children and their families; and commitment to working as a team member.

CHILDREN WHO NEED PALLIATIVE CARE

Potentially, all children with a life-limiting illness and their families can benefit from palliative care. Although this includes children with a wide range of different diagnoses, it is helpful in practice to consider four broad groups (1):

- life-threatening conditions for which curative treatment is feasible but may fail (e.g., cancer),

- conditions in which long periods of treatment aim to prolong good quality of life but in which premature death is anticipated (e.g., cystic fibrosis, human immunodeficiency virus/acquired immunodeficiency syndrome),
- progressive conditions in which treatment is palliative from diagnosis and may extend over many years (e.g., Batten disease, mucopolysaccharidoses),
- conditions of severe disability that, although not progressive, lead to extreme vulnerability to health complications and premature death is anticipated (e.g., severe cerebral palsy).

The number of children in the population falling into these categories has been underestimated in the past, but more recent data suggest a prevalence of at least one in 1,000 children (1,2).

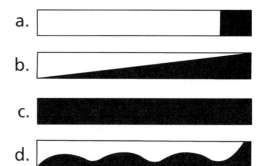

FIG. 30.1. Some models of the relationship between treatment aimed to cure and palliative care. The white areas represent treatment aimed to cure and the shaded area palliative care. (Adapted from Association for Children with Life-threatening or Terminal Conditions and Their Families and the Royal College of Paediatrics and Child Health. *A guide to the development of children's palliative care services. Report of a joint working party.* Bristol, U.K.: Association for Children with Life-threatening or Terminal Conditions and Their Families, 1997, with permission.).

PATTERNS OF CARE

These children ranging from newborn babies to young adults and with a variety of rare and often complex disorders present diverse symptoms and family problems. The illness may evolve over many years, and the needs of the child and family change with time. The pattern of managing the disease does not necessarily fit a simple and rigid model in which palliative care is introduced as a final resort, after all other treatment has been exhausted (Fig. 30.1A). A much more helpful approach clinically is a flexible system that introduces the concept of palliative care much earlier and incorporates it, when it is needed, with treatments that may still be aimed to cure. Numerous models illustrating this idea can be proposed (Fig. 30.1A–D) (1,3). Flexibility and awareness of the "gray areas" can help in the transition between treatments aimed to cure and palliative care, which is often difficult.

THE TRANSITION TO PALLIATIVE CARE

The transition to palliative care should be carefully considered, whether it is a gradual evolution or a clear-cut moment in time. It embodies an acknowledgment that the prime focus of care is increasingly, and eventually entirely, toward the child's quality of life. It is vital to emphasize to the family that choosing to withhold or withdraw treatments that aim to cure or prolong a child's life does not mean that the child will receive no care but rather that the focus of care changes. However, this can be difficult for many health care professionals. Just as for parents, it can also be painful for staff to acknowledge that doing the best for the child may not mean striving for life at all costs. Although they may recognize intellectually that to focus on palliative care is a valid, active, and specialized medical and nursing discipline, many continue emotionally to feel that it means they are giving up. This can result in a reluctance to consider a change in the focus of care or a delay, with the child enduring unnecessary suffering. Other barriers to the appropriate introduction of palliative care have been described (4–6). These include current arrangements for health care benefits, lack of knowledge, persistence of myths about pain relief, and fears by staff about whether it is ethical and legal to withhold treatments.

Nevertheless, progress in technology and the range of possible ways to sustain life without necessarily benefiting the child make decisions about the appropriateness of treatment unavoidable. In the United Kingdom, the Royal College of Paediatrics and Child Health's report (7) offers a framework of good medical practice to help doctors in making decisions in the child's best interest. They highlight five situations in which withholding and withdrawing treatments can be considered:

- the brain dead child,
- the permanent vegetative state,
- the "no chance" situation: life-sustaining treatment merely delays death without significant alleviation of suffering,
- the "no purpose" situation: although the child may survive with treatment, the degree of physical or mental impairment will be so great that it is unreasonable to expect him or her to bear it,
- the "unbearable" situation: the child and/or family feel that in the face of progressive and irreversible illness, further treatment is more than can be borne.

There are many levels of treatments including experimental therapies, mechanical ventilation, antibiotics, artificial nutrition, and intravenous fluids, and at different times the appropriateness of introducing or continuing to use any one of these may need to be addressed. Although ethically the withholding and withdrawal of treatments are equivalent, withdrawal can feel more difficult emotionally. Sometimes in children with chronic illness, there is time to consider whether it is appropriate to introduce a new aspect of treatment (e.g., initiating parenteral feeding or embarking on another cardiac transplant). This gives an opportunity to listen to the family, and child as well when possible, to explore the short- and longer term implications and to make a considered and mutual decision about withholding a treatment.

On other occasions, staff and families must face thinking about withdrawing established care. Adopting a flexible model (as in Fig. 30.1 B and D) can ease the transition to palliative care at these times. Treatments aimed to cure or prolong life and those directed at comfort are not mutually exclusive. This approach allows the philosophy of palliative care with concern for pain and symptom management, psychosocial support, and spiritual care to be introduced concurrently. Treatments that have been part of a child's and family's pattern for many years; for example, intensive physiotherapy or gastrostomy feeding can be continued but with a gradually decreasing emphasis. Forethought can also help to avoid sudden harsh decisions needing to be made at a time of crisis. A hospital admission for respiratory support or a transfusion can be used as an opportunity to clarify with the family their understanding of the child's deteriorating condition and the decreasing capacity of those treatments to improve the child's quality of life. Plans can be made calmly for the next time a crisis arises and the management of symptoms and the child's death anticipated and planned for.

PRINCIPLES FOR PAIN AND SYMPTOM MANAGEMENT

Excellent pain and symptom management at the end of life promotes control and frees the child, parent(s), and family members to deal with loss, grief, and changes in relationships and identity. Principles include

- aiming toward comfort for the child and family, optimizing quality of living and dying, and maintaining dignity;
- comprehensively assessing the physical, social, emotional, and spiritual factors contributing to each symptom;
- believing the child's report of pain, symptoms, and suffering;
- designing management based on this multidimensional assessment;
- incorporating pharmacologic and nonpharmacologic interventions;
- using a proactive approach and avoiding delay in treatment;
- keeping it simple and minimally invasive;
- considering the burden on the child and family;

- anticipating and treating common side effects vigorously;
- remaining flexible and reviewing regularly because goals are dynamic and the needs and desires of each child and family change;
- communicating and coordinating with other health care professionals involved;
- ensuring 24-hour availability of support for the family.

THE DEMOGRAPHICS OF PAIN IN PALLIATIVE CARE

Most of information available relates to children with cancer. In early studies, it is notable that procedure- and treatment-related pain was recorded as responsible for most of the pain that children with cancer experienced (8). Even though effective strategies to manage the pain are now available, recent studies still show a high incidence of procedure- and treatment-related pain compared with that caused by the disease itself (9). Disease-related pain is often described as short-lived because cancer therapy is effective in resolving pain at diagnosis (10) and because disease progression tends to be rapid during palliative care (11). However, the prevalence rate of pain and the need for regular strong analgesia are significant in children with cancer and was noted to be 89% in a recent Finnish study (12,13). Despite the high prevalence of pain and effective treatment strategies to provide significant relief (14,15), inadequate relief is still being documented (16).

Less information relating to other illnesses is available. The prevalence rate for significant pain in children with human immunodeficiency virus being treated as outpatients is 59%, with this rate increasing to 88% for pediatric inpatients. Parallel to the various causes of pain in childhood cancer, the origin of human immunodeficiency virus/acquired immunodeficiency syndrome–associated pain can be disease related, as in pancreatitis, or a consequence of an opportunistic infection, as in fungal enteritis (17). Procedure-related pain or other treatment-related effects such as peripheral neuropathy can be associated with antiretroviral treatment. The frequent presence of multiorgan involvement may cause pain to be present in several sites at the same time (18). The impact of the virus on normal childhood development can complicate the assessment of pain and other symptoms.

PAIN ASSESSMENT IN PALLIATIVE CARE

The general principles of careful and thorough assessment of pain and other symptoms apply equally to the child with advanced disease. It is important to keep in mind that some typical signs of acute pain such as increased heart rate, diaphoresis, and facial grimacing may not be helpful because they attenuate with time in chronic pain or may be altered in the very ill child. It is also essential to consider the contribution of psychologic factors such as sadness, fear, isolation, and the meaning of the pain because these are likely to contribute more than in a situation of acute pain. Flexibility and an individualized approach are important because children who have been living with a chronic illness may be more advanced in their understanding of their illness and their ability to report about it than usually healthy children. Conversely, some children regress emotionally with advanced illness and may not respond and interact in ways matching their developmental capabilities. Understanding the child's and family's coping skills and attitude should also be part of the assessment.

Formal pain measurement tools can help children and families to communicate about the location and intensity of the pain. This is helpful because the degree of relief afforded by therapeutic interventions can guide further therapy. Familiarity, preference, ease of use, and a child's energy level should be considered when choosing a pain intensity tool to prevent unnecessary burden on the child and family. For cognitively intact children older than 3 years of age, numerous options are available (Chapters 7 and 8). When children are cognitively impaired, nonverbal, or regressed, their pain can be more difficult to assess and the cause more difficult to identify. Parents are usually the most reliable observers and advocates for their child. They can identify their child's cues for pain, which usually include noting changes in their usual aspects of facial expression, vocalizations, posture, and tone, and patterns of sleeping, eating, and socializing.

PLANNING PAIN AND SYMPTOM MANAGEMENT

An individual plan of care designed in partnership with the child and his or her family is the cornerstone of management. Working in partnership with the family necessitates gathering a detailed history to identify fears and concerns about the illness, pain, symptoms, and the dying process. Anticipatory guidance can then be provided about options that exist to promote comfort, and teaching and planning can follow. It is important that the review of options for treating symptoms includes the impact of actions on quality of life and the burdens involved. Although it may be difficult, a forthright discussion enables a family to determine which choices fit with their goals. It should provide realistic information, can help allay anxiety and restore some sense of control to the family, offers reassurance that support will be available, and can help to give the parents confidence through this difficult time.

PHARMACOLOGIC APPROACHES FOR PAIN

Choosing the Drug

The World Health Organization analgesic ladder (Fig. 30.2) is well established in adult practice as a stepwise approach for choosing an analgesic in palliative care and is applicable to children (19,20). It is based on the severity of pain, which is broadly categorized as mild, mild to moderate, and moderate to severe. When used alone, nonsteroidal anti-inflammatory drugs or acetaminophen form the first step of the ladder for mild pain. Acetaminophen is proposed because of the associated low platelet counts in children living with cancer or acquired immunodeficiency syndrome. Nonsteroidal anti-inflammatory drugs

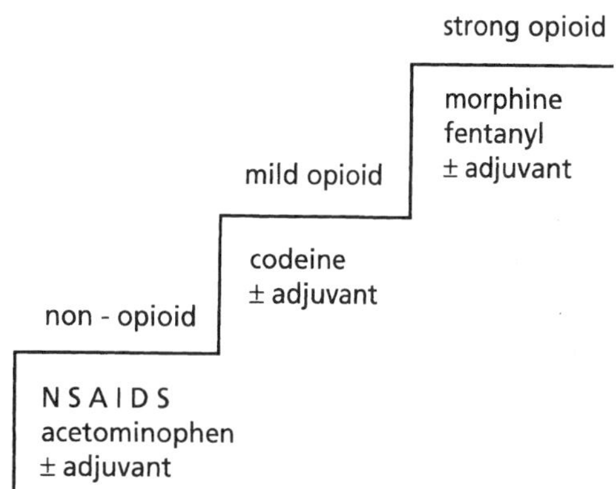

FIG. 30.2. The analgesic ladder. (Adapted from World Health Organization Ladder. *Cancer Pain Relief and Palliative Care. Technical Report Series 804.* Geneva: World Health Organization, 1990, with permission.)

and acetaminophen can be recommended at all steps in the ladder as concurrent medication with opioids. Other adjuvant medications can be used with any steps as coanalgesics or to counteract opioid-induced side effects.

After the clinician has determined which step of the ladder applies to the child, then the choice of opioid is determined by the child's opioid history, the clinician's experience, and the drugs available. The agonist–antagonist group of opioids are avoided because they have a ceiling effect. Meperidine (Demerol, pethidine) is not used in the setting of pain that is expected to last longer than a few days or if higher doses are anticipated because of its active and toxic metabolite normeperidine.

If a child experiences dose-limiting toxicity or an idiosyncratic adverse effect, an adjuvant medication can be added to counteract the side effect or to attempt to widen the therapeutic window and consequently reduce the opioid dose. Sometimes an alternative opioid offers a better side effect profile and is preferable to the addition of another agent.

Consider Stan (not his real name), a 6-year-old boy (weighing 20 kg) with refractory acute lymphocytic leukemia. For the past 2 weeks, he has had increasing pain thought to be secondary to marrow expansion. He initially had excellent relief with morphine. However, his analgesic requirements increased, and in the past 2 weeks, his parents have been finding it difficult to differentiate between pain inadequately relieved by the morphine or irritability induced or exacerbated by the morphine. Some information that helps in understanding the options to pursue include his parents' report of increased irritability at the peak onset of opioid action, approximately 30 minutes to 1 hour after his breakthrough dose of morphine. He is also having some difficulty with urinary retention. A decision is made to convert from morphine to hydromorphone with the intention of pain relief and a different side effect profile. Examples of this patient's earlier analgesic management are highlighted in the following sections.

To convert from one opioid to another, the equianalgesic table (Table 30.1) should be consulted after calculating the total dose of opioid being used regularly and for breakthrough doses. The phenomenon of incomplete cross-tolerance can be relevant clinically and should be considered when converting a child considered opioid tolerant from one opioid to another. This is accounted for after calculating the equianalgesic dose by administering the new opioid at a reduced dose (often 50% of the calculated equianalgesic dose) and subsequently titrating to effect.

Choosing the Route

Generally, the route should be one that is well tolerated and acceptable to the child. This is usually oral provided that the gastrointestinal tract is functional. The development of palatable and flexible preparations, including sustained-release products has greatly facilitated oral administration of opioids in children. The rectal route is not sustainable for more than a few doses. However, it may be helpful for a child who is transiently unable to tolerate the oral route because of vomiting or in the interval when a child at home is no longer able to take drugs orally and before a parenteral route is established. Neutropenia and/or thrombocytopenia are relative contraindications to the rectal route. The transdermal route for fentanyl can be valuable for children with reasonably stable analgesic needs but is not helpful for those with rapidly escalating pain because it takes 12 to 16 hours to reach steady state each time a dose adjustment is made. Clearance is also long (approximately 21 hours) should the fentanyl patch need to be removed for adverse effects or if pain resolves. Transmucosal fentanyl, available for adults for breakthrough pain, is not available for children except for the management of procedural pain in some countries; therefore, a different opioid should be prescribed.

In a severe acute pain crisis, the parenteral route would be most appropriate, ensuring the ability to titrate to analgesic effect. This route might also be required toward the end of life when the child's level of consciousness declines or when the oral route is no longer appropriate because of vomiting or inadequate absorption. Various devices can deliver opioids alone or in combination with other medications that may be required in palliative care. Drugs compatible with morphine are shown in Table 30.2. For children without intravenous access or in whom establishing intravenous access would be distressing, the subcutaneous route is appropriate and equivalent. A small (25 or 27 gauge) indwelling butterfly needle or plastic catheter is inserted in the upper arm, leg, or abdominal or chest wall and changed approximately every 5 days or sooner if redness develops. Often the simplest equipment such as a single syringe driver or patient-controlled analgesia pump is most appropriate at the end stage of life, enabling ambulation and manageability of the child cared for by the family at home.

The intramuscular route should not be used to deliver medication because it is painful and unnecessary when other options are available.

The epidural and intrathecal routes are rarely used because the indication of localized pain, inadequately relieved by systemic analgesics because of dose-limiting side effects, is uncommon in pediatric palliative care. Most children with advanced cancer have diffuse and disseminated disease. If it is indicated, an opioid can be used alone or in conjunction

TABLE 30.1. *Starting doses of opioids for opioid-naïve children*

Drug	Equianalgesic oral dose compared with morphine	Usual starting p.o. dose		p.o.:i.v./s.c. ratio	Equianalgesic parenteral dose compared with morphine	Usual i.v./s.c. starting dose		Biologic t√½ half-life
		<50 kg	>50 kg			<50 kg	>50 kg	
Codeine	190 mg, "usual" maximal dose is 120 mg	0.5–1 mg/kg q3–4h	15–30 mg q3–4h	1.5:1.0 s.c., *not* to be given intravenously	130 mg, "usual" maximal dose is 60 mg	0.25–0.5 mg/kg q3–4h s.c., *not* to be given intravenously	60 mg q3–4h s.c., *not* to be given intravenously	2.5–3 hr
Oxycodone (as in Percocet)	30 mg p.o. equianalgesic 1:1 with p.o. morphine	0.1–0.2 mg/kg q3–4h	5–10 mg q3–4h	Not available in parenteral form		N/A	N/A	2–3 hr
MORPHINE	30 mg	0.15–0.3 mg/kg q3–4h	5–10 mg q3–4h	3:1	10 mg	0.05–0.1 mg/kg q3–4h	5–10 mg q3–4h	2.5–3 hr
Hydromorphone (Dilaudid)	7.5 mg	0.05 mg/kg q3–4h	1–2 mg q3–4h	5:1	1.5 mg	0.1 mg/kg q3–4h	1–1.5 mg q3–4h	2–3 hr
Fentanyl[a]	Oral morphine of 45–134 mg/day = 25 µg/hr TD patch			N/A	Single dose of 100 µg By infusion: 100 µg/hr = 2.5 mg/hr, 2.6 morphine	0.5–1.5 µg/kg q30min	25–75 µg q30min	i.v.: 3–12 hr TD: 18–24 hr (elimination half-life) TD: i.v. ratio = 1:1, based on clinical experience

[a]*Caution:* Rapid infusion may cause chest wall rigidity.

When converting from one short half-life opioid to another, generally reduce the dose of the new opioid by 25% to 50% of the equianalgesic dose (because of incomplete cross-tolerance), then titrate as required.

Usual starting doses often are empiric and *not* necessarily calculated according to equianalgesic principles, i.e., the usual starting dose for hydromorphone may be 2 mg orally even though the parenteral:oral ratio is 1:5.

For infants 6 months of age, use one-third of the usual starting dose for infants younger than 6 months, then titrate to effect.

Transdermal fentanyl is not recommended for use in opioid-naïve patients.

Convert to sustained-release or long-acting preparation once approximate opioid requirements have been determined.

p.o., oral; i.v., intravenous; s.c., subcutaneous; N/A, not available; TD, transdermal.

Modified from Memorial Sloan–Kettering Cancer Center, Pain Service.

TABLE 30.2. *Parenteral drugs compatible when mixed with opioids*

Medication	Diamorphine alone[a]	Diamorphine with metoclopramide	Diamorphine with hyoscine hydrobromide	Diamorphine with dexamethasone	Diamorphine with methotrimeprazine
Dexamethasone	✓	✓	✓		×
Hyoscine hydrobromide	✓	✓		✓	✓
Cyclizine	✓, compatibility caution if >6.7 mg/mL cyclizine	× (at some concentrations)	✓	✓	✓
Ondansetron	✓				
Metoclopramide	✓		✓		✓
Haloperidol	✓, compatibility caution with higher concentrations of both >50 mg/mL diamorphine and >1.5 mg/mL haloperidol	✓	✓	✓	✓, up to concentrations of 50 mg/mL, diamorphine, 0.75 mg/mL haloperidol, 2.5 mg/mL methotrimeprazine
Midazolam	✓	✓	✓, up to concentrations of 70 mg/mL diamorphine, 0.5 mg/mL haloperidol, 4 mg/mL midazolam	✓	✓
Glycopyrrolate	✓	✓			✓
Methotrimeprazine	✓	✓	✓, up to concentrations of 4.5 mg/mL diamorphine, 120 μg/mL hyoscine hydrobromide, 7.5 mg/mL methotrimeprazine	×	

[a]Alternatively morphine or fentanyl.

The commonly used parenteral opioids (morphine, hydromorphone, and fentanyl) are generally considered to share equivalent compatibilities as documented in the *Palliative Care Formulary* for diamorphine.

Where specific incompatibilities are not noted, the medications would be considered compatible.

✓, compatible; ×, not compatible.

From Twycross R, Wilcock A, Thorp S. *PCF1-Palliative care formulary.* Oxford, UK: Radcliffe Medical Press Ltd., 1998:183–202, with permission.

with local anesthetic, baclofen, or ketamine (21). The switch from systemic to regional opioids in an opioid-tolerant child requires vigilant observation because there is a risk of acute respiratory depression from the systemic opioids when the pain is acutely reduced or relieved. The degree and rate at which the systemic opioids are reduced can prevent systemic toxicity and the effects of opioid withdrawal.

When changing routes, the child's 24-hour requirement of regular doses and breakthrough doses are totaled, and Table 30.1 referred to as a guide to the new dose needed. Frequent reassessments and adjustments can then be made as necessary.

Choosing the Dose

The initial weight-based calculation of a starting opioid dose for an opioid-naïve child is suggested in Table 30.1. Even with starting doses, there is a range of clinical practice. Some clinicians start at the higher end of the starting range to rapidly get pain under control, with the rationale that the child or family may refuse additional doses if immediate benefit is not obvious. Proponents of starting at the lower end of the dose range suggest that if acute, dose-related side effects are experienced, there may be reluctance to continue with the drug even if pain has been relieved.

Stan initially had excellent relief with immediate-release oral morphine at a starting dose of 4 mg (approximately 0.2 mg/kg per dose for his weight of 20 kg every 4 hours).

Choosing the Dose Interval

Pain should be prevented rather than treating as it recurs, so that if a child is having anything more than very intermittent, infrequent pain, an opioid should be given on an around-the-clock basis. To determine initial opioid requirements, doses of an immediate-release preparation are given every 4 hours, with additional doses for breakthrough pain. When the opioid requirements are determined (1 to 2 days), the preparation can be converted to a sustained-release preparation, always with the provision of breakthrough doses. This sustained-release preparation is generally administered orally but may be given transdermally. When choosing dose intervals and analgesic, the importance of enabling the child and family to have a good night's sleep should be kept in mind.

Providing Breakthrough or Rescue Doses

While the child is provided with an opioid regularly rather than waiting for the pain to recur, if pain recurs or breaks through the regular scheduled dose, then access should be provided for additional doses. It is best if the same opioid is used for both around-the-clock dosing or sustained-release dosing and the immediate-release preparations provided for breakthrough pain. In this way, estimation of the opioid requirements for titration is facilitated. Identifying the source of opioid-induced side effects is also more feasible. The dose range for this breakthrough medication is generally less than the amount of their regularly scheduled dose. A basic rule of thumb is to use one-fifth of the sustained-release preparation given every 12 hours or 10% of the 24-hour opioid requirements, available on an hourly basis. Another option for someone on a continuous infusion is to provide 50% to 200% of the hourly rate available at least hourly as a breakthrough dose. This is different from the dose ranges generally used in the acute, postoperative setting in which smaller, more frequent breakthrough doses are provided. The concept here is that children with persistent or continuous pain should not have to rely on frequently repeated doses for relief because this becomes exhausting and counterproductive to the goal of providing pain relief and maximizing function and quality of life.

Having done well on immediate-release morphine at a dose of 4 mg every 4 hours with rare breakthrough doses of 2 mg, Stan was changed to a sustained-release preparation of morphine, which was done by totaling his 24-hour analgesic requirements. Stan was changed to 15 mg sustained-release morphine of every 12 hours with a provision of 5 mg available every hour as needed for breakthrough doses. Although one-fifth of his every-12-hour dose is 3 mg, there is a fairly wide and appropriate dosing range and the convenience of dosing is one of the considerations when deciding among the options within this reasonable range.

Stan had been doing well on a sustained-release preparation of morphine. However, he developed gastroenteritis with diarrhea and vomiting and was unable to take his oral medications. Because Stan had a central line, he was changed to parenteral morphine. Referring to opioid table 30.1, the ratio when converting oral to parenteral hydromorphone was 3:1. However, many clinicians consider a 2:1 radio more appropriate. Stan's 24-hour morphine requirements of 15 mg every 12 hours and daily average of three additional breakthrough doses of 5 mg each was totaled (45 mg), divided by 3 to convert to a parenteral dose (15 mg) and divided by 24 to provide an approximate hourly infusion rate of 0.6 mg per hour of morphine. Breakthrough doses of 1 mg equal to roughly 50% to 200% of his hourly rate were provided on an hourly basis as needed. An alternative dosing regimen could have been to divide the 24-hour parenteral dose of morphine by 6 to provide 2.5 mg as intermittent dosing every 4 hours with approximately 50% of the every-4-hour dose as breakthrough. Had Stan not had a central line, the same dose could have been used as a continuous infusion or intermittent doses with breakthrough in the same manner but administered via a subcutaneous needle kept in place.

Opioid Titration

After the starting opioid doses have been used as a guide, ongoing titration to achieve pain relief is directed by the child's clinical response rather than a specific milligram dose. There is no ceiling or maximal dose with the opioids used for moderate to severe pain, and children with advanced disease such as cancer can require and tolerate huge doses of opioids (15). However, this is generally the exception; good pain control is achievable for most children with what would be considered more standard opioid dosing.

If the child has been requiring frequent breakthrough doses in a 24-hour period, then both the regularly scheduled or continuous dose is increased by 30% to 50% increments and the breakthrough dose proportionally titrated. Another option is to add up the scheduled and breakthrough doses in a 24-hour period and redistribute this increased dose over their regularly scheduled intervals, whether as a continuous infusion, an every-12-hour dose with a sustained-release preparation, or an every-4-hour dose with an immediate-release preparation.

Consider that for the first 24 hours on his intravenous morphine infusion of 0.6 mg per hour, Stan required a total of 7 additional mg of intravenous morphine as breakthrough doses. It would be reasonable to increase his hourly infusion by at least 0.3 mg per hour, which is what Stan had received as breakthrough doses or approximately a 50% increment to 0.9 mg per hour.

This approach is different from the acute, postoperative pain model in which many additional doses may be given in the course of a day and the basal or continuous dose is not increased. In this instance, the pain is not sustained but is decreasing and improving daily to resolution rather than the pattern of escalating pain and escalating requirements experienced by children living with and dying of advanced disease.

THE MANAGEMENT OF SIDE EFFECTS

Opioid-related side effects are not explored in detail in this chapter because they are well covered in Chapter 11. Potential side effects are best managed proactively by anticipating and avoiding them as much as possible. One such example is ensuring an adequate bowel regimen with a stool softener and a cathartic with the initiation of opioids. If side effects do occur, it is necessary to find out how bothersome, if at all, they are to the patient. For example, consider the child with a neurodegenerative process who has a marked and beneficial reduction in drooling with the initiation of morphine. If the side effects are bothersome, then they must be aggressively addressed or the child may elect to choose inadequate pain relief over the adverse effect.

THE USE OF ADJUVANTS IN PAIN MANAGEMENT

Specifics relating to the many options for adjunctive pharmacologic interventions are detailed elsewhere (20) and in Chapters 13 and 29. We provide here an overview of their use in children with advanced disease and in end-of-life care. The timing needs to be considered in the management plan in a child whose pain is partially controlled with an opioid but who is having some adverse effects that may be contributed to by the opioid, such as a child who is sleepier than he or she or the family would wish. In such an instance, the clinician may be reluctant to increase the opioid dose because of concern of worsening opioid-induced toxicity. It is then reasonable to either change to another opioid, particularly in the child who would prefer to take less medication.

Stan, who initially had excellent relief with morphine, transiently needed parenteral morphine and was subsequently titrated to relief. However, in the past 2 weeks, his blasts have increased markedly and with increasing analgesic requirements, he has urinary retention and irritability temporally related to the morphine, and the decision is made to change to an alternative opioid.

To convert the morphine to hydromorphone, the amount that Stan has been taking in the past 24 hours is added up. In the past 24 hours, Stan had sustained-release morphine, 60 mg every 12 hours with four additional breakthrough doses of 10 mg each. The equianalgesic table (Table 30.1) indicates that 30 mg oral morphine is roughly equianalgesic to 7.5 mg hydromorphone (a ratio of 0.25). To convert Stan's 160 mg morphine (60×2 and 4×10) to hydromorphone, multiply by 0.25, so that would roughly equal 40 mg hydromorphone. However, accounting for incomplete cross-tolerance, it would be prudent to reduce this by approximately 50% and provide 20 mg divided into six doses of immediate release. It would be reasonable to then provide 4 mg hydromorphone every 4 hours with a breakthrough dose of 2 mg as needed. After titration to relief and observing for adverse effects, a change to a sustained-release preparation would be appropriate. With this change, Stan achieved pain relief, with resolution of his irritability and urinary retention.

An alternative approach might be to add an adjuvant, such as a psychostimulant with the intent of providing enhanced pain relief and lessening the unwanted side effects (22). In some situations, a steroid could be used as an adjuvant for enhanced pain relief, permitting a reduced opioid dose. However, if the child's status is deteriorating and death is anticipated soon, then the addition of an adjuvant to try to maximize function is not likely to be helpful and only adds to the child's burden because more medicines must be taken.

INFORMATION ABOUT PAIN

It is critical to first address concerns about pain and its management with the child and family. The child should be included, as able, according to his or her level of understanding. The child should be helped to understand that the questions that he or she asks and answers about the pain helps the people caring for him or her to know how to lessen the pain and help him or her to feel better.

Parents need to hear their worries spoken, even if they would choose not to voice them; fears about pain and misperceptions about how it can be relieved are ubiquitous. They need to hear the information about the very reassuring and well-established facts about addiction, tolerance, and side effects rather than the approach that tends to be well meaning but is dismissive of their concerns.

Those who care for the dying want the child's personality and essence to remain in dying as in life. Clinicians must clearly communicate their intention that the purpose of the medications used is to relieve pain and other symptoms and not to hasten death.

Similarly, the team of health care professionals providing care may require an opportunity to discuss their concerns and review the facts. Inappropriate fear of side effects, particularly respiratory depression, can be a powerful factor in inadequate pain management.

NONPHARMACOLOGIC APPROACHES TO PAIN

Evaluating the total experience of pain and remembering the complexity of pain mechanisms mandate that health care providers use both pharmacologic and nonpharmacologic techniques to treat pain in the most effective, compassionate, and humane way. Similarly, other symptoms can be eased with a comprehensive focus that incorporates both medications and nonpharmacologic strategies.

Children have a natural affinity and a tremendous capacity and openness to these approaches. Nonpharmacologic strategies support the developmental work of children and contribute to their sense of well-being, personal control, and spirit.

Developmental stage influences the applicability of these approaches, which are reviewed in Table 30.3. Choice of techniques is also based on the child's energy level, interests, type of pain or symptoms, practicality, familiarity, cost considerations, and resource allocation. Cultural and spiritual practices can also influence a family's choices. An array of strategies can be naturally incorporated into palliative management.

Although many of these techniques have not been evaluated in rigorous controlled studies of end-of-life care, many of these techniques have been helpful clinically. For example, simple changes in the environment such as therapeutic positioning and using a fan helps to ease dyspnea. Loving family members and friends create a relaxed environment where distress may be diminished. Music has been found effective in promoting relaxation and assisting in the dying phase of life. Children familiar with cognitive-behavioral techniques, such as imagery, may find these skills useful to decrease physical symptoms such as pain, fear, and anxiety. Touch modalities, including massage, Kangaroo care, and swaddling, may ease symptoms and honor the parent–child relationship. It is valuable to remember that some children with neuropathic pain develop hypersensitivity and may prefer not to be touched. For these children, Therapeutic Touch may promote a relaxation response and be a helpful tool for parents and providers to learn. Other techniques (e.g., storytelling, art therapy, journal writing, animal-assisted therapies) may be helpful in eliciting memories and promoting life review before death.

As the illness progresses and death nears, these interventions may contribute to a quintessential combination of physical, social, psychologic, and spiritual benefits to enhance well-being and relieve suffering.

SYMPTOMS OTHER THAN PAIN

What Do We Know About Nonpain Symptoms in Pediatric End-of-Life Care?

Much of what has been published relating to the care of children at the end of life has been based on clinical experience with little or no formal evaluation or review of overall demographics. There has been a relatively recent interest in the study of a more formal approach to the care provided to children with advanced disease. For some progressive childhood illnesses, fairly specific symptoms are predictable. For example, progressive muscle weakness with eventual difficulty with eating, swallowing, and clearing secretions is a known pattern in advanced muscular dystrophy. Productive cough, possible hemoptysis, and breathlessness are prominent features in individuals with cystic fibrosis. Other illnesses have symptoms specific to the area involved, such as breathlessness secondary to pulmonary metastases in an adolescent with osteogenic sarcoma. Anticipating which symptoms are likely, reviewing with the child (as appropriate) and family any particular ones that they have concerns about,

TABLE 30.3. *Developmental approaches to non-pharmacologic strategies for pain management*

	Environmental modification	Distraction techniques	Cognitive-behavioral techniques	Sensory/physical modalities	Other strategies
Infants Developmental Age 0–1 yr	Decrease noise/light, calm demeanor, therapeutic positioning and containment, speak calmly and reassuringly, physical environment considerations, awareness of sleep-wake patterns, consider the anxiety level of child/parent(s) /practitioners	Audio: music (Transitions, Tibetan bells), soothing talk, soft novel voice; visual: mobiles, books for older; oral-motor stimulation: pacifiers, sucrose	Explanations: caregiver teaching	Physical/occupational therapy, swaddling/ containment, kangaroo care, positioning, developmental care, massage, oral-motor stimulation: pacifiers, sucrose, Therapeutic Touch	Music therapy, passive dance, prayer, Therapeutic Touch
Developmental Age 1–2 yr	As above	As above, consider variety below	As above	Rocking, positioning, physical/occupational therapy, massage, Therapeutic Touch	As above
Toddlers/ preschoolers Developmental Age 2–6 yr	Decrease noise/light, calm demeanor, therapeutic positioning, speak calmly and reassuringly, physical environment considerations, consider the anxiety level of child/ parent(s)/practitioners	Auditory: music, sing-along, ABCs; visual: pop-up books, puppets, kaleidoscopes, videos, counting tiles, flashlights; tactile: holding a favorite toy, squeezing and releasing a soft rubber ball; engaging: blow bubbles/party blowers/pinwheel; use of humor	Explanations: child and caregiver teaching, therapeutic play; imagery: magic circle/ magic game, stories use images familiar to child, storytelling; relaxation: "Go limp as a rag doll,"/yawn, "You are blowing your hurt away," "Pretend you are blowing out birthday candles," "choo-choo like a train"	Physical/occupational therapy/exercise, transcutaneous electrical nerve stimulation, heat/ cold application, massage, acupressure/acupuncture, Therapeutic Touch	Animal-assisted therapy, clowning, music/ art/dance therapies, prayer, Therapeutic Touch
School-age children Developmental Age 7–11 yr and teenagers: Developmental Age 12+ yr (techniques require greater sophistication with teens)	Decrease noise/light, calm demeanor, therapeutic positioning, speak calmly and reassuringly, physical environment considerations, consider the anxiety level of child/ parent(s)/practitioners	Auditory: Sony Walkman music; visual: videos, books; tactile: holding a Spinoza bear/ favorite toy, squeezing and releasing a Koosh ball; engaging: use of humor	Explanations: child, teen, and caregiver teaching; cognitive restructuring; imagery/hypnosis; storytelling; relaxation/ progressive muscle relaxation; biofeedback training; modeling; counseling	Physical/occupational therapy/ exercise, transcutaneous electrical nerve stimulation, heat/cold application, massage, acupressure/ acupuncture, Therapeutic Touch	Animal-assisted therapy, clowning, music/art/ dance, prayer, Therapeutic Touch

and having a proactive management plan regardless of location of care help to reduce the clinician's feelings of helplessness and the family's sense of vulnerability and reduces distress for the child.

Specific Symptoms

Some symptoms other than pain are discussed below, but more details are found in other sources (23). Symptoms can be assessed by observation and asking for input from the child, family members, or caregiver well known to the child. Collins et al. (24) developed an instrument for children to report their symptoms by modifying the adult-based Memorial Symptom Assessment Scale. They used a 30-item instrument for symptom self-report for both inpatient and outpatient children with cancer aged 10 to 18 years. Inpatients, children with solid tumors, and those having received chemotherapy in the previous 4 months were noted to rate higher symptom distress than groups not having these characteristics. Prevalent physical symptoms included lack of energy and appetite, pain, drowsiness, nausea, and cough. Worrying and feeling sad, nervous, and irritable were rated as common psychologic symptoms.

Although pain was reported as a frequent symptom of end-of-life children cared for at the first pediatric United Kingdom hospice, most of whom were cognitively impaired, muscle spasm and excessive secretions were reported as symptoms particularly difficult to control (25). Assessing the presence, location, and intensity of pain or other symptoms is a particular challenge in the cognitively impaired population. The parameters of distress are guided by behavioral observation by someone who knows the child best. Empiric trials of analgesia and other symptom management efforts are often necessary.

Respiratory Symptoms

A retrospective review was conducted over 11 years of all children dying of cancer who were cared for by a symptom care team at a large hospital in the United Kingdom. In the last 3 months of life, respiratory symptoms were noted in 40% of the case histories available for analysis (26). We know from adult-based studies of breathlessness at the end of life that this can be a symptom that is difficult to relieve without compromising cognitive function. Anecdotal evidence in children parallels this perspective.

Cystic fibrosis is a chronic progressive condition, with dyspnea acknowledged as a prominent symptom throughout advanced illness and at the end of life. However, until the work of Robinson et al. (27) in this area, virtually no studies had been undertaken about this very prominent and distressing symptom in this patient population. Caregivers are now alerted to the pattern of pain and breathlessness appearing with increased frequency in the last 2 years of life in individuals living with and dying of cystic fibrosis.

Breathlessness, like pain, is a subjective experience best measured by self-report. In children unable to report their degree of discomfort, the measurement of breathlessness is based on observation.

Clinicians should be guided in pursuing any investigations by assessing whether they might distress the child or improve the child's quality of life, to what degree they are required to direct therapy, and whether the timing is appropriate for potential therapy directed at the potential cause of the breathlessness. A standard symptom-reducing intervention is systemic opioids. The addition of benzodiazepines or other sedating medications can help to relieve the accompanying anxiety. Sedation may be required even when this intervention is acknowledged to potentially further compromise the child's cognitive function or respiratory status. Families and staff should be informed that these medications are given to help the child not mind the difficulty with breathing but that they may not change the breathing pattern.

Physical and environmental measures are often of benefit to the child and offer the family and staff some solace in providing "comfort care." Such maneuvers include position changes, a cold cloth and fan to the face, a favorite scent placed in the room, or supplemental oxygen.

Gina (not her real name) is 6 years old (weighing 20 kg) with multiply relapsed leukemia whose pain has been well controlled with 60 mg sustained-release morphine every 12 hours with an occasional breakthrough dose of 15 mg immediate-release morphine. She is now doing very poorly and playing only for a short time each day. In the past 3 days, she has become increasingly breathless and reports that she minds her breathing "very much." The family is concerned for her comfort and agrees that attempts at resuscitation would be inappropriate. Gina is treated with a 30% increase in her dose of morphine and a small initial dose of lorazepam (approximately 0.03 mg/kg starting dose) to help her not mind her breathlessness. In addition, a chest x-ray and check of her hemoglobin level to guide symptomatic therapy and treatment with antibiotics and blood transfusion were discussed with Gina and her family. The relative distress of investigations and treatment and the small chance of improvement in her quality of life at this time led the family to decline. Oxygen was tried to see whether it would bring Gina comfort but was not directed by blood gas levels or pulse oximetry.

Nausea and Vomiting

Nausea and vomiting are often multifactorial and have the best chance for relief if approached in a multifaceted way. Possible causes include the impact of the underlying disease process or the treatments of the illness. Electrolyte abnormalities and inadequate clearance of toxic metabolites from hepatic or renal insufficiency may play a role as well as opioids and other medications. Determining the most likely cause can help in choosing an antiemetic (Fig. 30.3). Small servings of preferred food or drink, avoiding bothersome odors, providing a well-ventilated space, and acupressure (28) can be helpful additional measures.

The prokinetic agents metoclopramide or domperidone are best considered if the nausea and vomiting are related to gastric stasis associated with eating or opioid therapy.

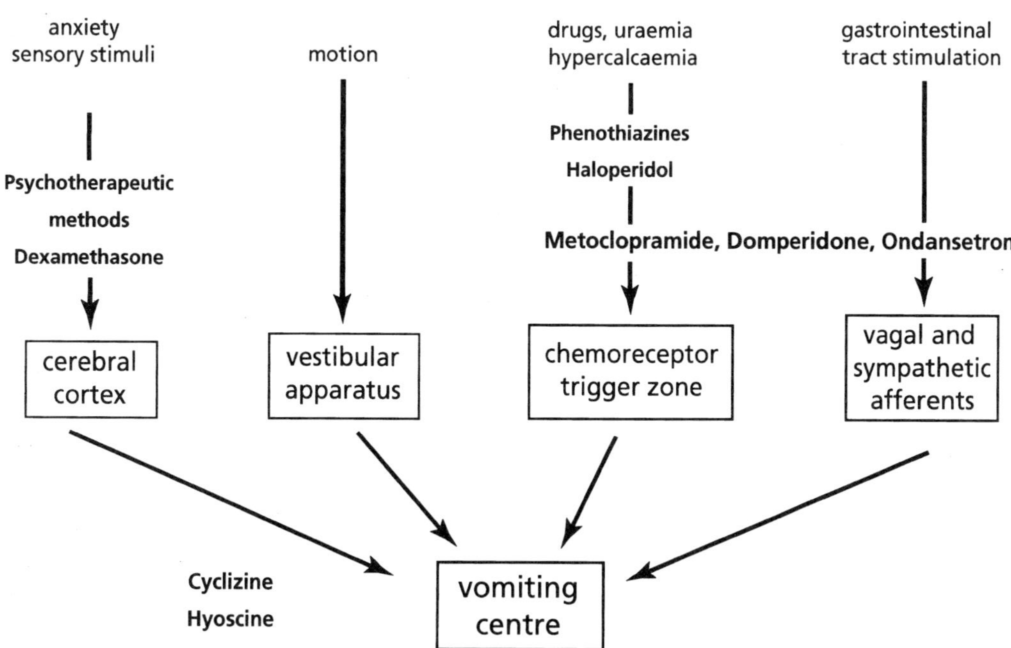

FIG. 30.3. Antiemetics and their sites of action.

Dystonia may be associated with these agents and, although reversible with 1.0 mg/kg diphenhydramine, is distressing. The recent concern about cisapride's numerous drug interactions and potential serious side effect profile has virtually eliminated its use as a prokinetic option (29). If nausea and vomiting are related to the peak onset of action after opioid administration, the opioid schedule can be changed to provide a smoother pharmacokinetic curve or an alternate opioid can be tried.

Anticipatory vomiting may be more selectively approached by a combination of pharmacologic anxiolysis with lorazepam and cognitive strategies; if movement is a trigger, an agent such as scopolamine (hyoscine) is appropriate.

The serotonin 5-HT_3 receptor antagonist ondansetron, typically used for the nausea and vomiting induced by chemotherapy, can also be helpful in other situations. When faced with increased intracranial pressure, as in the child with a brain tumor, the most helpful agent is dexamethasone or another steroid, although they are also of benefit for other causes of nausea. Deciding when to introduce steroids, how long to maintain them, and at what dose can be a challenge but must be considered because the adverse effects most frequently associated with prolonged use or higher doses can seriously affect quality of life. Cyclizine, from the neuroleptic class of agents, has been suggested to provide greater benefit than some of the other antiemetic options in the setting of increased intracranial pressure. This may be of particular help when combined with ondansetron in a child with increased intracranial pressure when the choice has been made to avoid steroids because of the side effect profile with continued use (23).

The cause is often unclear, and empiric trials of a range of antiemetics are used, often concurrently. When considering which neuroleptic to choose, one of the determining factors is whether sedation is a goal. Haloperidol is the least sedating of the group, which includes chlorpromazine and methotrimeprazine. Sometimes, particularly in the very end stages of life, sedation may be a beneficial effect.

Pruritus

Pruritus may be related to exogenous factors such as dry skin, the laundry or body soap, or medications including opioids. Endogenous causes may be the primary cause in liver or kidney failure. To some extent, the causes determine the intervention, although symptomatic relief may be provided by combined measures to moisten the skin and reduce irritation from clothes and sheets in addition to antihistamines.

Disturbed Sensorium

A child with an altered sensorium may present in an agitated and confused state or a sedated and confused state or may sometimes fluctuate between the two. Several concurrent factors contribute to this difficult symptom including opioids and other centrally acting medications, impaired kidney or liver function, or abnormalities in electrolytes or glucose metabolism. The degree of investigation is directed by the child's general condition and proximity to death, the likelihood of a reversible cause, and the tolerability of the possible interventions that attempt to reverse the cause. Concurrent strategies are directed at the relief of this symptom, which is always distressing to the family and sometimes to the patient. In a child unable to verbalize distress, pain or other distressing stimuli such as breathlessness and itch should be considered. Physical measures can also be used, particularly in instances of mild agitation, by incorporating routines that are comforting and familiar to the child, decreasing environmental stimulation, and having their favorite blanket or toy close at hand. A change to another opioid can be considered if dose reduction would cause increased distress and/or the addition of a neuroleptic. If the clinician thinks that it is unlikely that the child will live much longer, sedation would be preferable to a change of opioid.

Seizures

With the concurrent metabolic derangements that accompany the dying process, seizures may occur in children with no seizure history. They may also present in a child with previously well-controlled seizures in their new setting of hypoxemia or other biochemical disturbances. Some medications used for symptom relief may also decrease the child's threshold for seizures such as a neuroleptic used for the treatment of agitation. Seizures should be treated with anticonvulsants because they may be distressing to the child and certainly add to the stress of family members and other caregivers. The management of seizures at the end of life follows conventional anticonvulsant principles including treating the acute episode and providing ongoing anticonvulsant therapy with concurrent support and information for the family. Investigations into the possible cause or contributing factors should be considered in the context of the relative benefits and burdens of the investigations.

Bleeding

Correction of coagulopathy with platelets or other blood products should not be an automatic response to routine blood counts or minor petechiae but may be an appropriate preventive measure when the likelihood of bleeding is high. Additional treatments directed at preventing or reducing bleeding are tranexamic acid (25 mg/kg per dose orally or 10 mg/kg intravenously four times daily) or aminocaproic acid (100 mg/kg per dose intravenously or orally every 6 hours to a maximal daily dose of 30 g). The latter agent can also be applied as nose drops or a mouth rinse. When bleeding is anticipated, the staff and family should be helped to prepare physically and emotionally for this possibility. Health care workers can also prepare by having appropriate emergency medications such as analgesics and sedatives readily accessible to rapidly give to the child if he or she is conscious at the time of a massive bleed. Measures that help to reduce the visual impact include using dark towels and sheets.

THE TREATMENT OF REFRACTORY SYMPTOMS BY PROVIDING SEDATION AT THE END OF LIFE

Most of the time, pain and other symptoms both throughout the child's disease course and at the end of life can be adequately relieved with what would be considered usual or standard therapeutic measures (15). Infrequently, the symptoms may not be adequately relieved without significant compromise of consciousness. In such circumstances, albeit rare, it is essential to have an approach to management to ensure comfort in the face of a distressing symptom (30,31).

A suggested approach is that a discussion should take place with at least one other individual having extensive expertise in the management of pain and other symptoms occurring at the end of life. The discussion should include a review of which approaches have been tried to date with which adverse effects, the proximity of death, the presence of concurrent symptoms, and the child's, family's, and health professionals' understanding of the child's current condition. These factors assist with decisions about how comfort will be assured. Consider the child who has had repeated, sequential, and appropriate titration of systemic opioids including adjuvants for severe leg pain secondary to widely and locally invasive osteogenic sarcoma with inadequate pain relief despite intolerable toxicities of confusion and somnolence. The use of an epidural or comparable regional technique would be reasonable if the time frame is realistic. However, if death is anticipated or the child has concurrent breathlessness secondary to lung metastases, then such a technique would not be a beneficial intervention and sedation for the remainder of their end-of-life course would be more appropriate.

This issue of intervention is fraught with concerns and misperceptions. It is very important for health care professionals, the child (as appropriate), and the family to be aware of the intention of the intervention and that the intervention is not equivalent to euthanasia. Proactive discussion with staff about their potential concerns and what is referred to as the "principle of double effect" needs to be clarified. This refers to the concept that an action that has one intention, such as providing comfort to the child terminally ill with osteogenic sarcoma with refractory pain and breathlessness, may have the unintended but potential consequence of hastening death by contributing to further respiratory compromise. Even though health care professionals need to understand the concept, the reality is that this causal relationship is actually extremely unlikely in patients, such as this individual, with significant opioid tolerance and concurrent stimulation of the central nervous system because of their distressing symptoms. In fact, for this reason, in someone already on opioid therapy for symptom management, opioids are generally not the most effective agent for achieving sedation. Generally, adjuvants such as benzodiazepines or a sedating neuroleptic such as methotrimeprazine are added and titrated to provide relief through sedation. Tables indicating starting doses and titration are available (32).

The family and staff require ongoing guidance throughout this process, including supporting their continuing to talk with and to touch and hold the child and information about what, if any, vocalizations or other bodily responses should be expected to be present or absent.

PSYCHOLOGIC ISSUES

Caring for a child with a life-threatening illness presents a family with great emotional and practical burdens, which may exist over many years. The child's and family's level of anxiety and emotional distress, their coping skills, their past experiences of pain and illness, and the meaning that the symptoms and underlying illness have for them are intimately linked with the child's experience of the illness, both emotionally and physically.

Sensitive assessment of whether the child and the family are suffering is fundamental to palliative care. For providers, understanding the personal nature of suffering necessitates focusing not only on the body but understanding the whole person (32). Although pain and unrelieved symptoms may be a common cause of suffering and shared negative emotions, suffering is a very distinct, disturbing, complex, and individual experience (33–38). Physical pain can add to emotional distress, and emotional and psychologic suffering can influence physical pain.

Children and their parents fear dying in pain, and unrelieved symptoms heighten the degree of suffering. "Relentless pain and symptomatic distress and other causes of stress can drive a terminally ill person from coping, courage and integration to chaos and hopelessness" (36). To this end, palliative care specialists can address suffering proactively by treating potentially chronic pain and symptoms aggressively and promoting the psychosocial well-being of the patient at every opportunity (36).

In palliative care, a child's world changes and his or her sense of self is threatened as the condition progresses and debilitation occurs. Favorite activities may diminish, a sense of isolation may occur, and loss of autonomy may result from the inability to accomplish previously important purposes. Suffering or severe distress induced by loss of integrity, intactness, cohesiveness, or wholeness of the person (34) may result.

Carla (not her real name) was a 5-year-old girl in whom Burkitt lymphoma was progressing and, based on her family's preference, was receiving terminal care in a hospital. Despite ongoing titration of analgesics and anxiolytics, she continued to be distressed and agitated. The situation was resolved by recognizing that her distress was not solely related to increasing physical disease but to her emotional needs. She was suffering because her hope at this time of her life was to help care for her newborn premature brother that she had been anticipating. Successful intervention involved having her infant brother brought to stay in her room with her so she could help nurture and care for him. By pausing to understand Carla's profound suffering and needs, opportunities could be provided for her to regain a sense of meaning and worth and attain a sense of completion.

Over the past 20 years, the psychosocial dilemmas facing families with a child dying of cancer and their implications for looking after the families have been considered at some length (39–45). Several themes emerge repeatedly from the literature:

- the difficulty of living with uncertainty,
- that emotional needs and ways of coping vary among different family members and at different points through the illness,
- a family's need for information,
- the benefits of open and honest communication, both within the family and between the family and health care professionals,
- the importance to the family of retaining control and choices.

The specific needs of families with children with other life-threatening illnesses have not been as extensively explored, but there seems to be considerable common ground (1,2,46–48). The more extended time course for many of the children with nonmalignant diseases, their more intense nursing needs, and the many children with severe intellectual and physical handicap only intensify problems for families and increase the practical difficulties. Supportive techniques that help to alleviate suffering include questioning, attentive listening, being present, and compassion (33–35,49). These need to be part of flexible, coordinated, and prolonged multidisciplinary support for families that also addresses their practical problems and need for respite care. This is highlighted by a mother of a child with a neurodegenerative disease who, frustrated by the bureaucracy of accessing different professionals and departments for financial, medical, physiotherapy, and social help, said "If someone could coordinate my practical needs, I'd need a lot less psychological support."

SPIRITUAL ISSUES

Concern for a child's and family's spiritual needs is acknowledged as part of palliative care (1,6) but can be an aspect of care that health care professionals feel uneasy with and can find difficult to make sense of in practical terms.

The spiritual dimension in life is concerned with exploring its ultimate purpose and values. It focuses on our search for existential meaning in our life, relationships, experiences, and our attempts to transcend their material aspects. Spirituality may include religious belief, which addresses these questions through a particular system of faith and worship, but it is much broader. There is reason to believe that it is just as important to children and young people as it is to adults (50–53).

For children with life-threatening illnesses and the families facing their death, many powerful questions may arise: What is the purpose of my life? Why do children die? What is the meaning of pain and suffering? Why is life unfair? What is God's role? Are we being punished? These concerns can generate powerful feelings of anxiety, guilt, fear, isolation, and hopelessness. The anguish of spirit that results causes suffering in itself but can also contribute to the child's experience of physical pain and to the child's and family's ability to cope.

These worries and difficulties are often unspoken as parents, children, and health care workers evolve complex webs of avoidance, collusion, and mutual protection. To help, caregivers need to be open and receptive to the verbal and behavioral cues that children and families might give, both of their spiritual needs and religious beliefs (51,52). These may be overt:

> When Maya (not her real name), a 6-year-old girl with a progressive tumor, was asked what she did when she had pain, her father replied that they prayed together, but if that did not work, he would be prepared to use the pain medicine.

However, sometimes the cues that a child gives may be difficult even for a sensitive parent to interpret. Elizabeth's mother writes (54):

> My objective was to reach the best level of pain control with the minimum of sedation. If I'm honest I have to say I didn't always achieve this. I found it difficult to distinguish between

> confusion, anxiety and pain, indeed there were times when these were present together.

Staff also need the skill, confidence, and sometimes courage to act on the cues that they receive.

> Martin (not his real name), a 14-year-old boy with a progressive brain tumor and a serious history of depression, had become increasingly withdrawn, had taken to his bed, and complained of lack of energy and headaches that failed to respond to medication. His mother and grandmother did not want to risk deepening his depression by telling him of his tumor progression and prognosis. A trusted physician visited him at home and acknowledged his isolation and fears that his tumor had recurred and then answered his questions about his impending death honestly. Just 10 minutes later, he came down from his room saying "Thanks, I'd better get up now, I've got a lot of living to fit in."

Sometimes a family's belief system and interpretation of a situation can differ substantially from those of the people caring for them and potential conflict develops. Nursing and medical staff who have been brought up in the Western tradition tend to see little positive value in pain and suffering and only wish to alleviate them. However, some traditions hold a belief that pain and suffering are an inevitable, indeed necessary, part of this life. They may also believe that experiencing them is an essential contribution toward a better afterlife. Maya's father (above) was willing to use conventional analgesia to augment prayer, but other families may not be. It can be very challenging to negotiate a path of action when the family and health care team hold different beliefs about what is in the child's best interest.

A willingness to explore existential issues with mutual respect, finding opportunities for the child to express his or her own view, and acknowledging a shared effort to help the child provide a basis for working with the family. This approach may enable the child and family to express their feelings, perhaps verbally or symbolically such as through play or art. The opportunity may then develop to help them find some meaning in what is happening, to increase their sense of control, and to encourage them to find appropriate short-term goals and hopes. They can also be assured that staff will be along side them throughout the illness and will not abandon them.

PROVISION OF CARE

Palliative care is designed to promote comfort, trust, safety, closeness, and optimal quality of life. Venues for care, team dynamics, and anticipatory guidance and planning are important considerations that influence the quality of the living and dying experience for the child and the family.

Choice of Location of Care

Children can receive palliative care services in a variety of settings; home-based programs, a freestanding inpatient hospice, facilities located within a hospital, and district palliative care teams. The preference of the child and family and what they deem is the most supportive environment should guide which option is chosen. Regardless of the choice, families appreciate providers respecting their choice. In addition, if a family who has chosen home-hospice care and then returns to the hospital to receive care, the concept of "choosing what feels the most supportive" can allay a family's guilt that they failed as parents and family members.

Cultural preferences may make one option more suitable for a family and demands sensitivity and respect from providers (55,56). Logistic factors such as availability of services in a geographic area, different health care systems, resources, or a provider's familiarity with a setting may also influence the decision. Unfortunately, several barriers have been cited in the literature that may interfere with families accessing hospice and palliative care services. These include the provider's resistance to change, lack of equating a good death with success as a practitioner, propriety issues, and insurance issues. Awareness of and seeking solutions to address these issues are critical to ensure that palliative care and hospice services are presented as a viable option and to facilitate easier and earlier transition to supportive end-of-life care.

Types of Programs

Psychologic and emotional benefits for terminally ill children in the home environment have been well documented (57–65). Primary advantages include dying in a comfortable and familiar setting with a familiar and normal pattern of daily life and surrounded by loving family members. Although variations exist between types of home care–based programs, essential elements of these programs include

- 24-hour access to pediatric and family care expertise,
- 24-hour access to pediatric palliative care expertise,
- key worker to coordinate,
- immediate access to hospital if needed (62,66).

Specific inpatient palliative care facilities for children are still uncommon, and because the family home is often the preferred place for children and families, this is often where care and services are focused. Inpatient facilities include those primarily for respite care such as the freestanding children's hospices developed initially in the United Kingdom but now beginning to be established internationally (67,68). There are also hospital-based rooms devoted to palliative care and hospital-based comprehensive palliative care teams/programs that can facilitate a family's transition from a curative to a palliative approach to care (5,65,66,69). However, children are still cared for until death within acute and tertiary pediatric centers. This may be a positive choice by parents and children who know the staff well, feel supported, and do not wish to be at home. However, it requires a concerted effort in this setting to achieve a relaxed environment, flexibility in care, staff continuity, and ensuring that the family members are included. Education and support for health care staff in this situation are paramount. Ensuring that patients and parents are given control and have the opportunity for important and healing discussions must be emphasized and encouraged and can be achieved in all settings (G. Frager, personal communication).[1]

> Derrick was a 12-year-old boy with a background history of immune deficiency who then developed lymphoma. While being treated with the intent to cure, he developed progressive pulmonary compromise. His parents wished full investigative and supportive intervention, including ventilatory support and a lung biopsy to elucidate a possible infectious cause. Despite their decision about the degree of intervention, they were able to have an open discussion with Derrick before his intubation, subsequent deterioration, and death in the intensive care unit. In this conversation, Derrick told his parents how much he loved them, asked that they never forget him, and requested that if he did die, his mother should open their door at home to a cat, stating that he was going to "come back as a cat."

Planning Care as a Team

Planning comprehensive end-of-life care works best with a well-functioning multidisciplinary team in which each member can contribute his or her experience and expertise. However, it is also important to acknowledge that being a team member and working with children who are dying and their families can be a dynamic and a challenging task. Core tenets of a palliative care team include the following.

- Parents are the primary providers of care.
- A family-centered approach to care means the involvement of the child and family members as vested members of the team. Goals defined by the child and family direct the plan of care. Options for medicines, nonpharmacologic approaches, and other supportive and therapeutic approaches can be presented to the family. They in turn choose what fits with their values and family culture.
- The team is interdisciplinary in nature to meet the physical, psychosocial, spiritual, and practical needs of the child and family.

[1]With thanks to the family of Derrick Robinson, who died May 15, 1999, but whose strength of spirit lives on.

- A named coordinator of care for each child and family helps to respond quickly and effectively to changing needs, streamlines the process, and assists in mobilizing resources.
- Flexibility and creativity are essential to individualize care and to support the sense of control and autonomy to meet the needs, wishes, and goals of the child.
- The value of honest and ongoing communication and clarity of roles among and between team members cannot be overemphasized. Communication and collaboration among all team members create respect, prevent disruption in care, and avoid competition between health care professionals. This is of particular importance if a child's care takes place in more than one geographic setting and when care is transferred between providers.
- Being present, empathy, and listening are essential elements that bear witness to the child's and family's journey and reassure them that they will not be abandoned.

ANTICIPATION AND PLANNING AHEAD

It cannot be overstated that careful anticipation and planning for pain and symptom relief throughout palliative care and the active phases of dying can help to avoid crises and relieve suffering. In some geographic locations, pain and symptom algorithms for palliative care have been established to assist in promoting consistent, prompt care and in minimizing the time between identification and treatment of symptoms (70). The physician-approved algorithms function as standing orders that optimize comfort and quality of life.

One approach for helping parents to maintain control and to help reduce crisis management is to provide anticipatory guidance and information. Some of the information that parents appreciate most includes the likely progress of the disease with a description of potential symptoms and how they can be managed. Frequent discussions prepare parents for the natural changes in their child's condition. Making sure that medications and equipment are readily available even before symptoms occur and that possible changes of routes have been anticipated helps to avoid emergencies. Practical information for families includes how to administer medicines and general principles of loading, maintenance, and titration. They also value a description of physical signs that death is approaching, how death may occur, and what to do afterward. Through teaching, the family's knowledge, sense of control, confidence, and coping are strengthened, fear is reduced, symptoms are more readily managed, and crises are minimized. It is hoped that in this way the child can be helped to live with as little suffering as possible and die with dignity.

REFERENCES

1. Association for Children with Life-threatening or Terminal Conditions and Their Families and the Royal College of Paediatrics and Child Health. *A guide to the development of children's palliative care services. Report of a joint working party*. Bristol, U.K.: Association for Children with Life-threatening or Terminal Conditions and Their Families, 1997.
2. Lewis M. The lifetime service—a model for children with life-threatening illnesses and their families. *Pediatr Nurs* 1999;11:21–23.
3. Frager G. Pediatric palliative care: building the model, bridging the gaps. *J Palliat Care* 1996;12:9–12.
4. Liben S. Pediatric palliative care—obstacles to overcome. *J Palliat Care* 1996;12:24–28.
5. Levetown M. Pediatric hospice care: not the care of small adults. *Home Health Care Manage Practice* 1997; 9:36–42.
6. American Academy of Pediatrics Committees on Bioethics and Hospital Care. Palliative care for children. *Pediatrics* 2000;106:351–357.
7. Royal College of Paediatrics and Child Health. *Withholding or withdrawing life saving treatment in children—a framework for practice*. London: Royal College of Paediatrics and Child Health, 1997.
8. Cornaglia C, Massimo L, Haupt R, et al. Incidence of pain in children with neoplastic disease. *Pain* 1984;2 [Suppl]:S28.
9. Ljungman G, Gordh T, Sorensen S, et al. Pain in paediatric oncology: interviews with children, adolescents and their parents. *Acta Paediatr* 1999;88:623–630.
10. Miser AW, Mcalla J, Dothage JA, et al. Pain as a presenting symptom in children and young adults with newly diagnosed malignancy. *Pain* 1987;29:85–90.
11. Miser AW. Management of pain associated with childhood cancer. In: Schechter NL, Berde CB, Yaster M. eds. *Pain in infants, children, and adolescents*. Baltimore: Williams & Wilkins; 1993:411–424.
12. Sirkia K, Hovi L, Pouttu J, et al. Pain medication during terminal care of children, with cancer. *J Pain Symptom Manage* 1998;15:220–226.
13. Goldman A, Beardsmore S, Hunt J. Palliative care for

children with cancer—home, hospital or hospice? *Arch Dis Child* 1990;65:641–643.
14. Goldman A, Bowman A. The role of oral controlled-release morphine for pain relief in children with cancer. *Palliat Med* 1990;4:279–285.
15. Collins JJ, Grier HE, Kinney HC, et al. Control of severe pain in children with terminal malignancy. *J Pediatr* 1995;126:653–657.
16. Wolfe J, Grier H, Klar N, et al. Symptoms and suffering at the end of life in children with cancer. *N Engl J Med* 2000;342:326–332.
17. Hirschfeld S, Moss H, Dragisic K, et al. Pain in pediatric human immunodeficiency virus infection: incidence and characteristics in a single-institution pilot study. *Pediatrics* 1996;98:449–452.
18. Yaster M, Schechter N. Pain and human immunodeficiency virus infection in children. *Pediatrics* 1996;98: 455–456.
19. World Health Organization Ladder. *Cancer pain relief and palliative care. Technical report series 804.* Geneva: World Health Organization, 1990.
20. World Health Organization. *Cancer pain relief and palliative care in children.* Geneva: World Health Organization, 1998.
21. Galloway KS, Yaster M. Pain and symptom control in terminally ill children. *Pediatr Clin North Am* 2000;47: 711–747.
22. Yee JD, Berde CB. Dextroamphetamine or methylphenidate as adjuvants to opioid analgesia for adolescents with cancer. *J Pain Symptom Manage* 1994;9:122–125.
23. Goldman A. *Care of the dying child.* Oxford: Oxford University Press, 1998.
24. Collins JJ, Byrnes ME, Dunkel IJ, et al. The measurement of symptoms in children with cancer. *J Pain Symptom Manage* 2000;19:363–377.
25. Hunt AM. A survey of signs, symptoms and symptom control in 30 terminally ill children. *Dev Med Child Neurol* 1990;32:341–346.
26. Hain RD, Patel N, Crabtree S, et al. Respiratory symptoms in children dying from malignant disease. *Palliat Med* 1995;9:201–206.
27. Robinson WM, Ravilly S, Berde C, et al. End-of-life care in cystic fibrosis. *Pediatrics* 1997;100:205–209.
28. Dundee JW, Yang J, MacMillan C. Non-invasive stimulation of the P6 (Neiguan) antiemetic acupuncture point in cancer chemotherapy. *J Soc Med* 1991;84:221–212.
29. Shulman RJ, Boyle JT, Collett RB, et al. The use of cisapride in children. *J Pediatr Gastroenterol Nutr* 1999; 28:529–553.
30. Chemy NI, Portenoy RK. Sedation in the management of refractory symptoms. Guidelines for evaluation and treatment. *J Palliat Care* 1994;10:31–38.
31. Kenny NP, Frager G. Refractory symptoms and terminal sedation of children: ethical issues and practical management. *J Palliat Care* 1996;12:40–45.
32. Frager G. Palliative care and terminal care of children. *Child Adolesc Clin North Am* 1997;6:889–909.
33. Byock IR. The nature of suffering and the nature of opportunity at the end of life. *Clin Geriatr Med* 1996;12: 237–252.
34. Cassell EJ. *The nature of suffering and the goals of medicine.* New York: Oxford University Press, 1991.
35. Cassell EJ. Pain and suffering. In: Reich WT, ed. *Encyclopedia of bioethics.* New York: Simon & Schuster, 1995:1897–1905.
36. Chapman CR, Gavrin J. Suffering and its relationship to pain. *J Palliat Care* 1993;9:5–13.
37. Rogers BL, Cowles KV. A conceptual foundation for human suffering in nursing care and research. *J Adv Nurs* 1997;24:1048–1053.
38. Van Hooft A. The meaning of suffering. *Hastings Cent Rep* 1998;2813–2819.
39. Barbarin O, Chesler M. Coping as interpersonal strategy: families with childhood cancer. *Fam Syst Med* 1984;2:279–289.
40. Van Dongen-Melman J, Sanders-Woudstra J. Psychosocial aspects of childhood cancer—a review of the literature. *J Child Psychol Psychiatr* 1986;27:145–180.
41. Van Dongen-Melman J, Pruyn J, Van Zanen G, et al. Coping with childhood cancer: a conceptual view. *J Psychosoc Oncol* 1986;4:147–160.
42. Whittam EH. Terminal care of the dying child—psychosocial implications of care. *Cancer* 1993;71[Suppl]: 3451–3462.
43. Lauria M, Hockenberry-Eaton M, Pawletko T, et al. Psychosocial protocol for childhood cancer. *Cancer* 1996;78[Suppl]:1346–1356.
44. James L, Johnson B. The needs of parents of pediatric oncology patients during the palliative care phase. *J Pediatr Oncol Nurs* 1997;14:83–95.
45. Vickers J, Carlisle C. Choices and control: parental experiences of pediatric terminal home care. *J Pediatr Oncol Nurs* 2000;17:12–21.
46. While A, Citrone A, Cornish J. *Executive summary: a study of the needs and provisions for families care for children with life limiting incurable disorders.* London: Department of Health, Department of Nursing Studies, King's College London, 1996.
47. Mastroyannopoulou K, Stallard P, Lewis M, et al. The impact of childhood nonmalignant life threatening illness on parents: gender differences and predictors of parental adjustment. *J Child Psychol Psychiatry* 1997; 38:823–829.
48. Bluebond-Langner M. *In the shadow of illness.* Princeton: Princeton University Press, 1996.
49. Bretscher ME, Creagen ET. Understanding suffering: what palliative medicine teaches us. *Mayo Clin Proc* 1997;72:785–787.
50. Attig T. Beyond pain: the existential suffering of children. *J Palliat Med* 1996;12:20–23.
51. Hart H, Schneider D. Spiritual care for children with cancer. *Semin Nurs Oncol* 1997;13:263–270.
52. Fulton RA, Moore CM. Spiritual care of the school-age child with a chronic condition. *J Pediatr Nurs* 1995; 10:224–231.
53. Kenny G. The iron cage and the spiders web: children's spirituality and the hospital environment. *Pediatr Nurs* 1999;11:20–24.
54. Astelm J. Elizabeth and Alexandra's story. *Child Care Health Dev* 1995;21:369–375.
55. Martinson I. Hospice care for children: past, present and future. *J Pediatr Oncol Nurs* 1993;10:93–98.
56. Sagara M, Pickett M. Sociocultural influences and care of dying children in Japan and the United States. *Cancer Nurs* 1998;21:274–281.
57. Lauer ME. Ongoing challenges in paediatric hospice care. *Acta Paediatr* 1997;86:1037–1039.
58. Mulhern RK, Lauer ME, Hoffmann RG. Death of a child at home or in the hospital: subsequent psychological adjustment of the family. *Pediatrics* 1983;71:743–747.

59. Duffy CM, Pollock P, Levy M, et al. Home-based palliative care for children—Part II: the benefits of an established program. *J Palliat Care* 1990;6:8–14.
60. Collins JJ, Stevens MM, Sousens P. Home care for the dying child. *Aust Fam Physician* 1998;27:610–614.
61. Birenbaum LK, McCown DE, Nunneley C. *Nurses manual for family childhood cancer study*. Portland: Oregon Health Sciences University, 1986.
62. Goldman A. Home care of the dying child. *J Palliat Care* 1996;12:16–19.
63. Chambers EJ, Oakhill A. Models of care for children dying of malignant diseases. *Palliat Med* 1995;9: 181–185.
64. Sirkia K, Saarinen UM, Ahlgren B, et al. Terminal care of the child with cancer at home. *Acta Paediatr* 1997; 86:1125–1130.
65. Kopecky EA, Jacobson S, Joshi P, et al. Review of a home-based palliative care program for children with malignant and non-malignant diseases. *J Palliat Care* 1997;130:18–33.
66. Liben S, Goldman A. Home care for children with life-threatening illness. *J Palliat Care* 1998;14:33–38.
67. Worswick J. Helen House: a model of children's hospice care. *Eur J Palliat Care* 1995;2:17–20.
68. Eng B, Davies B. Canuck Place: a hospice for children. *Can Oncol Nurs J* 1992;2:18–20.
69. Campbell ML, Frank RR. Experience with end-of-life practice at a university hospital. *Crit Care Med* 1997; 25:197–202.
70. Pomietto M, ed. *Pediatric pain and symptom algorithms for palliative care*. Seattle: Children's Hospital and Regional Medical Center, 1999.

31

Sedation

G. Allen Finley and Neil L. Schechter

The use of sedation for diagnostic and treatment procedures in children has paralleled the increased recognition and treatment of pain that has occurred in the past 10 years. Unfortunately, many medical interventions involve procedures that penetrate the skin or body cavities in a way that causes pain. For most children, these necessary painful procedures are among the worst parts of being ill and, for many, cast an indelible shadow over their relationship with health care providers and institutions. Children anticipate some pain as a routine part of their visit based on past experience. This anticipation is magnified in children with chronic disease. There is now a strong literature that suggests that many children with chronic disease view diagnostic and treatment procedures as far worse than the disease for which they are being treated (1–3). For example, in 1990, McGrath and colleagues (3) reported experiences in an outpatient pediatric oncology clinic and found that the pain from repeated procedures was, for many children, the worst part of having cancer. Katz and colleagues (4) documented the level of distress in their study of 115 children undergoing oncology procedures (bone marrow biopsies) with local anesthetic infiltration but no systemic analgesia or sedation. They found that 97% of children demonstrated behavioral evidence of anxiety, 73% verbal expressions of pain, 65% cried, and 34% required restraint.

Despite this overwhelming concern, however, procedural pain has historically been ignored. Laceration repairs, bone marrow aspirations, lumbar punctures, and even venipunctures were accomplished by physically restraining the child so that the task could be performed with a minimum of movement by the child. This approach was unfortunately often cynically referred to as "brutane" (from halothane, a common general anesthetic). When sedation was offered, often inappropriate drugs were selected that either did not offer pain relief or were administered in a painful manner and the effects of which lasted far longer than was necessary to complete the procedure (5,6). There were often mishaps associated with sedation, such as excessive or prolonged side effects and even occasional deaths, which worked as a further disincentive for physicians to use it before procedures (7). Unfortunately, the pain and agitation that come with feeling helpless and physically restrained were often the only memories that children took from visits to the emergency department or the treatment room in hospitals. These memories often had an impact on subsequent procedures by increasing the perceived pain (8).

Much of this has changed in the past 15 years. New information about sedation as well as the increased recognition of the negative impact that inadequately treated pain has on children has led to a dramatic increase in the use of sedation (8–11). Unfortunately, problems persist. There remains no ideal, uniformly accepted approach to sedation, and there continue to be significant disciplinary biases about a variety of aspects of sedation. Recommendations by the pediatric (12), anesthesia (13), dental (14), and emergency medicine (15) societies differ on key elements, often determined by the needs and perspective of the specific discipline. There remains political controversy about who should be entitled to perform sedation, what credentials should be necessary, and who should control access to specific drugs.

Despite differences, there are many areas of agreement. The type of sedation that one uses clearly depends on the desired clinical effect. Noninvasive procedures that require only the child's cooperation and immobilization but that are not painful (i.e., computed tomography, electroencephalography, magnetic resonance imaging) require agents that induce sedation but not analgesia. Other procedures that require the child's cooperation but also may be associated with some pain (i.e., laceration repairs, lumbar punctures, phlebotomies, various dental procedures) that require different agents that offer localized analgesia in addition to sedation. Finally, there are procedures that are associated with a significant amount of pain and require immobilization. These include bone marrow aspirations, debridement, endoscopy, complex laceration repairs, and thoracostomy tube placements. These procedures may require even more potent agents. Regardless of the type of agent used, however, whether only for immobilization or for painful and complex procedures, all sedation requires adequate monitoring and preparation and should be performed by individuals skilled in airway maintenance. It is often not possible to predict what effect a specific drug might have, and, therefore, even if one is expecting to administer light sedation, one must be prepared for deep sedation or general anesthesia.

Many of the chapters in this book contain discussions about sedation for specific pain problems. This chapter emphasizes broader principles and generally reviews the strategies and methods of sedation. The reader is referred to chapters on specific problems for more individualized discussion.

DEFINITIONS

The terminology applied to the practice of sedation is clearly in flux. The American Academy of Pediatrics Subcommittee on Drugs (12,16), in a series of papers, offered the following definitions:

Conscious sedation: a medically controlled state of depressed consciousness that allows protective reflexes to be maintained, retains the patient's ability to maintain a patent airway independently and continuously, and permits appropriate response by the patient to physical stimulation or verbal command.

Deep sedation: a medically controlled state of depressed consciousness or unconsciousness from which the patient is not easily aroused, accompanied by partial or complete loss of protective reflexes. Patients may be unable to maintain a patent airway independently or respond purposely to physical stimulation or verbal command while deeply sedated.

General anesthesia: a medically controlled state of unconsciousness accompanied by the loss of protective reflexes, including the inability to maintain a patent airway and respond purposely to physical stimulation or verbal command.

Although these definitions attempt to create discrete categories of sedation, both the uniqueness of the categories that they describe and the usefulness of the categorization in general have recently been called into question by a number of authorities. Maxwell and Yaster (17) suggested that conscious sedation is in fact a myth. They state that individuals who are still responsive to voice will experience pain and typically will not be as immobile as is necessary to successfully complete a procedure. They state, therefore, that the level of sedation required for most procedures that require immobilization and cause pain is deep sedation. This opinion has been echoed by others as well. The Task Force on Sedation and Analgesia by Non-Anesthesiologists of the American Society of Anesthesiologists (13) offers the term *sedation analgesia* as the therapeutic goal that they believe is more precise than the term *conscious sedation*. The American College of Emergency Physicians (14) offers the term *procedural sedation* for the state associated with a depressed level of consciousness but one that allows the patient to maintain airway control independently and continuously.

In a review of sedation and analgesia for procedures in children, Kraus and Green (18) attempt to examine the 12 conflicting sets of guidelines for sedation that have been offered by professional organizations. They state that if a child is essentially cooperative, many procedures that are minimally invasive can be performed with the child in what they call a "primary sedation state." In this state, cardiorespiratory depression is unlikely, and this is the most common sedation level used by physicians. When the procedure is painful, however, such as a bone marrow aspiration or fracture reduction, and/or there is considerable anxiety, then deep sedation may be necessary. They state that this most likely should be accomplished by anesthesiologists, intensivists, or emergency department physicians who are extensively trained in advanced life support.

What emerges from any discussion about sedation, however, is the notion that there is an easy progression between states of sedation and any agent that can induce procedural or conscious sedation can also produce deep sedation. Therefore, most authorities on sedation believe that all individuals who perform sedation should be extremely vigilant and assume that any attempt at sedation may yield at least deep sedation and take appropriate precautions.

FACTORS THAT AFFECT THE PAIN EXPERIENCE DURING PROCEDURES

Numerous factors, both intrinsic and extrinsic to the child, have an impact on how the pain of procedures is experienced. These factors have been reviewed in detail earlier (Chapter 6) but are included here for sake of completeness.

Intrinsic Factors

It is quite clear that the age of the child has a significant impact on his or her perception of pain. In multiple studies (19,20), it has been demonstrated that younger children experience more pain from the same diagnostic and treatment procedures than do older children. The decrease in pain in older children seems to parallel the development of the Piagetian stage of concrete operations (often beginning between 5 and 7 years of age) when children develop the ability to generate hypotheses and recognize the possibility that short-term discomfort might have long-term benefit to them. An explanation of the benefits of an injection to a 2-year-old child is almost inevitably futile, whereas older children might understand such an explanation even though not necessarily relishing the experience. There is even a developmental progression in the response of infants to painful stimuli. Johnston and colleagues (21) examined the changes in pain expression in early infancy and found a predictable evolution of response from premature infants whose cries tended to alert caretakers of distress, to term babies, and to 2 and 4 month olds who demonstrated varying behavioral patterns in response to injection pain. It is clear, therefore, that the age of the child influences his or her response to painful procedures. Another key component of an individual's response to pain is that of personality or temperament. Several investigators have determined that children with different temperamental profiles (in particular, problems with adaptability or difficulty in general) are far more reactive to painful stimuli (22–24). Schechter and colleagues (22) found that the child's inherent temperament as rated by his or her parents in advance of an injection was the strongest predictor of responsiveness to the 5-year immunization. Another personality attribute involves coping styles. Several papers have reported that children have different styles of coping. One categorization suggests that children are either attenders or distractors (25). The attenders prefer to have information about the procedure in advance so they can reflect on the upcoming situation and master it, whereas distractors prefer to avoid focusing on the procedure and reduce preoccupation and anxiety. Other dimensions of personality that influence the perception of pain have also been identified, such as the tendency to amplify or reduce the size of a stimulus (26). These personality characteristics clearly have a role in determining types of cognitive-behavioral interventions that might be of maximal benefit (27).

Cognitive factors and personality characteristics have a role in pain perception. The context or meaning of the pain for the child is also important. For example, if a procedure is being contemplated to ascertain whether a cancer or other disease has spread, the anxiety about the information to be obtained will often amplify the pain associated with the procedure itself. Again, these issues are reviewed in depth elsewhere in this volume.

Finally, it appears that an individual's affective state affects on his or her perception of the pain associated with a procedure and the response to it. Anxiety and depression both can amplify nociception (28,29). Reducing anxiety through preparation, as is discussed below, clearly decreases overall pain perception. Other cognitive and psychologic factors associated with pain perception are described in Chapter 6.

Extrinsic Factors

Factors external to the child can also affect the pain experienced from a given procedure. It is quite clear that the skill of the operator is correlated with perceived pain (30,31). Although intuitively it would seem that the more experienced clinicians are with procedures, the more successful they are at completing them expeditiously and without unnecessary complications, studies have found no correlation between experience and successful completion of a procedure (such as completing a nontraumatic lumbar puncture) (30,31). Obviously, some procedures are more painful than others are, which is usually related to the length of time necessary to complete them and the amount of associated tissue damage (32). As previously mentioned, sedation strategies need to be developed based on the intensity of pain associated with a given procedure. Finally, the physical environment in which a procedure is performed may influence perceived pain. Procedures performed in comfortable surroundings such as a treatment room with developmentally appropriate decorations may be less anxiety producing than a more sterile room or a busy emergency department (33).

GOALS OF MANAGEMENT

The primary goal for management of painful procedures in children is the prevention (not treatment) of pain. All other outcomes are dependent on successful pain prevention—if pain is not prevented, then no other intervention will be sufficient. In fact, there is increasing evidence of long-term effects from incidental pain, at least in neonates, so it behooves us to make all possible efforts to avoid inflicting pain in children (34,35). The younger the child, the more important this is.

However, pain prevention alone may not solve all the problems, and specific goals include anxiolysis, lack of movement, and a rapid return to the "normal" (or at least preprocedure) state. Ideally, the child coming for a procedure, whether initial or repeat, should be relaxed and unafraid and able to cooperate with preparation. He or she should experience no pain during the procedure and should remain immobile for as long as is necessary. Recovery should be rapid and free of nausea, dysphoria, and pain, and normal eating and drinking should be possible within a few minutes of finishing. Subsequent recollection of the process should be at least of a "not unpleasant" experience, even if it was not exactly enjoyable.

Success in managing a program for procedural pain sedation requires flexibility and efficiencies of practice that make it acceptable not only to the oncologists, radiologists, and pediatricians using the service, but also to the providers, whether anesthesiologists or others. Although some practitioners initially view a formal preparation and sedation protocol as "interfering" with the smooth and rapid operation of their clinic, our experience suggests that most find that it improves efficiency and patient satisfaction.

PSYCHOLOGIC TECHNIQUES TO HELP CHILDREN COPE WITH PAINFUL PROCEDURES

Several strategies and techniques have been developed to help children cope with painful procedures. Obviously, the type of technique that one uses depends on the level of pain associated with the procedure and the degree of pharmacologic sedation that the child will receive. There are also significant individual differences depending on a child's age and personality style. All these must be taken into account when a treatment plan is developed, and therefore a "one size fits all" approach is inappropriate.

Many strategies to reduce pain have emerged from our increased understanding of the importance of psychologic factors in reducing or amplifying painful stimuli. The initial factors that we discuss are parental presence during sedation and preparation for procedures. We then discuss a variety of child-focused strategies including distraction, hypnosis, and rehearsal. During conscious sedation, by definition, children are awake enough to use these techniques, but if they are deeply sedated or have undergone general anesthesia, obviously these strategies are not appropriate. These strategies should be taught in advance of the procedure and, if possible, in an environment that is relaxed and calm.

Parental Presence

Historically, parents were excluded from the operating room, treatment room, or emergency department while their child was undergoing painful procedures. This was independent of whether the child was sedated. This policy developed because of concerns that parents' anxiety during this extraordinarily stressful time would increase the child's anxiety, which would subsequently increase his or her pain (36). In addition, it was thought that observation would be extremely stressful for the parents themselves as well as for individuals performing the procedure. In a number of papers, beginning in the late 1980s, it has become obvious that not only do children benefit from the parents' presence, but that parents want to be present (37–39). Recently, Boie et al. (40) surveyed 400 parents regarding their willingness and desire to be present during invasive procedures in the emergency department. Ninety-seven percent of the parents wanted to be present for venipunctures, 94% for laceration repairs, 86% for lumbar punctures, and 80% for endotracheal intubation. Eighty percent of parents wished to be present during resuscitation if their child were conscious, and 71% wanted to be present during resuscitation even if their child were unconscious. This work parallels the work of many other investigators who have identified the importance of parental presence in other situations. Parents are now often present during induction of anesthesia as well as in the treatment room during procedures, even ones in which the child is sedated. It is clear that parental presence decreases child anxiety and increases children's sense of security and comfort during a procedure, even one in which they are consciously sedated, although some research has started to define the specific parental behaviors that are actually helpful and those that decrease coping (41–43). Increasingly, it has been recognized that involving parents in the process by teaching them skills to distract and relax their child is of benefit to the parents and children (44).

Preparation

Preparation of children for painful procedures, operative procedures, and sedation has been discussed frequently throughout this volume. Helping children understand in a developmentally appropriate way what will be happening to them, how they will feel, and how long the procedure and the sensation will last clearly decreases anxiety, which has a direct impact on pain. The evolving literature on preparation, however, suggests strongly that there is no one model that makes sense for all children (45,46). As previously mentioned, some children are information seeking, and others are information rejecting. Some children become increasingly anxious when such information is offered, whereas others require repeated discussion to alleviate anxiety. It is most important to know the child while developing a strategy for preparing him or her. If the clinician does not know the child well, parents should be consulted about personality characteristics that may influence the style of preparation of the child.

Distraction/Hypnosis and Other Cognitive-Behavioral Strategies

Although many studies review the impact of cognitive and behavioral interventions on children's distress during painful procedures (Chapters 17 and 18), very few evaluate the combined impact of pharmacologic interventions with cognitive and behavioral strategies. Psychologic treatments can help to reduce anxiety before the onset of sedation, which may decrease the pharmacologic dose required for sedation. Kazak and colleagues (47) examined a combined intervention of pharmacologic and psychologic strategies and compared it to a pharmacologic-only intervention. Their group found benefit in combining pharmacologic and psychologic interventions for procedural distress. They stated that, after 18 months, the parents of the children randomized to the combined group perceived that their child's distress during procedures was lower than that for parents in the drug-only group. Nurses' rating supported this finding. Both groups, however, were lower than a control group that did not receive any systematic intervention.

In summary, a host of psychologic factors and strategies can have an impact on the pain that a child perceives during a painful procedure. Pharmacologic intervention clearly alleviates a significant amount of that discomfort, but combining pharmacologic strategies with psychologic strategies would seem to be the optimal approach toward controlling the burden of procedural pain.

PHARMACOLOGIC ALTERNATIVES

Local Anesthetics

For procedures involving tissue injury or nociceptive stimulation, it is most advantageous to use a local anesthetic agent to block sensory nerves before starting the procedure. Local anesthetic agents can be applied topically, injected into the tissue (infiltration), or injected in close proximity to a specific nerve, which may be relatively distant from the site of the procedure (nerve block). The advent of effective topical agents has been a tremendous boon to children undergoing medical procedures.

Lidocaine-Prilocaine Cream (EMLA)

Lidocaine-prilocaine cream [EMLA (eutectic mixture of local anesthetics)] is a cream composed of a mixture of two amide-type anesthetics, lidocaine and prilocaine (25 mg each per gram of cream), in an oil–water emulsion. When applied to the skin under an occlusive dressing, both drugs migrate into the epidermis and dermis, providing anesthesia. The depth and intensity of the anesthesia are dependent on the duration of exposure, with usual practice requiring 60 to 90 minutes for effective analgesia for skin punctures or incisions.

Lidocaine-prilocaine cream is used before venipuncture, intravenous catheter insertion, and minor dermatologic and plastic surgery procedures. It can also be used to reduce the discomfort of needle penetration through the skin when deeper anesthesia is required (48). An initial vasoconstriction is often noted during the first hour after application, which later becomes a vasodilation. Although there is a theoretic concern that excessive absorption of prilocaine could result in methemoglobinemia, this seems to be of little practical concern except with very large amounts of drug application or use on raw or mucosal surfaces (49–52).

Amethocaine (Ametop)

Amethocaine cream (40 mg tetracaine per gram of cream) is now available in a number of countries. It appears to provide benefits similar to those of lidocaine-prilocaine cream but with a shorter application time (53). Because tetracaine is an ester anesthetic, there is a risk of allergic reaction in those sensitive to paraaminobenzoic acid derivatives.

Infiltration and Nerve Block

The two commonly used and available local anesthetics are lidocaine and bupivacaine. Both provide effective anesthesia for procedures. Both drugs are available in preparations with epinephrine (usually 1:200,000), which may provide useful vasoconstriction for repair of lacerations. Naturally, epinephrine should not be used in areas where there is a terminal vascular supply, such as the fingers or penis.

Lidocaine (lignocaine) can be infiltrated or used for nerve block in concentrations from 0.5% to 2%. The higher the concentration is, the more intense the block. Lidocaine causes some pain (a stinging sensation) on injection, and buffering with a small amount of sodium bicarbonate (1% lidocaine:bicarbonate in a 9:1 ratio) dramatically reduces the discomfort in some situations (54), although not in all (55). Slow injection for infiltration also reduces discomfort (48), and effective anesthesia for intravenous cannula insertion can be provided with tiny amounts (0.05 mL) injected intradermally with a fine 27- or 30-gauge needle.

The toxicity of lidocaine is manifested as either central nervous system effects or cardiac conduction delay. It would be unusual to cause adverse effects from local infiltration of the skin, although rapid absorption from intravenous, intramedullary, or mucosal injection can cause dangerously high systemic levels at small doses. Use of local anesthetics for regional or intravenous nerve blocks is a specialized technique that should not be attempted without appropriate training and the personnel, ability, and equipment for cardiopulmonary resuscitation.

Bupivacaine is a longer lasting agent that can provide 6 hours or more of anesthesia, depending on the site of injection and the consequent blood supply and systemic absorption. A concentration of 0.25% is usually used for peripheral tissue anesthesia. However, it takes considerably longer to reach peak effect (10 to 20 minutes); therefore, it is less practical for immediate interventions. The toxic effects of overdose are similar to those of lidocaine but may be more dangerous because the cardiac effects are more difficult to reverse, probably owing to more assiduous binding of the drug to tissue.

Newer agents have been developed that may provide equivalent efficacy with less toxicity. Ropivacaine (Naropin) is not yet licensed for use in children, although some practitioners have used it successfully in neuraxial anesthesia for pediatric surgery.

Systemic Analgesics

When local anesthetics are insufficient for pain control during a painful procedure, systemic analgesics must be used instead or in addition. Although the pain from superficial skin surgery can be blocked effectively with local anesthetics, the deeper pain from, for example, bone marrow biopsy or aspiration, cannot be prevented without systemic analgesics (or major neuraxial or regional nerve block). There are three general approaches to brief systemic analgesia employed in procedural pain. In addition, sucrose or sweet taste has been shown to have a significant analgesic effect in neonates, probably mediated by endogenous opioids (because it can be reversed by naloxone) (56). Sucrose analgesia is discussed elsewhere in this text.

Opioids

All opioids can cause respiratory depression if used in doses greater than that needed for the immediate pain. Apnea is primarily a risk if the opioid is given rapidly or in a large dose, if other central nervous system depressants are used or if the painful stimulus is delayed or extremely brief. Itching, nausea, and vomiting are other side effects that occur occasionally, even with brief procedural use, but are usually transient or easily managed in this setting.

Fentanyl is a short-acting opioid that has been used for decades in general anesthesia for all ages. It is a potent lipophilic agent with a rapid onset and offset. Intravenous doses of 1 to 2 μg/kg can be an effective adjunct to other systemic sedatives within a minute or two of intravenous administration. More than 1 μg/kg given in a rapid bolus often causes a brief cough, and larger boluses can result in chest rigidity. In the United States, fentanyl is also available in an oral transmucosal formulation that has been used successfully for procedural pain management, although with a relatively high incidence of nausea and vomiting (57).

Remifentanil is a new ultrashort-acting synthetic opioid of the fentanyl family. Considerable interest has developed in some centers in its use for short painful procedures because of the rapid recovery. The corollary is that there is no residual analgesia after the patient has awakened, and alternative analgesics must be used if there is any ongoing pain. Because it is a very potent agent, respiratory depression to the point of apnea can develop quickly and at doses that are very close to those required for analgesia; therefore, it is not recommended for use except by experienced anesthesiologists (58,59).

Although morphine is the gold standard for management of continuing pain, it has a slower onset and longer duration of action than fentanyl, which make it less satisfactory for brief painful experiences. However, it has a wider margin for error than the shorter acting drugs.

Meperidine is a synthetic opioid that has been traditionally used for procedure sedation, usually in combination with one or more phenothiazines (see below for further discussion of drug combinations). No studies have shown any clear advantage of meperidine over other opioids for procedural pain, and side effects are at least as common. Prolonged use can result in the accumulation of normeperidine, resulting in central nervous system excitation and seizures. We do not see any particular reason for routine use of this drug, except in the rare case of true allergy to all other options.

Ketamine

Ketamine has been used for at least three decades in anesthesia. It is effective as an analgesia and general anesthetic agent and is still used as a sole agent in settings where sophisticated anesthesia equipment and supplies are unavailable, as in parts of sub-Saharan Africa. In the past decade, there has been a tremendous upsurge of interest in ketamine by emergency department physicians and pediatricians and promotion of its intravenous or intramuscular use for management of brief painful procedures, such suturing of lacerations in the emergency department (60,61). There is no question about its efficacy, but numerous studies also claim that it is "safe" based on small numbers or retrospective analysis (62–64).

Ketamine can result in unpleasant dysphoric effects during and after recovery, especially in adolescent and adult patients, although these are prevented to some extent by benzodiazepines. It blocks *N*-methyl-D-aspartate receptors in the spinal cord and elsewhere and thus is regarded as having a potentially synergistic effect with opioids for neuropathic and continuing pain treatment. Ketamine can provoke increased salivation, so concomitant use of an anticholinergic is often recommended. There is a traditional view that cardiac output and respiratory function are maintained under ketamine anesthesia, but there is no guarantee. A recent review of its use for gastroscopy in children found an 8% incidence of laryngospasm (the rate is higher in younger patients) with profound desaturation (65), and other respiratory complications have been reported (66). Conversely, nine cases of inadvertent ketamine overdose in healthy children (from 14 months to 7 years of age), ranging from five to 100 times the intended dose, resulted in no adverse effects other than very prolonged sedation, although ventilatory support was required in some cases (67). Even with appropriate dosing, no one should use the drug without advanced airway management and life support skills.

Nitrous Oxide

Nitrous oxide is a clear odorless gas that has been used for analgesia in minor surgical and dental procedures since 1844. During general anesthesia, it is administered at as much as 70% inspired concentration with oxygen, but usual guidelines for nonoperating room use limit it to 50%. It is a reasonable analgesic for minor procedures (68) but can make some children and adults disinhibited (it is commonly called "laughing gas") and can cause nausea and vomiting. Some patients become unconscious and lose control of their airways, especially when it is combined with other sedating drugs. The other issue of concern is the need to scavenge excess and exhaled gas from the room to prevent sedation of the staff.

Hypnotics and Anxiolytics

Hypnotic agents do not provide any analgesia and serve to manage only the anxiety, behavior, and memory components of pharmacologic procedure management. As discussed below, it is important to distinguish among the desired goals and the categories of stress that the patient will undergo. A pain-free procedure (e.g., magnetic resonance imaging or computed tomography scan) can be managed with a hypnotic alone, but it is a serious error to think that painful procedures can be managed without either local or systemic analgesia.

Benzodiazepines

Midazolam is now the only commonly used benzodiazepine for procedure-related sedation and anxiolysis in pediatrics. It is a relatively short-acting agent with a rapid elimination half-life and no active metabolites. It was originally licensed for intravenous use but has been administered orally, intranasally, intramuscularly, and rectally. An oral preparation is now available in some countries. Midazolam causes profound sedation and amnesia. As with any benzodiazepine, respiratory depression can occur and is a particular risk when combined with opioids (69), although the effects of midazolam overdose can be reversed with flumazenil.

Oral premedication with midazolam is used in many centers for sedation before anesthesia induction, but titration to a required sedation level during a procedure necessitates intravenous use. Numerous clinical studies have been done using midazolam as the primary sedating agent for children, and it is clear that there is no specific optimal dose. Most practitioners use increments of 0.05 mg/kg intravenously to a total dose of 0.1 or 0.2 mg/kg. Obviously the higher the dose is, the greater the need for prolonged postprocedure surveillance.

Midazolam has potent amnestic effects, but there is little research to show that amnesia is a desirable outcome. It may be simplistic to think that having no memory of a hospital experience is the best way to manage it. If the child was previously anxious or frightened, then he or she will not have any memory of the procedure going well and will remain frightened of future experiences.

Propofol

Propofol is a potent general anesthetic agent that is frequently used by anesthesiologists for deep sedation. It has antiemetic properties and generally results in a rapid recovery with a sense of well-being (and often hunger!). It has no significant analgesic effect and, in fact, can be quite painful when injected in a peripheral vein. Uncoordinated muscle movements and apnea can occur during induction, and it should only be used by those experienced in the administration of general anesthesia.

Chloral Hydrate

Chloral hydrate has a long history of use as a pediatric sedating agent since 1869 (70). Despite substantial clinical experience, questions remain concerning its safety (71). The American Academy of Pediatrics published recommendations in 1993 that emphasize, among other things, the importance of avoiding repetitive dosing (72). There is no reversal agent for chloral hydrate, and its effects and metabolites may persist for a long time. The plasma half-life of trichloroethanol, the active agent for which chloral hydrate is the prodrug, is 8 to 12 hours and substantially longer in infants and neonates (73).

Barbiturates

The barbiturates include several compounds that have been used for decades for sedation, anxiolysis, treatment of insomnia, and anesthesia: methohexital, pentobarbital, and thiopental are familiar names to most physicians. They have been given orally, rectally, intravenously, and intramuscularly and cause sedation or sleep with varying onset times and durations of action. It is well known that barbiturates can cause respiratory depression, especially when combined with opioids, inhaled agents like nitrous oxide, or other sedatives.

Intravenous methohexital and thiopental have been used as general anesthesia induction agents for many years. Recent studies have described their use for oncology procedures (74), although use for radiology procedures has usually involved rectal administration (75,76). It may be beneficial in avoiding the discomfort and anxiety produced by a venipuncture, but the rectal (or intramuscular) routes do not permit easy titration to effect. Conversely, Kain and colleagues (77) examined the costs of providing sedation for magnetic resonance imaging with propofol compared with a combination of thiopental and pentobarbital. They found that the extra drug cost of propofol was significantly offset by the prolonged nursing time required after barbiturate sedation.

Choosing Combinations

Most successful sedation techniques involve a combination of drugs, chosen to reach different goals. It is important to be intimately familiar with the effects, complications, and indications for each drug and class of drug and to think carefully about the specific problems of the procedure planned. Some of the concerns are as follows:

Duration and immobility: Will the procedure be extremely quick (bone marrow aspiration or lumbar puncture by an experienced oncologist) or very prolonged (burn debridement or dressing change)? Is the patient expected to remain immobile the whole time (as with magnetic resonance imaging) or is some movement acceptable or desirable (burns)? Long-acting drugs such as chloral hydrate or pentobarbital, although often easier to administer for long procedures with a wider margin of safety, usually result in a longer impairment of motor and neurologic function (78).

Environment: Is the room used for the procedure warm, quiet, and relatively dark, or will there be noise and bright lights?

Position and airway concerns: It is much easier to maintain a patent airway in someone in the lateral decubitus position in which secretions will drain out (as with a lumbar puncture) than the supine position. If there are airway concerns, then position may be a significant factor. A young child who is prone in a molded frame for radiotherapy may have the mandible pushed back by the face mask, resulting in airway obstruction. This then results in either arousal and movement or hypoxia.

Age: Age is always a factor for consideration. It may be feasible to provide conscious sedation with calm cooperation in a teenager or older child, but most experienced practitioners will say that a 2-year-old child must be either completely awake or completely asleep; the in-between state is disorienting and frightening and may, in fact, be impossible to achieve (17).

Pain: Finally, pain is the major influence on drug selection. Local and/or systemic analgesia is essential if successful procedure management is to be achieved for a painful inter-

TABLE 31.1. *Indications and strategies for procedural sedation and analgesia*[a]

Clinical situation	Indications	Procedural requirements	Common sedation strategies
Noninvasive procedures	Computed tomography, echocardiography, electroencephalography, magnetic resonance imaging, ultrasonography	Motion control	Comforting alone, oral chloral hydrate (in patients <3 yr of age), i.v. pentobarbital, p.r. methohexital, i.v. midazolam
Procedures associated with low level of pain and high anxiety	Dental procedures, flexible fiberoptic laryngoscopy, foreign body removal (simple), intravenous cannulation, laceration repair (simple), lumbar puncture, ocular irrigation, phlebotomy, slit-lamp examination	Sedation, anxiolysis motion control	Comforting and topical or local anesthesia, midazolam (p.o., i.n., p.r., or i.v.), nitrous oxide
Procedures associated with high level of pain, high anxiety, or both	Abscess incision and drainage, arthrocentesis, bone marrow aspiration, burn debridement, cardiac catheterization, cardioversion, central catheter placement, endoscopy, foreign body removal (complicated), fracture or dislocation reduction, hernia reduction, interventional radiology procedures, laceration repair (complex), paracentesis, paraphimosis reduction, sexual assault examination, thoracentesis, thoracostomy tube placement	Sedation, anxiolysis, analgesia, amnesia, motion control	Comforting and topical or local anesthesia, i.v. midazolam and fentanyl, i.m. or i.v. ketamine

[a]This table is intended as a general overview. Sedation strategies should be individualized. Although the pharmacopoeia is large, clinicians should familiarize themselves with a few agents that are flexible enough to be used in most procedures. In all cases, it is assumed that practitioners are fully trained in the technique, appropriate personnel and monitoring are used, and specific drug contraindications are absent.

p.o., oral; i.v., intravenous; i.m., intramuscular; p.r., rectal; i.n., intranasal.

vention. Conversely, it is potentially dangerous and certainly unnecessary to use opioids or ketamine for sedation for painless procedures such as computed tomography or magnetic resonance imaging.

Table 31.1 provides a general overview of indications and strategies for procedural sedation, taking into account the factors previously described.

Adverse Outcomes

Recently, there has been a welcome focus on evaluation of outcomes and collection of quality assurance data for procedural sedation by nonanesthesiologists. Comprehensive programs to audit results are essential in tracking rare adverse events because any one practitioner is unlikely to do enough procedures to recognize problems in his or her pattern of practice. Of course, it is essential that an accurate time-based record be completed for each sedation procedure so that subsequent evaluation of the quality of the sedation by audit can occur. Record keeping is also essential for each individual child in case problems arise in management. In addition, regular discussion of morbidity within a department or practice group should enhance the quality of care provided. Adverse events to be considered include oxyhemoglobin desaturation, apnea, stridor, laryngospasm, bronchospasm, hypotension, arrhythmias, paradoxical responses, emergence reactions, inadequate sedation, need for physical restraint, nausea, vomiting, and aspiration, among others. Prospective studies to assess safety have been impractical because of the many thousands of cases that would be required to provide a comparison with the extremely low mortality and morbidity of general anesthesia. It is generally assumed that the drugs and techniques available to anesthesiologists allow more precise titration of effect with faster onset, offset, and recovery than those used by nonanesthesia personnel. Even this may not be uncontested, however, because it has been suggested that more profound anesthesia, as administered by anesthesiologists, can result in enough transient atelectasis to impair radiologic diagnosis of chest computed tomography (79).

Malviya and colleagues (80) reported as many as 20% adverse events, including significant numbers of inadequate sedations, in a hospital-wide question/answer monitoring program involving more than 1,000 children. Peña and Krauss (81) had a much lower rate in the emergency department, with equal numbers of subjects. Coté et al. (82) reviewed adverse events reported to the U.S. Food and Drug Administration and the U.S. Pharmacopoeia and by pediatric specialists in the United States (82). By a process of independent review and consensus, they were able to attribute the cause of 95 incidents (51 deaths, nine permanent neurologic injuries, 21 prolonged hospitalizations, and 14 in which there were no consequences). Of course, there is no denominator for the data collection of Coté et al.; therefore, the incidence of problems is unavailable. However, it appeared that serious adverse outcomes (permanent injury or death) occurred more frequently at nonhospital facilities. Failure to use or respond to pulse oximetry was associated with bad outcomes wherever they occurred. Inadequate medical evaluation, medication errors, lack of adequate recovery procedures, and failure to have an independent observer monitoring the patient were all contributing factors as well.

PROVISION OF SERVICES

Sedation services are provided in different centers using nurse-, pediatrician-, and intensivist-led programs (83–85). Successful programs have been described with each model, but the common factors are that the practitioners involved are trained and experienced in patient selection, drug titration, and airway management and practice them frequently. In addition, a well-understood pathway must be provided to divert children to general anesthesia when appropriate (86,87). We believe that it is impossible to learn the appropriate techniques and skills for safe sedation of children from a textbook. Clinicians who wish to take on sedation services in their institution should seek training and mentorship from other experienced practitioners who will usually come from the disciplines of anesthesiology, emergency medicine, or intensive care medicine.

CONCLUSIONS

The quality of pediatric sedation has improved immensely, presumably because of the increased recognition of the importance of pain prevention and management in children, improved monitoring capabilities (particularly pulse oximetry), and increased attention to outcomes and morbidity. Many different organizations have produced standards for pediatric sedation, most of which contain common themes of presedation evaluation, monitoring equipment, experience and training of personnel, the use of different staff to monitor the patient and to perform the procedure, and protocols for care during recovery (12,13,88,89). Reports of complications should probably not be taken as evidence of poor management but rather as a result of a new intensity of focus on ensuring high-quality care. Anesthesiologists and anesthesiology departments should exemplify the standard of care and should demonstrate leadership in preventing pain, anxiety, and adverse outcomes during the many medical procedures that children must undergo.

REFERENCES

1. Miser AW, Dothage JA, Wesley RA, et al. The prevalence of pain in pediatric and young adult cancer population. *Pain* 1987;29:73–83.
2. Cornaglia C, Massimo L, Haupt R, et al. Incidence of pain in children with neoplastic diseases. *Pain* 1984;2:S28.
3. McGrath PJ, Hsu E, Capelli M, et al. Pain from paediatric cancer: a survey of an outpatient oncology clinic. *J Psychosoc Oncol* 1990;8:109–124.
4. Katz ER, Kellerman J, Siegel SE. Behavioral distress in children with cancer undergoing medical procedures: developmental considerations. *J Consult Clin Psychol* 1980;48:356–365.
5. Bernstein B, Schechter NL, Hickman T, et al. Premedication for painful procedures in children: a national survey. *J Pain Symptom Manage* 1991;6:190(abst).
6. Hockenberry MJ, Bologna-Vaughn S. Preparation for intrusive procedures using non-invasive techniques in children with cancer: state of the art vs new trends. *Cancer Nurs* 1985;8:97–102.
7. Coté CJ, Aldefer RJ, Notterman DA, et al. Sedation disasters: adverse drug reports in pediatrics—FDA, USP, and others. *Anesthesiology* 1995;83:A1183.
8. Weisman SJ, Bernstein B, Schechter NL. The consequences of inadequate analgesia during painful procedures in children. *Arch Pediatr Adolesc Med* 1998;152: 1467–1469.
9. Taddio A, Katz J, Ilersich AL, et al. Effect of neonatal circumcision on pain response during subsequent routine vaccination. *Lancet* 1997;349:599–603.
10. Fitzgerald M, Millard C, McIntosh N. Cutaneous hypersensitivity following peripheral tissue damage in newborn rats and its reversal with topical anaesthesia. *Pain* 1989;39:31–36.
11. Anand KJS, Sippell WG, Aynsley-Green A. Randomized trial of fentanyl anesthesia in preterm babies undergoing surgery: effects on the stress response. *Lancet* 1987;1:62–66.
12. Committee on Drugs, Section on Anesthesiology. Guidelines for the elective use of conscious sedation, deep sedation, and general anesthesia in pediatric patients. *Pediatrics* 1985;76:317–321.
13. Task Force on Sedation and Analgesia by Non-Anesthesiologists, American Society of Anesthesiologists. Practice guidelines for sedation and analgesia by non-anesthesiologists. *Anesthesiology* 1996;84:459–471.
14. Consensus Conference. Anesthesia and sedation in the dental office. *JAMA* 1985;254:1073–1076.
15. American College of Emergency Physicians. Clinical policy for procedural sedation analgesia in the emergency department. *Ann Emerg Med* 1998;31:663–677.
16. Committee on Drugs, American Academy of Pediatrics. Guidelines for monitoring and management of pediatric patients during and after sedation for diagnostic and therapeutic procedures. *Pediatrics* 1992; 89:1110–1115.
17. Maxwell LG, Yaster M. The myth of conscious sedation. *Arch Pediatr Adolesc Med* 1996;150:665–667.
18. Krauss B, Green SM. Primary care: sedation and analgesia for procedures in children. *N Engl J Med* 2000; 342:938–945.
19. Jay SM, Ozolins M, Elliott CH, et al. Assessment of children's distress during painful medical procedures. *Health Psychol* 1983;2:133–147.
20. Fradet C, McGrath PJ, Kay J, et al. A prospective survey of reactions to blood tests by children and adolescents. *Pain* 1990;40:53–60.
21. Johnston CC, Stevens B, Craig KD, et al. Developmental changes in pain expression in premature, full-term, two, and four-month-old infants. *Pain* 1993;52:201–208.
22. Schechter NL, Bernstein BA, Beck A, et al. Individual differences in children's response to pain: role of temperament and parental characteristics. *Pediatrics* 1991; 87:171–177.
23. Chen E, Craske MG, Katz ER, et al. Pain-sensitive temperament: does it predict procedural distress and response to psychological treatment among children with cancer? *J Pediatr Psychol* 2000;25:269–278.
24. Young MR, Fu VR. Influence of play and temperament on the young child's response to pain. *Child Health Care* 1988;18:209–217.
25. Rudolph KD, Dennig MD, Weisz JR. Determinants and consequences of children's coping in the medical setting: conceptualization, review, and critique. *Psychol Bull* 1995;118:328–357.
26. Petrie A. *Individuality in pain and suffering*. Chicago: University of Chicago Press, 1967.
27. Chen E, Joseph M, Zeltzer LK. Behavioral and cognitive interventions in the treatment of pain in children. *Pediatr Clin North Am* 2000;47:513–525.
28. Bijttebier P, Vertommen H. The impact of previous experience on children's reactions to venipunctures. *J Health Psychol* 1998;3:39–46.
29. Varni JW, Rapoff MA, Waldron SA, et al. Chronic pain and emotional distress in children and adolescents. *J Dev Behav Pediatr* 1996;17:154–161.
30. Schreiner RL, Kleinman MB. Incidence and effect of traumatic lumbar in the neonate. *Dev Med Child Neurol* 1979;21:483–487.
31. Carraccio C, Feinberg P, Hart LS, et al. Lidocaine for lumbar punctures: a help not a hindrance. *Arch Pediatr Adolesc Med* 1996;10:1044–1046.
32. Kurtis PS, DeSilva HN, Bernstein BA, et al. Comparison of the Mogen and Gomco clamps in combination with the dorsal penile nerve block in minimizing the pain of neonatal circumcision. *Pediatrics* 1999;103:E23.
33. Stephens BK, Barkey ME, Hall HR. Techniques to comfort children during stressful procedures. *Adv Mind Body Med* 1999;15:49–60.
34. Taddio A, Goldbach M, Ipp M, et al. Effect of neonatal circumcision on pain responses during vaccination in boys. *Lancet* 1995;345:291–292.
35. Taddio A, Katz J, Ilersich AL, et al. Effect of neonatal circumcision on pain response during subsequent routine vaccination. *Lancet* 1997;349:599–603.
36. Venham L. The effect of mother's presence on children's responses to dental treatment. *J Dent Child* 1979;46: 219–225.
37. Ross DM, Ross SA. Pain instruction with third and fourth grade children: a pilot study. *J Pediatr Psychol* 1985;10:55–63.
38. Shaw E, Routh D. Effects of mother presence on children's reaction to aversive procedures. *J Pediatr Psychol* 1982;7:33–42.
39. Bauchner H, Waring C, Vinca R. Parental presence during procedures in the emergency room. *Pediatrics* 1992; 87:544–548.
40. Boie ET, Moore GP, Brummet TC, et al. "Do parents want to be present during invasive procedures performed

on their children in the emergency department?" A survey of 400 parents. *Ann Emerg Med* 1999;34:70–74.
41. Haimi-Cohen Y, Amir J, Harel L et al. Parental presence during lumbar puncture: anxiety and attitude toward the procedure. *Clin Pediatr* 1996;35:2–4.
42. Blount RL, Corbin SM, Sturger JW, et al. The relationship between adults' behavior and child coping and distress during BMA/LP procedures: a sequential analysis. *Behav Ther* 1989;20:585–601.
43. Cohen LL, Manimala R, Blount RL. Easier said than done: what parents say they do and what they do during children's immunizations. *Child Health Care* 2000;29:79–86.
44. Bauchner H, Vinci R, Bak S, et al. Parents and procedures: a randomized controlled trial. *Pediatrics* 1996;98:861–867.
45. Fanurik D, Zeltzer LK, Roberts MC, et al. The relationship between children's coping sytles and psychological interventions for cold pressor pain. *Pain* 1993;53:213–222.
46. Peterson L. Coping by children undergoing stressful medical procedures: some conceptual, methodological, and therapeutic issues. *J Consult Clin Psychol* 1989;57:380–387.
47. Kazak A, Penati B, Brophy P, et al. Pharmacologic and psychologic interventions for procedural pain. *Pediatrics* 1998;102:59–66
48. Serour F, Mandelberg A, Zabeeda D, et al. Efficacy of EMLA cream prior to dorsal penile nerve block for circumcision in children. *Acta Anaesthesiol Scand* 1998;42:260–263.
49. Couper RT. Methaemoglobinaemia secondary to topical lignocaine/prilocaine in a circumcised neonate. *J Paediatr Child Health* 2000;36:406–407.
50. Law RM, Halpern S, Martins RF, et al. Measurement of methemoglobin after EMLA analgesia for newborn circumcision. *Biol Neonate* 1996;70:213–217.
51. Stevens B, Johnston C, Taddio A, et al. Management of pain from heel lance with lidocaine-prilocaine (EMLA) cream: is it safe and efficacious in preterm infants? *J Dev Behav Pediatr* 1999;20:216–221.
52. Touma S, Jackson JB. Lidocaine and prilocaine toxicity in a patient receiving treatment for mollusca contagiosa. *J Am Acad Dermatol* 2001;44[Suppl]:399–400.
53. Bishai R, Taddio A, Bar-Oz B, et al. Relative efficacy of amethocaine gel and lidocaine-prilocaine cream for Port-a-cath puncture in children. *Pediatrics* 1999;104:e31.
54. Bartfield JM, Ford DT, Homer PJ. Buffered versus plain lidocaine for digital nerve blocks. *Ann Emerg Med* 1993;22:216–219.
55. Serour F, Levine A, Mandelberg A, et al. Alkalinizing local anesthetic does not decrease pain during injection for dorsal penile nerve block. *J Clin Anesth* 1999;11:563–566.
56. Stevens B, Taddio A, Ohlsson A, et al. The efficacy of sucrose for relieving procedural pain in neonates—a systematic review and meta-analysis. *Acta Paediatr* 1997;86:837–842.
57. Schechter NL, Weisman SJ, Rosenblum M, et al. The use of oral transmucosal fentanyl citrate for painful procedures in children. *Pediatrics* 1991;95:335–339.
58. Litman RS. Conscious sedation with remifentanil during painful medical procedures. *J Pain Symptom Manage* 2000;19:468–471.
59. Litman RS. Conscious sedation with remifentanil and midazolam during brief painful procedures in children. *Arch Pediatr Adolesc Med* 1999;153:1085–1088.
60. Green SM, Nakamura R, Johnson NE. Ketamine sedation for pediatric procedures: part 1, a prospective series. *Ann Emerg Med* 1990;19:1024–1032.
61. Green SM, Johnson NE. Ketamine sedation for pediatric procedures: part 2, review and implications. *Ann Emerg Med* 1990;19:1033–1046.
62. McCarty EC, Mencio GA, Walker LA, et al. Ketamine sedation for the reduction of children's fractures in the emergency department. *J Bone Joint Surg Am* 2000;82:912–918.
63. Pellier I, Monrigal JP, Le Moine P, et al. Use of intravenous ketamine-midazolam association for pain procedures in children with cancer. A prospective study. *Paediatr Anaesth* 1999;9:61–68.
64. Pruitt JW, Goldwasser MS, Sabol SR, et al. Intramuscular ketamine, midazolam, and glycopyrrolate for pediatric sedation in the emergency department. *J Oral Maxillofac Surg* 1995;53:13–17.
65. Green SM, Klooster M, Harris T, et al. Ketamine sedation for pediatric gastroenterology procedures. *J Pediatr Gastroenterol Nutr* 2001;32:26–33.
66. Smith JA, Santer LJ. Respiratory arrest following intramuscular ketamine injection in a 4-year-old child. *Ann Emerg Med* 1993;22:612–615.
67. Green SM, Clark R, Hostetler MA, et al. Inadvertent ketamine overdose in children: clinical manifestations and outcome. *Ann Emerg Med* 1999;34:492–497.
68. Annequin D, Carbarjal R, Chauvin P, et al. Fixed 50% nitrous oxide mixture for painful procedures: a French survey. *Pediatrics* 2000;105:E47.
69. Bailey PL, Pace NL, Ashburn MA, et al. Frequent hypoxemia and apnea after sedation with midazolam and fentanyl. *Anesthesiology* 1990;73:826–830.
70. Butler T. The introduction of chloral hydrate into medical practice. *Bull History Med* 1970;44:168–172.
71. Steinberg AD. Should chloral hydrate be banned? *Pediatrics* 1993;92:442–461.
72. Committee on Drugs and Committee on Environmental Health. Use of chloral hydrate for sedation in children. *Pediatrics* 1993;92:471–473.
73. Mayers DJ. Sedative-hypnotic effects of chloral hydrate in the neonate. Trichloroethanol or parent drug? *Dev Pharmacol Ther* 1992;19:141–146.
74. Freyer DR, Schwanda AE, Sanfilippo DJ, et al. Intravenous methohexital for brief sedation of pediatric oncology outpatients: physiologic and behavioral responses. *Pediatrics* 1997;99:E8.
75. Pomeranz ES, Chudnofsky CR, Deegan TJ, et al. Rectal methohexital sedation for computed tomography imaging of stable pediatric emergency department patients. *Pediatrics* 2000;105:1110–1114.
76. Glasier CM, Stark JE, Brown R, et al. Rectal thiopental sodium for sedation of pediatric patients undergoing MR and other imaging studies. *AJNR Am J Neuroradiol* 1995;16:111–114.
77. Kain ZN, Gaal DJ, Kain TS, et al. A first-pass cost analysis of propofol versus barbiturates for children undergoing magnetic resonance imaging. *Anesth Analg* 1994;79:1102–1106.
78. Malviya S, Voepel-Lewis T, Prochaska G, et al. Prolonged recovery and delayed side effects of sedation for diagnostic imaging studies in children. *Pediatrics* 2000;105:E42.
79. Sargent MA, McEachern AM, Jamieson DH, et al. At-

electasis on pediatric chest CT: comparison of sedation techniques. *Pediatr Radiol* 1999;29:509–513.
80. Malviya S, Voepel-Lewis T, Tait AR. Adverse events and risk factors associated with the sedation of children by nonanesthesiologists. *Anesth Analg* 1997;85:1207–1213.
81. Peña BM, Krauss B. Adverse events of procedural sedation and analgesia in a pediatric emergency department. *Ann Emerg Med* 1999;34:483–491.
82. Coté CJ, Notterman DA, Karl HW, et al. Adverse sedation events in pediatrics: a critical incident analysis of contributing factors. *Pediatrics* 2000;105:805–814.
83. Sury MRJ, Hatch DJ, Deeley T, et al. Development of a nurse-led sedation service for paediatric magnetic resonance imaging. *Lancet* 1999;353:1667–1671.
84. Lowrie L, Weiss AH, Lacombe C. The pediatric sedation unit: a mechanism for pediatric sedation. *Pediatrics* 1998;102:E30.
85. Slonim AD, Ognibene FP. Sedation for pediatric procedures, using ketamine and midazolam, in a primarily adult intensive care unit: a retrospective evaluation. *Crit Care Med* 1998;26:1900–1904.
86. Morton NS, Oomen GJ. Development of a selection and monitoring protocol for safe sedation of children. *Paediatr Anaesth* 1998;8:65–68.
87. Keengwe IN, Hegde S, Dearlove O, et al. Structured sedation programme for magnetic resonance imaging examination in children. *Anaesthesia* 1999;54: 1069–1072.
88. Holzman RS, Cullen DJ, Eichhorn JH, et al. Guidelines for sedation by nonanesthesiologists during diagnostic and therapeutic procedures. *J Clin Anesth* 1994;6: 265–276.
89. Innes G, Murphy M, Nijssen-Jordan C, et al. Procedural sedation and analgesia in the emergency department. Canadian consensus guidelines. *J Emerg Med* 1999;17: 145–156.

32
Musculoskeletal Pain in Children

Donald T. Kulas and Laura E. Schanberg

Childhood musculoskeletal pain is a common complaint seen by general pediatricians. The 1995 to 1996 National Ambulatory Medical Care Survey performed in the United States showed that symptoms referable to the musculoskeletal system made up approximately 7% of all pediatric visits (1). Symptoms are mainly attributable to trauma (30%), overuse (28%), normal skeletal growth variants (18%), and growing pains (8%) (2). Other studies have shown that as many as 15% of all school-age children complain of musculoskeletal pain, with 4.5% of this group experiencing interference with normal activities for longer than 3 months (3). Although most musculoskeletal complaints in the pediatric population are of a benign nature, systemic diseases such as malignancies and rheumatologic diseases may present with pain as the primary symptom. In addition, chronic pain syndromes are the cause of significant morbidity, particularly in the teenage years. The differential diagnosis of musculoskeletal pain is extensive (Table 32.1), and the challenge for the general pediatrician is to identify when intervention is necessary, using a minimal amount of testing necessary to make the appropriate diagnosis.

Trauma and overuse injuries are often self-evident from the history and physical examination and are discussed only briefly here. Rather, this chapter focuses on the approach to the child with musculoskeletal pain, along with several specific causes of musculoskeletal pain, including arthritis and fibromyalgia.

DIAGNOSTIC EVALUATION OF MUSCULOSKELETAL PAIN

History

In the assessment of the child with musculoskeletal pain, the history and physical examination are of paramount importance. In fact, many of the diseases that may present with musculoskeletal complaints are diagnosed entirely on clinical grounds (e.g., juvenile rheumatoid arthritis, fibromyalgia, transient synovitis of the hip). Eliciting a comprehensive history and performing a complete physical examination are critical components in narrowing the differential diagnosis of musculoskeletal pain.

Even before the child is seen, the child's age can provide an initial framework from which to begin the evaluation, as outlined in Table 32.2 (4). Trauma occurs at all ages, but special attention to the possibility of child abuse should be made in the child younger than 2 years of age. Additionally, sprains and ligamentous injuries are unusual in the very young child. Particular mechanical problems, such as congenital dislocation of the hips, periostitis, and foreign objects (i.e., a piece of thread wrapped around a toe), are also more likely in that age group. Legg–Calvé–Perthes disease (LCP) is more often seen in 4- to 10-year-old children, whereas slipped capital femoral epiphysis (SCFE) is usually seen in children older than 10 years of age.

Infections can occur at any age, but the offending organisms vary throughout childhood (i.e., an adolescent with a septic knee may have a gonococcal infection). Neoplasms also

TABLE 32.1. *Differential diagnosis of the child with musculoskeletal pain*

- Traumatic
  - Fractures
  - Soft-tissue injury
  - Child abuse
  - Foreign body
  - Overuse injuries
- Orthopedic/mechanical
  - Legg–Calvé–Perthes disease
  - Slipped capital femoral epiphysis
  - Congenital hip dysplasia
  - Osgood–Schlatter disease
  - Hypermobility
- Infection
  - Osteomyelitis
  - Septic arthritis
  - Discitis
  - Soft-tissue infections/myositis
  - Lyme disease
  - Iliopsoas abscess
- Inflammatory
  - Juvenile rheumatoid arthritis
  - Spondyloarthropathies
  - Peri-infectious arthritis
  - Acute rheumatic fever
  - Dermatomyositis
  - Systemic lupus erythematosus
  - Mixed connective tissue disease
  - Transient synovitis of the hip
  - Henoch–Schönlein purpura
  - Inflammatory bowel disease
  - Psoriatic arthritis
  - Vasculitides
- Neoplasm
  - Leukemia
  - Lymphoma
  - Neuroblastoma
  - Ewing sarcoma
  - Osteoid osteoma
  - Osteogenic sarcoma
  - Chondrosarcoma
  - Histiocytosis X
- Idiopathic
  - Growing pains
  - Juvenile primary fibromyalgia syndrome
  - Complex regional pain syndrome
  - Localized pain syndrome
  - Low back pain
- Metabolic
  - Rickets (vitamin D deficiency)
  - Scurvy (vitamin C deficiency)
  - Osteoporosis
  - Hypothyroidism
  - Hyperparathyroidism
  - Hypervitaminosis A
  - Storage diseases
- Hematologic
  - Hemarthrosis
  - Hemophilia
  - Sickle cell disease
- Psychologic
  - Conversion reactions
  - Mood disorders
  - Anxiety disorders
  - School phobia
  - Posttraumatic stress disorder

TABLE 32.2. *Differential diagnosis of the child with limp by age*

- Toddler (age 1 to 3 years)
  - Developmental dysplasia of the hip
  - Torsional deformities
  - Discitis
  - Genu varum or genu valgum
  - Congenital leg length discrepancy
  - Toddler's fracture
  - Foreign bodies
  - Pauciarticular juvenile rheumatoid arthritis
- Child (age 4 to 10 years)
  - Toxic synovitis of the hip
  - Bacterial septic arthritis or osteomyelitis
  - Legg–Calvé–Perthes disease
  - Blount disease
  - Acquired leg length discrepancy (e.g., secondary to trauma)
  - Idiopathic toe walking
  - Osgood–Schlatter disease
- Adolescent
  - Slipped capital femoral epiphysis
  - Patellofemoral syndrome
  - Stress fracture
  - Tarsal coalition
  - Gonococcal arthritis
  - Septic arthritis
  - Idiopathic scoliosis
- Conditions occurring at all ages
  - Osteomyelitis
  - Septic arthritis
  - Tumors
  - Juvenile chronic arthritis

Adapted from Dabney KW, Lipton G. Evaluation of limp in children. *Curr Opin Pediatr* 1995;7:88–94, with permission.

occur at all ages, but specific malignancies characteristically present in particular age groups. Acute lymphoblastic leukemia and neuroblastoma are more frequent in children younger than 4 years old, whereas osteogenic sarcoma and Ewing sarcoma tend to occur in older children. Inflammatory processes such as juvenile rheumatoid arthritis (JRA) and reactive arthritis can present in all age groups, but it would be unusual to have a young child present with systemic lupus erythematosus.

When obtaining the history, pain characteristics such as symptom duration, intensity, alleviating and aggravating factors, progression, and radiation must be ascertained. Pain descriptors can also be useful (e.g., "deep" and "boring" for cancer type pain versus "aching" for arthritis pain). A full review of symptoms is essential with special care taken to determine the presence of fever (and its pattern) and growth failure. Inflammatory or neoplastic processes become important considerations in the face of steadily worsening symptoms, especially if associated with fever and/or weight loss. Growth interference is most often associated with a significant chronic systemic illness. The initiation of new athletic activity, conversely, may focus attention to an overuse syndrome as a cause. Preceding illnesses may suggest a postinfectious cause, commonly group A streptococcus and Epstein–Barr virus as well as others. Family history is also important, especially with regard to inflammatory or autoimmune disorders that may have a genetic component, such as HLA-B27 associated spondyloarthropathies and psoriasis.

Physical Examination

A complete physical examination is mandatory, with special attention to skin changes, new cardiac murmurs, and abdominal findings. A careful neurologic examination, including testing for muscle strength, is also important. The musculoskeletal examination should include determination of leg lengths, range of motion, gait, and assessment of spinal curvature. In particular, the distinction between arthralgia (pain in a joint) and arthritis (synovitis in a joint) is made based on a complete joint examination. The joint examination should be performed with attention to the presence of warmth, effusion or synovial thickening, erythema, tenderness or pain with range of motion, and other signs of inflammation. It should be emphasized that the presence of arthritis is ascertained by physical examination alone; laboratory studies are not helpful in determining whether arthritis is present.

Laboratory and Radiographic Testing

Deciding which laboratory tests to obtain at the first visit depends on the nature of the presenting complaints. A classic presentation of "growing pains" (discussed in detail below) may require nothing more than reassurance and close follow-up, whereas suspicion of an infected hip often leads to multiple blood tests, imaging studies, and hospitalization. The most commonly ordered tests for the workup of musculoskeletal pain include a complete blood count (CBC) with differential, erythrocyte sedimentation rate (ESR), and C-reactive protein (CRP). When infection is suspected, blood cultures and joint fluid aspiration may be appropriate. Although commonly ordered as part of a rheumatology panel, the antinuclear antibody (ANA) and rheumatoid factor are poor screening tests in children.

The ESR has been studied as a screening test for serious underlying disease in children with musculoskeletal complaints. In one study, serious underlying disease was seven times more likely in patients who presented with limp if their ESR was greater than 50 mm per hour compared with patients with an ESR less than 20 mm per hour (rates of 20 to 50 provided little additional information) (5). In fact, 78% of patients with an ESR greater than 100 had "significant diagnoses" (5). The ESR is commonly, but not always, elevated in infection, malignancy, and inflammatory disease, including systemic lupus erythematosus, some types of arthritis, and vasculitis. Although a normal ESR is reassuring, it cannot be used to exclude significant disease (5). Use of the CRP in conjunction with an ESR has been shown to be of particular value in the management of infectious disease (6). The CRP rises and falls much faster than the ESR because the half-life of fibrinogen is 3 days. A CRP that initially falls and then subsequently rises during treatment may indicate an inadequately treated infection (6). Either the ESR or CRP provides more diagnostic information than a CBC alone (6).

As noted above, the ANA and rheumatoid factor are not recommended as a screen for inflammatory processes. With recent increases in the sensitivity of this test (at the cost of specificity), a positive ANA can be found in 5% to 15% of the general population (7). Children who present with positive ANA titers and musculoskeletal pain but without other physical examination or laboratory findings of autoimmunity may go on to develop rheumatic disease (8). In the absence of other abnormal tests and physical findings, a positive ANA is of little diagnostic value and often leads to further, unnecessary testing (9). Rheumatoid factor is only present in 10% of children with arthritis and 30% of children with systemic lupus erythematosus; therefore, it is not helpful as screening test (10). Both the ANA and rheumatoid factor are part of the laboratory evaluation of children who have chronic arthritis but should not be used as a screen for the presence of arthritis. The diagnosis of chronic inflammatory arthritis in children is made entirely on clinical grounds (10).

If an infectious cause is being considered, cultures of both the blood and affected joint(s) should be obtained. Aspiration of joint fluid may be therapeutic as well as diagnostic. Because the hip joint is a closed space, moderate to large effusions of the hip may require aspiration to improve discomfort and prevent damaging the acetabular head from pressure. Joint fluid can also help differentiate infection from trauma from inflammatory disease (Table 32.3). The workup of an infected joint is discussed below, but joint fluid should be obtained for culture, cell count, and Gram stain.

Imaging studies may be helpful in making a diagnosis. These include plain films, bone scans, ultrasonography, and magnetic resonance imaging (MRI). In general, MRI provides a much better picture of the joint than does computed tomography. Fordham et al. (11) published an algorithm of imaging strategies for the child with an acute limp, as shown in Figure 32.1 (11). In the presence of a focal examination, obtain a radiograph of the affected area first. If this does not yield the diagnosis, obtain a radiograph of the limb both above and below the involved area. If the latter films are negative, then ultrasonography of the hip (if hip symptoms are present) or a bone scan (for nonhip symptoms) may be necessary. In the absence of a focal examination, radiographs are unlikely to be helpful, although a bone scan may be useful in delineating the extent of a multifocal process such as leukemia or multifocal osteomyelitis (11). Plain films are rarely useful in the initial evaluation of children who present with arthritis.

Choosing which tests to order depends on the physical examination and history. More specific recommendations for laboratory testing are made below as part of the discussion of specific causes of musculoskeletal pain.

TABLE 32.3. *Joint fluid characteristics*

Condition	Appearance	Viscosity	WBC (cells/mL)	%PMNs
Normal	Clear, yellow	High	<200	<25
Traumatic	Cloudy to bloody	Increased	<2,000	<25
Inflammatory	Cloudy	Low	10,000–50,000	25–75
Septic	Opaque	Low	>50,000	>75

WBC, white blood cell count; PMN, polymorphonuclear neutrophils.

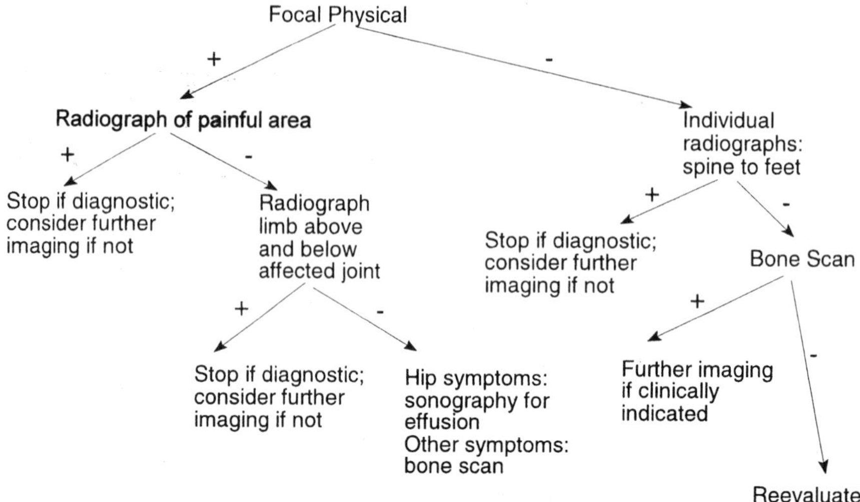

FIG. 32.1. Algorithm for imaging a child with a limp. (From Fordham L, Auringer ST, Frush DP. Pediatric imaging perspective: acute limp. *J Pediatr* 1998;132:906–908, with permission.)

SPECIFIC CAUSES OF MUSCULOSKELETAL PAIN

Mechanical/Trauma

Trauma or sport-related injuries are the most common cause of musculoskeletal pain in the pediatric patient (2). The diagnosis is usually self-evident by the history and physical examination. Sports and playground injuries have been shown to be the most common cause of limb pain, affecting 9% of all children (12). Overuse syndromes are caused by repetitive microtrauma (13). Sports-related injuries and overuse syndromes can be usefully classified by anatomic region (Table 32.4).

As with more overt evidence of trauma, overuse is elicited from the history, which reveals a pattern of repetitive physical activity. Examples of overuse injuries include stress fractures, Osgood–Schlatter syndrome (tibial tubercle apophysitis), shin splints, and Sever syndrome (calcaneal apophysitis). With a history of pain associated with trauma and/or overuse, plain films are usually ordered as an initial study, but a bone scan may be helpful in detecting subtle stress fractures. The child can be treated with nonsteroidal anti-inflammatory drugs (NSAIDs) and acetaminophen for

TABLE 32.4. *Common chronic sports-related pain syndromes by anatomic region*

Shoulder
Impingement syndrome
Elbow
"Little league" elbow
Panner disease
Avulsion fractures
Osteochondritis dissecans
Tennis elbow
Pelvis and hip
Avulsion injuries
Legg–Calvé–Perthes disease
Slipped capital femoral epiphysis
Knee
Osteochondritis dissecans
Osgood–Schlatter disease
Sindig–Larsen syndrome
Chondromalacia patella
Malalignment syndromes
Leg
Shin splints
Stress fractures
Compartment syndromes
Foot
Plantar fasciitis
Tarsal coalition
Stress fractures
Achilles tendinitis
Juvenile bunion
Spine
Musculoskeletal strain
Spondylolisthesis

Adapted from Sullivan JA. Recurring pain in the pediatric athlete. *Pediatr Clin North Am* 1984;31:1097–1112.

TABLE 32.5. *Pediatric dosing guidelines for selected medications used to treat musculoskeletal pain*

Medication	Daily dose	Frequency	Daily maximum
NSAIDs			
Salicylate	80–100 mg/kg	t.i.d.	Serum level 20–30 mg
Ibuprofen	30–40 mg/kg	t.i.d.	2,400 mg
Naproxen	20 mg/kg	b.i.d.	1,000 mg
Tolectin	40 mg/kg	t.i.d.	1,600 mg
Nabumetone	30 mg/kg	q.i.d.	2,000 mg
Remittive agents			
Sulfasalazine	40–60 mg/kg	b.i.d.	2–3 g
Methotrexate	10 mg/m^2	qwk	0.5–1.0 mg/kg
Etanercept	0.4 mg/kg	2 times/wk	25 mg
Analgesics			
Acetaminophen	10–15 mg/kg/dose	q4h	2.4 g
Hydrocodone	0.15 mg/kg	q4h	Limited by side effects
Oxycodone	0.05–0.2 mg/kg	q3–6h	Limited by side effects
Oxycodone SR	10 mg	q12h	Limited by tablet strength
Nortriptyline	10–30 mg	qhs	150 mg qhs

NSAIDs, nonsteroidal anti-inflammatory drugs; t.i.d., three times daily; b.i.d., twice daily; q.i.d., four times daily; SR, sustained release; qhs, at bedtime.

pain relief. Table 32.5 shows NSAIDs commonly used for children and the doses. Depending on the type of injury, immobilization may be considered. Initial plain films sometimes miss subtle stress fractures, and repeat imaging may be necessary if pain persists for more than 2 weeks. Avascular necrosis is a potential complication of overuse and may be demonstrated on imaging.

Another type of stress fracture is spondylolysis, which is a stress fracture of the pars interarticularis of the lower lumbar spine. Spondylolisthesis refers to the forward slippage of one vertebra over the inferior vertebra. Both of these lesions are rare before 5 years of age. If suspected, plain radiographs make the diagnosis.

Avascular Necrosis

Avascular necrosis can be either idiopathic (LCP) or a complication of another process (such as SCFE). Both of these processes are discussed below. The presence of avascular necrosis should be suspected when predisposing conditions such as sickle cell disease are present (14). Interestingly, antiphospholipid antibodies have also been found in association with avascular necrosis (15,16).

Legg–Calvé–Perthes Disease

LCP usually presents as a limp in children ages 4 to 8 years old, especially boys. It refers to avascular necrosis of the proximal femoral epiphysis, although the pathophysiology is still unknown. The pain associated with LCP is variable and may range from being asymptomatic (more likely) to severe pain involving the knee and/or thigh. When present, pain is often worsened by activity. Early in the disease process, plain films may not show abnormalities. Films should still be obtained, however, because they can be used to exclude other diagnoses (i.e., SCFE, see below). If LCP is suspected, MRI is recommended as follow-up imaging to negative plain films (11). Alternatively, a bone scan can be used to evaluate for avascular necrosis. Orthopedic consultation is recommended for further management. Treatment will vary depending on how far the necrosis extends, the age of the child, and the range of motion present on initial presentation.

Slipped Capital Femoral Epiphysis

SCFE is another diagnosis that must be considered when a child presents with either hip pain or a limp. As the name implies, SCFE refers to the displacement of the femoral epiphysis. Usually, SCFE occurs just before the adolescent growth spurt. The chief complaint is often limp. Pain is referred to the affected hip, with radiation to the knee or groin. The pain is usually unilateral. A typical case is an obese adolescent black male with an externally rotated leg on physical examination. Plain films will often provide the diagnosis, although computed tomography can also be used. If plain films are obtained, a frog-leg lateral view should be included.

The history and physical examination usually provide enough clues to make the diagnosis. Management cannot be delayed because delay in management could result in a worsening slippage. If untreated long enough, avascular necrosis may develop. An orthopedic surgery consultation is needed at the time of diagnosis. The child should avoid walking (placed on bed rest) until consultation is obtained, and the parents should be prepared for probable intervention/hospitalization.

INFECTIONS OF BONE AND JOINTS

Osteomyelitis

Bone and joint infections are serious pediatric concerns. Although the diagnosis of overuse syndromes, pain syndromes, or rheumatic disease is rarely a medical emergency, the diagnosis of bone and joint infections must be made quickly and therapy promptly started. The diagnosis may be straightforward or subtle. For example, a child with limp, fever, and a recent puncture wound to the bottom of the foot may not provide much of a diagnostic dilemma. However, more often the chief complaint is simply refusal to walk with fever of unknown origin. In fact, the most common presenting symptom of osteomyelitis is decreased use of an extremity (84%), with fever developing only 40% of the time (17). Therefore, clinical suspicion of bone and joint infections must always be high. Making the diagnosis of osteomyelitis can be challenging, and it should always be included on the differential of a child with limp especially in the presence of fever.

Osteomyelitis occurs via three different routes: direct inoculation (trauma), hematogenous seeding, and local invasion from an adjacent infection. In children, the hematogenous route is most common (13). Therapy is directed against the causative organism whenever possible. *Staphylococcus aureus*, coagulase negative staphylococci, *Pseudomonas aeruginosa*, *Streptococcus pyogenes*, *Streptococcus pneumoniae*, and *Salmonella* species are frequently isolated from children with osteomyelitis (18), with *S. aureus* being most commonly identified (17). *Haemophilus influenzae* used to be an important cause of osteomyelitis, but this has diminished markedly since the *H. influenzae* vaccination was introduced. A recent retrospective analysis failed to identify *H. influenzae* as a cause of osteomyelitis after 1990 (17).

Laboratory evaluation of suspected osteomyelitis should include a CBC with differential, ESR, and/or a CRP. As mentioned earlier, obtaining both an ESR and CRP allows a more refined approach to managing osteomyelitis. A rapid fall in the CRP can provide evidence that an infection is being adequately treated. Because the ESR can take weeks to months to decrease, some experts advocate that antibiotics be continued until the ESR normalizes. Blood cultures should be obtained, but bone biopsies or aspirates are more likely to identify the offending organism (17). Radiographs have been used to evaluate osteomyelitis, but they may be negative for the first 7 to 14 days of an infection. MRI and bone scans are more sensitive, particularly early in the course of disease. The technetium-99m bone scan has recently been shown to have a sensitivity of 94% for detecting osteomyelitis (17).

The treatment of osteomyelitis involves surgical debridement and antibiotic therapy. Ideally, antibiotic therapy is directed by the sensitivities of the isolated organism. As indicated above, length of treatment can be based on resolution of markers such as the ESR and CRP. In the past, inpatient hospitalization for 6 weeks of intravenous antibiotic therapy was a typical course. With home health care today, however, discharges can occur long before treatment is completed. In fact, some authors have suggested converting from intravenous to oral antibiotics as early as 4 days into therapy (19). Before switching to oral therapy, the child should show significant clinical improvement with resolution of fever, as well as decreasing markers of inflammation.

Septic Arthritis

The presence of joint pain, erythema, swelling, and fever is highly suggestive of septic arthritis and should be considered a medical emergency. The peak incidence occurs in children younger than 3 years old, with boys affected twice as often as girls. There is less often a history of trauma preceding the infection than seen in osteomyelitis (20). Several predisposing factors for septic arthritis have been identified including immunodeficiencies, hemoglobinopathies, and diabetes (20). Osteomyelitis and septic joints may coexist, as infection can travel from the bone to the joint. This is especially true in infants in whom a vascular connection exists between the metaphysis and epiphysis, allowing infections to pass from the metaphysis into the joint space (20).

Aspiration of the joint for culture (aerobic and anaerobic), Gram stain, and cell count should be quickly undertaken, usually after consultation with orthopedic surgeons. Synovial fluid from septic joints generally is purulent with greater than 50,000 white blood cells per milliliter (20). Blood cultures and a CBC should also be obtained. As discussed above, the ESR and/or CRP provide a means to follow the course of the illness. Further evidence for a septic joint can be procured through imaging studies, such as plain radiographs and ultrasonography (especially of the hip).

Treatment with antibiotics should begin as soon as infection is suspected. The offending organisms for septic arthritis are similar to those for osteomyelitis, with *S. aureus* again being the most common organism. In addition, *Neisseria gonorrhoeae* should always be considered in sexually active adolescents. Antibiotic treatment of the septic joint is similar to that for osteomyelitis, with antibiotic choice influenced by the identification and sensitivity of the isolated organism. Orthopedic intervention is also desirable for aggressive management.

Discitis

Children with discitis often present with limp or refusal to walk. As with osteomyelitis and septic joints, fever is frequently present. The older child will complain of back pain with a positive straight leg-raising test on examination, as well as localized tenderness over the site of the infection. Plain films may take 3 to 4 weeks to demonstrate the abnormality. If discitis is suspected, MRI is preferable to help make the diagnosis early in the course. A bone scan with single-photon emission computed tomography is an excellent diagnostic test and should be considered if the diagnosis of discitis is being entertained in the face of negative radiographic findings (11). As with other infections, obtaining a CBC and blood cultures is prudent. There are no specific guidelines on how to treat discitis, and orthopedic surgeons should be consulted for assistance.

Other Infections

Appendicitis can produce hip or thigh pain (and resultant limp) if the iliopsoas muscle is affected. Performing a thorough general physical examination (including abdominal examination) in addition to the musculoskeletal examination facilitates making this diagnosis. A psoas abscess can also present in a similar fashion. Both of these conditions require surgical consultation and referrals should be made as appropriate.

INFLAMMATORY ARTHRITIS

Juvenile Chronic Arthritis

Chronic inflammatory arthritis is the most common of the rheumatic diseases affecting children. It has been estimated that juvenile arthritis affects as many as 200,000 American children (21–23). With a reported incidence of 0.50 cases per 1,000 children, arthritis is the fifth most common chronic disease of childhood, behind only asthma, congenital heart disease, diabetes, and cleft lip/palate (24).

Although JRA may be self-limited with approximately two-thirds of patients having no active synovitis when reaching adulthood, many children experience potentially painful complications including joint deformities and destruction, osteoporosis, and growth abnormalities that may result in impairment of psychologic development and difficulty with daily activities (25,26). A minority of children has unremitting disease with mild to severe disease activity marked by chronic inflammation and pain. Although not well characterized in the pediatric literature, pain is generally considered to be a clinically significant symptom for many children with JRA.

JRA is actually a heterogeneous group of chronic inflammatory arthritides. There are several different classification schemes worldwide based on onset type and clinical course; however, the criteria established by the American College of Rheumatology is most commonly used in the United States (10). These criteria include the presence of persistent arthritis in one or more joints for a minimum of 6 weeks with onset before the sixteenth birthday and the exclusion of other causes of arthritis. Other types of chronic inflammatory arthritis include the juvenile spondyloarthropathies, psoriatic arthritis, and arthritis associated with inflammatory bowel disease. Figure 32.2 shows one classification scheme for juvenile chronic inflammatory arthritis.

The onset type of JRA is defined by the pattern of disease in the first 6 months (10). There are three onset types: systemic JRA, pauciarticular JRA (four or fewer involved joints), and polyarticular JRA (five or more involved joints). The subtype distinctions are made primarily on clinical grounds and are useful for guiding therapy and suggesting long-term outcome. Laboratory studies are not particularly helpful, with striking abnormalities found most reliably with systemic onset disease. These include anemia, thrombocytosis, leukocytosis, and high ESRs. Rheumatoid factor is present in fewer than 10% of children with JRA and is a poor prognostic indicator. The finding of a positive ANA indicates increased risk of inflammatory eye disease rather than suggesting a diagnosis. Table 32.6 compares the typical lab-

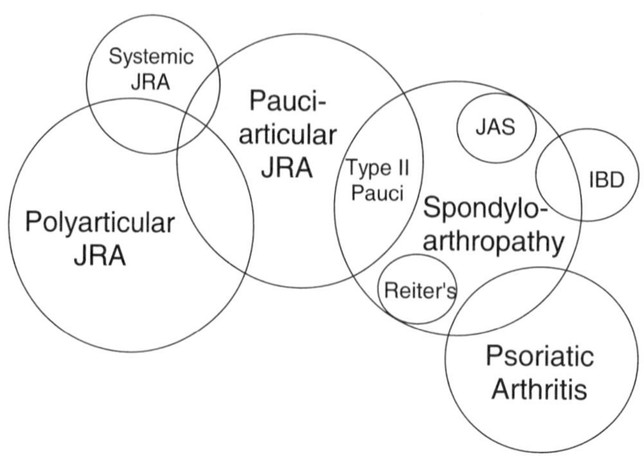

FIG. 32.2. Classification scheme for chronic arthritis in children. (From Schanberg LE, Sandstrom MJ. Causes of pain in children with arthritis. *Rheum Dis Clin North Am* 1999;25:31–53, with permission.)

TABLE 32.6. *Laboratory findings in arthritis in children*

	Systemic JRA	Polyarticular JRA RF positive	Polyarticular JRA RF negative	Pauciarticular JRA type I	Spondylo-arthropathy	Psoriatic arthritis
Gender	F = M	F > M	F > M	F > M	M > F	M = F
Onset age	Childhood to adulthood	Late childhood	Throughout childhood	Early childhood	Late childhood	Throughout childhood
Uveitis	Rare	Rare	Rare	Chronic	Acute	No
RF	No	100%	No	No	No	No
ANA	No	No	25%	>50%	No	No
HLA-B27	No	No	No	No	75%	50%
ESR	↑↑	Normal or ↑	Normal or ↑	Normal	Normal or ↑	Normal or ↑
HGB	↓↓	Normal or ↓	Normal or ↓	Normal	Normal or ↓	Normal

JRA, juvenile rheumatoid arthritis; RF, rheumatoid factor; F, female; M, male; ANA, antinuclear antibody; ESR, erythrocyte sedimentation rate; HGB, hemoglobin; ↑↑, markedly increased; ↓↓, markedly decreased; ↑, increased; ↓, decreased.

From Schanberg LE, Sandstrom MJ. Causes of pain in children with arthritis. *Rheum Dis Clin North Am* 1999;25:31–53, with permission.

oratory findings in various types of juvenile chronic arthritis. Clinical experience suggests that children with active systemic onset JRA and polyarticular JRA have the most significant pain complaints and are more likely to report cutting back on activities because of pain.

There are several forms of chronic inflammatory arthritis characterized as spondyloarthropathies. These conditions are often HLA-B27 associated and include Reiter disease, ankylosing spondylitis, arthropathies associated with illnesses such as Crohn disease and ulcerative colitis, reactive arthropathies, and psoriatic arthritis. Ankylosing spondylitis tends to affect adults more than children, although it should be considered in males presenting with sacroiliitis, especially if there is a positive family history. HLA-B27 is positive in greater than 90% of this population. Children with spondyloarthropathies may have pain complaints that are more generalized in nature and not limited to areas of active inflammation.

The course of disease is unpredictable in all types of juvenile chronic arthritis, but most often follows a fluctuating course with periods of flare and quiescence. Periods of flare are characterized by increased evidence of disease activity, marked by either a greater number of joints involved or increased inflammation in previously involved joints or both. The physical finding of more extensive arthritis is accompanied by worsening symptoms, particularly pain, but also fatigue and morning stiffness, as well as increased functional difficulties. During periods of flare, children may abruptly experience increased pain and more trouble completing routine activities, both at home and school. Children may also demonstrate more difficulty sleeping because of discomfort.

Clinically symptomatic disease flares in JRA may be accompanied by changes in biologic markers of total body inflammation and immune activation. Lower hemoglobin levels, elevations in the sedimentation rate, along with increases in serum levels of acute phase proteins and cytokines, have all been shown to correlate with clinical symptoms of disease activity in JRA (27–32). Increased total body inflammation results in local tissue damage that is directly responsible for increasing nociceptive pain through the cellular release of prostaglandins, leukotrienes, and kinins, all of which increase the activity of local primary afferent neurons in the periphery. Cytokines secreted by activated mononuclear cells are believed to modulate the initiation and perpetuation of systemic and localized inflammation. Cytokines play a direct role in nociception by activating or sensitizing C fibers (primary afferent neurons in the pain pathway).

Although the cause of disease flares in JRA continues to be unclear, current models invoke multiple possible triggers including infection, trauma, psychosocial stress, and mood imposed on a genetic predisposition (33). Infection by a virus or bacteria may induce the release of proinflammatory mediators (such as cytokines) from activated immune cells, resulting in an increase in disease activity and nociceptive pain. Stress and mood have also been shown to affect both immune activation and pain perception. Children with JRA are known to face numerous psychosocial stressors including increased dependence on family members, isolation from peers, physical disability, uncertainty about the future, and maintenance of complicated medical regimens, all of which may affect mood and pain perception.

Pain in Children with Juvenile Rheumatoid Arthritis

The pain related to juvenile chronic arthritis has been understudied despite the relatively extensive literature on pain experienced by adults with rheumatoid arthritis and osteoarthritis. Early studies comparing children's and adults' perceptions of arthritis-associated pain suggested that children with arthritis experienced less pain than their adult counterparts (34,35). These findings, however, were misleading because early studies failed to use age-appropriate measures of pain. Over the past 15 years, several pediatric pain researchers have developed age-appropriate measures of pain that appear to be reliable and valid throughout most of childhood.

Recently, these newly developed pediatric pain measures have been used to assess pain in children with arthritis. Several studies have been conducted, each of which suggests that pain is more prevalent than previously recognized. In contrast to earlier studies, Sherry and colleagues (36) found that 86% of 293 children with JRA reported pain during a routine pediatric rheumatology clinic visit. Data derived from the Cincinnati Juvenile Arthritis Databank looking at 462 children with JRA showed that 60% of children with JRA reported some degree of joint pain at onset, 50% still reported pain 1 year later, and 40% continued to report pain at 5-year follow-up (37). The level of pain reported by these children was in the mild to moderate range. In other studies, Varni and colleagues (38–40) comprehensively assessed pain experienced by children with JRA and other rheumatic diseases using the Pediatric Pain Questionnaire. These studies also showed that most children with JRA reported mild to moderate pain.

A recent study reported the pain experience of 56 children with juvenile chronic arthritis using several different pain instruments (41). Consistent with the other recent studies, these children on average reported pain in the low to middle ranges on all pain intensity measurement scales, although there was considerable variability in pain ratings. The results showed that pain is a significant problem for many children with juvenile chronic arthritis, with 25% reporting pain intensity in the middle or higher ranges of the pain measurement scales. This was particularly striking considering that all these children were established patients in a subspecialty clinic and presumably receiving appropriate medical care.

Pharmacologic Treatment of Pain in Juvenile Rheumatoid Arthritis

Historically, the treatment of pain in children with JRA has focused on controlling the underlying disease with medications and providing symptomatic relief with acetaminophen, heat or cold, splints, adaptive devices, and physical therapy. Various lines of research support this approach to pain management. Vandvik and Eckblad (42), in a study of 57 children admitted to the hospital with suspected rheumatic disease, found that disease severity was correlated with reports of pain intensity. Varni and colleagues (38–40) also showed a positive correlation between physicians' ratings of disease activity and pain intensity in children with JRA.

The mainstay of drug treatment for the pain of JRA continues to be NSAIDs with acetaminophen for acutely painful events (43). Although naproxen, ibuprofen, tolmetin sodium, and salicylates are the only NSAIDs formally approved by the U.S. Food and Drug Administration (FDA) to treat JRA, pediatric rheumatologists may choose to use other unapproved NSAIDs because of individual variations in efficacy and tolerance. Naproxen, ibuprofen, and trisalicylate are the only NSAIDs available in liquid form and therefore are most useful in young children. With twice-daily dosing, naproxen also offers convenience and may improve compliance. All children taking naproxen should be monitored for the development of pseudoporphyria, which is seen in 12% of children and is an indication to stop the medication (44,45). This most commonly occurs over the nasal bridge in fair-skinned children and usually recedes with discontinuation of the medication. In adolescents, long-acting preparations permitting once-daily dosing can greatly increase compliance. On occasion, indomethacin can be helpful in managing breakthrough pain.

In general, children tolerate NSAIDs better than adults do, and the occurrence of gastric ulcers is relatively uncommon (46). Dyspepsia, however, is not uncommon and often resolves with addition of an H_2 blocker. Although nabumetone and etodolac are not FDA-approved for use in children, they may be helpful in situations of gastrointestinal intolerance. Nabumetone tablets can be dissolved in a small amount of warm water and administered to even very young children. The cyclooxygenase-2–specific inhibitors have not yet been tested in children and should be reserved for teenagers and children with a history of peptic ulcers.

Remittive agents, particularly methotrexate, are indicated in children with multiple active joints and unremitting pain. Because of the ease of dosing, this has replaced gold as the remittive agent of choice in children. Methotrexate is generally dosed based on body surface area, starting at 7.5 to 10 mg/m^2 and titrating for efficacy. Doses as high as 1 mg/kg have been reported, but most patients respond at much lower levels (47). This may be dosed orally or via subcutaneous injection, especially at higher doses. It may be useful to prescribe the subcutaneous injection administered by a health care professional to ensure compliance. As with adults, monthly monitoring of blood counts and liver function testing is recommended, but clinically significant liver disease is rare in children. Most pediatric rheumatologists adjust doses for liver enzyme abnormalities that reach twice the normal level. Hydroxychloroquine and sulfasalazine are also commonly used in children, both alone and in combination.

Recently, a new biologic agent, etanercept, has received FDA approval for the treatment of juvenile arthritis. This agent is a soluble tumor necrosis factor receptor: Fc fusion protein and is recommended only for children with severe polyarticular arthritis. Etanercept blocks the binding of the inflammatory cytokine tumor necrosis factor α and has been shown effective in children who failed to respond to methotrexate (48). Interestingly, children taking etanercept, which is given twice weekly by subcutaneous injection, report resolution of pain and morning stiffness beyond what might be expected from the improvement seen in their joints. Studies using etanercept in children with systemic onset JRA are underway. Recommended pediatric doses for all these medications are shown in Table 32.3.

The use of systemic steroids should be avoided whenever possible. In particular, it is important to rule out malignancies before beginning even low-dose steroids in children presenting with symptoms of systemic onset JRA. It is safe practice to obtain a bone marrow on all children with fever, rash, anemia, and arthritis before starting steroids. To treat pain, steroids should only be used in low doses with the goal of restoring or maintaining function rather than completely relieving pain and should be limited to managing flares of disease while other interventions are put in place. It is often difficult to wean off steroids if used to treat more chronic symptomatology. The side effects of chronic steroid use in children include growth retardation and worsening of the osteoporosis associated with JRA even in the absence of corticosteroid therapy. Intra-articular steroids are a safe option to manage the inflammation in monoarticular or pauciarticular arthritis but may also be useful to treat a particularly painful joint in a child with polyarticular arthritis. Triamcinolone hexacetonide mixed with sterile lidocaine provides immediate relief of pain, with the procedure performed with conscious sedation in younger patients and topical anesthetic in older children.

Opioids are used to provide pain relief in acute situations as other medications and treatments are initiated. Oxycodone, a higher potency opioid, is often better tolerated than codeine with fewer side effects for the amount of pain relief. It is available in a liquid form; however, many small pharmacies will only carry oxycodone tablets in combination with other analgesics, such as acetaminophen or aspirin. In young children, one-half tablet every 4 to 6 hours will suffice. In older children with chronic pain, it is preferable to use a long-acting opioid preparation of either oxycodone or morphine, making short-acting opioid preparations available for breakthrough pain. As in adults, adjuvant medications are often useful for managing chronic pain. These most commonly include tricyclic antidepressants and selective serotonin reuptake inhibitors. The tricyclic antidepressants amitriptyline and nortriptyline are used in low doses given at night.

Psychosocial Variables and Pain in Juvenile Rheumatoid Arthritis

Obviously, the pharmacologic treatments for pain are geared toward reducing pain by managing the underlying disease process while simultaneously decreasing the manifest symptoms of physical discomfort. Several recent studies, however, suggest that disease severity is not the only relevant predictor of pain among children with JRA. In fact, when regression models are used to examine multiple predictors of present pain intensity in children with JRA, results suggest that the combination of medical status and disease severity variables explain only a small proportion of overall pain variance.

In a regression analysis conducted by Ilowite and colleagues (49), for example, joint inflammation explained only 10% of the variance in pain scores. There was no significant relationship between either the disease subtype or number of joints affected and pain scores. Similarly, Hagglund et al. (50) failed to show a statistically significant association between disease severity and pain ratings of children with JRA. Thompson et al. (39) found that medical status measures (arthritis subtype and disease activity) explained only modest amounts of variance (8% and 1%, respectively) in JRA subjects reports of pain.

The lack of robustness in the relationship between disease variables and pain variance reported by children with JRA recently prompted us to take a broader look at pain predictors. In addition to traditional disease variables, we examined the extent to which children's strategies for coping with pain related to variations in reported pain intensity (41). A model combining demographic variables, medical status variables, and coping variables explained more than 50% of the variance in reported pain intensity. Although disease activity clearly emerged as a significant predictor, our results indicated that the coping variable explained a significant and unique proportion of variance in these measures, even after controlling for important demographic and medical status measures. Specifically, children who rated their ability to control and decrease pain as high and who reported an infrequent tendency to catastrophize (i.e., engage in overly negative and unrealistic thinking about their pain) had significantly lower pain intensity ratings and reported having pain in fewer body locations. These findings are consistent with those of previous studies of children with fibromyalgia (51) and sickle cell disease (52,53).

A study investigating the interrelationships of daily stress, daily mood, and disease expression is currently underway, using multiple variables of disease expression including symptom report, severity of disease by examination, and biologic markers of disease activity, inflammation, and immune activation. Published data from a pilot study support the correlation of mood and daily event stress with pain and other disease symptoms, employing longitudinally repeated measures and within-person design to more accurately capture individual differences (54).

Taken together, it appears that psychosocial variables such as coping strategies and perceptions about disease are important to consider in the treatment of the pain of JRA. Addressing these issues while providing aggressive traditional medical management may help to reduce pain, elevate mood, and improve overall quality of life for children with arthritis.

Transient Arthritis

By definition, arthritis must be present in one joint for at least 6 weeks to make a diagnosis of any type of chronic childhood arthritis. The most common causes of painful arthritis in children are infectious or peri-infectious in nature and relatively short-lived. These may be during viral (e.g., Parvovirus, rubella, Epstein–Barr virus, Coxsackievirus) or bacterial infections (e.g., gonorrhea, staphylococci, streptococci) or 1 to 3 weeks after a presumed infection, such as poststreptococcal arthritis (including acute rheumatic fever) or toxic synovitis of the hip. Although the peri-infectious causes of arthritis in children may be acutely painful, they generally resolve in less than 6 weeks without specific therapy.

The classic example of a postinfectious arthritis is rheumatic fever. This illness follows a group A β-hemolytic streptococcal infection. The illness usually occurs 1 to 3 weeks after the original infection and affects predominantly children 5 to 15 years of age. The Jones criteria are used to make the diagnosis (55). In brief, a combination of major and minor criteria is needed. Major criteria include carditis, arthritis, erythema marginatum, chorea, and subcutaneous nodules. Minor criteria include fever, arthralgia, increased ESR or CRP, and a prolonged PR interval on an electrocardiogram. Critical to the diagnosis is identification of the organism (either by culture or appropriate titers). Therapy is directed at eradication of the original infection (if not already done) and prophylaxis against future outbreaks. If suspected, laboratory data should include an electrocardiogram, ESR, CRP, and streptococcal cultures. Although the Jones criteria are needed for a definitive diagnosis, some authors have suggested that any child with a sore throat or constitutional symptoms at presentation of arthritis be investigated with throat cultures and streptococcal antibodies (56). This is an important consideration because an echocardiogram to rule out carditis may be required if a streptococcal infection is (was) present (56).

Reactive arthritis is a sterile arthritis that occurs in a distant site and at a different time from the original infection (20). It can occur at any age and affects females as frequently as males. Often the onset of pain is sudden and has a tendency to affect lower limb joints. Frequently, there is history of a gastrointestinal illness. Organisms such as *Salmonella*, *Shigella*, *Campylobacter*, and *Yersinia* are frequently implicated. The arthritis usually resolves with minimal complications. The child who presents with gastrointestinal symptoms and arthritis should have stool studies done for the most common organisms. As indicated above, ulcerative colitis and Crohn disease should also be considered. NSAIDs can provide relief in reactive arthropathies. Usually the pain resolves with few complications.

Reiter disease is a specific subtype of reactive arthropathies. It is usually characterized by the triad of sterile urethritis, arthritis, and uveitis. The illness occurs more often in males. It frequently follows the gastrointestinal infections listed previously. In addition, sexually transmitted diseases such as chlamydial and gonococcal infections should always be considered as etiologic agents and appropriately ruled out. As with other reactive arthropathies, large joints are usually involved, especially the knees and ankles. Treatment involves NSAIDs and treatment of the underlying infection, if present. Most patients recover completely, although some will go on to develop more chronic problems. As with ankylosing spondylitis, HLA-B27 is seen in more than 90% of patients. Because sacroiliitis is a frequent complication of Reiter disease, follow-up of these patients should include careful spine examinations.

Transient Hip Synovitis

Transient hip synovitis is the most common cause of acute hip pain in children 2 to 10 years of age (57). The illness tends to affect boys more than girls. The presenting complaint is usually limp or refusal to walk. Most of the children are afebrile, and associated pain ranges from none to severe. When present, pain often has been present for only a short period (1 to 3 days). The physical examination is significant for decreased range of motion and a flexed, abducted, and externally rotated hip. Often a history of an upper respiratory infection is elicited.

Ultrasonography is an excellent diagnostic test and can demonstrate fluid in the hip with 95% accuracy. Plain films are generally not indicated, and bone scintigraphy is not helpful (57). One study looked at signal intensity in bone marrow on MRI to discriminate septic arthritis from transient synovitis (58). Interestingly, bone marrow changes were found in eight of nine patients with septic arthritis and none of 14 patients with transient synovitis (58). Future studies are needed to confirm these data before MRI is routinely recommended in this setting. Most often the diagnosis is made clinically without need for imaging studies.

The presence of fluid in the hip demonstrated by ultrasonography would be expected in children with either transient synovitis or a septic joint. This presents a diagnostic challenge because transient synovitis is a diagnosis of exclusion, and ruling out septic arthritis is absolutely necessary (13). As with a septic joint, transient hip synovitis is usually unilateral. Septic arthritis should be suspected if there is severe pain, fever, or an elevated ESR. Sometimes, with a septic joint, spasms may be present with palpation (57). Aspiration, of course, is mandatory if a septic joint is suspected. The difficulty is trying to decide which hips to aspirate. A recent study examining laboratory findings in cases of suspected transient synovitis addressed this question (59). Children with septic arthritis were found to have a hip effusion by ultrasonography (as expected) and at least two of the following criteria: fever higher than 38°C, ESR greater than 20 mm per hour, or CRP greater than 20 mg per liter ($p < 0.0001$ for each parameter). Sensitivity was 100%, but these markers were occasionally found in some patients with transient synovitis (which lowered the specificity to 89%). Leukocytosis was not a significant factor. Based on these findings, the authors suggested that hip joint aspiration be performed when effusion and two or more of the above criteria are found. Interestingly, radiographs were found *not* to have a significant impact on decision making in the initial evaluation of acute hip pain (59).

The treatment for transient hip synovitis is rest and NSAIDs (Table 32.5). The child must be closely followed, with re-evaluation if fever develops or pain or limping persists 7 to 10 days after initial presentation (57).

NEOPLASMS

Most worrisome to parents and pediatricians alike is the possibility of a neoplastic process underlying musculoskeletal complaints. It is the concern to exclude malignancy that often leads to extensive workups. Although neoplasms are an uncommon cause of musculoskeletal pain, they must at least be considered in all cases. A retrospective review of 29 children with malignancy illustrated many cases in which musculoskeletal pain was the predominant symptom of neoplasm (60). Numerous neoplasms were subsequently uncovered, including neuroblastoma, Ewing sarcoma, lymphoma, and leukemia (60). Limping in a child can be a presenting symptom of acute leukemia (61). Features of concern for neoplasm were back pain, night sweats, and nonarticular bone pain (60). Fever and weight loss are additional red flags. When malignancy is considered, CBC with peripheral smear, ESR, and lactate dehydrogenase are appropriate initial laboratory screening tests. Imaging studies are dictated by the type of complaint, i.e., plain films may be appropriate for localized bony symptoms, whereas MRI could be considered for soft-tissue findings and a bone scan for more generalized pain.

The pain associated with tumors can be owing to the lesion itself or associated pathologic stress fractures. This pain is often severe, waking the child from sleep. Growing pains are a much more common diagnosis in the pediatric population and may be difficult to discern from a more serious diagnosis on initial history. However, laboratory screening tests along with the presence of constitutional symptoms should help discriminate growing pains from a neoplastic process. The diagnosis of growing pains is discussed in detail below. Osteoid osteoma is an interesting benign tumor that occurs in children. The pain that occurs with osteoid osteoma is characteristically relieved with aspirin. Histiocytosis is another process that can present with musculoskeletal complaints. For example, an afebrile 3-year-old with a several-week history of limp and anterior right thigh pain was subsequently found to have Langerhans cell histiocytosis involving the fifth lumbar vertebra (62).

Referral to a hematologist/oncologist is necessary in cases of suspected neoplasm. Most often, specialists should direct the workup of these children. Obtaining bone marrow aspirations and extensive imaging studies before referral is costly and may delay diagnosis and treatment, especially if these tests need to be repeated by the specialist.

IDIOPATHIC MUSCULOSKELETAL PAIN SYNDROMES

Chronic pain syndromes are common in children, compromising approximately 25% of all new patients seen by pediatric rheumatologists. Of the children with chronic pain syndromes, 25% to 40% fulfills the Yunus criteria for juvenile primary fibromyalgia syndrome (63,64; L. Schanberg and D. Kredich, unpublished observation, 1991). Other diagnoses include growing pains, complex regional pain syndrome (CRPS, also known as reflex sympathetic dystrophy), localized pain syndromes, and low back pain. CRPS is discussed in detail in Chapter 34. This chapter focuses on two pain syndromes in children: growing pains and fibromyalgia.

Growing Pains

As mentioned previously, another interesting diagnostic dilemma for the pediatrician relates to growing pains. As with other pediatric musculoskeletal complaints, the challenge for the primary care doctor is to make the diagnosis with the least amount of testing, while identifying the less common, more significant diagnoses. This is not a trivial problem because the general pediatrician frequently encounters symptoms attributable to growing pains. Recent reports have suggested that growing pains represent the final diagnosis in 8% to 11% of all pediatric musculoskeletal pain (2,65). Because there is no diagnostic test, growing pains is a clinical diagnosis. This is not a straightforward issue because growing pains have been defined in a number of different ways.

Most authors would agree that a classic presentation consistent with growing pains is that of a child (6 to 10 years of age) who complains of pain in both legs that awakens him or her from sleep. The pain typically is symmetric in the thighs, knees, calves, or shins. The pain is of short duration, and the child usually falls back to sleep. The pain will wake the child only once per night, occurring as often as three to four nights every month, often on consecutive nights. Frequently, a history of increased physical activity during the day can be elicited (12,66).

Because the diagnosis is necessarily one of exclusion, attention must be paid to the history and physical examination. Neither morning stiffness nor a limp should be present, and there should be complete remission of symptoms between attacks (67). Pain-free intervals of days to months are common. Growing pains are nonarticular and short-lived. Progressively worsening symptoms should raise suspicion for other diagnoses. Possible red flags include any abnormal physical examination findings, including evidence of a limp, joint swelling, tenderness, abnormal gait, or limited range of motion. History significant for fever, malaise, weight loss, or night sweats should also trigger further evaluation. The term "growing pains" is actually a misnomer because there is no evidence to suggest that growing pains are, in fact, caused by growing. A classic history with the absence of worrisome findings, however, makes the possibility of other causes very remote (68).

Treatment can be simple, including the use of NSAIDs. A recent survey of treatment approaches to growing pains demonstrated that combinations of reassurance, massage, and analgesic therapy were most common (68). One small study has shown that muscle stretching may lead to a more rapid resolution of symptoms over time (69).

Interestingly, there is evidence suggesting that children with growing pains show an increase in other difficulties such as recurrent abdominal pain, negative mood, and behavioral problems, suggesting a possible psychosocial component to growing pains as seen in other pain syndromes (66). When confident of the diagnosis of growing pains, it is important to reassure the child and family. Symptoms of growing pains have been shown to become much less stressful to the child and family (and often abate) if concerns about cancer and rheumatic disorders are addressed (70).

An interesting corollary to growing pains is restless legs syndrome, which has been reported in children (71). The clinical features of restless legs syndrome share similarities with those of growing pains, including a desire to move the extremities and worsening of symptoms at rest, especially in the evening or night. A significant family history may suggest restless legs syndrome as a diagnosis. With a strong family history of restless legs and a high clinical suspicion, polysomnography can confirm the diagnosis (71). This is an important diagnosis to make distinct from growing pains because these children usually do not outgrow their symptoms.

Fibromyalgia

Fibromyalgia is a musculoskeletal pain syndrome of unknown cause characterized by widespread persistent pain, sleep disturbance, and the presence of multiple discrete tender points on physical examination. The pediatric form of this syndrome, juvenile primary fibromyalgia syndrome (JPFS), was first described in 1985 when Yunus and Masi (64) reported on 33 children who had symptoms of persistent pain and sleep difficulties. Of children with chronic pain syndromes, 25% to 40% fulfills criteria for JPFS (63,64). The prevalence of this syndrome in school-age children has been reported to be as high as 6.2%, using less stringent diagnostic criteria accepted by the American College of Rheumatology for adults (72).

JPFS is clearly more common in girls, with an average age at diagnosis of 13 years in the pediatric population (63,64,73). Although the cause remains unclear, many theories have been proposed. Disordered sleep physiology, abnormal levels of substance P causing enhanced central pain perception, disordered mood, dysregulation of the hypothalamic pituitary axis, poor physical fitness, microtrauma to muscles, and hypermobility have all been suggested as possible causes of this puzzling syndrome (74). Physiologic abnormalities are present in children and adults with fibromyalgia, but none explains the myriad symptoms described by people with fibromyalgia and seem to be epiphenomenal rather than truly causative. People with fibromyalgia have lower pain thresholds than matched controls and show decreased discrimination between pain and other noxious stimuli (75).

The diagnosis of JPFS is based on the criteria developed by Yunus and Masi (64). This includes the presence of diffuse musculoskeletal aching in at least three areas of the body for at least 3 months in the absence of an underlying condition. Laboratory tests are normal, and physical examination reveals the presence of five or more typical tender points, but no evidence of arthritis or other abnormalities. The location of the tender points is shown in Table 32.7. Unlike other chronic pain populations, patients with JPFS show few pain behaviors and move around with no apparent difficulty during examination (51, 76). Although showing few pain behaviors, children with fibromyalgia self-report characteristically high pain intensity and use unique descriptors, such as "miserable," "intense," and "unbearable" to describe their pain (53, 77).

Associated symptoms are common in JPFS, including nonrestorative sleep (100%), fatigue (91%), subjective soft-tissue swelling of the extremities (61%), chronic anxiety or tension (56%), chronic headaches (54%), tingling and numbness of the extremities (35%), and recurrent abdominal pain (27%) (64). Physical activity, weather, anxiety, or stress often modulates pain. In fact, the associated symptoms are so common that there is considerable overlap with other functional disorders such as irritable bowel disease, chronic fatigue syndrome, migraines, temporomandibular joint disorder, myofascial pain syndromes, premenstrual syndrome, and mood and anxiety disorders. All these disorders may be part of a spectrum of related syndromes (77).

TABLE 32.7. *Fibromyalgia tender points*[a]

1. insertion of nuchal muscles into occiput
2. upper border of trapezius–mid portion
3. muscle attachments to upper medial border of scapula
4. anterior aspects of the C5, C7 intertransverse spaces
5. second rib space ~ 3 cm lateral to the sternal border
6. muscle attachments to lateral epicondyle ~ 2 cm below bony prominence
7. upper outer quadrant of gluteal muscles
8. muscle attachments just posterior to greater trochanter
9. medial fat pad of knee proximal to joint line

[a]Recommended by the 1990 American College of Rheumatology (ACR) Criteria Committee for establishing diagnosis.

Points should be palpated with pulp of the thumb or forefinger using pressure equivalent to 4 kg. The presence of 11 or more tender points in conjunction with a history of widespread musculoskeletal pain (pain on both sides of the body, pain above and below the waist, and pain in an axial distribution) meets the ACR diagnostic criteria for fibromyalgia. These criteria have not been validated for use in children.

Although fibromyalgia is known to cause significant morbidity in adults (78,79), its impact in the pediatric population has only recently been addressed. Follow-up studies point out that many children with fibromyalgia continue to have persistent pain years after diagnosis (63,80). Thus, the illness has potential consequences not only on the health of the children but also on their psychosocial development (81,82). Many adolescents with untreated JPFS withdraw from both school and the social milieu, which has serious implications as they move into adulthood. Recent studies point to the coping ability of children with fibromyalgia as a significant predictor of health status. It has been shown that pain coping strategies significantly correlated with reported pain intensity, functional disability, and psychologic distress. Children who reported greater ability to control their pain had lower pain levels, less functional disability, and less psychologic distress (51).

Medical therapy to date has been largely unsuccessful. Medical alternatives for patients with JPFS, including NSAIDs, tricyclic antidepressants, and muscle relaxants, have proved to be of only modest and short-term benefit in adults and have not been studied in the pediatric population (83,84). Patients with JPFS seen at tertiary care centers are encouraged to pursue a combination of treatments (e.g., medication, aerobic exercise, pain coping skills training, stress management, and psychotherapy) with practitioners in their local communities (85). Such treatments, however, are difficult to coordinate, expensive, and often not reimbursed by insurance companies. In addition, children with JPFS are strongly encouraged to return to school and their normal activities once a diagnosis is made. A mainstay of therapy is education for both the family and child, including explanations of the syndrome and the interrelationships between mood, stress, poor sleep, pain, and lack of exercise. We emphasize the vicious cycle that many children with fibromyalgia find themselves in, even if we are unable to identify the cause of the problem. Of utmost importance in establishing a therapeutic relationship is reassurance that the pain is real and not imagined.

Children and adolescents with fibromyalgia actively attempt to cope but show less ability to manage their pain than healthy college students or people with other painful conditions such as arthritis and sickle cell disease (51). For this reason, treatment aimed at improving self-reliance through cognitive-behavioral therapy and a return to usual activities is encouraged (51,86). In fact, small studies in both children and adults show that cognitive behavioral therapies may be successful in this population (86–88). Aerobic exercise is another cornerstone of therapy (86–89). At presentation, children are generally inactive, participating in no physical activities at the current time, although they may have been involved in such activities in the past. In addition, patients complain of severe fatigue that prevents them from engaging in activity. Although increasing activity makes pain worse initially, there is gradual improvement over a several-week period and a paradoxical increase in energy. It is aerobic exercise, not stretching, strengthening, or manipulative techniques, that results in symptom improvement in fibromyalgia (86,88,90). Although alternative therapies may be helpful for patients with fibromyalgia, the data to support this assertion are still weak at best, and further studies are needed (90).

The nonrestorative sleep of children with fibromyalgia may be treated with careful sleep hygiene and low doses of amitriptyline or nortriptyline, which is often better tolerated. Dosing is begun at 10 mg every night and titrated for effect. Trazodone may be helpful occasionally if tricyclic antidepressants are ineffective. In addition, selective serotonin reuptake inhibitors can be added if there is evidence of a mood disorder. These are best dosed in the morning. In general, opioids are not useful in treating the pain of fibromyalgia, and chronic opioid therapy is not encouraged for these individuals.

CONCLUSION

The child presenting to the general pediatrician with complaints of musculoskeletal pain is a very common occurrence. The challenge is to make the appropriate diagnosis with a minimum of invasive tests. Usually, simple reassurance and analgesic advice can suffice for most complaints. Choosing the right specialist to whom to refer more difficult cases is important, as is immediately recognizing and initiating therapy of severe problems such as neoplasms or septic joints.

REFERENCES

1. Schappert S, Nelson C. National ambulatory medical care survey, 1995–1996 Summary. *Vital Health Stat* 1999;13:i–vi, 1–122.
2. de Inocencio J. Musculoskeletal pain in primary pediatric care: analysis of 1000 consecutive general pediatric clinic visits. *Pediatrics* 1998;102:E63.
3. Passo MH. Aches and limb pain. *Pediatr Clin North Am* 1982;29:209–219.
4. Dabney KW, Lipton G. Evaluation of limp in children. *Curr Opin Pediatr* 1995;7:88–94.
5. Huttenlocher A, Newman TB. Evaluation of the erythrocyte sedimentation rate in children presenting with limp, fever, or abdominal pain. *Clin Pediatr* 1997;36: 339–344.
6. Kallio MJ, Unkila-Kallio L, Aalto K, et al. Serum C-reactive protein, erythrocyte sedimentation rate and white blood cell count in septic arthritis of children. *Pediatr Infect Dis J* 1997;16:411–413.
7. Illei G, Klippel J. Why is the ANA result positive? *Bull Rheum Dis* 1999;48:1–4.
8. Cabral D, Petty R, Fung M, et al. Persistent antinuclear antibodies in children without identifiable inflammatory rheumatic or autoimmune disease. *Pediatrics* 1992; 89:441–444.
9. Deane P, Liard G, Siegel D, et al. The outcome of children referred to a pediatric rheumatology clinic with a positive antinuclear antibody test but without an autoimmune disease. *Pediatrics* 1995;95:892–895.
10. Brewer EJ, Bass J, Baum J. Current proposed revision of JRA criteria. *Arthritis Rheum* 1977;20:195–199.

11. Fordham L, Auringer ST, Frush DP. Pediatric imaging perspective: acute limp. *J Pediatr* 1998;132:906–908.
12. Abu-Arafeh I, Russell G. Recurrent limb pain in schoolchildren. *Arch Dis Child* 1996;74:336–339.
13. Renshaw TS. The child who has a limp. *Pediatr Rev* 1995;16:458–465.
14. Steinberg M. Management of sickle cell disease. *N Engl J Med* 1999;340:1021–1029.
15. Ura Y, Hara T, Mori Y, et al. Development of Perthes' disease in a 3-year-old boy with idiopathic thrombocytopenic purpura and antiphospholipid antibodies. *Pediatr Hematol Oncol* 1992;977–80.
16. Seleznick MJ, Silveira LH, Espinosa LR. Avascular necrosis associated with anticardiolipin antibodies. *J Rheumatol* 1990;18:297–298.
17. Karwowska A, Davies HD, Jadavji T. Epidemiology and outcome of osteomyelitis in the era of sequential intravenous-oral therapy. *Pediatr Infect Dis J* 1998;17: 1021–1026.
18. Lew D, Waldvogel F. Osteomyelitis. *N Engl J Med* 1997;336:999–1007.
19. Peltola H, Unkila-Kallio L, Kallio MJ. Simplified treatment of acute staphylococcal osteomyelitis of childhood. The Finnish Study Group. *Pediatrics* 1997;99: 846–850.
20. Shetty AK, Gedalia A. Septic arthritis in children. *Rheum Dis Clin North Am* 1998;24:287–304.
21. Cassidy JT, Nelson AM. The frequency of juvenile arthritis. *J Rheumatol* 1988;15:535–536.
22. Gewanter HT, Roghmann KJ, Baum J. The prevalence of juvenile arthritis. *Arthritis Rheum* 1983;26:599–603.
23. Towner SR, Michet CA O'Fallon WM, et al. The epidemiology of juvenile arthritis in Rochester, Minnesota 1960–1979. *Arthritis Rheum* 1983;26:1208–1213.
24. Gortmaker SL, Sappenfield W. Chronic childhood disorders: prevalence and impact. *Pediatr Clin North Am* 1984;31:3–18.
25. Hull RG. Outcome in juvenile arthritis. *J Rheumatol* 1988;27:66–71.
26. Ivey J, Brewer E, Giannini E. Psychosocial functioning in children with JRA. *Arthritis Rheum* 1981;24:S100.
27. De Benedetti F, Robbioni P, Massa M, et al. Serum interleukin-6 levels and joint involvement in polyarticular and pauciarticular juvenile chronic arthritis. *Clin Exp Rheumatol* 1992;10:493–498.
28. Endresen GKM, Hoyeraal HM, Kass E. Platelet count and disease activity in juvenile rheumatoid arthritis. *Scand J Rheumatol* 1977;6:237–240.
29. Hussein A, Stein J, Ehrich JHH. C-reactive protein in the assessment of disease activity in juvenile rheumatoid arthritis. *Scand J Rheumatol* 1987;16:101–105.
30. Lepore L, Pennesi M, Saletta S, et al. Study of IL-2, IL-6, TNFa, IFNg and b in the serum and synovial fluid of patients with juvenile chronic arthritis. *Clin Exp Rheumatol* 1994;12:561–565.
31. Mangge H, Kenzian H, Gallistl S, et al. Serum cytokines in juvenile rheumatoid arthritis: correlation with conventional inflammation parameters and clinical subtypes. *Arthritis Rheum* 1995;38:211–220.
32. Rooney M, David J, Symons J, et al. Inflammatory cytokine responses in juvenile chronic arthritis. *Br J Rheumatol* 1995;34:454–460.
33. Vandvik IH, Hoyeraal HM. Juvenile chronic arthritis: a biobehavioral disease. Some unsolved questions. *Clin Exp Rheumatol* 1993;11:669–680.
34. Laaksonen AL, Laine V. A comparative study of joint pain in adult and juvenile rheumatoid arthritis. *Ann Rheum Dis* 1961;20:386–387.
35. Scott PJ, Ansell BM, Huskisson EC. Measurement of pain in juvenile chronic polyarthritis. *Ann Rheum Dis* 1977;36:186–187.
36. Sherry DD, Bohnsack J, Salmonson K, et al. Painless juvenile rheumatoid arthritis. *J Pediatr* 1990;116: 921–923.
37. Lovell DJ, Walco GA. Pain associated with juvenile rheumatoid arthritis. *Pediatr Clin North Am* 1989;36: 1015–1027.
38. Gragg RA, Rapoff MA, Danovsky MB, et al. Assessing chronic musculoskeletal pain associated with rheumatic disease: further validation of the Pediatric Pain Questionnaire. *J Pediatr Psychol* 1996;21:237–250.
39. Thompson KL, Varni JW, Hanson V. Comprehensive assessment of pain in juvenile rheumatoid arthritis: an empirical model. *J Pediatr Psychol* 1987;12:241–255.
40. Varni JW, Thompson KL, Hanson V. The Varni/Thompson Pediatric Pain Questionnaire. Chronic musculoskeletal pain in juvenile rheumatoid arthritis. *Pain* 1987;28:27–38.
41. Schanberg LE, Keefe FJ, Lefebvre JC, et al. Pain coping and the pain experience in children with juvenile chronic arthritis. *Pain* 1997;73:181–189.
42. Vandvik IH, Eckblad G. Relationship between pain, disease severity and psychosocial function in patients with juvenile chronic arthritis (JCA). *Scand J Rheumatol* 1990;19:295–302.
43. Schanberg LE, Sandstrom MJ. Causes of pain in children with arthritis. *Rheum Dis Clin North Am* 1999;25: 31–53.
44. Lang BA, Finlayson LA. Naproxen-induced pseudoporphyria in patients with juvenile rheumatoid arthritis. *J Pediatr* 1994;124:639–642.
45. Levy ML, Barron KS, Eichenfield A, et al. Naproxen-induced pseudoporphyria: a distinctive photodermatitis. *J Pediatr* 1990;117:660–664.
46. Keenan GF, Giannini EH, Athreya BH. Clinically significant gastropathy associated with nonsteroidal anti-inflammatory drug use in children with juvenile rheumatoid arthritis. *J Rheumatol* 1995;22:1149–1151.
47. Wallace CA. The use of methotrexate in childhood rheumatic diseases. *Arthritis Rheum* 1998;41:381–391.
48. Lovell DJ, Giannini EH. Reiff A, et al. Etanercept in children with polyarticular juvenile rheumatoid arthritis. *N Engl J Med* 2000;342:763–769.
49. Ilowite NT, Walco GA, Pochaczevsky R. Assessment of pain in patients with juvenile rheumatoid arthritis: relation between pain intensity and degree of joint inflammation. *Ann Rheum Dis* 1992;51:343–346.
50. Hagglund KJ, Schopp LM, Alberts KR, et al. Predicting pain among children with juvenile rheumatoid arthritis. *Arthritis Care Res* 1995;8:36–42.
51. Schanberg LE, Keefe FJ, Lefebvre JC, et al. Pain coping strategies in children with juvenile primary fibromyalgia syndrome: correlation with pain, physical function, and psychological disability. *Arthritis Care Res* 1996; 9:89–96.
52. Gil KM, Williams DA, Thompson RJ, et al. Sickle cell disease in children and adolescents: the relation of child and parent pain coping strategies to adjustment. *J Pediatr Psychol* 1991;16:643–663.
53. Gil KM, Thompson RJ, Keith BR, et al. Sickle cell dis-

ease pain in children and adolescents: change in pain frequency and coping strategies over time. *J Pediatr Psychol* 1993;18:621–637.
54. Schanberg LE, Sandstrom MJ, Starr K, et al. The relationship of daily mood and stressful events to symptoms in juvenile rheumatic disease. *Arthritis Care Res* 2000; 13:33–41.
55. Anonymous. Guidelines for the diagnosis of rheumatic fever. Jones criteria, 1992 update. Special Writing Group of the Committee on Rheumatic Fever, Endocarditis, and Kawasaki Disease of the Council on Cardiovascular Disease in the Young of the American Heart Association. *JAMA* 1992;268:2069–2073.
56. Malleson PN. Management of childhood arthritis. Part 1: acute arthritis. *Arch Dis Child* 1997;76:460–462.
57. Hart JJ. Transient synovitis of the hip in children. *Am Fam Physician* 1996;54:1587–91, 1595–1596.
58. Lee SK, Suh KJ, Kim YW, et al. Septic arthritis versus transient synovitis at MR imaging: preliminary assessment with signal intensity alterations in bone marrow. *Radiology* 1999;211:459–465.
59. Eich GF, Superti-Furga A, Umbricht FS, et al. The painful hip: evaluation of criteria for clinical decision-making. *Eur J Pediatr* 1999;158:923–928.
60. Cabral D, Tucker L. Malignancies in children who initially present with rheumatic complaints. *J Pediatr* 1999;134:53–57.
61. Tuten HR, Gabos PG, Kumar SJ, et al. The limping child: a manifestation of acute leukemia. *J Pediatr Orthop* 1998;18:625–629.
62. Bodart E, Nisolle JF, Maton P, et al. Limp as unusual presentation of Langerhans' cell histiocytosis. *Eur J Pediatr* 1999;158:384–386.
63. Malleson PN, Al-Matar M, Petty RE. Idiopathic musculoskeletal pain syndromes in children. *J Rheumatol* 1992;19:1786–1789.
64. Yunus MB, Masi AT. Juvenile primary fibromyalgia syndrome: a clinical study of thirty-three patients and matched normal controls. *Arthritis Rheum* 1985;28: 138–145.
65. Oberklaid F, Amos D, Liu C, et al. "Growing pains": clinical and behavioral correlates in a community sample. *J Dev Behav Pediatr* 1997;18:102–106.
66. Manners P. Are growing pains a myth? *Aust Fam Physician* 1999;28:124–127.
67. Peterson H. Growing pains. *Pediatr Clin North Am* 1986;33:1365–1372.
68. MacArthur C, Wright JG, Srivastava R, et al. Variability in physicians' reported ordering and perceived reassurance value of diagnostic tests in children with 'growing pains'. *Arch Pediatr Adolesc Med* 1996;150:1072–1076.
69. Baxter MP, Dulberg C. "Growing pains" in childhood—a proposal for treatment. *J Pediatr Orthop* 1988;8: 402–406.
70. Menahem S. Understanding the management of the child with pain. *Med J Aust* 1983;1:579–582.
71. Walters AS, Picchietti DL, Ehrenberg BL, et al. Restless legs syndrome in childhood and adolescence. *Pediatr Neurol* 1994;11:241–245.
72. Buskila D, Press J, Gedalia A, et al. Assessment of nonarticular tenderness and prevalence of fibromyalgia in children. *J Rheumatol* 1993;20:368–370.
73. Schanberg LE, Keefe FJ, Lefebvre JC, et al. Pain coping strategies in children with juvenile primary fibromyalgia syndrome: correlation with pain, physical function, and psychological distress. *Arthritis Care Res* 1996;9: 89–96.
74. Simms R. Fibromyalgia syndrome: current concepts in pathophysiology, clinical features and management. *Arthritis Care Res* 1996;9:315–328.
75. Granges G, Littlejohn GO. Pressure pain threshold in pain-free subjects, in patients with chronic regional pain syndromes, and in patients with fibromyalgia syndrome. *Arthritis Rheum* 1993;36:642–646.
76. Sherry DD, McGuire T, Mellins E, et al. Psychosomatic musculoskeletal pain in childhood: clinical and psychological analyses of 100 children. *Pediatrics* 1991;88: 1093–1099.
77. Winfield J. Pain in fibromyalgia. *Rheum Dis Clin North Am* 1999;25:55–79.
78. Granges G, Zilko P, Littlejohn GO. Fibromyalgia syndrome: assessment of the severity of the condition two years after diagnosis. *J Rheumatol* 1994;21:523–529.
79. Ledingham J, Doherty S, Doherty M. Primary fibromyalgia syndrome—an outcome study. *Br J Rheumatol* 1993;32:139–142.
80. Rabinovich CE, Schanberg LE, Stein LD, et al. A follow up study of pediatric fibromyalgia patients. *Arthritis Rheum* 1990;33s:146.
81. Vandvik IH, Forseth KO. A bio-psychosocial evaluation of ten adolescents with fibromyalgia. *Acta Paediatr* 1994;83:766–771.
82. Thompson RJ, Gustafson KE, Gil KM. Psychological adjustment of adolescents with cystic fibrosis or sickle cell disease and their mothers. In: Wallander J, Siegel L, eds. *Advances in pediatric psychology: II. Behavioral perspectives on adolescent health*. New York: Guilford Press, 1995.
83. Goldenberg DL, Felson D, Dinerman H. A randomized, controlled trial of amitriptyline and naproxen in the treatment of fibromyalgia. *Arthritis Rheum* 1986;29: 1371–1377.
84. Leventhal L. Management of fibromyalgia. *Ann Intern Med* 1999;131:850–858.
85. Kimura Y. Fibromyalgia syndrome in children and adolescents. *J Musculo Med* 2000;17:142–158.
86. Sandstrom MJ, Keefe FJ. Self-management of fibromyalgia: the role of formal coping skills training and physical exercise training programs. *Arthritis Care Res* 1999;11:432–447.
87. Walco GA, Ilowite NT. Cognitive-behavioral intervention for juvenile primary fibromyalgia syndrome. *J Rheumatol* 1992;19:1617–1619.
88. Rossy LA, Buckelew SP, Dorr N, et al. A meta-analysis of fibromyalgia treatment interventions. *Ann Behav Med* 1999;21:180–191.
89. Sherry DD. Musculoskeletal pain in children. *Curr Opin Rheumatol* 1997;9:465–470.
90. Berman BM, Swyers JP. Complementary medicine treatments for fibromyalgia syndrome. *Baillieres Best Pract Res Clin Rheumatol* 1999;13:487–492.

33

Pain and Children with Developmental Disabilities

Tim F. Oberlander and Kenneth D. Craig

Pain is a frequent finding in children with developmental disabilities, yet its presentation can be confusing because it is frequently confounded by the child's functional disabilities and the underlying neurologic condition. When the expression of pain is ambiguous, decision making becomes highly subjective, and both the assessment and management of pain present tremendous challenges. This also raises many questions about our very understanding of pain itself, and one comes to recognize that there is a substantial lack of knowledge in this field. Measurement issues are of particular importance. The ability to communicate pain and distress is fundamental to seeking and obtaining health care. Regrettably, childhood developmental disabilities are associated with a variety of motor, cognitive, language, and social barriers that limit effective and timely communication of pain and distress. The special needs of these children also often make them highly vulnerable.

Health care professionals have observed and reported altered and blunted pain responses when working with children with developmental delays (1), adolescents with cerebral palsy (CP) (2), adults with mental retardation (3), and the frail elderly with dementia (4,5). To some, these findings suggest that neurologic impairment is associated with pain indifference or even insensitivity (6). Yet it is unclear how the neurologic impairment associated with the disability changes the neurologic substrate that is required for pain experience. Alternatively, the experience may remain undiminished, but there may be expressive limitations in speech or those motor skills ordinarily used to engage the care from others when hurt. In the absence of easily recognized verbal or motor-dependent forms of communication, it remains uncertain whether the pain experience itself is different or whether only the expressive manifestations are altered. How can pain be assessed and managed when typical means of verbal or nonverbal communication are altered or missing? Despite this confusing picture and the potential for pain to be processed, experienced, and expressed differently, there is no good evidence to date that cognitively or motor-impaired children are spared any of the miseries of pain. In the absence of good measures, it is reasonable to give the benefit of the doubt to the probability that injury, diseases, and procedures that would instigate pain in nondisabled people also create pain in children with disabilities.

Admittedly, congenital insensitivity to pain does exist, but the incidence of true insensitivity is rare (7) and usually not difficult to recognize because these children experience complications of untreated diseases and injuries because they lack the protective functions of pain. In other children, these complications are not present, even though the children consistently fail to display common pain behaviors when injured or ill. Rather than concluding that they are insensitive or experience reduced pain, we should look beyond the diminished pain behavior to understand the pain experience of these children.

A significant neurologic impairment, whether from multifactorial causes (CP), genetic/metabolic disorders (Down syndrome), traumatic brain injury, or disorders of unknown origin, presents complex clinical pain problems that until recently have attracted little systematic study. Given that the term *significant neurologic impairment* (SNI) can be used to describe clinical conditions with diverse causes, anatomic lesions, and functional limitations, a considerable research effort remains. This chapter focuses on pain in children with a variety of developmental disabilities to illustrate the spectrum of cognitive, motor, and communication limitations that are common in varying degrees in children with significant neurologic impairment. We review our current understanding of pain in children with such conditions, the possible impact that significant neurologic impairment may have on a pain experience, sources of chronic and acute pain, and strategies for pain assessment and management. Because this is a relatively new area of investigation, the chapter both examines our current understanding of pain in this setting and attempts to stimulate further discussion and work in the field.

EPIDEMIOLOGY AND FUNCTIONAL IMPACT OF PAIN

Developmental disabilities represent a large proportion of childhood illnesses (Table 33.1), and all are potentially associated with an increased incidence of pain. It has been estimated by the World Health Organization that this broad category represents 15% to 20% of all children (8). Developmental disabilities result from a variety of known acquired, metabolic, and genetic disorders as well as unknown etiologic factors. The prevalence of particular pathophysiologic conditions (estimates of the probability of a person having the disease/condition at a specific time) in this heterogeneous group of conditions varies; however, the destructive, additive effects of pain in the presence of a disability is common to all conditions. At present, there are no satisfactory epidemiologic data regarding the incidence or prevalence of chronic or acute pain in populations of children with disabilities. Estimates must be derived from indirect measures. There is good reason to believe that pain is much more a part of the daily lives of most of these children than is the case for children without disabilities. Children with disabilities certainly suffer from the same sources of pain that afflict the general child population (9). In the domain of acute pain, injuries, childhood diseases, and surgery can be expected. Chronic pain is also commonplace. As many as 30% to 40% of children and adolescents complain of recurrent pain (headaches, abdominal and musculoskeletal pain) occurring at least once a week (10,11). The prevalence of weekly episodes of bad

TABLE 33.1. *Estimated prevalence of developmental disabilities and other chronic conditions of childhood*

Developmental disorder or chronic disease	Cases per 1,000
Attention deficit disorder	100
Speech and language disorder	70
Asthma	29.3
Mental retardation (mild and severe)	20
Cerebral palsy	2
Severe hearing impairment	1.5
Autism	0.4
Visual impairment	0.4
Diabetes mellitus	1
Sickle cell anemia	0.9
Cystic fibrosis	0.3

Adapted from Gortmaker SL, Walker DK, Weitzman M, et al. Chronic conditions, socioeconomic risks, and behavioral problems in children and adolescents. *Pediatrics* 1990;85:267–276, with permission.

stomach pain and back pain has been reported to be 15% to 20% of school-age children (10,12). Migraine headaches range in prevalence from 8% to 11% (13–15) in children, and musculoskeletal pain may occur in more than 30% of children at least once a week (16).

In addition, many childhood disabilities result in painful conditions that require recurrent painful and invasive procedures, resulting in pain during activities of daily living. This is compounded by frequent difficulties in communicating distress and soliciting help to reduce pain and discomfort, which in turn lead to an increased incidence, severity, and duration of pain in children with disabilities. Therefore, even by crude indirect methods estimating the level and extent of pain in children with developmental disabilities, pain must have a higher incidence and prevalence than among children in general and must be considered a serious problem.

Efforts to understand pain in this setting require an evaluation of the functional impact of the pain, its role in the quality of life, and its interaction with the disability itself. Some systematic work characterizing functional disability associated with various childhood disabilities has been accomplished (17–19), and recently Palermo (20) reviewed work characterizing the deleterious impact of pain on child and family functioning.

Studies of childhood pain typically focus on describing pain symptoms, duration, and intensity without accounting for their functional consequences, even though they are likely to have a major impact on child and family well-being, broadly defined. The measurement of functional disability related to adult pain outcomes has received considerable attention because of issues related to work and cost-related effects; however, little analogous work has been done in pediatric populations. Walker and Greene (21) provide four reasons for assessing a child's functional disabilities and, by extension, the impact of pain: (a) to examine impact of disease on a child's everyday function, (b) to investigate the extent to which illness and symptoms create a burden for the family, (c) to describe changes in children's function as a result of treatment interventions, and (d) to study individual differences in function within patient populations.

Several groups have proposed multidimensional approaches to defining the disabling processes. Nagi (17) and Butler and Campbell (19) propose models that combine aspects of the World Health Organization's system of impairment, disability, and handicap. Butler and Campbell called for careful attention to five dimensions: pathophysiology, impairment, functional limitations/activity, disability/participation, and societal limitations/context factors (Table 33.2a). Using this schema, the impact of CP has been described in Table 33.2b. Taking this one step further, Table 33.2c describes the functional consequences of chronic pain in a child with a developmental disability.

A 13-year-old boy with CP, spastic diplegia, mild cognitive impairment, a ventriculoperi-

TABLE 33.2a. *National Center for Medical Rehabilitation Research model of disablement: five dimensions of human functioning*

Dimension	Description
Pathophysiology	Interruption or interference of normal physiology and developmental processes or structures
Impairment	Loss or abnormality of body structure or body function
Functional limitation	Restriction of ability to perform activities
Disability	Inability to participate in typical societal role functions
Societal limitation	Barriers to full participation in society that result from attitudes, architectural barriers, and social policies

Adapted from Butler C, Campbell S, AACPDM Treatment Outcomes Panel. Evidence for the effects of intrathecal baclofen for spastic and dystonic cerebral palsy. *Dev Med Child Neurol* 2000;42:634–645.

TABLE 33.2b. *Examples of selected effects of cerebral palsy on dimensions of human functioning*

Dimension	Examples
Pathophysiology	Cystic lesions and white matter loss as a result of periventricular leukomalacia of the premature infant's brain
Impairment	Spasticity, contractures, low endurance, perceptual dysfunction
Functional limitation	Awkward walking with fatigue, difficulty dressing, poor concentration and sustained listening, reading problems
Disability	Learning delays, education in restricted environment, limited sports participation, interference with dating and sexuality, not able to take communion at church, cannot participate in family activity by doing chores at home, unable to achieve independent living
Societal limitation	Exclusion from school/city team sports, denial of medical treatment or equipment by insurer, government action that blocks the building of independent living units for people with disabilities, failure of voters to support funding of wheelchair lifts for public buses

toneal shunt for hydrocephalus and recurrent headaches describes his headaches as throbbing, ever present, and "very big," and rates the pain as "10 out of 10!" He attends a local secondary school in a modified program; however, because of the pain, he has missed a substantial number of days in school. When his pain is at its worse, the boy remains in a dark room in bed, is unable to care for himself, and becomes highly dependent on his mother. With the pain, he reports feeling "angry" and is described by his mother as prone to shouting and screaming when the pain is present. His sleep is interrupted because of the pain, and his social contact has become limited. He does not feel that his pain is well understood by his family or physicians.

The Butler and Campbell framework can be used to assess the functional impact of pain for this child (Table 33.2c). On one hand, the *pathophysiology* of the disability would be the central lesions (presumably prenatal ischemic neurologic injury), as well as the chronic headaches, which may or may not be related to factors associated with the disease (e.g., hydrocephalus/shunt malfunction or a concurrent migraine disorder). Note that both the disease and pain receive consideration as potentially interrelated but separate pathophysiologic entities. The *impairment* includes the neuromotor impairment (spasticity) and frequency and intensity of the symptom (head pain), regardless of the cause. Compounding this impairment are the cognitive and communication impairments that are a concurrent consequence of the central lesions. The *functional limitations* that follow are a consequence of his motor, cognitive, and communication limitations and the impact that the pain may have on activities of daily living (e.g., sleep, self-care, relationship with his mother, peer relationships). The subject's *disability* is his difficulty in carrying on his life as an adolescent attending school or in age-appropriate social relationships. Finally, the *societal limitations* are those barriers placed by society which limit his participa-

TABLE 33.2c. *Examples of selected effects of pain in a child with cerebral palsy on dimensions of human functioning*

Dimension	Examples
Pathophysiology	Altered pain system function (?neurotransmitters, ?reduced descending inhibition, ?increased excitatory neurochemicals)
Impairment	Technologic assistive devices (gastrointestinal tube, epidural pumps), spasticity, contractures, low endurance, perceptual dysfunction
Functional limitation	Increased incidence of pain-related invasive procedures, awkward walking/seating/communication, difficulty activities of daily living
Disability	Headaches prevent/limit attendance/performance at school
Societal limitation	Exclusion from school, denial of appropriate pain management (i.e., others might assume that individual is not in pain because of difficulty communicating distress)

tion, where, even in a modified classroom setting, his teachers had difficulty understanding, managing, and coping with his pain. The boy may also be denied appropriate and timely pain management because his caregivers may not accept that he experiences pain in the same fashion as nonimpaired youths.

This model of disabling processes has important implications for understanding pain in the child with a developmental disability. It separates the functional consequences of pain and its measurement (frequency, duration, and intensity) from the measurement of functional limitations that might be related to the neurologic condition. It also helps to distinguish between children who experience pain with little or no functional limitations from those who are more severely restricted in function. Although the two may be separate in an etiologic sense, our assessment and management of pain in this setting are invariably influenced by the functional limitations imposed by neurologic impairment. For instance, in the case described, pain assessment and management have to consider his limited capacity to communicate pain and other events. The model also illustrates the potential for an additive effect of chronic pain on the underlying disability and the role of the disability in the family. The model, however, does have its limitations. The development of appropriate measures of the impact of chronic and acute pain in children with disabilities and its additive influence on quality of life remains to be done. Further, there is little room in this model for assessment and delineation of the strengths and resources available to children, yet these often provide a basis for development of comprehensive care programs for these children.

THE CHALLENGE OF DEFINING PAIN

How Do We Define Pain When Typical Expression Is Impaired?

The study of pain in individuals with a disability offers an opportunity to re-examine our understanding of what constitutes the effectively universal but highly personal human experience of pain. In general, pain, or the "afferent component," must be perceived or experienced before any "efferent responses" can be generated, such as self-report or other behavioral changes (22). Feeling pain and reporting pain are often parallel and closely related phenomena, but they cannot be considered equivalent (23).

Self-report, nonverbal expression, and evidence of tissue damage may be highly discordant (24,25), suggesting that differences between the perception and expression of pain depend on the environmental and biologic (i.e., an individual's neurologic condition) context in which it occurs. The potential for dissociation between pain experience and the various signs of its presence make understanding the nature of the subjective experience even more difficult.

Although all people share basic aspects of the pain experience, there also are dramatic variations, which almost invariably give pain a unique character for the individual person. The shared features are well described by the definition of pain by the International Association for the Study of Pain, which states that it is "an unpleasant sensory and emotional experience associated with actual or potential tissue damage, or described in terms of such damage" (26). Characterization of the experience of pain as an unpleasant sensory and emotional experience with actual or potential tissue damage appears to be applicable to people with and without neurologic impairment. However, emphasis in this definition on self-report presumes a capacity for effective verbal communication of this highly personal, subjective experience. In an editorial, Anand and Craig (27) point out that this characterization of pain does not adequately provide for pain experience in preverbal infants or nonverbal elderly adults. Signals of acute distress in these and other individuals with communication limitations may be discounted or ignored because of a lack of a capacity for self-report, and, as a consequence, pain may remain poorly treated (28,29). (See also the Addendum on page 616.)

All features of the behavioral response to pain need to be accepted as evidence of its presence. None should be discounted as a "surrogate measure" of pain (22). Whatever the behavioral and physiologic repertoire that is available to the individual, including those with a developmental disability, the expression should be seen as sufficient to index pain. Current standards of practice, care guidelines, and accreditation standards mandate continuous monitoring of pain. For example, the Joint Commission on Accreditation of Healthcare Organizations in the United States has issued standards requiring explicit pain assessment in hospitals, ambulatory care facilities, health care networks, home care, and long-term care organizations (30). The American Pain Society has vigorously campaigned to have pain included in routine chart assessments as the "fifth vital sign" to denote its importance for the psychologic well-being of the individual. It behooves clinicians and others responsible for individuals with communication impairment to specify for the individual the evidence of pain that they consider clinically significant and warranting intervention (Joint Commission on Accreditation of Healthcare Organizations standards). In this setting, an individual's response to a noxious event needs to be considered the pain measure, irrespective of whether they can complain.

It is also asserted in the International Association for the Study of Pain definition of pain that the experience of pain is dependent on previous experience (26). The presence of nociceptive, biologic systems and vigorous, specific reactions to tissue insult from birth (31,32) indicate that the perception of pain is inherent to all organisms with a nervous system and therefore the capability for pain perception should not be construed as dependent on previous painful experience (27). Pain is a primordial and fundamental sensory system that guards the organism against damage from its external or internal environment. There is no reason to believe that the first experience of tissue injury is any less painful than subsequent experiences, although the interpretation and meaning of these events will transform during maturation and reflect the impact of contextual factors associated with the individual's cumulative history of pain experiences. Just as Anand and Craig (27) have argued this case for preverbal infants, this applies equally to nonverbal children. Neurologic damage, however, may be associated with functional impairment in learning skills, the capacity to cognize experience, and memory in varying degrees. It is in the domain of understanding the meaning and the capacity to use pain to guard one's safety that there are likely to be qualitative variations in the experience of pain between individuals with and without disabilities. The cognitive capabilities of the individual are likely to be primary determinants of the individual differences that are superimposed on the shared qualities of pain that all people experience.

THE PAIN EXPERIENCE

Children with a developmental disability may have impairment that arises from events during embryogenesis, at delivery, or by a condition that presents itself after delivery, with all these potentially resulting in a wide spectrum of functional disabilities. Regardless of the source of disability, common to them all is the experience of pain in daily life, but the nature of this experience is open to conjecture. Pain experience in this context may be changed by damage or other changes in the neurologic substrates that subserve the pain system, including its sensory, affective, cognitive, and communicative parameters, or as a result of the social and other environmental contexts in which the pain occurs. The available literature on pain in people with significant neurologic impairment mostly has not been helpful, other than to questionably imply insensitivity or indifference, as noted above. Pain has been poorly quantified, studied with methodologically limited techniques, and typically reported in anatomic/surgical terms (33–37) rather than in terms of the complex, phenomenologic experiences of this population.

Fortunately, a body of literature is beginning to emerge using fine-grain measures appropriate to infants (38) and children. First, it is significant that children and adults with disabilities frequently display deficits in typical pain behaviors associated with calls or appeals to others for care and treatment (39). These deficits appear to have led to the belief that children and adults with neurologic impairments have an increased likelihood of pain insensitivity (i.e., a decreased sensory pain experience) or pain indifference (i.e., a decreased emotional response to pain) (40,41). Beliefs that children with SNI who fail to display common pain behaviors experience no or reduced pain put them at risk for substandard health care. There is no evidence substantiating claims that, in the presence of cognitive or communication impairments, there is insensitivity or indifference to pain.

A useful distinction can be made between involuntary, relatively reflexive reactions to pain and the learned skills that people acquire to capture the attention and care available from others. We propose that a condition leading to impaired cognitive functioning would limit acquisition of the complex skills, including the effective use of language, ordinarily deployed to access care from others, but would leave the inherent, unlearned reaction patterns intact. Studies focusing on the latter indicate minimal differences in pain behavior between people subjected to ordinarily painful invasive procedures who have cognitive and communication impairments and those who are not impaired (2,4,42). One exception would be findings that adolescents with profound neurologic impairment were only minimally responsive to immunization injections (2). No detailed studies of pain in this pediatric population with SNI have been reported. It seems likely that there have been failures to address the pain needs of children with SNI as a result of their difficulty with communication, caregivers' misperceptions of the children, and a lack of systematic study of the problem.

Central Neurologic Lesions and the Pain System

Currently, there are no published data establishing a direct link between the damaged neurologic substrate that underlies a developmental disability and an altered pain system (Table 33.3). Further, we have no evidence indicating how abnormal development would alter subsequent growth and function of the pain system. However, study of several related phenomena may lead to an understanding of possible relationships between neurologic lesions and the pain system. Indirect evidence of possible relationships between central lesions and altered pain reactivity comes from emerging research in diverse clinical settings that include degenerative and hypoxic, ischemic injuries.

The relationship between pain and the motor system has been well described (43). The response to pain in an awake individual is frequently an immediate and obvious motor reaction, a biologically inherent and protective necessity. Essential to this reaction pattern is the sensorimotor integration that occurs in the

TABLE 33.3. *Possible relationships between central neurologic lesions, mechanisms, and altered pain states*

Condition	? Location/mechanisms	Pain system function
Stroke/degenerative conditions	Basal ganglia lesion	? Persistent pain state ± pain reactivity
Cerebral palsy	Altered sensory integration/ decreased central downregulation	? Decreased modulation of pain signals
Spinal cord injury	Hypoxia, *N*-methyl-D-aspartate receptor upregulation	? Decrease in pain modulation/ transmission
? Autism/Down syndrome	Altered central serotonin activity	? Altered pain reactivity

basal ganglia (43). The basal ganglia play a role in integration of a variety of sensory/affective/cognitive components of pain and the modulation of nociceptive information. Study of the effects of lesions to the basal ganglia and frontal lobe has implications for understanding interactions between neurologic impairment and pain. Severe neuropathic and persistent central pain states, as well as motor impairment, have been described in case reports of adults with pathologic conditions that involve the basal ganglia, including Huntington disease (44), stroke, and trauma (45,46). Similar lesions in children also may result in altered pain states, yet these remain to be described.

The impact of the neurologic disturbances that affect motor function in CP on the pain system is less clear. In CP, neuronal damage is rarely confined to one anatomic or functional region or neurotransmitter system. Therefore, alterations to the pain experience in individuals with CP may be a result of many interrelated factors that affect sensory, motor (i.e., spasticity) and cognitive/affective components of the pain system. These possibilities require detailed research.

A similar source of research that may yield some understanding of how an acute neurologic injury alters pain signals comes from work investigating pain after a stroke or spinal cord injury (47). Several well-described chronic pain syndromes are associated with spinal cord damage and stroke. These pain conditions may be related to altered neurotransmitter function (e.g., *N*-methyl-D-aspartate, γ-aminobutyric acid, ion changes, peptide release), loss of descending inhibition, excitotoxicity, or anatomic factors. Whether these processes are responsible for complex pain syndromes in children with central lesions at birth or acquired brain injuries remains to be determined. It is noteworthy that the impact of these pathophysiologic processes on the modulation of pain is one of hyperexcitable presence of pain rather than its absence.

A possible link between the neurologic substrate that comprises genetic developmental disabilities, such as phenylketonuria, Down syndrome, or Rett syndrome, and an altered pain system may be the monoamine neurotransmitter serotonin. It has been demonstrated that many genetic disorders associated with cognitive impairment also are associated with altered levels and function of biologic amines (e.g., serotonin) (48–51). Given that these neurochemicals also are involved in the transmission and modulation of pain signals, it is conceivable that an altered capacity to modulate pain is present in these conditions. Although it is unclear whether developmental disabilities are the consequence of genetic or epigenetic phenomena, the possible relationship between altered monoaminergic structure/function, developmental disability, and altered pain systems warrants further investigation.

There has been considerable historic debate about the sensory impairment that may accompany CP. Earlier in the past century, Freud and Osler [quoted in Crothers and Paine (52)] reported that sensation was rarely disturbed in CP. In contrast, research over the past 40 years has closely examined this question and has identified significant numbers of children with spastic and athetoid CP with tactile agnosia (53–56). Using subjective, self-report measures of temperature, pain, and stereognosis, 40% to 50% of children with CP had sensory disturbances (57). How these findings are associated with nociception and their impact on the pain experience in this setting remain unclear, but one cannot categorically reject the proposition that the mechanisms responsible for CP do not also affect pain.

Recent work suggests there may be a reduced cardiac autonomic response to acute pain among frail elderly with dementia (4). Similarly, cardiac autonomic (heart rate) and facial response to acute pain were also blunted in a study of adolescents with SNI during a vaccination procedure (2). Although the relationship between central lesions, autonomic regulation, and an altered pain system remains to be determined, these findings raise fascinating questions about the changes that may accompany neurologic injury that also influence pain reactivity.

Influence of Cognition and Communication

The ability to communicate pain and distress is an integral part of human existence and a necessary component of the assessment and management of pain (58). Children with impaired communication skills are more vulnerable than other children to pain and suffering as a consequence of failure to diagnose underlying diseases and injuries. Gaffney (59,60) and others (61) have described the age-related developmental course that children follow in their understanding of pain and in the use of language to communicate pain/distress during childhood. Typically, a child's understanding of pain progresses from vague, nonspecific terms in the preschool period to abstract concepts of pain causality in adolescence. Similarly, words used to describe pain become increasingly specific, differentiated, and informative with increasing age (59,61). This work highlights the importance of accounting for developmental level when attempting to understand childhood pain. The principle is no less applicable to the child with SNI.

In the presence of SNI, cognitive and language development are frequently disrupted, and typical means of communication are frequently altered or unavailable. Some children with SNI do not have language skills that are recognizable by even familiar communication partners. This difficulty in language/communication, coupled with the multitude of potential pain sources, makes identifying the presence of pain, its source, and a useful treatment extremely challenging. Some children with mild cognitive impairment may be able to use language to report pain intensity (62); however, the overall usefulness of self-report in this population remains uncertain. Similarly, observational assessments may also be problematic because many children with impairment have idiosyncratic behaviors, vocalizations, and facial responses that may be either overinterpreted as pain/distress cues or dismissed as representing other emotional states. Concurrent motor impairments (e.g., coordination disorders, paralysis) may also interfere with assessing pain in this setting. Subtle variations in social skills also appear to contribute to communication deficits. Gilbert et al. (41) observed that preschool-age children with developmental delays responded to everyday sources of pain such as the bumps and bruises encountered in free play with other children. However, they reacted with less intense distress (e.g., they cried less often) and were less likely to display a social response (e.g., seeking the help of nearby adults).

These limitations on the use of standard or typical measures impose a considerable onus on those accepting responsibility for the care of these children to specify in advance the measures that they will use to determine pain in these children. Careful attention to cognitive, motor, motivational, social, and expressive strengths and limitations is needed to ascertain optimal measurement.

Work by McGrath et al. (63) identified pain behavior specific to children with severe physical and cognitive impairments. Although the items generated were not always specific to pain (i.e., they could not distinguish depression or other illness) or were paradoxical indicators of pain reactions, this work provides an empiric basis for the development of valid and reliable pain scales in this population. Some items used by caregivers to determine whether their child was in pain included moaning, crying, eating less, increased sleep, crankiness, irritability, and reduced or increased activity.

Frequently, children unable to use speech rely on nonverbal communication. Various augmentative and alternative communication techniques are available that use picture symbols, eye gaze, vocalizations, signs, and computer technology. Although this approach enhances communication, the lack of pain-related vocabulary/language might significantly limit their ability to effectively express distress. Oberlander et al. (64) found that adolescents with CP who were capable users of augmentative and alternative communication reported that pain was a common occurrence in daily life; however, technical aspects of augmentative and alternative communication use and a limited pain vocabulary reduced their ability to obtain relief when pain was present. Descriptions of pain were long, and considerable effort and patience were required to communicate distress. They were often obliged to use nonspecific words such as "cry" and "upset" to describe pain. Further, the options available for pain treatment were described by the adolescents as consisting of "Tylenol" or the option to "just live with it." These preliminary data suggest that, even with communication through technologically sophisticated devices, functional use of language to obtain timely and appropriate pain relief remained lacking. This is an important area for further research and clinical work.

Environmental and Social Influences

Beyond the alterations to the pain system caused by neurologic injury, and its impact on daily life, the pain experience can also be adversely influenced by the social context in which it occurs. Considerable evidence demonstrates that recognition and management of pain is influenced by the beliefs and attitudes of health care professionals (65–67). Nurse sophistication is often of particular importance as they usually represent the final common pathway for analgesic administration in studies of postoperative pain management in adults (68) and children (69). Incorrect assumptions about the quantity and qualities of pain and risk of addiction have led to the widespread undertreatment of pain in children (70). Over the past decade, the recognition of this process has led to improved pain management across the age spectrum, from the youngest nonverbal neonate to the frail elderly. It is notable that the increasing use of day surgery and early discharge practices shifts the responsibility for pain control to family members and other nonprofessional caretakers who should become as well informed in pain management as sophisticated health care professionals.

There are very few studies of caretakers' understanding of pain in children and adults with significant neurologic impairment or of how these views influence pain management. However, evidence of the impact of caretakers' pain beliefs can be gained from a number of related studies. In a study of caretakers' reports of injury/illness incidents, used as a measure of apparent pain sensitivity, adults with severe mental retardation were seen as more likely to display signs of pain insensitivity or indifference (3). In a study of occupational therapists' knowledge of pain in children, pain was commonly associated with a particular condition such as arthritis, acquired immunodeficiency syndrome, or cancer, already seen as painful, rather than in a nonspecific clinical setting, such as individuals with CP or mental retardation (71). This study of professionals also reported a low level of awareness and use of pain assessment measures or behavioral cues suggestive of pain. In a single study of the understanding of pain among health care professionals working with children with SNI, Oberlander and O'Donnell (72) found that the presence of pain could be easily recognized, but the location was not readily identified. Even experienced caregivers were uncertain that an expression of distress was related to a pain experience, and they had difficulties differentiating pain from other affective states.

SOURCES OF PAIN

Pain arises from many typical and uncommon sources in children with developmental disabilities. Beyond the everyday pain associated with bumps and scrapes of childhood, the consequences of neurologic impairment include an increased number of sources of discomfort that are typical or more common to specific conditions. For example, in CP, these include pain associated with activities of daily living, pain sources related to high tone, and sources associated with invasive procedures.

The activities of daily living for a child with developmental disabilities often are achieved through means other than those available to the nondisabled child. This may be the result of having to cope with coordination disorders or diplegic gaits or of using assistive devices for positioning and mobility (e.g., walkers, seating systems, manual and power wheelchairs) that frequently bring new and different sources of pain. Dislocated hips, pressure sores from skin breakdown, and repetitive-use injuries occur and must be considered in the distressed child. Splinting and casting that are required for the prevention and treatment of contractures can be associated with additional potential pain. For some, eating and swallowing are difficult, and special feeding techniques or enterostomy feeds are required. Although feeding tubes can be very successful for nutritional supplementation, gastric distention, tugging or pulling on the site, or skin breakdown at the tube site are potential causes of pain on an everyday basis. Constipation also can be a common source of discomfort. Even efforts at communication (either verbal or through the use of a mechanical device), although not typically thought of as painful, have been reported by adolescents using such devices as a source of discomfort (72).

Most children with CP experience motor changes with a constellation of positive signs that include increased tone, spasms, increased deep tendon reflexes, and clonus coupled with the negative signs of weakness and loss of dexterity. The challenge for the child, family, and caregiver is to achieve a goal of comfort and maximized performance. Spasticity and spasms can cause significant discomfort through waking and sleeping hours. The management of spasticity can be challenging and includes a combination of physiotherapy, orthopaedic surgery, neurosurgery (selective dorsal rhizotomy), and pharmacologic management.

Individuals with developmental disabilities may undergo more invasive and frequent procedures to manage the consequences of their underlying condition. These are additional sources of acute and everyday pain. In children with CP, high tone/spasticity may be treated through surgical intervention (selective dorsal rhizotomy) or by surgical implantation of an intrathecal baclofen pump. The longer term consequences of high tone, such as contractures or scoliosis, may require aggressive orthopedic treatment or surgery. Pharmacologic management of tone may include intramuscular injection with botulinum toxin, a procedure that may successfully relieve hypertonia but is also associated with pain. The placement of gastric and jejunostomy tubes may be clearly indicated but again may be a source of acute procedural discomfort. Together, neurologic impairment and its management can present impressive sources of acute and ongoing pain.

Pain in this setting is typically thought to be nociceptive in origin; however, after repeated injury or surgery, neuropathic pain may also occur. To the best of our knowledge, there are no documented cases of neuropathic pain in the child with CP; however, anecdotally, individuals have been reported with swelling, redness, and extreme tenderness in the extremities (T. F. Oberlander, personal observation), suggestive of neuropathic pain. Because of the confusing neurologic and clinical picture, identification of the neuropathic pain has been challenging. It is conceivable that neuropathy may be another source of ongoing and poorly treated pain in this setting.

PAIN ASSESSMENT

Effective assessment of pain is an essential step toward establishing a diagnosis, determining treatment efficacy, and relieving pain (see review of pain assessment in children in Chapters 7 and 8). Given that pain assessment in children without disabilities can be subjective and limited by age-specific cognitive and language capacities, there is an even greater challenge in working with children with disabilities. In the past 20 years, several pain assessment scales have been developed that include physiologic, behavioral, and self-report measures (73). These scales have been both unidimensional and multidimensional measures, and several have established psychometric properties and clinical utility. Measures range from cry, facial expression, body movement, and self-report responses to visual analog scale and questionnaires; however, these scales only offer an imprecise guide to possible domains for assessing pain in children with developmental disabilities.

Assessment of pain in children with limited communication skills is challenging for both the child and caregiver (74). A child's limited repertoire of distress signals may become evident during a normally very painful event or be difficult to discriminate from fear, sadness, or even contentment. Until recently, there have been few published works addressing pain assessment of children with developmental disabilities. Emerging reports provide some description of the expression of pain in the case of particular disabilities and provide scales that have face validity, some empiric validity, and perhaps clinical utility. In a case report, Collignon et al. (75) described the difficulty of pain assessment in three children with CP. Giusiano et al. (76) reported on the development of a 22-item scale focusing on observations made during the response to physical examination and thought to be indicative of pain in this setting. McGrath et al. (77) reported on the pain responses observed by parents and caregivers of cognitively and physically impaired children. The account provided illustrates the vast and at times conflicting behaviors that are thought to be pain related in developmentally disabled children. Considerable work must be done before we have valid and reliable tools for pain assessment in children with developmental disabilities.

A 9-year-old boy presented to the pain service 1 year after a severe head injury incurred during a motor vehicle accident. This accident left the boy with significant motor, cognitive, and language impairments, and he became dependent on his family for all aspects of daily care. He is able to communicate only with eye movements, facial grimaces, crying, and gross body movement.

Despite these impairments, the boy had achieved stable health until 1 month before his visit. At that time, his mother noticed an increased frequency and duration of crying, and facial grimacing. This occurred at the same time that his gastric feeding tube was replaced, and he had been treated for a urinary tract infection. There were no associations with other aspects of his daily life. No other signs or symptoms were present. The "pain" behavior was worse in the supine position. The pain was described by his mother as paroxysmal, "crampy," lasting 2 to 3 hours, and worse at night, disturbing his sleep. During the pain episodes, he would cry, grimace, and kick his legs. Nothing seemed to relieve the pain or shorten the episodes. These symptoms led to a prolonged admission to hospital for extensive and sometimes painful investigations of possible neurologic and infectious sources. None was found, and the "pain" behaviors continued.

This case illustrates the confusing and nonspecific presentation of pain in this setting. In the absence of specific pain assessment measures, a comprehensive pain history is essential. This should include an account of known baseline behaviors or physical conditions, known stresses, and an understanding of the typical repertoire of verbal and nonverbal cues used to communicate pain and a variety of affective states. Could a distress/pain behavior be confused with anxiety or even pleasure? How have others responded to these cues in the past? The influence of the caregiver's perceptions, social setting, and the individual's tolerance to change/stress are key to understanding the child's current situation. Together, this background will prevent the clinician from being derailed at the outset by the false assumption: "I can't assess, therefore I'm stuck" (Table 33.4).

The next step would be to choose pain-related markers that make sense to the individual child's disease, disability, and possible

TABLE 33.4. *Factors to consider in assessment of pain in children with a significant neurologic impairment*

Underlying neurologic condition/process
Developmental level
Usual behavioral and health condition: baseline condition
Usual means of communication
Caregivers' views and understanding of what is happening
Role of intercurrent illness
Differential diagnosis: what else is going on?

sources of pain. Understanding how these markers have changed over time and as a result of analgesia can be helpful. Because these measures may reflect pain or other phenomena, one must always consider what else an acute behavioral change could reflect, such as an underlying organic condition or acute concurrent illness. The child's typical means of communication must be considered and used. Sometimes, either a person or mechanism that facilitates communication is inadvertently removed. For example, postoperative distress can be avoided if a laptop computer or hearing aids are not removed to a "safe" place on admission.

It may be necessary to consider novel approaches to assessment. For example, if an individual is not be able to cooperate with sensory testing to assess the level of a local anesthetic block, the pain service physician or nursing staff may have to provide an alternate assessment technique appropriate for the patient. For example, the placement of ice on a patient's skin may elicit a grimace that would permit testing of skin sensation during regional analgesia.

In the absence of widely available and clinically meaningful pain measures for the populations of concern here, our best appreciation of pain should be guided by a variety sources of information over multiple time points. Work is urgently needed to develop useful and reliable pain assessment instruments for use in this setting to improve the subjective impressions currently employed out of necessity. From our experience, the most significant barrier to effective pain management remains the absence of effective pain assessment tools.

PAIN MANAGEMENT

Pain management in these children shares many goals with other pediatric settings (see Chapter 11–13 for review of common pediatric pain management pharmacologic options). Pain management requires objectives that are specific to the child and the current clinical condition and a comprehensive plan that frequently includes combinations of pharmacologic and nonpharmacologic options. In the first instance, pain management needs to focus on identifying the underlying pathology, thereby reducing distress and facilitating a return to baseline function. However, even with all diagnostic avenues explored, a diagnosis may not be possible. Then, careful empiric evaluation of the pain and the exacerbating and mediating factors, clinical judgment, an empiric medication trial, and careful follow-up may be the only available management options. Overall, the success of pain management in this setting requires a clearly identified plan and coordinated communication and decision making between the child, caregivers, and clinicians.

Management of the pain may only relieve the symptom, leaving the functional impairment unaltered. For example, in using an antispasticity agent to improve neuromuscular tone in a child with spastic quadriplegia, the drug may reduce pain and reduce tone; however, reduced tone may in fact lead to diminished fine motor skills, reduced ability to stand and transfer, and apparent loss of muscle strength. This leads to even broader effects of increased distress and decreased independence. It is crucial to recognize that improved pain symptoms do not always mean improved function, and continued evaluation of both the symptom and functional outcomes is an essential component of any pain management intervention (M. O'Donnell, personal communication).

Everyday Pain

As in other pediatric settings, typical medical options such anti-inflammatory drugs (e.g., aspirin, acetaminophen, nonsteroidal anti-inflammatory drugs) and opioids (e.g., codeine) should be considered for everyday pain. Selection of appropriate medications should ideally follow an appreciation of likely pathophysiology of the pain (i.e., acute inflammatory pain may respond to nonsteroidal anti-inflammatory drugs). The World Health Organization analgesic ladder provides a graduated analgesic approach to treating pain with steps ranging from nonopioids to opioids plus adjuvant medications for increasing or persisting pain (78). Medications given on an as-needed basis may be used to optimize treatment, but some form of pain self-report and caretaker judgment is required. The risks of underestimating a child's pain are considerable (79). In this setting, in which assessment is uncertain, as-needed dosing may lead to either under- or overtreatment and therefore should be *avoided*. The route of medication administration should be the least invasive and appropriate for the patient and sources of pain. The oral or gastric tube route is preferable. With the added pain of injections and reduced muscle mass, intramuscular injections should also be avoided. In working up the analgesic ladder, subcutaneous medications delivered via indwelling catheters may be an appropriate way to administer opioids. Transdermal analgesics such as lidocaine-prilocaine cream [EMLA (eutectic mixture of local anesthetics)] or other topical agents should be considered before injections, venipuncture, refills of intrathecal baclofen pumps, and other cutaneous procedures. Silver nitrate and 3% sucralfate in Desitin ointment (37% zinc oxide) can be very effective topical agents for controlling local irritation at gastric tube sites.

In addition to the analgesic ladder, pharmacologic options specific to the underlying condition or source of pain should be considered. Spasticity and spasms may be common sources of pain and should be approached with a treatment plan specific to the pathophysiology of the condition. Treatment of the child or adult with spasticity typically includes physical therapy, orthopedic surgery, neurosurgery, and pharmacologic options. The latter has a number of advantages over surgical treatments. The ability to titrate the dose to clinical effect as well as to reverse the effects if necessary is an important advantage.

Various pharmacologic agents are available for managing spasticity that leads to discomfort. Appropriate knowledge and awareness of the child's condition are essential to effective and successful use of these medications. Many drugs have been reported as having potential antispasticity effects, including diazepam, dantrolene, baclofen (oral and intrathecal), botulinum toxin A, tizanidine, vigabatrin, clonidine, morphine, intrathecal fentanyl, and lidocaine. Of these medications, diazepam, baclofen, dantrolene, and botulinum toxin A have received the most attention in children (80).

Diazepam was one of the earliest antispasticity medications used. Benzodiazepines enhance presynaptic inhibition of primary afferent input in the spinal cord by facilitating or potentiating the effects of γ-aminobutyric acid. The effect is a reduction in the release of excitatory neurotransmitters. There is randomized clinical trial evidence of the efficacy of diazepam on tone in adults (81,82); however, the benefits in children are limited by unwanted side effects (80).

Dantrolene has been available and considered for use in spasticity management since the early 1970s. This drug's action is at the level of the muscle by decreasing calcium influx from the sarcoplasmic reticulum. The reduced calcium flux decreases excitation–contraction coupling and essentially weakens the muscle (83). The adult and pediatric literature suggests that dantrolene may have an effect on spasticity derived at a supraspinal level, but the effect often occurs in the presence of muscle weakening (84–86).

Oral baclofen is a synthetic γ-aminobutyric acid agonist that appears to act at postsynaptic terminals, resulting in a decrease in neuronal activity by increasing potassium conductance (87). Adult (82,88–91) and pediatric (92–95) randomized clinical trials demonstrated a reduction in tone; however, the effect is greater for spasticity of spinal origin with no demonstrated improvement in function. Intrathecal administration of baclofen involves delivery of the drug at minute doses through a subarachnoid catheter via a pump delivery system. There is evidence from double-blind, placebo-controlled, randomized trials that intrathecal baclofen decreases tone (96–99), although changes in functional abilities have not been clearly delineated.

Botulinum toxin A, the neurotoxin produced by *Clostridium botulinum*, has been used therapeutically for a variety of neurologic conditions. It exerts its paralyzing effect on target muscles by preventing the release of acetylcholine from presynaptic axons at motor endplates. The toxin is injected into the muscle, causing paralysis through a reversible chemical denervation, which for some individuals has led to improved tone and gait (100,101).

Although drug management of spasticity may have a role to play in reducing everyday pain associated with CP, the standard treatment remains physical and occupational therapy (102).

Frequently, children and infants with degenerative conditions such as a metabolic/genetic disease or human immunodeficiency virus encephalopathy present with pain behaviors and irritability of an unclear origin that appears to be refractory to typical analgesic or sedative medications. This is a particularly frustrating and unsatisfying situation for the children families and clinicians. Judicious medication trials with anticonvulsants such as gabapentin or carbamazepine may be helpful adjuncts.

Acute Procedural Pain

Acute procedural or postoperative pain management for children with developmental disabilities also is challenging and requires the same imaginative approach used in other settings (Tables 33.5 and 33.6). Simple management strategies may be helpful. At the outset, keeping the usual caregivers at hand may help in assessment and allow differentiation of nonspecific arousal behavior from pain behavior. Similarly, communication and consultation with the usual primary care and subspecialty physicians and other professionals (physical therapist, occupational therapist, speech and language pathologist, child life worker) are helpful in the management of ongoing or preexisting problems. Medications used before surgery, such as anticonvulsant and muscle relaxants, should be continued. Nursing staff involved in managing postoperative pain require ongoing support from the pain management team, and a customized assessment–management protocol should be developed for each child.

Children with developmental disabilities traditionally have not been considered candidates for demand techniques (patient-controlled analgesia) or regional analgesic techniques because of difficulties with motor function and communication. An alternative approach to continuous systemic opioids involves the use of both lay caregiver- and nurse-controlled analgesia. In clinical experience (C. Montgomery, personal communication), demand techniques have been used successfully and safely in selected children with CP. Without the use of a continuous opioid background, the caregiver administers opioid

TABLE 33.5. *Guidelines for pain management*

1. Keep usual caregivers at hand to assist in management.
2. Maintain typical means of communications (e.g., computer, eye gaze device).
3. Maintain typical means of comfort and mobility (e.g., seating system, form board, wheelchair).
4. Use behavioral and nonpharmacologic interventions appropriate to child and pain condition.
5. Medication should be matched to type of pain (e.g., neuropathic, inflammatory, nociceptive).
6. Use analgesic ladder with nonopioid adjuvant medications.
7. Note that improved symptoms are not always associated with improved function.
8. Maintain communication and consultation with usual primary care and subspecialty health care professionals for management of ongoing and preexisting conditions.
9. In the case of surgical procedures, maintain all usual preoperative medications [anticonvulsant and muscle relaxants (e.g., baclofen, diazepam)].
10. Nursing staff who are managing postoperative epidural require significant support from the pain management team and a customized assessment protocol for each case.
11. Consider novel approaches to sensory assessing effect of management strategy.

TABLE 33.6. *Typical analgesics and adjuvant medications for pain management in children with disabilities*

Class	Medication	Indications	Dose	Disadvantages	Advantages
Weak NSAID	Acetaminophen	Nonopiod to coanalgesic	10–15 mg/kg/dose p.o. q4–6h p.r.n. Post Op: 20 mg/kg/dose p.o., q6h or 35 mg/kg p.r. q8h × 48 hr, then reassess, (max 90 mg/kg/day)	Risk of hepatorenal, toxicity, mild analgesic effect	Opioid sparing
NSAIDs	Naproxen	Nonopioid coanalgesic, anti-inflammatory, bony pain	5–7 mg/kg/dose p.o./p.r. q8–12h	GI upset, GI bleeding, platelet dysfunction, risk of hepatorenal toxicity	Oral and rectal formulation, b.i.d. dosing, extensive pediatric experience
NSAIDs	Ketorolac	Nonopioid coanalgesic, anti-inflammatory, bony pain	0.3–0.5 mg/kg/dose q6h i.v. for 48 hr (for short term use only)	GI bleeding, platelet dysfunction, risk of hepatorenal toxicity	Parenteral, may be used i.v.
NSAIDS (COX2 selective)	Rofecoxib	Nonopioid coanalgesic, anti-inflammatory, bony pain	0.5 mg/kg/dose p.o. (max 50 mg/24 hr)	Possible less analgesic efficacy than nonselective NSAIDs	Liquid formulation, decreased risk of platelet dysfunction, GI and renal toxicity
α_2 agonists	Clonidine	Nonopioid coanalgesic	2–4 μg/kg p.o. q4–6h	Sedation, hypotension	Opioid sparing, sedation
Benzodiazepines	Diazepam		0.1–0.8 mg/kg/24 hr p.o. *div* q6–8h	Sedation, respiratory depression, paradoxical agitation	Improved tone, nonopioid adjuvant
GABA agonists	Baclofen	Spasticity of spinal or central origin	5 mg p.o. t.i.d. (increased to 80–120 mg/day)[a] increase slowly to desired clinical effect	Drowsiness, dizziness, nausea, hypotonia, hypotension	Improved tone, nonopioid adjuvant; intrathecal route available
Anticonvulsant	Gabapentin	Neuropathic pain	5 mg/kg/24 hr p.o. qhs initially, then increase to b.i.d. and then increase to t.i.d. and titrate to effect Maintenance: 8–35 mg/kg/24 hr p.o. div t.i.d.[a]	Somnolence, dizziness, fatigue, nystagmus	Sedation, neuropathic pain
Calcium flux agent	Dantrolene	Spasticity of spinal or central origin	0.5 mg/kg/dose p.o. b.i.d., then increase to max 3 mg/kg/dose p.o. b.i.d.–q.i.d. (max 400 mg/24 hr)[a]	Monitor transaminases to detect hepatic injury	Reduces tone by reducing muscle strength

[a]Dose titrated to effects.

p.o., oral; p.r., rectal; NSAIDs, nonsteroidal anti-inflammatory drugs; p.r.n., use as needed; GI, gastrointestinal; b.i.d., twice daily; i.v., intravenous; GABA, γ-aminobutyric acid; qhs, at bedtime; t.i.d., three times daily; q.i.d., four times daily.

Adapted from O'Donnell ME, Armstrong R. Pharmacologic interventions for management of spasticity in cerebral palsy. *MRDO Res Rev* 1997;3:204–211.

boluses, typically morphine 20 μg/kg per bolus as frequently as every 5 minutes at the times when the patient requires analgesia. This allows relatively precise linking of opioid use with times of need such as during dressing and cast changes or before mobilization. This administration should be closely monitored by a team that includes the pain service, attending physicians, and ward nurses. The use of patient-controlled opioid analgesia in combination with regularly scheduled nonopioid coanalgesics can provide effective systemic analgesia and minimize opioid side effects.

The use of epidural analgesia with either an opioid alone or an opioid/local anesthetic combination (e.g., fentanyl, bupivacaine) can provide excellent analgesia without systemic sedation. This technique can successfully provide analgesia during dressing changes and physiotherapy. Postoperative pain management can be confounded by spasticity that frequently follows orthopedic procedures. Adjunctive use of spasmolytic medications, such as benzodiazepines alone or in combination with clonidine, may help break a vicious pain–spasticity cycle. The use of adjunctive medications may also reduce the need for opioid analgesia.

The potential for significant and undesired side effects of many analgesics may limit their use in children with developmental disabilities. Historically, these children have been denied the benefits of systemic opioids for acute pain because of a perceived decreased margin of safety related to reduced pulmonary function. Their limited cognitive and communication capabilities are contributing factors, but medical considerations have been more important because of a greater risk of unwanted side effects. With decreased cardiorespiratory reserve owing to coexisting neuromuscular weakness, scoliosis, delayed gastric emptying, and poor nutrition, usual opioid side effects are frequently less well tolerated. Pulmonary aspiration may be the consequence of postoperative delayed gastric emptying, ileus, and vomiting, aggravated by opioids and already impaired by bulbar reflexes and gastrointestinal motility. Altered airway reflexes and decreased respiratory reserve, limited accuracy of assessment of pain, and the use of concurrent sedatives may put the child at higher risk of respiratory depression when systemic opioids are used. Careful, frequent clinical monitoring of arousal state and respiratory activity are required when opioids are used. For this reason, monitoring with continuous pulse oximetry and appropriate nursing and pain service coverage is recommended. Opioid-induced constipation may also complicate preexisting gastrointestinal problems and add another source of pain. Excessive sedation from systemic opioids or drugs used to treat nausea or pruritus may interfere with communication and appropriate titration of analgesia and reporting of side effects. Increased sedation may prevent early opportunities for seating and mobility, possibly contributing to positioning complications such as pressure sores.

Finally, the treatment of generalized aroused behavior with intravenous opioids, on the assumption that the behavior is all pain related, may result in inappropriate sedation and respiratory depression. When there is persistent arousal behavior in the presence of appropriate pain management, a possible new diagnosis should always be considered. Surgical complications, such as postoperative pneumonia, pressure sores, or compartment syndrome, may also be evolving, particularly in this population that often undergoes orthopedic procedures. Careful, frequent re-examination of these patients and consideration of a broad differential diagnosis are indicated, particularly when pain assessment and treatment of pain may be uncertain.

As with all children, behavioral interventions can be particularly helpful options for managing acute pain. Depending on the child's ability to communicate or responsiveness to external stimulation, distraction and imagery may be a helpful adjunctive therapy. From clinical experience, physical measures such as massage, touch, heat or cold therapy can be considered, although to date there have been no published studies evaluating these measures for this population.

SUMMARY

Regardless of the cause or functional limitations, understanding pain in children with developmental disabilities is an area that requires urgent attention. There is evidence of unnecessary pain and suffering. The pain experience in the child with a developmental disability often is complex and confusing and raises many questions about the very nature of pain itself. Early work in this field suggested that the pain experience of children with developmental disabilities may be blunted. Although neurologic impairment associated with conditions such as CP or genetic disorders such as Down syndrome may alter the neurologic system and hence the ability to comprehend and communicate pain, there is no evidence that this reflects pain insensitivity or indifference. It must be concluded that disabled children suffer the miseries of pain shared by all humans.

There is an emerging body of evidence to support a relationship between the pain system and the motor, sensory, and autonomic systems impaired in children with developmental disabilities. Changes in these systems may have a profound and unique impact on the pain experience, although there is little direct evidence of this to date. Beyond the altered neurologic substrates responsible for disabilities, communication disabilities and social/environmental factors also influence the pain experience. Pain may arise from common activities of daily living, spasticity, procedures, and surgery. In the presence of cognitive and communication impairments, pain assessment can be challenging. Establishing a clear pain history, including baseline information of child-specific patterns of behaviors and ongoing comparative use of this information over time, can provide clinically meaningful measures. Pain management should be directed at the underlying sources of pain, when possible, and include the analgesic ladder for everyday pain, opioids for acute/procedural pain (with or without nonsteroidal anti-inflammatory drug adjuvants), and anticonvulsants and antispasticity medications for high muscle tone. With appropriate monitoring, demand and regional analgesic techniques can provide effective and safe postoperative pain control.

The lack of basic and clinical knowledge in this field continues to challenge clinicians, patients, and families. As work in the field of pain progresses, continued collaborative research is urgently needed to understand the epidemiology, to investigate the neurologic basis for the unique pain experience, and to develop appropriate pain assessment and management strategies for children with developmental disabilities.

ACKNOWLEDGMENT

The authors acknowledge the valuable clinical insights and contributions of Drs. Maureen O'Donnell and Carolyne Montgomery. Dr. Craig's contributions were supported by grants from the Social Sciences and Humanities Research Council of Canada and the Canadian Institutes of Health Research.

ADDENDUM

Since this chapter was written, the International Association for the Study of Pain's (http://www.iasp-pain.org/terms-p.html, 2001) definition of pain now recognizes that "The inability to communicate in no way negates the possibility that an individual is experiencing pain and is in need of appropriate pain-relieving treatment." While this definition acknowledges the needs of the individuals described in this chapter and recognizes the importance of communication limitations in diverse populations, it characterizes these individuals as unable to communicate. In this way, the definition fails to recognize that people who may be impaired in self-report often communicate very effectively if attention is devoted to nonverbal behavior as a source of information.

REFERENCES

1. Gilbert CA, Lilley CM, Craig KD, et al. Postoperative pain expression in preschool children: validation of the

Child Facial Coding System. *Clin J Pain* 2000;15: 192–200.

2. Oberlander TF, Gilbert CA, Chambers CT, et al. Biobehavioral responses to acute pain in adolescents with a significant neurologic impairment. *Clin J Pain* 1999;15:201–209.
3. Biersdorff KK. Incidence of significantly altered pain experience among individuals with developmental disabilities. *Am J Mental Retard* 1994;98:619–631.
4. Porter FL, Malhotra KM, Wolf CM, et al. Dementia and response to pain in the elderly. *Pain* 1996;68: 413–421.
5. Hadjistavropoulos T, LaChapelle DL, MacLeod FK, et al. Measuring movement-exacerbated pain in cognitively impaired frail elders. *Clin J Pain* 2000;16:54–63.
6. Thrush DC. Congenital insensitivity to pain: a clinical, genetic and neurophysiological study of four children form the same family. *Brain* 1973;96:369–386.
7. Yanagida II. Congenital insensitivity and naloxone. *Lancet* 1978;2:520–521.
8. Boyle CA, Decoufle P, Yeargin-Allsopp M. Prevalence and health impact of developmental disabilities in US children. *Pediatrics* 1994;93:399–403.
9. McGrath PJ, Rosmus C, Canfield C, et al. Behaviors caregivers use to determine pain in non-verbal, cognitively impaired individuals. *Dev Med Child Neurol* 1998;40:340–343.
10. Kristjansdottir G. Prevalence of pain combinations and overall pain: a study of headache, stomach pain and back pain among school-children. *Scand J Soc Med* 1997;25:58–63.
11. McGrath PA. *Pain in children: nature, assessment, and treatment*. New York: Guilford Press, 1990.
12. Borge AI, Nordhagen R, Moe B, et al. Prevalence and persistence of stomach ache and headache among children. Follow-up of a cohort of Norwegian children from 4 to 10 years of age. *Acta Paediatr* 1994;83:433–437.
13. Lee LH, Olness KN. Clinical and demographic characteristics of migraine in urban children. *Headache* 1997;37:269–276.
14. Abu-Arefeh I, Russell G. Prevalence of headache and migraine in schoolchildren. *BMJ* 1994;309:765–769.
15. Sillanpaa M. Prevalence of headache in prepuberty. *Headache* 1983;23:10–14.
16. Mikkelsson M, Salminen JJ, Kautiainen H. Non-specific musculoskeletal pain in preadolescents. Prevalence and 1-year persistence. *Pain* 1997;73:29–35.
17. Nagi S. Concepts revisited: implications for prevention. In: Pope A, Taylor A, eds. *Disability in America: toward a national agenda for prevention*. Washington, DC: National Academy Press, 1991:309–327.
18. World Health Organization. *International classification of impairments disabilities and handicaps*. Geneva: World Health Organization, 1980.
19. Butler C, Campbell S. Evidence for the effects of intrathecal baclofen for spastic and dystonic cerebral palsy. AACPDM Treatment Outcomes Committee Review Panel *Dev Med Child Neurol* 2000;42: 634–645.
20. Palermo TM. Impact of recurrent and chronic pain on child and family daily functioning: a critical review of the literature. *J Dev Behav Pediatr* 2000;21:58–69.
21. Walker LS, Greene JW. The functional disability inventory: measuring a neglected dimension of child health status. *J Pediatr Psychol* 1991;16:39–58.
22. Anand KS, Grunau RE, Oberlander TF. Developmental character and long-term consequences of pain in infants and children. *Child Adolesc Psychiatr Clin North Am* 1997;6:703–724.
23. Craig KD. The facial expression of pain: better than a thousand words? *Am Pain Soc J* 1992;1:153–162.
24. Emde RN, Harmon RJ, Metcalf D, et al. Stress and neonatal sleep. *Psychosom Med* 1971;33:491–497.
25. Manne SL, Jacobsen PB, Redd WH. Assessment of acute pediatric pain: do child self-report, parent ratings, and nurse ratings measure the same phenomenon? *Pain* 1992;48:45–52.
26. Merskey H, ed. Classification of chronic pain: descriptions of chronic pain syndromes and definitions of pain terms. *Pain* 1986[Suppl 3]:51.
27. Anand KJS, Craig KD. New perspectives on the definition of pain. *Pain* 1996;67:3–6.
28. Anand KJS, McGrath PJ. An overview of current issues and their historical background. In: Anand KJS, McGrath PJ, eds. *Pain in neonates*. Amsterdam: Elsevier Science, 1993:1–18.
29. Walco GA, Cassidy RC, Schechter NL. Pain, hurt, and harm: the ethics of pain control in infants and children. *N Engl J Med* 1994;331:541–544.
30. Joint Commission on Accreditation of Healthcare Organizations. *Pain assessment and management standards*. Oakbrook Terrace, IL: Joint Commission on Accreditation of Healthcare Organizations, 2000.
31. Grunau RV, Craig KD. Pain expression in neonates: facial action and cry. *Pain* 1987;28:395–410.
32. Anand KJ, Hickey PR. Pain and its effects in the human neonate and fetus. *N Engl J Med* 1987;317: 1321–1329.
33. Root L, Goss JR, Mendes J. The treatment of painful hip in cerebral palsy by total hip replacement or hip arthrodesis. *J Bone Joint Surg Am* 1986;68:590–598.
34. Trainer N, Bowser BL, Dahm L. Obturator nerve block for painful hip in adult cerebral palsy. *Arch Phys Med Rehabil* 1986;67:829–830.
35. Pritchett JW. Treated and untreated unstable hips in severe cerebral palsy. *Dev Med Child Neurol* 1990;32:3–6.
36. Harris MM, Kahana MD, Park TS. Intrathecal morphine for postoperative analgesia in children after selective dorsal root rhizotomy. *Neurosurgery* 1991;28: 519–521.
37. Sparkes ML, Klein AS, Duhaime A-C, et al. Use of epidural morphine for control of postoperative pain in selective dorsal rhizotomy for spasticity. *Pediatr Neurosci* 1989;15:229–232.
38. Blackman JA. Crying in the child with a disability: the special challenge of crying as a signal. In: Barr RG, Hopkins B, Green JA, eds. *Crying a sign and symptom and signal*. London: Cambridge University Press, 2000.
39. Gilbert-MacLeod CA, Craig KD, Rocha EM, et al. Everyday pain responses in children with and without developmental delays. *J Pediatr Psychol* 2000;25: 301–308.
40. Biersdorff KK. Pain insensitivity and indifference: alternative explanations for some medical catastrophes. *Ment Retard* 1991;29:359–362.
41. Gilbert-MacLeod CA, Craig KD, Rocha EM, et al. Everyday pain responses in children with and without developmental delay. *J Pediatr Psychol* 2000;25: 301–308.

42. Hadjistavropoulos T, LaChapelle DL, MacLeod FK, et al. Measuring movement-exacerbated pain in cognitively impaired frail elders. *Clin J Pain* 2000;16:54–63.
43. Chudler EH, Dong WK. The role of the basal ganglia in nociception and pain. *Pain* 1995;60:3–38.
44. Albin RL, Young AB. Somatosensory phenomenal in Huntington's disease. *Mov Disord* 1988;3:343–346.
45. Lee JL, Wang AD. Post-traumatic basal ganglia hemorrhage: analysis of 52 patients with emphasis on the final outcome. *J Trauma* 1991;31:376–380.
46. Yang Y. Pure sensory stroke confirmed by CT scan. *Chin Med J* 1991;104:595–598.
47. Yezierski RP. Pain following spinal cord injury: the clinical problem and experimental studies. *Pain* 1996; 68:185–194.
48. Curtius HC, Niederwieser A, Viscontini M, et al. Serotonin and dopamine synthesis in phenylketonuria. *Adv Exp Med Biol* 1981;133:277–291.
49. Becker LE. Synaptic dysgenesis. *Can J Neurol Sci* 1991;18:170–180.
50. Nielsen JB, Lou HC, Andresen J. Biochemical and clinical effects of tyrosine and tryptophan in the Rett syndrome. *Brain Dev* 1990;12:143–147.
51. Riederer P, Weiser M, Wichart I, et al. Preliminary brain autopsy findings in progredient Rett syndrome. *Am J Med Genet Suppl* 1986;1:305–315.
52. Crothers B, Paine RS. *The natural history of cerebral palsy*. Cambridge, MA: Harvard University Press, 1959.
53. Monfraix C, Tardieu G, Tardieu C. Disturbances of manual perception in children with cerebral palsy. *Cerebr Palsy Bull* 1961;3:544–552.
54. Lesny I. Disturbance of two-point discrimination sensitivity in different forms of cerebral palsy. *Dev Med Child Neurol* 1971;13:330–334.
55. Lesny I, Stehlik A, Tomasek J, et al. Sensory disorders in cerebral palsy: two-point discrimination. *Dev Med Child Neurol* 1993;35:402–405.
56. Yekutiel M, Guttman E. A controlled trial of the retraining of the sensory function of the hand in stroke patients. *J Neurol Neurosurg Psychiatry* 1994;56: 241–244.
57. Tachdjian MO, Minear WL. Sensory disturbances in the hands of children with cerebral palsy. *J Bone Joint Surg Am* 1958;40:85–90.
58. Craig KD. Ontogenetic and cultural influences on the expression of pain in man. In: Kosterlitz HW, Terenius LY, eds. *Pain and society, Dahlem Konferenzen 1980*. Weinheim: Verlag Chemie Gmbh, 1980:37–52.
59. Gaffney A, Dunne EA. Developmental aspects of children's definitions of pain. *Pain* 1986;26:105–117.
60. Gaffney A. How children describe pain: a study of words and analogies used by 5–14- year-olds. In: Dubner R, Gebhart GF, Bond MR, eds. *Proceedings of the Vth World Congress on Pain*. Amsterdam: Elsevier Science, 1988:341–347.
61. Tesler M, Savedra M, Ward JA, et al. Children's language of pain. In: Dubner R, Gebhart GF, Bond MR, eds. *Proceedings of the Vth World Congress on Pain*. Amsterdam: Elsevier Science, 1988:348–352.
62. Fanurik D, Koh JL, Schmitz ML, et al. Children with cognitive impairment: parent report of pain and coping. *J Dev Behav Pediatr* 1999;20:228–234.
63. McGrath PJ, Rosmus C, Canfield C, et al. Behaviors caregivers use to determine pain in non-verbal, cognitively impaired individuals. *Dev Med Child Neurol* 1998;40:340–343.
64. Oberlander TF, Dhanani S, Dupuis J, et al. Description of language available to communicate pain among adolescents and young adults with significant neurologic impairment. In: Jensen T, Turner J, Wiesenfeld-Hallen Z, eds. *Proceedings of the 8th World Congress on Pain*. Seattle: IASP Press, 1997.
65. Watt-Watson JH. Nurses' knowledge of pain issues: a survey. *J Pain Symptom Manage* 1987;2:207–211.
66. Vortherms R, Ryan P, Ward S. Knowledge of, attitudes toward, and barriers to pharmacologic management of cancer pain in a statewide random sample of nurses. *Res Nurs Health* 1992;15:459–466.
67. Schechter NL. The undertreatment of pain in children: an overview. *Pediatr Clin North Am* 1989;36:781–794.
68. Cohen FL. Postsurgical pain relief: patients' status and nurses' medication choices. *Pain* 1980;9:165–174.
69. Mather L, Mackie J. The incidence of postoperative pain in children. *Pain* 1983;15:271–282.
70. Gadish HS, Gonzalez J. Factors affecting nurses' decisions to medicate pediatric postoperative patients in pain. First International Symposium on Pediatric Pain, Seattle, 1988.
71. Turnquist KM, Engel JM. Occupational therapists' experiences and knowledge of pain in children. *Phys Occup Ther Pediatr* 1994;14:35–51.
72. Oberlander TF, O'Donnell ME. Beliefs about pain among professionals working with children with significant neurologic impairment. *Dev Med Child Neurol* 2001;43:138–140.
73. Finley GA, McGrath PA, eds. *Measurement of pain in infants and children: progress in pain research and management, volume 10*. Seattle: IASP Press, 1998.
74. Hadjistavropoulos T, von Baeyer C, Craig KD. Pain assessment in persons with limited ability to communicate. In: Turk DC, Melzack R, eds. *Handbook of pain assessment*, 2nd ed. New York: Guilford, 2001.
75. Collignon P, Guisiano B, Porsmoguer E, et al. Difficultés du diagnostic de la douleur chez l'enfant polyhandicapé. *Ann Pediatrie (Paris)* 1995;42:123–126.
76. Giusiano B, Jimeno MT, Collignon P, et al. Utilization of neural network in the elaboration of an evaluation scale for pain in cerebral palsy. *Methods Inf Med* 1995; 34:498–502.
77. McGrath PJ, Rosmus C, Canfield C, et al. Behaviors caregivers use to determine pain in non-verbal, cognitively impaired individuals. *Dev Med Child Neurol* 1998;40:340–343.
78. World Health Organization. *Cancer pain relief and palliative care: technical report series 804*. Geneva: World Health Organization, 1990.
79. Chambers CT, Reid GJ, Craig KD, et al. Agreement between child and parent reports of pain. *Clin J Pain* 1999;14:336–342.
80. O'Donnell ME, Armstrong R. Pharmacologic interventions for management of spasticity in cerebral palsy. *MRDD Res Rev* 1997;3:204–211.
81. Cook JB, Nathan PW. On the side of action of diazepam in spasticity in man. *J Neurol Sci* 1967;5:33–37.
82. Young RR, Delwaide PJ. Drug therapy: spasticity. *N Engl J Med* 1981;304:96–99.
83. Pinder RM, Brogden RN, Speight TM, et al. Dantrolene sodium: a review of its pharmacologic properties and therapeutic efficacy in spasticity. *Drugs* 1977;13:3–23.

84. Denhoff E, Feldman S, Smith MG, et al. Treatment of spastic cerebral-palsied children with sodium dantrolene. *Dev Med Child Neurol* 19775;17:736–742.
85. Haslam RHA, Walcher JR, Lietman PS, et al. Dantrolene sodium in children with cerebral palsy. *Arch Phys Med Rehabil* 1974;55:384–388.
86. Katrak PH, Cole AMD, Poulos CJ, et al. Objective assessment of spasticity, strength and function with early detection of dantrolene sodium after cerebrovascular accident: a randomized double-blind study. *Arch Phys Med Rehabil* 1992;73:4–9.
87. Zieglgansberger W, Howe JR, Sutor B. The neuropharmacology of baclofen. In: Muller H, Zierski J, Penn RD, eds. *Local spinal therapy of spasticity*. Berlin: Springer, 1988.
88. Hudgson P, Weightman D. Baclofen in the treatment of spasticity. *BMJ* 1971;4:15–17.
89. Duncan GW, Shahani BT, Young RR. An evaluation of baclofen treatment for certain symptoms in patients with spinal cord lesions: a double-blind crossover study. *Neurology* 1976;26:441–446.
90. Whyte J, Robinson KM. Pharmacological management. In: Glenn MB, Whyte J, eds. *The practical management of spasticity in children and adults*. Philadelphia: Lea & Febiger, 1990.
91. Hattab JR. Review of European clinical trials with baclofen. In: Feldman RG, Young RR, Koella WP, eds. *Spasticity: disordered motor control*. Chicago: Yearbook Medical Publishers, 1980.
92. Schwartzman JS, Tilberz GP, Kogler E, et al. Effects of Lioresal in cerebral palsy. *Folia Med (Cracov)* 1976;72: 297–302.
93. Calia RG, Santomauro E, Traldi S. The use of baclofen in children with cerebral palsy. *Folia Med (Cracov)* 1976;73:199–202.
94. Milla PJ, Jackson ADM. A controlled trial of baclofen in children with cerebral palsy. *J Int Med Res* 1977;5: 398–404.
95. Ebbutt AF, Jukes AM. United Kingdom therapeutic trial of Lioresal in the treatment of spasticity of cerebral origin. In: *Baclofen: spasticity and cerebral pathology*. Cambridge: Cambridge Medical Publications, 1978:109–115.
96. Coffee RJ, Cahil D, Steers W, et al. Intrathecal baclofen for intractable spasticity of spinal origin: results of a long-term multi-center study. *J Neurosurg* 1993; 78:226–232.
97. Hugenholtz H, Nelson RF, Dehoux E, et al. Intrathecal baclofen for intractable spinal spasticity: a double-blind cross-over comparison with placebo in 6 patients. *Can J Neurol Sci* 1992;19:188–195.
98. Penn RD. Intrathecal baclofen for spasticity of spinal origin: seven years of experience. *J Neurosurg* 1992; 77:236–240.
99. Albright AL, Cervi A, Singletary J. Intrathecal baclofen for spasticity in cerebral palsy. *JAMA* 1991;265: 1418–1422.
100. Koman LA, Mooney JF, Smith B, et al. Management of cerebral palsy with botulinum A toxin: preliminary investigation. *J Pediatr Orthop* 1994;13:489–495.
101. Cosgrove AP, Corry IS, Graham HK. Botulinum toxin in the management of the lower limb in cerebral palsy. *Dev Med Child Neurol* 1994;36:386–396.
102. O'Donnell ME, Armstrong R. Pharmacologic interventions for management of spasticity in cerebral palsy. *MRDD Res Rev* 1997;3:204–211.
103. Gortmaker SL, Walker DK, Weitzman M, et al. Chronic conditions, socioeconomic risks, and behavioral problems in children and adolescents. *Pediatrics* 1990;85:267–276.

34
Neuropathic Pain in Children

Charles B. Berde, Alyssa A. Lebel, and Gunnar Olsson

Neuropathic pain conditions are those associated with injury, dysfunction, or altered excitability of portions of the peripheral, central, or autonomic nervous system (1). Implied in this definition is that the painful sensation is not nociceptive, i.e., pain persists independent of ongoing tissue injury or inflammation. In this chapter, we review (a) biologic bases of persistent neuropathic pain, (b) clinical diagnostic evaluation of patients with neuropathic pain, (c) general approaches to treatment, (d) epidemiology, and (e) clinical features of common neuropathic pain conditions in childhood.

Nociceptive pain refers to pain associated with acute tissue injury or acute inflammation. Nociceptive pain is an expected result of tissue injury. It is associated with normal neural transmission, is well localized, and usually resolves with healing. Conversely, when the somatosensory system is damaged, sensory loss, a negative symptom, may be accompanied by unexpected positive sensations, felt as mild or excruciating pain. If the generator of pain remains obscure and untreated, pain becomes chronic and intractable, often resistant to medical and interventional therapies. Chronic nociceptive stimulation of the peripheral and central nervous systems, as occurs with infection, arthritis, and chemical irritation of peripheral tissues, may also ultimately produce sustained pain and altered excitability in the peripheral and central nervous systems with some features in common with neuropathic injury.

Common clinical characteristics of neuropathic pain disorders are summarized in Table 34.1. Nociceptive pain typically improves steadily after injury, whereas neuropathic pain may persist or even intensify over periods of weeks, months, or even years.

The clinical sensory features of neuropathic pain are cutaneous hypesthesia; hyperalgesia (lowered sensory threshold) to noxious, thermal, and mechanical stimuli; allodynia (a normally nonnoxious stimulus, such as light touch, produces pain); and hyperpathia (summation of stimuli ultimately reduce threshold and intensify response). Associated features are neurogenic inflammation, autonomic dysregulation, and motor phenomena, such as dystonia and weakness.

Failure to understand that neuropathic pain may persist despite healing of a site of surgery or trauma has commonly led unsophisticated clinicians to falsely diagnose malingering or somatoform disorders.

Nociceptive pains are often protective in the sense that they may protect the subject from further damage to tissues. In the absence of nociceptive sensation, patients might walk too soon after a fracture or a sprain, for ex-

TABLE 34.1. *Common features of neuropathic pain conditions*

Pain descriptors
Burning, electrical, stabbing, shooting
Spontaneous and evoked
Sensory disturbances
Allodynia, hyperpathia/hyperalgesia
Dysesthesia, paresthesia
Focal sensory deficits in some or all modalities
Hypersensitivity to cold
Motor findings
Spasms, dystonia, tremor
Fasciculations, weakness, atrophy
Autonomic disturbances
Cyanosis, erythema, mottling
Increased sweating, swelling
Poor capillary refill

ample. In contrast, neuropathic pain rarely serves to keep the subject from harm because it involves erroneous generation and transmission of information. Because the pain is just as "real" as the pain of fractures and sprains, it is a challenge to clinicians to convince patients and their parents that it is generally not injurious to move or bear weight on an extremity with neuropathic pain because of this difference between protective and nonprotective pain. Educational materials used in our clinic are provided in the Appendix.

MECHANISMS

The mechanisms that generate or perpetuate neuropathic pain are varied and complex. Injuries to peripheral nerves may involve crush, transection, compression, demyelination, axonal degeneration, inflammation, ischemia, or a variety of other processes. (For a detailed discussion of the pathophysiology of damaged nerve, see reference 2.) The loci of increased excitability after peripheral nerve transection, for example, may include several levels in the nervous system, including axon sprouts or neuroma at the cut end of the nerve, the dorsal root ganglion cell bodies, cell bodies in the spinal dorsal horn, or a variety of more rostral cites in the central nervous system.

The pathophysiologic mechanisms associated with chronic inflammatory (nociceptive) and neuropathic pain are now being elucidated through basic science at a molecular level. This new understanding is just starting to produce novel clinical therapies, targeting cloned ion channel proteins, neurotrophins (3) and their receptor sites, cytokines and other inflammatory mediators of hyperalgesia (4), and specific opioid receptor subtypes.

Central sensitization is the pathophysiologic hallmark of neuropathic pain. It is defined by a variety of nociceptive mechanisms involving molecules, receptors, and neural networks that produce neuronal plasticity, a neuronal reorganization within the central nervous system after peripheral tissue damage or nerve injury (5).

Central sensitization is primarily initiated by sustained C-fiber discharge projecting to the superficial layers of the dorsal horn. These nociceptive fibers produce slow excitatory postsynaptic potentials that, when summated, induce "windup" in central pain projection neurons. C-fiber nociceptor discharge is increased by both inflammatory and neuropathic processes. Soft-tissue injury releases algesic molecules (bradykinins, adenosine triphosphate, hydrogen ions) and induce cytokines and prostanoids. Soft-tissue and neural injury increase local production and retrograde transport of nerve growth factors (tumor necrosis factor α, nerve growth factor, leukemia inhibitory factor), which alter dorsal root ganglion and dorsal horn function and ion channel induction and expression. Other mechanisms that induce central neural changes include ectopic firing of dorsal root ganglion (DRG) cells and neurites, proliferation of DRG satellite cells, phenotypic change of afferent Aβ fibers and DRG cells to facilitate algesia, and changes in gene expression of sodium channels and neuropeptides in the nociceptive terminals and DRG. Within the dorsal horn, sustained C-fiber input decreases the magnesium blockade of the activity-dependent *N*-methyl-D-aspartate receptor in association with increased intracellular calcium influx. Calcium-dependent second messenger cascades perpetuate central pain transmission neuron activity. Aδ-fiber activation depresses analgesic, inhibitory, γ-aminobutyric acid and glycinergic interneurons in lamina II. Structural changes include sprouting of touch fiber afferents into nociceptive fiber territory and sympathetic nerve sprouting around large-diameter touch neurons in the DRG. Most significantly, experimental chronic pain ultimately results in death of inhibitory interneurons of lamina II in the dorsal horn, increasing central pain transmission, and limiting pharmacologic efficacy. Concurrent with central sensitization, gene expression of ion channels and neuropeptides is altered at nociceptive terminals and the DRG. Immediate early genes regulating opioid receptor classes and peptides are also altered. This complex array of pain mechanisms after focal injury, made more complicated after multifocal and variable injury, may explain the comparatively poor success with medication management and regional nerve blockade in chronic pain states (6).

Although central sensitization is commonly associated with persistently increased peripheral afferent activity, particular in C fibers, it is sometimes, but not always, dynamically maintained by ongoing peripheral hyperexcitability (7).

An essential and potent descending analgesic system originates in the midbrain periaqueductal gray (8). This pathway is densely populated with endogenous opioids, opioid receptors, and analgesic biogenic amines (norepinephrine and serotonin). It projects to the rostral ventromedial medulla and spinal dorsal horn. It is modulated by input from the prefrontal and insular cortex, cingulate cortex and amygdala, hypothalamus, reticular formation, and locus ceruleus. The rostral ventromedial medulla has two major neuronal populations, on and off cells, both projecting to laminae I, II, and V of the spinal cord. On cells are inhibited and off cells are activated by morphine (9). Off cells contribute to constitutive descending facilitation of responsiveness to pain. This descending pathway travels through the rostral ventrolateral medulla to the spinal cord and contributes to the seemingly paradoxical morphine-induced hyperalgesia with intrathecal opioid therapy.

Much of the mechanistic study of neuropathic pain has initially focused on peripheral, spinal, and brainstem mechanisms, in part because of the ability to study identified groups of neurons in animal models using electrophysiologic and immunohistochemical techniques. It is apparent, however, that nerve injury also generates plastic changes in higher brain structures (10), including the thalamus and primary sensory cortex, and in a variety of brain regions involved in emotion and attention. Recent work using functional magnetic resonance (11,12), positron emission tomography (13), and magnetic source imaging has documented some of these changes; examples are described below.

DIAGNOSTIC APPROACH

A careful history and physical examination are essential to diagnostic evaluation. Classically, adults with neuropathic pains often describe their pain as "burning," "shooting," or "electrical." Children may provide similar descriptors, but we have been impressed with the variety of descriptors used. The history should include a detailed description of the inciting event or injury when present. Along with a history of the presenting complaint, a broad-based assessment of the impact of the pain on individual and family functioning is important.

Neurologic examination must be thorough and systematic. It is important to establish the overall integrity of neurologic functioning by a complete evaluation of motor, sensory, cerebellar, cranial nerve, reflex, cognitive, and emotional functioning. Although the clinician may regard the causes of pain as obvious from the history, thorough examination is mandatory to avoid missing uncommon but severe conditions, including malignancies and degenerative disorders.

Commonly, evaluation for strength may be limited by pain, and careful and repeated evaluation may be needed to distinguish true deficits from limitations owing to pain. Sensory examination should establish dermatomal deficits and abnormalities in distinct sensory modalities, including light touch, pinprick, temperature sense, and proprioception. The term hyperalgesia is used to mean an increased sensitivity to pain (a left-shifted stimulus–response curve).

Allodynia refers to normally innocuous stimuli such as light stroking of the skin provoking intense pain. Allodynia is an extremely significant clinical sign in supporting the diagnosis of neuropathic pain. Although extreme sensitivity to touch may be associated with conditions that injure the skin directly (e.g., obvious burns), allodynia in the absence of severe skin pathology generally implies disordered sensory processing. Deep-tissue pathology affecting bones, joints, and muscles cannot account for allodynia.

A considerable percentage of children with complex regional pain syndrome (CRPS) (see below) exhibit mechanical allodynia and hyperalgesia to cold in a distribution that crosses peripheral portions of several dermatomes and instead involves a "stocking" or "glove" distribution of the affected limb. In these cases, a nondermatomal distribution does not always imply psychogenic or conversion pain syndromes. Conversely, some patients with truly psychogenic conditions may have distress with light touch.

The sensory examination may be quantified with formal quantitative sensory testing (QST) (14,15). QST measures subjective sensory thresholds to nonpainful and painful stimuli, indicative of small sensory neuronal function, C-, Aδ-, and Aβ-fiber function. Aδ fibers respond to cool stimuli, pinprick, and cool/heat pain. C fibers respond to heat stimuli and cool/heat pain. Aβ fibers respond to vibrotactile stimuli and suggest central sensitization when testing demonstrates mechanical allodynia. QST is indicated when the clinical examination shows slight sensory fiber dysfunction (e.g., numbness, allodynia, hyperalgesia, summation). It is particularly useful in pediatric practice because it is noninvasive and painless, eliminating the need for sedation.

Nerve conduction studies measure the function of myelinated large- and medium-size nerve fibers, abnormal in hereditary sensorimotor neuropathies and severe, nonselective nerve injury but unaffected in small-fiber neuropathy and selective injury. A normal nerve conduction study does not preclude the diagnosis of neuropathy or neuralgia. Sedation may be required for nerve conduction study because of pain or anxiety associated with electrical stimulation. Appropriate choices with minimal effect on baseline nerve conduction include benzodiazepines, nitrous oxide, and barbiturates.

Other diagnostic testing for patients with neuropathy may include laser Doppler fluximetry to assess capillary flow in affected limbs with sympathetic dysfunction (16) and generalized autonomic nervous system evaluation (papillary reflexes, tilt-table testing for orthostasis, cardiac R-R interval variability, gastroesophageal motility, sudomotor function). If the history and examination suggest metabolic or toxic neuropathy, then specific studies may be obtained for toxins (e.g., heavy metals), metabolic abnormalities (e.g., vitamin B_{12} deficiency, thyroid dysfunction, storage diseases), or other biochemical abnormalities.

EPIDEMIOLOGY

The incidence of neuropathic pain in adults is estimated to be between 0.6% and 1.4% (based on a U.S. population of 270 million) and includes, in order of most frequent to least frequent diagnoses: diabetic neuropathy, postherpetic neuralgia, cancer-associated causalgia and reflex sympathetic dystrophy (CRPS types I and II), spinal cord injury, phantom limb pain, multiple sclerosis, stroke, human immunodeficiency virus–associated peripheral nerve disease (Guillain–Barré, lead and other toxic neuropathies, vasculitis), and trigeminal neuralgia. Patients with a neuropathic component of low back pain, such as arachnoiditis, may increase estimates.

A recent review of the epidemiology of chronic pain in children (17) presents the following prevalence data for several chronic or recurrent painful disorders: arthritis, 3 to 460 per 100,000; sickle cell disease, 28 to 120 per 100,000; limb pain, 4.2% to 33.6%; knee pain, 3.9% to 18.5%; recurrent abdominal pain, 6% to 15%; nonmigraine headache, 6.3% to 29%.

In contrast, the incidence and prevalence of neuropathic pain conditions in children and adolescents are unknown: population-based epidemiologic studies are largely unavailable. Several conditions that are common in adults, such as diabetic peripheral neuropathy, trigeminal neuralgia, postherpetic neuralgia, and stroke, are quite rare among children.

At the Pain Clinic at Boston Children's Hospital, painful disorders with a neuropathic component comprise more than 40% of outpatient referrals. Among these patients, the more common neuropathic conditions include posttraumatic and postsurgical peripheral neuropathic pains, CRPS types I and II (see below), and neuropathic pain owing to tumor involvement of the peripheral or central nervous system. Metabolic and toxic neuropathies, neurodegenerative disorders, and pain after central nervous system injury are all seen but with a lower frequency than the previous group of conditions. It is hoped that in the future, large-scale, population-based epidemiologic studies of neuropathic pain will be conducted.

GENERAL CONSIDERATIONS FOR TREATMENT OF NEUROPATHIC PAIN

The management of neuropathic pain may be frustrating for patients and their caregivers. Unlike many forms of nociceptive pain, such as postoperative pain, it is rarely possible to predict high success rates for any single therapy for neuropathic pain. Much of the treatment involves trial and error, titration of medications as limited by side effects, and weighing of risks and benefits. Because of these difficulties, it becomes especially important to develop a solid therapeutic alliance with patients and their parents. Functional rehabilitation with return to school or work and palliation are often the treatment goals because, in many cases, definitive resolution of the pain is not feasible.

Psychologic/Cognitive-Behavioral Treatments for Neuropathic Pain

Many patients with neuropathic pain, in our experience, benefit from relaxation training, biofeedback training, and structured counseling regarding coping strategies and stress management. Supportive individual or family counseling has provided great benefit to many of our patients. School avoidance, depression, alexithymia, anxiety, and family dysfunction are common and require active intervention. The reader is referred to Chapter 17 for more details.

Some patients or their parents may believe that return to school or other normal activities should be delayed until recovery is complete. This belief can amplify or perpetuate a disabled condition. In most cases, it is helpful to encourage continued full participation in school and other activities whenever possible. As noted above, the view of neuropathic pain as nonprotective pain is crucial.

Physical Therapy for Neuropathic Pain

Physical therapy (PT) interventions may be useful for many children with neuropathic pain; these approaches are discussed in detail in Chapter 24. Cutaneous desensitization and transcutaneous electrical nerve stimulation may be symptomatically helpful for patients with allodynia. Aerobic exercise training, strength training, and postural exercises may restore function in patients who have become deconditioned because of their painful condition. PT also appears to have a primary "cycle-breaking" role in patients with CRPS, as outlined below.

Drug Therapy for Neuropathic Pain

Most of the pharmacologic treatment of neuropathic pain in children and adolescents is based on extrapolation from adult studies. In selected conditions, several classes of drugs, including antidepressants, anticonvulsants, local anesthetic–like drugs, and opioids have shown varying degrees of effectiveness in the treatment of a number of neuropathic conditions in adults. More detailed discussion of the pharmacology of several of these drug classes is included in Chapter 13.

Pediatric prescribing for neuropathic pain is largely based on limited case reports or case series. For antidepressants and anticonvulsants, there are more extensive pediatric safety and pharmacokinetic data from clinical trials of their use for treatment of nonpainful conditions such as depression, epilepsy, and enuresis.

For most drugs used in the treatment of neuropathic pain, slow titration is recommended to minimize development of side effects and to detect adverse reaction when they are mild rather than severe. Children and parents need proper anticipatory guidance regarding assessment of central and peripheral side effects and should recognize that a trade-off between moderate analgesia and some side effects is often necessary. A side effect such as sedation may be more or less desirable for an individual patient. For example, the side effect of sedation may be harmful to a patient unable to focus during school but may be helpful to a patient unable to fall asleep at night.

Tricyclic Antidepressants

Tricyclic antidepressants are among the oldest and best established analgesics for a number of neuropathic pain conditions (18) including diabetic neuropathy (19), postherpetic neuralgia (20), and central poststroke pain. Prospective, controlled studies have shown effectiveness both in reducing pain intensity and in improving related measures of well-being (e.g., sleep quality, work attendance, mood) in several neuropathic conditions in adults (18).

Studies in adults have found effectiveness with a range of tricyclic antidepressants that have predominant actions on both serotonin and norepinephrine reuptake (21,22). In most cases, our preference is to start first with nortriptyline because of a suggestion of slightly less bothersome anticholinergic side effects than with amitriptyline. For selected patients who are oversedated with very small doses of nortriptyline, desipramine may be considered as an alternative. Our general titration schedule for nortriptyline is depicted in Table 34.2. Titration is based on both the patient's analgesic response and on the occurrence of side effects. The dosing scheme listed here refers to ambulatory outpatients. For occasional inpatients with severe neuropathic pain (e.g., from spinal metastases owing to cancer), a more rapid titration scheme may be used.

In a small number of children treated with tricyclic antidepressants (especially desipramine) for depression, behavioral disorders, or enuresis, there have been case reports of sudden death attributed to rhythm disturbances. It has not been established whether these children had an underlying predisposition to arrhythmias, such as abnormal conduction pathways or abnormal excitability, and epidemiologic studies would suggest that the overall risk of sudden death is quite low (23, 24). Before initiating treatment with a tricyclic antidepressant, a careful history should be elicited for suggestive symptoms, such as palpitations or presyncope. It is accepted practice in many centers to obtain an electrocardiogram before initiating a tricyclic antidepressant and again if there is dose escalation to a full antidepressant therapeutic range. The cardiovascular effects of tricyclic antidepressants in therapeutic doses in children are overall fairly mild (25). Tricyclic antidepressants should be used with extreme caution among patients with preexisting rhythm disturbances and patients with cardiomyopathies, including those owing to Adriamycin.

Common side effects of tricyclic antidepressants include sedation, dry mouth, orthostatic hypotension, constipation, urinary retention, and tachycardia. If tricyclics are to be discontinued, tapering over 1 to 2 weeks is recommended to avoid symptoms such as irritability and bothersome vivid dreaming at night owing to rapid eye movement rebound.

Other Antidepressants

In general, data supporting other classes of antidepressants in the treatment of neuropathic pain is much less robust than for tricyclic antidepressants. There have been occasional positive trials for selective serotonin reuptake inhibitors such as paroxetine (26), but negative results have been more common. Nevertheless, they can be considered for trials for individual patients and for treatment of associated depressed mood, anxiety, and sleep disturbance. In general, selective serotonin reuptake inhibitors are preferable to benzodiazepines in the long-term treatment of anxiety. Other agents, such as bupropion, venlafaxine, and nefazodone, have insufficient study to recommend them as first-line analgesics for patients with neuropathic pain. For occasional patients with apparent visceral neuropathic pain owing to motility disorders, selective serotonin reuptake inhibitors or a tetracyclic such as trazodone may be beneficial because these drugs have fewer of the anticholinergic constipating effects of tricyclics.

Anticonvulsants

Anticonvulsants are first-line agents for many forms of neuropathic pain (27). Earlier studies in adults showed some effectiveness of phenytoin, carbamazepine, clonazepam, and valproic acid in clinical trials. In recent years, gabapentin has emerged as the most widely prescribed anticonvulsant for neuropathic pain because of its effectiveness (28,29), a comparatively low side effect profile, and a very low frequency of severe adverse reactions. In particular, gabapentin lacks most of the hematologic, hepatic, dermatologic, immunologic, periodontal, and maxillofacial complications of the older agents listed above. Gabapentin also exhibits beneficial effects on mood and is now commonly used in the treatment of anxiety disorders. As with use of anticonvulsants in treatment of epilepsy, sudden discontinuation should be avoided (30).

Pediatric experience with gabapentin is extensive in its use for epilepsy but is largely confined to case reports or very small case series in the treatment of pain in children (31,32). Dosing of gabapentin must be individualized. Recommendations vary widely for a titration scheme. Our practice is listed in Table 34.2.

Gabapentin is generally well tolerated. Occasional patients report a wide range of mood or behavioral changes.

Carbamazepine, valproic acid, and clonazepam are also commonly used for management of neuropathic pain in adults. Carbamazepine, valproic acid, and phenytoin all require monitoring for their individual spectra of hematologic, hepatic, pancreatic, or dermatologic (33) toxicities.

Phenytoin and valproic acid have the unique advantage that in the setting of severe neuropathic pain (e.g., a "cancer pain emergency"), one can rapidly (i.e., within 1 to 2 hours) achieve therapeutic effect by an intravenous loading procedure identical to that used for treatment of status epilepticus. There is little experience available with a similar rapid loading procedure for most oral agents such as gabapentin.

Second-Line Anticonvulsants: Pregabalin, Topiramate, and Lamotrigine

Pregabalin, topiramate, and lamotrigine are being used increasingly for adults with neuropathic pain who have not responded to other agents. Pediatric experience is largely confined to the treatment of refractory epilepsy.

TABLE 34.2. Sample dose titration regimen for medications used for neuropathic pain

I. Nortriptyline dose escalation schedule

A. For ambulatory outpatients

	<50 kg	>50 kg
Day 1–4	0.2 mg/kg q.h.s.	10 mg q.h.s.
Day 5–8	0.4 mg/kg q.h.s.	20 mg q.h.s.

Increase as tolerated every 4–6 days until:
1. good analgesia occurs
2. limiting side effects occur, or
3. dosing reaches 1 mg/kg/day (<50 kg) or 50 mg (>50 kg). In condition 3, consider measuring plasma concentration and ECG before further dose escalation. Consider twice-daily dosing (25% in the morning; 75% in the evening).

B. For inpatients or others with severe and uncontrolled pain, for whom a more rapid escalation is needed, begin at 0.2 mg/kg (10 mg for patients >50 kg) and titrate upwards every 1–2 days in steps outlined for ambulatory outpatients listed above.

II. Gabapentin dose escalation schedule

A. For ambulatory outpatients

	<50 kg	>50 kg
Day 1	2 mg/kg q.h.s.	100 mg q.h.s.
Day 2	2 mg/kg b.i.d.	100 mg b.i.d.
Day 3	2 mg/kg t.i.d.	100 mg t.i.d.
Day 4	2 mg/kg a.m. and midday, 4 mg/kg q.h.s.	100 mg a.m. and midday, 200 mg q.h.s.

Continue to increase by 2 mg/kg (<50 kg) or 100 mg (>50 kg) each day, alternating the timing of the increased dose so that at least half of the daily dose is at nighttime.

B. For inpatients or others with severe and uncontrolled pain for whom a more rapid escalation is needed, a similar scheme can be used with threefold larger dose steps for each increment. For example, a 50-kg inpatient with severe neuropathic cancer pain might escalate as follows:

Day 1	300 mg q.h.s.
Day 2	300 mg b.i.d.
Day 3	300 mg t.i.d.
Day 4	300 mg q a.m. and midday, 600 mg q.h.s.

Continue to escalate by 300 mg/day

C. Dose escalation continues until:
1. good analgesia is achieved
2. side effects are experienced
3. a total daily dose of 60 mg/kg is reached

Note that in regimen A, a maximal dose would be reached in 30 days, whereas with regimen B, a maximal dose is achieved in 10 days.

q.h.s., every night; b.i.d., twice daily; t.i.d., three times daily.

The mechanisms of these agents overlap and involve voltage-gated ion channels, glutamate release, *N*-methyl-D-aspartate receptors, γ-aminobutyric acid receptors, and glycine receptors. Second-generation agents have a more significant effect on amino-3-hydroxy-5-methyl-4-isoxazoleproprionic acid subtype glutamate and *N*-methyl-D-aspartate receptors.

Lamotrigine limits repetitive firing of sodium channels and inhibits neurotransmitter release (glutamate, aspartate, γ-aminobutyric acid, and acetylcholine). The therapeutic range is 300 to 500 mg per day. It has minimal drug interactions but a potentially serious side effect: Stevens–Johnson reaction. This adverse effect is most likely in patients younger than 6 years of age, on multiple antiepileptic drugs, with developmental delay and a history of hypersensitivity.

Topiramate inhibits voltage-gated sodium and calcium channels, amino-3-hydroxy-5-methyl-4-isoxazoleproprionic acid subtype glutamate receptors, and carbonic anhydrase. The therapeutic dose range is 50 to 400 mg per day. Adverse reactions include dizziness, somnolence, mild cognitive impairment (including confusion and difficulty with word finding), and renal calculi. Weight loss is a potential side effect, although this side effect is used for therapeutic benefit in patients with neurologic or psychologic disorders who are significantly overweight.

Local Anesthetic–Like Drugs

Lidocaine and its oral analogs, including mexiletine, have some evidence for effectiveness for several types of neuropathic pain (34). In many centers, an intravenous lidocaine infusion (35) is used to predict response to either oral mexiletine or to chronic subcutaneous (36) lidocaine infusion. The predictive value of the lidocaine test is imperfect. Several initial case series described fairly rapid infusion of large doses that were likely to have transiently produced plasma concentrations greater than 5 to 10 μg/mL. A positive analgesic response, in our opinion, is much more specific and predictive of future effectiveness if analgesia can be achieved either by a brief infusion of 2 mg/kg over 20 minutes or by a targeted, computer-controlled infusion set to achieve plasma concentrations of 2 to 4 μg/mL. Mexiletine dosing is very commonly limited by the occurrence of gastrointestinal side effects (37). Lidocaine infusions are used most commonly in our practice for inpatients with refractory pains owing to cancer (36).

Opioids

The effectiveness of opioids for neuropathic pain has been a subject of considerable controversy. It was common clinical teaching that opioids were ineffective for neuropathic pain. This view was supported in some degree by a study by Arner et al. (38) using a fixed dose of morphine in patients classified by clinical examination as having nociceptive, neuropathic, or idiopathic pain conditions. Other studies suggest modifying this view and report that a considerable percentage of patients with neuropathic pain owing to cancer (39), phantom limb (40), postherpetic neuralgia (41), and other causes may find good analgesic benefit with tolerable side effects.

Acupuncture and Other Complementary Therapies for Neuropathic Pain

Acupuncture and other complementary therapies are being used with increasing regularity for children as well as adults with neuropathic pain. Readers are referred to Chapters 18, 24, 25, and 26 for detailed discussions of these therapies. The safety of acupuncture appears well established, and children in general exhibit surprisingly little distress over the procedure (42) if it is explained and demonstrated in an appropriate manner. Because of its low risk and low side effect profile, acupuncture can be considered for patients who do not improve with a range of other treatments. Anecdotally, there are clearly patients in our clinic who have found considerable improvement with acupuncture after lack of improvement with several medication trials.

Conversely, the status of evidence for the effectiveness of acupuncture in controlled trials for a range of pain conditions is comparatively weak (43,44). Design of clinical trials for acupuncture is difficult; there is considerable disagreement regarding the best scientific and ethical practices for inclusion of sham, placebo, or untreated control groups. Expectation of benefit has a substantial effect on effectiveness (45). Cost, availability of services, and the requirement for repeated visits can be practical limitations to acupuncture for many patients.

Herbal medications are widely used by children and adults (46). It is important for clinicians to ask patients and their parents about use of these formulations because many have significant interactions with prescribed medications. The status of evidence regarding herbal treatments for pain is weak. Lack of standardization of formulations is an ongoing concern.

NEUROPATHIC PAIN SYNDROMES

Pain After Amputation

Amputation necessarily involves sectioning of major nerve trunks. Patients experience nociceptive pain shortly after the surgery. Nociceptive stump pain may persist owing to a variety of causes, including wound breakdown, superficial or deep-tissue infection, or mechanical pain owing to pressure from a poorly fitting prosthesis. Stump pain may also have neuropathic characteristics, including allodynia, autonomic changes, and dysesthesias. The indications for exploration of a stump and for "burying a neuroma" are controversial.

Phantom phenomena refer to pain and other sensations experienced by the patient as if they are occurring in the missing distal extremity. The term *phantom limb pain* was apparently introduced by S. Weir Mitchell during the American Civil War (47). Phantom limb sensations are variable. The limb may be perceived to be present, often in a foreshortened, plastic, and distorted position. Over time, approximately 1 to 6 months, the sensations may be less anatomic and more transient, kinesthetic, and paresthetic. The phantom may be felt to telescope into the stump and eventually fade away. A subgroup of patients reports persistent itching in the phantom.

Functional magnetic resonance imaging has recently provided a fascinating window into the biologic traces (tissue oxygen consumption ratio of oxyhemoglobin to deoxyhemoglobin) of cortical reorganization underlying these phenomena (11,40,48). Patients with phantom pain show a change in the somatotopic map of the parietal cortex. Cortical regions that previously were activated via stimulation of the missing limb subsequently become activated by stimulation of adjacent body regions. In the case of upper extremity amputation, stimulation of the face may activate parietal cortex previously mapped to the distal upper extremity.

Phantom limb pain, as with phantom sensations, may vary in intensity, localization, frequency, and duration. It is not restricted to limbs, possibly occurring after the removal of any body part. For example, phantom breast sensation is well described after mastectomy. Prevalence estimates in the adult literature vary widely (49), but more recent prospective studies suggest that approximately half of amputees will experience moderate to severe phantom limb pain (50).

Several case series of pediatric amputees have been reported in recent years; these have described some of the clinical characteristics of children with phantom limb pain.

Krane and Heller (51) retrospectively surveyed a cohort of children 5 to 19 years of age who had undergone amputation over a 10-year period. In their series, 100% of patients reported phantom sensations. Although most subjects reported phantom limb pain, fewer than 40% had this documented in the medical record, suggesting that there was underrecognition of the problem by medical and nursing staff. Among those with preoperative pain, 75% experienced phantom limb pain.

Wilkins et al. (52) reported on a retrospective survey of 42 pediatric patients with a missing limb secondary to a congenital deficiency or surgery/trauma reported phantom pain in 29% of the total sample: 3.7% of the congenital group and 48.5% of the surgical group.

Smith and Thompson (53) at the Mayo Clinic retrospectively reviewed 75 pediatric patients with amputations; 67 were cancer related and eight trauma associated. Phantom limb pain was reported in 48% of patients with cancer-related amputations compared with 12% of patients with trauma-associated amputations. "Among patients with cancer, phantom limb pain was experienced by 74% who were exposed to chemotherapy before or at the time of amputation, 44% who received chemotherapy after amputation, and 12% who never received chemotherapy." Patients with trauma-related amputation and those who did not receive chemotherapy reported phantom limb pain at a mean of 6 days after surgery; 76% of patients with cancer and exposure to chemotherapy reported phantom pain within 72 hours after surgery.

Prevention and treatment of phantom pain have received some recent study. Early and active use of a prosthesis appears to reduce the persistence and severity of phantom pain. The benefits appear to be related to use of the prosthesis in functional activities (48), not the mere presence of an artificial appendage because patients who used nonfunctioning prostheses were more likely to experience phantom limb pain (54).

Ramachandran and colleagues (55) described a novel approach to treatment of phantom limb pain in which a vertical mirror is positioned so that movement of the contralateral (intact) limb is seen by the patient as if it were in the expected position of the amputated limb. This approach is fascinating. In view of its safety and simplicity, it should be considered more widely for these patients.

Drug therapy of phantom limb pain has received limited study. Despite the common view that opioids are ineffective, Huse et al. (40) recently reported on a controlled prospective trial of sustained-release oral morphine for adults with phantom limb pain and showed both a significant analgesic response and a significant effect in reversing amputation-induced cortical reorganization, based on magnetic source imaging. A prospective trial by Panerai et al. (22) included patients with phantom limb pain along with other diagnoses collectively labeled as "central pain." This study showed effectiveness of tricyclic antidepressants, especially clomipramine compared with placebo. Case reports and small case series have reported some effectiveness of anticonvulsants, including clonazepam and gabapentin.

Rusy and colleagues (32) treated seven children and adolescents with gabapentin with relief of pain in six of the seven at approximately 1-year follow-up.

Because of the widely reported association of preamputation pain with subsequent phantom limb pain, several investigators have examined whether regional anesthesia via the peripheral perineural, plexus, epidural, or subarachnoid route might reduce the incidence, severity, or persistence of phantom limb pain. Results have been somewhat inconsistent. A series by Bach and co-workers (56) showed a substantial reduction in phantom limb pain at 6 months after intensive pre-, intra-, and postoperative epidural infusions of opioids and local anesthetics (56). Similar results were reported by Jahangiri et al. (57). Subsequent studies have yielded mixed results. Nikolajsen et al. (58,59) compared groups of patients receiving pre-, intra-, and postoperative epidural bupivacaine-morphine infusions with control subjects that received epidural saline pre- and intraoperatively, and epidural bupivacaine-morphine postoperatively. In their studies, there was no difference between groups on QST measures (59) in the stump at 1 week and at 6 months, nor was there a difference in the incidence or severity of stump pain or phantom limb pain (58). A study by Lambert et al. (60) compared epidural analgesia with a perineural infusion of bupivacaine. Postoperative analgesia was significantly better in the epidural group, although there were no differences in the incidence of phantom limb pain at 6 and 12 months.

It remains unclear whether the differences in findings in different studies relate to differences in patient population, duration of infusions, drug selection for infusions, placebo effects that are better controlled in some studies than others, or other factors. It is possible that increased understanding of the essential generators of central hyperexcitability (pre-, intra-, and postoperative factors) will lead to more effective approaches to preemptive or preventive treatments for phantom limb pain and other forms of postsurgical neuropathic pain (61).

Because the immediate pain of amputation can be quite severe, we continue to make use of epidural infusions in our practice, and our practice is to try to achieve very dense degrees of afferent blockade before the onset of surgery.

Plexus Injuries and Other Plexopathies

Adults who have major stretch or avulsion injuries of the brachial plexus frequently experience prolonged neuropathic pain that may be difficult to treat. Traumatic plexopathies may occur in adolescents after motorcycle or bicycle accidents. Additional deafferentation syndromes resulting in central pain include spinal cord injury (congenital and posttraumatic) and nerve root avulsion.

Brachial plexus injury at the time of delivery owing to shoulder dystocia is not uncommon in obstetric practice. A large epidemiologic study from Sweden reports an incidence of 4.6 per 1,000 livebirths (62). Neonatal brachial plexus traction injury presents with a variable spectrum of motor and sensory deficits. Most infants show spontaneous recovery of function over the first 6 months of life, with no apparent signs of distress or guarding with touch or limb movement suggestive of neuropathic pain. A subgroup of infants, probably less than 5%, appear to experience guarding or distress with touch or movement of the limb. In rare cases, infants may manifest self-injurious behavior, such as biting their insensate hand. This may be a possible human correlate of autotomy, the self-mutilating behavior observed in animals after partial and focal nerve injury.

Fortunately, the neonatal presentation is rarely complicated by pain (63), but limitations of pain assessment in this population may falsely reassure investigators. A study from Riyadh reviewed 127 consecutive cases of obstetric brachial plexus injury and found six cases (4.7%) with clinical evidence of self-mutilation (64).

McCann and colleagues in our group (manuscript in preparation) recently reviewed the medical records of 281 infants and young children with neonatal brachial plexus injury cared for in our center in Boston by orthopedic surgeons and neurosurgeons with a specialized interest in pediatric reconstructive surgery. Seven cases were identified with evidence for self-mutilation and, in some cases, distress with touch or PT. Interestingly, in six of seven cases, self-mutilation began only after surgical reconstructive procedures, which involved a diverse spectrum of nerve dissection, sural nerve grafting, shoulder joint release, tendon transfer, and osteotomy procedures.

Painful plexus injury associated with trauma and malignancy is anecdotally recognized in children, increasingly with the use of directed neurologic examination and QST.

Neuropathic Pain in Childhood Cancer

Neuropathic pain may result from tumor itself as well as from aspects of tumor therapy. Primary central nervous system tumors, particularly of the spinal cord, can produce pain owing to local compression or irritation. Metastases from extramedullary tumors often invade the spine, with involvement of individual roots, plexuses, or cauda equina, or with epidural tumor masses producing spinal cord compression. These patients may have severe pain that resists treatment with extremely large opioid infusion rates, even more than 1,000 mg morphine per hour (65,66). General issues of treatment of cancer pain are discussed in Chapter 29.

The optimal choice of treatments for tumor-related neuropathic pain must be individualized. Tricyclic antidepressants and anticonvulsants should be considered. Opioids should be tried; dosing can be escalated as needed and as limited by side effects (67,68). If opioid dose escalation appears ineffective, consideration should be given to a trial of a second opioid, particularly methadone. Methadone's combined action as a μ opioid agonist and an *N*-methyl-D-aspartate receptor antagonist may render it uniquely effective for some patients with neuropathic cancer pain (69), although calculation of equipotent dosing is complex (70,71); much smaller initial doses should be used than would be predicted from potency ratios derived from opioid-naïve subjects. Corticosteroids such as dexamethasone can be very useful, particularly in short-term use in patients with spinal involvement of tumor; with more prolonged use, adverse effects become more prevalent. Regional anesthetic techniques can provide good analgesia in selected cases involving widespread spinal invasion of tumor. Drug selection and technical issues are described elsewhere (66) and in Chapter 22.

Chemotherapeutic agents, such as vincristine, can produce injury to the peripheral or central nervous system. In the majority of cases, vincristine produces a painless peripheral and autonomic neuropathy with reduced proprioceptive sense, hyporeflexia, and constipation as common features. In a subgroup of patients, however, there are considerable burning or shooting pain and dysesthesia. Tricyclic antidepressants and anticonvulsants have been effective for several patients with these symptoms.

Complex Regional Pain Syndromes (Reflex Sympathetic Dystrophy and Causalgia)

CRPS types I and II refer to conditions in which there is pain in an arm or leg with neuropathic pain and sensory characteristics (e.g., spontaneous and evoked pain, burning, allodynia, hyperalgesia, dysesthesia, paresthesia) along with neurovascular abnormalities, including coldness, mottling, abnormal sweating, poor capillary refill, and nonarticular swelling (Fig. 34.1). CRPS type I/reflex sympathetic dystrophy refers to this constellation of findings in patients with no demonstrable injury to a particular peripheral nerve. CRPS type II/causalgia refers to this group of findings occurring in association with signs and symptoms of partial or complete peripheral nerve injury, with a well-defined area of sensory abnormalities. The terms CRPS-1 and CRPS-2 were developed by a consensus conference with at least a partial aim of relying on clinical features and avoiding presumptions regarding specific mechanisms or treatment responses in diagnosis (72). The diagnostic criteria from this consensus group may have some drawbacks, including relatively poor specificity (73,74), and some clinicians object to the choice of the term CRPS, which they regard as too vague to be helpful.

The term *sympathetically maintained pain* (SMP) became popular in the late 1980s; pain relief by sympathetic block was considered essential to diagnosis. The positive effect of sympathetic block, at least in the early stages of the disorder, was emphasized by Bonica (75). In pediatrics, the emphasis on confirming SMP versus sympathetically independent pain (SIP) seems less crucial for diagnosis than for adults, in part because of the high percentage of children who will show excellent recovery using a regimen that combines PT and cognitive-behavioral treatment (CBT) (76–79) and will therefore never receive or require sympathetic blockade (see below).

CRPS was regarded as rare in children until several case series were reported in the 1970s and 1980s (76,78). It is probable that this was owing to underrecognition of this group of disorders. For example, in our series from 1991 (79), the median time from onset of symptoms to seeking medical attention was 2 weeks; the median time to a diagnosis of reflex sympathetic dystrophy/CRPS/causalgia was 11 months. Our impression is that over the past 10 years, clinicians have become much more aware of this group of diagnoses, and most children are now being diagnosed much earlier after the onset of signs and symptoms.

CRPS in children and adolescents has a unique set of epidemiologic features. These disorders are very rare before 6 years of age. Onset of symptoms occurs more frequently at approximately 10 to 12 year of age, and new onset cases continue to be frequent throughout adolescence and young adulthood. Pediatric CRPS is predominantly a condition of the lower extremities (approximately 6 to 8:1 compared with upper extremities), and girls are affected at least six times as often as boys. These

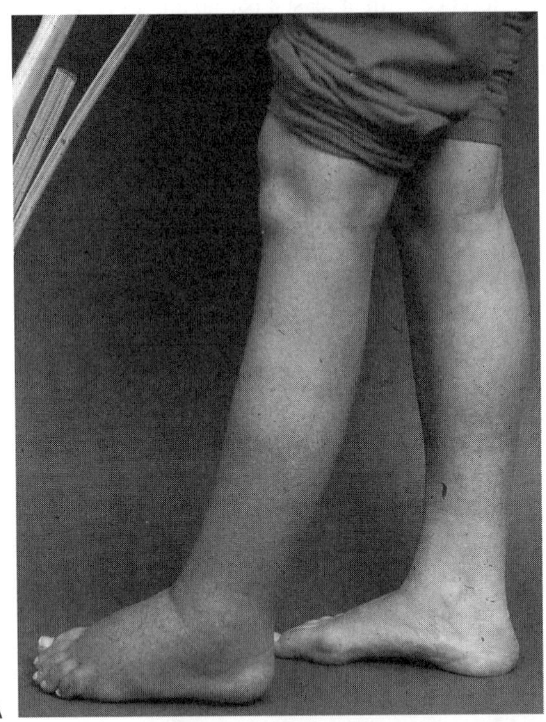

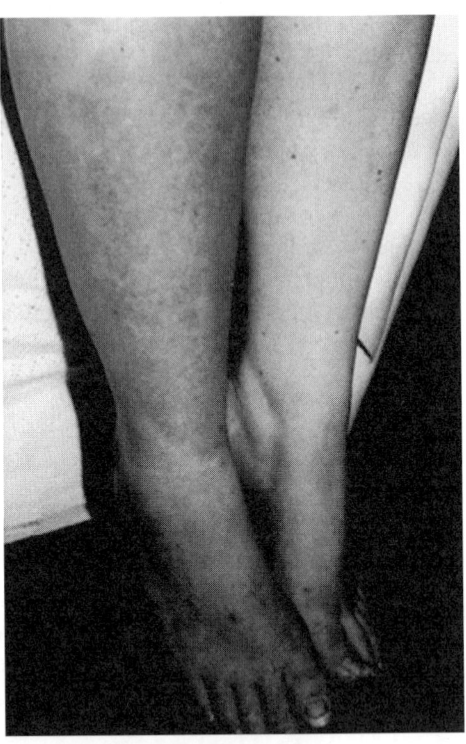

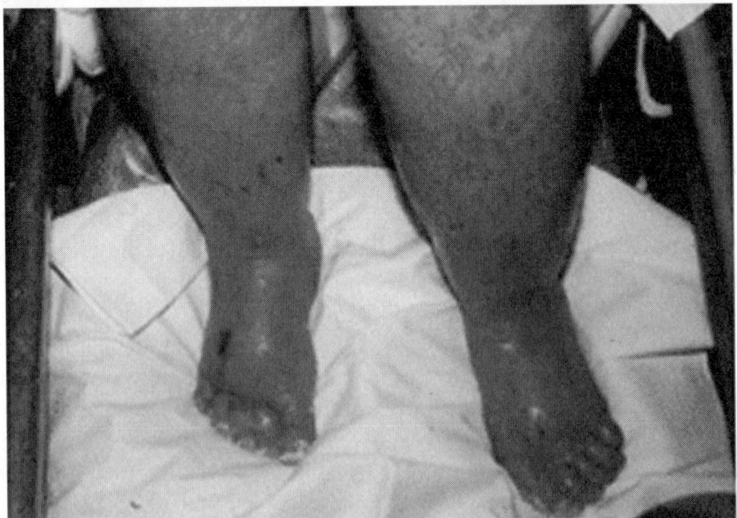

FIG. 34.1. A–C: The lower extremities of three patients with complex regional pain syndrome type I/reflex sympathetic dystrophy. Each shows a spectrum of clinical features including varying degrees of mottling, swelling, cyanosis or erythema, muscle atrophy, and abnormal limb posture. (**B** and **C** are courtesy of Dr. Robert Wilder, with permission.)

features are different from those of CRPS in adults, in which the gender ratio is less marked, and upper and lower extremity cases occur with approximately the same frequency.

Most published case series on CRPS in children have been retrospective. Recently, our group in Boston completed two prospective, randomized, controlled trials for treatment of CRPS in children: (a) a prospective "rehabilitative" trial of PT and CBT for the treatment of CRPS in children and adolescents and (b) a prospective trial of sympathetic blockade in children and adolescents with CRPS. We also included a standardized assessment profile that included pain measures, quantitative gait measures, a structured neurologic examination, autonomic measurements, psychologic measures, and QST. Findings of the PT/CBT trial are summarized in Table 34.3.

Overall, there was excellent improvement in both pain scores and measures of gait and stair-climbing impairment. All patients were ambulating without assistive devices by the end of the 6-week study protocol.

A cohort of patients with persistent pain and limb dysfunction after treatment with PT and CBT underwent a prospective, controlled trial of lumbar sympathetic blockade using combined infusions via lumbar epidural and lumbar paravertebral sympathetic indwelling catheters. In most cases, the decision to perform blockade was made based on persistent pain rather than on persistent inability to bear weight or tolerate PT. The initial dosing of the lumbar sympathetic catheter was performed using a double-blind, double-dummy comparison of intravenous saline plus lumbar sympathetic lidocaine versus intravenous lidocaine plus lumbar sympathetic saline. Patients then received an intensive 1-week inpatient treatment that utilized open-label continuous infusions of local anesthetics via either epidural or lumbar sympathetic catheters, along with PT, CBT, and a therapeutic milieu. Blinded administration showed that lumbar sympathetic administration of lidocaine was more effective than placebo plus intravenous lidocaine, and most of the patients with persistent pain and dysfunction on admission showed good improvement over the course of a 1-week hospitalization. A small subgroup of patients showed good improvement of limb function but little or no improvement in their pain score during this treatment regimen. Even among this more refractory subgroup, reductions in pain scores were shown over subsequent

TABLE 34.3. *Rehabilitative treatment trial for pediatric complex regional pain syndrome*

Design
- 6-week randomized comparison between
  - Group A: Physical therapy three times weekly + cognitive-behavioral treatment once weekly
  - versus
  - Group B: Physical therapy once weekly + cognitive-behavioral treatment once weekly

Measures (detailed assessment by observers blinded to group performed three times)
1. enrollment
2. short-term (after 6 weeks)
3. long-term (6–12 months): pain, gait, stair climbing, psychological inventories, regional and systemic autonomic signs and symptoms, quantitative sensory testing
4. end-of-study telephone follow-up assessments of pain and functional status

Outcomes
- 28 patients completed protocol
- At enrollment, all required assistive devices (wheelchair, crutches, cast boots)
- Psychologic scores within normal ranges for age
- Normal cardiovascular autonomic regulation despite prevalent regional signs and systemic autonomic symptoms
- Neurologic examinations showed 18 cases with CRPS1, ten with CRPS2
- Quantitative sensory testing abnormalities were common and varied
  - CRPS1 most commonly showed cold hyperalgesia
  - CRPS2 most commonly showed vibration hypoesthesia
- Visual analog scale spontaneous pain scores (median) improved in both groups
  - Group A: pre, 6.3; short term, 0; long term, 0
  - Group B: pre, 6.7; short term, 1.4; long term, 1.8
- Gait and stair climbing function scores improved in both groups
- No between-group differences in pain or motor function scores
- 42% experienced at least one recurrent episode
- At end of study, none of the patients required assistive devices

CRPS1, CRPS2, complex regional pain syndrome types I, II.

Data from Lee BH, Scharff L, Sethna NF, et al. Physical therapy and cognitive-behavioral treatment of complex regional pain syndromes. *J Pediatr* 2002;141:135-140.

weeks and months, with a diverse spectrum of other individualized treatment trials.

Several response patterns to nerve blockade have been noted in patients with CRPS. A subgroup of patients exhibits one or both of the following two anomalous responses:

1. a marked right shift in epidural or spinal local anesthetic dose response curves, i.e., much larger than normal doses are required to produce clinical signs of sensory, motor, and sympathetic blockade,
2. even with apparent very dense sensory, motor, and sympathetic blockade of the lower body (including lack of response to tetanic stimulation), pain is undiminished.

Medications that have been used for pediatric CRPS include antidepressants, anticonvulsants, local anesthetic–like drugs, calcitonin, corticosteroids, and opioids. Responses to each of these are quite variable. Individual patients have had excellent analgesic responses to gabapentin, nortriptyline, and prednisone; others have not. Experience with a series of pediatric patients with CRPS at St. Gorans's Children's Hospital in Stockholm (abstract presentation, International Symposium on Pediatric Pain, London, June 2001) found that amitriptyline produced a high frequency of side effects and little evidence of effectiveness.

From 1985 to 2001, more than 650 pediatric patients with CRPS have been evaluated and treated at Boston Children's Hospital. Over this period, we have referred only one patient for operative sympathectomy and two for phenol chemical sympathectomy (for circulatory insufficiency rather than for pain relief). A few patients (fewer than eight, based on available records) have either self-referred for operative, chemical, or radiofrequency sympathectomy or have had sympathectomy before referral to our center. One patient with causalgia after limb-sparing resection of an osteosarcoma of the femur chose above-the-knee amputation and a prosthesis for both pain and functional improvement after removal of two infected bone allografts and multiple reconstructive procedures. No other patients with CRPS have received limb amputation at our center in Boston. Approximately one to two patients annually receive temporary trials of either spinal cord stimulation or peripheral nerve stimulation for CRPS; an additional one to two patients with other diagnoses receive spinal cord stimulation trials or implantation annually. Implantable spinal opioid infusions for pediatric CRPS have been tried for only a few patients at our center over this 16-year period; they are used more frequently for patients with malignancies or with spasticity of cerebral origin.

Based on experience in centers worldwide, including our own, as summarized above, we believe that it is absolutely critical to reassure patients and families that CRPS in the overwhelming majority of children and adolescents should *not* be regarded as a diagnosis that implies long-term pain and/or disability. Because the experience in the adult literature appears so much less optimistic, it is common for families to come to physicians with a very worried and pessimistic attitude. A systematic Internet search for sites related to pediatric CRPS or reflex sympathetic dystrophy (O. Arenas, personal communication) revealed a high preponderance of very pessimistic impressions regarding prognosis and potential for long-term disability. Reassurance, avoidance of catastrophizing, and development of a positive rehabilitative outlook are essential aspects of our treatment approach.

Toxic and Metabolic Neuropathies

Painful peripheral neuropathy secondary to metabolic and toxic disorders is uncommon in children (i.e., secondary to diabetes, lead or mercury intoxication, alcohol, and occupational exposures). However, patients with unexplained limb pain, abnormal sensory examination, and autonomic dysfunction warrant evaluation for infection (acquired immunodeficiency syndrome, Lyme borreliosis, postinfectious autoimmune polyneuropathy), malignancy (paraneoplastic neuropathy, nerve and plexus infiltration, herpes zoster in immunocompromised host), vasculitides (rheumatoid arthritis, lupus erythematosus, Sjögren syndrome), and congenital sensory neuropathy (variants of familial dysautonomia and chronic sensory gangliopathy). Other pediatric populations that manifest sensory neuropathy include patients with uremia, a history of chemotherapy, and malabsorption syndromes with hypovitaminosis and some patients with restless legs syndrome.

Hereditary Neurodegenerative Disorders

The incidence of neuropathic pain associated with heredodegenerative disorders and inborn errors of metabolism is unknown. We frequently receive referrals of patients with severe neurodegenerative disorders who have long-standing severe irritability or even persistent crying and screaming, despite thorough efforts to identify recognizable sources of pain. Anecdotal reports of successful treatment of irritability in patients with leukodystrophies and pain in patients with mitochondrial encephalomyopathy using anticonvulsants/ion channel blockers are provocative. Channelopathy is found after nerve injury, in association with multiple sclerosis, and in an experimental mouse model deficient in myelin basic protein (81).

Mitochondrial Disorders

There is a spectrum of metabolic disorders that involve mitochondrial dysfunction, with associated impairments in energy metabolism. These disorders have enormous variability in clinical presentation, ranging from minimal symptoms to progressive deterioration of multiple organ systems including the peripheral and central nervous systems, skeletal muscle, heart, and gastrointestinal tract. Methods of molecular diagnosis are rapidly evolving. If these diagnoses are suspected, clinicians are encouraged to consult with tertiary pediatric neurogenetics and metabolism centers before drawing diagnostic or prognostic conclusions with families.

A growing number of children with mitochondrial disorders is being recognized as having chronic pain. Among the patients we have treated, the most common form of pain has been an apparent visceral neuropathic pain/visceral hyperalgesia associated with gastrointestinal dysmotility. We presume that, in some cases, this is associated with degeneration of autonomic innervation of the gastrointestinal tract. Other patients with mitochondrial disorders have had rapid progression of extremity neuropathic pain coincident with progressive axonal or demyelinating deterioration of peripheral nerves.

In individual cases, both visceral pain and extremity pain have improved with trials of anticonvulsant or antidepressant therapy. Tricyclic antidepressants often exacerbate constipation and should be used with caution (or with an increased laxative regimen) in patients with recurrent constipation.

In a small number of extreme cases in which patients experienced severe visceral pain and long-standing retching, celiac plexus neurolytic blockade has been of benefit. We restrict consideration of celiac neurolysis to patients who have failed other medical approaches, who have a clearly favorable response to temporary celiac plexus blockade with local anesthetics, and whose overall disease trajectory clearly predicts a short life span.

Erythromelalgia

Erythromelalgia is an uncommon syndrome of recurrent severely painful and warm, erythematous distal extremities. The characteristic feature of these patients is that their pain is exacerbated by heat and improved by cold. Several of these patients first present to physicians with the affected hands or feet kept in a bucket of ice. For some patients, these findings occur in isolation (primary erythromelalgia); in others, it may be associated with autoimmune and collagen vascular disorders (secondary erythromelalgia). Hypertension and thrombocythemia are commonly associated. The mechanisms that produce erythromelalgia are poorly understood. Abnormal platelet–endothelium interaction has been cited as a cause, and some patients do respond to treatment with aspirin. Some patients have features suggestive of a peripheral neuropathic process, and some of these may improve with medical therapies used for neuropathic pain such as anticonvulsants. One study shows a genetic locus at chromosome 2q31-32 (82). One retrospective review of 168 adult cases found that 4.2% of cases presented in childhood (83). Several case reports and small series of children and adolescents are reported, some cases in association with acute hypertension and some in association with autoimmune disorders and thrombocythemia. Prevalence data are not available. The condition is generally refractory to medical management, but some patients respond to antihypertensive agents, epidural anesthetics, and ion channel blockers. It is to be excluded from acrosyndromes of Fabry disease (deficiency of α-D-galactosidase type A activity), connective tissue disorders, and mercury toxicity (84).

Neuropathic Pain as a Secondary Component of Other Disorders

It is worth noting that many acute and chronic pain conditions not generally regarded as neuropathic can result in secondary nerve dysfunction and may have clinical features underlying peripheral and central mechanisms and responses to drug therapy that resemble the better recognized neuropathic disorders. For example, scleroderma and mixed connective tissue disease are properly regarded as collagen vascular disorders, with autoimmune and vasculopathic processes as the primary sources of pathology, leading initially to nociceptive pain owing to joint inflammation and ischemia of distal extremities. However, repetitive or ongoing ischemia of the vasa nervorum can lead to ischemic peripheral neuropathy, whereas fibrosis of the connective tissues enveloping the brachial plexus can cause a painful plexopathy. In many of these patients, drug therapies used traditionally for neuropathic pain, such as tricyclic antidepressants and anticonvulsants, may be effective.

In a similar fashion, although burn injury can produce active nociceptive pain, this form of injury is also a potent and sustained sensitizer of primary cutaneous nociceptive afferents. Third degree burns, which destroy dermal terminals of sensory fibers, produce a multifocal neural trauma, leading to central sensitization. Chronic neuropathic pain, as well as eschars and contractures, may limit functional rehabilitation in the recovery period.

CONCLUSIONS

Neuropathic pain conditions are a comparatively common source of persistent pain among children referred to tertiary centers. Much of the treatment is currently extrapolated from that for similar disorders in adults, although age-related biologic differences may be relevant to disease mechanisms, natural history, and responses to treatment. Prospective clinical trials, in most cases involving multiple pediatric centers, are needed to better define the pathophysiology, epidemiology, and optimal treatments for pediatric neuropathic pain disorders.

ACKNOWLEDGMENT

Supported by National Institutes of Health grant RO1 HD35737 and by grants from the Bradley Foundation and Advocates for Children's Pain Relief to Dr. Berde.

REFERENCES

1. Bennett G. Neuropathic pain: an overview. In: Borsook D, ed. *Molecular neurobiology*. Seattle: IASP Press, 1997:109–113.
2. Devor M. The pathophysiology and anatomy of damaged nerve. In: Wall W, Melzack R, eds. *Textbook of pain*. Edinburgh: Churchill-Livingstone, 1984.
3. McArthur JC, Yiannoutsos C, Simpson DM, et al. A phase II trial of nerve growth factor for sensory neuropathy associated with HIV infection. AIDS Clinical Trials Group Team 291. *Neurology* 2000;54:1080–1088.
4. Watkins LR, Goehler LE, Relton J, et al. Mechanisms of tumor necrosis factor-alpha (TNF-alpha) hyperalgesia. *Brain Res* 1995;692:244–250.
5. Woolf CJ, Salter MW. Neuronal plasticity: increasing the gain in pain. *Science* 2000;288:1765–1769.
6. Schwartzman RJ, Grothusen J, Kiefer TR, et al. Neuropathic central pain: epidemiology, etiology, and treatment options. *Arch Neurol* 2001;58:1547–1550.
7. Gracely RH, Lynch SA, Bennett GJ. Painful neuropathy: altered central processing maintained dynamically by peripheral input. *Pain* 1992;51:175–194.
8. Fields HL. Pain modulation: expectation, opioid analgesia and virtual pain. Progress in *Brain Res* 2000; 122:245–253.
9. Heinricher MM, Schouten JC, Jobst EE. Activation of

brainstem N-methyl-D-aspartate receptors is required for the analgesic actions of morphine given systemically. *Pain* 2001;92:129–138.
10. Flor H. The functional organization of the brain in chronic pain. *Prog Brain Res* 2000;129:313–322.
11. Borsook D, Becerra L, Fishman S, et al. Acute plasticity in the human somatosensory cortex following amputation. *Neuroreport* 1998;9:1013–1017.
12. Hofbauer RK, Rainville P, Duncan GH, et al. Cortical representation of the sensory dimension of pain. *J Neurophysiol* 2001;86:402–411.
13. Rainville P, Duncan GH, Price DD, et al. Pain affect encoded in human anterior cingulate but not somatosensory cortex. *Science* 1997;277:968–971.
14. Yarnitsky D, Sprecher E, Zaslansky R, et al. Heat pain thresholds: normative data and repeatability. *Pain* 1995;60:329–332.
15. Meier PM, Berde CB, DiCanzio J, et al. Quantitative assessment of cutaneous thermal and vibration sensation and thermal pain detection thresholds in healthy children and adolescents. *Muscle Nerve* 2001;24: 1339–1345.
16. Irazuzta JE, Berde CB, Sethna NF. Laser Doppler measurements of skin blood flow before, during, and after lumbar sympathetic blockade in children and young adults with reflex sympathetic dystrophy syndrome. *J Clin Monit* 1992;8:16–19.
17. McGrath P. Chronic pain in children. In: Crombie IK, Linton SJ, LeResche L, et al., eds. *Epidemiology of pain*. Seattle: IASP Press, 1999:81–102.
18. McQuay HJ, Tramer M, Nye BA, et al. A systematic review of antidepressants in neuropathic pain. *Pain* 1996;68:217–227.
19. Max, MB, Culnane M, Schafer SC, et al. Amitriptyline relieves diabetic neuropathy pain in patients with normal or depressed mood. *Neurology* 1987;37:589–596.
20. Bowsher D. The effects of pre-emptive treatment of postherpetic neuralgia with amitriptyline: a randomized, double-blind, placebo-controlled trial. *J Pain Symptom Managet* 1997;13:327–331.
21. Max MB, Lynch SA, Muir J, et al. Effects of desipramine, amitriptyline, and fluoxetine on pain in diabetic neuropathy. *N Engl J Med* 1992;326:1250–1256.
22. Panerai AE, Monza G, Movilia P, et al. A randomized, within-patient, cross-over, placebo-controlled trial on the efficacy and tolerability of the tricyclic antidepressants chlorimipramine and nortriptyline in central pain. *Acta Neurol Scand* 1990;82:34–38.
23. Varley CK. Sudden death related to selected tricyclic antidepressants in children: epidemiology, mechanisms and clinical implications. *Paediatr Drugs* 2001;3: 613–627.
24. Biederman J, Thisted RA, Greenhill LL, et al. Estimation of the association between desipramine and the risk for sudden death in 5- to 14-year-old children. *J Clin Psychiatry* 1995;56:87–93.
25. Wilens TE, Biederman J, Baldessarini RJ, et al. Cardiovascular effects of therapeutic doses of tricyclic antidepressants in children and adolescents. *J Am Acad Child Adolesc Psychiatry* 1996;35:1491–1501.
26. Sindrup SH, Gram LF, Brosen K, et al. The selective serotonin reuptake inhibitor paroxetine is effective in the treatment of diabetic neuropathy symptoms. *Pain* 1990;42:135–144.
27. Ross EL. The evolving role of antiepileptic drugs in treating neuropathic pain. *Neurology* 2000;55:S41–S46.
28. Backonja MM. Gabapentin monotherapy for the symptomatic treatment of painful neuropathy: a multicenter, double-blind, placebo-controlled trial in patients with diabetes mellitus. *Epilepsia* 1999;40:S57–S59.
29. Rowbotham M, Harden N, Stacey B, et al. Gabapentin for the treatment of postherpetic neuralgia: a randomized controlled trial. *JAMA* 1998;280:1837–1842.
30. Cora-Locatelli G, Greenberg BD, Martin JD, et al. Rebound psychiatric and physical symptoms after gabapentin discontinuation. *J Clin Psychiatry* 1998;59: 131(abst).
31. McGraw T, Kosek P. Erythromelalgia pain managed with gabapentin. *Anesthesiology* 1997;86:988–990.
32. Rusy LM, Troshynski TJ, Weisman SJ. Gabapentin in phantom limb pain management in children and young adults: report of seven cases. *J Pain Symptom Manage* 2001;21:78–82.
33. Tennis P, Stern R. Risk of serious cutaneous disorders after initiation of use of phenytoin, carbamazepine, or sodium valproate: a record linkage study. *Neurology* 1997;49:542–546.
34. Kalso E, Tramer MR, McQuay HJ, et al. Systemic local-anaesthetic-type drugs in chronic pain: a systematic review. *Eur J Pain* 1998;2:3–14.
35. Galer BS, Harle J, Rowbotham MC. Response to intravenous lidocaine infusion predicts subsequent response to oral mexiletine: a prospective study. *J Pain Symptom Manage* 1996;12:161–167.
36. Brose W, Cousins M. Subcutaneous lidocaine for treatment of neuropathic cancer pain. *Pain* 1991;45:145–148.
37. Wallace MS, Magnuson S, Ridgeway B. Efficacy of oral mexiletine for neuropathic pain with allodynia: a double-blind, placebo-controlled, crossover study. *Reg Anesth Pain Med* 2000;25:459–467.
38. Arnér S, Meyerson BA. Lack of analgesic effect of opioids on neuropathic and idiopathic forms of pain. *Pain* 1988;33:11–23.
39. Portenoy RK, Foley KM, Inturrisi CE. The nature of opioid responsiveness and its implications for neuropathic pain: new hypotheses derived from studies of opioid infusions. *Pain* 1990;43:273–286.
40. Huse E, Larbig W, Flor H, et al. The effect of opioids on phantom limb pain and cortical reorganization. *Pain* 2001;90:47–55.
41. Rowbotham MC, Reisner-Keller LA, Fields HL. Both intravenous lidocaine and morphine reduce the pain of postherpetic neuralgia. *Neurology* 1991;41:1024–1028.
42. Kemper KJ, Sarah R, Silver-Highfield E, et al. On pins and needles? Pediatric pain patients' experience with acupuncture. *Pediatrics* 2000;105:941–947.
43. Smith LA, Oldman AD, McQuay HJ, et al. Teasing apart quality and validity in systematic reviews: an example from acupuncture trials in chronic neck and back pain. *Pain* 2000;86:119–132.
44. Moore RA, McQuay HJ, Oldman AD, et al. BMA approves acupuncture. BMA report is wrong. *BMJ* 2000; 321:1220–1221.
45. Kalauokalani D, Cherkin DC, Sherman KJ, et al. Lessons from a trial of acupuncture and massage for low back pain: patient expectations and treatment effects. *Spine* 2001;26:1418–1424.
46. Gardiner P, Kemper KJ. Herbs in pediatric and adolescent medicine. *Pediatr Rev* 2000;21:44–57.
47. Mitchell SW, Morehouse CR, Keen WW. *Gunshot wounds and other injuries of the nerves*. Philadelphia: JB Lippincott, 1864.

48. Lotze M, Grodd W, Birbaumer N, et al. Does use of a myoelectric prosthesis prevent cortical reorganization and phantom limb pain? *Nat Neurosci* 1999;2:501–502.
49. Kalauokalani D, Loeser JD. Phantom limb pain. In: Crombie IK, Linton SJ, LeResche L, et al., ed. *Epidemiology of pain*. Seattle: IASP Press, 1999:143–153.
50. Kooijman CM, Dijkstra PU, Geertzen JH, et al. Phantom pain and phantom sensations in upper limb amputees: an epidemiological study. *Pain* 2000;87:33–41.
51. Krane EJ, Heller LB. The prevalence of phantom sensation and pain in pediatric amputees. *J Pain Symptom Manage* 1995;10:21–29.
52. Wilkins KL, McGrath PJ, Finley GA, et al. Phantom limb sensations and phantom limb pain in child and adolescent amputees. *Pain* 1998;78:7–12.
53. Smith J, Thompson JM. Phantom limb pain and chemotherapy in pediatric amputees. *Mayo Clin Proc* 1995;70:357–364.
54. Weiss T, Miltner WH, Adler T, et al. Decrease in phantom limb pain associated with prosthesis-induced increased use of an amputation stump in humans. *Neurosci Lett* 1999;272:131–134.
55. Ramachandran VS, Rogers-Ramachandran D. Synaesthesia in phantom limbs induced with mirrors. *Proc R Soc Lond B Biol Sci* 1996;263:377–386.
56. Bach S, Noreng M, Tjellden N. Phantom limb pain in amputees during the first twelve months following limb amputation after preoperative lumbar epidural blockade. *Pain* 1988;33:297–301.
57. Jahangiri M, Jayatunga AP, Bradley JW, et al. Prevention of phantom pain after major lower limb amputation by epidural infusion of diamorphine, clonidine and bupivacaine. *Ann R Coll Surg Engl* 1994;76:324–326.
58. Nikolajsen L, Ilkjaer S, Christensen JH, et al. Randomised trial of epidural bupivacaine and morphine in prevention of stump and phantom pain in lower-limb amputation. *Lancet* 1997;350:1353–1357.
59. Nikolajsen L, Ilkjaer S, Jensen TS. Effect of preoperative extradural bupivacaine and morphine on stump sensation in lower limb amputees. *Br J Anaesth* 1998; 81:348–354.
60. Lambert A, Dashfield A, Cosgrove C, et al. Randomized prospective study comparing preoperative epidural and intraoperative perineural analgesia for the prevention of postoperative stump and phantom limb pain following major amputation. *Reg Anesth Pain Med* 2001; 26:316–321.
61. Kissin I. Preemptive analgesia. Why its effect is not always obvious. *Anesthesiology* 1996;84:1015–1019.
62. Hoeksma AF, Wolf H, Oei SL. Obstetrical brachial plexus injuries: incidence, natural course and shoulder contracture. *Clin Rehabil* 2000;14:523–526.
63. Rossitch E Jr, Oakes WJ, Ovelmen-Levitt J, et al. Self-mutilation following brachial plexus injury sustained at birth. *Pain* 1992;50:209–211.
64. Al-Qattan MM. Self-mutilation in children with obstetric brachial plexus palsy. *J Hand Surg [Br]* 1999;24: 547–549.
65. Collins JJ, Grier HE, Kinney HC, et al. Control of severe pain in children with terminal malignancy. *J Pediatr* 1995;126:653–657.
66. Collins JJ, Grier HE, Sethna NF, et al. Regional anesthesia for pain associated with terminal pediatric malignancy. *Pain* 1996;65:63–69.
67. Cherny NI, Thaler HT, Friedlander-Klar H, et al. Opioid responsiveness of cancer pain syndromes caused by neuropathic or nociceptive mechanisms: a combined analysis of controlled, single-dose studies. *Neurology* 1994;44:857–861.
68. Mercadante S, Portenoy RK. Opioid poorly-responsive cancer pain. Part 3. Clinical strategies to improve opioid responsiveness. *J Pain Symptom Manage* 2001;21: 338–354.
69. Crews JC, Sweeney NJ, Denson DD. Clinical efficacy of methadone in patients refractory to other mu-opioid receptor agonist analgesics for management of terminal cancer pain. Case presentations and discussion of incomplete cross-tolerance among opioid agonist analgesics. *Cancer* 1993;72:2266–2272.
70. Ripamonti C, Groff L, Brunelli C, et al. Switching from morphine to oral methadone in treating cancer pain: what is the equianalgesic dose ratio? *J Clin Oncol* 1998; 16:3216–3221.
71. Gagnon B, Bruera E. Differences in the ratios of morphine to methadone in patients with neuropathic pain versus non-neuropathic pain. *J Pain Symptom Manage* 1999;18:120–125.
72. Stanton-Hicks M, Janig W, Hassenbusch S, et al. Reflex sympathetic dystrophy: changing concepts and taxonomy. *Pain* 1995;63:127–133.
73. Harden RN, Bruehl S, Galer BS, et al. Complex regional pain syndrome: are the IASP diagnostic criteria valid and sufficiently comprehensive? *Pain* 1999;83: 211–219.
74. Bruehl S, Harden RN, Galer BS, et al. External validation of IASP diagnostic criteria for Complex Regional Pain Syndrome and proposed research diagnostic criteria. International Association for the Study of Pain. *Pain* 1999;81:147–154.
75. Bonica JJ. Causalgia and other reflex sympathetic dystrophies. *Postgrad Med* 1973;53:143–148.
76. Bernstein BH, Singsen BH, Kent JT, et al. Reflex neurovascular dystrophy in childhood. *J Pediatr* 1978;93: 211–215.
77. Sherry DD, Wallace CA, Kelley C, et al. Short- and long-term outcomes of children with complex regional pain syndrome type I treated with exercise therapy. *Clin J Pain* 1999;15:218–223.
78. Dietz FR, Mathews KD, Montgomery WJ. Reflex sympathetic dystrophy in children. *Clin Orthop* 1990;258: 225–231.
79. Wilder RT, Berde CB, Wolohan M, et al. Reflex sympathetic dystrophy in children. Clinical characteristics and follow-up of seventy patients. *J Bone Joint Surg Am* 1992;74:910–919.
80. Lee BH, Scharff L, Sethna NF, et al. Physical therapy and cognitive-behavioral treatment of complex regional pain syndromes. *J Pediatr* 2002;141:135–140.
81. Waxman SG. Acquired channelopathies in nerve injury and MS. *Neurology* 2001;56:1621–1627.
82. Drenth JP, Finley WH, Breedveld GJ, et al. The primary erythermalgia-susceptibility gene is located on chromosome 2q31-32. *Am J Hum Genet* 2001;68:1277–1282.
83. Davis MD, O'Fallon WM, Rogers RS 3rd, et al. Natural history of erythromelalgia: presentation and outcome in 168 patients. *Arch Dermatol* 2000;136:330–336.
84. Drenth JP, Michiels JJ, Ozsoylu S. Acute secondary erythermalgia and hypertension in children. Erythermalgia Multidisciplinary Study Group. *Eur J Pediatr* 1995; 154:882–885.

34. Appendix
Neuropathic Pain (Nerve Pain)
An Information Sheet for Patients and Their Parents[1]

You/your child has been diagnosed with a form of nerve pain (neuropathic pain). The purpose of this handout is to explain why these kinds of pain are different from ordinary pain, and what this means for your treatment.

Ordinary Pain (Nociceptive Pain)

Ordinary pain is a very useful form of sensation because it protects us from hurting ourselves. If we did not feel ordinary pain, we might burn our fingers on the stove, step on a tack, or not know when we had some serious problem, such as appendicitis. *Ordinary pain is what you feel when normal nerves send messages from injured or inflamed body tissues.*

Ordinary pain from a single injury, like that from an operation or from breaking your leg, usually gets better over a few days to, at most, one to two weeks. Sometimes, ordinary pain can last longer if tissues continue to be chronically injured or inflamed. For example, arthritis produces long-lasting ordinary pain, because there is repeated or ongoing inflammation of the joints.

Milder forms of ordinary pain respond well to medicines such as acetaminophen (Tylenol) or ibuprofen (Advil). More severe ordinary pain, like that from major surgery, is usually made better by stronger pain medicines like morphine, meperidine (Demerol) or oxycodone (Percocet).

[1]Pain Treatment Service, Children's Hospital.

Nerve Pain (Neuropathic Pain)

Some other kinds of pain are not caused by normal nerves reporting that tissues are injured. *Instead, these other kinds of pain, called nerve pain or neuropathic pain, are caused by abnormal messages being sent by the nerves, even when tissue injury has healed.* For example, people who have had a foot amputated often feel that their missing foot still hurts ("phantom pain") even though the foot is gone. Although we don't know all the details about how this works, we think that some of the reason people hurt for long periods after an amputation is that the nerves that ended in the stump were injured and they continue to fire messages, and the brain and spinal cord continue to interpret these messages as painful. In addition, certain areas of the spinal cord can become "sensitized" or "activated," so that they have abnormal "gating" of pain messages and perpetuate a pain cycle.

The important things to remember about nerve pain are:

a. *Nerve pain is real.*

Nerve pain feels just as intense, or perhaps even more intense than ordinary pain. That is, it really hurts.

b. *People with nerve pain are not crazy.*

People don't fake or make up nerve pain: it's not "all in their heads." Although people with nerve pain aren't crazy, there is no doubt that for all kinds of health problems, including nerve pain, how bad it feels may be affected by stress, fatigue, diet and general health. Pain is harder to cope with if you are tired, depressed, anxious or having family troubles. (For example, if you had an ulcer, along with giving you antacids and other medications, we would treat you with stress reduction, alterations in diet, avoidance of coffee, etc. The same considerations apply to nerve pain).

c. *Nerve pain is real, but it is telling your brain wrong information.*

For people with nerve pain in the leg, even though the leg hurts when they move it, they won't damage it by moving it. This is very important but hard for people to believe, because we are all used to listening to our pain.

d. *Much of the treatment of nerve pain involves working through the pain, since the pain is not protecting us from harm.*

e. *Other parts of the treatment of nerve pain involve "reprogramming the nerves" to send messages properly.* Common treatments include:

- exercises, mobilization, physical therapy
- transcutaneous electrical nerve stimulation (TENS)
- medications
- behavioral medicine techniques including relaxation training, stress management, biofeedback training and counseling in life-style alterations

Questions People Commonly Ask

a. *If the nerves are working wrong, why can't you just cut out the confused nerves?*

Although a few people require surgery for nerve pain, this is rare. For most people, cutting a nerve will create a new area of nerve injury and new kinds of pain. Nerve surgery should be undertaken only after conservative treatments have been tried and only by specialists in nerve surgery, such as specialized neurosurgeons, plastic and reconstructive surgeons and orthopedic surgeons.

b. *Is nerve pain very rare, and why haven't I heard of it before?*

Nerve pain is fairly common, and it is often under-recognized. The following conditions are examples of types of nerve pain:

- phantom pain (nerve pain in a missing foot or hand)
- diabetic neuropathy (nerve pain from diabetes)
- post-herpetic neuralgia (nerve pain following shingles)
- neuroma pain (nerve pain from a cut nerve that is trying to regenerate)
- reflex sympathetic dystrophy (RSD-nerve pain of an arm of leg along with signs of abnormal activity of the sympathetic nerves, including coldness, blue or purple color changes, increased sweating, abnormal hair growth, swelling, loss of muscle bulk, etc.)

c. *What kinds of medications are helpful?*

Although some patients are relieved by simple medications such as acetaminophen or ibuprofen, many are not. In fact, some kinds of neuropathic pain are not easily relieved by stronger medications such as morphine, although others are. Interestingly, medications that work on "nerve hyperexcitability" or "descending pain-inhibiting pathways in the spinal cord" often work better. These include:

- tricyclic antidepressants
- anticonvulsants (seizure medications)
- vasodilators (blood pressure medications)

d. *If you are prescribing an antidepressant, doesn't that mean you think I or my child is crazy?*

No, you are not crazy, and the pain is not "in your head." Antidepressants are probably the most useful group of drugs for nerve pain, and they help great numbers of patients. Although having chronic pain makes some people feel a bit depressed, frustrated or angry, these medications work on nerve pain in ways that are separate from their antidepressant actins. In addition, they are effective for nerve pain in doses much lower than those used for depression.

e. *Why will behavioral medicine be effective if the pain is real and not just "in my head?"*

Although the pain is "real" and "not just in your head," it is certainly true that mood, attention, stress and related factors can influence how bothersome the pain is. Behavioral medicine techniques can help:

- create a state of relaxation
- teach you how to deal with stressful situations
- modify nerve input with biofeedback

Behavioral medicine techniques are of proven value in a number of "physilogic" disorders, including migraine headaches and high blood pressure. We have found them all very useful for reflex sympathetic dystrophy as well.

f. *Where are nerve block injections, and what are they for?*

The majority of patients with neuropathic pain do not *need nerve block injections.* As mentioned earlier, one particular type of neuropathic pain in the arms or legs is also associated with coldness, mottling, sensitivity to touch, swelling and blue or purple discoloration. This type is often called reflex sympathetic dystrophy or RSD. A newer name for this condition is complex regional pain syndrome type 1, or CRPS 1.

Most patients with RSD get better with physical therapy, behavioral medicine treatment, TENS and non-narcotic medications. A small subgroup continues to make slow progress, or they have severe problems with the circulation in their arm or leg. For these more severely affected patients, local anesthetic medications are injected either by a needle or by a tiny tube that is left in place near a group of nerves. This procedure is called a nerve block. Nerve blocks improve the pain and circulation, and they can help break the cycle for many but not all patients. The choice of injections through a needle or a tube depends on a number or factors that differ among different patients' conditions. Your doctors will describe the details of this. Although a needle and a numbing medication are involved, your doctors have ways of making these procedures comfortable and quite safe. Your doctors are use to caring for children and adults who are afraid of needles, and they are use to making the injections not hurt. Side-effects and adverse reactions can occur, but they are quite rare and can be treated effectively.

Even though the local anesthetics only remain active for a period of hours, they can break the cycle for days, weeks, or even permanently in many patients with RSD. Although the majority of patients with RSD are helped considerably by these nerve blocks, it is very difficult to predict how long the pain relief will last, and what factors make the pain go away entirely for some patients.

It is important to emphasize that nerve blocks work best if they are combined with physical therapy and behavioral medicine treatment.

35

Burn Pain Management

Avoiding The "Private Nightmare"

Madelyn D. Kahana

Burn injury is one of the most painful of all human ailments, regardless of the age of the patient. Each year in the United States approximately 80,000 people are hospitalized with significant burns. One-third to one-half of those admitted are children (1). All have pain and disfigurement. Characteristically, the pain is relentless, punctuated with the need for procedural intervention and more pain. Pain need not be an integral part of the burn experience. Analgesia is not only possible but is mandatory to ensure optimal patient outcome.

Because the burn injury can be hemodynamically challenging, even immediately life threatening, pain management is sometimes the secondary concern of the burn surgeon (2). Yet, without immediate analgesic intervention, these children are very likely to be victim to the pathologic processes that later are responsible for chronic neuropathic pain states. Effective pain management involves much more than the administration of sufficient analgesics. A coordinated multidisciplinary approach to provide physical and emotional support for patients and their families is also imperative. This problem is simply enormous.

Complicating this issue is the fact that there is relatively little in the way of rigorous pediatric burn pain research. The recommendations that follow are largely experiential or are derived from adult clinical trials or bench research in pain physiology. The opportunity for investigation in this area is also enormous.

THE ACUTE BURN INJURY: EPIDEMIOLOGY AND PATHOPHYSIOLOGY

In children, a disproportionate number of burn injuries occurs from birth through 4 years of age. The most frequent injuries are scalds, often occur in the home, and frequently are preventable. Typical agents responsible for the burn wound are hot liquids from the stove, the microwave (3), or hot tap water. Home hot water heater temperature is usually set between 40°C and 55°C. At 70°C, a set point commonly found in large apartment buildings, water can produce a full thickness burn in a small child in less than 1 second.

The environment outside the home is also dangerous. From cigarette lighters to hot coal remnants of a beach grill, the potential for injury is anywhere and everywhere. In addition, nonaccidental burns are all too common in children. Intentional burns now represent 9% of injuries in the child abuse records (3). Those clinicians involved in the care of the burned child must be aware that child abuse is a distinct possibility and take the required steps to report suspicious injury to child protective authorities.

Thermal injury produces a complex injury of the integument that follows a reproducible pattern of tissue response. With deep wounds, there is an area of tissue necrosis surrounded by an area of ischemia. Tissue in the ischemic region is vulnerable and survival depends on

TABLE 35.1. *Characteristics of burn wounds*

Type of burn	Physical characteristics	Healing process
Superficial (first degree)	Red, no blisters, dry, blanches, painful	No intervention necessary
Partial thickness (second degree)	Pink, blanches, blisters, painful	Dermal appendages repopulate epidermis
Full thickness (third degree)	White, dry, leathery, no blanching, insensate	Grafting essential for healing

the restoration of blood flow. Surrounding the zone of ischemia is an area of hyperemia. Numerous mediators liberated by the inflammatory process support increased blood flow in this tissue. This tissue is generally viable.

Burn wounds are classified as partial thickness or full thickness depending on their depth. A superficial partial thickness wound involves only the epidermis (first degree) or the upper dermis (second degree). Epidermal injuries are painful but self-limited and do not require hospital care. Dermal injuries frequently require hospital care and are consistently painful because sensory nerves residing in the dermis are affected. These wounds may heal without surgical intervention by proliferation of the preserved epidermal elements of the skin appendages, hair follicles, and sweat glands. Deep dermal injury and wounds that destroy the entire dermis are classified as functional full thickness and full thickness wounds, respectively. The dermal appendages are compromised in these wounds such that grafting is necessary for healing to occur without excessive scarring. Contrary to classic teaching, full thickness wounds are also painful. Pain is produced in these areas by the spared nerve endings in the deep dermis and by the periphery of the wound where nerve destruction is incomplete and inflammation is active (Table 35.1).

MECHANISMS OF BURN PAIN

There is acute pain at the site of burn injury immediately. In addition, there is a rapid neuronal upregulation at multiple levels of the sensory pathway that may amplify the acute pain experience and also provide fertile ground for the development of chronic pain pathology. The amount of acute local pain is a function of the depth of the wound. In partial thickness wounds, nerve endings are damaged and sensitized. In deeper wounds, this process occurs at the periphery of the injury and in the nerve endings spared in the wound itself. Both Aδ- and C-fiber nociceptors are activated by thermal stimuli and transmit information to the spinal cord and ultimately to the sensory cortex. Activated nerve terminals also participate in the inflammatory process through the release of neuropeptides such as substance P. This results in vasodilation, edema, and erythema. Thermal peripheral neuronal sensitization leads to nociceptor activation in the immediate region of the injury (primary hyperalgesia).

With the increase in activity of the Aδ and C fibers, there is sensitization of the second-order dorsal horn neurons in the spinal cord (secondary hyperalgesia). The activation of the second-order neurons occurs by the action of neurotransmitters such as glutamate and tachykinins. There are resultant upregulation and sensitization to pain outside the region of original injury. The threshold for activation of the dorsal horn is reduced; normally nonnociceptive neurons can produce pain and nonnociceptive stimuli can be interpreted as pain, e.g., mechanosensory information. To interrupt this process, prompt effective receptor blockade is required. Analgesia must be a priority of care to avoid the potential neuropathology of secondary hyperalgesia (4,5).

Shortly after injury, healing begins. Nerve regeneration and tissue reinnervation occur, which provide additional opportunities for the development of chronic pain states. Nerve growth factor levels are elevated in the injured dermis leading to collateral sprouting of nerve terminals and the proliferation of sympathetic neurons. Sprouted ends of the regenerating axons show heightened sensitivity to a variety of humoral factors such as cytokines, present in abundance in the burn wound (6). Thermal hyperalgesia occurs along with collateral sprouting (7). In the dorsal horn, peripheral injury causes sprouting of A afferent nerve from lamina III into laminae I and II, the sites of nociceptive synapses. Sympathetic postganglionic neurons also sprout in response to peripheral burn injury and innervate the dorsal root ganglion. This neuronal reorganization leads to the production of pain by nonnociceptive mechanosensory stimulus and can ultimately result in the development and maintenance of chronic pain states.

Thus, the burn injury itself and the healing process that must occur are both important in the pathophysiology of burn pain. Neuronal upregulation and the promotion of a pathologic chronic pain process are almost inevitable. Meticulous attention to rapid effective analgesia is crucial to the optimal management of these patients and to their ultimate quality of life.

THERAPEUTIC APPROACHES TO BURN PAIN

Unique about the management of burn pain is the need for patients to undergo frequent, intensely painful procedures (e.g., dressing changes, debridement) as well as the presence of relentless "rest pain" (8,9). Opioids remain the mainstay of acute burn pain management in children and adults. Analgesic doses must be titrated to the desired effect and administered on a schedule that accommodates both rest pain and procedural pain. The dose of analgesic required to control rest pain is almost never sufficient to accommodate painful procedures. Additional medications or alternative analgesic techniques, such as dissociative anesthesia, must be employed to manage procedural pain effectively. Pain management strategies must also accommodate the multitude of other medical problems that plague these complex patients. When pain is refractory to opioids, options to treat neuropathic pain need to be entertained. In fact, in all phases of treatment, alternatives and adjuncts to classic pain management with opioid administration can be very useful and are reviewed (10).

PAIN ASSESSMENT IN THE BURNED CHILD

A detailed discussion of the pain assessment scales is beyond the scope of this chapter and is reviewed elegantly elsewhere (11). Well-validated, age-appropriate measurement tools are readily available and should be a ritual part of patient assessment. In fact, pain/comfort documentation should be recorded as the fifth vital sign in the burned child in whom pain is so prevalent (9).

THE INJURY: IMPACT ON PHARMACOLOGY

The first few days after serious burn injury are marked by the need for significant intravascular volume replacement therapy. This generally results in the dilution of the plasma proteins including the serum albumin concentration. The free fraction of the protein-bound narcotics and sedative agents increases as a result, particularly the benzodiazepines (12). Simultaneously, the extracellular space is expanded with interstitial fluid accumulation, a result of the capillary leak that accompanies the generalized inflammatory response after burn injury. With the increase in the extracellular space, the volume of distribution of many pharmacologic agents may also increase. Even after successful resuscitation, the release of cytokines after burn injury results in the maintenance of the systemic inflammatory response syndrome. Cardiac output is elevated, systemic vascular resistance is reduced, and the patient's metabolic rate is markedly increased. The clearance of opioids and sedatives should increase as well, although data exploring this issue are sparse and inconsistent.

There are no data examining the pharmacology of the sedatives and opiates in the burn patient population early in the clinical course of this injury. Furman et al. (13) studied the pharmacokinetics of morphine in adult burn patients 2 weeks after injury, well after initial

TABLE 35.2. *The burn injury: a timeline*

Time after injury	Pathophysiology/clinical priorities
First 12 hours	Carbon monoxide poisoning, cyanide poisoning, burn shock (low cardiac output), hypovolemia, disseminated intravascular coagulation, myoglobinuria
Second 12 hours	Increased cardiac output, inhalation injury (airway sloughing), capillary leak, increasing metabolic rate
1–7 days	Pulmonary edema, surgical excision and grafting, increased metabolic rate, infection risk, ulcer risk
7–14 days	More excision and grafting, continued infection risk, continued ulcer risk, metabolic rate variable
14 days	More wound coverage, rehabilitation

resuscitation. They described a reduction in the volume of distribution and an increase in the terminal elimination half-life of intravenous morphine. However, two other studies found similar morphine pharmacokinetics in burned and nonburned adults, at a similar time point after injury (14,15). In all these studies, there was inadequate control for comorbidity, making interpretation of the data difficult and confusing. In pediatric patients, there simply are no data that address this issue.

Clearly, with the data lacking and the clinical condition of the affected child rapidly changing, individual patient assessment must dictate the appropriate end point of analgesic and sedative therapy. In children with premorbid hepatic or renal dysfunction or in whom organ system dysfunction occurs as a result of this profound insult, drug metabolism and elimination may be altered. That too must be considered in planning the choice of analgesic and the dosing regimen. Careful titration of the appropriate agent is key to successful alleviation of pain and suffering (Table 35.2).

MANAGEMENT STRATEGIES

Burn injuries produce significant background or baseline/rest pain (16). This persists for the entire treatment period. Of interest, pain perception is proportional to the size and depth of the wound only in the first week after injury. Thereafter, it varies widely regardless of the magnitude of the wound (17,18). Analgesic strategies must therefore include a plan to address this constant discomfort. In addition, there is the need to provide relief for regular procedures that punctuate the day of a burn victim with intense pain, e.g., burn wound dressing changes and physical therapy.

During the initial resuscitation period, the intravenous administration of narcotics in high doses is required for baseline and procedural pain management. Morphine and fentanyl are the most commonly used agents. Agonist–antagonist combinations are limited by the ceiling effect of these drugs (19). Meperidine is not recommended because of the potential for accumulation of the toxic metabolite normeperidine over the extended treatment period. Intramuscular administration of analgesics is *not* recommended because absorption is erratic and delayed (Table 35.3).

The course of burn pain varies considerably. In general, as the wound is closed surgically, as the percentage of open body surface area decreases, so the pain decreases. However, the donor sites harvested for skin closure are new painful wounds to consider. The emergence of skin buds with healing is accompanied by cutaneous neuronal sprouting another new source of thermal hyperalgesia. Therefore, during the first few days and weeks after injury the liberal use of intravenous narcotics is warranted, often in a continuous infusion with additional agent administered for procedures.

Pain resistant to opiates may signal narcotic tolerance or the early onset of a neuropathic process that would respond better to tricyclic antidepressants or anticonvulsants. Tolerance is managed simply by increasing the dose of narcotic administered, titrating to effect.

TABLE 35.3. *Pain management strategies*

Drug	Route	Dose	Onset
Morphine	Intravenous	0.2–0.4 mg/kg q1–2h, infusion: 0.2–0.4 mg/kg/hr	5–8 min
	PCA	Bolus dose: 0.1 mg/kg, lockout: 6–8 min, 4-hr limit: none (titrate to effect)	
	Oral: prompt release	0.3–0.6 mg/kg q4h	0.5–1 hr
	Controlled release	0.3–0.6 mg/kg q8–12h	0.5–1 hr
Fentanyl	Intravenous	2–4 μg/kg q1–2h, infusion: 1–4 μg/kg/hr (titrate to effect)	1–2 min
	Transmucosal	10–20 μg/kg	8 min
	Transdermal	Adjust individually, minimal dose: 25 μg	6–12 hr
Acetaminophen	Oral	10–15 mg/kg q4–6h	0.5 hr
	Rectal	Initial: 30–40 mg/kg, subsequent: 20 mg/kg q6–8h	1 hr
Codeine	Oral	0.5–1 mg/kg q6h	0.5–1 hr
Ibuprofen	Oral	10 mg/kg q8h	0.5 hr
Ketorolac	Oral	0.2 mg/kg q8h	0.5 hr
	Intravenous	0.5 mg/kg q8h (48-hr use only)	10 min

PCA, patient-controlled analgesia.

When a neuropathic pain state is suspected or when escalating doses of narcotics are ineffective, alternative agents can be employed. An infusion of intravenous lidocaine has been a useful adjunct in this situation in the acute injury setting (20). Even with a plasma concentration of 1 μg/mL lidocaine, by which motor and sensory function should be little affected, there is significant reduction of the spontaneous firing of neurons, both peripherally and at the dorsal horn, that is characteristic of neuropathic pain (21) (Table 35.4).

In less severe injury or as time progresses, patient- and parent/nurse-controlled analgesia are very effective for the management of procedural and rest pain, even in small children (22). If the patient is enterally fed, oral administration of immediate- and sustained-release opioid preparations can also be appropriate and effective (23). Transmucosal (24, 25) and transcutaneous fentanyl preparations are also reasonable choices in this setting, as is acetaminophen or nonsteroidal anti-inflammatory agents (26,27). Nonsteroidal anti-inflammatory agents should be reserved for use after the initial resuscitation and stabilization period when the relative risks of bleeding and renal insufficiency are more tolerable (Table 35.3).

The most useful adjunct class of drugs for sedation and anxiolysis in this setting is the benzodiazepines. Midazolam and lorazepam are equally effective. Both agents can precipitate respiratory depression and hemodynamic instability when used in combination with an opioid; therefore, caution is recommended. Because anxiety always accompanies burn injury, the liberal administration of benzodiazepines is suggested for both the patient at rest and the patient undergoing a therapeutic procedure (Table 35.5).

Ketamine has also been used extensively in the burned child as an intravenous anesthetic and amnestic, particularly for the daily burn procedure. Ketamine can be exploited as an analgesic and a dissociative anesthetic. Ketamine acts at the *N*-methyl-D-aspartate subtype of the glutamate receptor (28,29). This recep-

TABLE 35.4. *Treatment for neuropathic pain*

Drug	Route	Dose
Amitriptyline	Oral	0.1–2 mg/kg qhs, start at low dose and increase slowly; may be given in divided doses q8h
Gabapentin	Oral	3–5 mg/kg q8h, begin with one dose qhs, increase frequency as tolerated
Lidocaine	Intravenous	20 μg/kg/min (adjust for level 1–2 μg/mL)

TABLE 35.5. *Adjuncts for sedation, analgesia, and pruritus*

Drug	Route	Dose	Onset
Midazolam	Intravenous	0.1 mg/kg q1h infusion: 0.05–0.2 mg/kg/hr	2–5 min
	Oral	0.5–1.0 mg/kg (single dose)	10–20 min
Lorazepam	Intravenous	0.05 mg/kg q6–8h	10–20 min
	Oral	0.05 mg/kg q6h	0.5–1 hr
Propofol	Intravenous	30–150 μg/kg/min (must be titrated) 5–10 μg/kg/min for itching	2–3 min
Ketamine	Intravenous	0.5–2.0 mg/kg q20min	1–2 min
	Oral	5–10 mg/kg (one dose)	15–30 min
Diphenhydramine	Oral, intravenous	1–2 mg/kg q4–6h	15–30 min
Hydroxyzine	Oral, intravenous	0.5–1.0 mg/kg q4–6h	15–30 min
Cyproheptadine	Oral	2–4 mg/dose q8h (maximum, 16 mg/day)	30–60 min
Ondansetron	Oral, intravenous	0.15 mg/kg q8h	15–30 min
Naloxone	Intravenous	0.5–1.0 μg/kg/hr infusion	1–2 min

tor is thought to be particularly important in the pain caused by tissue and nerve injury, which may account for the efficacy of ketamine in the burn care setting. Patients are comfortable and amnestic; however, side effects can be problematic. Respiratory depression is uncommon as is hemodynamic instability. Hallucinations are common and disturbing, particularly if no benzodiazepine pretreatment is given (30). As significant side effects can occur with ketamine, it is best used under the supervision of an anesthesiologist (Table 35.5).

Although less often described in relation to the burned child, propofol infusion in combination with an analgesic is another reasonable alternative for management of painful daily procedures in this patient population. Hypotension and respiratory depression may occur so that patient selection and monitoring are imperative (31). Propofol infusion as a long-term sedative in the burned child may also help to moderate the anxiety that accompanies this injury, but, as with all children, the potential induction of serious metabolic acidosis limits its safety (32). In the spontaneously breathing child, propofol should be used only under the direction of an anesthesiologist (Table 35.5).

Inhalation of nitrous oxide and oxygen is a useful tool to control procedural pain (33). Scavenging can be problematic and in combination with narcotics, the patient may be induced into a state of general anesthesia with the risk of significant respiratory depression. The supervision of an anesthesiologist is mandatory.

The induction of general anesthesia has been demonstrated to be safe and very effective for debridement and dressing changes when given in a treatment room of a burn unit under the direct care of an anesthesiologist (34). A well-designed general anesthetic results in a completely comfortable child and a recovery period that can be quite brief. Logistics and resources make this the gold standard, but it is not often feasible.

The use of α_2 agonist therapy has not been described in the burn patient except as a tool to facilitate withdrawal of narcotic therapy. Clearly, as a class of drugs, these agents are potent analgesics. However, there are animal data that suggest that in sepsis, mortality is dramatically increased after the administration of α_2 agonists (35). In the acute setting, when infection is a real risk to these children, α_2 agonist therapy should be withheld and opiates substituted.

Local and regional anesthetic techniques can be used before harvesting skin for grafting and are effective for donor site pain management (36,37). The postoperative application of topical local anesthetic solutions to donor sites or the intraoperative subcutaneous injection of donor sites with dilute local anesthetic solutions can reduce narcotic requirements (38,39). In addition, the early use of biologic dressings to close wounds alleviates the pain associated with new skin growth (40). Although there are no data exploring the use of paraspinal opiates in burn injury, this modality of treatment, employed by the author frequently in this patient population, can be very effective and can facilitate more rapid weaning from mechanical ventilation.

Nonpharmacologic adjuncts can be very useful in the acute phase of burn injury. The patient must be able to cooperate with the process chosen. The use of distraction therapy with video virtual reality and hypnosis has been tested in a limited number of adolescents with large burns. Each has proven effective in reducing narcotic requirements and pain perception scores (41–44). These are limited experiences, although results are encouraging. In the young child, parental participation can reduce the child's experience of pain during invasive procedures and may also improve parental understanding and compliance with long-term care goals (45).

In the healing phase of burn injury, itching can plague the patient, and in the acute phase of burn injury, it can complicate the generous use of narcotics. The cause of pruritus is not well understood. The sensation is initiated by chemical, mechanical, and thermal stimuli and transmitted by nonmyelinated C fibers in the epidermis and the dermoepidermal junction. These fibers travel to the dorsal horn of the spinal cord, synapse with the spinothalamic tract, and ultimately terminate in the postcentral gyrus (46).

The prototypical chemical itch mediator is histamine, although there are many others. Serotonin, proteases, prostaglandins, and a variety of peptides (e.g., substance P, endorphins) all can produce or enhance itching. All are present in the acute and the healing burn wound. Effective therapy can be difficult and frustrating for the patient and the clinician. Antagonists targeting the chemomediators of itching are useful in this setting (i.e., the antihistamines, antiserotonin agents, and the low-dose narcotic antagonists). Low-dose propofol infusion (5 to 10 μg/kg per minute) has also been given with some success (Table 35.5).

Permanent pain is unusual in burn patients, but healing and rehabilitation often take years. Physical therapy and pressure garments, worn to reduce scarring, produce pain and discomfort. Dysesthesias within the burn scar are seen in 80% of patients at 1 year postburn (47). However, this is a patient population that has not been well studied. Recommendations for treatment must be derived from those made for other pathologic conditions. Psychologic evaluation needs to parallel the physical evaluation. Biofeedback, hypnosis, antidepressants, and anticonvulsants may all be useful. A multidisciplinary approach is essential. Regular re-evaluation and follow-up are crucial to a successful intervention as is true for other neuropathic pain states.

ADDICTION AND TOLERANCE

There are no data to suggest that burned children are any more likely than other hospitalized patients to become addicted to the narcotics that they require for their painful injuries (48). More precisely, there are no data. Tolerance to narcotics and opioid abstinence syndromes are both seen in these children, and the clinician must be careful to taper the doses of opiates slowly to avoid symptoms of withdrawal. Reduction of drug dose by 20% per week is prudent.

CONCLUSIONS

The first dressing change for a burned child and each one thereafter should be perfect. Adequate analgesia and amnesia should be given by a dedicated provider to avoid the haunting of that child, preserve his or her trust, and avoid the "private nightmare" that burn care can become. That is the ideal world. Less than that can change the quality of his or her life for long after the burn scar is formed. These are some of the most vulnerable and challenging children in pain that there are in health care today, and they are often all but forgotten.

REFERENCES

1. Brigham PA, McLoughlin E. Burn incidence and medical care use in the United States: estimate, trends and data sources. *J Burn Care Rehabil* 1996;17:95–107.
2. Ryan CM, Schoenfeld DA, Thorpe WP, et al. Objective estimates of the probability of death from burn injuries. *N Engl J Med* 1998;338:362–366.
3. Hansbrough J, Hansbrough W. Pediatric burns. *Pediatr Rev* 1999;20:117–120.
4. Pedersen JL, Kehlet H. Hyperalgesia in a human model of acute inflammatory pain: a methodological study. *Pain* 1998;74:139–151.
5. Treede RD, Meyer RA, Raja SN, et al. Peripheral and central mechanisms of cutaneous hyperalgesia. *Prog Neurobiol* 1992;38:397–421.
6. Devor M. Neuropathic pain and injured nerve-peripheral mechanisms. *Br Med Bull* 1991;47:619–630.
7. Tanelian DL, Monroe S. Altered thermal responsiveness during regeneration of corneal cold fibers. *J Neurophys* 1995;73:1568–1573.
8. Choiniere M, Melzack R, Rondeau J, et al. The pain of burns: characteristics and correlates. *J Trauma* 1989;29: 1531–1539.
9. Jonsson CE, Holmsten A, Dahlstrom L, et al. Background pain in burn patients: routine measurement and recording of pain intensity in a burn unit. *Burns* 1998;24:448–454.
10. Henry DB, Foster RL. Burn pain management in children. *Pediatr Clin North Am* 2000;47:681–698.
11. Franck LS, Greenberg CS, Stevens B. Pain assessment in infants and children. *Pediatr Clin North Am* 2000;47: 487–512.
12. MacLennan N, Heimbach DM, Cullen BF. Anesthesia for major thermal injury. *Anesthesiology* 1998;89: 749–766.
13. Furman WR, Munster AM, Cone EJ, Morphine pharmacokinetics during anesthesia and surgery with burns. *J Burn Care Rehabil* 1990;11:391–394.
14. Perry S, Inturrisi C. Analgesia and morphine disposition in burn patients. *J Burn Care Rehabil* 1983;4:276–279.
15. Herman RA, Veng Pedersen P, Miotto J, et al. Pharmacokinetics of morphine sulfate in patients with burns. *J Burn Care Rehabil* 1994;15:95–103.
16. Kealey GP. Pharmacologic management of background pain in burn victims. *J Burn Care Rehabil* 1995;15: 358–362.
17. Choiniere M, Melzack R, Rondeau J, et al. The pain of burns: characteristics and correlates. *J Trauma* 1989;11: 1531–1539.
18. Jonsson CE, Holmsten A, Dahlstrom L, et al. Background pain in burn patients: routine measurement and recording of pain intensity in a burn unit. *Burns* 1998; 24:448–454.
19. Ashburn MA. Burn pain: the management of procedure related pain. *J Burn Care Rehabil* 1995;16:365–371.
20. Jonsson A, Cassuto J, Hanson B. Inhibition of burn pain by intravenous lignocaine infusion. *Lancet* 1991;338: 151–152.
21. Chaplan SR, Bach FW, Shafer SL, et al. Prolonged alleviation of tactile allodynia by intravenous lidocaine in neuropathic rats. *Anesthesiology* 1995;83:775–785.
22. Gaukroger P, Chapman J, Davey R. Pain control in pediatric burns—the use of patient controlled analgesia. *Burns* 1995;17:396–399.
23. Alexander L, Wolman R, Blache C, et al. Use of morphine sulfate (MS Contin) in patients with burns: a pilot study. *J Burn Care Rehabil* 1992;13:581–583.
24. Lind G, Marcus M, Mears S, et al. Oral transmucosal fentanyl citrate for analgesia and sedation in the emergency department. *Ann Emerg Med* 1991;20: 1117–1120.
25. Kahana, MD. Analgesia with oral transmucosal fentanyl citrate for burn wound dressing changes in children. *Pediatr Pain* 1995(abst).
26. Meyer WJ, Nichols RJ, Cortiella J, et al. Acetaminophen in the management of background pain in children post burn. *J Pain Symptom Manage* 1997;13:50–55.
27. Birmingham PK, Tobin MJ, Fisher DM, et al. Initial and subsequent dosing of rectal acetaminophen in children. *Anesthesiology* 2001;94:385–389.
28. Tverskoy M, Oren M, Vaskovich M, et al. Ketamine enhances local anesthetic and analgesic effects of bupivacaine by peripheral mechanism: a study in postoperative patients. *Neurosci Lett* 1996;215:5–8.
29. Jackson DL, Graff CB, Richardson JD, et al. Glutamate participates in the peripheral modulation of thermal hyperalgesia in rats. *Eur J Pharmacol* 1995;284:321–325.
30. Reich DL, Silvay G. Ketamine: an update on the first twenty-five years of clinical experience. *Can J Anaesth* 1989;36:186–197.
31. Kataria BK, Ved SA, Nicodemus BF. The pharmacokinetics of propofol in children using three different data analysis approaches, *Anesthesiology* 1994;80:104–122.
32. Strickland RA, Murray MJ. Fatal metabolic acidosis in a pediatric patient receiving an infusion of propofol in the intensive care unit: is there a relationship? *Crit Care Med* 1995;23:2:405–409.
33. Filkin SA, Cosram P, Marvin JA. Self-administered analgesia: a method of pain control. *J Burn Care Rehabil* 1981;2:33–44.
34. Dimick P, Helvig E, Heimbach D, et al. Anesthesia assisted procedures in a burn intensive care unit procedure room: benefits and complications. *J Burn Care Rehabil* 1993;14:446–449.
35. Conran A, Wischmeyer P, Wolfson R, et al. Alpha 2 agonists increase anesthetic mortality in a rat model of endotoxemia, *Anesthesiology* 2000(abst).
36. Pedersen JL, Crawford ME, Dahl JB. Effect of preemptive nerve block on inflammation and hyperalgesia after human thermal injury. *Anesthesiology* 1996;84: 1020–1026.
37. Beausang E. Subcutaneous adrenaline infiltration in paediatric burn surgery. *Br J Plast Surg* 1999;52:480–481.
38. Jellish WS, Gamelli RL, Furry PA. Effect of topical local anesthetic application to skin harvest sites for pain management in burn patients undergoing skin grafting procedures. *Ann Surg* 1999;229:115–125.
39. Brofelt B, Cornwell P, Doherty D, et al. Topical lidocaine in the treatment of partial thickness burns. *J Burn Care Rehabil* 1989;10:63(abst).
40. Barret JP, Dziewulski P, Ramzy PI, et al. Biobrane versus 1% silver sulfadiazine in second degree pediatric burns. *Plast Reconstr Surg* 2000;105:62–65.
41. Hoffman HG, Doctor JN, Patterson DR, et al, Virtual reality as an adjunctive pain control during burn wound care in adolescent patients. *Pain* 2000;85305–309.
42. Patterson DR. Non-opioid based approaches to burn pain. *J Burn Care Rehabil* 1995;16:372–376.
43. Patterson D, Everett J, Burns G, et al. Hypnosis for the

treatment of burn pain. *J Consult Clin Psychol* 1992;60: 713–717.

44. Miller A, Hickman L, Lemasters G. A distraction technique for control of burn pain. *J Burn Care Rehabil* 1992;13:576–580.
45. George A, Hancock J. Reducing pediatric burn pain with parent participation. *J Burn Care Rehabil* 1993;14: 104–107.
46. Koblenzer C, Atopic dermatitis—an update for the next millennium, itching and the atopic skin. *J Allergy Clin Immunol* 1999;104:3.
47. Choiniere M, Melzack R, Papillon J. Pain and paresthesia in patients with healed burns: an exploratory study. *J Pain Symptom Manage* 1991;6:437–444.
48. Hedderich R, Ness TJ. Analgesia for trauma and burns. *Crit Care Clin* 1999;15:167–184.

36

Sedation and Analgesia in the Emergency Department

Steven M. Selbst and William T. Zempsky

Children frequently seek care in the emergency department for the relief of pain from traumatic injuries and other painful medical conditions. Acute pain serves a useful function and is necessary for survival. Acute pain warns children to avoid particular stimuli and tells the individual that tissue damage has occurred (1). Acute pain also helps the emergency department physician to localize an injury or infection and often helps to confirm a diagnosis. For instance, the diagnosis of cellulitis depends on finding a tender, erythematous lesion on a child's skin. Likewise, the diagnosis of appendicitis is characteristically determined by localized tenderness in the right lower abdominal quadrant, along with symptoms of vomiting and fever. Although acute pain and tenderness are important, chronic pain serves no useful function. Thus, efforts must be made to quickly alleviate a child's pain and suffering.

In some cases, an emergency department physician must inflict pain on an already uncomfortable child to make a correct diagnosis or appropriately manage a child's injury or illness. Laboratory tests and painful repositioning of a child are frequently necessary and unavoidable in the emergency department. Although such procedures and maneuvers cannot realistically be eliminated, efforts must be made to minimize the associated pain.

The field of emergency medicine has assumed a leadership role in pain management. Research in the area of pediatric pain control in the acute care setting has increased dramatically in recent years. Despite the progress made, pain control is still neglected for many children in the emergency department (2–5). In 1990, Selbst and Clark (2) reported that 60% of adult patients in the emergency department setting received analgesia for burns and fractures compared with 28% of pediatric patients with similar conditions. In that study, emergency department physicians and pediatricians were equally unlikely to give analgesics to children. Since then, there have been great advances in the recognition, assessment, and management of pain in children. The care of infants and children who undergo painful procedures in the emergency department has improved considerably. However, two more recent studies (3,4) showed that children still do not receive appropriate analgesia for painful conditions. Inadequate dosing of medications for children on discharge from the emergency department remains a significant problem (2,4).

The reasons for inadequate pain control of children in the emergency department have not been established with certainty. One can speculate that many pediatricians and emergency department physicians expect babies and young children to cry, so this nonspecific response to pain is usually tolerated and not controlled. Also, because young children and infants often cannot verbalize or localize their pain, physicians may ignore their pain or assume it does not exist (6). This may explain why children younger than 2 years of age are less likely than older children to receive analgesic medications (2). In addition, fear of addiction to opiate medications may cause some physicians to keep them from young children even in an acute situation. This fear is unfounded, and addiction from short-term use of opiates to treat acute pain is extremely rare

(7–9). Emergency department physicians may also withhold opiate analgesics because they fear side effects such as respiratory depression and hypotension. These side effects are less likely if drugs are used in appropriate doses. Such adverse effects should be manageable in the emergency department, and the potential problems do not justify leaving a child in severe pain (6). Other physicians withhold analgesics because they fear this will mask symptoms. Although pain and tenderness play an important role in diagnosis, children should not be left to suffer once evaluated. Finally, many physicians are still not familiar with techniques for pain control or medication doses for children. Thus, they avoid their use in pediatric patients. Instead of giving analgesics, emergency department physicians may use brute force to complete a painful procedure or evaluation, while convincing the young child that "this will only hurt for a minute" (1). Table 36.1 lists possible reasons why children do not receive adequate analgesia in the emergency department.

The most common indications for procedural sedation and analgesia in one emergency department were orthopedic fracture and dislocation reduction (30%), diagnostic imaging studies (22%), repair of lacerations (27%), abscess drainage (4%), arthrocentesis (3%), lumbar puncture (3%), and other (11%) (10). This chapter addresses several methods for pain management in the emergency department. Analgesic medications are the mainstay for controlling pain, but other techniques and nonpharmacologic means of reducing pain are discussed. Table 36.2 lists the desired characteristics of the ideal analgesic in the emergency department.

TABLE 36.1. *Reasons for inadequate pain control in the pediatric emergency department*

Pain is not recognized
Infants and young children do not verbalize
Babies are "supposed" to cry
Misconception that infants cannot feel pain
Misconception that children will not remember pain
Misconception that children will get addicted to narcotics
Fear of respiratory depression, hypotension
Fear of masking symptoms
Other conditions take priority
Unfamiliarity with analgesics, doses

TABLE 36.2. *Ideal analgesic in the emergency department*

Rapid onset
Short duration of effect
Easily administered
Effective analgesia
Minimal side effects

MINOR INJURIES: STRAINS AND SPRAINS

Children frequently present to the emergency department with painful conditions such as contusions, strains, and sprains. Most often, resting and splinting the injured body part can reduce pain from minor injuries. In addition, pain control is usually accomplished with orally administered, nonopiate medications such as acetaminophen, ibuprofen, and aspirin. Opiate medications such as codeine are also good alternatives.

Acetaminophen is an excellent choice to treat pain from sprains and minor injuries. Acetaminophen acts on nonopioid receptors in the brain to inhibit prostaglandin synthetase. Acetaminophen is somewhat expensive but is well tolerated and comes in liquid form, so it can be more easily administered to young children. One study of postpartum pain showed that 1,000 mg acetaminophen is equal to 60 mg codeine (11). Acetaminophen does not cause bleeding and does not cause bronchospasm in asthmatics (12,13). It is best dosed at 15 mg/kg every 4 hours. It exhibits an effect in 20 to 40 minutes, with a peak effect in 2 hours. Acetaminophen has no anti-inflammatory effects. Therapeutic doses are rarely associated with side effects, but overdose can cause liver toxicity (13).

Nonsteroidal anti-inflammatory drugs such as ibuprofen are extremely valuable to treat minor pain from musculoskeletal injuries. Ibuprofen is believed to be more potent than aspirin and has a longer half-life (14). Nonsteroidal anti-inflammatory drugs are thought to interfere with the formation of cyclooxygenase

TABLE 36.3. *Analgesics for painful minor injuries*

Analgesic	Advantages	Disadvantages
Acetaminophen	Well tolerated, safe	Liver toxicity if overdosed
Ibuprofen	Long duration of action	Gastrointestinal irritation
Codeine	Potent opioid analgesia	Nausea, constipation

products produced in injured tissues. These products sensitize nerve endings and produce pain (13). The usual dose is 10 mg/kg given orally every 6 hours (13). The recommended dose for older children is 400 mg every 4 to 6 hours for mild to moderate pain. Ibuprofen is available in liquid form, making it suitable for use in very young children. Ibuprofen is nonaddictive and does not cause respiratory or cardiac depression. It may cause gastrointestinal bleeding, but this risk is small (15). These agents also cause renal and hepatic dysfunction and should be used with caution in children with renal or hepatic disease. Their effect on platelets (acetylation) is reversible. Nonsteroidal anti-inflammatory drugs can cause sodium retention, and they have cross-reactivity with aspirin, so they should not be used with patients who have aspirin sensitivity (14).

The use of aspirin for pain management in children has declined in recent years. Aspirin has been associated with Reye syndrome when used to treat varicella and flu-like illnesses. This has not been noted when the medication is used to control pain from minor trauma. However, other medications mentioned above have gained popularity.

Finally, codeine is a safe, effective narcotic analgesic that can be given to children to control pain from minor injuries. Codeine has a low addiction potential. It is usually given orally at a dose of 0.8 to 1.5 mg/kg every 4 to 6 hours (14). Codeine can be made into a liquid for use with young children. It is helpful to combine the drug with acetaminophen to produce an even greater analgesic effect than when either agent is used alone (12). Codeine has the potential to cause respiratory depression, but this rarely occurs. It has no renal or hepatic toxicity and does not alter platelet function. Like other opiates, it can cause nausea and vomiting, which limits its usefulness.

The benefits of the above analgesics far outweigh the few side effects involved with their use in young children. Table 36.3 summarizes the advantages and disadvantages of these analgesics for treating painful minor injuries in children.

FRACTURES

Children with fractures are often in obvious pain when they present to the emergency department. Older children are particularly distressed because they quickly recognize the disability associated with their injury. Younger children seem to tolerate pain from fractured extremities surprisingly well. As with minor injuries discussed previously, splinting and resting the injured extremity can reduce pain. Oral analgesics are useful to control mild pain, but intravenous opiate medications are ideal for those with displaced fractures. Further treatment will be required before attempted reduction of the fracture by an orthopedic surgeon.

Most opiate medications used to alleviate pain from fractures can cause important adverse effects such as respiratory depression and hypotension. However, these side effects are often dose related and may be reversed with naloxone, making opioids safe for use in the emergency department setting. These drugs should be used cautiously with infants younger than 6 months of age who are not ventilated because pharmacokinetic differences in young infants may predispose them to respiratory depression. Such infants should receive one-fourth to one-third of the initial calculated dose recommended for older children and should be closely monitored (14). Opioid analgesics can be given by various routes. In general, the intramuscular route should be avoided because the injection itself is quite painful and causes delayed drug absorption, and the dose given cannot be titrated. The intravenous route is more advantageous because titration is possible, although some pain is involved in starting the intravenous line (15).

Morphine is perhaps the gold standard for controlling severe pain from a fracture or other serious injury. The usual dose of morphine is 0.1 to 0.15 mg/kg given intravenously over a few minutes (17,18), and this can be safely repeated every 2 to 4 hours. In some cases, when a child is in severe pain, the dose is escalated. However, the patient must be carefully monitored for adverse effects. Fortunately, most children reach analgesia before the onset of respiratory depression (18). The maximal recommended dose is 10 mg for opioid-naïve subjects. The higher dose and a dosing interval of every 1 to 2 hours are suggested for those who receive narcotics often and perhaps have some tolerance to the drug. Subsequent doses may be reduced to 0.05 mg/kg if the patient is moderately sedated. When given intravenously, its effect is almost immediate, and the peak effect occurs in approximately 20 minutes. Morphine may cause pooling of blood by decreasing peripheral vascular resistance, which sometimes results in hypotension (19). However, this is only a great concern if the patient has a severe injury and shows signs of hypovolemia. The fluid status of an injured child requires careful attention from the emergency department staff. However, morphine need not be withheld once intravenous fluids have corrected volume depletion. If a child is awake, alert, and screaming in pain, morphine can be safely administered while the patient is carefully monitored.

Fentanyl is another useful agent for treating severe pain owing to fractures. This synthetic opioid is given slowly (over 3 to 5 minutes) at a dose of 2 to 3 μg/kg intravenously (14,18). It has a very rapid onset of action (a few minutes) and a short duration of action (30 to 40 minutes), which makes it quite useful in the emergency department. Fentanyl is a relatively safe drug. It rarely causes hypotension, making it an excellent choice for injured children with severe pain. A study of adult patients found that the drug caused hypotension in only 0.4% (alcohol intoxication may have been responsible for some of those cases). Hypotension may be unusual because histamine is not released when the drug is given (20).

Respiratory depression can occur within minutes of fentanyl administration, but this has been reported in only 0.7% of adult patients, (some of these may have also been intoxicated with alcohol) (20). Fentanyl-induced apnea occurs even less often and may be related to the rate of infusion rather than the dose (21). These adverse effects are serious; however, they can be reversed with naloxone and are less likely when dosage guidelines are followed and the drug is given slowly (21,22). It is always best to individualize dosing and titrate the drug to a desired effect to reduce side effects. Equipment and personnel to manage an obstructed airway should be nearby whenever fentanyl is used.

The most serious side effect, which is uncommonly caused by fentanyl, is neuromuscular blockade. This rare but frightening effect results in thoracic and abdominal muscle rigidity. This circumstance is expected only when high doses (>15 μg/kg) are used, and thus should not occur in the emergency department if dosing regimens are followed (21,22). Most often, this side effect is reversible with naloxone, but succinylcholine may be required. Despite the problems noted, fentanyl remains a valuable analgesic that should be used liberally in the emergency department when a child presents with severe pain.

Meperidine is another opioid agent that can be used to treat moderate to severe pain owing to a fracture. It can be given intravenously or intramuscularly at a dose of 0.5 to 1 mg/kg every 2 to 3 hours. The maximal recommended dose for opioid-naïve patients is 125 mg (23). Meperidine has few significant advantages over morphine. However, side effects include nervousness, tremors, disorientation, and even seizures when the medication is administered intravenously (24). Thus, morphine may be a better choice for severe pain unless a patient specifies that meperidine works better for him or her.

Ketorolac has not been well studied for treating pain caused by fractures in the emergency department. It is a parenteral nonsteroidal anti-inflammatory drug that inhibits prostaglandin synthesis and is considered a peripherally acting analgesic. It is not yet approved by the U.S. Food and Drug Administration for intravenous administration, but multiple studies have demonstrated this route to be safe and efficacious in children. It is generally given as a loading dose of 1 mg/kg intravenously to a maximum of 60 mg, followed by 0.5 mg/kg intravenously (30 mg maximum) every 6 hours (25). Ketorolac has been shown in children to be comparable with opiates for treatment of postoperative pain and orthopedic injuries, with less sedation and fewer side effects (25–27). Because it has no central action, it does not cause respiratory depression, nausea, or vomiting. In a recent study of children with isolated forearm fractures, ketorolac showed a trend toward pain relief (not statistically significant, small patient sample size). It did not have an opioid-sparing effect (25). Table 36.4 summarizes the medications commonly used to treat severe pain owing to fractures in children.

Fracture reduction in the emergency department is likely to be associated with significant pain. The child's anxiety will further exacerbate the pain. Thus, it is often useful to combine an anxiolytic with an analgesic medication before the painful procedure. Morphine or fentanyl is often combined with a short-acting sedative such as 0.1 to 0.2 mg/kg diazepam (28) or 0.05 to 0.2 mg/kg midazolam given slowly, intravenously every 15 minutes as needed. Midazolam may be preferable to diazepam because it has a shorter onset of action (approximately 5 minutes) and a more rapid recovery (approximately 1 to 4 hours). Combining a benzodiazepine and an opiate analgesic produces amnesia, sedation, and muscle relaxation, which is preferred for orthopedic procedures. One retrospective study of children undergoing orthopedic procedures found the combination of fentanyl and diazepam to be safe (28). The likelihood of respiratory depression increases with the use of a sedative, and proper precautions to protect the airway must be taken.

Nitrous oxide has been used for analgesia in emergency settings for more than 30 years. A few studies with pediatric patients showed it to be an effective agent for reducing discomfort while performing painful procedures including fracture reduction and reduction of dislocated radial head injuries (29,30). Nitrous oxide has numerous advantages for use in the emergency setting. For instance, it can be delivered in a painless way. In addition, it has a short duration of action and a sedative, dissociative effect on the patient. The child may complain of pain but does not seem to be experiencing pain (dissociative effect) and does not remember the pain later (amnesic effect). Patients who receive this gas feel like they are floating, drowsy, or euphoric. Effects are noted after 4 minutes with a nitrous oxide–oxygen mixture and dissipate approximately 4 to 5 minutes after the gas is removed. Nitrous oxide–oxygen mixture has been used on children as young as 16 months, but it is certainly more difficult to use in young, uncooperative children. It may be best for children 8 years of age and older (30). Masks for administering the gas can be flavored to help gain acceptance with young patients.

When used in a 50/50 mixture with oxygen, nitrous oxide provides analgesia, not anesthe-

TABLE 36.4. *Analgesics for severe pain owing to fractures*

Analgesic	Advantages	Disadvantages
Morphine	Rapid onset, potent analgesia	Respiratory depression, hypotension
Fentanyl	Potent analgesia, less hypotension	Respiratory depression, apnea
Meperidine	Potent analgesia	Respiratory depression, seizures
Ketorolac, tromethamine	Nonnarcotic	Not well studied in children

sia. The patient remains awake during a procedure and is able to follow instructions. When used properly in a mixture with more than 20% oxygen, nitrous oxide does not produce serious side effects (29,30). Nitrous oxide affects the cerebral cortex (not the brainstem); therefore, circulatory and respiratory depression does not occur and there is little relaxation of skeletal muscle. The gas is nonallergenic and not flammable or explosive but must be used with oxygen and will support combustion if a fire develops. A fail-safe system that shuts off the flow of nitrous oxide when there is no oxygen flow is imperative (30). A child can hold the mask on his or her face, so that it will fall off should the child become unresponsive. It can also be given with a nasal mask, enabling the patient to breathe through the mouth during the procedure. These precautions will avoid possible anoxia, which could be catastrophic. Some patients experience vomiting with nitrous oxide, but this effect is usually an inconvenience rather than a danger because the patients maintain their cough and gag reflexes. In one study (31), 7% of patients fell asleep with the gas, but they could all be easily aroused. Bone marrow suppression, testicular dysfunction, and liver and central nervous system disorders are only seen with chronic exposure to the gas (32).

One study showed that for suturing of facial wounds in young children (2 to 6 years old), regimens including continuous-flow 50% nitrous oxide were more effective in reducing distress than midazolam. This approach also had fewer adverse effects and shorter recovery times than oral midazolam. Although vomiting occurred more often in the group receiving nitrous oxide, there were no episodes of aspiration (33).

However, there are some limits to use of nitrous oxide (29,30). Personnel demands are great because there should be staff present who can manage an obstructed airway in an unconscious patient. In addition to the orthopedist who will reduce the fracture, an emergency department physician must be present to assist and deliver the gas. It is not recommended for children who are already sedated, unconscious, or intoxicated or who have head or chest injuries. In addition, the required equipment costs several thousand dollars. This equipment must be inspected daily to ensure safety. In addition, a scavenger device is needed to eliminate nitrous oxide from the emergency department so that workers and other patients do not experience the effects of the gas. A simple device can be attached to the machine to accomplish this (32).

Finally, not all patients report complete pain relief with nitrous oxide. Some studies have shown it to be very helpful in 80% to 95% of patients. There may be marked pain relief in one-third of patients and partial pain relief in the remaining two-thirds (30,31). Table 36.5 reviews the advantages and disadvantages of nitrous oxide–oxygen analgesia.

Ketamine hydrochloride has recently gained popularity for limiting pain during orthopedic procedures. It can provide intense analgesia at subanesthetic doses. It causes dissociative amnesia and a trance-like state in which the child can follow commands but cannot respond verbally (17,34–36). Thus, it is an excellent agent to reduce pain during reduction of even significantly displaced fractures. The drug can be given intramuscularly at a dose of 4 to 5 mg/kg (37). Preferably, the drug is given intravenously at a dose of 0.5 to 2 mg/kg (usually 1 mg/kg). Ketamine has the advantage of rapid onset of action: 1 minute if given intravenously, 5 to 10 minutes if given intramuscularly. It does not cause prolonged sedation, and a single intravenous dose has an effect for approximately 15 minutes (38). Ke-

TABLE 36.5. *Nitrous oxide–oxygen analgesia*

Advantages
- Rapid onset, short duration of action
- Produces sedation, amnesia, dissociation
- Useful when local anesthesia is impractical
- May be used for young children
- Safe when mixed with oxygen

Disadvantages
- Fail-safe system required
- Equipment is expensive
- Scavenger device needed
- Not all patients benefit
- Requires patient cooperation
- Requires more personnel

tamine can also be given orally (10 mg/kg), and sedation occurs in 30 to 45 minutes with duration of effect approximately 2 hours. A recent study in children found intravenous ketamine with midazolam was a more effective combination than fentanyl with midazolam for pain and anxiety relief during orthopedic procedures in the emergency department. Patients in that study had less respiratory depression than those receiving fentanyl (39).

Ketamine has few disadvantages beyond the pain of injection. Unusual, unpleasant sensations and dreams with subsequent flashbacks are rarely reported (38). Benzodiazepines given concomitantly with ketamine may decrease the likelihood of this reaction (40). However, a recent study showed midazolam given concurrently with ketamine had no beneficial effect in preventing mild agitation and may be unnecessary (41). In another prospective study, none of the children who received ketamine experienced nightmares (35). Ketamine can also cause increased production of saliva (11%) and vomiting on awakening (in approximately 6%). Excess salivation can be effectively prevented by previous administration of atropine (0.01 mg/kg) or glycopyrrolate (0.005 mg/kg) (38). Ketamine does not generally impair pharyngeal or laryngeal function or protective airway reflexes such as cough or swallowing. Thus, the risk of airway compromise is less with ketamine than some other agents. This is perhaps the major advantage of ketamine and the most important reason for its popularity in the emergency department. However, laryngospasm is a rare adverse effect, and precautions should be taken to manage the airway if this develops (42). Neonates and those with upper respiratory infection are more likely to have laryngospasm, and they should not get ketamine. Ketamine can also elevate blood pressure, intracranial pressure, and pulmonary artery pressure; therefore, those with head trauma, central nervous system malformations, and cardiovascular or respiratory disease should not receive this drug (18).

Propofol is a nonopioid, nonbarbiturate sedative-hypnotic agent generally given intravenously for sedation during short procedures. Propofol does not have analgesic properties of its own. This agent has been used infrequently in the emergency department, but one report found it effective when used in combination with fentanyl for fracture reduction in adult patients (43). Another recent study found that propofol (when combined with morphine analgesia) induced sedation as effectively as midazolam but with shorter recovery time when used while reducing fractures in children (44). Induction doses range from 1.0 to 3.0 mg/kg, with maintenance infusion rates for total intravenous anesthesia ranging from 75 to 300 μg/kg per minute. [Pediatric patients generally require bolus doses as much as 50% greater than those used for adults and maintenance rates 25% to 50% greater than those effective in adult patients (44).] Propofol is advantageous because it has a rapid onset of action, a rapid recovery phase, and amnesic properties. It is a potent sedative, associated with significant respiratory depression, and therefore great caution should be exercised with its use. Complication rates were low in the study by Havel et al. (44) but the patient sample size was small; therefore, routine use cannot yet be recommended. Mild transient hypoxemia was found in 11% (similar to a group receiving midazolam instead of propofol), and this was rapidly corrected with noninvasive measures (44). Green et al. (45) recommended great caution in the use of this agent in the emergency department. The *Physicians Desk Reference* (46) recommends that this agent be administered only by persons trained in administration of general anesthesia.

Other sedative agents are less desirable for fracture reduction in the emergency department. *Pentobarbital* is an agent that induces sedation rapidly after intravenous administration, and the effect dissipates in 30 to 60 minutes (18). Pentobarbital has no analgesic properties of its own and may increase pain perception and therefore is not ideal for painful procedures. When opiates are combined with 4 to 5 mg/kg pentobarbital, prolonged sedation may result, making the combination less convenient in a busy emergency department. It has greatest use for nonpainful procedures such as sedation for children undergoing imaging studies. Likewise, *chloral hydrate* is a pure sedative hypnotic with no analgesic properties. It is a relatively safe drug, but its sedation effect is variable and sometimes long lasting, making it less desirable for use in the emergency department (18). It is generally unhelpful for fracture reduction.

Combining opioids with phenothiazines is also not recommended. For years, the combination of 2 mg/kg meperidine, 1 mg/kg promethazine, and 1 mg/kg chlorpromazine was used to provide sedation and analgesia. However, this combination requires a painful intramuscular injection and may promote the sedative effect of the opiate without the analgesic effect (6,18). Moreover, this combination can produce prolonged sedation, and its use is not recommended in the emergency department (47,48).

In some emergency departments, fractures are reduced with a *mini-Bier-block* using lidocaine for regional anesthesia (49). The mini-Bier block involves a double pneumatic tourniquet or two blood pressure cuffs placed above the elbow (49–51). The child is attached to a cardiac monitor, and an intravenous line is started in both upper extremities. One of these intravenous lines is established for administration of medications that may be needed to stop a seizure. Diazepam, midazolam, and thiopental should be available for use if complications develop. The affected limb is elevated and exsanguinated as the upper cuff is inflated to occlude the arterial blood supply. Then lidocaine (without epinephrine) is infused into the intravenous line of the affected extremity at a dose of 1.5 mg/kg (100 mg maximum). Tourniquet pressure must be maintained, and the injection of local anesthetic into the limb should be performed slowly to avoid generating supra-arterial pressure in the limb venous system, leading to escape of the drug under the tourniquet. The injured extremity will receive a significant amount of anesthetic in an isolated compartment. Next, the lower cuff is inflated. Once inflated, the upper cuff is deflated so the lower cuff is wrapped around an anesthetized part of the extremity. After the procedure and at least 15 minutes after infusion of the lidocaine, the lower blood pressure cuff can be slowly deflated. The child should be observed for as long as 1 hour in the emergency department (51). Some prefer to reserve this technique for use in more controlled circumstances such as the operating room.

LACERATION REPAIR

Repair of lacerations in the emergency department should be essentially painless (Table 36.6). Tetracaine, adrenaline, and cocaine (TAC) was the first topical anesthetic useful in laceration repair. TAC provides excellent and painless anesthesia for facial lacerations. TAC is comparable with lidocaine infiltration in that repair of facial lacerations can be accomplished approximately 90% of the time without additional anesthetic (52–54). The efficacy of TAC in extremity and trunk lacerations is reduced to approximately 50% (54,55). This is likely owing to the decreased vascularization of the extremities, which decreases uptake of the anesthetic through the wound. Unfortunately, TAC use has been associated with disorientation, seizures, and death secondary to the systemic absorption of cocaine (56,57). In these cases, TAC was placed near mucous membranes or dripped into the eye. The toxicity and expense of cocaine have caused TAC to be replaced by other formulations that are both safer and less

TABLE 36.6. *Reducing pain of wound closure*

Topical anesthetics
TAC (tetracaine, adrenaline, and cocaine)
LET (lidocaine, epinephrine, and tetracaine)
EMLA (lidocaine, prilocaine)
Bupivanor (bupivicaine with norepinephrine)
Lidocaine infiltration
Tissue adhesives
Dermabond
Histoacryl blue
Steri-strips

expensive. TAC should no longer be used as an anesthetic for wound repair.

A topical anesthetic suitable for wound anesthesia should contain both a local anesthetic and a vasoconstrictor. LET (lidocaine, epinephrine, and tetracaine) can be made by a hospital pharmacy as a liquid or gel preparation and provides wound anesthesia comparable with that of TAC (58,59). This anesthetic takes 20 to 30 minutes to be effective (58,59). The liquid preparation can be placed on a cotton ball and held or taped into the wound that requires anesthesia. LET gel is prepared by mixing the LET solution with methylcellulose (60). The gel is placed in the wound and then covered with an occlusive dressing. LET gel is at least as efficacious as the solution (60). LET should not be used on the digits or genitalia because of the vasoconstrictive nature of epinephrine nor should it be placed on mucous membranes because of the increased risk of anesthetic absorption at these sites. Wounds amenable to topical anesthesia should be clean, carry a low risk of infection, and be less than 5 cm in length. Another topical anesthetic, Bupivanor, a combination of bupivacaine and norepinephrine, has also been shown as effective as TAC or lidocaine infiltration for facial and scalp wound anesthesia (61).

For those centers where LET or other similar solutions are not available, eutectic mixture of local anesthetics [EMLA (lidocaine-prilocaine cream)], which is commercially available, also provides topical anesthesia for laceration repair (55,62). Lidocaine-prilocaine cream is superior to TAC for extremity laceration anesthesia where it can be used without adjunctive anesthesia in approximately 80% of cases (55). Unfortunately, lidocaine-prilocaine cream takes an hour to be effective even in open wounds (55). It should be placed on amenable wounds after triage to allow anesthesia to occur while maintaining adequate patient flow in the emergency department.

Other means of wound closure that are less painful should also be considered. Tissue adhesives, such as octylcyanoacrylate (Dermabond) and butylcyanoacrylate (Histoacryl Blue), cause significantly less pain during application than simple interrupted sutures for repair of low tension wounds, while providing equivalent cosmetic outcome (63–65). Steri-Strips provide similar painless closure and are underutilized.

For those wounds not amenable to or not sufficiently anesthetized by topical anesthetics, infiltration with either 0.5% or 1.0% lidocaine is necessary. The dose should not exceed 3 to 5 mg/kg. Lidocaine with epinephrine can also be used (7-mg/kg dose), which will decrease the bleeding associated with wound repair. As with the topical anesthetics containing a vasoconstrictor, lidocaine with epinephrine should not be used in areas supplied by end arteries such as the digits, genitalia, or ear pinna.

Lidocaine can be injected in an almost painless manner (Table 36.7). The clinician should shield the patient from visualizing the needle during preparation of the medication as well as the injection. Pain of injection can be minimized by buffering the anesthetic with bicarbonate, warming the lidocaine before injection, and injecting slowly into the wound with a small gauge needle (66–70). Buffering lidocaine decreases the pain of injection by neutralizing the acidic pH of lidocaine (66,69), which is done by mixing lidocaine and bicarbonate in a 9:1 ratio (66). Buffered lidocaine can be made as needed in the emergency department or in advance and will remain stable for approximately 30 days (71,72). Warming lidocaine to body temperature before injection has also been shown to decrease the pain of injection (67). By slowly administering small amounts of lidocaine and then advancing the needle through the anesthetized area, the pain associated with tissue

TABLE 36.7. *Techniques to decrease the pain of lidocaine infiltration*

Buffer with bicarbonate (9 mL lidocaine/1 mL $NaHCO_3$)
Warm to body temperature
Inject slowly
Use small needle (30 gauge)
Inject into wound

distention during infiltration can be minimized (68). The needle should be inserted into the open wound, which is less painful than injecting through the intact dermis (70).

VENIPUNCTURE AND INTRAVENOUS ACCESS

The child who requires venipuncture, intravenous access, injection, or other percutaneous procedures in the emergency department poses a dilemma for the clinician who wishes to make this a painless procedure. The urgent or emergent nature of these procedures limits the use of adequate pain control. Recent advances have demonstrated that many percutaneous procedures can be performed painlessly even in the emergency department (Table 36.8).

Ample evidence exists that lidocaine-prilocaine cream is an excellent transdermal anesthetic for procedures such as venipuncture, intravenous placement, and injection (73–76). This is a combination of 2.5% lidocaine and 2.5% prilocaine that is placed under an occlusive dressing over the site to be anesthetized (62). However, it requires at least 1 hour to provide adequate analgesia, which has been a barrier to its effective use in the busy emergency department. Fein et al. (77) showed that in large children's hospital's emergency department, 90% of patients wait more than an hour from the time of triage to have intravenous access attempted. Using a combination of clinical criteria and an experienced triage nurse's assessment, it is possible to predict which patients will need venous access with some degree of accuracy (78). The lidocaine-prilocaine cream can then be placed on patients in triage minimizing the inappropriate use of the anesthetic while maximizing the number of painless procedures.

TABLE 36.8. *Reducing pain of percutaneous procedures*

EMLA (lidocaine-prilocaine cream)
Amethocaine
Lidocaine iontophoresis
Lidocaine infiltration
Vapocoolant sprays

Amethocaine (tetracaine) 4% gel appears be a superior alternative to lidocaine-prilocaine cream for the emergency setting in that it has a 30- to 45-minute application time and provides superior anesthesia before venous cannulation (79,80). The comparison study of Romsing et al. (80) of 60 children showed those receiving amethocaine for 45 minutes had significantly lower pain scores for venous cannulation than those with lidocaine-prilocaine cream applied for 1 hour (80). Although available in Britain and Canada, amethocaine is not currently available in the United States. Amethocaine gel is placed over the site to be anesthetized and then covered with an occlusive dressing similar to the placement of lidocaine-prilocaine cream (79,80).

Lidocaine iontophoresis (Numby Stuff) uses a low-level electric current to deliver an ionized form of 2% lidocaine with epinephrine into the skin before invasive procedures (81). During iontophoresis, a positively charged drug such as lidocaine is repelled through the skin by a positively charged electrode. The iontophoretic unit is powered by a 9-V battery connected to the patient by two oppositely charged electrodes (81). Lidocaine with epinephrine is instilled into the positive hydrogel electrode; this electrode is placed over the area to be anesthetized and connected to the iontophoretic unit by a wire carrying the positive charge (81). A negative or "dispersive" electrode formulated from karaya gum is placed on the patient at least 4 to 6 cm away from the drug delivery electrode. A 1- to 4-mA current is then turned on allowing drug delivery to occur. The iontophoretic dose is calculated as a product of current and time and recorded in the unit milliampere-minutes. Effective anesthesia requires a total iontophoretic dose of 30 to 40 milliampere-minutes (81).

Two pediatric emergency department trials found lidocaine iontophoresis effective for reducing the pain of venous cannulation compared with a placebo (82,83). The major advantage of lidocaine iontophoresis is its speed; anesthesia can be achieved in approximately 10 minutes (82). Success in providing venous access is unaffected by this method of anesthesia (82). The depth of anesthesia achieved with iontophoresis is 8 to 10 mm versus approximately 3 to 5 mm with lidocaine-prilocaine cream (84,85). No systemic lidocaine levels are detected during routine use of this device (86). A major complaint concerning iontophoresis is the tingling associated with drug delivery. Many children report no sensation; however, some complain of itching or burning with drug delivery. Zempsky et al. (82) found that the iontophoresis can be completed successfully in approximately 95% of children by gradually increasing the current to allow accommodation to the sensation and using distraction techniques (82). Partial thickness burns are a rare but significant side effect of iontophoresis (87).

Lidocaine injected intradermally with a small-gauge needle can rapidly provide anesthesia before venous cannulation (88). Lidocaine used for this technique should be buffered, as discussed in the wound anesthesia section (66). With proper technique, anesthesia can be achieved painlessly, decreasing the pain of venous cannulation without affecting the success of venous access (39). Alternatively, saline with benzyl alcohol preservative injected intradermally has been shown to provide equivalent anesthesia to 1% lidocaine before intravenous line placement (89).

Ethyl chloride and other refrigerant or vapocoolant sprays can be sprayed on the skin to produce rapid cooling and anesthesia before painful procedures. Reis and Holobukov (90) showed that a vapocoolant spray plus distraction provides anesthesia equivalent to that with lidocaine-prilocaine cream before immunization in the 4- to 6-year-old age group. The advantage of this technique is that it works quickly (in approximately 30 seconds) and is inexpensive (90). Unfortunately, it does not seem to be effective in decreasing the pain of venous cannulation (91). If a refrigerant spray is used, the procedure should be performed quickly because the anesthesia provided by this method is fleeting.

LUMBAR PUNCTURE

Lumbar puncture is a commonly performed procedure in the emergency department. Unfortunately, it has been traditional practice in many centers to perform this procedure on infants without any local anesthesia out of fear that it will interfere with the success of the procedure. However, lidocaine infiltration before lumbar puncture does not affect the procedure success rate and has been shown to decrease the struggling of infants during the procedure (92,93). Lidocaine for this procedure can be buffered and infiltrated with a small-gauge needle as previously discussed.

Lidocaine-prilocaine cream also provides effective anesthesia before lumbar punctures and may be used in conjunction with lidocaine infiltration to minimize patient discomfort (94,95). The lidocaine-prilocaine cream patch provides equivalent efficacy and offers ease of application before lumbar puncture as a benefit; thus, it may be more easily placed in a busy triage area (96). Other methods of topical anesthesia such as amethocaine and lidocaine iontophoresis have not been studied. At our institution, lidocaine iontophoresis has been used before lumbar puncture with success.

Some patients require sedation before a lumbar puncture is performed. In the emergency department, the intravenous route is the most efficacious and expedient method of sedation for the patient requiring diagnostic lumbar puncture.

Midazolam is the drug of choice for this procedure (see section on fracture reduction). Midazolam provides anxiolysis and sedation, which are essential for lumbar puncture, and can be used in conjunction with local anesthesia. In rare cases, fentanyl may be used in conjunction with midazolam to provide adequate sedation. This combination carries with it a higher risk of respiratory complications (21). Propofol can also be used for this procedure, but more data regarding its use in the emergency setting is necessary before it can be recommended (45,46). Ketamine should not be used for diagnostic lumbar puncture because of the potential for increased intracranial pressure associated with the use of this medication (18).

ABDOMINAL PAIN

Children presenting with undifferentiated abdominal pain create a difficult dilemma for the practitioner. A myth believed by many clinicians is that pain management is contraindicated in these patients because it may mask the patient's symptoms, thereby preventing the appropriate diagnosis. There are no data to support this claim. Meanwhile, the child with abdominal pain is often allowed to remain in pain while routine studies are performed, appropriate consults are obtained, and a diagnosis is made.

Several studies of adult patients have demonstrated that opiates can be used in these patients without altering the clinical result (97,98). In a double-blind, placebo-controlled study of morphine use for adult patients presenting to the emergency department with abdominal pain, those patients who received morphine had lower pain scores than those receiving placebo, but diagnostic accuracy was unchanged (99). A similar pediatric study of 52 children also showed decreased pain in the morphine group but no change in diagnostic accuracy (100). Additionally, this study showed that there were no changes in the location of pain or percussion tenderness in the morphine group (100). Clinical experience with this patient group shows that the use of pain medications not only makes the child more comfortable but often makes the examination of the child's abdomen and radiologic studies such as ultrasonography easier and thus aids in diagnosis. Further study with larger groups of children is necessary but should not hinder the use of analgesics in selected patients with abdominal pain.

GUIDELINES FOR SEDATION AND ANALGESIA

Because the sedative and analgesic agents discussed above have the potential for respiratory depression, it is imperative that emergency departments institute protocols for their use. Several organizations including the American Academy of Pediatrics, the American College of Emergency Physicians, and the Joint Commission on Accreditation of Healthcare Organizations have developed guidelines for sedation of children, but each emergency department of an institution should modify these for safety (101–103). Table 36.9 summarizes precautions for use of sedative agents in the emergency department.

Conscious sedation generally refers to a state in which patients have a minimally depressed level of consciousness and can maintain protective airway reflexes, respond to physical stimuli, and follow commands (e.g., "open your eyes"). *Deep sedation* refers to the state in which patients have a more depressed

TABLE 36.9. Precautions needed for use of sedation/analgesia in the emergency department

Appropriate personnel present
Must be capable of airway management
Must be familiar with equipment
Must be trained in cardiopulmonary resuscitation
Monitoring (continuous or frequent)
Cardiac monitor
Blood pressure
Pulse oximeter
Needed equipment
Oxygen source
Suction
Oral airways, nasal airways
Bag and mask device
Various size endotracheal tubes
Laryngoscope (various size blades)
Stylets
Intravenous catheters and fluids
Medications
Epinephrine
Sodium bicarbonate
Atropine
Lidocaine
Succinylcholine
Naloxone
Flumazenil

level of consciousness, may not have protective airway reflexes, and are difficult to arouse. They may not respond purposefully to physical stimulation or verbal commands. In reality, most procedures in the emergency department, such as fracture reduction, require a deep level of sedation.

The American Academy of Pediatrics guidelines for conscious sedation recommend that emergency equipment be available for patients of all ages and sizes (101). This includes a suction device and a positive pressure oxygen delivery system capable of delivering greater than 90% FiO_2 for at least 60 minutes. Personnel trained in pediatric life support and at least one additional support person to monitor the patient should be available. The personnel should have knowledge of the sedative agents used and their potential complications. Patients should have continuous monitoring of oxygen saturation and heart rate with at least intermittent monitoring of blood pressure and respiration during and after the procedure. Pulse oximetry is essential because of the proven difficulty in recognizing hypoxemia even by experienced personnel.

If a patient is expected to achieve deep sedation, the above requirements remain. In addition, an intravenous line should be established before sedation. Furthermore, frequent monitoring of the child's blood pressure, cardiac rhythm, and temperature is advised. It is recommended that a defibrillator and medications for resuscitation be kept nearby. Reversal agents such as naloxone and flumazenil are also useful. Restraining devices used during a procedure should be checked periodically to be sure that there is no airway obstruction or chest restriction. Finally, a third person, trained in pediatric resuscitation, should be present to assist the patient.

The American Academy of Pediatrics (101) recommends several *dietary precautions* before sedation. Infants should not have milk or solids for several hours before elective sedation (not within 4 hours for infants younger than 5 months, 6 hours for those 6 to 36 months, and 8 hours for older children). Intake of clear liquids may continue but should cease in all cases within 2 hours of the scheduled sedation. Those at risk for aspiration of gastric contents (such as those with history of gastroesophageal reflux, extreme obesity, pregnancy, previous esophageal dysfunction) may benefit from appropriate pharmacologic treatment to reduce gastric volume and increase gastric pH.

For the emergency patient, sedation should still be preceded by an evaluation of food and fluid intake (101). It is prudent to assume that all patients in the emergency department have a full stomach when planning the use of sedatives or analgesics. The increased risks of sedation must be weighed against the benefits, and the lightest effective sedation should be used. Some patients may benefit from delaying the procedure or administration of appropriate pharmacologic treatment to reduce gastric volume and increase gastric pH. Consider airway protection before sedation.

Before discharge, any child who has received conscious sedation, should be awake enough to sit and speak without assistance and preferably able to ambulate. Younger children should be able to perform age-appropriate functions. The child should also have stable cardiovascular function, an adequate airway, and adequate hydration status before leaving the emergency department. The child's condition must be carefully documented before, during, and after the procedure.

RESTRAINT AND REASSURANCE

It is sometimes necessary to restrain a young child to perform a painful procedure. Physical restraint should be used sparingly because the usual goal is to provide enough sedation and pain relief that restraint is unnecessary. Brute force and restraint should never be the method chosen to avoid appropriate medications. It has been said that "the goal of pain management therapy is to ease the child's suffering rather than to make things easy for the clinician" (18). When restraint is used, it may initially increase the child's anxiety. However, it will ultimately reduce their pain by allowing the physician to better perform the task in as short a time as possible (1). Rather than attempting a technical procedure on a moving target, one might secure the child in hospital sheets wrapped around the extremities or papoose boards with Velcro straps. The need for such restraint should be explained to parents, but there are only rare complications such as bruising, edema, or transient vascular compromise to be concerned with (6). Parents may have a calming influence on the child and should be nearby but should not be involved in restraining the child.

Of course, even in a busy emergency department, uncooperative children should not be treated abruptly or harshly. The staff's desire to finish the procedure must be tempered by the need to reassure the child and make the experience as pleasant as possible. Words of explanation should be chosen carefully, keeping in mind that the toddler and young schoolchild understand more than they say (1,6). A child should be warned honestly about possible pain, but it is wise to allow for the possibility that it may not hurt as much as anticipated. The explanation of the task should not include casual teasing, condescension, or talk about the child without including him or her in the discussion (6). Nonexistent choices should not be offered to the child (6). Keep in mind that older children may be more understanding of the need to do a procedure and may tolerate the pain better than a younger child. However, they are more likely to be depressed about an injury because they quickly anticipate the future disability. Thus, they may not tolerate pain related to trauma as well as a younger child (8). It was shown previously that an empathic, age-appropriate explanation about an impending needle stick will help to reduce pain behavior compared with cold, impersonal instructions (104). Likewise, role-playing or allowing a child to read about a procedure will reduce physiologic markers and behavioral responses to pain (105). Although these attempts may be time-consuming, they will prove worthwhile. Finally, once the child has been told of the procedure, do not allow a long delay before it is accomplished. The anticipation may be the worst part.

BEHAVIORAL APPROACH TO PAIN IN THE EMERGENCY DEPARTMENT

When one addresses the nonpharmacologic approach to pain in the emergency department, the effect of the environment itself must be considered. The patient should be placed in a private, preferably soundproof room where the cries of other children, which can only serve to heighten the patients anxiety and pain response, can be muffled.

Simple distraction techniques such having the child blow bubbles or use a pinwheel during a painful procedure have been shown to decrease the pain associated with procedures (106,107). The presence of child life therapists in the department is a helpful adjunct to assist in the use of distraction and imagery in reducing pain, whether it is procedural or illness related. Other members of the staff may also be trained in the techniques of guided imagery and hypnosis (108).

Hypnosis has been used for a wide range of conditions including the pain associated with fracture and dislocation reduction, needle phobias, burn pain, vasoocclusive crisis, and the pain associated with laceration repair (109–113). Hypnosis is not difficult to learn. Many physicians use some of the basic techniques such as calm reassurance, steady speech cadence, and a laying on of hands in their daily practice (109). Involving a child in a detailed story has been shown to be more helpful than simple distraction techniques during a procedure (114). Although hypnosis is not likely to replace pharmacologic means of pain control, it can be a useful adjunct helping children to cope with the pain associated with medical conditions and procedures, whether short or long term.

Making the emergency department "child friendly" is an essential component of any effort to minimize patient distress. Providing the child with age-appropriate games, books, and other materials will help to provide distraction. Outfitting each procedure room with videocassette recorders for watching a favorite video will help to engage the child in pain. Giving the child and adolescent a range of music to choose from, to be delivered via headphones, will also assist in reducing pain and distress while in the emergency department.

Bauchner et al. (115) demonstrated the positive effect that parental presence during procedures had on parental anxiety without affecting the procedure success rate. However, this presence did not reduce the pain experienced by the child (115). Parental presence during procedures was found to be helpful to both parent and child in a pediatric intensive care unit study (116). Parents seem to markedly favor being present for emergency department procedures and should receive guidance on how best to calm and distract their child during a painful period (117).

SPECIAL CIRCUMSTANCES IN THE EMERGENCY DEPARTMENT

Some pediatric patients in the emergency department should receive systemic analgesics with great caution, if at all. Patients with altered mental status or with injuries that place the airway at risk are considered unstable and are not candidates for systemic analgesia. Likewise, patients who are hemodynamically unstable also present a challenge in the emergency department. Once these injuries are identified and stabilized, pain should be addressed.

Furthermore, many children present to the emergency department with injuries that occurred just after they have eaten. These children pose a difficult dilemma. Unless the most recent meal is known, it is best to consider every child in the emergency department to have a full stomach. Sedation and analgesia are often given for urgent and emergent procedures even for patients who have not been instructed to receive nothing by mouth according to standard guidelines. However, one must use caution in these situations and weigh the need of accomplishing a procedure with proper sedation versus the risk of vomiting and aspiration (118). Some recommend giving analgesia but delaying a procedure for 3 to 4 hours unless it is a true emergency. For instance, a child with a fracture can be given morphine for pain, but deep sedation for fracture reduction can be delayed.

One should consider altering the agents used for sedation when a child may have eaten recently. For instance, ketamine may be of benefit because protective airway reflexes will be maintained with this agent should vomiting occur. In one large study of adverse events with ketamine sedation in children, data on the time of the last meal were not collected (119). However, pooled data from multiple ketamine studies did not demonstrate an association between fasting state and emesis (32). Still, some recommend not using ketamine if the child has had a full meal within 3 hours of the procedure (120). Finally, others recommend the use of prokinetic, antiemetic drugs to increase gastric emptying and reduce gastric volume. For instance, metoclopramide may be given at a dose of 0.1 to 0.2 mg/kg intravenously or orally and has an onset time of 1 to 3 minutes. This agent will not reduce the possibility of vomiting and aspiration but may limit the damage (121).

In summary, it is best to individualize decisions about sedation based on the needs of the patient, resources, and expertise available.

SUMMARY

In the emergency department, medical staff frequently treat children in pain. Unfortunately, pain may be unavoidably inflicted on children while they are in the emergency department. The emergency department staff must recognize a child in pain and use a variety of medications, local anesthetics, and nonpharmacologic techniques to manage this pain.

REFERENCES

1. Selbst SM. Managing pain in the pediatric emergency department. *Pediatr Emerg Care* 1989;5:56–63.

2. Selbst SM, Clark M. Analgesic use in the emergency department. *Ann Emerg Med* 1990;19:1010–1013.
3. Friedland LR, Pancioli AM, Duncan KM. Pediatric emergency department analgesic practice. *Pediatr Emerg Care* 1997;13:103–106.
4. Petrack EM, Christopher NC, Kriwinsky J. Pain management in the emergency department: patterns of analgesic utilization. *Pediatr,* 1997;99:711–714.
5. Friedland LR, Kulick RM. Emergency department analgesic use in pediatric trauma victims with fractures. *Ann Emerg Med* 1994;23:203–207.
6. Selbst SM, Henretig FM. The treatment of pain in the emergency department. *Pediatr Clin North Am* 1989; 36:965–978.
7. Paris PM. Pain management in children. *Emerg Med Clin North Am* 1987;5:699–707.
8. Schechter NL. Pain and pain control in children. *Curr Prob Pediatr* 1985;15:1–67.
9. Paris PM. Narcotics. *Emerg Med* 1986;18:66–73.
10. Pena BM, Krauss B. Adverse events of procedural sedation and analgesia in the emergency department. *Ann Emerg Med* 1999;34:483—491.
11. Amadio P. Peripherally acting analgesics. *Am J Med* 1989;77:17–23.
12. Weinberger M. Analgesic sensitivity in children with asthma. *Pediatrics* 1978;62:910–915.
13. Means W. Pain relief for children: new concepts, new methods. *Contemp Pediatr* 1994;11:70–91.
14. Lynn AM, Ulma GA, Spieker M. Pain control for very young infants: an update. *Contemp Pediatr* 1999;16: 39–66.
15. Lesko SM, Mitchell AA. An assessment of the safety of pediatric ibuprofen: a practitioner-based randomized clinical trial. *JAMA* 1995;273:929–933.
16. Selbst SM. Analgesia in children—why is it underused in emergency departments? *Drug Saf* 1992;7:8–13.
17. Yaster M, Deshanpande KJ. Management of pediatric pain and opioid analgesics. *J Pediatr* 1988;113: 421–429.
18. Sacchetti A, Schafermeyer R, Gerardi M, et al. Pediatric analgesia and sedation. *Ann Emerg Med* 1994;23: 237–250.
19. Joseph MH, Brill J, Zeltzer LK. Pediatric pain relief in trauma. *Pediatr Rev* 1999;20:75–83.
20. Chudnofsky CR, Wright SW, Dronen SC, et al. The safety of fentanyl use in the emergency department. *Ann Emerg Med* 1989;18:635–639
21. Yaster M, Nicholas DG, Deshpand JK, et al. Midazolam fentanyl intravenous sedation in children: case report of respiratory arrest. *Pediatrics* 1990;86:463–466.
22. Krauss B. Practical aspects of procedural sedation and analgesia. In: Krauss B, Brustowicz RM, eds. *Pediatric procedural sedation and analgesia*. Philadelphia: Lippincott Williams & Wilkins, 1999:223–236.
23. Cole TB, Sprinkle RH, Smith SJ, et al. Intravenous narcotic therapy for children with severe sickle cell pain crises. *Am J Dis Child* 1986;140:1255–1259.
24. Tang R, Shimomura S, Rotblatt M. Meperidine induced seizures in sickle cell patients. *Hosp Formal* 1980;76:764–772.
25. Pierce MC, Fuchs S. Evaluation of ketorolac in children with forearm fractures. *Acad Emerg Med* 1997;4:22–26.
26. Watcha MF, Jones MB, Lagueruela RG, et al. comparison of ketorolac and morphine as adjuvants during pediatric surgery. *Anesthesia* 1992;76:368–372.
27. Koenig KL, Hodgson L, Kozak R, et al. Ketorolac vs meperidine for the management of pain in the emergency department. *Acad Emerg Med* 1999;1:544–549.
28. Pohlgeers AP, Friedland LR, Keegan-Jones L. Combination fentanyl and diazepam for pediatric sedation. *Acad Emerg Med* 1995;2:879–883.
29. Griffin GC, Campbell VD, Jones R. Nitrous oxide-oxygen sedation for minor surgery, experience in a pediatric setting. *JAMA* 1981;245:2411–2413.
30. Gamis AS, Knapp JF, Glenski JA. Nitrous oxide analgesia in a pediatric emergency department. *Ann Emerg Med* 1989;18:177–181.
31. Stewart RD. Nitrous oxide sedation/anesthesia in emergency medicine. *Ann Emerg Med* 1985;114: 139–148.
32. Dula DJ, Skiendzielewski J, Snover SW. The scavenger device for nitrous oxide administration. *Ann Emerg Med* 1983;12:759–762.
33. Luhmann JD, Kennedy RM, Porter FL, et al. A randomized clinical trial of continuous-flow nitrous oxide and midazolam for sedation of young children during laceration repair. *Ann Emerg Med* 2001;37:20–27.
34. Green SM, Johnson NE. Ketamine sedation for pediatric procedures. Part 2. Review and implications. *Ann Emerg Med* 1990;19:1033–1046.
35. Green SM, Rothrock SG, Lynch EL, et al. Intramuscular ketamine for pediatric sedation in the emergency department. Safety profile with 1022 cases. *Ann Emerg Med* 1998;31:688–697.
36. Green SM, Rothrock SG, Harris T, et al. Intravenous ketamine for pediatric sedation in the emergency department. Safety and efficacy with 156 cases. *Acad Emerg Med* 1998;5:971–976.
37. Green SM, Hummel CB, Wittlake WA, et al. What is the optimal dose of intramuscular ketamine for pediatric sedation. *Acad Emerg Med* 1999;6:21–26.
38. Dachs RJ, Innes GM. Intravenous ketamine sedation of pediatric patients in the emergency department. *Ann Emerg Med* 1997;29:146–150.
39. Kennedy RM, Proter FL, Miller JP, et al. Comparison of fentanyl-midazolam with ketamine-midazolam for pediatric orthopedic emergencies. *Pediatrics* 1998; 102:956–963.
40. Green SM, Nakamura R, Johnson NE. Ketamine sedation for pediatric procedures: part I, a prospective series. *Ann Emerg Med* 1990;19:1024–1032.
41. Sherwin TS, Green SM, Khan A, et al. Does adjunctive midazolam reduce recovery agitation after ketamine sedation for pediatric procedures? A randomized, double-blind, placebo-controlled trial. *Ann Emerg Med* 2000;35:229–238.
42. Pena BMG, Krauss B. Adverse events of procedural sedation and analgesia in a pediatric emergency department. *Ann Emerg Med* 1999;34:483–491.
43. Swanson ER, Seaberg DC, Mathias S. The use of propofol for sedation in the emergency department. *Acad Emerg Med* 1996;3:234–238.
44. Havel CJ, Strait RJ, Hennes H. A clinical trial of propofol vs. midazolam for procedural sedation in a pediatric emergency department. *Acad Emerg Med* 1999;6:989–997.
45. Green SM. Propofol for emergency department proce-

dural sedation—not yet ready for prime time. *Acad Emerg Med* 1999;6:975–978.
46. *Physicians Desk Reference*, 54th ed. Montvale, NJ: Medical Economics, 2000:543–544.
47. Terndrup TE, Cantor RM, Madden CM. Intramuscular meperidine, promethazine, chlorpromazine: analysis of use and complications of 487 pediatric emergency department patients. *Ann Emerg Med* 1989;18: 528–533.
48. Terndrup TE, Dire DJ, Madden CM, et al. A prospective analysis of intramuscular meperidine, promethazine, and chlorpromazine in pediatric emergency department patients. *Ann Emerg Med* 1991;20: 431–435.
49. Bolte R, Steven SS, Scott J, et al. Mini-dose Bier block intravenous regional anesthesia in emergency department treatment of pediatric upper-extremity injuries. *J Pediatr Orthop* 1994;14:534–537.
50. Blasier RD, White R. Intravenous regional anesthesia for management of children's extremity fractures in the emergency department. *Pediatr Emerg Care* 1996; 12:404–406.
51. Kennedy R, Jaffe D. Musculoskeletal problems. In: Krauss B, Brustowicz RM, eds. *Pediatric procedural sedation and analgesia*. Philadelphia: Lippincott Williams & Wilkins, 1999:285–292.
52. Pryor G, Kilpatrick WR, Opp DR. Local anesthesia in minor lacerations. Topical TAC versus lidocaine infiltration. *Ann Emerg Med* 1980;9:568–571.
53. Bonadio WA, Wagner V. Efficacy of TAC topical anesthetic for repair of pediatric lacerations. *Am J Dis Child* 1988;142:203–205.
54. Hegenbarth MA, Altieri MF, Hawk WH, et al. Comparison of topical tetracaine, adrenaline and cocaine anesthesia with lidocaine infiltration for repair of lacerations in children. *Ann Emerg Med* 1990;4:319–322.
55. Zempsky WT, Karasic RB. EMLA versus TAC for topical anesthesia of extremity wounds in children. *Ann Emerg Med* 1997;30:163–166.
56. Daily D. Fatality secondary to misuse of TAC solution. *Ann Emerg Med* 1988;17:159–160.
57. Mofenson HC, Caraccio TR. Tack up a warning on TAC [Letter]. *Am J Dis Child* 1989;143:519–520.
58. Schilling CG, Bank DE, Borchert BA, et al. Tetracaine, epinephrine and cocaine (TAC) versus lidocaine, epinephrine, and tetracaine (LET) for anesthesia of lacerations in children. *Ann Emerg Med* 1995; 25:203–208.
59. Ernst AA, Marvez E, Nick TG, et al. Lidocaine, adrenaline, tetracaine gel versus tetracaine, adrenaline, cocaine gel for topical anesthesia in linear scalp and facial lacerations in children aged 5 to 17 years. *Pediatrics* 1995;95:255–258.
60. Resch K, Schilling C, Borchert BD, et al. Topical anesthesia for pediatric lacerations: a randomized trial of lidocaine-epinephrine-tetracaine solution versus gel. *Ann Emerg Med* 1998;32:693–697.
61. Smith GA, Strausbaugh SD, Harbeck-Weber C, et al. Comparison of topical anesthetics without cocaine to tetracaine-adrenaline-cocaine and lidocaine infiltration during repair of lacerations: bupivacaine-norepinephrine is an effective new topical anesthetic agent. *Pediatrics* 1996;97:301–307.
62. Steward DJ. Eutectic mixture of local anesthetics (EMLA): what is it? What does it do? *J Pediatr* 1993;122:S21–S23.
63. Simon HK, McClario DJ, Bruns TJ, et al. Long-term appearance of lacerations closed with a tissue adhesive. *Pediatrics* 1997;99:193–195.
64. Bruns TB, Robinson BS, Smith RJ, et al. A new tissue adhesive for laceration repair in children. *J Pediatr* 1998;132:10–12.
65. Quinn J, Wells G, Sutcliffe T, et al. A randomized trial comparing octylcyanoacrylate tissue adhesive and sutures in the management of lacerations. *JAMA* 1997;277:1527–1530.
66. Bartfield JM, Gennis P, Barbera J, et al. Buffered versus plain lidocaine as a local anesthetic for simple laceration repair. *Ann Emerg Med* 1990;19:1387–1390.
67. Davidson JAH, Boom SJ. Warming lidocaine to reduce pain associated with injection. *BMJ* 1992;305: 617–618.
68. Krause RS, Moscati R, Filice M, et al. The effect of injection speed on the pain of lidocaine infiltration. *Acad Emerg Med* 1997;4:1032–1035.
69. Scarfone RJ, Jasani M, Gracely EJ. Pain of local anesthetics: rate of administration and buffering. *Ann Emerg Med* 1998;31:36–40.
70. Bartfield JM, Sokaris SJ, Raccio-Robak N. Local anesthesia for lacerations: pain of infiltration inside versus outside the wound. *Acad Emerg Med* 1998;5: 100–104.
71. Bartfield JM, Homer PJ, Ford DT, et al. Buffered lidocaine as a local anesthetic: an investigation of shelf life. *Ann Emerg Med* 1991;21:16–19.
72. Meyer G, Henneman PL, Fu P. Buffered lidocaine [Letter]. *Ann Emerg Med* 1991;20:218–219.
73. Robieux I, Kumar R, Radhakrishan S, et al. Assessing pain and analgesia with a lidocaine-prilocaine emulsion in infants and toddlers during venipuncture. *J Pediatr* 1991;118:971–973.
74. Manner T, Kanto J, Iisalo E, et al. Reduction of pain at venous cannulation in children with a eutectic mixture of lidocaine and prilocaine (EMLA cream): comparison with placebo cream and no local premedication. *Acta Anaesthesiol Scand* 1987;31:735–739.
75. Halperin DL. Topical skin anesthesia for venous, subcutaneous drug reservoir and lumbar puncture in children. *Pediatrics* 1989;84:281–284.
76. Uhari M. A eutectic mixture of lidocaine and prilocaine for alleviating vaccination pain in infants. *Pediatrics* 1993;92:719–721.
77. Fein JA, Callahan JM, Boardman CR. Intravenous catheterization in the ED: is there a role for topical anesthesia? *Am J Emerg Med* 1999;17:624–625.
78. Fein JA, Callahan JM, Boardman CR, et al. Predicting the need for topical anesthetic in the pediatric emergency department. *Pediatrics* 1999;104:E19.
79. Lawson RA, Smart NG, Gudgeon C, et al. Evaluation of an amethocaine gel preparation for percutaneous analgesia before venous cannulation in children: *Br J Anaesth* 1995;75:282–285.
80. Romsing J, Henneberg SW, Walther-Larsen S, et al. Tetracaine gel vs EMLA cream for percutaneous anaesthesia in children. *Br J Anaesth* 1999;82: 637–638.
81. Zempsky WT, Ashburn MA. Iontophoresis: noninvasive drug delivery. *Am J Anesthesiol* 1998;25:158–162.

82. Zempsky WT, Anand KS, Sullivan KM, et al. Lidocaine iontophoresis for topical anesthesia before intravenous line placement in children. *J Pediatr* 1998;132: 1061–1063.
83. Kim MK, Kini NM, Troshynski TJ, et al. A randomized clinical trial of dermal anesthesia by iontophoresis for peripheral intravenous catheter placement in children. *Ann Emerg Med* 1999;33:395–399.
84. Ashburn MA. The iontophoresis of lidocaine with epinephrine: an evaluation of the depth and duration of skin anesthesia following short delivery times. *Anesthesiology* 1994;81:A391(abst).
85. Bjerring D, Arendt-Nielson L. Depth and duration of skin analgesia to needle insertion after topical application of EMLA cream. *Br J Anaesth* 1990;64:173-–177.
86. Ashburn M, Love G, Gaylord B, et al. Iontophoretic administration of 2% lidocaine HCl and 1:100,000 epinephrine in man. *Clin J Pain* 1997;13:1322–1326.
87. Rattenbury JM, Worthy E. Is the sweat test safe? Some instances of burns received during pilocarpine iontophoresis. *Ann Clin Biochem* 1996;33:456–458.
88. Klein EJ, Shugerman RP, Leigh-Taylor K, et al. Buffered lidocaine. Analgesia for intravenous line placement in children. *Pediatrics* 1995;95:709–712.
89. Fein JA, Boardman CR, Stevenson S, et al. Saline with benzyl alcohol as intradermal anesthesia for intravenous line placement in children. *Pediatr Emerg Care* 1998;14:119–122.
90. Reis EC, Holobukov R. Vapocoolant spray is equally effective as EMLA cream in reducing immunization pain in school-aged children. *Pediatrics* 1997;100:E5.
91. Ramsook CA, Kozinetz C, Moro-Sutherland D. The efficacy of ethyl chloride as a local anesthetic for venipuncture in an emergency room setting. Presented at the 39th meeting of the Ambulatory Pediatric Association, San Francisco, 1999:93.
92. Carraccio C, Feinberg P, Hart LS, et al. Lidocaine for lumbar punctures. A help not a hindrance. *Arch Pediatr Adolesc Med* 1996;150:1044–1046.
93. Pinheiro JM, Furdon S, Ochoa LF. Role of local anesthesia during lumbar puncture in neonates. *Pediatrics* 1993;9:379–382.
94. Juarez Gimenez JC, Oliveras M, Hidalgo E, et al. Anesthetic efficacy of eutectic prilocaine-lidocaine cream in pediatric oncology patients undergoing lumbar puncture. *Ann Pharmacother* 1996;30:1235–1237.
95. Halperin DL, Koren G, Attias D, et al. Topical skin anesthesia for venous, subcutaneous drug reservoir and lumbar punctures in children. *Pediatrics* 1989;84: 281–284.
96. Calamandrei M, Messeri A, Busoni P, et al. Comparison of two application techniques of EMLA and pain assessment in pediatric oncology patients. *Reg Anesth* 1998;21:557–5560.
97. LoVecchio F, Oster N, Sturmann K, et al. The use of analgesics in patients with acute abdominal pain. *J Emerg Med* 1997;15:775–779.
98. Attard AR, Corlett MJ, Kidner NJ, et al. Safety of early pain relief for acute abdominal pain *BMJ* 1992;30: 5554–5556.
99. Pace S, Burke TF. Intravenous morphine for early pain relief in patients with acute abdominal pain. *Acad Emerg Med* 1996;3:1086–1092.
100. Kim MK, Strait RT, Sato TT. A randomized clinical trial of analgesia for children with acute abdomen. Presented at the Pediatric Academic Societies meeting, Boston, May 2000.
101. American Academy of Pediatrics, Committee on Drugs. Guidelines for monitoring the management of pediatric patients during and after sedation for diagnostic and therapeutic procedures. *Pediatrics* 1992;89: 1110–1115.
102. ACEP Pediatric Emergency Medicine Committee. The use of pediatric sedation and analgesia policy statement. *Ann Emerg Med* 1993;22:626–627.
103. Joint Commission on Accreditation of Healthcare Organizations. *Comprehensive accreditation manual for hospitals: the official handbook.* Chicago: JCAHO, 1997:15–17, 76–80.
104. Fernald C, Corry J. Empathic vs directive preparation of children for needles. *Child Health Care* 1981;10:44–47.
105. Fassler D. The fear of needles in children. *Am J Orthopsychiatr* 1985;55:371–377.
106. French GM, Painter EC, Coury DL. Blowing away shot pain: a technique for pain management during immunization. *Pediatrics* 1994;93:384–388.
107. Fowler-Kerry S, Lander J. Management of injection pain in children. *Pain* 1987;30:169–175.
108. Kutner L. *No tears no fears: children with cancer coping with pain* (video). Vancouver: Canadian Cancer Society, 1986.
109. Serson KV. Hypnosis for pediatric fracture reduction. *J Emerg Med* 1999;17:53–56.
110. Bierman SF. Hypnosis in the emergency department. *Am J Emerg Med* 1989;7:238–242.
111. Ewin DM. Emergency room hypnosis for the burned patient. *Am J Clin Hypn* 1986;29:1–12.
112. Zeltzer L, Dash J, Holland JP. Hypnotically induced pain control in sickle cell anemia. *Pediatrics* 1979; 64:533–536.
113. Ambrose G, Newbold G. *A handbook of medical hypnosis*. London: Bailliere Tindall, 1980.
114. Zeltzer L, Lebaron S. Hypnosis and non-hypnotic techniques for reduction of pain and anxiety during painful procedures in children and adolescents with cancer. *J Pediatr* 1982;101:1032–1035.
115. Bauchner H, Waring C, Vinci R. Parental presence during procedures in an emergency room: results from 50 observations. *Pediatrics* 1991;87:544–588.
116. Powers KS, Rubenstein JS. Family presence during invasive procedures in the pediatric intensive care unit: a prospective study. *Arch Pediatr Adolesc Med* 1999; 153:955–958.
117. Sacchetti A, Lichenstein R, Carracio CA, et al. Family member presence during pediatric emergency department procedures. *Pediatr Emerg Care* 1996;12: 268–271.
118. Krauss B, Green SM. Sedation and analgesia for procedures in children. *N Engl J Med* 2000;342:938–945.
119. Green SM, Kupperman N, Rothrock SG, et al. Predictors of adverse events with intramuscular ketamine sedation in children. *Ann Emerg Med* 2000;35:35–42.
120. Green S. Dissociative agents: Ketamine protocol—Loma Linda University emergency department [appendix]. In: Krauss B, Brustowicz RM, eds. *Pediatric procedural sedation and analgesia*. Philadelphia: Lippincott Williams & Wilkins, 1999:55–58.
121. Yaster M, Krane EJ, Kaplan RF, et al. *Pediatric pain management and sedation handbook.* St. Louis: Mosby, 1997:402–405.

37

The Pain (and Stress) in Infants in a Neonatal Intensive Care Unit

C. Mae Wong, Neil McIntosh, Gopi Menon, and Linda S. Franck

WHY BOTHER ABOUT PAIN (AND STRESS) IN INFANTS IN A NEONATAL INTENSIVE CARE UNIT?

A small proportion of newborns requires highly invasive care. Such care is obviously distressing and may be obviously painful, and yet, until the past few years, there has been little acceptance that this is of any clinical importance. Eland and Anderson (1) in 1977 first showed that pain was largely ignored in children (and particularly so in the preverbal infant), reporting that only half of the children who were prescribed postoperative analgesia actually received any, and those who did received only small amounts compared with adults with similar conditions. Many authors have since repeated their studies but, with the possible exception of operative and postoperative management, little has changed. Franck (2), in a survey of nurses in U.S. neonatal units in 1987 demonstrated that 79% thought that analgesia was underused, with 34% of infants still receiving none postoperatively. In addition, 34% had no analgesia before invasive procedures and no opioid analgesia was ever used in 5% of units. A seminal study by Porter et al. (3) showed that although pain is now acknowledged to be a significant problem, all too frequently little is done about it.

Anatomy/Physiology

Before Anand and Hickey (4) first drew attention to the developmental neurobiology of pain in 1987, there was little in the clinical literature that brought together any reasons why pain should be acknowledged as important in infants. In 1931, Tilney and Rosett (5) described the incomplete myelination of nerves in infancy. This anatomic feature combined with the clinical inability of infants to localize pain, the perception that a high threshold to pain was necessary to tolerate birth, and an apparent absence of memory of pain conditioned clinicians to ignore even the possibility of pain. A detailed description of the developmental neurobiology of pain in the human is outside the scope of this chapter, and the reader is referred to the review of Fitzgerald (6). The neuroanatomic and neurophysiologic requirements for pain reception and perception are present in even the most preterm infants. It is possible that, because of deficient spinal inhibitory control and other regulatory mechanisms, the preterm infant may even be supersensitive to pain compared with the term infant, who in turn may be more sensitive than the older child and adult.

Early Outcome for Operative Analgesia

It was the work of Anand et al. (7) that changed people's views on pain and analgesia related to surgical procedures in newborns. They demonstrated that newborns having a thoracotomy for persistent ductus arteriosus had a distinctly worse outcome when given no operative analgesia. Not only were there obvious surrogate metabolic measures of stress in the newborns receiving no analgesia but also major postoperative clinical problems in this group.

Anand and Hickey (8) followed this up with a study on neonates needing cardiac surgery. Comparing deep intraoperative anesthesia using high-dose sufentanil and postoperative infusions of morphine for 24 hours with lighter operative anesthesia (halothane and morphine) followed by postoperative morphine and diazepam on an intermittent basis, there were more clinical complications and evidence of physiologic stress in the light anesthesia group.

Attitudes

Attitudes subtly but regularly affect practice in medicine. The attitudes of medical, nursing, and allied professionals involved in the care of the newborn require attention so that there can be better management of pain in the future. Porter et al. (3) showed that although there is a general acceptance by these professions that the newborn feels pain, they still receive inadequate analgesia for procedural and subacute pain. In the long term, the consequences of therapy need to be explored, but with ongoing research, an appropriate balance of problem and therapy will be possible. In the meantime, nonpharmacologic management, such as nonnutritive sucking and sucrose, should be instituted for all painful neonatal procedures (9).

DEFINITIONS IN THE NEWBORN: DIFFERENTIATING STRESS, DISTRESS, AND PAIN

An understanding of the specific definitions used in this chapter is important for effective management. The International Association for the Study of Pain defined pain as "an unpleasant sensory and emotional experience associated with actual or potential tissue damage.... Pain is always subjective. Each individual learns the application of the word through experiences related to injury in early life." Anand and Craig (10) discussed the problems of this definition, which are essentially twofold. First, the limited ability of the newborn, and in particular the preterm infant, to communicate makes judgments by caregivers about the degree of pain or discomfort quite difficult. Second, the intrinsic unlikelihood that it is only with the second and subsequent painful experiences that pain becomes a phenomenon of significance. If the first potentially painful stimulus to a newborn is a circumcision, is it not painful? Anand and Craig argue, with considerable justification, that pain is a fundamental characteristic of life in higher beings and has an important biologic protection value. Similarly, it seems irrational to believe that just because an infant cannot describe or remember his or her experience it is not real pain at the time (10).

Stress is the term applied to physiologic responses generated by some external stimuli. These are adaptive responses and may cause no harm. There may be no conscious awareness of them, and there is no associated suffering. *Distress* is the suffering resulting from the effects of excessive stress. It may be physical or emotional, and its perception requires higher consciousness. It is often affected by past experience. Its recognition by the observer depends on either a verbal description by the subject or, in the younger subject, the inference of suffering from behavioral cues. *Pain* is a description of a particular form of distress to which we all easily relate. Many pain responses are common to distress from other causes. *Nociception* is a term used to describe the effects (e.g., metabolic, neurobehavioral) of a noxious stimulus independent of any judgment of higher consciousness, memory, or possible emotional effects or suffering. This is what is often measured, directly or indirectly, in studies of neonatal pain.

Acute pain is the immediate pain resulting from a procedure or operation. In a neonatal unit, such pain arises frequently from the many and varied procedures that are required. Such repeated acute episodes (*repetitive pain*) can increase the sensitivity of the newborn to painful stimuli (hyperalgesia) and can lead to stimuli that are not normally painful becoming so (allodynia). *Chronic* pain, as defined by the International Association for the Study Pain, is pain of several months' duration. By this definition, the newborn in the first month of life cannot yet be subject to chronic pain, but inflammatory pain from meningitis, osteomyelitis, or a chemical burn from a tissued intravenous drip is of a different nature and can last longer than the usual acute pain. As such they may be classified as *subacute*.

In neonatal intensive care, babies are regularly exposed to noxious influences. Any intrusive procedure may create an undesirable stress response. The morbidity related to stress probably depends on its severity and duration and the maturity of the infant. Therefore, it is important to continually review the relief of stress as part of the problem list of these infants.

WHAT CAUSES PAIN (AND STRESS) IN NEWBORNS IN A NEONATAL INTENSIVE CARE UNIT?

Newborns in neonatal intensive care are subjected to frequent invasive diagnostic and therapeutic interventions (11) that result in the physiologic, endocrine, and behavioral responses associated with pain in individuals capable of verbal recall (12). These interventions include endotracheal intubation and suction, heel puncture, arterial and venipuncture, nasogastric tube insertion, chest drain insertion, lumbar puncture, suprapubic aspiration of urine, x-rays, diaper changes. Barker and Rutter (11) identified that the most common procedure in the neonatal intensive care unit (NICU) was heel puncture followed by endotracheal suction. Although individually short-lived, their frequency may make them unrelenting.

Other highly invasive and painful procedures include ophthalmologic examination and treatment for retinopathy. The pain of these procedures is more prolonged as is the postoperative wound pain of patients after surgery for persistent ductus arteriosus and hernia repair.

Infants with some medical and surgical conditions probably also experience chronic distress. This may be related to prolonged intubation, labored respiration, physical restraint or exposure, bright artificial lighting, and noise. The presence and severity of chronic distress are difficult to measure, although there is some evidence that interventions that reduce chronic distress may improve outcome (13,14). Some inflammatory conditions may also result in chronic or persistent pain (e.g., necrotizing enterocolitis, meningitis) (15).

CLINICAL ASSESSMENT OF PAIN

At present, no easily administered, widely accepted, uniform technique exists for assessing pain in infants, although it is an area of active research. Assessment techniques can be based on behavioral observations or physiologic and hormonal measures. A multidimensional assessment of pain in infants is more accurate than dependence on a single parameter (16), and such composite measures usually use both physiologic and behavioral indicators. The following discussion highlights some of the important features of each type of pain assessment.

Behavioral Pain Assessment

Pain assessment tools that measure pain-related behavior in preverbal infants are used alone or to supplement physiologic measures. One problem with using such tools is that health care providers consistently underestimate pain in infants who, because of illness or immaturity, display less pain behavior than healthy, full-term infants do, even when the painful stimulus is the same (17). The use of standardized, multidimensional assessment tools and staff education leads to pain assessments that more closely reflect the actual pain intensity.

Another problem with behavioral observations is the inability to discriminate between distress and agitation from causes other than pain (e.g., hunger, wet diaper). Assessment methods such as the COMFORT scale (18) measure the infant's global behavioral distress, which may be pain related. In situations in which the source of pain is clearly identifiable (e.g., procedural pain), global distress scales may be a better indicator of the overall impact of the experience than a specific measure of pain intensity. In other situations in which the source of pain is not clear, measures of distress may confound the assessment of pain.

Physiologic Measures of Pain

Pain activates the autonomic nervous system. Sympathetic stimulation produces the fight-or-flight response of tachycardia, peripheral vasoconstriction, sweating, and pupil dilation together with increased secretion of catecholamines and adrenocortical hormones (19). Although sensitive to changes in pain intensity, these parameters reflect a global response to pain-related stress and are not unique to pain. For example, alterations in these parameters can occur in infants because of crying or handling. The precise measurement of physiologic and hormonal responses to pain is generally invasive, expensive, and slow; therefore, it is not appropriate for clinical assessment of pain. Thus, although clinicians generally associate pain with changes of 10% to 20% in noninvasively measured physiologic parameters (e.g., heart rate, blood pressure, respiratory rate), there are no standard pain assessment tools that rely exclusively on these parameters.

Selection of an appropriate clinical assessment method should be based first on the developmental age of the infant and second on the type of pain or medical condition. Where specific pain assessment tools exist (e.g., for procedural or postoperative pain), these should be used. The validity and reliability of the measures, the specific dimensions of pain that are measured (e.g., intensity, location, quality), and the feasibility of use in the clinical setting are equally important considerations. In the subsequent sections, published infant-specific pain assessment tools that may be useful in a variety of clinical settings are listed in Table 37.1. The reader is also referred to reviews of these pain assessment tools (20–22).

Pain Assessment Tools for Infants

In the absence of self-report, behavioral and physiologic parameters are used to infer pain in infants. Behavioral indicators of pain include facial expression, cry, gross motor movement, changes in behavioral state, or changes in behavior patterns such as sleep. Because the preterm infant's response to pain is less robust than that of a full-term infant, the care provider needs to understand and recognize their more subtle pain cues. They display less crying, weaker facial grimacing, and limp, flaccid, listless posturing.

Facial expression has been the most comprehensively studied behavioral pain assessment measure. It is the most reliable and consistent indicator of pain across populations and types (23) and as such should be considered the gold standard of behavioral responses for pain in infants. An infant experiencing acute pain has eyes that are forcefully closed, a brow that is lowered and furrowed, nasal roots that are broadened and bulged with a deepened nasolabial furrow, and a square mouth with a taut, cupped tongue (24).

An evaluation of procedural pain in infants using facial expression can be performed using the Neonatal Facial Coding System, which is a valid and reliable coding system for quantifying facial actions associated with acute pain in infancy. Grunau and colleagues (25) recently established the feasibility of using the complete Neonatal Facial Coding System in real time at the bedside. The Infant Body Coding System (26) is a behavioral measure for assessing gross motor activity in infants. However, body activity appears less specific to pain than facial expression in the preterm and full-term infant (27).

Other behavioral assessment tools with preliminary validity in preterm and/or full-term infants include the Postoperative Pain Score (28) and the Liverpool Infant Distress Scale (29) for postoperative pain, and the Neonatal Infant Pain Scale (30) for procedural pain. Behavioral assessment tools developed from studies of older infants include

TABLE 37.1. *Clinical assessment of infant pain*

Measure and author	Age level	Indicators	Pain stimulus
Behavioral Pain Score, Pokela (37)	Preterm and full-term neonates	Facial expression, body movements, response to handling/consolability, rigidity of limbs	Procedural pain in ventilated neonates
Clinical Scoring System	Infants 1–7 mo	Sleep facial expression, cry motor activity, excitability, digit flexion, sucking, tone, consolability, sociability	Postoperative pain
CRIES, Krechel and Bildner (34)	Full-term neonates	Crying, oxygen saturation, heart rate, blood pressure, expression, sleeplessness	Postoperative pain
Distress Scale for Ventilated Newborn Infants, Sparshott (38)	Preterm and full-term neonates	Facial expression, body movement, color, heart rate, blood pressure, oxygen saturation	Procedural pain in ventilated neonates
Neonatal Facial Coding System, Grunau et al. (25)	Preterm and full-term neonates, infants up to 4 mo	Facial muscle group movement: brow bulge, eye squeeze, nasolabial furrow, open lips, stretch mouth, lip purse, taut tongue, chin quiver	Procedural pain
Infant Body Coding System, Craig et al. (27)	Preterm and full-term neonates	Hand, foot, arm, leg, head, torso motor activity	Procedural pain
Liverpool Infant Distress Scale, Horgan and Choonera (29)	Full-term infants	Spontaneous movements, spontaneous excitability, flexion of fingers and toes, facial expression, quantity of crying, quality of crying, sleep	Postoperative pain
Modified Behavioural Pain Scale, Taddio et al. (31)	Infants 2–4 mo of age	Facial expression, cry, gross motor movement	Immunization pain
Neonatal Assessment of Pain Inventory, Joyce et al. (32)	Infants 1–36 mo	Smiling, sleeping, response to touch, sleeping, crying, respirations	Postoperative pain
Neonatal Infant Pain Scale, Lawrence et al. (30)	Preterm and full-term neonates	Facial expression, cry, breathing patterns, arms, legs, state of arousal	Procedural pain
Pain Assessment Tool, Hodgkinson et al. (35)	Full-term infants	Posture/tone, sleep pattern, expression, color, cry, respirations, heart rate, oxygen saturation, blood pressure, nurses' perception of infant pain	Postoperative pain
Premature Infant Pain Profile, Stevens et al. (39)	Preterm and full-term neonates	Gestational age, behavioral state, heart rate, oxygen saturation, brow bulge, eye squeeze, nasolabial furrow	Procedural pain
Scale for Use in Newborns, Blauer and Gerstmann (36)	Preterm and full-term neonates	Movement, tone, facial expression, behavioral state, breathing, heart rate, blood pressure	Procedural pain

From Franck LS, Greenberg CS, Stevens B. Pain assessment in infants and children. *Pediatr Clin North Am,* 2000;47:487–512, with permission.

the Modified Behavioral Pain Scale (31) for use in infants 4 to 6 months of age undergoing immunizations and the Neonatal Assessment of Pain Inventory (32,33) for use with children 1 to 36 months of age.

Multidimensional tools that include behavioral observations and quantification of physiologic parameters include the CRIES (34) and the Pain Assessment Tool (35) developed for postoperative pain and the Scale for Use in Newborns (36) developed for procedural pain. The Behavioral Pain Score (37) and the Distress Scale for Ventilated Newborn Infants (38) were specifically developed to assess the responses of ventilated newborn infants to procedural pain.

The infant pain assessment tool that has been most widely validated in premature and full-

TABLE 37.2. *Premature infant pain profile*

Procedure	Indicator	0	1	2	3	Score
Observe infant for 15 sec	Gestational age (wk)	>36	32–35 + 6	28–31 + 6	<28	
Baseline: HR ...... S_aO_2 .... RR	Behavioral state	Active/awake, eyes open, facial movements, crying	Quiet awake, eyes open, no facial movements	Active sleep, eyes closed, facial movements	Quiet sleep, eyes closed, no facial movements	
Observe infant for 30 sec	Heart rate increase: Max	0–4 bpm	5–14 bpm	15–24 bpm	>25 bpm	
	S_aO_2 decrease: Min	0–2.4%	2.5–4.9%	5.0–7.4%	>7.5%	
	Brow bulge	None (0%–9% of time)	Minimum (10%–39% of time)	Moderate (40%–69% of time)	Maximum (>70% of time)	
	Eye squeeze	None	Minimum	Moderate	Maximum	
	Nasolabial furrow	None	Minimum	Moderate	Maximum	
TOTAL SCORE						

HR, heart rate; S_aO_2, arterial oxygen percent saturation; RR, respiratory rate; bpm, beats per minute.
From Stevens B, Johnston C, Petryshen P, et al. Premature Infant Pain Profile: development and initial validation. *Clin J Pain* 1996;12:13–22, with permission.

term infants during procedural pain is the Premature Infant Pain Profile (PIPP) (39). The PIPP (Table 37.2) is a seven-indicator measure that includes behavioral, physiologic, and contextual indicators. The gestational age and behavioral state of the infant are taken into consideration in the scoring. This measure had initial validity and reliability determined using four retrospective data sets. Clinical validation, which included the establishment of interrater and intrarater reliability, was determined prospectively (40). Clinical utility has been established by comparing the PIPP and the CRIES (41). The PIPP has been used primarily to evaluate procedural pain in preterm neonates older than 28 weeks' gestational age. Recently, the PIPP has been validated for evaluating postoperative pain in neonates (42) and for determining the efficacy of pain-relieving interventions in premature infants (43,44).

Factors That Influence Pain

Pain is unique among neurologic functions because of the degree of plasticity in pain neurophysiology. Although structural and functional maturity are reached at an early age, anatomic and functional changes occur throughout life that are related to the effects of each pain experience. This plasticity means that the perception and meaning of pain are unique to each individual and are determined not by maturation alone but also by previous experience. Currently available methods to assess pain in infants do not adequately incorporate the context of pain. Thus, the clinician needs to subjectively incorporate them into the assessment of pain. These factors do not influence pain in isolation but are listed below separately for clarity.

Biologic Factors

Genetic variation leads to differences in the amounts and types of neurotransmitters and receptors that are available to mediate pain. Recent advances in molecular biology have investigated the genes responsible for pain perception and modulation. Gender may also influence pain perception. Reports of gender differences in pain response in the newborn period are inconsistent (44,45).

Previous pain experience leads to alterations in pain signal processing that may be reversible or permanent. Studies of premature infants (44,46) suggest that previous pain experience is the most important factor accounting for differences in response to the acute pain of heel puncture. Newborn infants who were subjected to more frequent painful procedures in the NICU had decreased behavioral and increased cardiovascular responses compared with infants who experienced less pain, even after controlling for gestational age–related differences in pain expression.

Behavioral State

The behavioral state of the infant, ranging from deep sleep to awake and crying, acts as a moderator of behavioral pain responses. The behavioral state of the infant immediately before the painful stimulus affects the extent of the response. Infants in awake states demonstrate more obvious reactions to pain than infants in sleep states. Infants in a deep sleep state show less vigorous facial expression in response to heel puncture than infants who are alert or aroused before the heel puncture (24,47). Term and healthy preterm newborns who are handled or immobilized before heel puncture exhibit greater physiologic and behavioral reactivity, indicating that previous stress may result in greater instability in response to pain (48).

Gestational Age

Gestational age affects infant pain responses, with most preterm infants displaying fewer and less vigorous behavioral responses to pain (24,39,44,47). However, the interaction between gestational age and pain experience has not been well studied. Because younger infants are often subjected to painful procedures more frequently, the pain responses of more preterm infants may represent more of an effect of pain experience than of age (44).

Pain Characteristics

Pain characteristics such as the source or cause, location, and timing of pain influence the perception and response to pain. Most research has focused on the responses to acute pain caused by single noxious stimuli. However, pain commonly occurs over a prolonged period or is recurrent in nature. Because of the tremendous plasticity within pain processing systems, these factors significantly affect the infant's experience of pain (49).

Parents

Nurses caring for the infant in pain must care for the infant's family as well. Parents have many concerns and fears about their infant's pain and about the drugs used in the treatment of pain (50). Parents may fear the effects of pain on their child's development. They may also fear that their infant may become addicted to the analgesics (51). Nurses must be prepared to respond to questions from parents and encourage parent participation in providing nonpharmacologic comfort measures to their infant. Parents must be reassured that they are expected to ask questions about their infant's pain management (52).

Practitioner Factors

The attitudes, beliefs, and lack of knowledge of health care professionals have been a major factor in the undertreatment of pain in both adults and children. Fear of addiction and a disproportionate concern for side effects have resulted in severe underutilization of opioid analgesics for acute postoperative pain for infants and children (53).

Lack of education about pain in nursing and medical education is a major cause of myths and biases that impede appropriate assessment and management of pain in infants. Research has shown that infant pain management is strongly influenced by a nurse's biases (54), personal experiences with pain (55), and area of specialization (17). Nurses must closely examine their own beliefs and attitudes about pain, explore the impact that their attitudes might have on their patient care, and challenge their beliefs to determine whether they are science or tradition-based. Hester et al. (56) described an "illusion of certainty" in which providers assume that they know the level of a patient's pain without having to measure it, simply based on the type of illness or procedure, without regard to the individual patient's experience. The use of validated pain assessment tools results in greater consistency in provider ratings of pain and may reflect more accurately pain experienced by preverbal infants.

Pain Assessment in Conjunction with Pain Treatment

In the light of the multiple diverse factors that may influence pain experience and pain behavior, it is probably not surprising that there are no clear pain score thresholds at which particular treatments are warranted. To give fixed numbers to represent pain in all infants would be unreasonable. Each individual infant's responses should be evaluated and changes in these responses in relation to pain and its treatment assessed. For example, if an infant's pain score increases by 20%, interventions to relieve pain would be expected to bring the score back to baseline. An alternative interpretation of aiming to maintain all infants with a pain score in the lowest 20% to 25% of the scale is feasible, but care must be taken that more naturally alert infants are not sedated or treated unnecessarily. In any case, even the percentage thresholds cited here are arbitrary because no studies have yet determined these.

Implementing Clinical Assessment of Pain in Infants

Despite the substantial evidence that the pain experience of infants can be assessed in the clinical setting, pain assessment is not routinely performed in most NICU settings. Implementing an effective pain assessment program is more complex than simply selecting an appropriate assessment tool. Pain assessment must be viewed by the health care team as an integral component of quality patient care and numerous organizational, provider, and patient barriers must be overcome (57,58). Successful implementation is determined by the degree of collaboration between the health care team and family to achieve the shared goal of reduced pain for the infant (59). It requires resources for education, team building, development of processes and documentation of outcomes, and management change. For these reasons, continuous quality improvement strategies are useful for successful implementation of pain assessment for infants in the clinical setting (57,60–62).

Common themes are noted in reports of successful implementation of all clinical pain assessment programs related to the content of the program, the organizational structure to support improved pain assessment, and the process by which the change process is initiated and sustained. These factors are relevant to implementation of pain assessment programs in inpatient and outpatient settings. The fundamental elements include (a) multidisciplinary collaboration; (b) staff education about pain pathophysiology, assessment, and management; (c) staff participation in the development of setting-specific protocols; (d) simple to use, standardized, routine pain assessment for all patients; (e) formal documentation of pain assessment in the medical record; (f) mutual goal setting for pain control between the health care provider and family; and (g) monitoring of adherence and effect of pain assessment on pain management. Research is needed to evaluate the cost and effectiveness of pain assessment on an organizational as well as on an individual level because there are no data in the NICU setting.

MANAGEMENT OF STRESS AND DISTRESS

Prevention Is Better Than Cure

There is good reason to believe that pain and distress cause physiologic upset, which may be detrimental in sick and preterm infants. The possible effects are hypoxia (37), coagulopathy (8), respiratory incoordination (63), catabolism (7), increased blood pressure (64), and increased intracranial pressure (65). The use of nonpharmacologic, environmental techniques to improve the comfort of infants receiving intensive care is becoming more widespread. These techniques include nesting or swaddling, dimming of lights, and lessening noise. These maneuvers are empowering to the nurse but must be applied with as much care as any medication. Dimming lights and covering incubators reduces the good visibility that is needed for the observation of the high-risk infant (9).

The routine use of medications to provide "background cover" for infants receiving intensive care has also become more common, in line with practice in other intensive care areas. This has happened despite some real concerns about the risks of routine analgesia and sedation, particularly in the immature and rapidly developing brain. There is evidence of marked variability in practice, and a lack of good scientific information on the balance of risk to benefit.

Are Sedatives Enough for Distress?

The relative influence of analgesia, sedation, and abolition of undesirable spontaneous activity (e.g., with muscle relaxation) in ventilated babies has not been clear. This has been reflected in variable practice and confused language (e.g., referring to paralyzed infants "waking up").

There is increasing literature on the physiologic stability resulting from the use of opioid infusions (mainly morphine and fentanyl) with their analgesic and sedative effects (63–67) and their short-term safety if used carefully (68,69). There is also a small amount of data on the use of midazolam in the neonate (70,71) as well as some anxiety after the NOPAIN study (13). Although opioids and midazolam are effective for perioperative pain and sedation, there is insufficient evidence in terms of long-term outcome to support their use for prolonged sedation of ventilated neonates not experiencing operative pain. The NOPAIN and NEOPAIN trials are attempting to answer this question.

The NOPAIN multicenter pilot study was designed to assess the feasibility of a trial testing the effect of analgesia or sedation on mortality and neurologic morbidity. Sixty-seven preterm infants of 24 to 32 weeks' gestation who were ventilated in the first 3 days of life were randomized within 8 hours of ventilation to an infusion of morphine, midazolam, or placebo (10% dextrose). The primary outcome studied was a composite adverse outcome of death or major neurologic abnormality on ultrasonography (grade 3 or 4 intraventricular hemorrhage or periventricular leukomalacia). This outcome was reduced in infants receiving morphine (4%) compared with placebo (24%) or midazolam (32%) ($\chi^2 = 7.04$, $p = 0.03$). In terms of physiologic responses, the responses to endotracheal suction were reduced with morphine ($p < 0.001$) and midazolam ($p < 0.002$) compared with placebo. The study suggested that at best there was no benefit from midazolam and at worst there could be a higher incidence of periventricular leukomalacia (13). A definitive randomized, double-blind, placebo-controlled study is now underway comparing morphine with placebo (the NEOPAIN Study).

Practical difficulties with opioid infusions include the tolerance (see below) that develops after use for more than a few days and the effects, especially with morphine, on gut motility. One might therefore consider weaning and stopping morphine in preterm infants once the acute phase of their illness is ended and the risk of major new intraventricular hemorrhage is small (after 5 days), even if the baby was still ventilator dependent. This may alleviate some of the problems with weaning from intravenous fluids onto milk feeds, a difficult but important transition for very preterm infants. At this stage, although the frequency of invasive procedures may be reduced, there is no reason to believe that the chronic distress of intensive care is any less, and environmental measures to reduce distress and efforts to minimize handling and procedural pain are important.

Sedative agents such as chloral hydrate or triclofos also cause tolerance and are thus not the perfect solution but may be of use in selected infants when there are overt signs of distress. Some nonventilated infants with chronic lung disease appear to be very distressed by the effort of breathing, and occasionally sedation with a small dose of chloral hydrate or triclofos helps in their management.

In situations associated with severe pain in infants likely to be tolerant to morphine, fentanyl with its wider therapeutic ratio should be used at increasing doses. It has been suggested that fentanyl should be the analgesic of choice in infants with chronic lung disease because it has fewer histaminic effects (72) and in infants predisposed to pulmonary hypertension because it has been shown to reduce pulmonary vascular resistance (67).

MANAGEMENT OF PAIN

The treatment of pain in neonates has been hindered by a lack of knowledge about the pharmacologic effects and adverse consequences of analgesics in this age group as well as by the difficulty of pain assessment. Only in recent years has increasing research in this field allowed more evidence-based guidelines to be formed concerning the type of analgesia, dosing regimens, and evaluation of efficacy. These have been advanced on and summarized with the recent publication of a new international consensus statement with recommendations on the management of pain in newborn infants (73).

Suggested guidelines for the management of procedural pain are featured in Figures 37.1 and 37.2. Drug treatments used in neonates are summarized in Table 37.3.

Procedural Pain

Anticipate and Prevent

The SOPAIN study comprised a week-long study of procedures and analgesia administration from patient charts from North American and European NICUs (74). The results from the 14 Canadian units were fully reported in 1997 (75): 2,134 invasive procedures were performed on 239 patients; specific treatment was only given for 0.8% of procedures, and in another 6% of procedures the patient was already on analgesia for other reasons. Conversely, perioperative pain was consistently treated and primarily with opioids.

Procedural pain is often not deemed severe or chronic enough to justify the use of pharmacologic analgesic interventions that may have adverse effects, but with the recent realization that pain may be damaging to infants, there has been the development of effective nonpharmacologic analgesia.

Nonpharmacologic

Methods of Blood Sampling

Blood samples should be obtained from indwelling central venous or arterial lines whenever feasible to prevent further skin punctures. Heel punctures, although quick for small volumes of blood, are comparatively painful. Venipuncture has been shown to be less painful than heel punctures (76,77). When a heel puncture is necessary, using a spring-loaded lance has been shown to reduce distress (78).

Comforting/Swaddling

Comfort measures and swaddling have been shown to help reduce crying and heart rate after procedures such as heel punctures and injections (79). Parents should be encouraged to participate in these actions so that they may play an active role in relieving the distress of their infants.

Nonnutritive Sucking

Sucking a pacifier can help ameliorate pain in both term and preterm infants (79–83). The action is not opioid mediated and terminates almost immediately on sucking completion

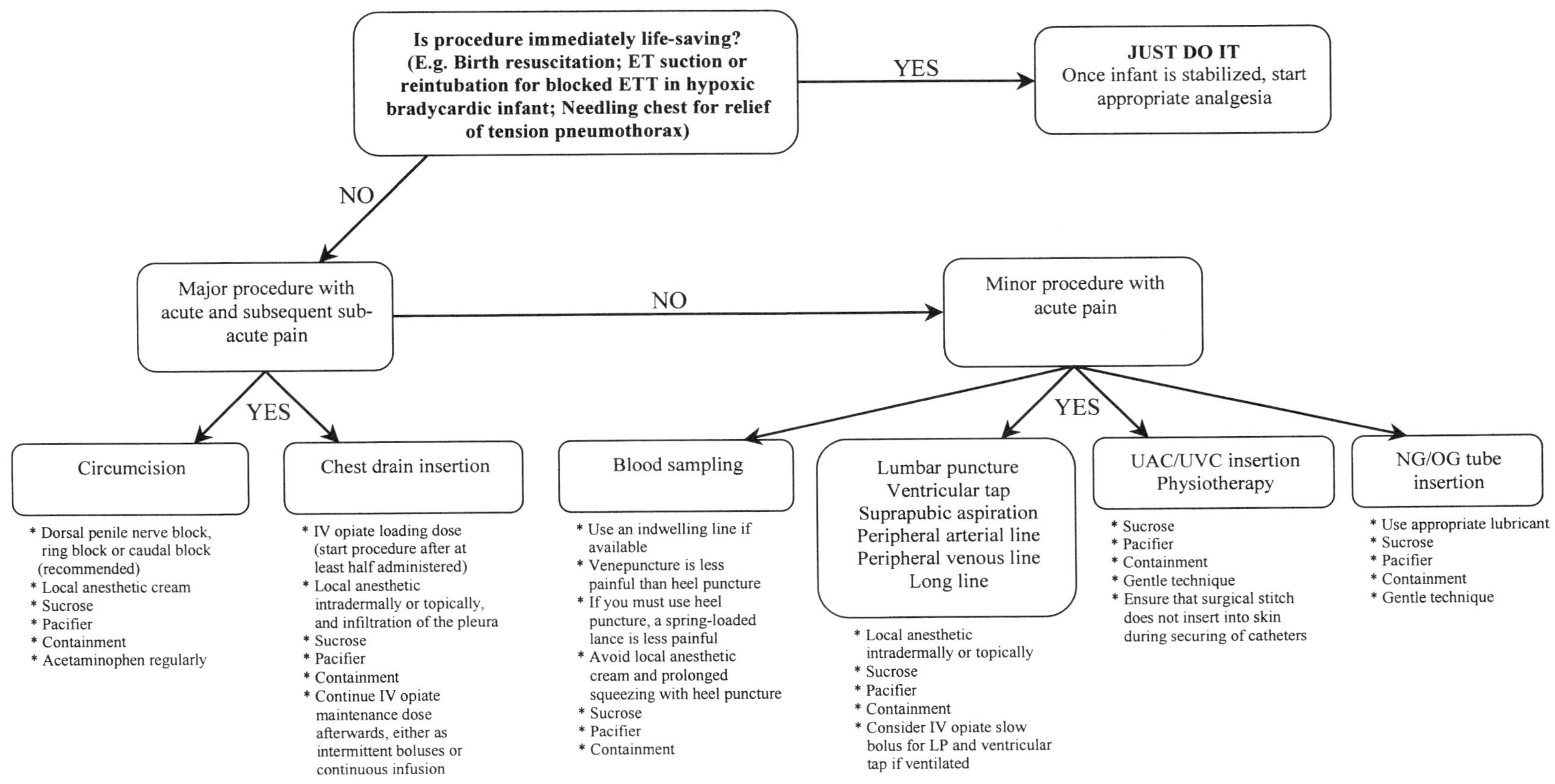

FIG. 37.1. An algorithm for the multimodal management of procedural pain in neonates. Operative procedures including ophthalmic laser/cryotherapy require general or epidural anesthesia. Ventilatory procedures are outlined in Figure 37.2. *ET*, endotracheal; *ETT*, endotracheal tube; *UAC*, umbilical arterial catheter; *UVC*, umbilical venous catheter; *NG*, nasogastric; *OG*, orogastric; *L*, lumbar puncture.

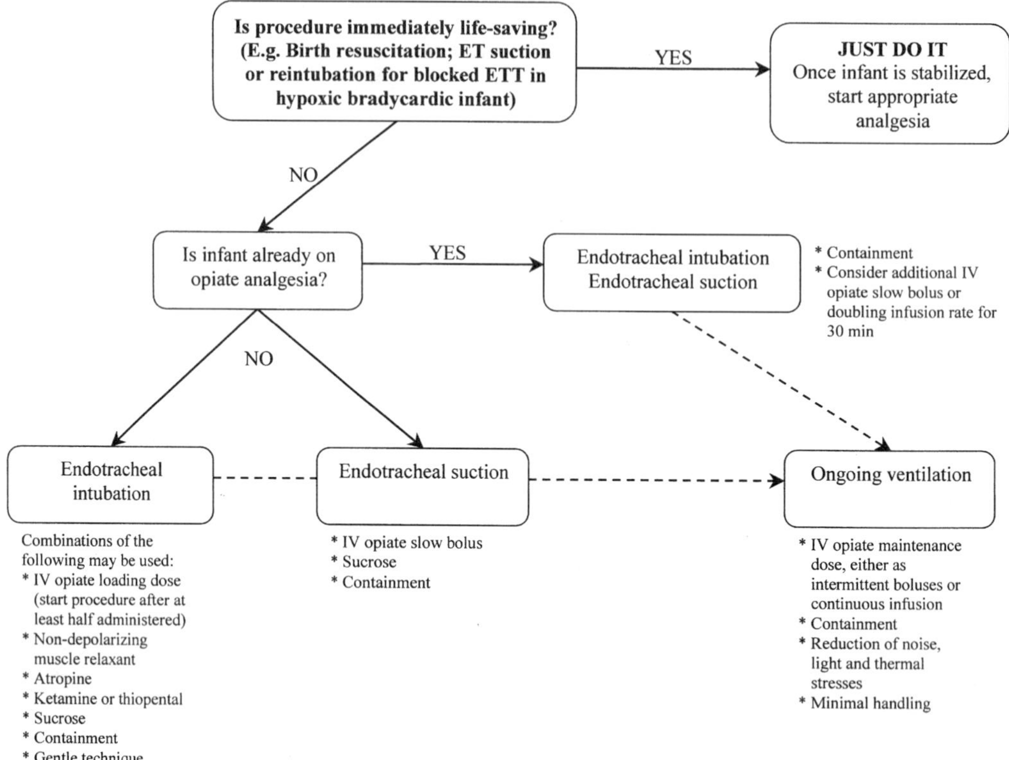

FIG. 37.2. An algorithm for the multimodal management of pain from ventilatory procedures in neonates. (Important: The routine use of opiates in ventilated neonates is currently being investigated in the NEOPAIN Trial.)

(84). Nonnutritive sucking attenuates not only behavioral responses to pain but also physiologic (83) and hormonal (85). Although Carbajal et al. (82) found that pacifiers alone were more effective than sucrose analgesia alone, Blass and Watt (81) found the opposite. However, both groups agreed that a pacifier and sucrose together were most effective.

Milk

Although milk reduces pain via opioid pathways in animal studies (86,87), in the human newborn, there are conflicting results. Formula milk has some effect (88,89), while breast milk does not (90,91). In all cases, sucrose or glucose had a greater effect than milk.

Sweet-Tasting Substances

Perhaps the most widely investigated form of neonatal analgesia, apart from opioids, has been the use of sweet-tasting substances such as sucrose. Blass et al. (92) showed in 1987 that intraoral sucrose given to newborn rats resulted in an increase in pain threshold and that this finding was reversed by the administration of an opioid antagonist, indicating that the analgesic effect was mediated by the endogenous opioid system. Similar results were also obtained in newborn rats using fructose and glucose (93). Human newborn studies confirmed that glucose had the same effect (82,87,91,94); therefore, strictly speaking, "sucrose" analgesia is a misnomer. For convenience, however, we use the term in this chapter.

TABLE 37.3. *Drugs used for sedation and analgesia*

Drug name	Dose: Intermittent	Dose: Infusion	Side effects and important notes
12%–24% sucrose		0.5–1 mL on tongue	Not effective given via nasogastric tube; risk of hyperglycemia
Local anesthesia			
2.5% lidocaine/2.5% prilocaine (EMLA cream)		0.5 g (0.5 mL) topically for 30 min	Risk of methemoglobinemia; also local pallor, erythema, blistering, and edema; avoid inflamed or traumatized skin surfaces
4% amethocaine (Ametop cream)		Dose not defined yet	local erythema, edema, and pruritus; avoid inflamed skin surfaces
Lidocaine 0.5%–1% infiltration		0.5 mL intradermally/subcutaneously	Avoid preparations combined with epinephrine; respiratory depression, convulsions, hypotension, heart block, bradycardia, and cardiac arrest if administered intravenously or intrathecally; avoid inflamed tissue
Epidural anesthesia			
Morphine	25–50 μg/kg bolus q6h	3–4 μg/kg per hr used in older infants	Respiratory depression, hypotension, bradycardia
Bupivacaine		0.5 mL/kg of 0.25% solution bolus, then 0.2 mL/kg per hr of 0.125% solution	As for lidocaine
Chloroprocaine		1 mL/kg of 3% solution bolus, then 1 mL/kg per hr of 3% solution	As for lidocaine
Systemic			
Sedative			
Chloral hydrate	30 mg/kg p.o./p.r. q8h		Vomiting, abdominal distention, rash, eosinophilia, leukopenia, dependence if prolonged use
Triclofos	30 mg/kg p.o. q6h		As for chloral hydrate
Midazolam		≤33/40: 60 μg/kg per hr i.v. for 24 hr, then 30 μg/kg per hr >33/40: 60 μg/kg per hr i.v. >1 mo postnatal age: 100 μg/kg per hr i.v.	Respiratory depression, hypotension, bradycardia, seizures, dependence if prolonged use
Phenobarbitone	5–10 mg/kg i.v./p.o. q12h		Respiratory depression, rash, megaloblastic anemia, hyperkinesia
Analgesic			
Opioid			
Morphine	50–100 μg/kg i.v.	150 μg/kg i.v. loading dose, then 10–30 μg/kg per hr i.v.	Respiratory depression, hypotension, bradycardia, tachycardia, constipation, urinary retention, sweating, and seizures
Fentanyl	2–5 μg/kg i.v.	10–15 μg/kg i.v. loading dose, then 1–4 μg/kg per hr i.v.	As for morphine; also muscle rigidity and hypothermia
Alfentanil	0.05–0.3 μg/kg i.v.	0.05–0.2 μg/kg per hr i.v.	As for fentanyl
Sufentanil	0.05–0.3 μg/kg i.v.	0.05–0.2 μg/kg per hr i.v.	As for fentanyl
Meperidine	500–1,000 μg/kg i.v.	500–4,000 μg/kg per hr i.v.	As for fentanyl
Nonsteroidal anti-inflammatory drugs			
Acetaminophen	10–15 mg/kg p.o. q6h 20–25 mg/kg p.r. q6h		Rash, liver damage if overdose
Indomethacin	0.2–0.3 mg/kg i.v. q8h		Gastrointestinal bleeding, necrotizing enterocolitis, oliguria, hematuria, acute renal failure, cerebral vasoconstriction, thrombocytopenia, systemic and pulmonary hypertension
Ibuprofen	10–15 mg/kg p.o. q6h 20–25 mg/kg p.r. q6h		Oliguria; fewer side effects than indomethacin
Anesthetic agents			
Thiopentone	5 mg/kg i.v.	1–5 mg/kg per hr i.v.	Hypotension, hypothermia, airway hyperreactivity; potentiated by sulfonamides
Ketamine	0.5–1 mg/kg i.v./i.m. 2–5 mg/kg p.o.	10–45 μg/kg per min i.v. used in anesthesia	Increased muscle tone, tachycardia, hypertension
Propofol	3–4 mg/kg i.v.	2–4 mg/kg per hr i.v.	Metabolic acidosis, myocardial depression

p.o., orally; i.v., intravenously; p.r., rectally; i.m., intramuscularly.

Numerous randomized, controlled trials have now been conducted in human newborns investigating the efficacy of sucrose analgesia in procedures such as heel punctures (81,90,91,95–99), venipuncture (81,82,100) and immunization injections (101–103). Various doses have been explored, ranging from 0.05 to 2 mL of 7.5% to 50% sucrose solution, and different outcomes measured (e.g., crying times, behavioral pain scores, physiologic parameters). Sucrose has also been compared with milk (90,91) and nonnutritive sucking (81,82) for procedural pain and also with lidocaine-prilocaine cream (EMLA cream) and nerve blockade for circumcision. The differences in trial methodology and outcome measurements make a meta-analysis difficult, although this was attempted by Stevens et al. (104) in 1997. All trials have found that sucrose has a positive analgesic effect for term and preterm infants with the exception of one study (99) in which 7.5% sucrose, a relatively low concentration, was no better than water.

The meta-analysis by Stevens et al. (104) reviewed 13 randomized, controlled, blinded trials published between 1991 and 1996 with respect to reduction in cry duration. Seven trials were excluded because the data were not extractable and another because cry duration was not an outcome measure. The meta-analysis only looked at whether increasing amounts of sucrose provided an increasing degree of analgesia. The groups were stratified according to the absolute sucrose dose administered in grams, calculated from the volume and concentration of sucrose given. Pacifier use and other comfort measures involved were not taken into account, and, although other outcomes were not formally assessed, it was noted in three studies that sucrose also caused a significant decrease in heart rate and in two a reduction in facial expression. The conclusion was that an absolute sucrose dose of 0.24 g or greater is effective in reducing cry duration, but there is little difference between 0.24 g and larger doses. Since this meta-analysis was published, Ramenghi et al. (105) have shown that the mode of action appears to be taste mediated rather than absorptive, which indicates that sucrose concentration may be more important than absolute sucrose dose. Now a subsequent larger meta-analysis by Stevens et al. (161) has confirmed that sucrose is effective for reducing procedural pain.

When compared with an equal volume of milk, two studies found that sucrose and glucose were effective, whereas breast milk was no better than water (90,91). Others have found that infant formula is effective but not to the same extent as sucrose (81,88). The disaccharide lactose has been found to have no effect in both animal (93) and human studies (88).

Sucrose certainly appears to have a place in procedural analgesia for neonates. It is effective, easily available, and inexpensive. However, it should be used as an adjunct to, and not a substitute for, more effective analgesic agents, particularly during more painful procedures such as circumcision. None of the studies has reported adverse effects, but these have not yet been looked at in detail, and this must be borne in mind when sucrose is used. Although sucrose seems to be effective and relatively safe in preterm neonates (95,97, 100) (earliest gestational age studied is 27 weeks), there remains the risk of predisposing this group of infants to hyperglycemia or necrotizing enterocolitis.

Pharmacologic

Acetaminophen/Paracetamol

Acetaminophen is commonly used for treating mild to moderate pain in children and adults. With standard doses, accumulation does not occur in neonates because their limited ability to conjugate phenolic drugs with glucuronic acid is compensated somewhat by a well-developed capability for sulfate conjugation (106). However, acetaminophen can only be delivered orally or rectally, and poor absorption can result in widely varying serum concentrations in both term and preterm neonates (107,108). A randomized, double-blinded, controlled trial found acetaminophen to be of no use in alleviating heel puncture pain (109). It can be used, however, to treat other pain in neonates such as postcircumcision pain.

Topical Local Anesthesia

This is available in various forms such as lidocaine ointment or gel and amethocaine cream, but the most commonly used in pediatric practice is lidocaine-prilocaine cream (EMLA), which is a eutectic mixture of 2.5% lidocaine and 2.5% prilocaine. It is effective when used to minimize pain from venipuncture in children. Its use has been restricted in infants because of a potential risk of methemoglobinemia from the prilocaine moiety (110). In 1999, Essink-Tjebbes et al. (111) published an efficacy and safety review of studies involving the use of lidocaine-prilocaine cream in neonates (excluding circumcision) and found that lidocaine-prilocaine cream was safe when used once a day in both term and preterm neonates. They subsequently showed that using 0.5 g as many as four times a day on heels of preterm infants did not raise methemoglobin levels (112). A study of term neonates using 1 g lidocaine-prilocaine cream on intact skin found that methemoglobin concentrations were significantly higher in the lidocaine-prilocaine cream group in the intervals from 3.5 to 13 hours after application but were well below potentially harmful levels (113).

Topical local anesthetics seem to be of benefit on some occasions but not in others. Lidocaine-prilocaine cream reduces existing hyperalgesia (114) in a punctured heel but does not provide analgesia for a heel puncture (78,115). This may be because prilocaine causes vasoconstriction and reduced heel blood flow, and hence blood collection is more difficult. Another trial of lidocaine-prilocaine cream for venipuncture in healthy preterm infants showed no benefit in behavioral or physiologic outcome (116). In their review, Essink-Tjebbes et al. (112) proposed that poor efficacy might be owing to application for too short a time because neonates have thinner skin than children and thus absorb the drug more quickly. They recommended a dose of 0.5 g applied for no longer than 30 minutes. Trials examining the efficacy of topical local anesthetics during circumcision have given rise to more consistent positive results (see below).

Awake Versus Anesthetized Neonatal Tracheal Intubation

Awake tracheal intubation, which is direct laryngoscopy and intubation without premedication, is commonly performed on neonates in NICUs because it is usually an emergency procedure on an unstable newborn. This contrasts with intubation after anesthesia induction before surgery, when the newborn is relatively well. The arguments for and against awake intubation were recently reviewed (117). Anesthetic agents such as thiopentone, propofol, and ketamine reduce the severity of acute adverse physiologic reactions to tracheal intubation. However, the long-term effects of both the physiologic changes and the anesthetic agents in neonates remain to be determined. Despite common use at the time of going to press, there is no evidence of a positive benefit from morphine for intubation in the NICU, although there are no data to suggest adverse effects.

Operative and Postoperative Management

Until the 1960s, the standard management for a thoracotomy for persistent ductus arteriosus ligation consisted of a sedative such as nitrous oxide and a paralyzing agent such as curare, but not analgesia. In the survey mentioned earlier involving 76 tertiary NICUs (2), it was found that although 50% of centers commonly used analgesia after major abdominal surgery, only approximately 10% did so for ventriculoperitoneal shunts, persistent ductus arteriosus ligations, and gastrostomies. In the same year, Anand et al. (7) showed that neonates are capable of mounting potentially detrimental physiologic, hormonal, and metabolic stress responses to pain, effects reversible with analgesia.

This awoke the medical and nursing professions to the realization that neonates experience pain and that adverse consequences might not be uncommon. It is therefore in perioperative pain management that the major improvements in neonatal pain have been made in the past decade. No newborn should ever undergo, without anesthesia or analgesia, major surgery for which an older child or adult would be given anesthesia.

In the general treatment of operative pain, nonpharmacologic interventions are less appropriate, although they may be used as adjuncts to standard drugs. Nonsteroidal anti-inflammatory drugs are generally avoided in neonates because of reports of intracranial and other hemorrhages as well as convulsions. Nonsteroidal anti-inflammatory drugs can also result in renal toxicity, necrotizing enterocolitis, inhibition of platelet aggregation, and Reye syndrome. Opioids have therefore been the mainstay of perioperative analgesia in neonates. Anesthetic agents such as thiopentone, ketamine, and propofol are used intraoperatively. Thiopentone has been investigated for use in the newborn more than other anesthetic agents have, but there is still scant literature on its safety, especially in the preterm infant.

Opioids: Morphine Versus Fentanyl

Morphine has been regarded as the gold standard with which other opioids are compared. Because of the immaturity of the hepatic glucuronidation system, the half-life of morphine is prolonged in neonates when compared with older infants (6.8 versus 3.9 hours) (118). It is further prolonged with decreasing gestational age (10 hours at 30 weeks' gestational age versus 6.7 hours at term) (119). Morphine clearance reaches adult values by the age of 1 to 3 months (120,121). There is also interindividual variability in morphine metabolism (119,122,123) and approximately 80% of the drug is unbound to plasma proteins. In adults, the main metabolites of morphine sulfate are morphine-6-glucuronide, which has stronger analgesic properties than morphine itself, and morphine-3-glucuronide, which is responsible for the side effects of morphine. These metabolites are usually present in plasma at higher concentrations than morphine. In neonates, morphine-6-glucuronide is hardly detectable, the dominant metabolite being morphine-3-glucuronide; thus, neonates are predisposed to more of the adverse effects of morphine such as decreased intestinal motility, hypotension, bradycardia, and urinary retention, with less analgesic benefit.

Fentanyl is a synthetic opioid that is equipotent to morphine at a dose 100 times less. Because it is relatively short acting, it needs to be administered by continuous infusion or frequent boluses. More than 90% of this drug is metabolized by the liver, and hence excretion is delayed in neonates (124). Fentanyl has significant respiratory depressant effects, and tolerance is a major problem with long-term administration. Another serious side effect, especially when fentanyl is given rapidly, is muscle rigidity, which has been occasionally fatal when chest wall rigidity has led to failure of ventilation.

In 1999, a randomized trial comparing morphine (20 μg/kg per hour) and fentanyl (1.5 μg/kg per hour) for analgesia in neonates undergoing mechanical ventilation in the first 2 days of life showed that fentanyl at this dose was as effective as morphine as an analgesic (125). Fentanyl also caused fewer gastrointestinal side effects and appeared to decrease β endorphin levels significantly in contrast to morphine. A separate trial in 1998 showed that during extracorporeal membrane oxygenation, neonates who received morphine (20 μg/kg per hour) required less supplemental analgesia, had a lower prevalence of withdrawal, and were discharged sooner than neonates who received fentanyl (10 μg/kg per hour) (126). This finding might be explained by the higher dose of fentanyl used in this trial. Another small study showed that fentanyl increased the incidence of perioperative hypothermia when compared with morphine or epidural bupivacaine (127). The hypothermia is probably owing to the inhibition of nonshivering thermogenesis by fentanyl (128). The evidence for and against either morphine or fentanyl therefore remains in limbo, and their use depends on the individual practitioner.

Diamorphine is not used in neonates, probably because of its potency. The data to support the use of other opioids (e.g., alfentanil, sufentanil, remifentanil, meperidine) in neonates, particularly if born preterm, are minimal, especially with regard to safety profile and long-term consequences. Alfentanil, sufentanil, and remifentanil all have side effects similar to those of fentanyl, of which the most unpleasant is muscle and chest wall rigidity.

Opioid Tolerance, Dependence, and Withdrawal

Opioid tolerance and dependence are iatrogenic complications of analgesia and sedation in the NICU (129,130). Neonates can become tolerant to the sedative effects of opioids, requiring increasing doses to maintain the same levels of analgesia or sedation over time. Neonates also develop physical dependence leading to opioid withdrawal after abrupt discontinuation of the drug.

Neonatal opioid withdrawal is a generalized disorder characterized by central nervous system hyperirritability, gastrointestinal dysfunction, respiratory distress, and autonomic hyperfunction that, if untreated, can lead to seizures. After prolonged fentanyl administration, abnormal movements not usually associated with opioid withdrawal have also been observed in infants (131). Withdrawal symptoms associated with long-term benzodiazepine treatment are less well defined (132).

The incidence and severity of withdrawal symptoms may be greater for fentanyl than for morphine. The risk of clinically significant opioid withdrawal symptoms with abrupt discontinuation or rapid tapering increases significantly after 5 days of continuous infusion or frequent bolus doses (126,133). The probability of withdrawal symptoms approaches 100% when the drugs are administered for more than 9 days (134).

Objective assessment of the clinical severity of opioid withdrawal symptoms is important for determining appropriate treatment. Opioid blood levels are poor indicators of symptom severity (135), and the degree of withdrawal is best measured by the number and severity of behavioral signs. Scales to assess the severity of iatrogenic opioid withdrawal symptoms have been derived from measures of neonatal abstinence syndrome in the otherwise healthy full-term infant with in utero opioid exposure (136). These scales have been modified because some of the signs of opioid withdrawal cannot be assessed in the critically ill or preterm infant (129,137). Signs of withdrawal may take as long as 48 hours to manifest after discontinuation of opioids.

Tapering the drug dose before discontinuation will prevent or lessen the severity of withdrawal. However, guidelines for effective weaning of infants from opioids are not well established (Table 37.4). Caron and Maguire

TABLE 37.4. *Opioid and benzodiazepine tapering guidelines for the prevention of withdrawal symptoms*

If opioids and benzodiazepines have been in use for more than 5 days:

1. Initiate withdrawal symptom scoring for all patients who receive opioids or benzodiazepines for more than 5 days. Score every 4 hours. Continue to monitor for signs of withdrawal for at least 48 hours after the drug has been stopped.
2. Reduce opioid and/or benzodiazepine infusion rate by 20% of the last maintenance dose every 24 hours. For intermittent bolus administration, reduce total daily dose by 20% per day.
3. If withdrawal symptoms develop, reduce weaning rate to 10% per day or consider not weaning for a 24-hour period, then resume weaning.
4. If withdrawal scores do not decrease, consider the following options:
   a. Reinitiate or add benzodiazepine therapy
   b. Increase opioid to previous dose (especially if gastrointestinal symptoms noted)
   c. If symptoms do not resolve, initiate clonidine
   d. Consider consultation with the pain control service at any point

(138) reported prevention of withdrawal with an initial decrease of 25% of the opioid dose, followed by decreases of 10% every 4 hours. Another method of weaning consists of decreasing the infusion by 20% to 40%, then by 10% every 12 to 24 hours, depending on symptoms (139). Infants demonstrating severe withdrawal symptoms may need a taper of no more than 10% per day to avoid rebound withdrawal and delays in progress toward discharge (129). During the weaning period, painful procedures should be actively managed by using appropriate analgesia.

Mild symptoms may be managed effectively with environmental and behavioral interventions such as minimizing light, noise, and handling or by prone positioning (140). Agitation and hyperirritability may be reduced by swaddling or rocking. Severe behavioral disturbances or gastrointestinal symptoms require pharmacologic treatment. Use of longer acting opioids such as methadone may reduce the symptom severity during the weaning process (130). The α-adrenergic agonist clonidine may be effective in controlling central nervous system symptoms during the tapering of opioids. Clonidine has been used to treat opioid withdrawal in neonates (141,142). It partially ameliorates the symptoms of withdrawal by decreasing the central nervous system noradrenergic activity and is a useful adjunct in the treatment of withdrawal symptoms that are not resolved by slowing the weaning or reinstituting benzodiazepine or opioid therapy. However, clonidine is ineffective in reducing the gastrointestinal symptoms associated with opioid withdrawal.

Epidurals and Early Extubation Strategies

Morphine can also be administered by the epidural route. This provides adequate analgesia with fewer doses and lower total doses than the intravenous route (143). Unfortunately, apnea and desaturation still occur with epidural administration. Alternative epidural analgesics include bupivacaine and chloroprocaine.

Previously, the fear of infections and lack of appropriate-size catheters limited the use of epidural analgesia in neonates. In skilled hands, however, the use of epidural analgesia after major surgery allows even 32-week gestation neonates to be successfully extubated at completion of surgery with no subsequent respiratory depression or apnea (144,145). Postoperative analgesia can be maintained by either intermittent top-ups or continuous infusions. A review of epidural analgesia in 240 neonates found only three cases of complications (dural puncture, convulsion, intravascular migration of catheter) (146). Another report cited difficulty with placing lumbar catheters in two of 20 patients, but this was overcome by using the caudal route (145). Epidural analgesia is a promising alternative to general anesthesia or systemic analgesia for various surgical procedures. The advantages of earlier extubation (e.g., reduced ventilator-induced lung injury and pulmonary infections) and the avoidance of systemic administration of powerful analgesics probably outweigh the minimal risks when used carefully.

Painful Medical Conditions

The use of analgesics in inflammatory conditions that would be expected to cause pain such as necrotizing enterocolitis, meningitis, osteomyelitis, peritonitis, and possibly large periventricular hemorrhage is variable, but it is logical in infants in whom some of the pathologic effects may be compounded by stress (e.g., diaphragmatic splinting and apnea caused by pain).

Swaddling and minimal handling may help in such situations. Reduction of ambient light and other sensory input may help in babies with meningitis or central nervous system irritability for other reasons (e.g., large intraventricular hemorrhage, hypoxic ischemic encephalopathy). Decompression of the stomach with continuous drainage in babies with necrotizing enterocolitis may reduce the discomfort of abdominal distention. The most appropriate analgesia for necrotizing enterocolitis is a parenteral analgesic effective for severe pain (i.e., an opioid infusion). This should be started after assessment and resuscitation to ensure that the potential hypotensive and respiratory suppressant effects of opioids will not create further complications. Opioids are probably the drug of choice in severe pain from any cause.

Acetaminophen or a nonsteroidal anti-inflammatory agent such as ibuprofen may be appropriate in mild to moderate pain but should be used with caution in preterm infants because of undesirable antiplatelet and vascular effects (more pronounced with indomethacin).

Circumcision

The most ancient painful ritual in the newborn infant is the circumcision of the male. In the United States, it is commonly carried out for nonmedical reasons. Although a dorsal penile nerve block provides effective analgesia, circumcision without analgesia is still the norm. Yet even the rabbis of the old testament used a mixture of sweet wine and honey to ameliorate the pain, agents known now from "scientific studies" to be analgesic. There is now a large body of evidence showing that circumcision is painful (147–157) and that long-term effects may result if carried out without analgesia (158). Analgesia is of proven benefit (147—149,151–157); hence, it is no longer ethical to perform circumcision without analgesia. The American Academy of Pediatrics has issued a policy statement endorsing analgesia for the procedure (159). Ring blocks or dorsal penile nerve blocks are the gold standard analgesia for circumcision (147–149,151,152,154,156). Lidocaine-prilocaine cream is also beneficial but to a lesser extent (147,149,151,152,154). Sucrose analgesia is effective but less so than lidocaine-prilocaine cream (148,153), although the two methods can be used concurrently. Acetaminophen is not adequate (150) but may be used postoperatively. Side effects to be aware of with nerve blocks include hematoma formation and penile edema, and lidocaine-prilocaine cream can produce local erythema or blistering.

EVALUATION OF THE EFFICACY OF TREATMENT

Evaluation of the efficacy of pain treatments used for infants in the NICU should be at the level of the individual patient and at the unit level. The decision that a pain treatment is effective should be based on a demonstrated reduction in pain response measured by a validated pain assessment tool. However, research in the area of neonatal pain assessment has not progressed sufficiently to provide specific guidelines for clinicians regarding how to judge the effectiveness of pain interventions for neonatal patients; therefore, unit specific protocols should be developed.

A general principle derived from the research on procedural pain is that a 10% to 20% decrease in behavioral responses, physiologic responses, or composite assessment scores is usually judged to be a clinically significant decrease in pain (34,39). However, if the objective of the treatment is pain prevention, then there should be no increase in any of the measures during the treatment. Furthermore, lack of responsiveness can occur with repeated pain, and provision of comfort measures and analgesia may allow increased responsiveness so that it might appear that pain increased in the presence of pain treatment. Thus, the evaluation of the efficacy of treatment is context dependent and must be individualized. Clarifying the objectives and desired outcomes of the pain treatment among the members of the infant's care team before initiation facilitates evaluation of the efficacy of the treatment and enables prompt recognition and response to any desired or adverse effects.

The efficacy of pain treatment within the entire NICU must also be evaluated. A periodic and systematic clinical audit should be performed to track the nature and prevalence of pain within each unit, with the practice patterns of nonpharmacologic and pharmacologic interventions and the incidence and severity of adverse effects related to the intervention. Review of patient outcomes and practice patterns facilitates continuous improvement of the quality of pain management on the unit (61). Recently, the Joint Commission on Accreditation of Health Care Organizations in the United States set standards for pain management (160). These standards are intended to ensure that all hospitalized patients receive optimal pain management. The standards emphasize the importance of the audit and evaluation of pain management, particularly in the areas of (a) patient (parent) information; (b) staff competency; (c) routine, standardized pain assessment; (d) appropriate use of pain treatments; and (e) monitoring of adverse effects of pain treatment. Clinicians can also expect greater scrutiny from regulating bodies. This increased emphasis on a systematic clinical audit and benchmarking of individual and unit level practices will provide researchers with improved preliminary data on which to base future studies of the relative efficacy of different approaches to neonatal pain management.

CONCLUSIONS

Good management of neonatal pain starts with the recognition that newborn infants can feel pain, which is often undertreated. A procedure deemed painful to an adult should also be considered painful to a newborn infant. Neonatal pain management includes the consistent treatment of procedural and other forms of pain and distress using principles of anticipation and prevention and alleviation or eradication. Pain must be adequately assessed (the most difficult task) and the effectiveness of treatments must be adequately monitored. The importance of this in the short term is in the reduction of morbidity. In the long term, the eradication of prolonged behavioral changes may be more important than we currently appreciate.

ACKNOWLEDGMENTS

C. Mae Wong is on a Neonatal Pain Research Fellowship provided by the Rivendell Trust.

REFERENCES

1. Eland JM, Anderson JE. The experience of pain in children. In: Jacox AK, ed. *Pain: a source book for nurses and other health professionals*. Boston: Little, Brown, 1977.
2. Franck LS. A national survey of the assessment and treatment of pain and agitation in the neonatal intensive care unit. *J Obstet Gynecol Neonatal Nurs* 1987; 16:387–393.
3. Porter FL, Wolf CM, Gold J, et al. Pain and pain management in newborn infants: a survey of physicians and nurses. *Pediatrics* 1997;100:626–632.
4. Anand KJ, Hickey PR. Pain and its effects in the human neonate and fetus. *N Engl J Med* 1987;317: 1321–1329.
5. Tilney F, Rosett J. The value of brain lipoids as an index of brain development. *Bull Neurol Inst N Y* 1931; 1:28–71.
6. Fitzgerald M. Neurobiology of fetal and neonatal pain. In: Wall PD, Melzack R, eds. *Textbook of pain*. London: Churchill-Livingstone, 1994:46–52.
7. Anand KJ, Sippell WG, Aynsley-Green A. Randomised trial of fentanyl anaesthesia in preterm babies undergoing surgery: effects on the stress response. *Lancet* 1987;1:62–66.
8. Anand KJ, Hickey PR. Halothane-morphine compared with high-dose sufentanil for anesthesia and postoperative analgesia in neonatal cardiac surgery. *N Engl J Med* 1992;326:1–9.
9. Franck LS, Lawhon G. Environmental and behavioral strategies to prevent and manage neonatal pain. In: McGrath PJ, Anand KJ, Stevens B, eds. *Pain in neonates*. Amsterdam: Elsevier, 2000:205–218.
10. Anand KJ, Craig KD. New perspectives on the definition of pain. *Pain* 1996;67:3–6.
11. Barker DP, Rutter N. Exposure to invasive procedures in neonatal intensive care unit admissions. *Arch Dis Child Fetal Neonatal Ed* 1995;72:F47–F48.
12. Anand KJ. Neonatal stress responses to anesthesia and surgery. *Clin Perinatol* 1990;17:207–214.
13. Anand KJ, Barton BA, McIntosh N, et al. Analgesia and sedation in preterm neonates who require ventilatory support: results from the NOPAIN trial. Neonatal outcome and prolonged analgesia in neonates. *Arch Pediatr Adolesc Med* 1999;153:331–338.
14. Als H, Lawhon G, Duffy FH, et al. Individualized developmental care for the very low-birth-weight preterm infant. Medical and neurofunctional effects. *JAMA* 1994;272:853–858.
15. Kidd S, Stephen R, Midgley P, et al. Stress, distress and pain in the newborn. *Pediatr Res* 1997;42:392.
16. Stevens B. Composite measures of pain. *Prog Pain Res Measure* 1998;10:161–178.
17. Page GG, Halvorson M. Pediatric nurses: the assessment and control of pain in preverbal infants. *J Pediatr Nurs* 1991;6:99–106.
18. Ambuel B, Hamlett KW, Marx CM, et al. Assessing distress in pediatric intensive care environments: the COMFORT scale. *J Pediatr Psychol* 1992;17:95–109.
19. Fitzgerald M, Anand KJ. Developmental neuroanatomy and neurophysiology of pain. In: Schechter NL, Berde CB, Yaster M, eds. *Pain in infants, children and adolescents*. Baltimore: Williams & Wilkins, 1993:11–31.

20. Abu-Saad HH, Bours GJ, Stevens B, et al. Assessment of pain in the neonate. *Semin Perinatol* 1998;22: 402–416.
21. Franck LS, Miaskowski C. Measurement of neonatal responses to painful stimuli: a research review. *J Pain Symptom Manage* 1997;14:343–378.
22. Finlay GA, McGrath PJ. *Measurement of pain in infants and children*. Seattle: IASP Press, 1998.
23. Craig KD. Behavioural measures of pain. *Prog Pain Res Measure* 1998;10:103–121.
24. Grunau RV, Craig KD. Pain expression in neonates: facial action and cry. *Pain* 1987;28:395–410.
25. Grunau RE, Oberlander T, Holsti L, et al. Bedside application of the Neonatal Facial Coding System in pain assessment of premature neonates. *Pain* 1998;76: 277–286.
26. Craig KD, McMahon RJ, Morison JD, et al. Developmental changes in infant pain expression during immunization injections. *Soc Sci Med* 1984;19: 1331–1337.
27. Craig KD, Grunau RV. Neonatal pain perception and behavioural measurement. In: Anand KJ, McGrath PJ, eds. *Pain in neonates*. Amsterdam: Elsevier, 1993: 67–106.
28. Barrier G, Attia J, Mayer MN, et al. Measurement of post-operative pain and narcotic administration in infants using a new clinical scoring system. *Intensive Care Med* 1989;15[Suppl 1]:S37–S39.
29. Horgan M, Choonara I. Measuring pain in neonates: an objective score. *Paediatr Nurs* 1996;8:24–27.
30. Lawrence J, Alcock D, McGrath P, et al. The development of a tool to assess neonatal pain. *Neonatal Network* 1993;12:59–66.
31. Taddio A, Nulman I, Koren BS, et al. A revised measure of acute pain in infants. *J Pain Symptom Manage* 1995;10:456–463.
32. Joyce BA, Schade JG, Keck JF, et al. Reliability and validity of preverbal pain assessment tools. *Issues Compr Pediatr Nurs* 1994;17:121–135.
33. Schade JG, Joyce BA, Gerkensmeyer J, et al. Comparison of three preverbal scales for postoperative pain assessment in a diverse pediatric sample. *J Pain Symptom Manage* 1996;12:348–359.
34. Krechel SW, Bildner J. CRIES: a new neonatal postoperative pain measurement score. Initial testing of validity and reliability. *Paediatr Anaesth* 1995;5:53–61.
35. Hodgkinson K, Bear M, Thorn J, et al. Measuring pain in neonates: evaluating an instrument and developing a common language. *Aust J Adv Nurs* 1994;12:17–22.
36. Blauer T, Gerstmann D. A simultaneous comparison of three neonatal pain scales during common NICU procedures. *Clin J Pain* 1998;14:39–47.
37. Pokela ML. Pain relief can reduce hypoxemia in distressed neonates during routine treatment procedures. *Pediatrics* 1994;93:379–383.
38. Sparshott M. The development of a clinical distress scale for ventilated infants: identification of pain and distress based on validated behavioural scores. *J Neonatal Nurs* 1996;2:5–11.
39. Stevens B, Johnston C, Petryshen P, et al. Premature Infant Pain Profile: development and initial validation. *Clin J Pain* 1996;12:13–22.
40. Ballantyne M, Stevens B, McAllister M, et al. Validation of the premature infant pain profile in the clinical setting. *Clin J Pain* 1999;15:297–303.
41. Schiller C, Stevens B, Sidani S. Determining the clinical utility of two measures of neonatal pain. *Pain Res Manage* 1999;4:60.
42. McNair C, Ballantyne M, Dionne K. Postoperative pain assessment in the neonatal intensive care unit. International Pediatric Nursing Research Symposium: Clinical Care of the Child and Family. Montreal, 1999.
43. Eriksson M, Gradin M, Schollin J. Oral glucose and venepuncture reduce blood sampling pain in newborns. *Early Hum Dev* 1999;55:211–218.
44. Stevens B, Johnston C, Franck L, et al. The efficacy of developmentally sensitive interventions and sucrose for relieving procedural pain in very low birth weight neonates. *Nurs Res* 1999;48:35–43.
45. Davis M, Emory E. Sex differences in neonatal stress reactivity. *Child Dev* 1995;66:14–27.
46. Johnston CC, Stevens BJ. Experience in a neonatal intensive care unit affects pain response. *Pediatrics* 1996;98:925–930.
47. Stevens BJ, Johnston CC, Horton L. Factors that influence the behavioral pain responses of premature infants. *Pain* 1994;59:101–109.
48. Porter FL, Wolf CM, Miller JP. The effect of handling and immobilization on the response to acute pain in newborn infants. *Pediatrics* 1998;102:1383–1389.
49. McIntosh N. Pain in the newborn, a possible new starting point. *Eur J Pediatr* 1997;156:173–177.
50. Lawson JR. Pain in the neonate and fetus. *N Engl J Med* 1988;318:1398–1399.
51. Franck LS, Scurr K, Couture S. Parent views on infant pain and pain management in the NICU. *Newborn Infant Nursing Reviews* 2001;1:106–113.
52. *It is critical that you know.... What you should do when your baby is in the neonatal intensive care unit.* Newport Beach, CA: American Association of Critical Care Nurses, 1987.
53. Schechter NL. The undertreatment of pain in children: an overview. *Pediatr Clin North Am* 1989;36:781–794.
54. McCain GC, Morwessel NJ. Pediatric nurses' knowledge and practice related to infant pain. *Issues Compr Pediatr Nurs* 1995;18:277–286.
55. Burokas L. Factors affecting nurses' decisions to medicate pediatric patients after surgery. *Heart Lung* 1985; 14:373–379.
56. Hester NO, Foster RL, Jordan-Marsh M. Putting pain measurement into clinical practice. *Prog Pain Res Measure* 1998;10:179–198.
57. Agency for Healthcare Policy and Research. *Acute pain management: medical procedures and trauma, part 2*. Rockville, MD: Department of Health and Human Services, 1992.
58. Max MB. Improving outcomes of analgesic treatment: is education enough? *Ann Intern Med* 1990;113:885–889.
59. Schechter NL, Blankson V, Pachter LM, et al. The ouchless place: no pain, children's gain. *Pediatrics* 1997;99:890–894.
60. Friedrichs JB, Young S, Gallagher D, et al. Where does it hurt? An interdisciplinary approach to improving the quality of pain assessment and management in the neonatal intensive care unit. *Nurs Clin North Am* 1995; 30:143–159.
61. Furdon SA, Eastman M, Benjamin K, et al. Outcome measures after standardized pain management strategies in postoperative patients in the neonatal intensive care unit. *J Perinatal Neonatal Nurs* 1998;12:58–69.

62. Miaskowski C, Jacox A, Hester NO, et al. Interdisciplinary guidelines for the management of acute pain: implications for quality improvement. *J Nurs Care Quality* 1992;7:1–6.
63. Dyke MP, Kohan R, Evans S. Morphine increases synchronous ventilation in preterm infants. *J Paediatr Child Health* 1995;31:176–179.
64. Brazy JE, Kinney HC, Oakes WJ. Central nervous system structural lesions causing apnea at birth. *J Pediatr* 1987;111:163–175.
65. Friesen RH, Honda AT, Thieme RE. Changes in anterior fontanel pressure in preterm neonates during tracheal intubation. *Anesth Analg* 1987;66:874–878.
66. Vacanti JP, Crone RK, Murphy JD, et al. The pulmonary hemodynamic response to perioperative anesthesia in the treatment of high-risk infants with congenital diaphragmatic hernia. *J Pediatr Surg* 1984; 19:672–679.
67. Hickey PR, Hansen DD, Wessel DL, et al. Blunting of stress responses in the pulmonary circulation of infants by fentanyl. *Anesth Analg* 1985;64:1137–1142.
68. Quinn MW, Otoo F, Rushforth JA, et al. Effect of morphine and pancuronium on the stress response in ventilated preterm infants. *Early Hum Dev* 1992;30: 241–248.
69. Orsini AJ, Leef KH, Costarino A, et al. Routine use of fentanyl infusions for pain and stress reduction in infants with respiratory distress syndrome. *J Pediatr* 1996;129:140–145.
70. Burtin P, Jacqz-Aigrain E, Girard P, et al. Population pharmacokinetics of midazolam in neonates. *Clin Pharmacol Ther*1994;56:615–625.
71. Jacqz-Aigrain E, Daoud P, Burtin P, et al. Placebo-controlled trial of midazolam sedation in mechanically ventilated newborn babies. *Lancet* 1994;344:646–650.
72. Rosow CE, Moss J, Philbin DM, et al. Histamine release during morphine and fentanyl anesthesia. *Anesthesiology* 1982;56:93–96.
73. Anand KJ. Consensus statement for the prevention and management of pain in the newborn. *Arch Pediatr Adolesc Med*2001;155:173–180.
74. Anand KJ, Salanikio JD, SOPAIN Study Group. Routine analgesic practices in 109 neonatal intensive care units (NICUs). *Pediatr Res* 1996;39:192A.
75. Johnston CC, Collinge JM, Henderson SJ, et al. A cross-sectional survey of pain and pharmacological analgesia in Canadian neonatal intensive care units. *Clin J Pain* 1997;13:308–312.
76. Larsson BA, Tannfeldt G, Lagercrantz H, et al. Venipuncture is more effective and less painful than heel lancing for blood tests in neonates. *Pediatrics* 1998;101:882–886.
77. Shah VS, Taddio A, Bennett S, et al. Neonatal pain response to heel stick vs veniepuncture for routine blood sampling. *Arch Dis Child Fetal Neonatal Ed* 1997;77: F143–F144.
78. McIntosh N, van Veen L, Brameyer H. Alleviation of the pain of heel prick in preterm infants. *Arch Dis Child Fetal Neonatal Ed* 1994;70:F177–F181.
79. Campos RG. Soothing pain-elicited distress in infants with swaddling and pacifiers. *Child Dev* 1989;60: 781–792.
80. Blass EM, Hoffmeyer LB. Sucrose as an analgesic for newborn infants. *Pediatrics* 1991;87:215–218.
81. Blass EM, Watt LB. Suckling- and sucrose-induced analgesia in human newborns. *Pain* 1999;83:611–623.
82. Carbajal R, Chauvet X, Couderc S, et al. Randomised trial of analgesic effects of sucrose, glucose, and pacifiers in term neonates. *BMJ* 1999;319:1393–1397.
83. Field T, Goldson E. Pacifying effects of nonnutritive sucking on term and preterm neonates during heelstick procedures. *Pediatrics* 1984;74:1012–1015.
84. Blass EM, Ciaramitaro V. A new look at some old mechanisms in human newborns: taste and tactile determinants of state, affect, and action. *Monogr Soc Res Child Dev* 1994;59:1–81.
85. Gunnar MR, Fisch RO, Malone S. The effects of a pacifying stimulus on behavioral and adrenocortical responses to circumcision in the newborn. *J Am Acad Child Psychiatry* 1984;23:34–38.
86. Blass EM, Fitzgerald E. Milk-induced analgesia and comforting in 10-day-old rats: opioid mediation. *Pharmacol Biochem Behav* 1988;29:9–13.
87. Blass EM, Shide DJ, Weller A. Stress-reducing effects of ingesting milk, sugars, and fats. A developmental perspective. *Ann N Y Acad Sci* 1989;575:292–305.
88. Blass EM. Milk-induced hypoalgesia in human newborns. *Pediatrics* 1997;99:825–829.
89. Blass EM. Infant formula quiets crying human newborns. *J Dev Behav Pediatr* 1997;18:162–165.
90. Ors R, Ozek E, Baysoy G, et al. Comparison of sucrose and human milk on pain response in newborns. *Eur J Pediatr* 1999;158:63–66.
91. Skogsdal Y, Eriksson M, Schollin J. Analgesia in newborns given oral glucose. *Acta Paediatr* 1997;86: 217–220.
92. Blass E, Fitzgerald E, Kehoe P. Interactions between sucrose, pain and isolation distress. *Pharmacol Biochem Behav* 1987;26:483–489.
93. Blass EM, Shide DJ. Some comparisons among the calming and pain-relieving effects of sucrose, glucose, fructose and lactose in infant rats. *Chem Senses* 1994;19:239–249.
94. Ramenghi LA, Griffith GC, Wood CM, et al. Effect of non-sucrose sweet tasting solution on neonatal heel prick responses. *Arch Dis Child Fetal Neonatal Ed* 1996;74:F129–F131.
95. Bucher HU, Moser T, von Siebenthal K, et al. Sucrose reduces pain reaction to heel lancing in preterm infants: a placebo-controlled, randomized and masked study. *Pediatr Res* 1995;38:332–335.
96. Haouari N, Wood C, Griffiths G, et al. The analgesic effect of sucrose in full term infants: a randomised controlled trial. *BMJ* 1995;310:1498–1500.
97. Johnston CC, Stremler R, Horton L, et al. Effect of repeated doses of sucrose during heel stick procedure in preterm neonates. *Biol Neonate* 1999;75:160–166.
98. Overgaard C, Knudsen A. Pain-relieving effect of sucrose in newborns during heel prick. *Biol Neonate* 1999;75:279–284.
99. Rushforth JA, Levene MI. Effect of sucrose on crying in response to heel stab. *Arch Dis Child* 1993;69:388–389.
100. Abad F, Diaz NM, Domenech E, et al. Oral sweet solution reduces pain-related behaviour in preterm infants. *Acta Paediatr* 1996;85:854–858.
101. Allen KD, White DD, Walburn JN. Sucrose as an analgesic agent for infants during immunization injections. *Arch Pediatr Adolesc Med* 1996;150:270–274.

102. Barr RG, Young SN, Wright JH, et al. "Sucrose analgesia" and diphtheria-tetanus-pertussis immunizations at 2 and 4 months. *J Dev Behav Pediatr* 1995;16: 220–225.
103. Lewindon PJ, Harkness L, Lewindon N. Randomised controlled trial of sucrose by mouth for the relief of infant crying after immunisation. *Arch Dis Child* 1998; 78:453–456.
104. Stevens B, Taddio A, Ohlsson A, et al. The efficacy of sucrose for relieving procedural pain in neonates—a systematic review and meta-analysis. *Acta Paediatr* 1997;86:837–842.
105. Ramenghi LA, Evans DJ, Levene MI. "Sucrose analgesia": absorptive mechanism or taste perception? *Arch Dis Child Fetal Neonatal Ed* 1999;80: F146–F147.
106. Levy G, Khanna NN, Soda DM, et al. Pharmacokinetics of acetaminophen in the human neonate: formation of acetaminophen glucuronide and sulfate in relation to plasma bilirubin concentration and D-glucaric acid excretion. *Pediatrics* 1975;55:818–825.
107. Lin YC, Sussman HH, Benitz WE. Plasma concentrations after rectal administration of acetaminophen in preterm neonates. *Paediatr Anaesth* 1997;7:457–459.
108. van Lingen RA, Deinum JT, Quak JM, et al. Pharmacokinetics and metabolism of rectally administered paracetamol in preterm neonates. *Arch Dis Child Fetal Neonatal Ed* 1999;80:F59–F63.
109. Shah V, Taddio A, Ohlsson A. Randomised controlled trial of paracetamol for heel prick pain in neonates. *Arch Dis Child Fetal Neonatal Ed* 1998;79: F209–F211.
110. Frey B , Kehrer B. Toxic methaemoglobin concentrations in premature infants after application of a prilocaine-containing cream and peridural prilocaine. *Eur J Pediatr* 1999;158:785–788.
111. Essink-Tjebbes CM, Hekster YA, Liem KD, et al. Topical use of local anesthetics in neonates. *Pharm World Sci* 1999;21:173–176.
112. Essink-Tjebbes C, Wuis EW, Liem KD, et al. Safety of lidocaine-prilocaine cream application four times a day in premature neonates: a pilot study. *Eur J Pediatr* 1999;158:421–433.
113. Brisman M, Ljung BM, Otterbom I, et al. Methaemoglobin formation after the use of EMLA cream in term neonates. *Acta Paediatr* 1998;87:1191–1194.
114. Fitzgerald M, Millard C, McIntosh N. Cutaneous hypersensitivity following peripheral tissue damage in newborn infants and its reversal with topical anaesthesia. *Pain* 1989;39:31–36.
115. Larsson BA, Jylli L, Lagercrantz H, et al. Does a local anaesthetic cream (EMLA) alleviate pain from heel-lancing in neonates? *Acta Anaesthesiol Scand* 1995; 39:1028–1031.
116. Acharya AB, Bustani PC, Phillips JD, et al. Randomised controlled trial of eutectic mixture of local anaesthetics cream for venipuncture in healthy preterm infants. *Arch Dis Child Fetal Neonatal Ed* 1998;78:F138–F142.
117. Duncan HP, Zurick NJ, Wolf AR. Should we reconsider awake neonatal intubation? A review of the evidence and treatment strategies. *Paediatr Anaesth* 2001; 11:135–145.
118. Lynn AM, Slattery JT. Morphine pharmacokinetics in early infancy. *Anesthesiology* 1987;66:136–139.
119. Bhat R, Chari G, Gulati A, et al. Pharmacokinetics of a single dose of morphine in preterm infants during the first week of life. *J Pediatr* 1990;117:477–481.
120. Lynn A, Nespeca MK, Bratton SL, et al. Clearance of morphine in postoperative infants during intravenous infusion: the influence of age and surgery. *Anesth Analg* 1998;86:958–963.
121. McRorie TI, Lynn AM, Nespeca MK, et al. The maturation of morphine clearance and metabolism. *Am J Dis Child* 1992;146:972–976.
122. Bhat R, Abu-Harb M, Chari G, et al. Morphine metabolism in acutely ill preterm newborn infants. *J Pediatr* 1992;120:795–799.
123. Jacqz-Aigrain E, Burtin P. Clinical pharmacokinetics of sedatives in neonates. *Clin Pharmacokinet* 1996;31: 423–443.
124. Collins C, Koren G, Crean P, et al. Fentanyl pharmacokinetics and hemodynamic effects in preterm infants during ligation of patent ductus arteriosus. *Anesth Analg* 1985;64:1078–1080.
125. Saarenmaa E, Huttunen P, Leppaluoto J, et al. Advantages of fentanyl over morphine in analgesia for ventilated newborn infants after birth: a randomized trial. *J Pediatr*1999;134:144–150.
126. Franck LS, Vilardi J, Durand D, et al. Opioid withdrawal in neonates after continuous infusions of morphine or fentanyl during extracorporeal membrane oxygenation. *Am J Crit Care* 1998;7:364–369.
127. Okada Y, Powis M, McEwan A, et al. Fentanyl analgesia increases the incidence of postoperative hypothermia in neonates. *Pediatr Surg Int* 1998;13:508–511.
128. Plattner O, Semsroth M, Sessler DI, et al. Lack of nonshivering thermogenesis in infants anesthetized with fentanyl and propofol. *Anesthesiology* 1997;86:772–777.
129. Franck L, Vilardi J. Assessment and management of opioid withdrawal in ill neonates. *Neonatal Network* 1995;14:39–48.
130. Suresh S, Anand KJ. Opioid tolerance in neonates: mechanisms, diagnosis, assessment, and management. *Semin Perinatol* 1998;22:425–433.
131. Lane JC, Tennison MB, Lawless ST, et al. Movement disorder after withdrawal of fentanyl infusion. *J Pediatr* 1991;119:649–651.
132. Bergman I, Steeves M, Burckart G, et al. Reversible neurologic abnormalities associated with prolonged intravenous midazolam and fentanyl administration. *J Pediatr* 1991;119:644–649.
133. Arnold JH, Truog RD, Orav EJ, et al. Tolerance and dependence in neonates sedated with fentanyl during extracorporeal membrane oxygenation. *Anesthesiology* 1990;73:1136–1140.
134. Katz R, Kelly HW, Hsi A. Prospective study on the occurrence of withdrawal in critically ill children who receive fentanyl by continuous infusion. *Crit Care Med* 1994;22:763–767.
135. Mack G, Thomas D, Giles W, et al. Methadone levels and neonatal withdrawal. *J Paediatr Child Health* 1991;27:96–100.
136. Finnegan LP, Connaught JF, Kron KE. A scoring system for the evaluation and treatment of the neonatal abstinence syndrome: a new clinical and research tool. In: Marselli PLL, Garanttini SL, Serini F, eds. *Basic and therapeutic aspects of perinatal pharmacology*. New York: Raven Press, 1975:139–152.

137. Doberczak TM, Kandall SR, Wilets I. Neonatal opiate abstinence syndrome in term and preterm infants. *J Pediatr* 1991;118:933–937.
138. Caron E , Maguire DP. Current management of pain, sedation, and narcotic physical dependency of the infant on ECMO. *J Perinatal Neonatal Nurs* 1990;4: 63–74.
139. Anand KJ, Ingraham J. Pediatric. Tolerance, dependence, and strategies for compassionate withdrawal of analgesics and anxiolytics in the pediatric ICU. *Crit Care Nurse* 1996;16:87–93.
140. Maichuk GT, Zahorodny W, Marshall R. Use of positioning to reduce the severity of neonatal narcotic withdrawal syndrome. *J Perinatol* 1999;19:510–513.
141. Hoder EL, Leckman JF, Ehrenkranz R, et al. Clonidine in neonatal narcotic-abstinence syndrome. *N Engl J Med* 1981;305:1284.
142. Hoder EL, Leckman JF, Poulsen J, et al. Clonidine treatment of neonatal narcotic abstinence syndrome. *Psychiatry Res* 1984;13:243–251.
143. Haberkern CM, Lynn AM, Geiduschek JM, et al. Epidural and intravenous bolus morphine for postoperative analgesia in infants. *Can J Anaesth* 1996;43: 1203–1210.
144. Murrell D, Gibson PR, Cohen RC. Continuous epidural analgesia in newborn infants undergoing major surgery. *J Pediatr Surg* 1993;28:548–552.
145. Vas L, Naregal P, Sanzgiri S, et al. Some vagaries of neonatal lumbar epidural anaesthesia. *Paediatr Anaesth* 1999;9:217–223.
146. Bosenberg AT. Epidural analgesia for major neonatal surgery. *Paediatr Anaesth* 1998;8:479–483.
147. Butler-O'Hara M, LeMoine C, Guillet R. Analgesia for neonatal circumcision: a randomized controlled trial of EMLA cream versus dorsal penile nerve block. *Pediatrics* 1998;101:E5.
148. Herschel M, Khoshnood B, Ellman C, et al. Neonatal circumcision. Randomized trial of a sucrose pacifier for pain control. *Arch Pediatr Adolesc Med* 1998;152: 279–284.
149. Holliday MA, Pinckert TL, Kiernan SC, et al. Dorsal penile nerve block vs topical placebo for circumcision in low-birth-weight neonates. *Arch Pediatr Adolesc Med* 1999;153:476–480.
150. Howard CR, Howard FM, Weitzman ML. Acetaminophen analgesia in neonatal circumcision: the effect on pain. *Pediatrics* 1994;93:641–646.
151. Howard CR, Howard FM, Fortune K, et al. A randomized, controlled trial of a eutectic mixture of local anesthetic cream (lidocaine and prilocaine) versus penile nerve block for pain relief during circumcision. *Am J Obstet Gynecol* 1999;181:1506–1511.
152. Lander J, Brady-Fryer B, Metcalfe JB, et al. Comparison of ring block, dorsal penile nerve block, and topical anesthesia for neonatal circumcision: a randomized controlled trial. *JAMA* 1997;278:2157–2162.
153. Mohan CG, Risucci DA, Casimir M, et al. Comparison of analgesics in ameliorating the pain of circumcision. *J Perinatol* 1998;18:13–19.
154. Olson TL, Downey VW. Infant physiological responses to noxious stimuli of circumcision with anesthesia and analgesia. *Pediatr Nurs* 1998;24:385–389.
155. Russell CT, Chaseling J. Topical anaesthesia in neonatal circumcision: a study of 208 consecutive cases. *Aust Fam Physician* 1996 Jan;Suppl 1:S30–S34.
156. Spencer DM, Miller KA, O'Quin M, et al. Dorsal penile nerve block in neonatal circumcision: chloroprocaine versus lidocaine. *Am J Perinatol* 1992;9: 214–218.
157. Taddio A, Stevens B, Craig K, et al. Efficacy and safety of lidocaine-prilocaine cream for pain during circumcision. *N Engl J Med* 1997;336:1197–1201.
158. Taddio A, Goldbach M, Ipp M, et al. Effect of neonatal circumcision on pain responses during vaccination in boys. *Lancet* 1995;345:291–292.
159. Circumcision policy statement. Task Force on Circumcision. *Pediatrics* 1999;103:686–693.
160. Joint Commission on Accreditation of Healthcare Organizations. *Accreditation manual for hospitals*. Oakbrook Terrace, IL:JCAHO, 2001.
161. Stevens B, Yamada J, Ohlsson A. Sucrose for analgesia in newborn infants undergoing painful procedures (Cochran Review). In: *The Cochran Library*, Issue 2, Oxford: Update Software, 2002.

38

Management of Common Pain Problems in the Primary Care Pediatric Setting

Neil L. Schechter

Pain problems are frequently encountered in pediatric health care settings. Pain is often the presenting symptom in common childhood illnesses such as otitis media, pharyngitis, and viral infections of the mouth. Pain is also a concern in normative problems such as teething, and the health care provider is often asked for advice about possible interventions. Finally, pain and anxiety are frequently associated with injections and needlesticks, which are common occurrences in most pediatric settings.

Unfortunately, however, there is an enormous disparity between the frequency with which these problems are encountered and the research that exists to help understand and alleviate them. One would assume that, given the fact that millions of needlesticks occur on a daily basis in the United States and that many children are deeply disturbed by them, there would be an outpouring of research aimed at understanding how to make injections and blood draws less painful. This is, unfortunately, not the case. Similarly, despite the fact that otitis media and pharyngitis are among the most common causes of visits to a physician, there are only a handful of articles that address the considerable pain associated with these entities.

The disparity between the frequency of the symptom and available research is, in part, explained by the strong tendency in medicine to focus on cure and not on symptom control. For example, when a child with otalgia stemming from otitis media visits the physician, the assumption is made that by treating the underlying disease (otitis), the presenting symptom (otalgia) will gradually dissipate. The provider, therefore, treats the underlying cause of the problem but does not directly address the symptom that brought the child to the doctor in the first place, i.e., discomfort. This phenomenon highlights a basic tenet of medical anthropology (1)—that patients seek medical care for illnesses (a change in their state of being, i.e., not feeling well or worrying about a new symptom), whereas doctors tend to treat diseases (abnormalities in structure or function). For the patient, the pain is an integral part of the illness, whereas for the doctor, the pain may be a peripheral concern, not necessarily requiring direct intervention.

This chapter reviews the available information on the incidence, cause, and treatment of pain associated these relatively common pediatric problems. The limited research, both well controlled and anecdotal, is reviewed, but it should be rapidly clear that these problems need for rigorous additional research.

OTITIS MEDIA

Otitis media is an inflammation in the middle ear. Subcategories of this diagnosis include acute otitis media, otitis media with effusion, recurrent acute otitis media, and otitis media with residual or persistent effusion. Another common source of ear pain is otitis externa, inflammation of the external ear canal, which is not the major focus of this chapter and therefore is only briefly mentioned.

After health supervision visits, otitis media is the most common cause of visits to physicians for children. It is the most common reason for outpatient antimicrobial treatment in the United States, and epidemiologic studies suggest that more than 50% of the courses of antibiotics prescribed for children younger than 5 years of age are prescribed for otitis media (2,3). In the United Kingdom, 30% of children younger than 3 years of age visit their physician with acute otitis media each year, and one in ten children has an episode of acute otitis media by 3 months of age (4). In the United States, by 2 years of age, 70% of children have had three or more episodes of otitis media (5).

Ear pain is a common complaint associated with otitis media. Hayden and Schwartz (6) found that 42% of children diagnosed with otitis media had severe pain, 40% had mild to moderate pain, and 17% had no pain. Their research suggests that younger children tended to have less pain, a finding that is not supported by other pain research in children and that may have resulted from the inadequacy of measurement techniques in the era in which the study was performed.

The frequency and severity of otalgia in otitis are understandable, given the sensory innervation of the ear. The ear is well innervated with pain-sensitive structures and thus sensitive to pain associated with inflammation. Pain-sensitive structures in the external ear include the skin at the external auricle, the external auditory canal, the perichondrium of the auricle, and the outer portion of the external auditory canal. In the middle ear, pain-sensitive structures include the tympanic membrane, periosteum, and mucoperiosteum of the mastoid. Inflammatory processes that stimulate nociceptors through stretching, irritation, or toxic products may result in pain.

Pain associated with external otitis results when the pinnae of the ear are moved, but such pain does not occur in middle ear disease. Pain associated with otitis media often results from increased pressure in the middle ear secondary to Eustachian tube dysfunction, which stretches pain-sensitive structures. There are certainly other causes for otalgia in children (7) that may represent either alternative otologic diagnoses or pain referred from an area supplied by the same nerves as the ear (the fifth and ninth cranial nerves) (8). Many authors have commented on the complexity of the diagnosis of acute otitis and its overdiagnosis (5,8).

Antibiotics

Although otitis media is commonly treated with antibiotics, there remains significant controversy about their efficacy in its overall treatment. There is, however, some support for the value of antibiotic treatment in decreasing the symptoms associated with otitis. In a placebo-controlled study of children with otitis, Burke et al. (9) randomly assigned children to an antibiotic or placebo group. The group that received antibiotics cried significantly less than the placebo group. Pain ceased at an average of 2.8 days in the antibiotic group and 3.2 days in the placebo group, and the children in the antibiotic group used fewer analgesics over the course of their illness. More recent studies, however, offer a less optimistic picture (10). Delmar et al. (10) suggest that the early use of antibiotics provides only modest benefit for pain relief in acute otitis media. In their study, 60% of all children were pain free within 24 hours of presentation, and antibiotic administration did not appear to alter this situation. At 2 to 7 days after presentation, however, when only 14% of children in the control group had pain, early use of antibiotics reduced that risk by 41%. Delmar et al. calculated that to prevent one child from experiencing pain 2 to 7 days after otitis presentation, 17 children must be treated initially with antibiotics. Damoiseaux et al. (11) likewise found a modest effect from antibiotic administration on the symptoms of otitis. Finally, O'Neill (4), in a review examining clinical evidence for use of antibiotics, suggested that there was an equal balance between benefit and harm associated with antibiotic administration.

Systemic Analgesia

Regardless of the degree of efficacy of antibiotics in reducing discomfort in otitis, it is clear that most children experience significant pain for some period during the course of their illness, and therefore additional methods of pain control should be considered as a routine part of treatment.

Despite the high frequency of otitis media in children and the fact that it causes significant distress in children, the data on analgesia use in children for this problem are extremely limited. In the one randomized clinical trial that compared the efficacy of analgesics in otitis media, Bertin and colleagues (12) compared ibuprofen, acetaminophen, and placebo for symptom control in acute otitis media. At 48 hours, in the 219 children 1 to 6 years of age with otoscopically proven otitis media, all of whom had been given antibiotics, pain was present in 7% of children who had received ibuprofen three times daily compared with 10% of children receiving acetaminophen and 25% of children given placebo. Ibuprofen was significantly more effective than placebo, but acetaminophen was not. Although the study was limited by inadequacies of pain measurement in the children, it does suggest that nonsteroidal anti-inflammatory drugs are preferable to acetaminophen for analgesia in children with otitis.

For more severe pain, opioids may be required to supplement acetaminophen or ibuprofen. Common choices include oxycodone, hydrocodone, and codeine. Regardless of the regimen selected, analgesics should be administered around the clock for the first few days after the diagnosis of otitis media, which is the time when pain is most prominent and least likely to be influenced by antibiotic administration.

Local Treatment

In addition to systemic analgesics, local treatments are often used to provide pain relief in otitis media. In a review of the historic treatment of earache among Laplanders, Stenforth and Henriksen (13) reported that warm compresses using oatmeal or warm stones or breathing into the child's ear have been found effective. Lapps also would place drops of animal or child urine into the ear canal. Such treatments had the effect of warming the ear, which decreases pain but clearly might not meet the hygiene requirements of modern medicine. Local anesthetic agent combinations such as Auralgan (antipyrine, benzocaine, and oxyquinoline sulfate dissolved in dehydrated glycerine) have also been used for many years but have only recently been subjected to rigorous evaluation. Several mechanisms have been postulated for the analgesic activity of Auralgan including the hygroscopic activity of the glycerine, which decreases the pressure in the middle ear through osmosis through the tympanic membrane, analgesic activity of antipyrine, and the local anesthetic action of benzocaine. Hoberman et al. (14) compared Auralgan administration with an olive oil placebo in the management of moderate to severe pain in children with acute otitis. They found that Auralgan provided additional relief at 30 minutes beyond that of olive oil. It may well be that in the future that additional techniques of providing local anesthesia more directly to the tympanic membrane and middle ear, such as through the use of iontophoresis or local anesthetic combinations such as lidocaine-prilocaine cream (EMLA), which are both currently used for anesthesia of the tympanic membrane before surgery, will be more routinely used for the pain of acute illness as well (15,16).

Otitis externa is routinely and successfully treated with local anesthetic, local antibiotic, and local anti-inflammatory solutions. The addition of systemic antibiotics may increase the cost and side effects and reduce patient compliance without improving outcome (17).

Summary

In summary, it is clear that otitis media is associated with significant pain in most children. Antibiotics may provide some relief after a few days, but initially, systemic, nonsteroidal anti-inflammatory agents should be used after the diagnosis is made, and more potent analgesic agents should be used in children whose pain is not responsive to nonsteroidal anti-inflammatory drugs. Local anesthetic agents also should be considered.

PHARYNGITIS

Acute pharyngitis is a common pediatric problem and accounts for as many as 5% of office visits yearly. In studies of the general population, upper respiratory infections, which include pharyngitis, are responsible for almost 200 visits to the physician per 1,000 individuals in the population annually, by far the most frequent category of infectious disease (18). Inflammation of the pharynx and surrounding lymphoid tissue may be caused by a myriad of agents, including bacteria (often *Streptococcus*) and a variety of viral agents, including Epstein–Barr virus, adenoviruses, and Coxsackievirus. Depending on the study, it appears that pharyngitis of streptococcal origin represents 15% to 30% of cases in children and 5% to 10% of cases in adults (19). In a study by Bertin et al. (20), 80% of children with streptococcal pharyngitis initially rated their pain as 4 or 5 of a possible10. Regardless of its origin, pharyngitis may cause continuous pain or pain associated with swallowing. In addition, with streptococcal pharyngitis, there is often associated headache and abdominal pain.

Antibiotics

As with otitis, there remains continued controversy about the impact of antibiotic treatment on pharyngitis. In the *Cochrane Review* of symptom relief associated with antibiotics for pharyngitis (21), 90% of all patients, both treated and untreated, were well 1 week after the onset of symptoms. Those treated with the antibiotics, however, had reduced symptoms by day 3 (22). There is, however, significant variability among studies. Randolph et al. (23), for example, suggest that within 48 hours of initiating antibiotic therapy, there is a dramatic decrease in pain associated with pharyngitis. Other authors, however, such as Middleton et al. (24), suggest that there was a slight decrease in the continuous pain associated with pharyngitis at 48 hours when antibiotics were used but no significant improvement in a host of other variables, such as malaise and pain on swallowing. Their group suggests that the value of early prescription of penicillin for symptom relief is questionable. Appropriate diagnostic procedures for this entity (cultures versus rapid antigen tests versus clinical observation) continue to be debated and have recently been reviewed (19,25).

Systemic Analgesics

Regardless of the diagnostic process and the initiation of antibiotics, pain remains a problem in individuals with pharyngitis and, at least the first few days of illness, requires symptom management. There has been limited research that has addressed pain associated with pharyngitis however. Bertin et al. (20) compared the analgesic efficacy of acetaminophen, ibuprofen, and placebo during the first 48 hours after antibiotic administration for pharyngitis. They found that spontaneous pain resolved in 80% of the children who took ibuprofen, 70% of the children who took acetaminophen, and 55% of the children who were given the placebo. The differences between the ibuprofen and placebo proved to be statistically significant, supporting the relative advantage of ibuprofen over acetaminophen for pain relief in pharyngitis. In a study of adults with sore throat pain, Schachtel et al. (26) found that aspirin with caffeine provided more pain relief more rapidly than aspirin alone or with placebo. He postulated that the caffeine may increase aspirin absorption and enhance gastromucosal microcirculation. O'Brien et al. (27) and Marvez-Valls et al. (28) evaluated the impact of steroids on providing pain relief for pharyngitis. O'Brien et al. studied the addition of intramuscular dexamethasone, whereas Marvez-Valls et al. reported on intramuscular betamethasone. In both of these reports, patients who received a steroid injection reported significant pain relief within 6 hours compared with those receiving placebo. In the work by Marvez-Valls et al., the steroid administration was more successful in alleviating symptoms in patients who had culture-positive streptococcal pharyngitis. Their data suggest that it might be advantageous to consider the use of rapid streptococcal antigen tests to help direct steroid use. This area clearly deserves more study, but it may well be that oral steroids have a role in acute pharyngitis in the future.

Local Treatment

Several other treatments have been suggested that decrease symptoms associated with pharyngitis. Macknin et al. (29) have suggested that zinc gluconate lozenges may significantly reduce symptoms associated with pharyngitis in adults. The lozenges, however, did not appear to have similar effect in children (30).

Other local treatments may have some efficacy in children. Salt water gargles, lozenges, and local anesthetic sprays have been used, although no formal studies have examined their value.

Summary

In summary, it does appear that the pain associated with pharyngitis of bacterial or viral origin requires analgesic therapy. Nonsteroidal anti-inflammatory drugs or, in the future, steroids, may be beneficial. Anecdotal evidence also supports the efficacy of local treatments.

VIRAL INFECTIONS OF THE MOUTH

Numerous viral infections cause painful mouth ulcers that can make eating or drinking extremely uncomfortable. Primary herpetic gingivostomatitis (herpes simplex virus 1) typically occurs in children in the preschool years. It is characterized by fever and other constitutional symptoms in addition to vesicles on the gingiva, palate, lips, and tongue that eventually develop into mouth ulcers. Herpangina ulcers develop in the oropharynx in the posterior oral cavity. It may be caused by a number of different viruses, but Coxsackievirus A is the most common agent associated with it. Because of the mouth's rich innervation, these lesions are often extremely painful. If inadequately treated, the pain of herpetic gingivostomatitis and herpangina can decrease oral intake sufficiently to cause dehydration and may necessitate hospitalization.

Although there is now literature that suggests that acyclovir suspension may be beneficial in the treatment of herpetic gingivostomatitis (31), for the most part, the treatment of these entities is symptomatic. The most common treatments are local anesthetic sprays and solutions. Viscous lidocaine is often prescribed for the symptomatic treatment of these lesions. It should be swished and spit by children older than 3 years of age and applied with a cotton-tipped applicator in children younger than 3 years because overdose has been reported in children who were prescribed viscous lidocaine for viral mouth infections (32). A 2% viscous lidocaine solution contains 100 mg/5 mL lidocaine hydrochloride. Because doses of more than 5 mg/kg per dose every 3 hours are potentially toxic in small children, care must be taken to describe accurately to parents the exact amount of lidocaine to be placed in the child's mouth. In addition, the half-life of viscous lidocaine in younger children is prolonged and clearance is decreased compared with adults, thus compounding further the potential for life-threatening lidocaine overdose.

Another local anesthetic that has been commonly used is benzocaine, which has poor absorption by mucous membranes and is therefore safer than lidocaine. However, methemoglobinemia has been reported, particularly in younger children as a rare side effect associated with benzocaine administration.

In addition to local anesthetic solutions, several "magic mouthwashes" have evolved that reportedly relieve mouth ulcer pain. In general, each mouthwash has at least two components: one intended to adhere to the lesion and at least one to provide local pain relief. One such preparation includes equal parts of diphenhydramine, viscous lidocaine, and aluminum and magnesium hydroxide suspension (Maalox). Another mouthwash contains equal parts of diphenhydramine and attapulgite suspension (Kaopectate). There is limited literature on the efficacy of these mouthwashes, yet anecdotal experience supports their use.

A final pharmacologic strategy that has some anecdotal support is the use of sucralfate suspension. This strategy was developed initially for radiation therapy–induced mucositis but has been reported for use in ulcers associated with viral infections. Sucralfate suspension plus diphenhydramine and attapulgite suspension solutions that coat the lesions have been used with some efficacy (33).

Finally, it is essential that children with these viral infections be adequately hydrated. Frequently, the pain in their mouth is associated with refusal to eat or drink, and occasionally they become dehydrated and require hospitalization. An often successful strategy is to have them swish with local anesthetic solution just before drinking and then use a straw to minimize the area of contact of the mouth with the liquid. This must be done with caution because local anesthetics may impair swallowing and increase the possibility of aspiration.

TEETHING

Many symptoms have been associated with teething in infancy. These include irritability, drooling, sleep disturbances, fever, diarrhea, and increased susceptibility to infection. Despite this perception, it remains unclear the extent to which these symptoms are the result of teething or are normative phenomena that tend to occur in infancy and are not necessarily associated with tooth eruption. Wake and colleagues (34), in a prospective cohort study of 21 children, did not confirm associations between tooth eruption and symptoms traditionally associated with teething. Despite this, however, they identify strong parental and professional beliefs to the contrary.

As regards pain, the assumption has been that inflammation or irritation of the gingiva as the tooth erupts is responsible for discomfort in children. Concern about the pain associated with teething has a long history, and gum lancets, blistering, bleeding, leeches on the gums, and cautery were all used in the past to reduce pain (35). In a number of studies, teething infants were reported to show more mouthing and drooling than nonteething infants. In one double-blind, randomized controlled study, for example, a solution containing lignocaine, benzyl alcohol, and myrrh tincture was compared with placebo (36). Mothers reported that the teething solution provided more relief than placebo, although the relief was independent of the stage of eruption of the tooth and was only present in males.

In the Wake et al. study, parents were asked to report on the degree of discomfort thought to be associated with their infants' teething. Eighty-one percent of parents thought that their infants' distress during teething was mild to moderate, whereas 14% thought it was severe. Eighty-six percent of the group used acetaminophen, and 52% of the group used some type of teething gel to relieve symptoms.

It should be evident, therefore, that given the lack of clarity about whether teething is associated with pain, it is unlikely that suggested remedies have been formally studied. In general, several teething solutions are available, most of which contain benzocaine, a topical anesthetic thought to be relatively safe in babies. Unfortunately, available studies do not suggest that benzocaine penetrates the gingival mucous membrane and therefore will not relieve pain in the gingiva or teeth (37). This casts serious doubt on its ability to relieve the pain associated with teething. Cold or frozen teething rings appear to help based on the well-documented efficacy of cold in relieving pain. Others have suggested that hard crackers or bread also bring about some pain relief. None of these techniques has been formally studied, however, and their use stems from decades of anecdotal experience.

INJECTIONS

For many children, needle punctures symbolize their encounters with pediatric health care providers. Everyone who works with children in a health care setting has entered a room and encountered an anxious child whose only concern is whether he or she will be receiving a "shot." Such preoccupations are unfortunately not inappropriate. The recent immunization schedule of the American Academy of Pediatrics calls for at least 19 injections in the first 6 years of childhood (38). There are multiple visits at which children receive four and sometimes five injections. In addition, parenteral antibiotics are commonly administered in emergency departments, and phlebotomy is at least an every day occurrence for children who are hospitalized. Menke (39) found that hypodermic needles were the most stress-producing stimulus when a series of stimuli were presented to hospitalized children. Although all children are concerned about needles, there is variation in the degree of their concern and their response pattern. It is clear, for example, that there are significant developmental trends associated with the fear of needles. For the most part, the younger the child is, the more pain is experienced (40). In addition, it appears that one's biologically determined temperamental style and a host of environmental and experiential factors form an individual's concern about injections and response to them (41).

It is not only the response of the injectee that is problematic. Reis and colleagues (42) found that providers are less likely to complete the full complement of immunizations when children are scheduled to receive three or more injections at a visit compared with situations in which they are scheduled to receive two or fewer. Parents express concerns about immunization pain as well, and, accordingly, pain associated with immunizations is considered an important barrier to compliance.

Although there is significant effort underway to identify alternative routes of administration and devices (43), at present, parenteral administration of medications and blood drawing remain an essential part of pediatric medicine. It behooves us, therefore, to identify techniques that minimize the pain associated with injections.

Preparing the Child

Approaches to preparing the child for a pending needle procedure obviously vary according to the age of the child. For infants, this involves primarily preparing the parents, whereas for toddlers and older children, the procedure must be discussed with the child as well.

Preparation clearly decreases anxiety, promotes cooperation, and allows the child a sense of mastery. It helps to diminish distorted ideas or fantasies that the child may have. For infants, preparation involves primarily telling the parent what the infant will experience and explaining how the parent can help. Making sure that the infant is relaxed and calm and has been adequately fed is also important. For toddlers, discussion should take place a short time (1 to 2 minutes) before the actual administration. A prolonged waiting period often increases anxiety. For preschoolers, the use of dolls and play materials to help to explain the procedure and to allow them to rehearse the procedure is often helpful. School-age children can potentially appreciate the value of the injection to them. Therefore, time should be taken to explain the purpose of the injection and how it will feel. Techniques that can be used to reduce pain, such as distraction, also may be taught. Finally, in adolescents, the long-term health benefits of the procedure can be emphasized. Adolescents still benefit from detailed discussion of the sensations associated with the injection as well as the exact nature of the procedure that will occur.

In general, preparation should empower the child to control his or her anxiety by emphasizing information sharing and support. Fernald and Corry (44) compared empathic preparation, which is supportive and child centered, and described the child's sensations and fears with directive preparation, in which the child is instructed to be big and brave and to try not to cry. They found that supportive preparation with statements such as "this is going to hurt a little and I don't mind if you cry," coupled with the description of what will actually take place and the reason for the injection reduced pain.

Site Selection

An ideal site is one that has adequate muscle mass to accommodate the injection but no major nerves or vessels running through it. As a result of changing patterns of muscle mass in children, selection of the site for an intramuscular injection depends on the age of the child. Several potential sites have been described: the anterolateral thigh, various gluteal sites, and the deltoid muscle. In children younger than 1 year of age, the anterolateral thigh is most commonly used because the gluteal muscles enlarge when walking begins and the deltoid muscles are inadequately developed. For children older than 18 months of age, the deltoid muscle is frequently suggested, in particular, for the DTP (diphtheria toxoid, tetanus toxoid, and pertussis) immunization. Ipp and colleagues (45), comparing DTP immunization in the thigh with that in the deltoid, reported that two-thirds of the group that had a thigh injection limped for 24 to 48 hours after the immunization, and 30% reported severe pain compared with 8% who had an injection in the deltoid. Several gluteal sites have been identified: the dorsal gluteal area (the upper outer aspect of the buttocks) and the ventrogluteal area, the center of a triangle whose boundaries are the anterior superior iliac spine, a tubercle of the iliac crest, and the upper border of the trochanter. Although studies comparing the dorsal gluteal area with the lateral thigh have suggested that injections in it are less painful, this area contains the sciatic nerve, and there have been numerous reports of nerve injuries from intramuscular injections at this site. The dorsal gluteal area is therefore not recommended. There is now evolving nursing literature that suggests that the ventrogluteal site is less painful for intramuscular injections than the vastus lateralis muscle and, as a result, is the preferred site for intramuscular injections (46). Although some individuals have sug-

TABLE 38.1. *Intramuscular injections*[a]

	Location	Needle length (in.)	Needle gauge	Needle angle (deg)
Infant <4 mo	Vastus lateralis, ventrogluteal	5/8	25 gauge for immunizations, 23 gauge for viscous drugs	90 unless very thin or emaciated
Infant >4 mo	Vastus lateralis, ventrogluteal	1	25 gauge for immunizations, 23 gauge for other injections, 22 gauge for viscous drugs	90 unless very thin or emaciated
Toddler (1–2 yr)	Deltoid, ventrogluteal, vastus lateralis	5/8 1 1	25 gauge for immunizations, 23 gauge for other injections, 22 gauge for viscous drugs	90 unless very thin or emaciated
Preschool/ school-age (3–11 yr)	Deltoid, ventrogluteal	5/8 1	25 gauge for immunizations, 23 gauge for other injections, 22 gauge for viscous drugs	90 unless very thin or emaciated
Adolescent (12–18 yr)	Deltoid, ventrogluteal	5/8 1	25 gauge for immunizations, 23 gauge for other injections, 22 gauge for viscous drugs	90 unless very thin or emaciated

[a]Significant controversy remains regarding needle length. Needle lengths presented are those most commonly accepted and do not include techniques that require bunching of the skin and muscle.

Adapted from *Reducing the anxiety and pain of injections: a guide for managing the pediatric patient.* Franklin Lakes, NJ: Becton Dickinson, 2000.

gested that this site is not appropriate for children younger than 3 years of age, this remains controversial. Table 38.1 contains a developmental approach to location selection and needle length. In general, however, because of the limitations of the literature, these data remain primarily anecdotal and recommendations cannot be wholly evidence based.

A host of potential complications of intramuscular injections exists. These include fibrosis, contracture, abscess, nerve injury, and, very rarely, gangrene. Factors that affect the complication rate include the injection site, the injectate itself, needle length, and the frequency of injection. Beecroft and Redick (47) surveyed more than 600 pediatric nurses regarding intramuscular injection practice complications. Nine percent of nurses reported that they had cared for a child admitted to the hospital for complications from an intramuscular injection. Twenty-five percent of nurses reported that they observed a complication from an injection that they had administered, most commonly secondary to selection of an inappropriately sized needle or patient movement. Twenty-seven percent reported hitting a blood vessel during an injection.

In summary, then, site selection is an important aspect of intramuscular injection. Complications are not infrequent. At this time, the vastus lateralis would appear to be the appropriate site for young children and the deltoid the appropriate site for older children. The ventrogluteal site appears to have significant anecdotal support, although limited supporting research literature at this time.

Injectate Properties

Characteristics of the Injectate

Specific properties of the injectate, such as its pH, may affect the associated pain of administration. Lyons and Howell (48) compared Pluserix measles, mumps, and rubella vaccine with the measles, mumps, and rubella 2 vaccine. They found a clear difference between pain at the site between these two, with the Pluserix being far less painful. Children who received the measles, mumps, and rubella 2 were twice as likely to cry as those receiving the Pluserix. The authors speculate that the increased acidity of the measles, mumps, and rubella 2 may be responsible for its burning or stinging at the site. There is increased pharmaceutical interest in developing parenteral medications that are equally effective in terms of immunogenicity and reactogenicity but that may be less painful, given the increased public concern about pain during immunizations. At present, we are unable to identify published work that compares existing formulations of similar immunizations regarding pain associated with their injection.

Temperature

Warming the injectate clearly reduces associated discomfort. Both Cragg and colleagues (49) and Finkel and Berg (50) reported that warming lidocaine prevents some of the pain associated with its injection. Although warming medication to room temperature seems beneficial, there has been some work that suggests warming the injectate to body temperature even reduces the pain more. There are no data on the affect of warming immunizations, especially regarding their biologic availability. One can speculate, however, given the fact that the immunization will rapidly climb to body temperature on injection, that warming before injection may have a limited impact. Formal research is clearly necessary before routine warming of injected substances can be recommended.

Diluent Choice

Finally, some evidence exists that using lidocaine as a diluent may reduce some of the discomfort associated with intramuscular injections. Schichor et al. (51) compared ceftriaxone injections using sterile water as a diluent with those using lidocaine at the time of injection, 10 minutes, 20 minutes, 6 hours, and 24 hours later. At all assessment points, there was significantly more pain in the group that had sterile water as the diluent compared with the group that had lidocaine as the diluent. This finding may have relevance to other intramuscular injections that require dilution.

Analgesic and Anesthetic Approaches

Several pharmacologic and physical approaches have been developed to attempt to reduce pain at the injection site. Some combination of these approaches should be used for all needle procedures.

Physical Approaches

Holmes (52) developed a syringe ice pushup that has ice emerging from the portal of the syringe that is then rubbed on the skin for 10 seconds. He suggests that this technique offers 2 seconds of anesthesia during which a needle may be relatively painlessly inserted. Other investigators examined the impact of pressure at the injection site (53). They found that 10 seconds of pressure at the injection site dramatically reduced the pain associated with needle insertion.

Pharmacologic Strategies

Several pharmacologic approaches also have been found to reduce pain associated with needle insertion. In infants, administration of a 24% solution of oral glucose placed on the pacifier or the tongue has been shown to dramatically reduce the pain of procedures in babies (54). Such a solution can be made by adding a packet of sugar to 10 mL of water, which yields approximately a 30% solution. Barr et al. (55) and others have shown that this effect gradually decreases over time and is most potent in the first few months of life and essentially gone by 6 months. Other investigators have determined that the effect of sucrose is not only one of distraction but may be mediated through opioid pathways. They found that sucrose analgesia can be reversed with naloxone (56).

Numerous topical agents also have demonstrated the ability to anesthetize skin. Lidocaine-prilocaine cream (EMLA) has been well studied (57,58). Use of this cream approximately 1 hour before needle insertion correlates with significantly reduced pain during phlebotomy, reservoir access, and immunizations. A study by Uhari (59) reveals that application of lidocaine-prilocaine cream is associated with reduced pain after 24 hours after intramuscular injection. Various other agents are also available. Lidocaine can be injected through a small-caliber needle. This reduces the pain of subsequent needle insertion; however, the lidocaine administration itself is associated with both the needlestick and the burning sensation associated with lidocaine. If lidocaine is buffered in a 9:1 solution (lidocaine:sodium bicarbonate), the burning of lidocaine can be somewhat alleviated (60). An alternative method of lidocaine administration is through iontophoresis. Several devices are available in which lidocaine is driven through the skin using an electric current (61). A deeper level of anesthesia is obtained (8 to10 mm) compared with that obtained with lidocaine-prilocaine cream, and anesthesia occurs after only 10 minutes. Some children have reported that the iontophoretic process is uncomfortable for them, and a number of burns have been reported. Amethocaine has been reported to have dramatic success in reducing pain of needle procedures as well (62). Although amethocaine is not universally available at present, it has the advantages of not causing vasoconstriction, which sometimes complicates lidocaine-prilocaine cream use, and a more rapid onset of action (63).

Finally, the use of a simple freeze spray has been reported to reduce the pain of needle insertion. Eland (64) and Reis and Holubkov (65) both reported on the value of vapocoolant spray in reducing the pain associated with needle insertion. Reis and Holubkov soaked a cotton ball in a dichlorodifluoromethane and trichloromonofluoromethane (Fluori-methane) solution and then pressed it on the injection site for 10 seconds. They reported efficacy equal to that of lidocaine-prilocaine cream in reducing injection pain.

Cognitive and Behavioral Techniques

As discussed previously, preparation is essential to reduce the anxiety associated with injections. Parental presence is another key element. The importance of parental presence has been described previously in this volume. Parents should be employed as coaches and distractors and not necessarily as restrainers. They should be given materials to help them in distracting the child. Distraction techniques themselves, as well as hypnosis, are reviewed in other chapters. The use of bubble solutions, party blowers, and pinwheels have dramatically reduced sharp pain. Hypnosis is also extremely effective. Other strategies include the use of favorite stories, kaleidoscopes, listening to music, and other types of meditation. They have all demonstrated efficacy in relieving the pain associated with needlesticks.

Technique

Anecdotally, injections given by some individuals hurt more than those given by others. There has been limited focused research investigating the unique aspects of technique that contribute to those differences.

Holding Techniques

It is important that the muscle that will receive the injection be relaxed. If the injection is to be placed in the deltoid, the arm must be flexed at the elbow. In the vastus lateralis, bending the knee will relax the muscle. In the ventrogluteal area, the child can be placed on one side with the upper leg flexed in front of the lower leg. If immobilization is necessary to prevent the child from moving, several techniques are available. There remains controversy about whether parents should hold the child during procedures. Many parents are uncomfortable participating, whereas others want to participate and children are often more comfortable when parents hold them. This certainly should be an individual decision made by the providers and the parents jointly. Techniques include the "big hug," in which an individual crosses the child's arms in front of his or her body and is in effect hugging them (66). Another technique involves having the child sit sideways in the lap of the provider or parent. Both of these techniques are described in nursing textbooks. Before the child is restrained, the injectate should be drawn into a syringe. Controversy continues to exist regarding the need to change needles after the puncture of the rubber stopper before injecting the child. Manufacturers suggest that current techniques of producing needles assure that there is essentially no blunting of the needle with a single puncture of a rubber stopper. Many clinicians believe, however, that the needle is less sharp after it has been used previously to obtain the injectate.

Injection Technique

As regards the technique of injection, the Z-track method of injection appears to be associated with the least pain (67). In this method, cutaneous tissue is laterally displaced before site cleansing and needle insertion. Keen (68), comparing Z-track intramuscular injections with standard injection technique in 50 adults receiving multiple injections of meperidine, reported less pain associated with the Z track. Concern was raised in this study that there may be more pain initially with this technique but less pain overall. Many nursing authorities, however, suggest that this technique is the one that most effectively minimizes the pain and discomfort of intramuscular injection. This technique appears superior because it minimizes leakage of the injected material back along the track into subcutaneous fat. In effect, it seals the injectate in the muscle. The needle should be inserted quickly, using a darting motion and stabilized so that it does not move. Usually, the needle angle should be approximately 90 degrees. Aspiration for blood should be routine.

Finally, because of the increased number of immunizations that must be given at a single visit, there has been some preliminary research on sequential versus simultaneous injections. With simultaneous injections, multiple providers coordinate their injection of the child to occur at the same time in contrast to sequential injections in which one individual gives one injection followed by another. Anecdotally, many believe that because there is no anticipation of subsequent shots with simultaneous injections, there is less anxiety and therefore less pain. However, simultaneous injections can overwhelm the child and be perceived as an assault. One study (69) examined this question in 4- to 6-year-old children and found that although a child's rating of pain was independent of whether injections were simultaneous or sequential, both parents and providers thought that simultaneous injections were less painful.

Summary

Needlesticks, unfortunately, remain an essential part of pediatric practice. Although efforts are underway to develop needleless injection units, to date they have not been successful, and all are plagued with technical problems. There has been an active effort to create orally administered immunizations, but these are not yet available. Finally, there are efforts underway to create vaccine combinations. In the interim, however, multiple injections remain necessary as part of well child supervision and sick child care for the foreseeable future. By appropriately selecting the site, preparing the child, and teaching him or her distraction techniques, using local anesthetics, and techniques designed to reduce pain, the overall burden of needlesticks can be somewhat reduced.

OVERALL SUMMARY

Encountering pain is common in pediatric practice. The frequently occurring pediatric infectious diseases are associated with pain that often brings the child to the doctor initially and dissipates gradually over the course of the illness. Pain is also attributed to normative processes such teething. Finally, injections are woven into the fabric of everyday pediatric practice and present significant challenges for children depending on their age, temperament, and previous experience.

Pain in all these problems should be addressed even if it cannot be entirely eliminated. Expecting the pain is the first step toward treating it. Routine use of local anesthetics and systemic analgesics for disease-related pain and developing a plan to reduce injection-related pain will go a long way toward reducing the anxiety often associated with a visit to the doctor.

REFERENCES

1. Kleinman A, Eisenberg L, Good B. Culture, illness and care. *Ann Intern Med* 1978;88:251–258
2. Nelson WL, Kuritsky JN, Kennedy DL. Outpatient pediatric antibiotic use in the US: trends and therapy for otitis media, 1976–1986. Abstracts of the 27th Interscience Conference on Antimicrobial Agents and Chemotherapy. American Society for Microbiology, 1987.
3. Teele DW, Klein JO, Rosner B, et al. Burdens in the practice of pediatrics: middle ear disease during the first five years of life. *JAMA* 1983;249:1026–1029.
4. O'Neill P. Clinical evidence: acute otitis media. *BMJ* 1999;319:833–835.
5. Berman S. Otitis media in children. *N Engl J Med* 1995; 332:1560–1565.
6. Hayden GF, Schwartz RH. Characteristics of earache among children with acute otitis media. *Am J Dis Child* 1985;139:721–723.
7. Ingvarsson L. Acute otalgia in children—findings and diagnosis. *Acta Paediatr Scand* 1982;71:705–710.
8. Browning GG. Childhood otalgia: acute otitis media. *BMJ* 1990;300:1005–1006.
9. Burke P, Bain J, Bovinson D, et al. Acute red ear in children: controlled trial of non-antibiotic treatment in general practice. *BMJ* 1991; 303:558–562.
10. Del Mar C, Glasziou P, Hayem M. Are antibiotics indicated as initial treatment for children with acute otitis media. *BMJ* 1997;314:1526–1529.
11. Damoiseaux RA, van Balen FA, Hoes AW, et al. Primary care based randomised double blind trial of amoxicillin versus placebo for acute otitis media in children aged under 2 years. *BMJ* 2000;320:350–354.
12. Bertin L, Pons G, D'Athis P, et al. A randomized double blind multicentre controlled trial of ibuprofen versus acetaminophen and placebo for symptoms of acute otitis media in children. *Fundam Clin Pharmacol* 1996;10: 387–392.
13. Stenforth LE, Henriksen AO. Treatment of earache among the Lappish people. *J Largyngol Otol* 1990;104: 109–111.
14. Hoberman A, Paradise JL, Reynolds EA, et al. Efficacy of Auralgan for treating ear pain in children with acute otitis media. *Arch Pediatr Adolesc Med* 1997;151: 675–678.
15. Bingham B, Hawke M, Halik J. The safety and efficacy of EMLA cream topical anesthesia for myringotomy

and ventilation tube insertion. *J Otolaryngol* 1991;20: 93–95.

16. Ramsden RT, Gibson WP, Moffat DA. Anesthesia of the tympanic membrane using iontophoresis. *J Laryngol Otol* 1977;91:779–785.
17. Halpern MT, Palmer CS, Seidlin M. Treatment patterns for otitis externa. *J Am Board Fam Pract* 1999;12:1–7.
18. Armstrong GL, Pinner RW. Outpatient visits for infectious diseases in the United States, 1980 through 1996. *Arch Intern Med* 1999;159:2531–2536.
19. Bisno AL. Acute pharyngitis. *N Engl J Med* 2001;344: 205–211.
20. Bertin L, Pons G, d'Athis P, et al. Randomized double-blind, multicenter, controlled trial of ibuprofen versus acetaminophen and placebo for treatment of symptoms of tonsillitis and pharyngitis in children. *J Pediatr* 1991; 119:811–814,
21. Del Mar CB, Glasziou PP. Do antibiotics shorten the illness of sore throat? The Cochrane Library. In: Douglas R, Berman S, Black RE, et al., eds. *Acute respiratory infectious module of the Cochrane Database of Systematic Reviews*. Oxford: Update Software, 1997.
22. Graham A, Fahey T. Sore throat: diagnostic and therapeutic dilemmas. *BMJ* 1999;319:173–174.
23. Randolph MF, Gerber MA, DeMeo KK, et al. Effect of antibiotic therapy on the clinical course of streptococcal pharyngitis. *J Pediatr* 1985;106:870–875.
24. Middleton DB, D'Amico F, Merenstein JH. Standardized symptomatic treatment versus penicillin as initial therapy for streptococcal pharyngitis. *J Pediatr* 1988; 113:1089–1094.
25. Tsevat J, Kotagal UR. Management of sore throats in children: a cost-effectiveness analysis. *Arch Pediatr Adolesc Med* 1999;153:681–688.
26. Schachtel BP, Fillingim JM, Lane AC, et al. Caffeine as an analgesic adjuvant. *Arch Intern Med* 1991;151: 733–737.
27. O'Brien JF, Meade JL, Falk JL. Dexamethasone as adjuvant therapy for severe acute pharyngitis. *Ann Emerg Med* 1993;22:212–215.
28. Marvez-Valls EG, Ernst AA, Gray J et al. The role of betamethasone in the treatment of acute exudative pharyngitis. *Acad Emerg Med* 1998;5:567–572.
29. Mossad SB, Macknin ML, Medendorp SV, et al. Zinc gluconate lozenges for treating the common cold. *Ann Intern Med* 1996;125:81–88.
30. Macknin ML, Piedmonte M, Calendre C, et al. Zinc lozenges for treating the common cold in children: a randomized controlled trial. *JAMA* 1998;279: 1962–1967.
31. Amir J, Harel L, Smetana Z, et al. Treatment of herpes simplex gingivostomatitis with acyclovir in children. *BMJ* 1997;314:1800–1803.
32. Gonzalez del Rey J, Wason S, Druckenbrod RW. Lidocaine overdose: another preventable case? *Pediatr Emerg Care* 1994;10:344–346.
33. Barker G, Loftus L, Cuddy P, et al. The effects of sucralfate suspension and diphenhydramine syrup plus kaolin-pectin on radiotherapy-induced mucositis. *Oral Surg Oral Med Oral Pathol* 1991;71:288–293.
34. Wake M, Hesketh K, Lucas J. Teething and tooth eruption in infants: a cohort study. *Pediatrics* 2000;106: 1374–1379.
35. Dally A. The lancet and the gum-lancet: 400 years of teething babies. *Lancet* 1996;348:1710–1711.
36. Seward MH. The effectiveness of a teething solution in infants: a clinical study. *Br Dent J* 1969;127:457–461.
37. United States Food and Drug Administration. Oral health care products for over the counter human use. *Fed Reg* 1982;47:22809.
38. Committee on Infectious Diseases, American Academy of Pediatrics. *Two thousand red book: report of the Committee on Infectious Disease*, 25th ed. Elk Grove Village, IL: American Academy of Pediatrics, 2000:22.
39. Menke E. School aged children's perception of stress in the hospital. *Child Health Care* 1981;9:80–86.
40. Fradet C, McGrath PJ, Kay J, et al. A prospective survey of reactions to blood tests in children and adolescents. *Pain* 1990;40:53–60
41. Schechter NL, Bernstein BA, Beck A, et al. Individual differences in children's response to pain: role of temperament and parental characteristics. *Pediatrics* 1991; 87:171–177.
42. Reis EC, Jacobson RM, Tarbell S, et al. Taking the sting out of shots: control of vaccination-associated pain and adverse reactions. *Pediatr Ann* 1998;27:375–386.
43. Richards CA. Alternative vaccination strategies aimed at decreasing number of injections. *Infect Dis Child* 1998;June:34, 47.
44. Fernald CD, Corry JJ. Empathic versus directive preparation of children for needles. *Child Health Care* 1981; 10:44–46.
45. Ipp MM, Gold R, Goldbach M, et al. Adverse reaction to diphtheria, tetanus, pertussis-polio vaccination at 18 months of age: effect of injection site and needle length. *Pediatrics* 1989;83:679–682.
46. McCaffery M, Beebe A. *Pain: clinical manual for nursing practice*. St. Louis: Mosby, 1989.
47. Beecroft PC, Redick SA. Intramuscular injection practices of pediatric nurses: site selection. *Nurse Educator* 1990;15:23–28.
48. Lyons R, Howell F. Pain and measles, mumps, and rubella vaccination. *Arch Dis Child* 1991;66:346–347.
49. Cragg AH, Berbaum K, Smith TP. A prospective blinded trial of warm and cold lidocaine for intradermal injection. *AJR Am J Roentgenol* 1988;150:1183–1184.
50. Finkel LI, Berg DJ. Heating lidocaine appears to prevent painful injection. *AJR Am J Roentgenol* 1987;148: 651.
51. Schichor A, Bernstein B, Weinerman H, et al. Lidocaine as a diluent for ceftriaxone in the treatment of gonorrhea: does it reduce the pain of injection? *Arch Pediatr Adolesc Med* 1994;148:72–77.
52. Holmes HS. Options for painless local anesthesia. *Postgrad Med* 1991;89:71–72.
53. Barnhill BJ, Holbert MD, Jackson NM, et al. Using pressure to decrease the pain of intramuscular injections. *J Pain Symptom Manage* 1996;12:52–58.
54. Blass E, Hoffmeyer LB. Sucrose as an analgesic for newborn infants. *Pediatrics* 199187:215–218.
55. Barr RG, Young SN, Wright JH, et al. "Sucrose analgesia" and diphtheria-tetanus-pertussis immunizations at 2 and 4 months. *J Dev Behav Pediatr* 1995;16:220–225.
56. Blass EM, Cramer CP, Fanselow MS. The development of morphine-induced antinociception in neonatal rats: a comparison of forepaw, hindpaw, and tail retraction from a thermal stimulus. *Pharmacol Biochem Behav* 1993;44:643–649.
57. Halperin DL, Koren G, Attias D, et al. Topical skin anesthesia for venous subcutaneous drug reservoir and

lumbar punctures in children. *Pediatrics* 1989;84: 281–284.
58. Robieux I, Kumar R, Radhakrishnan S, et al. Assessing pain and analgesia with a lidocaine-prilocaine emulsion in infants and toddlers during venipuncture. *J Pediatr* 1991;118:971–973.
59. Uhari M. A eutectic mixture of lidocaine and prilocaine for alleviating vaccination pain in infants. *Pediatrics* 1993;92:710–721.
60. Cheney PR, Molzen G, Tandberg D. The effect of pH buffering on reducing the pain associated with subcutaneous infiltration of bupivacaine. *Am J Emerg Med* 1991;9:147–148.
61. Zempsky WT, Anand KJS, Sullivan KM, et al. Lidocaine iontophoresis for topical anesthesia before intravenous line placement in children. *J Pediatr* 1998;132: 1061–1063.
62. Lawson RA, Smart NG, Gudgeon C, et al. Evaluation of amethocaine gel preparation for percutaneous analgesia before venous cannulation in children. *Br J Anaesth* 1995;75:282–285.
63. Bishai R, Taddio A, Bar-Oz B, et al. Relative efficacy of amethocaine and lidocaine-prilocaine cream for Port-a-Cath puncture in children. *Pediatrics* 1999;104: E31.
64. Eland JM. Minimizing pain associated with pre-kindergarten intramuscular injections. *Issues Comp Pediatr Nurs* 1981;5:361–372.
65. Reis EC, Holubkov R. Vapocoolant spray is equally effective as EMLA cream in reducing immunization pain in school-aged children. *Pediatrics* 1997;100:E5.
66. Wong DL, Hockenberry-Eaton M, Wilson D, et al. *Whaley and Wong's nursing care of infants and children*, 6th ed. St. Louis: Mosby, 1999.
67. Taylor HJ. Patients deserve painless injections. *RN* 1992;55:25–26.
68. Keen MF. Comparison of intramuscular injection techniques to reduce site discomfort and lesions. *Nurs Res* 1988;35:207–210.
69. Horn MI, McCarthy AM. Children's responses to sequential versus simultaneous immunization injections. *J Pediatr Health Care* 1999;13:18–23.

39

Diagnosis, Classification, and Medical Management of Headache in Children and Adolescents

Mirja Hämäläinen and Bruce J. Masek

In this chapter, we review approaches to the diagnosis and treatment of headaches in children. Along with diagnostic and therapeutic evaluation in a medical framework, we emphasize a biopsychosocial model that emphasizes wellness and minimizes the impact of recurrent headaches on daily functioning.

EPIDEMIOLOGY

Occasional headaches are quite common in children; 20% of those younger than 5 years of age have them, and their frequency increases with age (1). Approximately 10% to 20% of children younger than 10 years have recurrent headaches (2,3). Before puberty, migraine and other headaches are equally common in boys and girls: 3% to 7% of children have migraine (4). At puberty, migraine becomes more common in girls: 10% to 27% of adolescent girls and 4% to 20% of adolescent boys have migraine (4). There is some evidence that the prevalence of migraine and other headaches has increased (5,6). A significant proportion of nonmigraine headache is probably tension-type headache. Sometimes it is difficult to differentiate migraine and tension-type headache, especially when headaches occur frequently (7). It is also possible that the inherited migraine trait becomes evident earlier owing to burdensome lifestyle. Approximately 60% of those who had migraine as children continue to have migraine attacks as adults (8).

MEDICAL EVALUATION

Sufficient time should be reserved for a careful history and examination, on which the clinical diagnosis of headache is based. Both parents and the child should be interviewed to find out the character and special features of the child's headache, associated symptoms, possible triggers, and relieving factors. Subjects such as school, friends, hobbies, eating and sleeping habits, the child's way of reacting in stressful situations, other diseases, and drug treatments should be discussed. Family conflicts may cause the child to have psychosomatic symptoms, such as headache. If the child's headache history is long, it is wise to inquire whether a suspicion of a particular disease made the parents bring their child to a physician.

A careful clinical and neurologic investigation should be performed that includes taking the blood pressure, checking visual acuity, and performing an ophthalmoscopic examination. Growth should be evaluated, and a growth curve of cranial circumference should be drawn for those younger than school age. Signs of infection or systemic disorders may be revealed in the clinical examination. It is necessary to palpate cranial and cervicobrachial muscles.

Data obtained from the history and clinical examination determine whether and which further investigations are indicated. In otherwise healthy children with migraine or tension-type headachc, no laboratory tests are necessary. More investigations are required if symptoms have recently increased, the child's behavior has changed, or headaches occur in the mornings with vomiting. Investigations should also be continued if the clinical examination reveals strabismus, decrease of visual acuity, papilledema, balance or coordination abnormalities, or clonic tendon reflexes, which may be signs of increased intracranial pressure.

Laboratory investigations may be necessary to rule out infections. Ophthalmologic consultation may be necessary to diagnose astigmatism or other vision problems. Increased intracranial pressure can be detected by brain imaging or direct measurement. Electroencephalography is not warranted as a routine diagnostic investigation for headaches in children. A electroencephalogram is often abnormal immediately after a complicated migraine attack, and there are often minor changes between the attacks that are not diagnostic. Electroencephalography should therefore be recorded only if epilepsy is suspected.

Headache in children can be caused by various reasons (Table 39.1). In a recent retrospective review of patients who presented with a chief complaint of headache at a pediatric emergency department, 39% had viral illness, 16% had sinusitis, 16% had migraine, more than 6% had posttraumatic headache, 5% had streptococcal pharyngitis, and 5% had tension-type headache (9). Other causes of headache include systemic diseases, arteriovenous malformations, disturbances in cerebrospinal fluid flow or absorption or both, intracranial hemorrhages, ocular and dental diseases, psychogenic causes, obstructive sleep apnea, bacterial infections, and brain tumors. Metabolic causes such as hypoxia or hypoglycemia can cause headache, and cranial neuralgias are very rare in children.

TABLE 39.1. *Causes of headache in children*

Migraine and tension-type headache
Psychogenic headache
Heterophoria and refractive errors
Dental braces
Sequelae to accidents
Sinusitis and other cranial infection or inflammation
Increased intracranial pressure
Systemic disorders
Epileptic attacks
Drugs
Obstructive sleep apnea (snoring)
Hypertension (rare)

HEADACHE MECHANISMS AND TYPES

Migraine

Migraine is inherited. Often one of the parents or family members has migraine. There is an inborn trait to develop migraine attacks that becomes visible at different periods of life. This migraine activity is thought to be generated by neurons in the brainstem (10). There may be cyclical variation in how easily the migraine generator can be activated, and many factors working together may contribute to this migraine threshold. A migraine attack starts as a disorder in the neurons in the brainstem that leads to release of numerous neurotransmitters that may cause cerebral vasoconstriction, extracranial vasodilation, and other migraine symptoms.

In most children, migraine attacks begin at school age. There are also descriptions of a very early onset. Syndromes that are thought to precede migraine or to be associated with migraine pathogenesis are sometimes called migraine equivalents. According to the International Headache Society criteria (12), these are benign paroxysmal vertigo and alternating hemiplegia of childhood. There is no consensus on whether recurrent abdominal pain and cyclic vomiting are migraine equivalents. It has not been confirmed whether spells of vomiting and pallor in infants precede migraine. Young children with such symptoms must be thoroughly investigated.

Most parents who themselves have migraine can recognize typical features of these attacks in their children. The most recent diagnostic criteria for migraine were published by the International Headache Society (Table 39.2). These criteria require that in children younger than 15 years of age, the attacks last 2 to 48 hours, which includes sleep. Other-

TABLE 39.2. *Diagnostic criteria for migraine in children (Headache Classification Committee, 1988)*

At least one of the following:

I. History and physical and neurologic examinations do not suggest any other type of headache
II. History and/or physical and/or neurologic examinations do suggest such a disorder, but it is ruled out by appropriate investigations
III. Such a disorder is present, but migraine attacks do not occur for the first time in close temporal relation to the disorder

A. Migraine without aura
   1. At least five attacks fulfilling criteria 2 through 4 below
   2. Headache attacks lasting 4 to 72 hours (untreated or unsuccessfully treated). In children younger than age 15, attacks may last 2 to 48 hours. If the patient falls asleep and wakes up without migraine, duration of attack is until time of awakening
   3. Headache has at least two of the following characteristics:
      a. Unilateral location
      b. Pulsating quality
      c. Moderate or severe intensity (inhibits or prohibits daily activities)
      d. Aggravation by walking stairs or similar routine physical activity
   4. During headache, at least one of the following:
      a. Nausea and/or vomiting
      b. Photophobia and phonophobia

B. Migraine with aura
   1. At least two attacks fulfilling criterion 2a through d
   2. At least three of the following four characteristics:
      a. One or more fully reversible aura symptoms indicating focal cortical and/or brainstem dysfunction
      b. At least one aura symptom develops gradually over more than 4 minutes or two or more symptoms occur in succession
      c. No aura symptom lasts more than 60 minutes; if more than one aura symptom is present, accepted duration is proportionally increased
      d. Headache follows aura with a pain-free interval of less than 60 minutes (it may also begin before or simultaneously with the aura)

Others have proposed additional modifications to the International Headache Society criteria for pediatric headaches (53,54).

wise, the International Headache Society criteria are the same for children and adults (12). During a migraine attack, the child appears ill and often likes to withdraw into a darkened and quiet room. Many children fall asleep during a migraine attack and may wake symptom free. The most disturbing symptom in migraine is usually severe pain, which may be similar to that of headache associated with subarachnoid hemorrhage or an infection of the central nervous system.

Diagnosis of migraine in children requires exclusion of other causes of headache. Some physicians prefer a headache history of at least 6 months to confirm the diagnosis, although the 6-month criteria is not a prerequisite in the International Headache Society criteria. After migraine attacks, children should completely improve and otherwise remain well. Between migraine attacks, a clinical and neurologic examination must be normal. Approximately half of children with migraine have aura, which usually includes visual or sensory symptoms that may be frightening. Further investigations are warranted if aura symptoms are prolonged (lasting longer than 1 hour) or include motor weakness, dysphasia, or symptoms of basilar migraine (ataxia, dizziness, dysarthria, and confusion). Aura symptoms are to be distinguished from milder and more prolonged prodromal symptoms that include more subtle changes in mood, activity level, or appetite and may precede the onset of headache by as long as a day.

In familial hemiplegic migraine, the aura includes some degree of hemiparesis and may be prolonged. At least one first-degree relative has identical migraine attacks, which may be precipitated by insignificant trauma. In some families with familial hemiplegic migraine, a mutation of a brain-specific calcium channel subunit gene has been mapped to chromosome 19 (13). Ophthalmoplegic migraine and retinal migraine are rare forms of migraine.

Tension-Type Headache

Attacks of tension-type headache typically are shorter and do not fulfill the diagnostic criteria for migraine. They are not associated with vomiting or simultaneous photo/phonophobia. The International Headache Society criteria permits either photo- or phonophobia but not both. Clinical features of tension-type headache are not well defined in adolescents. Tension-type headache is usually mild or moderate; there may very short bouts of severe headache, sometimes background headache, and often pressing feeling in the temples or a "tight band around the head." Part of tension-type headache is associated with abnormal tension in cranial muscles. Muscular tenderness and tightness can often be palpated in the neck muscles. Sometimes there is tightness in the shoulder and dorsal and posterior femoral muscles as well. The exact pathogenesis of tension-type headache is not known. It may be difficult to differentiate migraine and tension-type headache in some patients (7,11) because at times the two may coexist and symptoms are overlapping, especially if headache attacks occur frequently. Tension-type headache typically occurs in the afternoon or evening after school.

Chronic Daily Headache

A small subgroup of children report continuous, daily, or near-daily headache with no specific cause determined by history, physical examination, and laboratory investigation. In some cases, this can develop after a history of more typical episodic migraine or tension-type headaches. Specific psychologic issues, including depression, trauma, school difficulties, and various stressors, may be identified in some cases; in others, no specific psychologic factors are identified.

A common and treatable cause of chronic daily headache is medication overuse with rebound. This may occur with prolonged daily use of acetaminophen, nonsteroidal anti-inflammatory drugs, or barbiturate/caffeine/analgesic combinations. Tapering off these agents may often produce a reduction in headache severity and frequency.

CAUSES OF HEADACHES

Epilepsy

Most common type of headache associated with epilepsy is postictal headache, i.e., the headache after an epileptic attack. Sometimes headache can occur before or during an attack, especially in rolandic or benign occipital epilepsy. Differential diagnosis between migraine and epilepsy may be difficult if dizziness, dysarthria, or visual disturbances accompany a headache attack. In epilepsy, neurologic symptoms present with headache, whereas in migraine, an aura should disappear at the onset of a headache.

Ophthalmologic and Dental Causes

Heterophoria or refractory errors can cause headache in the ocular, frontal, or temporal region. This type of headache will disappear after correction with spectacles. Dental braces may cause daily headache, which will cease after their removal. Patients with bruxism and malocclusion who have daily or mild recurrent headaches should be referred to a dentist. A more detailed discussion of evaluation and treatment of facial pain and headache of dental origin can be found in Chapter 43.

Sinusitis

Sinusitis may cause frontal and maxillar or a generalized headache. Other symptoms may be mild. In children with allergic rhinitis, asthma, or recurrent respiratory infections, scanning of sinuses is indicated. On occasion, migraine may be misdiagnosed as chronic sinusitis and vice versa.

Brain Tumors and Increased Intracranial Pressure

Brain tumors cause headache by obstructing the circulation of the cerebrospinal fluid and stretching the pain-sensitive areas, including the dura mater. Headache caused by malignant tumors is usually rapidly progressive. Benign brain tumors, which are often located in the posterior fossa or in the midline in children, may grow slowly and therefore also gradually block the circulation of the cerebrospinal fluid. In this case, the children may partly adapt to the increase of the intracranial pressure, which may continue for several months before a correct diagnosis is made. Increased intracranial pressure should be suspected if the headache is nocturnal or occurs early in the morning with vomiting, if there are nocturnal attacks of restlessness and crying with vomiting, if the child becomes clumsier and develops problems with balance and coordination, or if visual acuity decreases.

Nocturnal or morning headache and vomiting, acute progressive headache, and headache worsened by straining or coughing are symptoms of increased intracranial pressure. Headache as the only symptom of a brain tumor is rare (14,15).

Signs and symptoms of increased intracranial pressure may also develop after hemorrhage or meningitis. Congenital hydrocephalus owing to a narrow mesencephalic aqueduct usually develops within the first months of life and causes macrocephaly. Because the cranial sutures have been ossified by the age of 2 to 3 years, increased intracranial pressure does significantly affect cranial growth, and thereafter slowly developing hydrocephalus causes headache.

Children with shunted hydrocephalus and recurrent headaches should be thoroughly investigated with brain imaging and shunt radiographs, which may not, however, show any signs of increased intracranial pressure. In selected cases, investigation should be continued with measurement of intracranial pressure.

In pseudotumor cerebri, which is a rare cause of headache in children, intracranial pressure is increased without a mass lesion or obstruction of the ventricular system. Benign intracranial hypertension has been associated with hormonal therapies or their withdrawal and mastoiditis owing to chronic otitis media. Acetazolamide, corticosteroids, diuretics, repeated lumbar punctures, and surgery have been used as treatments. Most patients respond to nonsurgical treatment (16).

Abnormalities around the craniocervical junction, including Chiari 1 malformations, atlanto-occipital subluxations and C2 root impingement, may cause headache. Although Chiari 1 malformations commonly produce occipital headache, most patients with this disorder (which involves caudal displacement of the cerebellar tonsils through the foramen magnum) will have additional findings on neurologic examination, including sensory and motor changes in the limbs and unsteadiness of gait. Occipital neuralgia is more commonly recognized in adults. Children rarely have true occipital neuralgia, although occipital headache in children is much more commonly muscular in origin.

Sleep Apnea

In children, chronic snoring is abnormal and a sign of a too narrow pharynx and airway. This usually results in oxygen deficiency during sleep, which may cause morning tiredness, daytime attention deficit, and headache. Children who have syndromes associated with midfacial and mandibular hypoplasia are especially prone to sleep apnea. Treatments include removal of the adenoids and then the tonsils, and sometimes investigations in a sleep laboratory. In few of cases, other surgical interventions or nighttime use of continuous positive airway pressure may be required.

FOLLOW-UP AND INVESTIGATIONS

Children with occasional mild headaches do not require medical follow-up. If the child

TABLE 39.3. *Indications for brain imaging in children with headache*

Age 5 years or younger
Nocturnal or morning headache accompanied with vomiting
Disturbances of consciousness with headache
Physical exercise or straining or cough worsens headache
Progressively worsening or treatment-resistant headache
Child's behavior changes
Retardation of normal growth or development
Accelerated growth of cranial circumference
Abnormal clinical findings

has recurrent severe or moderate headaches at least once or twice a month, he or she should be seen by a doctor. If the history of headache is short, the child should be followed for at least 6 months to make sure that the symptoms do not progress and that the child's development and growth continue normally. If the headache is severe, invariably unilateral, or nocturnal or occurs early in the morning with vomiting or if the child has seizures or focal neurologic symptoms or signs, imaging should be performed to exclude intracranial pathology, especially in young children (Table 39.3). A recent study analyzed the cost-effectiveness of different strategies for imaging of children with suspected brain tumor and characterized several factors that can help to stratify risk (17).

ENVIRONMENTAL, LIFESTYLE, AND DIETARY FACTORS

Several factors may contribute to tension-type headache and migraine. Flickering or bright light, smells, fasting, and sleep deprivation may trigger migraine attacks. Children with headache should be advised to eat regular meals (especially breakfasts) and get enough sleep. It is wise to protect the eyes and the head against sunlight and not to head the ball when playing soccer. Balance between exercise, rest, and sleep is individual and varies greatly among adolescents. If demands set by the child or parents seem to be too high and the child's tolerance to disappointment low, guidance may be necessary to make them adopt a more realistic attitude toward schoolwork and hobbies.

There is a minority of patients with migraine in whom specific food items or additives trigger headache. These are cheese, chocolate, processed meats, citrus fruit, nuts, colored sweets, aspartame, caffeine, monosodium glutamate, benzoic acid, tartrazine, and spices. Most migraine patients do not have any certain food as a trigger.

SYMPTOMATIC DRUG TREATMENT OF MIGRAINE (ACUTE TREATMENT)

Symptomatic treatment is targeted against the moderate or severe migraine pain (18,19) and to alleviate other symptoms such as nausea and vomiting. Drugs should be given at the very onset of a migraine attack, and the child should be allowed to rest in a quiet room. Recommended doses are shown in Table 39.4. A dose may be repeated after 2 hours. Liquid forms and effervescent tablets are easier to swallow than ordinary tablets. Suppositories usually absorb quite slowly and should be used only in prolonged attacks. In children aged 4 to 15 years, single doses of liquids of acetaminophen (15 mg/kg) and ibuprofen (10 mg/kg) are well-tolerated and effective treatments (20). Acetaminophen has a more rapid onset than ibuprofen, but ibuprofen is twice as effective as acetaminophen to abort migraine within 2 hours. Other non-steroidal anti-inflammatory drugs, except ibuprofen, have not been investigated in the treatment of a migraine attack in children.

Epidemiologic studies indicate that the risk of Reye syndrome is associated with aspirin use and viral infections (varicella and influenza). Therefore, aspirin is not recommended for migraine attacks in children and adolescents if they have symptoms or signs of infection. Some over-the-counter analgesics contain a combination of barbiturate, acetaminophen, and caffeine or barbiturate, aspirin, and caffeine. They are used and have been investigated in mild to moderate migraine attacks in adults, but they have not

TABLE 39.4. *Drugs that can be used in the treatment of migraine in children*

Attack treatment	Single dose (mg/kg)	Maximal daily dose (mg/kg)	
Analgesic			
Ibuprofen	10	40	
Acetaminophen (paracetamol)	15	60	
Antiemetic			
Metoclopramide	0.15–0.30	0.5–1.0	Mixture, tablet, suppository
	0.1	0.3	Intramuscular/intravenous
Prochlorperazine	0.1–0.3	0.4–0.5	Tablet, suppository
Prophylactic treatment	**Daily dose (mg/kg)**	**Maximal daily dose (mg)**	
Propranolol	0.5–2	160	
Amitriptyline	0.1–2 (doses >1 mg/kg daily divided into two doses)	100	

been investigated in children. It should be remembered that caffeine and barbiturates are habit forming and can lead to rebound headaches and overuse of analgesics. They should not be used for tension-type headache because the risk of drug-induced headache is even greater.

Sumatriptan selectively stimulates serotonin 5-HT_1 receptors that constrict affected vessels and blocks nociceptive impulses. It is used only for migraine and should relieve migraine symptoms at all phases of a migraine attack after the headache has begun, but it has no benefit at the aura phase. Although numerous studies have shown that sumatriptan in tablet form is effective treatment of migraine in adults, it has been difficult to show a difference as compared with placebo in children and adolescents (21). Intranasal sumatriptan showed promising results in 14 6- to 9-year-old children (22) and in several other recent studies (23–25).

Subcutaneous sumatriptan is packed in 6-mg syringes for adults. Sumatriptan (0.06 mg/kg) was injected subcutaneously to 50 6- to 18-year-old children and adolescents with migraine attacks in an outpatient clinic (26). The safety of sumatriptan has been shown in 12- to 17-year-old adolescents, but more data on its safety and efficacy are needed in younger children. Other 5-HT_1-agonists have not yet been adequately investigated in children and adolescents.

Early administration of analgesics seems to decrease nausea as well. Metoclopramide or prochlorperazine may be used to alleviate nausea and vomiting (Table 39.4), but there are no controlled trials on their use in children. They may sometimes cause extrapyramidal and dystonic reactions, which may require treatment with anticholinergics such as diphenhydramine or benztropine; one might also try diazepam (fluid) rectal solution for quick relief.

Prophylactic Drug Treatment of Migraine

In adults, amitriptyline, various beta-blockers, and valproic acid have proven effective in migraine prophylaxis. Prophylactic drug treatments for migraine have not been shown very effective in children in clinical trials (Table 39.5), and no single drug is superior when potential adverse effects are considered (27).

The results obtained with the beta-blocker propranolol are inconsistent (28,29). In one trial, 82% of the children (23 of 28) significantly benefitted from propranolol (20 to 40 mg three times daily) and 14% (four of 28) benefitted from placebo (28), but in another trial, propranolol (40 mg two to three times daily) did not differ from placebo (29). One trial found clonidine to be effective (30), but another study did not show a difference between clonidine and placebo (31). Papaverine

TABLE 39.5. *Outcome of double-blind, placebo-controlled studies on the prophylactic drug treatment of migraine in children*

Drug and dose [ref.]	N	Result	Drug	Placebo	Therapeutic gain	Number needed to treat
Propranolol 20–40 mg × 3 [Ludvigsson (28)]	28	+	82%	14%	68%	1.5
Propranolol 40 mg × 2 [Forsythe et al. (29)]	39	–	?	?		
Propranolol 3 mg/kg/d, self-hypnosis [Olness et al. (29a)]	28	–	?	?		
Clonidine 25–75 μg/d [Sills et al. (31)]	43	–	?	?		
Clonidine 25–50 μg/d [Sillanpää (30)]	57	±	57%	42%	15%	6.7
5-HT 5 mg/kg/d [Santucci et al. (30a)]	21	±	?	?		
Pizotifen 1–1.5 mg/d [Gillies et al. (36)]	39	–	?	?		
Pizotifen 2.5–3.75 mg/d (abdominal migraine) [Symon and Russell (35)]	14	+	?	?		
Flunarizine 5 mg/d [Sorge et al. (37)	63	+	?	?		
Nimodipine 10–20 mg × 3 [Battistella et al. (33)]	30	±	?	?		
Papaverine 5–10 mg/kg/d [Sillanpää and Koponen (32)]	37	+	58%	17%	41%	2.44
Trazodone 1 mg/kg/d [Battistella et al. (34)]	35	±	±	?	?	

+, effective; –, no effect; ±, some effect; ?, unknown.

(32), nimodipine (33), and trazodone (34) have each been evaluated in a single trial with some efficacy reported. Pizotifen was found effective in abdominal migraine (35) but not in migraine (36). Flunarizine has been shown effective (37), but its use has been questioned because of side effects such as drowsiness and weight gain. Valproic acid has been effective in migraine prophylaxis in adults, but it has not been studied in children. In long-term use, valproic acid may cause weight gain, hair loss, and cytopenia; rare side effects such as hepatic toxicity and pancreatitis can occur. Amitriptyline, nortriptyline, and imipramine have been used as migraine prophylaxis, mainly in the United States. They are effective in relieving chronic pain in adults, but their efficacy in children with migraine has received only limited evaluation (38); amitriptyline significantly decreased school absences (38). Despite this lack of controlled trials, nortriptyline and other tricyclics are prescribed as first-line agents for migraine prophylaxis by the physicians in the Pain Treatment Service as well as the Neurology Clinic at Children's Hospital, Boston.

Prophylactic drug treatment may be indicated for patients whose attacks are long and incapacitating or occur several times per month and are not relieved by symptomatic treatment. Children who are 7 years or older may sometimes benefit from 0.5 to 2 mg/kg propranolol daily, divided into two or three doses (Table 39.4). Before drug therapy, blood pressure should be measured and electrocardiography performed. Propranolol may cause hypoglycemia, bradycardia, bronchospasm (in children with reactive airways disease), and hypotension and may decrease tolerance to physical exercise. For those who are active in sports, a starting dose of propranolol should be very low. Propranolol may exacerbate depressive symptoms in susceptible children. Electrocardiography should be performed and blood pressure should be controlled before amitriptyline (0.1 to 2 mg/kg daily) is prescribed. The dose of amitriptyline should be increased slowly (every 2 weeks), and doses of more than 1 mg/kg daily should be divided into two doses. Any drug used for prophylactic treatment should be evaluated for approximately 6 to 12 weeks before it can be considered ineffective. If effective, a break is recommended after 6 months. Drug prophylaxis should be an individually tailored monotherapy with parents and possibly the child being involved in the choice of drug.

NONPHARMACOLOGIC TREATMENT

Biobehavioral Intervention

Biobehavioral intervention for pediatric headache refers to a collection of procedures that can be divided into two general categories. In one category are procedures to teach patients self-control skills to prevent headache. Biofeedback techniques and relaxation training are included in this category. In the other category are procedures designed to modify behavior patterns that increase the risk of headache occurrence or reinforce headache activity. Contingency management of pain behavior and cognitive-behavioral stress management techniques are the main examples.

Behavioral Assessment

Gaining an understanding of the antecedents and consequences of headache pain is an important component of treatment. The headache diary is the most useful instrument in this regard. The diary should allow the child to record the time of onset, activities before the onset, any worries or concerns as far back as 24 hours before the onset, severity and duration of pain, pain medication taken, and activity pattern during headache (39). The information reported in the diary serves several functions. It provides additional clues about possible behavioral antecedents and consequences temporally linked to headache activity, thereby identifying areas of possible intervention. In addition, ongoing monitoring of headache activity will indicate more accurately the effects of the intervention and guide treatment planning. The validity of children's headache diaries has been investigated in at least one instance, and a significant correlation was found between child and parent ratings of headache activity (40).

Biofeedback

In clinical practice, biofeedback techniques rarely are used alone in the treatment of chronic headache in children. Biofeedback training involves providing a visual or auditory analogue of physiologic activity to teach the individual to manipulate that activity. The two most common modalities are thermal and electromyographic biofeedback. Thermal biofeedback consists of measuring surface skin temperature (usually from a finger) so that the child can learn to increase peripheral skin temperature. Electromyographic biofeedback of facial or neck muscle activity allows the child to learn to relax these muscle regions. In our view, biofeedback training is a technology-based form of relaxation therapy. Biofeedback is also useful to motivate the child who is reluctant to practice relaxation techniques. It is also useful to assess arousal to various stimuli and to gauge the relaxation learning curve during practice trials in the office. In the hands of a properly trained clinician, biofeedback can be used adeptly as an assessment tool and to reinforce learning and application of relaxation skills.

Relaxation Training

Many techniques are available to develop relaxation skills in children. There is no evidence to support one technique over another in terms of acceptance or efficacy. In fact, they may all result in the same physiologic effect if practiced regularly (41). The most commonly employed techniques are progressive muscle, deep breathing, imagery, and autogenics (42,43). They are easily taught to children as young as 7 years of age, can be used in various combinations, and can be tailored to the child's situation or personality. With 2 to 3 weeks of practice, the child is able to decrease the time needed to achieve relaxation and may then use the method in their natural environment to cope with stress and pain.

Pain Behavior Management

Pain behavior management is the component of biobehavioral treatment that parents implement. Based on principles of behavior modification, guidelines have been developed for parents to follow when their child's behavior indicates that a headache is present (39). These guidelines encourage parents to (a) eliminate the sources of reinforcement maintaining headache pain behavior and (b) promote active coping and normal activity (to the extent possible) if a headache is present. These guidelines can be taken a step further, if necessary, by having parents implement a contingency that rewards their child if they try to maintain normal activity patterns (e.g., school) when reporting headache. What this means in a practical sense is for parents to avoid giving excessive attention to their child's headache. Parents can be instructed to respond matter-of-factly to pain behavior and requests for special attention. Parents sometimes inadvertently focus the child on pain and negate attempts by the child to cope by asking about headaches. Parents should also be prepared to question whether school or social performance demands are being avoided because of headache. If the child must miss an important activity such as school, then bed rest should be the rule. This helps parents avoid feeling guilty about doubting the veracity of their child's reports of headache and inadvertently reinforcing pain behavior. Probably the most significant thing that parents can do is to go about their business and let their child manage headache pain, except where the administration of pain medication is concerned. Moreover, parents can focus attention on adaptive coping that is evident in their child's behavior, such as the use of relaxation techniques and maintenance of normal activity patterns, perhaps employing sensible modifications depending on pain intensity.

Cognitive-Behavioral Stress Management

Cognitive-behavioral strategies employed in the management of headache target recurrent negative stressful thoughts that interfere with coping and appear to be associated with increased headache activity (44). The basic method involves first identifying negative thoughts and situations that may be associated with increased risk for headache. Then the child is taught to activate a positive thought when in this situation and, if indicated, engage in adaptive behavior appropriate to the situation. This sequence is rehearsed repeatedly in treatment sessions and reinforced contingent on successful practice and application. Assessment of the types of coping strategies already in use is helpful before teaching additional strategies. This can be done using hypothetical situations based on headache diary information or from the child's history or by administering an instrument designed to assess coping strategies in children such as the Kidcope (45).

Efficacy Of Biobehavioral Intervention

Reviews of the efficacy of biobehavioral treatment of pediatric headache disorders indicate improvement rates ranging from 60% to 100% (46,47). There are at least 31 reports (47) in the literature from case studies to placebo-controlled investigations. Relaxation training combined with biofeedback is the most frequent intervention employed, and migraine the most common diagnosis. In control group outcome studies, sample size ranges from 20 to 99 patients, with group membership varying considerably from five to 37 children. Follow-up intervals extend up to 2 years after the end of treatment.

Evidence for the efficacy of relaxation alone or combined with biofeedback training comes from 11 randomized waiting list control group investigations (47). An additional four placebo-controlled group studies have yielded contradictory results. Two studies found that cognitive-behavioral and relaxation training (48) and relaxation alone (49) were effective in reducing headache in children and adolescents versus an attention placebo intervention, which had no effect. However, two other studies found that a credible placebo control intervention was as effective as relaxation alone, relaxation combined with biofeedback, or a single session to educate the patient about strategies to modify suspected headache precipitants (50; N. L. Hoag, unpublished).

Pain behavior management alone has not been systematically investigated in control group outcome studies. However, it has been found to effectively reduce headache and restore functioning (e.g., school attendance) in case studies. To our knowledge, cognitive-behavioral procedures alone have not been investigated in the treatment of pediatric headache. These are areas of research that need more attention.

CONCLUSION

There is sufficient evidence that biobehavioral intervention is effective in treating pediatric headache. Treatment is cost-effective and, importantly for most parents, an effective way to control headache without medication for long periods (51). Future research efforts should focus on testing single components of treatment versus credible placebo alternatives and comparing biobehavioral interventions with pharmacologic interventions. The efficacy and cost-efficiency of minimal contact biobehavioral treatment for headache in children is another promising approach that requires further investigation (52).

REFERENCES

1. Sillanpää M, Piekkala P, Kero P. Prevalence of headache at preschool age in an unselected child population. *Cephalalgia* 1991;11:239–242.
2. Bille B. Migraine in school children. *Acta Paediatr* 1962;51[Suppl 136]:13–151.
3. Carlsson J. Prevalence of headache in schoolchildren: relation to family and school factors. *Acta Paediatr* 1996;85:692–696.
4. Abu-Arafeh I, Russell G. Prevalence of headache and migraine in schoolchildren. *BMJ* 1994;309:765–769.
5. Sillanpää M, Anttila P. Increasing prevalence of headache in 7-year-old schoolchildren. *Headache* 1996;36: 466–470.
6. Stang PE, Yanagihara T, Swanson JW, et al. Incidence of migraine headache: a population-based study in Olmsted County, Minnesota. *Neurology* 1992;42: 1657–1662.
7. Rossi LN, Cortinovis I, Bellettini G, et al. Diagnostic criteria for migraine and psychogenic headache in children. *Dev Med Child Neurol* 1992;34:516–523.
8. Bille B. A 40-year follow-up of school children with migraine. *Cephalalgia* 1997;17:488–491.
9. Burton LJ, Quinn B, Pratt-Cheney JL, et al. Headache etiology in a pediatric emergency department. *Pediatr Emerg Care* 1997;13:1–4.
10. Weiller C, May A, Limmroth V, et al. Brain stem activation in spontaneous human migraine attacks. *Nat Med* 1995;1:658–660.
11. Metsähonkala L, Sillanpää M, Tuominen J. Headache diary in the diagnosis of childhood migraine. *Headache* 1997;37:240–244.
12. Headache Classification Committee of the International Headache Society. Classification and diagnostic criteria for headache disorders, cranial neuralgias and facial pain. *Cephalalgia* 1988;8[Suppl 7]:1–96.
13. Ophoff RA, Terwindt GM, Vergouwe MN, et al. Familial hemiplegic migraine and episodic ataxia type-2 are caused by mutations in the Ca2+ channel gene CACNL1A4. *Cell* 1996;87:543–552.
14. Tal Y, Dunn HG, Chrichton JU. Childhood migraine—a dangerous diagnosis. *Acta Paediatr Scand* 1984;73: 55–59.
15. Medina LS, Kuntz KM, Pomeroy S. Children with headache suspected of having a brain tumor: a cost-effectiveness analysis of diagnostic strategies. *Pediatrics* 2001;108:255–263.
16. Soler D, Cox T, Bullock P, et al. Diagnosis and management of benign intracranial hypertension. *Arch Dis Child* 1998;78:89–94.
17. Rossi LN, Vassella F. Headache in children with brain tumors. *Child Nerv Syst* 1989;5:307–309.
18. Mortimer MJ, Kay J, Jaron A. Childhood migraine in general practice: clinical features and characteristics. *Cephalalgia* 1992;12:238–243.
19. Hämäläinen ML, Hoppu K, Santavuori P. Pain and disability in migraine or other recurrent headaches as reported by children. *Eur J Neurol* 1996;3:528–532.
20. Hämäläinen ML, Hoppu K, Valkeila E, et al. Ibuprofen or acetaminophen for the acute treatment of migraine in children—a double-blind, randomized, placebo-controlled, crossover study. *Neurology* 1997;48:103–107.
21. Hämäläinen ML, Hoppu K, Santavuori P. Sumatriptan

for migraine attacks in children: a randomized placebo-controlled study. Do children with migraine respond to oral sumatriptan differently from adults? *Neurology* 1997;48:1100–1103.
22. Ueberall MA, Wenzel D. Intranasal sumatriptan for the acute treatment of migraine in children. *Neurology* 1999;52:1507–1510.
23. Winner P, Rothner AD, Saper J, et al. A randomized, double-blind, placebo-controlled study of sumatriptan nasal spray in the treatment of acute migraine in adolescents. *Pediatrics* 2000;106:989–997.
24. Hershey AD, Powers SW, LeCates S, et al. Effectiveness of nasal sumatriptan in 5- to 12-year-old children. *Headache* 2001;41:693–697.
25. Rothner AD, Winner P, Nett R, et al. One-year tolerability and efficacy of sumatriptan nasal spray in adolescents with migraine: results of a multicenter, open-label study. *Clin Ther* 2000;22:1533–1546.
26. Linder SL. Subcutaneous sumatriptan in the clinical setting—the first 50 consecutive patients with acute migraine in a pediatric neurology office practice. *Headache* 1996;36:419–422.
27. Hermann C, Kim M, Blanchard EB. Behavioral and prophylactic pharmacological intervention studies of pediatric migraine: an exploratory meta-analysis. *Pain* 1995;60:239–255.
28. Ludvigsson J. Propranolol used in prophylaxis of migraine in children. *Acta Neurol Scand* 1974;50:109–115.
29. Forsythe WI, Gillies D, Sills MA. Propranolol ('Inderal') in the treatment of childhood migraine. *Dev Med Child Neurol* 1984;26:737–741.
29a. Olness K, MacDonald JT, Uden DL. Comparison of self-hypnosis and propranolol in the treatment of childhood migraine. *Pediatrics* 1987;79:593–597.
30. Sillanpää M. Clonidine prophylaxis of childhood migraine and other vascular headache. A double blind study of 57 children. *Headache* 1977;17:28–31.
30a. Santucci M, Cortelli P, Rossi PG, et al. L-5-hydroxytryptan versus placebo in childhood migraine prophylaxis: a double-blind crossover study. *Cephalalgia* 1986;6:193–202.
31. Sills M, Congdon P, Forsythe I. Clonidine in childhood migraine: a pilot and double-blind study. *Dev Med Child Neurol* 1982;24:837–841.
32. Sillanpää M, Koponen M. Papaverine in the prophylaxis of migraine and other vascular headache in children. *Acta Paediatr Scand* 1978;67:209–212.
33. Battistella PA, Ruffilli R, Moro R, et al. A placebo-controlled crossover trial of nimodipine in pediatric migraine. *Headache* 1990;30:264–268.
34. Battistella PA, Ruffilli R, Cernetti R, et al. A placebo-controlled crossover trial using trazodone in pediatric migraine. *Headache* 1993;33:36–39.
35. Symon DN, Russell G. Double blind placebo controlled trial of pizotifen syrup in the treatment of abdominal migraine. *Arch Dis Child* 1995;72:48–50.
36. Gillies D, Sills M, Forsythe I. Pizotifen (Sanomigran) in childhood migraine. A double-blind controlled trial. *Eur Neurol* 1986;25:32–35.
37. Sorge F, De Simone R, Marano E, et al. Flunarizine in prophylaxis of childhood migraine. A double-blind, placebo-controlled, crossover study. *Cephalalgia* 1988; 8:1–6.
38. Hershey AD, Powers SW, Bentti AL, et al. Effectiveness of amitriptyline in the prophylactic management of childhood headaches. *Headache* 2000;40:539–549.
39. Masek BJ, Russo DC, Varni JW. Behavioral approaches to the management of chronic pain in children. *Pediatr Clin North Am* 1984;31:1113–1131.
40. Andrasik F, Burke EJ, Attanasio V, et al. Child, parent, and physician reports of a child's headache pain: relationships prior to and follow-up treatment. *Headache* 1985;25:421–425.
41. Everly GS, Benson H. Disorders of arousal and the relaxation response: speculations on the nature and treatment of stress-related disease. *Int J Psychosom* 1989; 36:15–21.
42. Cautela J, Grodin J. *Relaxation: a comprehensive manual for adults, children, and children with special needs.* Champaign, IL: Research Press, 1978.
43. Poppen R. *Behavioral relaxation training and assessment.* Elmsford, NY: Pergamon, 1988.
44. Richardson GM, McGrath PJ. Cognitive-behavioral therapy for migraine headaches: a minimal therapist contact approach versus a clinic-based approach. *Headache* 1989;29:352–357.
45. Spirito A, Stark L, Williams C. Development of a brief coping checklist for use with pediatric populations. *J Pediatr Psychol* 1988;13:555–574.
46. Holroyd KA, Penzien DB. Pharmacological versus nonpharmacological prophylaxis of recurrent migraine headache: a meta-analytic review of clinical trials. *Pain* 1990;42:1–13.
47. Holden EW, Deichmann MM, Levy JD. Empirically supported treatments in pediatric psychology: recurrent pediatric headache. *J Pediatr Psychol* 1999;24:91–109.
48. Richter IL, McGrath PJ, Humphries PJ, et al. Cognitive and relaxation treatment of paediatric migraine. *Pain* 1986;25:195–203.
49. Larsson B, Helm L. Chronic headaches in adolescents: treatment in a school setting with relaxation training as compared with information—contact and self-regulation. *Pain* 1986;725:325–336.
50. McGrath PJ, Humphries P, Goodman JT, et al. Relaxation prophylaxis for childhood migraine: a randomized placebo-controlled trial. *Dev Med Child Neurol* 1988; 30:626–631.
51. Masek BJ. Commentary: the pediatric migraine connection. *J Pediatr Psychol* 1999;24:110.
52. Scharff L, Etherage J. The role of minimal-and no-contact behavioural treatments in migraine. *Dis Manage Health Outcomes* 2000;8:313–325.
53. Winner P, Wasiewski W, Gladstein J, et al. Multicenter prospective evaluation of proposed pediatric migraine revisions to the I.H.S criteria. Pediatric Committee of the American Association for the Society of Headache. *Headache* 1997;37:545–548.
54. Maytal J, Young M, Schechter A, et al. Pediatric migraine and the International Headache Society criteria. *Neurology* 1997;48:602–607.

40

Recurrent Abdominal Pain

Lisa Scharff, Alan M. Leichtner, and Leonard A. Rappaport

Each age group throughout childhood and adolescence seems to have a pain complaint that is shared by a significant number of children. These pain complaints cause considerable anxiety for parents and sometimes the child, and their evaluation demands significant resources from society. In infancy, the pain complaint is colic, in the preschool-age child, it is "growing pains" of the lower extremities, in the preschool- and school-age child, the complaint is abdominal pain, and in the adolescent, it is headache.

Some common themes are relevant to each of these pain complaints. First, the discomfort appears to be real and interferes with the activities of the child. Second, the nature of the complaint is such that there is a possibility that the complaint represents a significant organic disease, and this possibility, although small, can prompt extensive evaluation. Finally, the cause of these pain complaints of childhood and adolescence remains unclear, and the care of these children and adolescents remains fraught with anxiety for parents and physicians.

This chapter focuses on recurrent abdominal pain in school children, but the overall model applies to the other pain complaints of childhood and adolescence.

DEFINITION AND PREVALENCE

Recurrent abdominal pain (RAP) is currently defined by a description first proposed by Apley (1). The abdominal pain must occur at least once per month for 3 consecutive months, be accompanied by pain-free periods, and be severe enough to interfere with a child's normal activities.

Studies investigating the prevalence of RAP have reported variable findings, with population prevalence rates ranging from 9% to nearly 25% (2–5) depending on the age and gender of the children sampled as well as the criteria used to define RAP. Apley and Naish (2) reported a prevalence rate of 10.8% in a primary and secondary school sample of 1,000 children, with girls affected more often than boys (12.3% compared with 9.5%). They also reported similar incidence rates in girls and boys up to 8 years of age, after which the incidence increased sharply in girls (peaking at a 25% incidence rate at 9 years of age) and tended to decrease in boys up to the mid-teens. Girls also reported an older age of onset than boys. Faull and Nicol (3) conducted an epidemiologic study of RAP in 5 and 6 year olds who were living a new town in the north of England (presumed to be a highly stressful place to live) and identified a 25% prevalence rate.

RAP has been reported to frequently coexist with other types of recurrent pain such as chronic headache or migraine. Apley and Naish (2) reported that 14% of school-age children with RAP complained of headaches compared with 5% of a nonmedical control group. Alfven (6) observed that 58% of a group of patients with RAP reported frequent headaches compared with 21% of controls.

One of the greatest difficulties in researching RAP is the definition of RAP itself. The most commonly used operational definition (at least three episodes of pain occurring within 3 months that are severe enough to affect the child's activities) lacks a set of symptom-focused diagnostic criteria. Altered bowel habits, vomiting, and migraine may accompany abdominal pain in some of these children. Samples of children with RAP used in various research studies may in reality represent a heterogeneous population. Few studies have investigated the prevalence of accompanying symptoms in children with RAP, and none has determined whether accompanying symptoms have an association with prognosis or treatment indications. There has been growing recognition that a valid and reliable set of symptom-based diagnostic criteria is sorely needed for this population of recurrent pain sufferers (7). A recent meeting of experts in childhood gastrointestinal disorders developed criteria for the diagnosis of multiple pediatric functional gastrointestinal complaints but did not develop new diagnostic criteria for RAP. The consensus was that this diagnosis was too vague and that there was a great deal of overlap between RAP and the established criteria for irritable bowel syndrome (IBS) and functional dyspepsia. In addition, research regarding the pathogenesis of abdominal pain in children continues to identify different causes for RAP (8). A diagnostic category "functional abdominal pain" was included in the new criteria, with the following diagnostic criteria: at least 12 weeks duration of

1. continuous or nearly continuous abdominal pain in a school-age child or adolescent,
2. no or only occasional relationship of pain with physiologic events (e.g., eating, menses, or defecation),
3. some loss of daily functioning,
4. the pain is not feigned (e.g., malingering),
5. insufficient criteria for other functional gastrointestinal disorders that would explain the abdominal pain.

This new functional abdominal pain diagnosis was not intended as a substitute for Apley's RAP definition. Pediatric abdominal pain sufferers who previously met Apley's RAP criteria would, under the new set of diagnostic criteria, be categorized into multiple categories including IBS, functional dyspepsia, functional abdominal pain, and abdominal migraine. The term RAP itself will likely be abandoned because of its vague definition, but it is used in this chapter because Apley's definition and term are the ones used in most of the previous research reviewed here.

COMMON SIGNS AND SYMPTOMS

Children with RAP usually present with characteristic signs and symptoms. The pain is usually periumbilical and difficult for the child to describe. It usually lasts less than 1 hour and almost never lasts longer than 3 hours. The pain can often be associated with autonomic symptoms such as pallor, sweating, nausea, and occasionally vomiting. There is rarely an intervention that is always successful in decreasing the pain, and the pain does not wake the child up from sleep. Some children with RAP also report headaches. As indicated by the name, the pain is intermittent and recurrent with asymptomatic periods.

RED FLAGS

Most reviews, in an attempt to aid the evaluating physician, have outlined a number of "red flags" that have been associated with organic pathology (Table 40.1). Each of these indicates an increased likelihood of organic disease, and the concurrence of a number of these symptoms or signs should significantly increase a physician's suspicion of a definable cause for the pain. The most common red flag

TABLE 40.1. *Red flags for pathology*

Weight loss
Pain awakening the child at night
Fevers
Pain far from umbilicus
Dysuria
Guaiac-positive stools
Anemia
Elevated erythrocyte sedimentation rate

is deviation from the typical historic presentation of RAP. For example, a child with abdominal pain that occurs far from the umbilicus is more likely to have a diagnosable cause of the abdominal pain (termed Apley's law because of his original description of this association) (Table 40.1).

CAUSES OF RECURRENT ABDOMINAL PAIN

Despite considerable controversy concerning the underlying cause of RAP, almost all studies have found that only approximately 10% of children seem to have a recognizable organic disease that explains the pain complaint (2,9). Ultimate proof requires that treatment of the proposed etiologic agent alleviate the abdominal pain.

The range of organic disease that causes RAP represents a textbook of pediatrics in that almost any disease can and does cause abdominal pain. However, when the identified causes in previous studies are examined by system, at least a third of the organic disease is referable to the gastrointestinal or genitourinary system. Therefore, a particular focus of the history and physical examination must be directed toward these systems.

Several putative gastrointestinal causes of RAP merit specific mention because of their relatively recent description, high prevalence in the pediatric age group, and controversial relationship to the symptom of RAP. These include lactose intolerance, malabsorption of other carbohydrates, and infection with *Helicobacter pylori*.

Many authors have implicated lactose malabsorption as a cause of RAP. Malabsorbed lactose is fermented in the colon by the normal bacterial flora. Gas produced as a result of the fermentation and water obligated by the osmotic activity of malabsorbed carbohydrate and its metabolites may lead to bowel distention and diarrhea, although the latter is not always present. Furthermore, fermentation products may directly stimulate colonic motility. However, it is clear that some individuals may malabsorb lactose and yet have no symptoms of lactose intolerance. Additional factors such as the exact nature of the colonic flora and the form in which the lactose is ingested probably account for this variability in symptomatology (10).

The clinical relationship of lactose malabsorption and RAP in children is controversial. Barr et al. (11) and others (12) reported a 40% to 50% incidence of lactose malabsorption in children with RAP. When these children were instructed to follow a lactose-free diet, 25% of them reported a more than 50% reduction in pain. Other investigators have found a lower incidence of lactose intolerance in these children and a significant placebo effect of dietary restriction (13). Most recently, studies in populations with a high incidence of primary acquired lactose intolerance have again demonstrated that lactose malabsorption accounts for symptoms in a significant proportion of children with RAP (14). In summary, lactose intolerance probably accounts for RAP in only a small subset of patients, but it should be especially considered in children of susceptible racial and ethnic backgrounds.

In the same manner, malabsorption of other carbohydrates has been implicated in the pathogenesis of RAP in a small number of children. The sugar alcohol sorbitol is found in a variety of different fruits, especially prunes and pears, and is used as a sweetener in candy and chewing gum. Some children may develop symptoms with the ingestion of as little as two pieces of sorbitol-sweetened gum (15,16). Intolerance of the widely occurring sugar fructose has also been described in children (17), and it is likely that there are other carbohydrates in the Western diet that are malabsorbed in some individuals, resulting in abdominal pain. Although such causes of RAP are exceedingly unusual, they merit emphasis because of the relative ease of treating them by dietary restriction alone.

H. pylori is a gram-negative, spiral-shaped bacteria that is able to colonize the gastric mucosa in humans with resulting gastritis. Risk factors for infection include familial overcrowding, endemic country of origin, and low socioeconomic status. Accordingly, estimates of the incidence of infection in developing countries are between 3% and 10% per year versus 1% per year in the United States (18). In adults, this organism causes antral gastritis and gastric and duodenal ulcers. The strongest association is between duodenal ulcers and infection with *H. pylori*, and eradication of the organism prevents recurrence of the ulcer (19). However, the role of treatment in patients with dyspepsia who do not have mucosal ulceration is disputed (20). The role of *H. pylori* in causing RAP in children is also controversial. Although many studies have been conducted, interpretation of their results is confounded by several factors including widely different patient populations (ranging from healthy children to children referred to a pediatric gastroenterologist specifically for upper endoscopy), imprecise definitions of RAP, and the use of diagnostic techniques of varying sensitivity and specificity (21). The weight of evidence suggests that *H. pylori* infection is very unlikely to be the cause of classic RAP in children whose symptoms meet the Apley definition. Therefore, screening for *H. pylori* infection is not recommended for these patients. In contrast, in children with documented duodenal ulcers and *H. pylori* infection, the organism should certainly be considered the cause of the abdominal symptoms. The question of whether severe *H. pylori*–induced gastritis, in the absence of ulceration, can cause RAP awaits further study (22). Until more information is available, treatment of such patients should be individualized.

PATHOPHYSIOLOGY

Much of the difficulty in determining the cause of RAP is a result of peculiarities in the innervation of the abdominal viscera (for a review, see reference 23). The pain receptors, or nociceptors, are located in the submucosa, muscular layers, and serosa of hollow viscera and in the capsule of solid organs. In addition, similar receptors are found in the parietal peritoneum. The sensory afferent fibers are largely of the C type, and the pain sensation transmitted by them tends to be relatively dull, poorly localized, gradual in onset, and of long duration. Visceral pain fibers in the intestine are activated in response to stretching or an increase in the tension of the wall rather than by other mechanical stimuli. Inflammation or ischemia may also cause pain, probably via the action of tissue mediators that directly stimulate the nociceptors or lower their threshold for activation.

Stimulation of visceral pain fibers generally results in dull, poorly localized abdominal pain, so-called visceral pain. Such pain is usually felt in the midline because the sensory nerves travel to both sides of the spinal cord. Pain from the stomach and duodenum is felt in the epigastrium, pain from the distal small intestine and proximal colon in the periumbilical region, and pain from the distal colon and rectum in the hypogastrium. Visceral pain may be accompanied by *referred pain* felt in the skin or deeper tissues because the somatic and visceral nerves from the different sites travel together to the central nervous system. Pain resulting from stimulation of nociceptors in the parietal peritoneum is more intense and better localized, usually to one side of the abdomen. It has become increasingly evident that the perception of pain can be modified by higher cortical centers, and these centers may in turn affect gastrointestinal function. These observations have led to the notion of a "brain–gut axis," with a bidirectional flow of information.

Functional gastrointestinal disorders are defined as conditions in which chronic or recurrent symptoms occur in the absence of any readily identified structural or biochemical abnormalities (24). It has been hypothesized that functional gastrointestinal disorders result from perturbations in the brain–gut axis. The two primary functional gastrointestinal disorders identified in adults are IBS and functional dyspepsia. Both disorders also occur in children. Idiopathic RAP meeting the Apley definition might also be considered a functional gastrointestinal disorder, and none of the diagnoses for functional gastrointestinal disorders is exclusive. The comorbidity of such diagnoses significantly contributes to the confusion in the research literature regarding assessment and treatment. Of particular note is the overlap between IBS and RAP.

IBS is diagnosed by using one of two established sets of criteria (25,26). It is characterized by abdominal pain and disordered defecation, resulting in constipation, diarrhea, or a variable consistency of bowel movements. Hyams and colleagues (27) conducted a community-based study of RAP and IBS in school-age children and identified a 13% to 17% prevalence rate of RAP. In addition, the authors estimated that 6% of middle school–age children and 14% of high school–age children would qualify for a diagnosis of IBS. The same investigators (28) applied IBS diagnostic criteria to children presenting at a gastroenterology clinic meeting the Apley criteria for RAP. Of the 171 patients without an organic diagnosis for pain, 117 (68%) fulfilled criteria for a diagnosis of IBS.

The overlap between IBS and RAP has also led to some speculation that RAP may be a manifestation of IBS without the altered bowel habits that accompany this syndrome in adults. The many similarities between IBS and RAP include prevalence rate, prognosis, psychiatric comorbidity, family history of somatic and psychiatric symptoms, and stressful life events as symptom triggers (29). It is possible that the presence or absence of altered bowel habits is related to developmental changes that affect intestinal motility.

Autonomic nervous system dysregulation has been suspected as a cause of both IBS (30) and RAP (31). The studies investigating autonomic nervous system functioning in RAP have reported conflicting results, however, and much of the research was conducted without control groups or with small sample sizes. Research does indicate that children with RAP may exhibit prolonged transit time (32) and higher rectosigmoid motility (33) than control populations, and these are similar to findings in adult patients with IBS (34). Other measures of autonomic functioning have been identified as altered in patients with IBS compared with normal controls (35); however, none of this research has been conducted with a sufficient sample of children with RAP.

The phenomenon of visceral hyperalgesia has also been considered a significant issue in both IBS and RAP. Visceral hyperalgesia is thought to be associated with hyperexcitability of neurons of the dorsal horn in response to either peripheral tissue irritation or in response to descending influences originating in the brain stem (36). This results in a lowered pain threshold in the gut as well as altered reflexes associated with digestion. Multiple studies have demonstrated that people with IBS have lower pain thresholds to painful stimuli applied in the area of the rectosigmoid junction and the rectum (37,38). These studies have not been replicated in children with RAP, mostly owing to ethical concerns regarding the invasive nature of the testing required to assess visceral hyperalgesia.

Functional dyspepsia is another functional gastrointestinal disorder identified in adults that may overlap with RAP of childhood. Dyspepsia is characterized by episodic or persistent symptoms in the upper abdomen or epigastrium (39). In ulcer-like dyspepsia, the predominant complaint is pain. In dysmotility-like dyspepsia, the predominant symptoms are early satiety, bloating, or nausea. The cause of functional dyspepsia is thought to be disordered motility or visceral hyperalgesia, and it must be differentiated from dyspepsia resulting from mucosal disease such as esophagitis, gastritis, or ulcer disease and from pancreatic and hepatobiliary disease. Functional dyspepsia has been noted in children, but it has not been well studied (40). Although the location of pain in classic RAP of childhood is periumbilical, it is possible that some children with this diagnosis might be better characterized as having functional dyspepsia.

Although multiple pathophysiologic avenues have been explored to account for RAP, currently our best understanding of the cause of RAP is that the pain complaint represents a physiologic stimulus combined with a vulnerability to that stimulus. That is, a child has actual pain that might be from, for example, constipation or an increased intake of lactose relative to the child's ability to break that lactose down. Both would cause a painful stimulus in most children, but some would ignore it and some would complain of the pain. Therefore, the pain is a necessary but not a sufficient cause for the RAP complaint.

In fact, the child must indeed repeatedly engage in pain behavior or verbally complain to his or her caretakers for attention to be drawn to the pain. Things that can influence the presence or absence of such complaints would include characteristics of the child such as temperament in addition to forces outside the child such as how well he or she is integrated into the social milieu of life and how focused the child's parents are on somatic symptoms. Thus, multiple variables have important roles in determining whether he or she focuses on the pain or is distracted by involvement in life. The interaction between the physiologic stimuli and the child's internal and external life experiences determines the presence or absence of a pain complaint. Therefore, theoretically, altering any or all parts of the formula can alleviate the pain experience.

ASSESSMENT OF RECURRENT ABDOMINAL PAIN

Physical Examination and History

When confronted with a child with RAP, the physician's first responsibility is to identify those organic diseases that could be causing the pain symptom, while protecting the child and family from both the excessive trauma and expense of a nonproductive invasive evaluation. The physician must therefore be primarily concerned with determining the most efficient and productive approach to the evaluation of abdominal pain.

Most clinicians who evaluate many children with abdominal pain believe that the most essential facets of the workup are a complete history and physical evaluation. When confronted with such a child, a busy physician must slow down his or her pace or make a return appointment to get an adequate history and to complete a full physical examination. With both of these in hand, organic diseases can almost always be uncovered without extensive laboratory evaluation. To supplement the history and physical evaluation, the previously described red flags (Table 40.1) are quite helpful. An extensive workup unguided by a suggestive history or physical examination is rarely productive.

The appropriate laboratory evaluation for RAP is rather minimal. A complete blood count with an erythrocyte sedimentation rate can be quite useful in screening for anemia or nonspecific inflammation. Because most studies have shown that approximately one-third of organic diseases causing RAP derive from the genitourinary tract, a urinalysis in all children and a urine culture in females is appropriate. A rectal examination with stool guaiac test is also indicated.

Varying suggestions have been made for other tests to be included in the basic workup for RAP. For example, it has been suggested that abdominal ultrasonography is an atraumatic and productive test for these children (41); however, several studies have demonstrated the lack of its utility in the evaluation of RAP. Other researchers have suggested the use of lactose breath tests for children who are at risk for having low lactase levels in middle childhood or children with a history suggestive of lactose intolerance. However, the usefulness of such a test in the general population remains unclear. Finally, a stool test for ova and parasites has been proposed by some physicians in populations who are at risk for *Giardia* or other common parasites, but there has been no empiric support for its general use. It remains our opinion that all supplementary studies should be used only when the standard evaluation indicates an increased likelihood of an organic cause.

Psychologic Factors and Treatment

Pain is a very complex phenomenon, affected by multiple physiologic, affective, behavioral, and cognitive factors, all of which need to be assessed. A psychologic evaluation can reveal many possible contributory factors in RAP. Anxiety and acute stressors are often identified as triggers of RAP episodes. Case studies of children with RAP often describe these children as anxious, with precipitating episodes of extreme stress such as the breakup of their parents' marriage. The relationship between anxiety, acute stressors, and pain episodes, however, is not clearly cause and effect. A stressful event may be related to the onset of a particular RAP episode but does not explain a long-standing history or a high frequency of such episodes.

A through psychologic assessment includes a pain interview and an evaluation of psychosocial factors that may influence pain. Information about characteristics of the child's pain including pain descriptions, patterns of pain, intensity of pain, accompanying symptoms, potential pain triggers, disability owing to pain, and current pain management methods and the child's understanding of the diagnosis need to be assessed. Psychosocial issues such as family conflict and problems with peers or school also need to be investigated because such stressors may serve as repeated triggers of pain episodes.

Multiple studies assessing psychologic characteristics in patients with RAP have identified that children with RAP also tend have high levels of anxiety (42–44) and depression (45,46). Such findings have often led to the conclusion that RAP is mainly an expression of psychologic distress, a conclusion supported by the fact that a significant percentage of children with anxiety disorders also report frequent bouts of abdominal pain (47). Subsequent controlled studies have challenged this hypothesis by demonstrating that children with organic abdominal pain such as gastritis and peptic ulcer disease also have levels of anxiety higher than those in nonmedical controls (48–50). These studies suggest that psychologic distress may be related to the presence of gastrointestinal pain and not the cause of the pain. Elevated anxiety is to be expected in children with RAP and is sometimes associated with the onset of a pain episode but should not be assumed to be causally related to RAP unless evidence can support that assumption.

Another aspect of RAP that has received some attention in the psychology literature has been the influence of parental behavior in the encouragement of somatic symptoms. Parents may affect a child's pain behavior through direct encouragement of pain behavior by rewarding complaints or by modeling pain behavior themselves. When parents react to abdominal pain by relieving the child of responsibilities or giving special privileges, they may be inadvertently using reinforcement to encourage pain responses. One study reported that parents of patients with RAP and peptic ulcer were more likely to encourage illness behavior associated with gastrointestinal symptoms compared with nonmedical controls and psychiatric patients (51). Parents in general do not consciously encourage their children to complain about pain: most parents behave as they always have when their child is sick. After several months, it may become clear that the pain complaints are serving as a long-term coping strategy, and parents need to be encouraged to reinforce active coping behaviors and non–pain-related verbalizations and actions.

One important behavioral consideration in any chronic pediatric pain case is school attendance. Excessive school absence is a significant problem for many children with RAP who can miss as much as half of the school year (52). Some children who report abdominal pain may do so out of a desire to avoid school. These children may be highly anxious or fearful of school situations, have learning disabilities that may make school aversive to them, or may be subject to aggressive teasing and taunting at school.

Another factor to assess for is a possible history of physical or sexual abuse. Somatic symptom reporting is common in abused children (53); however, only a minority of children with somatic complaints have been abused (54). Case studies have shown such associations, but there is no available information regarding the comorbidity of RAP and abuse. Thus, it is wise to assess children with RAP for a history of abuse as well as for current abuse.

Stressful life events such as marital problems between the child's parents are often attributed to be causal factors in RAP (44,55). However, most studies investigating life events in children with RAP compared with controls have found no significant differences in life events or marital problems among the parents (50,56,57). Recently, more attention has been paid to how children's skills in coping with pain and stress mediate the influence of these stressors on pain. A stressful life event may not be a sufficient trigger of a pain episode, but how that child copes with the stressor and subsequent stressors may be an important factor in the development of a recurrent pain problem. Walker et al. (58) conducted a prospective study that examined how several variables may mediate the influence of life stress on pain in both patients with RAP and those with organic abdominal pain. They reported that continued pain reports were significantly related to life stress but only in children with low levels of social competence or in children whose parents also reported high levels of somatic symptoms.

Analytic Model of Recurrent Pain

As previously stated, only 10% of children with RAP have a clearly definable cause. This leaves 90% of children with frequent pain complaints that occur without an identified cause. For physicians to evaluate and treat such children successfully, they must approach these children with a theoretic model that provides adequate guidance for initial workup, treatment, and long-term management if necessary. One such theoretic model is proposed in Figure 40.1. The model describes the role of causal and mediating factors in RAP as well as disability resulting from child and environmental factors or how pain is interpreted (Fig. 40.1).

TREATMENT OF RECURRENT ABDOMINAL PAIN

Management of RAP should be individualized to reflect the proposed causes of the pain and the psychosocial needs of the child and family. There is no formula for the treatment of RAP, and the best intervention includes an amalgam of an excellent clinical assessment and a clear understanding of the child's family and environment, integrated into a working model of the cause and treatment of RAP.

Feedback to Patient and Family

It is key from the beginning of the clinical contact to share your model of RAP with the family. At the first visit, it is essential to include the following information in your discussion before beginning any workup of the pain.

1. RAP is common is children.
2. Only 10% of children with RAP have an identifiable organic cause for their pain symptom.
3. Despite the fact that we cannot find a cause of the pain, we believe that the pain is real.
4. We will do a directed medical workup dictated by the child's symptoms and signs in combination with what we know about the most common organic causes of RAP.
5. If an organic cause is found, we will treat it appropriately.
6. Usually the abdominal pain goes away, but sometimes the problem that we find was not the actual cause of the pain, and even after treatment, the pain may persist.
7. In one-third of children with RAP, the pain persists, in another third, it is replaced by another pain symptom, and in the final third, the pain goes away.
8. After the initial workup, we will make a plan jointly for treatment and follow-up.
9. This plan will include regular follow-up at a 3- to 4-month interval and a list of

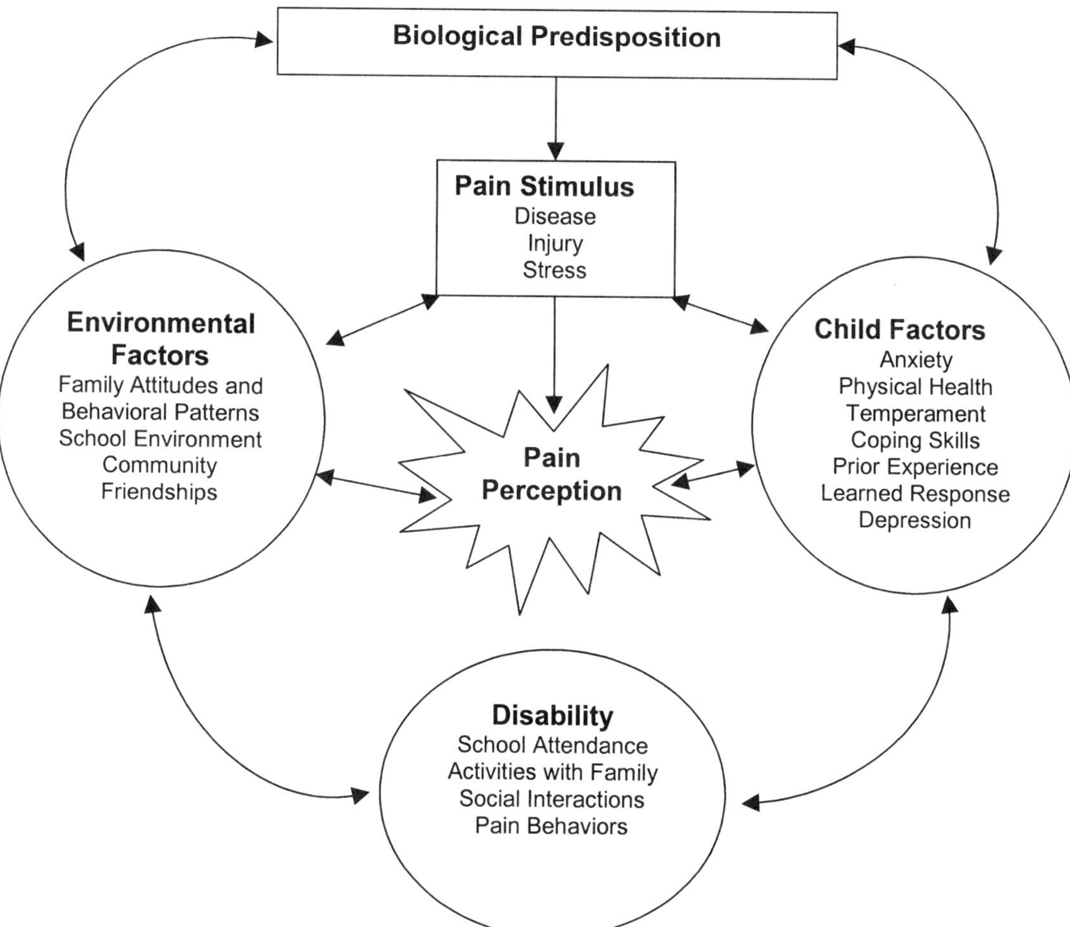

FIGURE 40.1. Interactions between precipitating, child, and environmental factors affect both pain perception and disability. Note that pain itself is not directly related to disability: the extent to which pain interferes with activity is highly variable.

symptoms that should be cause for earlier contact.

10. This plan may also include consultation with professionals experienced in teaching a child biobehavioral pain management techniques, which seem helpful in treating RAP (such techniques are discussed in the following section).
11. Our job together is to limit the impact that the pain has on the child's and family's lives.

If this model is shared after the workup is complete and the clinician is comfortable that there is no recognizable organic problem, the family will often feel that the clinician is dismissing or giving up on them. The perception of an unsuccessful workup with no resolution is very different from experiencing the medical workup as an initial step in the treatment of a common childhood problem.

Biobehavioral Treatment of Recurrent Abdominal Pain

In many cases, despite assurance and support from the treating physician, the child continues to suffer from pain and impairment. Biobehavioral treatment strategies administered by a trained professional such as psychologists and social workers can significantly aid in decreasing a child's pain complaints. Such treatments address how the child understands pain, variables that may be reinforcing pain such as school anxiety, and parental reinforcement of pain complaints. A thorough behavioral and psychologic assessment is necessary to determine which specific treatment approaches are needed. As shown in Figure 40.1, there are multiple variables that influence the expression of pain and the presence of disability.

Biobehavioral treatment of children with RAP has unfortunately not been well researched, and the literature on this subject generally involves uncontrolled treatments as well as small sample sizes (59). In general, there are two categories of biobehavioral treatment studies: those that use operant approaches to reduce pain complaints and behaviors (i.e., encouraging or reinforcing well behavior, ignoring pain behavior) and those that use stress-management approaches to reduce subjective reports of pain and teach the child to cope with stressful triggers of pain and to cope with the pain itself.

Treatment programs based on operant theory have resulted in many cases in decreased verbal reports of abdominal pain in children diagnosed with RAP. In one case study, Miller and Kratochwill (60) implemented a time-out procedure in the home of a 10-year-old girl with RAP, and although pain behavior decreased at home, it subsequently increased at school. When time out was implemented at her school, all reports of pain decreased. Single case reports of token systems (61) and positive reinforcement (62) have also reported successful use of operant-based treatments to reduce abdominal pain complaints. The use of such operant treatment modalities alone is not generally recommended; pain behaviors may be decreased while the subjective discomfort of the child is not taken into account. Operant procedures used alone may result in teaching children to not report pain that may require medical attention.

Stress management and cognitive-behavioral strategies have also been investigated and found to be successful, although the conclusions that can be drawn from the results of such studies are limited. Such treatment programs for RAP often add an operant component in the form of parent training in how to avoid positive reinforcement of sick behaviors and focus on rewarding healthy behaviors.

In a case series design, Finney et al. (63) used a multicomponent behavioral treatment with 16 children meeting Apley's criteria for RAP. Treatment consisted of a varying number of sessions over 1 to 6 months and included various components such as monitoring of symptoms, limited parent attention, relaxation training, increased dietary fiber, and required school attendance. At the end of the treatment, 25% of the participants demonstrated no abdominal pain symptoms, and 56% were rated as improved.

Sanders and colleagues (64) used a wait list control group to assess the utility of a cognitive-behavioral treatment consisting of stress management and parent training with patients with RAP. Over the course of eight sessions, the children's parents were provided with education about RAP as well as how to distinguish between sick and well behaviors, a reward system was put in place for well behaviors, and relaxation and stress coping skills were taught to the children for pain management. Both the treatment and wait list groups demonstrated symptom improvement; however, the controls were significantly less improved. Seventy-five percent of the treated group and 25% of the controls were pain free at the end of treatment.

In another study, Sanders et al. (65) used a larger sample size of 44 children and a control treatment group of "assurance" that nothing was physically wrong with the child and that symptoms would likely improve. Both the cognitive-behavioral and control treatments resulted in a significant decrease in symptoms. However, the cognitive-behavioral treatment resulted in significantly more pain-free children at the end of treatment and at the 12-month follow-up. Of the patients receiving cognitive-behavioral therapy, 55.6% were reportedly pain free at the end of treatment compared with 23.8% of the standard care patients.

Certainly a percentage of children improve with little or no treatment; however, the studies that have used psychologic treatment strategies have demonstrated the efficacy of these modalities. Continued research in the area is called for, with an emphasis on larger controlled studies and a more clearly definable study population.

Other biobehavioral treatment modalities such as biofeedback have yet to be researched in a controlled manner in children with RAP. Clinically, biofeedback is a useful treatment approach because the instrumentation involved interests and motivates a school-age population and also because it teaches children that they have a great deal of control over their own bodies.

From a practical standpoint, it continues to be difficult to identify individuals trained in using these techniques with children. Pediatric psychologists and other mental health professionals with training in biobehavioral treatment strategies can often be found in children's hospitals or the child psychiatry department at local hospitals. In addition, a growing number of nurses is being trained in how to use these treatment techniques. The number of gastroenterology departments in local hospitals that use biofeedback has increased exponentially in recent years, and school-based programs have introduced these techniques to an ever-growing number of school nurses.

CONCLUSION

RAP is a common complaint in childhood that is amenable to successful treatment using a family-centered model based on research findings. Such collaborative work with a family helps the child and cements a relationship between a family and a clinician. Jointly, the health care providers involved and the family can facilitate the child's growth and development while appropriately attending to the child's pain symptom. The traumatic and expensive workup that some children with RAP experience is no longer necessary with current knowledge when used appropriately.

ACKNOWLEDGMENT

Preparation of this chapter was supported in part by a grant from the National Institutes of Health (HD38647) to Dr. Scharff.

REFERENCES

1. Apley J. *The child with abdominal pains*. Oxford: Blackwell Scientific Publications, 1975.
2. Apley J, Naish N. Recurrent abdominal pains: a field study of 1,000 schoolchildren. *Arch Dis Child* 1958;33: 165–170.
3. Faull C, Nicol AR. Abdominal pain in six year olds: an epidemiological study in a new town. *J Child Psychol Psychiatry* 1986;27:251–260.
4. Oster J. Recurrent abdominal pain, headache, and limb pains in children and adolescents. *Pediatrics* 1972;50: 429–436.
5. Zuckerman B, Stevenson J, Bailey V. Stomachaches and headaches in a community sample of preschool children. *Pediatrics* 1987;79:677–682.
6. Alfven G. The covariation of common psychosomatic symptoms among children from socio-economically differing residential areas. An epidemiological study. *Acta Paediatr* 1993;82:484–487.
7. Von Baeyer CL, Walker LS. Children with recurrent abdominal pain: issues in the selection and description of research participants. *Dev Behav Pediatr* 1999;20: 307–312.
8. Bury RG. A study of 111 children with recurrent abdominal pain. *Aust Paediatr J* 1987;24:117–119.
9. Saavedra JM, Perman JA. Current concepts in lactose malabsorption and intolerance. *Annu Rev Nutr* 1989;9: 475–592.
10. Barr RG, Levine MD, Watkins JB. Recurrent abdominal pain of childhood due to lactose intolerance. *N Engl J Med* 1979;300:1449–1452.
11. Barr RG, Francoeur TE, Westwood M, et al. Recurrent abdominal pain due to lactose intolerance revisited. *Am J Dis Child* 1986;140:302.
12. Wald A, Chandra R, Fisher SE, et al. Lactose malabsorption in recurrent abdominal pain of childhood. *J Pediatr* 1982;100:65–68.
13. Ceriani R, Zuccato E, Fontana M, et al. Lactose malabsorption and recurrent pain in Italian children. *J Pediatr Gastroenterol Nutr* 1988;7:852–857.
14. Hyams JS. Chronic abdominal pain caused by sorbitol malabsorption. *J Pediatr* 1982;100:772–773.

15. Hyams JS. Sorbitol intolerance: an unappreciated cause of functional gastrointestinal complaints. *Gastroenterology* 1983;84:30–33.
16. Wales JK, Primhak RA, Rattenbury J, et al. Isolated fructose malabsorption. *Arch Dis Child* 1990;65: 227–229.
17. Ernst PB, Gold BD. *Helicobacter pylori* in childhood: new insights into the immunopathogenesis and gastric disease and implications for managing infection in children. *J Pediatr Gastroenterol Nutr* 1999;28:462–473.
18. Coghlan JG, Gilligan D, Humphries H, et al. *Campylobacter pylori* and recurrence of duodenal ulcers—a 12-month follow-up study. *Lancet* 1987;2:1109–1111.
19. McColl K, Murray L, El-Omar E, et al. Symptomatic benefit from eradicating *Helicobacter pylori* infection in patients with nonulcer dyspepsia. *N Engl J Med* 1998;339:1869–1874.
20. Macarthur C, Saunders N, Feldman W. *Helicobacter pylori*, gastroduodenal disease, and recurrent abdominal pain in children. *JAMA* 1995;273:729–734.
21. Drumm B, Koletzko S, Oderda G. *Helicobacter pylori* infection in children: a consensus statement. *J Pediatr Gastroenterol Nutr* 2000;30:207–213.
22. Gormally J, Drumm B. *Helicobacter pylori* and gastrointestinal symptoms. *Arch Dis Child* 1994;70: 165–166.
23. Way LW. Abdominal pain. In: Sleisenger MH, Fordtran JS, eds. *Gastrointestinal disease: pathophysiology, diagnosis, management.* Philadelphia: WB Saunders, 1989:238–250.
24. Drossman DA, et al. Identification of subgroups of functional gastrointestinal disorders. *Gastroenterol Int* 1990;3:653–654.
25. Manning AP, Thompson WG, Heaton KW, et al. Towards positive diagnosis of the irritable bowel. *BMJ* 1978;2:653–654.
26. Thompson WG, et al. Irritable bowel syndrome: guidelines for diagnosis. *Gastroenterol Int* 1989;2:92–95.
27. Hyams JS, Burke G, Davis PM, et al. Abdominal pain and irritable bowel syndrome in adolescents: a community-based study. *J Pediatr* 1996;129:220–226.
28. Hyams JS, Treem WR, Justinich C, et al. Characterization of symptoms in children with recurrent abdominal pain: resemblance to irritable bowel syndrome. *J Pediatr Gastroenterol Nutr* 1995;20:209–214.
29. Burke R, Elliott M, Fleissner R. Irritable bowel syndrome and recurrent abdominal pain: a comparative review. *Psychosomatics* 1999;40:277–285.
30. Clauw DJ. The pathogenesis of chronic pain and fatigue syndromes, with special reference to fibromyalgia. *Med Hypotheses* 1995;44:369–378.
31. McGrath PJ, Feldman W. "On `Clinical approach to recurrent abdominal pain in children"': response. *J Dev Behav Pediatr* 1986;7:63.
32. Dimson SB. Transit time related to clinical findings in children with recurrent abdominal pain. *Pediatrics* 1971;47:666–674.
33. Kopel FB, Kim IC, Barbero GJ. Comparison of rectosigmoid motility in normal children, children with recurrent abdominal pain, and children with ulcerative colitis. *Pediatrics* 1967;39:539–545.
34. Camilleri M. Motor function in irritable bowel syndrome. *Can J Gastroenterol* 1999;13[Suppl A]: 8A–11A.
35. Tougas G. The autonomic nervous system in functional bowel disorders. *Can J Gastroenterol* 1999;13[Suppl A]:15A–17A.
36. Mayer EA, Gebhart GF. Basic and clinical aspects of visceral hyperalgesia. *Gastroenterology* 1995;107: 271–293.
37. Chun A, Desautels S, Slivka A, et al., Visceral algesia in irritable bowel syndrome, fibromyalgia, and sphincter of Oddi dysfunction, type III. *Dig Dis Sci* 1999;44: 631–636.
38. Rossel P, Drewes AM, Petersen P, et al. Pain produced by electric stimulation of the rectum in patients with irritable bowel syndrome: further evidence of visceral hyperalgesia. *Scand J Gastroenterol* 1999;34:1001–1006.
39. Talley NJ, et al. Functional dyspepsia: a classification with guidelines for diagnosis and management. *Gastroenterol Int* 1991;4:145–160.
40. Hyams JS. Functional gastrointestinal disorders. *Curr Opin Pediatr* 1999;11:375–378.
41. Shannon A, Martin DJ, Feldman W. Ultrasonographic studies in the management of recurrent abdominal pain. *Pediatrics* 1990;86:35–38.
42. Davison IS, Faull C, Nicol AR. Research note: temperament and behaviour in six-year-olds with recurrent abdominal pain: a follow-up. *J Child Psychol Psychiatry* 1986;27:539–544.
43. Hodges K, Kline JJ, Barbero G, et al. Anxiety in children with recurrent abdominal pain and their parents. *Psychosomatics* 1985;26:859–866.
44. Wasserman AL, Whitington PF, Rivara FP. Psychogenic basis for abdominal pain in children and adolescents. *J Am Acad Child Adolesc Psychiatry* 1988;27:179–184.
45. Hodges K, Kline JJ, Barbero G, et al. Depressive symptoms in children with recurrent abdominal pain and in their families. *J Pediatr* 1985;107:622–626.
46. Hughes MC. Recurrent abdominal pain and childhood depression: clinical observations of 23 children and their families. *Am J Orthopsychiatry* 1984;54:146–155.
47. Livingston R, Taylor JL, Crawford SL. A study of somatic complaints and psychiatric diagnosis in children. *J Am Acad Child Adolesc Psychiatry* 1988;27:185–187.
48. Kaufman K, et al. Recurrent abdominal pain in adolescents: psychosocial correlates of organic and nonorganic pain. *Child Health Care* 1997;26:15–30.
49. Walker LS, Greene JW. Children with recurrent abdominal pain and their parents: more somatic complaints, anxiety, and depression than other patient families? *J Pediatr Psychol* 1989;14:231–243.
50. Walker LS, Garber J, Greene JW. Psychosocial correlates of recurrent childhood pain: a comparison of pediatric patients with recurrent abdominal pain, organic illness, and psychiatric disorders. *J Abnorm Psychol* 1993; 102:248–258.
51. Walker LS, Zeman JL. Parental response to child illness behavior. *J Pediatr Psychol* 1992;17:49–71.
52. Robinson JO, Alverez JH, Dodge JA. Life events and family history in children with recurrent abdominal pain. *J Psychosom Res* 1990;34:171–181.
53. Rimsza ME, Berg RA. Sexual abuse: somatic and emotional reactions. *Child Abuse Neglect* 1988;12:201–208.
54. Kinzl JF, Traweger C, Biebl W. Family background and sexual abuse associated with somatization. *Psychother Psychosom* 1995;64:82–87.
55. Liebman WM. Recurrent abdominal pain in children: a retrospective survey of 119 patients. *Clin Pediatr* 1978; 17:149–153.

56. McGrath PJ, Goodman JT, Firestone P, et al. Recurrent abdominal pain: a psychogenic disorder? *Arch Dis Child* 1983;58:888–890.
57. Walker LS, Greene JW. Negative life events and symptom resolution in pediatric abdominal pain patients. *J Pediatr Psychol* 1991;16:341–360.
58. Walker LS, Garber J, Greene JW. Somatic complaints in pediatric patients: a prospective study of the role of negative life events, child social and academic competence, and parental somatic symptoms. *J Consult Clin Psychol* 1994;62:1213–1221.
59. Janicke DM, Finney JW. Empirically supported treatments in pediatric psychology: recurrent abdominal pain. *J Pediatr Psychol* 1999;24:115–127.
60. Miller AJ, Kratochwill TR. Reduction of frequent stomach complaints by time out. *Behav Ther* 1979;10:211–218.
61. Sank LI, Biglan A. Operant treatment of a case of recurrent abdominal pain in a 10-year-old boy. *Behav Ther* 1974;5:677–681.
62. Wasserman T. The elimination of complaints of stomach cramps in a 12-year-old child by covert positive reinforcement. *Behav Ther* 1978;1:13–14.
63. Finney JW, et al. Pediatric psychology in primary health care: brief targeted therapy for recurrent abdominal pain. *Behav Ther* 1989;20:283–291.
64. Sanders MR, Rebgetz M, Morrison M, et al. Cognitive-behavioral treatment of recurrent nonspecific abdominal pain in children: an analysis of generalization, maintenance, and side effects. *J Consult Clin Psychol* 1989; 57:294–300.
65. Sanders MR, Shepherd RW, Cleghorn G, et al. The treatment of recurrent abdominal pain in children: a controlled comparison of cognitive-behavioral family intervention and standard pediatric care. *J Consult Clin Psychol* 1994;62:306–314.

41
Chest Pain

Maureen Strafford

Chest pain is a well-respected symptom, ominous in its implications for serious cardiac disease for both the lay public and medical personnel. Chest pain is a common complaint responsible for urgent medical evaluation in adults. However, patients between 10 and 21 years of age also account for 650,000 annual physician visits, representing 0.25% to 0.30% of pediatric patient visits (1,2). Chest pain is the second most common cause of referral to a pediatric cardiologist and the seventh most common health problem reported among urban African-American adolescents (3). Although it should be reassuring that chest pain is more common in healthy children than in children with cardiac disease; nevertheless, chest pain often prompts urgent medical attention and creates anxiety for patient and family. Chest pain results in physical distress, anxiety, sleep disturbances, school absences, and extensive utilization of medical resources for the pediatric patient. As with any complaint of pain, the cause of the symptom must be clarified and treated appropriately.

However, the complaint of chest pain may be acute, semiacute, or chronic, and, therefore, the evaluation may be urgent, extensive, and/or prolonged and may involve multiple subspecialists. The pediatric patient with chest pain may present to a primary care family practitioner or pediatrician, an emergency department physician, cardiologist, or gastroenterologist. Therefore, the approach to diagnosis, management, and treatment may vary, and often guidelines for assessment and treatment are lacking. Because a definitive cause may remain elusive or be defined as idiopathic, anxiety and dysfunction, both physical and psychologic, may unnecessarily persist for the patient and family.

This chapter reviews the various causes of chest pain in the pediatric patient and discusses the literature on this topic that has resulted in the general recommendation that the pediatric patient with chest pain usually has a benign, self-limited condition that should be treated conservatively in terms of diagnostic evaluation, treatment, and follow-up.

GENERAL CONSIDERATIONS

Because chest pain may be caused by disease or abnormalities in a variety of organ systems, it is helpful to review briefly the anatomy of this area and the multiple systems that may refer pain to the chest area. Pain may originate from somatic structures (muscles, ligaments, fascia, spine) or visceral structures in the thorax and/or abdomen. Because the afferent nerves of the heart, aorta, esophagus, lungs, and upper chest wall all share a common pathway in the spinal cord, it is not surprising that many different lesions from a variety of locations may cause chest pain with the same quality.

The thoracic surface from the neck to xiphoid process and along the anteromedial aspects of the arms is covered by dermatomes T1 to T6. The thoracic viscera, which include the myocardium, pericardium, great vessels, esophagus, and mediastinum, receive sensory innervation from T1 to T4 fibers. Therefore, pain from these organs produces a similar sensation of deep, poorly localized retrosternal or pericardial pain.

Fibers from T5 and T6 are responsible for sensory innervation of the lower thoracic wall, diaphragmatic muscles, peritoneal surfaces, gallbladder, pancreas, duodenum, and stomach. Abnormalities in these organs can result in deep, poorly localized pain in the xiphoid area, back, or infrascapular region on the right side.

EVALUATION OF THE PEDIATRIC PATIENT WITH CHEST PAIN

As with any complaint of pain, a thorough history, including family history, and physical examination are required.

History

Chest pain occurs in children of all ages, although the typical patient is a preadolescent or adolescent (mean age, 11.9 years), but it has been described as a complaint in a 2-year-old child. Approximately 50% of patients are younger than 12 years of age, and the cause in this group is more likely to have a cardiac or pulmonary origin, whereas the older adolescent patient is more likely to have a psychogenic cause (4,5). In addition to a routine medical history, including a comprehensive review of systems, the patient with chest pain needs careful attention paid to the description of the pain. The most common narrative is the complaint of sharp, midsternal pain without radiation lasting less than 15 minutes but usually occurring more than once a day. In various studies, 7% to 36% of patients have a chronic complaint of chest pain lasting longer than 6 months (2,5–7). It is often helpful to permit the child, even a young child, to describe in his/her own words the nature and quality of the pain. Parental observations are important but should be elicited after the child has the opportunity to describe the pain. The temporal nature of the chest pain is important and should include time of onset, number of episodes, frequency, and duration. The location and radiation as well as associated activities (e.g., eating, physical exertion, trauma, foreign body ingestion, use of cigarettes and/or drugs) should be noted. Pain that awakens a child from sleep, causes him or her to miss school or desirable social activities, or is associated with systemic symptoms (e.g., fever, cough, dizziness, palpitations, vomiting) are important historic facts to obtain. A thorough history of past evaluations, treatments, and diagnoses in the patient who has had recurrent chest pain can be helpful. In one study, 15% of patients had visited an emergency department more than once (5).

A family history should not only include attention to cardiac disease but also questioning about chest pain and recent family cardiac illness and/or death of family member or even family friend. Screening practices to detect cardiovascular disease in college-age athletes have been reviewed and were described as inadequate on 40% of intake history forms, including the recording of a history of chest pain, in the questionnaires reviewed from the National Collegiate Athletic Association members (8). Finally, asking the young patient and his or her family members about their fears and concerns regarding the symptom of chest pain is often revealing and extremely helpful when a treatment plan is being formulated.

Physical Examination

Because there is an association between an abnormal physical examination in children with chest pain and the presence of organic disease (4), the importance of a thorough physical examination cannot be minimized.

Patients anxiously expect immediate and detailed attention paid to the cardiac examination because of the feared association of chest pain with serious cardiac disease. It is beneficial to be thorough but not abnormally focused initially on the cardiac examination. Obviously, initial assessment includes the degree of acute distress present. Review of vital signs and the general "wellness" of the patient is important. Initial inspection should rule out generalized evidence of trauma and/or bruising, skin infections, or evidence of chronic, possible multisystem disease.

Careful examination of the chest should include inspection, palpation, percussion, and auscultation. Inspection of the chest wall should rule out asymmetry, abnormal respiratory pattern, and abnormal breast enlargement or gynecomastia in males. Palpation may reveal abnormal cardiac impulse, localized swelling or tenderness, breast enlargement and/or tenderness, and fremitus or subcutaneous air. Percussion may also localize an area of pain or reveal underlying pulmonary disease.

Finally, auscultation should be thorough and complete. The cardiac auscultatory examination should search for dysrhythmias, murmurs, and/or clicks, which often may be elicited only with a change in posture or position. Auscultation of the lungs should obviously examine all areas for the possibility of infection, asthma, effusions, or consolidation. The remainder of the physical examination should be equally thorough. Abdominal pathology may result in referred pain to the chest. The presence of abnormal physical findings in other areas of the body may point to a multisystem problem, of which chest pain is one symptom. In general, studies of chest pain in children have supported the finding that an abnormal physical finding is more likely to be associated with organic disease (2).

Studies of children with chest pain are not numerous, but some observations and recommendations regarding diagnosis, evaluation, and treatment can be made from the studies over the past two decades. Before discussing the findings of these retrospective and prospective studies, it is helpful to review the most common causes of chest pain in children.

CARDIAC CAUSES OF CHEST PAIN

Cardiac causes are not the most common causes of chest pain in children but are the most common causes of concern for patients, families, and occasionally physicians. Therefore, it is worthwhile to review the rare but possible causes of heart disease responsible for chest pain in pediatric patients.

Patients and families may be unduly alarmed about the possible association of serious cardiac disease in an otherwise healthy child with chest pain. Similarly, the physician evaluating a child with chest pain may be concerned that previously unrecognized cardiac disease is the cause of chest pain. An extremely rare but frightening presentation of unrecognized heart disease is sudden, unexpected death in an otherwise healthy individual. However, media attention to the rare event of sudden death from unrecognized cardiac disease in an active, successful athlete does create fear for young adolescents and families.

Therefore, the physician may believe that extensive laboratory evaluation and/or referral to a cardiologist is the best form of reassurance for all concerned (9). However, chest pain has not been found to be a common premorbid complaint in studies examining sudden death in young patients. Lambert et al. (10) reported on eight patients with sudden death who had previously unrecognized heart disease (four had myocarditis, three had hypertrophic obstructive disease, and one had left coronary artery calcification). Twenty-nine athletes who died suddenly and unexpectedly had postmortem examinations that noted an identifiable cardiac structural abnormality in 28 patients (11). However, only seven patients had suspected cardiac disease and only two patients had complained of chest pain that was not evaluated. Six of these seven patients had abnormal electrocardiograms with evidence of left ventricular hypertrophy. Syncope, extreme light-headedness, dizziness, or a positive family history of sudden death in young adults are all more worrisome historic facts to take note of.

Certainly when an abnormal cardiac murmur, dysrhythmia, or other abnormal finding is noted, appropriate evaluation and referral are needed. In general, it should be reassuring to physicians that the cardiac causes of chest pain in children are not numerous and can usually be ruled out after careful history and physical examination.

Cardiac pain is a result of coronary artery ischemia (from an imbalance of myocardial oxygen supply and demand) or from irritation of the pericardial and pleural serosa. Patients with structural abnormalities, acquired heart disease such as myocarditis or pericarditis, and dysrhythmia may all experience chest pain under particular conditions.

Structural Abnormalities

Before discussing those specific structural lesions that may lead to an imbalance of myocardial oxygen supply and demand, children with previously diagnosed congenital heart disease should be discussed. It is rare to see chest pain in children with cardiac disease. Children with severe left ventricular outflow tract obstruction (discussed below) or pulmonary vascular obstructive disease (Eisenmenger complex) and cyanotic congenital heart disease from a variety of causes may all be at greater risk of ischemia because of their underlying pathophysiology. However, although these lesions also represent a group at high risk of sudden death, reviews have not shown chest pain to be a common preterminal symptom or a predictor of sudden death in patients with recognized heart disease.

Fyfe and Moodie (12) reviewed 57 patients with idiopathic chest pain in a review of 67 patients presenting for evaluation of chest pain in a pediatric cardiac clinic. Twenty of these 57 children were also found to have a cardiac lesion, but a causal relationship between the symptom of chest pain and the underlying defect could not be made.

Chest pain will be a symptom of cardiac dysfunction in patients with only a few specific structural abnormalities of the heart and often only under particular physiologic conditions. These abnormalities include lesions resulting in left ventricular outflow tract obstruction, mitral valve prolapse (MVP), and coronary artery anomalies.

Left Ventricular Outflow Tract Obstruction

Obstruction to left ventricular output can result in an increase in myocardial oxygen demands, especially during exercise or tachycardia. Lesions such as aortic stenosis at the subvalvar, valvar, or supravalvar level are associated with chest pain and/or dysrhythmias under particular physiologic conditions. Hypertrophic obstructive cardiomyopathy is an additional cause of left ventricular outflow tract obstruction. Because of the autosomal dominant inheritance seen with this lesion, a thorough family history is helpful.

The patient with any of these lesions should have distinctive physical findings. In addition, it should be reassuring that mild degrees of left ventricular outflow tract obstruction, no matter what the anatomic reason, should not be associated with ischemic chest pain.

The murmur of aortic obstruction is usually a harsh ejection murmur (grade II or higher) heard best in the aortic area (right upper sternal border) with radiation to the carotids. A thrill may be palpated.

Hypertrophic obstructive cardiomyopathy or idiopathic hypertrophic subaortic stenosis may have a more variable murmur because it is a dynamic condition and the murmur will vary with the degree of left ventricular filling (i.e., the "fuller" the left ventricle, the less intense the murmur). Therefore, increased afterload (supine position, squatting, isometric exercise) will decrease the degree of dynamic obstruction and decrease the murmur. When left ventricle filling is impeded, such as during a Valsalva maneuver or by standing, the murmur will increase in intensity. The finding of a murmur suggestive of left ventricular outflow tract obstruction should result in referral to a cardiologist to define the level and degree of obstruction.

Mitral Valve Prolapse

Recent attention has been made to the association between MVP and chest pain. Since the first description in 1963 by Barlow et al. (13) and especially since the advent of echocardiographic technology, MVP has been increasingly diagnosed. Studies in children have shown the incidence to vary from 1.2% to 35% (14–16), depending on the method of diagnosis (auscultation and/or echocardiography) or the age group examined. Overall, there is probably an incidence of MVP in less than 5% of the pediatric population.

Vague, usually nonexertional chest pain has been described in children with MVP. A study in 119 children with MVP showed that only 18% of children presented with chest pain (17). Most patients were asymptomatic and had been referred for cardiac evaluation because a murmur or click had been detected, especially during a febrile illness.

Chest pain in patients with MVP probably results from papillary muscle dysfunction and subendocardial ischemia. Angina-type chest pain is less common in these patients; pain is usually described as vague and nonexertional discomfort. In a Polish study of 67 children referred for evaluation of MVP, 31% complained of chest pain, but often more than one symptom was present including palpitations, fatigue, and dyspnea (18). The association of MVP and anxiety symptoms may be overestimated. A study was done in which 19 patients with known MVP from a cardiology practice who complained of chest pain were compared with patients with chest pain but no known cardiac disorder. The MVP group did not show any increase in panic disorder or anxiety compared with the patients with chest pain alone (19). The association of MVP with dysrhythmias is well known and may contribute to symptoms of chest pain. Ventricular ectopy has been described in children with MVP with an incidence as high as 50% (10). Serious ventricular dysrhythmias have been described in 19% of children with MVP who underwent a treadmill exercise test (20). However, there is no clear association between symptoms of chest pain and/or palpitations and dysrhythmias detected on Holter monitoring or during exercise testing. Although sudden death has been described in patients with MVP, probably based on a serious dysrhythmia or embolic phenomenon, sudden death is extremely rare in children with MVP.

MVP is usually detected when a midsystolic click and/or late systolic murmur is heard. Because there are significant changes in the quality of the click and/or murmur with changes in posture and position, it is important to perform a careful and thorough physical examination and to understand the effects of a variety of maneuvers on the physical findings.

A maneuver that will increase left ventricular volume will result in a decrease in MVP and therefore a decrease in the murmur of mitral regurgitation. On auscultation, this results in a shorter murmur and the click moving closer to the second heart sound. Therefore, changing the patient from the sitting to supine position or from standing to squatting, passive leg raising or isometric exercise are all maneuvers that result in a decrease in the murmur's intensity.

Decreasing left ventricular size and volume will result in an increase in prolapse and regurgitation and therefore a louder murmur. Maneuvers such as changing from sitting to standing, squatting to standing, inspiration, and Valsalva maneuver will all result in more mitral regurgitation and a louder murmur.

The murmur of idiopathic hypertrophic subaortic stenosis as reviewed above also changes with these maneuvers. In both conditions, a careful physical examination must include these maneuvers or the murmur and/or click may be missed.

In addition to abnormalities on cardiac examination, it may be observed that children with MVP often have a characteristic tall, slender habitus; pectus carinatum and pectus excavatum and scoliosis and kyphosis have also all been described in this group of patients. Patients with Marfan syndrome and other mesenchymal dysplastic syndromes such as Ehlers–Danlos and von Willebrand have a well-recognized incidence of MVP.

Noncardiac causes of chest pain in children and adolescents with MVP have been reviewed and should be considered in an evaluation of any patient with chest pain and MVP. In one study, 17 patients with MVP and chest pain underwent comprehensive gastrointestinal evaluation. Evaluation consisted of esophageal manometry, Bernstein test, esophageal pH probe, and esophagogastroscopy. Fourteen of the 17 patients had at least one abnormal finding. Resolution of chest pain followed appropriate treatment for the gastrointestinal condition that was detected (21). A patient with MVP with chest pain may need to have other conditions considered during an evaluation and not a quick assumption that chest pain is part of the mitral valve clinical constellation.

Coronary Artery Anomalies

Because chest pain can result from myocardial ischemia, abnormalities in coronary arteries are a rare but possible cause of cardiac-derived chest pain. Anomalous origin of the left coronary artery from the pulmonary artery, coronary artery fistulae, and an abnormal course of the left coronary from the anterior sinus of Valsalva between the aorta and pulmonary artery (potentially resulting in compression during high output states such as exercise) are all unusual but well-described causes of true angina in young patients. Left coronary ostial stenosis and atresia and anomalies of the right coronary artery have also been described. All these anomalies, although rare, result in myocardial ischemia, typically during exercise or other periods of high output. The chest pain observed in these situations is often identical in description and radiation to the anginal pain observed in adults with coronary artery disease. Chest pain in these patients often is associated with exercise, cold, stress, and anxiety.

Patients with these rare lesions may have a totally normal physical examination. However, murmurs may be present and are a result of continuous flow through a fistula, mitral regurgitation from papillary muscle dysfunction, or gallops from myocardial dysfunction. The history of pain during exercise or stress is often an important clue in these patients.

Acquired Myocardial Disease

Acquired myocardial disease represents a subgroup of cardiac causes of chest pain, often associated with acute symptoms. Pericarditis, myocarditis, coronary arteritis (Kawasaki disease), and acute pulmonary processes with pleural/pericardial irritation may all cause chest pain. Pericarditis may be seen in a variety of processes: viral and bacterial infection, rheumatic, and autoimmune (including post-cardiac surgery, known as postcardiotomy syndrome). Acute blunt chest trauma may result in a posttraumatic pericardial effusion, and symptoms may not appear for weeks or months after trauma.

Myocarditis may present acutely with chest pain or later as a result of deteriorating myocardial function and ischemia, especially during exercise.

Kawasaki disease is an acute febrile syndrome of unknown origin, most commonly seen in children (especially of Japanese descent) younger than 4 years of age. Although 50% of patients will have dilation of the coronary arteries owing to vasculitis, only 15% of patients will have persistent arterial aneurysms after the acute phase (22). However, these patients with persistent coronary artery aneurysms are at increased risk of thromboembolic events and myocardial infarction. Chest pain may be a symptom of myocardial infarction in older children, but asymptomatic acute myocardial infarction has been described in 37% of patients with persistent aneurysms. In a retrospective study of patients with Kawasaki disease with cardiac sequelae, 61% had chest pain and myocardial infarction as presenting symptoms (23).

Dysrhythmias

If a dysrhythmia alters cardiac output or coronary artery perfusion, then chest pain may result. Usually the alteration in coronary perfusion seen with a dysrhythmia must be sustained before causing symptoms, especially in a patient with normal cardiac function. It is important to differentiate true ischemic pain from discomfort caused by the sensation of a dysrhythmia, i.e., palpitations or a "skipped beat" sensation. These unusual sensations can predispose the patient to additional anxiety and hyperventilation can often result.

Because of the feared association of chest pain with cardiac disease, the patient and family need reassurance that the child has a healthy heart and that most chest pain in pediatric patients is benign and self-limited in nature. In fact, in most healthy children with chest pain, no organic cause will be found. Before discussing idiopathic chest pain and reviewing the studies examining chest pain in pediatrics, it is helpful to review other noncardiac causes of chest pain. These include musculoskeletal, pulmonary, gastrointestinal, and psychogenic causes.

MUSCULOSKELETAL CAUSES OF CHEST PAIN

Musculoskeletal causes of chest pain are common in pediatric patients, representing approximately 30% of cases (4,5). Chest pain of musculoskeletal origin has particular characteristics. Pain is usually insidious, often sharp, nagging, and localized, although radiation is not uncommon. Repetitive trauma or unusual physical activity usually precedes the onset of the pain. There are several well-defined syndromes responsible for chest pain from musculoskeletal sources, and the most common ones seen clinically are the following.

Costochondritis. Chest pain owing to costochondritis may be mild to severe, localized, and reproducible with palpation, coughing, and movement of the tender area. A history of a recent upper respiratory infection is often obtained.

Trauma, muscle spasm, or overuse. In healthy, active athletes, various painful conditions may cause chest pain. Muscle tears and/or spasms are not infrequent in weight lifters. Direct trauma may result from active contact sports, but stress fractures may also be seen in tennis or sports such as baseball or basketball in which repetitive throwing actions occur and may cause overuse pain or spasm. Blunt trauma such as seen in child abuse should also be considered, especially in a younger child with chest pain.

Precordial catch or Texidor twinge. This benign condition clinically presents as characteristic chest pain in an otherwise healthy child. Precordial catch syndrome pain is typically sudden, brief, periapical, easily localized, nonradiating, nonexertional, and, importantly, intensified by inspiration (24). Because of the severity with deep inspiration, the patient will often begin to breathe shallowly and rapidly. The frequency varies from once a day to only occasionally. The cause is unclear.

Tietze syndrome. This clinical syndrome is observed after minor trauma. The pain is usually localized, moderate, and associated with visible swelling. The swelling is helpful in differentiating this syndrome from costochondritis. The swelling may remit and recur over months or years and may be seen with an elevated erythrocyte sedimentation rate.

Slipping rib syndrome. When the tip of the eighth, ninth, or tenth rib overrides the rib above, chest pain can often result. The onset is sudden and aching and may radiate to chest or abdomen. Bending over, deep breathing, and arm hyperextension may reproduce the pain. "Hooking" the affected costal margin and pulling anteriorly usually reproduces the pain also. The diagnosis of slipping rib syndrome can be made on physical examination alone, and more costly and invasive evaluations can be avoided (25). Occasionally surgical resection of the affected rib is required to alleviate symptoms.

Xiphoid cartilage syndrome. This painful condition involving the xiphoid is more common in adults. Occasionally, after vigorous running, children will report a "stitch" or pain at the insertion of the xiphoid into the abdominal musculature. Pressure on the xiphoid process may spontaneously reproduce the pain.

Herpes zoster. Although rare in children, the intense pain of this intercostal neuralgia can be seen days preceding the diagnostic appearance of vesicles. Although postherpetic neuralgia is less common in pediatric patients, early acyclovir therapy and sympathetic block have an important role in the treatment of the intense pain usually seen with herpes zoster and the possible prevention of the development of postherpetic neuralgia.

Fibromyalgia and other myofascial pain syndromes. Also known as fibrositis or diffuse myofascial pain syndrome, generalized muscle pain that involves the chest can be seen with these syndromes. The cause is unknown. Children are less commonly affected than adults. Pain is usually continuous and lasts longer than 3 months. Tenderness can be elicited on palpation over multiple points. Anterior chest pain associated with local tenderness may represent a type of myofascial pain. Trigger points can be present, especially involving the pectoralis, scaleni, sternalis, and intercostal muscles. Similar myofascial pain syndromes may involve lateral chest wall musculature such as the anterior serratus and intercostals. Treatment has included heat, massage, low-dose amitriptyline, injection of local anesthetic into trigger point areas, and/or sympathetic blocks.

Other musculoskeletal causes. Other less common causes of chest pain include tumor or connective tissue disorders. Patients with sickle cell anemia or cystic fibrosis may also present with acute chest pain during exacerbations of their diseases. Chronic pain is a common problem in patients with cystic fibrosis, seen especially in aging patients with cystic fibrosis (26). Patients with cystic fibrosis may complain of chest pain as a result of chest wall muscle fatigue after prolonged episodes of coughing. Although other diagnoses, including pneumothorax, should be considered, chest pain in patients with cystic fibrosis may also be owing to rib fractures. Patients with negative rib films for fractures have been found to have positive bone scans, indicating multiple rib fractures. Improved pulmonary toilet can be achieved with the use of epidural analgesia in these patients with rib fractures and severe chest pain.

Patients with sickle cell anemia may present with acute chest pain as a manifestation of their vaso-occlusive disease (see Chapter 28).

A discussion of chest wall and musculoskeletal causes of chest pain should include the breasts as a potential cause of pain. In females, puberty, menstruation, pregnancy, and mastitis may all be associated with the symptom of chest pain. In males, concerns regarding gynecomastia, especially in the adolescent male, raise anxiety and attention to this condition.

PULMONARY CAUSES OF CHEST PAIN

Respiratory disorders may account for 2% to 21% of cases of chest pain in children (4,5,7). When acute chest pain is present, especially with fever, cough, or other systemic symptoms, an acute pulmonary process should obviously be considered. Chronic diseases such as cystic fibrosis, sickle cell anemia, and asthma may all be associated with chest pain from underlying pulmonary disease as well as musculoskeletal reasons (see previous discussion). Other less common conditions that may present with chest pain include foreign body aspiration, pneumothorax, chemical pneumonitis, diaphragmatic irritation from intraabdominal pathology, Mediterranean fever, and acute pulmonary embolism, which should be considered in the adolescent female who may be using oral contraceptives. Exercise-induced asthma with chest pain as the primary complaint has been studied and should be considered. In a study of 147 children with chest pain with exercise with normal cardiovascular examinations, maximal exercise tests helped confirm exercise-induced asthma in 10% (14 patients) (27). Another study examining pulmonary function testing with exercise in children with chest pain revealed a higher incidence of exercise-induced asthma than previously reported. In this study, 72.7% had evidence of exercise-induced asthma and inhaled albuterol resulted in a subjective improvement in 97% and objective improvement in 70% of patients (28).

GASTROINTESTINAL CAUSES OF CHEST PAIN

The abdominal organs and esophagus are major sources of referred pain to the chest. Visceral pain is usually deep, difficult to localize or reproduce, and radiates away from the source of pathology. Esophageal disease may cause retrosternal or epigastric pain, whereas intra-abdominal pathology may be substernal or epigastric.

Causes of chest pain owing to esophageal disorders include esophagitis and reflux, foreign body ingestion, achalasia, hiatal hernia, esophageal spasm, and gastric distension especially during hyperventilation. Unusual causes of esophagitis in children include medication-induced esophagitis. A report describing esophageal ulcers in children after ingestion of antibiotic capsules documented chest pain as a common presenting symptom (29).

Berezin et al. (30) used the intraesophageal acid perfusion (Bernstein) test as a provocative test in 60 children with chest pain. None of these patients had any other symptom of esophagitis. Of these 60 patients, 45 were shown to have esophagitis, and symptoms were reproducible in 18 patients during the test. Another study, Berezin et al. (31) investigated 27 children with idiopathic chest pain. In 21 of the 27 children (78%), a gastrointestinal cause of the chest pain was found. These included esophagitis (16 patients), gastritis (four patients), and esophageal spasm (one patient). All patients responded to appropriate therapy for these conditions, and chest pain disappeared. These studies raise an interesting question: Do many children with idiopathic chest pain have undiagnosed gastrointestinal pathology? A study of 83 children with chest pain who were referred for esophageal manometry and esophagogastroscopy showed that 57% had both normal esophageal histology and normal motility. Thirteen patients had dysmotility by either diffuse esophageal spasm or achalasia. Fifteen patients had esophagitis alone. Eight patients had both esophagitis and motility problems. Patients with esophagitis responded to therapy, but those with dysmotility were relatively refractory to therapy. Many of these gastrointestinal conditions may resolve over time, even without treatment, similar to the resolution of symptoms often seen in patients with idiopathic chest pain. In addition, the use of nonsteroidal anti-inflammatory drugs, which are often prescribed in patients with idiopathic chest pain, may aggravate, exacerbate, or cause persistent symptoms if unrecognized gastrointestinal pathology is the cause of the chest pain (32). Finally, the coexistence of gastrointestinal pathology in patients with asthma has also been examined. Rather than attributing chest pain to asthma alone, further examination of the gastrointestinal system can be revealing in some patients. Sixteen patients with asthma and chest pain for more than 2 months were studied using esophagogastroduodenoscopy, esophageal manometry, and Bernstein testing. Eleven of the 16 patients (75%) had evidence of esophagitis.

Seven patients had gastroesophageal reflux. Chest pain was associated with an episode of gastroesophageal reflux in all these patients. Chest pain and esophagitis resolved in 82% of patients after medical treatment. The coexistence of these two different reasons for chest pain may be less common but should certainly be considered in patients with prolonged symptoms. Treatment can be effective (33).

PSYCHOGENIC CAUSES OF CHEST PAIN

When an organic cause for chest pain cannot be found, it is practice to label this condition as idiopathic chest pain. This diagnosis should not imply that psychogenic issues are the basis for the pain. In fact, psychogenic pain is real pain and associated dysfunction, including missed school time and family dysfunction, is commonly seen. In addition, patients with organic disease causing chest pain such as cystic fibrosis or asthma may have a component of psychogenic pain when they complain of chest pain.

Hyperventilation syndrome is the most common manifestation of psychogenic chest pain. Often, hyperventilation is not recognized, especially if the patient is not seen during an acute episode. Hyperventilation syndrome may also be a cause of chronic chest pain. Herman et al. (34) reviewed records of

34 hyperventilating children and found that at follow-up 40% still had evidence of hyperventilation syndrome as adults, often with the addition of other somatic symptoms of chronic anxiety.

Globus hystericus may present as substernal pain or discomfort, suggestive of esophageal disease. An invasive gastrointestinal workup may delay the diagnosis of severe anxiety and/or depression that underlies this complaint.

Reviews of children with chest pain have found a range of incidence with respect to psychogenic causes. Kashani et al. (35) reported on 100 children who attended a pediatric cardiology clinic. Four of the 100 patients presented with chest pain. All four met criteria for major depression disorder (according to the *DSM-III*). However, Driscoll et al. (36) reviewed 40 children with chest pain (45% with idiopathic chest pain) and found none to have a psychogenic cause for the chest pain. Asnes et al. (37) reviewed 123 children who presented with chest pain and found that 29% had psychogenic causes for chest pain. A careful history of family members or friends with chest pain, cardiac disease, or recent deaths is critically important. Asnes et al. noted a family history of chest pain in 47% and a history of recurrent somatic complaints other than chest pain in 56%.

A retrospective review of chest pain in young adults was designed to assess the relationships between chest pain, psychiatric disorders, and early experiences of ill health used data from the Medical Research Council National Survey of Health and Development in the United Kingdom. Chest pain (especially exertional chest pain) is strongly associated with psychiatric disorders in young adults. Childhood experiences, including illness in parents, are associated with subsequent chest pain complaints (38).

OTHER CAUSES OF CHEST PAIN

Although less common, there are interesting reports of chest pain in adolescents and young adults who ingested cocaine (39,40), marijuana or ephedrine (41), and overdoses of caffeine (42) or accidentally ingested or inhaled mercury vapor (43) and trichloroethane aerosol (44). In addition, Friedman et al. (45) studied a large group of adolescents and adults and found cigarette smoking to be associated with chest pain. A history of either active or passive smoking is often not obtained in a pediatric history. An unusual complication of syrup of ipecac emesis has been pneumomediastinum and retropneumoperitoneum presenting with chest pain after the use of ipecac hours earlier (46). Chest epilepsy and spinal cord meningioma have been described as very unusual causes of chest pain (47,48). Patients with anorexia nervosa may complain of chest pain. In a pain survey of 54 patients with anorexia nervosa, 87% reported a complaint of chest pain, and 38% of these patients were diagnosed as idiopathic chest pain (49).

TREATMENT AND FOLLOW-UP OF THE PEDIATRIC PATIENT WITH CHEST PAIN

A discussion of chest pain in children must include recommendations for treatment and follow-up. There is limited literature on pediatric patients with chest pain. However, it is helpful to review both the prospective, retrospective, and follow-up studies that have examined chest pain in children. From these studies, recommendations can be made regarding evaluation, treatment, and follow-up. When an organic cause can be found, treatment is fairly straightforward: treat the underlying problem, e.g., the pneumonia or costochondritis. However, a review of the studies in the literature will reveal that idiopathic chest pain remains the most common "cause" of chest pain in pediatric patients. In this group of patients, treatment and follow-up may be poorly defined, and patients often feel frustrated with recommendations and the slow resolution of symptoms. This approach may be, in part, responsible for the multiple evaluations that some patients with idiopathic chest pain continually seek out.

PROSPECTIVE STUDIES

Since 1976, six prospective studies have examined chest pain in children (Table 41.1). Although these studies vary in clinical settings, patient demographics, and results, some common observations are made and are worth reviewing. Driscoll et al. (36) reviewed all patients seen over a 9-week period in the outpatient department, emergency department, or cardiac clinic with a primary complaint of chest pain. Forty-three patients were identified (0.288% occurrence rate). Three patients refused inclusion in the study. The gender distribution was 22 boys and 18 girls (average age, 12 years; range, 5 to 19 years). The most common diagnoses represented were idiopathic (45%), costochondritis (22.5%), muscle strain/chest trauma (10%), and coughing and bronchitis (12.5%). Of note, no cases of psychogenic chest pain were described. When chest pain had been present for less than 6 months, a cause could be defined in 65% of these patients. In contrast, chronic chest pain of longer than 6 months' duration was more likely to be idiopathic; only 33% of patients with chronic chest pain had an identifiable cause of the pain.

TABLE 41.1. *Prospective studies of chest pain in pediatric patients*

Study	Clinical setting	Patient demographics	Cause	Additional observations
Driscoll et al. (36)	Outpatient, ED, cardiac clinic over 9-wk period	*N*=43 (3 refused inclusion);22 boys/18 girls; mean age, 12 yr; range, 5–19 yr	Idiopathic (45%) Costochondritis (22.5%) Muscle strain/trauma (10%) Cough/bronchitis (12.5%)	No psychogenic cause; 18/41 positive family history of CP, but did not predict diagnosis; 4/13 with idiopathic CP had resolution of symptoms; 14/17 resolved symptoms when CP owing to other causes; 14/31 interviewed by psychiatrist perceived psychologic problems; 52% interpreted CP to be owing to cardiac disease; chronic CP (>6 mo) more likely to be idiopathic
Pantell and Goodman (5)	Adolescent clinic, 1-yr period	*N*=100; 37 boys/63 girls; mean age, 16.4 yr; 91 blacks	Idiopathic (39%) Musculoskeletal (31%) Hyperventilation (20%) 46 pts had single specific cause; 11 had multiple causes	Chronic, stable CP most common presentation; 41% missed school; 69% restricted physical activity; hyperventilation commonly seen when multiple causes; adverse life events, 31%
Labibidi and Wankum (50)	Pediatric cardiac clinic	*N*=98; 36/98 had idiopathic CP; 56% girls (9–19 yr); mean, 12 yr; 44% boys (10–18 yr); mean, 13 yr	Idiopathic (37%)	Study examined pts with idiopathic CP; 83% felt pain owing to cardiac disease; 100% of pts expressed "great concern" over CP; extensive cardiac evaluation, including CXR, ECG, echocardiogram, and stress test; 1-mo and 2-yr follow-up reported 97% of pts had symptom resolution
Selbst et al. (4)	Urban pediatric ED, 1-yr period	*N*=407; 55% girls/90% black; mean age, 11.9 yr; range, 2–18.9 yr	Idiopathic (21%) Musculoskeletal (15%) Cough (10%) Asthma/pneumonia (11%) Costochondritis (9%) Gastrointestinal disorders (4%) Cardiac (4%)	Younger children more likely to have organic cause; nonorganic disease more common in chronic CP (>6 mo); psychogenic pain more likely if positive family history of chest pain; 31% had disturbed sleep; 30% reported school absence
Rowe et al. (51)	Urban pediatric ED, 1-yr period	*N*=336 (325 completed questionnaire); M/F, 1.0; mean age, 11.6 yr; range, 2–28 yr	Chest wall (28%) Pulmonary (19%) Traumatic (15%) Idiopathic (12%) Psychogenic (5%)	27% reported school absence; physical examination notable for chest wall tenderness in 41%; lab: CXR and ECG not extremely helpful
Evangelista et al. (52)	Pediatric cardiac clinic	*N*=50; mean age, 13 yr; range, 5–21 yr	Musculoskeletal (76%) Exercise-induced asthma (12%) Gastrointestinal disorders (8%) Psychogenic (4%) Cardiac (0%)	Systematic history; physical examination, ECG excluded cardiac disorders

ED, emergency department; CP, chest pain; pts, patients; CXR, chest x-ray; ECG, electrocardiogram

The description of the chest pain varied, but the largest group with idiopathic chest pain had more chronic symptoms. Most children described the pain as sharp, but dull, pressing, and pounding were also common descriptors. Eighteen of 41 children related a memory of a relative or acquaintance with cardiac-related chest pain. However, there was no clear relationship between diagnostic category and a positive family history of heart or lung disease. Of interest, only four of 13 patients (31%) with idiopathic chest pain had resolution of symptoms on follow-up compared with 14 of 17 (82%) in other diagnostic categories.

Thirty-one of the 40 children had an interview by a psychiatrist who was unaware of the patient's diagnosis. Fourteen of these patients had abnormal psychologic findings and one required hospitalization. Fourteen of 31 children perceived problems in their environment, either home or school. Fifty-two percent of patients and family members thought that the chest pain was related to cardiac disease at the time of presentation.

Pantell and Goodman (5) prospectively studied 100 adolescents seen in an adolescent clinic with a primary or secondary complaint of chest pain. This was a not an emergency department setting, and therefore these patients were generally not acutely ill. Ninety-one percent of the study population was black, and 63% were female (average age, 16.4 years). These demographic findings were similar to the clinic population in general. Most patients (64%) had chest pain for 6 months or less and had experienced more than six episodes. The character of the pain was described as sharp, nonradiating, felt over the left precordium or substernal area, and lasting less than 1 hour. Sixty-nine percent of patients had restricted activity, and 41% missed school because of the pain. A family history for cardiac or lung disease was positive in 57%.

The cause of the chest pain was determined in 46 patients; 11 had multiple causes. The most common causes noted were idiopathic (39%), musculoskeletal (31%), and hyperventilation syndrome (20%). Psychologic issues were reviewed; 31% reported significant negative life events within 6 months; 26% within 3 months. Twelve core family members were recently hospitalized for serious illness, and four had had heart attacks (one fatal). However, significant life events were reported equally in each of the diagnostic categories. Patients were also asked two interesting questions about their understanding of chest pain (Table 41.2). The results of these questions support the idea that patients with chest pain frequently worry about the possibility of underlying heart disease.

Lababidi and Wankum (50) reviewed findings in children with idiopathic chest pain; 98 patients with a complaint of chest pain were seen in a pediatric cardiology clinic. Extensive evaluation was performed on most of these children, including a chest x-ray, electrocardiogram, M-mode echocardiogram, and exercise stress testing. Thirty-six of 98 (37%) patients had idiopathic chest pain. Of patients with idiopathic chest pain, 56% were girls (mean age, 12 years; range, 9 to 19 years) and 44% were boys (mean age, 13 years; range, 10 to 18 years). The pain was characterized as mild, recurrent, lasting a few minutes, occurring mostly during activity, and over the whole precordium in most patients.

Significant life events were noted in many patients: divorce in the family (39%) and recent death from heart attack (33%). Eighty-three percent of the patients felt that the heart was the source of pain, and 100% of these patients' parents expressed great concern over the symptom of chest pain. This group of patients with idiopathic chest pain, unlike those

TABLE 41.2. *Patients' concerns about meaning of chest pain*

	What do you *think* caused your pain?	What were you *afraid* caused your pain?
Heart	4	44
Heart disease	6	12
Cancer	2	12
Gas	7	0
Don't know	61	23
Miscellaneous	20	9

in other studies in children, had more extensive laboratory evaluations than are routinely done. All children had normal electrocardiograms and 29 of 36 had normal exercise tests at maximal levels; the seven of 36 who were not physically fit enough to reach maximal levels were nevertheless reassured that their heart function was normal.

All patients received follow-up telephone calls, and 97% of patients had resolution of symptoms within 1 week of cardiac evaluation. No further reports of chest pain were noted in a 2-year follow-up. One patient initiated psychiatric therapy because of repeated somatic complaints. The follow-up data are interesting. The quick and prolonged resolution of symptoms in this group of patients with idiopathic chest pain is striking compared with other studies. Does extensive cardiac evaluation, although costly, more effectively reassure the healthy but worried patient with idiopathic chest pain?

Selbst et al. (4) prospectively reviewed all emergency department visits during a 1-year period in patients through age 19 years with a chief complaint of chest pain. Four hundred seven children were evaluated (approximately 70,000 emergency department visits). The age range was 2 to 18.9 years (mean, 11.9 years); 55% were girls and 90% were black. The nature of the pain was less chronic than in other studies (43% had an acute onset of less than 48 hours), but this may be a reflection of the study being done in an emergency department setting. Thirty-one percent of patients had disturbed sleep and 30% reported school absence because of pain. The pain was described as sharp in 41%, mainly in the sternal area (49%) and either constant or lasting less than 5 minutes in most of the patients.

Physical examination was remarkable for chest wall tenderness detected in 51% of those patients who had an abnormal physical finding on examination. Laboratory results of note included chest x-ray, electrograms, and echocardiograms, with normal results being the significant finding in all patients who had these tests performed. Diagnoses in these patients showed an idiopathic origin to be most common (21%) followed by musculoskeletal (15%), cough (10%), costochondritis (9%), and psychogenic causes (9%).

Selbst et al. (4), as a result of the findings in this study, made these interesting observations and suggestions regarding the evaluation of the child with chest pain. In the younger child, look for organic disease. Organic disease was related to pain that awakened the child and was of acute onset and associated with an abnormal physical finding, especially fever. Nonorganic disease was related to having chronic pain for more than 6 months and a positive family history of chest pain and heart disease. Psychogenic pain was 3.7 times more likely if there was a positive family history of chest pain.

In 1990, Rowe et al. (51) reviewed 336 consecutive patients with a primary or secondary complaint of chest pain seen during a 2-year period in an urban emergency department setting. Of the 336 patients, 325 completed a questionnaire and had a complete physical examination. The age range was 2 to 18 years (mean age, 12 years). The male-to-female ratio was 1.0. The pain was described as being in the anterior chest wall, moderate to severe, interfering with normal activity, and exacerbated by breathing in most patients.

The causes of pain were chest wall (28%), pulmonary (19%), traumatic (15%), idiopathic (12%), and psychogenic (5%). This study showed a much lower incidence of idiopathic and psychogenic causes than other studies.

In 2000, Evangelista et al. (52) prospectively studied specific factors in the history and physical examination that permitted accurate diagnosis. In 50 patients referred to a pediatric cardiac clinic, accurate diagnosis was made based on history, physical examination, and electrocardiogram, and no patient had a cardiac cause for their complaint. The breakdown of causes is listed in the Table 41.1.

RETROSPECTIVE AND FOLLOW-UP STUDIES

Four retrospective studies (Table 41.3) and two follow-up studies (Table 41.4) also examined chest pain in pediatric patients.

TABLE 41.3. *Retrospective studies of chest pain in pediatric patients*

Study	Clinical setting	Patient demographics	Cause	Additional observations
Fyfe and Moodie (12)	Cardiology clinic, 4-yr period	*N*= 67; 40 male pts/27 female pts; mean, 12.3 yr; range, 8–19 yr	Cardiac (6%) Idiopathic (85%)	20 to 57 pts with idiopathic chest pain also had a cardiac diagnosis, but no causal connection could be made between symptom of chest pain and underlying defect; 34/37 pts with chest pain and no underlying cardiac defect had telephone follow-up 13 mo later, 29/34 pts had no or reduced symptoms
Selbst (7)	Urban pediatric emergency department	*N*= 267; 129 male pts/138 female pts; 135 children <12 yr, 132 children 12–19 yr	Idiopathic (28%) Functional (anxiety) (17%) Costochondritis (10%) Musculoskeletal (15%) Gastrointestinal (7%) Cough/upper respiratory infection (6%) Asthma/pneumonia (6%)	Teenagers had higher incidence of functional chest pain, females pts secondary to anxiety more than male pts; laboratory evaluations not helpful; follow-up (10 mo after study) 22% follow-up questionnaire completed; 35/60 respondents still had chest pain; 34/60 either parent or child was worried about the pain
Zavaras-Angelidou et al. (53)	Pediatric emergency department	*N*=134; 180 episodes	Cardiac (15%)	History/physical; examination best approach
Tunaoglu et al. (54)	Pediatric cardiac clinic	*N*=100; 54 female pts (mean, 11.3 yr); 46 male pts (mean, 9.9 yr)	Cardiac (22%) Recent family death (19%) Idiopathic (92%)	Chest pain left precordium; no radiation 60%–66%; Psychiatric symptoms common (74% of 55 pts interviewed)

pts, patients

In 1985, Selbst (7) retrospectively reviewed 267 children with chest pain who were seen in an emergency department over a 26-month period (occurrence rate = 0.249%); there were 129 boys and 138 girls. Ages ranged from 21 months to 19 years; 135 children were younger than 12 years of age and 132 children were 12 to 19 years of age. There were 166 Hispanic patients and 87 black patients.

TABLE 41.4. *Follow-up studies of chest pain in pediatric patients*

Study	Clinical setting	Patient demographics	Cause			Additional observations
Rowland and Richards (55)	Pediatric cardiac clinic, 8-yr period, average 4-yr follow-up	*N*=44 pts; 23 male pts/8 female pts; mean age, 12.2 yr; range, 8–18 yr	Idiopathic (100%)			31/44 had telephone follow-up; duration of symptoms 1 mo to 10 yr; 45% still had symptoms, 55% had no further symptoms; no specific disease was detected during the follow-up period
Selbst et al. (56)	Pediatric urban emergency department, 2-yr follow-up	Initial data present in 1985; original *N*=407 children, *N*=149/407; 54% female pts; 86% black; mean age, 11.34 yr	*Diagnosis* Idiopathic Musculoskeletal Psychogenic Costochondritis Asthma/cough	*Initial* 13% 16% 9% 9% 3%	*FU* 34% 11% 11% 6% 17%	34% of the original changed in follow-up; idiopathic increased the most; only 1 cardiac lesion was uncovered (mitral valve prolapse); chest pain resolved in 57% of pts at 2 yr follow-up; resolution of symptoms not related to age, gender, diagnosis, physical examination
Kaden et al. (57)	Pediatric cardiac clinic	*N*=25; adolescents	Cardiac (22%) Noncardiac or insignificant cardiac disease(84%)			Chest pain has emotional impact but most have resolution of symptoms

pts, patients; F/U, follow-up

The pain was acute or semiacute (1 day to 1 month) in onset in 69% of patients. Recurrent visits were noted in 22% of patients. Family history was obtained in only 33% of patients; 38 patients had a positive family history of heart disease, lung disease, or chest pain. Laboratory evaluations were generally not helpful. Seventy-one of 76 had a normal chest x-ray; 91 of 100 had a normal electrocardiogram.

Diagnoses included idiopathic (28%), functional (anxiety) (17%), musculoskeletal (15%), costochondritis (10%), cough, upper respiratory infection, asthma, pneumonia (12%), and gastrointestinal (7%). In general, teenagers had a higher incidence of functional chest pain compared with younger children. Female patients had pain secondary to anxiety more than males.

Follow-up (10 to 36 months after visit) showed that only 22% completed a questionnaire. Of these, 36 of 60 respondents still had chest pain, and 34 of 60 (either the parent or child) were still worried about the pain. Obviously, this limited response may have been biased toward those who still had chest pain.

In 1984, Fyfe and Moodie (12) retrospectively reviewed 67 patients with a primary complaint of chest pain who were evaluated in a pediatric cardiology clinic over a 4-year period. This study was also interested in addressing the frequency of associated cardiac disease in pediatric patients with chest pain. As expected, a small number (only 6%) of patients had underlying cardiac disease that could be associated with chest pain; 57 patients (85%) had chest pain and no clear cause could be determined. Of these 57 patients, 20 patients (35%) had isolated cardiac anomalies, but a causal relationship could not be established between chest pain and the underlying cardiac defect.

Thirty-four of the 37 patients with idiopathic chest pain without cardiac anomalies were evaluated by telephone at a mean of 13 months after the initial assessment; 29 of 34 were asymptomatic or had reduced symptoms. It is interesting that of the 37 patients with idiopathic chest pain, 32 had echocardiograms and 23 had exercise treadmill testing in addition to a chest x-ray and electrocardiogram. This dramatic resolution in symptoms is similar to Lababidi (50) who found 98% resolution in symptoms after a more extensive cardiac evaluation than is usually performed in the patient with idiopathic chest pain.

A review of 180 episodes of chest pain in 134 patients who presented to a pediatric emergency department demonstrated a relationship between the chest pain and cardiac disease in 15% of patients. This study emphasized the importance of a good history and physical examination as the diagnostic key to proper diagnosis. Treatment was reassurance in many patients (53).

Tunaoglu et al. (54) reviewed 100 consecutive patients referred to a cardiac clinic in Turkey. There were 54 girls (mean age, 11.3 years) and 46 boys (mean age, 9.9 years); 22% had heart disease and 19% of the children had a recent death in the family. Symptoms persisted for longer than 1 week in 92% of patients. Idiopathic was the diagnosis in 92%. Seventy-four patients had a psychiatric interview and 55 patients had psychiatric symptoms, and five required psychiatric care of anxiety, conversion disorder, or depression.

FOLLOW-UP STUDIES

There is truly a paucity of data on follow-up of pediatric patients with chest pain. Rowland and Richards (55) reported on the follow-up of patients with idiopathic chest pain who were initially evaluated in a pediatric cardiology clinic with the chief complaint of chest pain. Follow-up averaged 4.1 years. During an 8-year period, 44 patients were seen who were thought to have idiopathic chest pain; 31 of the 44 (70%) patients had follow-up by telephone or letter, and 17 (55%) had no further symptoms. No specific disease was uncovered during follow-up.

In 1990, Selbst et al. (56) reported on a 2-year follow-up of a group of previously reported patients with chest pain seen in an emergency department. Of the original 407 patients, 149 were studied for 6 months or longer. The group lost to follow-up did not differ demographically from the group that was followed except that more idiopathic or psychogenic pain was represented in the group lost to follow-up. The mean age of patients in the follow-up group was 11.3 years; 54% female and 86% were black. Thirty-four percent of the original diagnoses changed during the follow-up. Although idiopathic chest pain was still the most common cause, the diagnosis of idiopathic pain increased from 13% to 34% at the end of the follow-up period. Only one child was found to have a heart abnormality (MVP). The diagnosis of psychogenic chest pain changed from 9% to 11% over the follow-up period.

Chest pain resolved in 57% of patients during the 2-year follow-up period. Resolution of symptoms was not related to child's age, gender, initial diagnosis, or findings on physical examination. Therefore, these authors concluded that chest pain does abate but slowly, and although organic disease is rarely uncovered in follow-up, it is more likely for a diagnosis to change to idiopathic or psychogenic over time.

An interesting questionnaire follow-up study of adolescents seen in a pediatric cardiology clinic for the evaluation of chest pain revealed that adolescents with and without chest pain (healthy control group) know that chest pain does not usually signify a heart problem (89% of group) and that heart attacks were rare in their age group (67%). They were aware that asthma and gastrointestinal causes could account for the chest pain (72% to 78%). Although this group of adolescents appeared knowledgeable about the cause of chest pain and felt healthy, they were nevertheless "more concerned" about their hearts than controls were (80% versus 55%). They also thought that they should visit a doctor more often than the healthy controls (77% versus 59%). In fact, 44% of patients changed their behavior in some way even though they had been reassured that they were healthy. Reassurance was helpful, but 19% still had heightened concern after a visit to a cardiologist. Symptoms had resolved in 22% of patients within 2 to 9 months and in 73% by 9 months' follow-up. This study confirms the older studies that adolescents with chest pain are healthy and need clear, concrete explanations and reassurance to avoid ongoing psychogenic distress (57).

SUMMARY

In a review of chest pain in the pediatric patient, idiopathic chest pain has generally gained the most attention. The pediatric patient with idiopathic chest pain is usually a young adolescent female who complains of specific, localized precordial pain with symptoms occurring over months to years. The pain can wake the patient from sleep and cause school or work absence. The pediatric patient with idiopathic chest pain makes repeated visits to health care providers, usually in emergency department settings, and keeps follow-up appointments or referral appointments more faithfully than other pediatric patients with chest pain. During follow-up, occult disease is rarely found. Rather, the diagnosis of idiopathic disease is usually confirmed or changed to a psychogenic diagnosis. Symptoms will diminish or resolve but usually over months or even years. Often, conservative treatment, including repeated reassurance to a young patient who might be especially afraid of heart disease, is most beneficial. Conservative measures include comfort measures such as heat, massage, nonsteroidal anti-inflammatory drugs, and transcutaneous electrical nerve stimulation. Behavioral treatment programs using biofeedback and relaxation mental imagery techniques have shown a decrease in the complaint of chest pain in pediatric patients with symptomatic MVP (58). However, patients with idiopathic chest pain or chest pain from other causes may also benefit from such behavioral treatment plans.

In general, based on the literature discussed above, one is advised to follow a conservative approach to invasive evaluation and treatment. Laboratory evaluations such as chest x-ray and electrocardiograms are overwhelmingly normal in these patients. However, the patient with acute chest pain and an abnormal finding on physical examination should have treatment and follow-up directed toward the appropriate diagnosis. When an acute process is present such as pneumonia or costochondritis, treatment should result in resolution of symptoms.

As this discussion has suggested, cardiac disease is extremely rare as a cause of chest pain, and often physical examination, history of exertional chest pain, or family history of idiopathic hypertrophic subaortic stenosis will identify patients with cardiac disease. The primary care provider should make appropriate referral to a cardiologist when one of these factors is identified or an abnormal cardiac finding is discovered.

Follow-up studies suggest that missed diagnoses are rare in children with chest pain. However, in the larger group of patients with more chronic, idiopathic chest pain, it is helpful for care providers to have recommendations regarding long-term treatment plans. Chest pain represents one of the more common chronic pain complaints seen among pediatric patients. As studies have shown, the complaint of chest pain often prompts the patient and family to seek urgent evaluation outside the primary care setting. In addition, adolescents are an age group that often does not seek routine health care, but they also represent the majority of patients with chronic, idiopathic chest pain. For pediatricians or family practitioners, the adolescent with chest pain may seek further medical evaluation and treatment after an initial acute assessment in the emergency department setting. Repeated emergency assessments may be minimized if the primary care provider plays an active and necessary role in follow-up care. The patient with idiopathic chest pain may feel frustrated and anxious if symptoms continue despite reassurance and conservative treatment. Often the physician feels equally frustrated. As with any chronic pain complaint, missed school or work is a critical marker of serious dysfunction. The patient who exhibits evidence of social dysfunction, i.e., missed school or work, and evidence of family stress as a result of the chronic complaint of chest pain might benefit from a closer and more extensive evaluation.

A careful and thoughtful assessment of the "meaning" of chest pain to the patient and family cannot be minimized. If the patient and family express unresolved concern regarding undiagnosed cardiac disease, cardiac referral in a select group of idiopathic chest pain patients may help allay anxiety and continued symptoms as some studies have suggested (27). The possibility of unrecognized gastrointestinal pathology should be reassessed. Finally, the primary care provider should consider the role of behavioral techniques in helping the patient cope with recurrent symptoms. Often introduction to behavioral medicine techniques with a psychologist is a nonthreatening way to introduce psychotherapy as part of treatment. Clearly, the ongoing relationship that a patient and family has with a pediatrician or family practitioner can make a psychologic referral more acceptable as time passes and a chronic symptom persists.

In summary, the pediatric patient with chest pain is often a challenge to physicians. The principles and treatment approaches that we use in all patients with chronic pain should find increasing application to the pediatric patient with chest pain. As a result, we may also learn more about the nature of idiopathic chest pain in children and better define an effective evaluation and treatment plan for these patients in the future.

REFERENCES

1. Ezzati T. *Ambulatory care utilization patterns of children and young adults: vital and health statistics*, series 13, no. 39 [publication no (PHS) 78-1790]. Washington, DC: U.S. Dept of Health, Education and Welfare, 1978.
2. Feinstein RA, Daniel WA Jr. Chronic chest pain in children and adolescents. *Pediatr Annu* 1986;15:685–686, 691–694.
3. Brunswick AF, Boyle JM, Tarica C. Who sees the doctor? A study of urban black adolescents. *Soc Sci Med* 1979;13A:45–56.
4. Selbst SM, Ruddy RM, Clark BJ, et al. Pediatric chest pain: a prospective study. *Pediatrics* 1988;82:319–323.
5. Pantell RH, Goodman BW. Adolescent chest pain: a prospective study. *Pediatrics* 1983;71:881–887.
6. Gutgesell HP, Barst RJ, Humes RA, et al. Common cardiovascular problems in the young Part 1: murmurs,

chest pain, syncope and irregular rhythms. *Am Fam Phys* 1997;56:1825–1830.
7. Selbst SM. Chest pain in children. *Pediatrics* 1985;75: 1068–1070.
8. Pfister GC, Puffer JC, Maron BJ. Pre-participation cardio-vascular screening for US college student-athletes. *JAMA* 2000;283:1597–1599.
9. Billups D, Martin D, Swain RA. Training room evaluation of chest pain in the adolescent athlete. *South Med J* 1995;88:667–672.
10. Lambert EC, Menon VA, Wagner HR. Sudden, unexpected death from cardiovascular disease in children. *Am J Cardiol* 1974;34:89–96.
11. Maron BJ, Roberts WC, McAllister HA, et al. Sudden death in young athletes. *Circulation* 1980;62:218–229.
12. Fyfe DA, Moodie DS. Chest pain in pediatric patients presenting to a cardiac clinic. *Clin Pediatr* 1984;23: 321–324.
13. Barlow JB, Pocock WA, Marchand P. The significance of late systolic murmurs. *Am Heart J* 1963;66:443.
14. Warth DC, King ME, Cohen JM. Prevalence of mitral valve prolapse in normal children. *J Am Coll Cardiol* 1985;5:1173–1177.
15. Greenwood RD. Mitral valve prolapse incidence and clinical course in a pediatric population. *Clin Pediatr* 1984;23:318–320.
16. Sbarbara JA, Mehlman DJ, Wu L, et al. A prospective study of mitral valvular prolapse in presumably healthy young men. *Chest* 1979;75:555–559.
17. Bissett GS, Schwartz DC, Meyer RA, et al. Clinical spectrum and long-term follow-up of isolated mitral valve prolapse in 119 children. *Circulation* 1980;62: 423–429.
18. Rokicki W, Krzystolik-Ladzinska J, Goc B. Clinical characteristics of primary mitral valve prolapse syndrome in children. *Acta Cardiol* 1995;50:147–153.
19. Bowen RC, D'Arcy C, Orchard RC. The prevalence of anxiety disorders among patients with mitral valve prolapse syndrome and chest pain. *Psychosomatics* 1991; 32:400–406
20. Kavey RE, Sondheimer JH, Blackman MS. Detection of dysrhythmia in pediatric patients with mitral valve prolapse. *Circulation* 1980;62:582–587.
21. Woolf PK, Gewitz MH, Berezin S, et al. Non-cardiac chest pain in adolescents and children with mitral valve prolapse. *J Adolesc Health* 1991;12:247–250.
22. Kato H, Ichinose E, Kawasaki T. Myocardial infarction in Kawasaki disease: clinical analyses in 195 cases. *J Pediatr* 1986;108:923–927.
23. Burns JC, Shike H, Gordon JB, et al. Sequelae of Kawasaki disease in adolescents and young adults. *J Am Coll Cardiol* 1996;28:253–257
24. Reynolds JL. Precordial catch syndrome in children. *South Med J* 1989;82:1228–1230.
25. Taubman B, Vetter VL. Slipping rib syndrome as a cause of chest pain in children. *Clin Pediatr* 1996;35: 403–405.
26. Ravilly S, Robinson W, Suresh S, et al. Chronic pain in cystic fibrosis. *Pediatrics* 1996;98:741–747.
27. Nudel DB, Diamant S, Brady T, et al. Chest pain, dyspnea on exertion, and exercise induced asthma in children and adolescents. *Clin Pediatr (Phila)* 1987;26: 388–392.
28. Weins L, Sabath R, Ewing L, et al. Chest pain in otherwise healthy children and adolescents is frequently caused by exercise-induced asthma. *Pediatrics* 1992;90: 350–353.
29. Kato S, Komatsu K, Harada Y. Medication-induced esophagitis in children. *Gastroenterol Jpn* 1990;25: 485–490.
30. Berezin S, Medow M, Glassman M, et al. Use of the intraesophageal acid perfusion test in provoking nonspecific chest pain in children. *J Pediatr* 1989;115: 709–712.
31. Berezin S, Medow M, Glassman M, et al. Chest pain of gastrointestinal origin. *Arch Dis Child* 1988;63: 1457–1460.
32. Glassman MS, Medow MS, Berezin S, et al. Spectrum of esophageal disorders in children with chest pain. *Dig Dis Sci* 1992;37:663–666.
33. Berezin S, Medow MS, Glassman MS, et al. Esophageal chest pain in children with asthma. *J Pediatr Gastroenterol Nutr* 1991;12:52–55.
34. Herman SP, Stickler GB, Lucas AR. Hyperventilation syndrome in children and adolescents: long-term follow-up. *Pediatrics* 1981;67:183–187.
35. Kashani JH, Lababidi Z, Jones RS. Depression in children and adolescents with cardiovascular symptomatology: the significance of chest pain. *J Am Acad Child Psychol* 1982;21:187–189.
36. Driscoll DJ, Glicklich LB, Gallen WJ. Chest pain in children: a prospective study. *Pediatrics* 1976;57:648–651.
37. Asnes RS, Santulli R, Bemporad JR. Psychogenic chest pain in children. *Clin Pediatr* 1981;20:788–791.
38. Hotopf M, Mayou R, Wadsworth M, et al. Psychosocial and developmental antecedents of chest pain in young adults. *Psychosom Med* 1999;61:861–867.
39. Shannon M, Lacouture PG, Roa J, et al. Cocaine exposure among children seen at a pediatric hospital. *Pediatrics* 1989;83:337–342.
40. Selbst SM. Chest pain in an adolescent: think of cocaine! *Pediatrics* 1989;84:582.
41. James LP, Farrar HC, Komoroski EM, et al. Sympathomimetic drug use in adolescents presenting to a pediatric emergency department with chest pain. *J Toxicol Clin Toxicol* 1998;36:321–328
42. Leson CL, McGuigan MA, Bryson SM. Caffeine overdose in an adolescent male. *Clin Toxicol* 1988;26: 407–415.
43. Lien DC, Todoruk D, Rajani H, et al. Accidental inhalation of mercury vapor: respiratory and toxicologic consequences. *CMAJ* 1983;129:591–594.
44. Woo OF, Healey K. Chest pain and hypoxemia from inhalation of a trichloroethane aerosol product. *J Toxicol Clin Toxicol* 1983;20:333–341.
45. Friedman G, Sieglaub A, Dales L. Cigarette smoking and chest pain. *Ann Intern Med* 1975;83:1–7.
46. Wolowodiuk OJ, McMicken D, O'Brien P. Pneumomediastinum and retropneumoperitoneum: an unusual complication of syrup-of-ipecac-induced emesis. *Ann Emerg Med* 1984;13:1148–1151.
47. Gulati S, Kumar L. "Chest epilepsy" is a child. *Postgrad Med J* 1992;68:369–370.
48. Marseglia GL, Savasta S, Ravelli A, et al. Recurrent chest pain as the presenting manifestation of spinal meningioma. *Acta Paediatr* 1995;84:1086–1088.
49. Birmingham CL, Stigant C, Goldner EM. Chest pain in anorexia nervosa. *Int J Eat Disord* 1999;25:219–222.

50. Lababidi Z, Wankum J. Pediatric idiopathic chest pain. *Mo Med* 1983;80:306–308.
51. Rowe BH, Dulberg CS, Peterson RG, et al. Characteristics of children presenting with chest pain to a pediatric emergency department. *CMAJ* 1990;143:388–394.
52. Evangelista JA, Parsons M, Renneburg AK. Chest pain in children: diagnosis through history and physical examination. *J Pediatr Health Care* 2000;14:3–8.
53. Zavaras-Angelidou KA, Weinhouse E, Nelson DB. Review of 180 episodes of chest pain 134 children. *Pediatr Emerg Care* 1992;8:189–193.
54. Tunaoglu FS, Olgunturk R, Akcabay S, et al. Chest pain in children referred to a cardiology clinic. *Pediatr Cardiol* 1995;16:69–72.
55. Rowland TW, Richards MM. The natural history of idiopathic chest pain in children: a follow-up study. *Clin Pediatr* 1986;25:612–614.
56. Selbst SM, Ruddy R, Clark BJ. Chest pain in children. Follow-up of patients previously reported. *Clin Pediatr* 1990;29:374–377.
57. Kaden GG, Shenker IR, Gootman N. Chest pain in adolescents. *J Adolesc Health* 1991;2:251–255.
58. Smith MS, Womack WM. Stress management techniques in childhood and adolescence. *Clin Pediatr* 1987;26:581–585.

42

Colic: The Pain Perplex

Ronald G. Barr and M. Alex Geertsma

Despite the fact that the noun "perplex" is considered obsolete (1), we have coined the term to describe the uncomfortable relationship between the clinical entity of "colic" and the experience of pain in infants. As a noun, it denotes "entanglement"; in its more common use as a transitive verb, it indicates "filling a person with uncertainty as to the nature or treatment of a thing by reason of its involved or intricate nature." Both forms of the term define the clinical problem, namely, to treat or manage a condition that is involved and intricate and about which we are uncertain. We are uncertain exactly because our understanding of colic syndrome is deeply entangled, in this instance, with our understanding of pain in infants.

Indeed, if we could solve the question of whether colic syndrome is a pain syndrome of infancy, we would probably know almost all that we need to know about pain. This is because the syndrome of colic provides a challenge that is different from most of the paradigms used to understand pain in infants. In most paradigms, the pain stimulus is known (e.g., phenylketonuria testing or inoculations) or at least proximal in time (e.g., postoperative). However, in infants with colic, there is no identifiable pain stimulus, and the experience, painful or otherwise, is recurrent and prolonged. Although the phenotypic similarity of the behavior of an infant with colic and an infant responding to a pain stimulus may be striking, it does not constitute a demonstration that the infant is in pain, only that it might be. The behavioral similarities do make it clear, however, why the behavior of infants with colic arouses such concern for parents.

THE SYNDROME OF COLIC

In pediatrics, the term colic is usually reserved for a behavioral syndrome of recurrent crying that occurs during the first 3 months of life that is characterized by three typical behavioral dimensions (2–4). First, the crying typically occurs in a pattern characterized by an increase in overall daily duration of distress behaviors into the second month of life, followed by a decline to lower and more stable levels by the fourth month. The crying typically, but not universally, tends to cluster in the late afternoon and evening hours (2–5), and the increase and decrease across ages are almost completely accounted for by the changes in late afternoon and evening crying. Second, there are several associated behaviors that cluster together with the crying bouts. The most prominent features of the crying bouts are that they are prolonged and difficult to soothe. The most often mentioned associated behaviors include those thought to indicate hypertonia, such as an arched back posture, legs being drawn up over the abdomen, flushed face, and clenched fists. Contributing to the impression that something must be wrong is the facial grimacing, sometimes referred to as a "pain facies" because of its phenotypic similarity to the facial appearance when an infant is undergoing a pain experience (6). All these features contribute to the impression that infants with colic are undergoing a pain experience during their crying bouts. Third, at least some of the crying bouts are described as occurring in paroxysms, that is, the bouts are typically acute, unpredictable, unexplained, and seem to begin and end unrelated to anything that goes on in the environment. Whether there are crying paroxysms that are specific to infants with colic remains unclear. It is more likely that they just have more of these bouts in proportion to the overall amount of crying that they do (4,5,7,8). In a smaller proportion of infants (on the order of 30%), the symptoms may persist into the fourth or fifth month (2,3). In a few infants, the crying may not decrease at all, and the earlier colic syndrome gets perpetuated in a mutual breakdown of caregiver–infant regulation, sometimes referred to as "persistent mother–infant distress syndrome" (9,10).

Although most clinicians consider crying to be the predominant defining characteristic of the syndrome, there is no consensus about the quantity or quality of crying that is needed nor whether other behaviors should be included in the definition of the syndrome (4,11,12). By far the most widely used criterion is the so-called "rule of threes" of Wessel et al. that defines colic as crying or fussing that continues for more than 3 hours per day for more than 3 days per week and that is considered "serious" colic if this lasts longer than 3 weeks (2). However, there is no obvious cutoff amount of crying that describes a uniquely different group of infants who meet these criteria. Rather, the criteria appear to delineate the upper end of a continuous spectrum of crying behavior (13). The quality of crying is sometimes described as different, often as "high-pitched" and/or a "pain" cry. Exactly what those differences might be acoustically and whether they are specific to infants with "colic" remains controversial (14–16).

On current evidence, it remains the case that the cause must be considered unknown, although several attributions of causality have been considered. By far the most common attribution is that the crying bouts represent episodes of gastrointestinal pain. In part, this is because of the frequent presence of symptoms thought to be gastrointestinal in origin, including what is interpreted as diarrhea (looser stools) and vomiting (usually regurgitation). By far the most commonly reported is the presence of gas (per rectum) and abdominal distention (4). Indeed, the lay description of the syndrome is often "colic and gas" or just "wind" (3,17,18). However, even if gas and distention are present, good evidence that they represent a primary role for gastrointestinal dysfunction as a cause is not available. The symptoms probably reflect expulsion of gas that is normally present owing to the increased intra-abdominal pressure occurring during crying episodes (4,19–21). The evidence with regard to cow's milk protein intolerance is somewhat more convincing (for a review, see reference 4). However, the evidence also suggests that, even if cow's milk protein is a cause of colic, it accounts for approximately 5% or less of the cases (22,23).

Precise definition of the syndrome is complicated further by the fact that the crying of infants who do not have colic is similar in almost all respects to that of infants who do meet clinical criteria for the syndrome, except that they have quantitatively more of it. In particular, the pattern of crying (i.e., the evening clustering and the peak crying during the second month of age) is identical in both (24–27). Indeed, the early peak pattern is also characteristic of normal infants of the !Kung San, a hunter–gatherer society with radically different caretaking practices than those typical of Western industrialized societies. This implies that this pattern is a behavioral universal of infancy (28). In addition, the critical difference is not that infants with colic cry more frequently than those without but rather that the longer total daily duration of crying is owing primarily to the fact that the crying bouts that they do have last longer (6,29).

COLIC AS A MANIFESTATION OF INFANT BEHAVIORAL STATE ORGANIZATION

To appreciate how crying in infants with and without colic may reflect the same organizational principles unrelated to underlying pathology, it is useful to consider crying behavior as a reflection of infant behavioral state. The concept of a behavioral state refers to the notion that infant behavior is organized as a set of discontinuous and distinct modes of activity representing central nervous system conditions rather than as a continuum of arousal. A behavioral state is (a) self-organizing in the sense that it is maintained until the pattern of necessary and/or sufficient conditions occurs that results in a "shift" to another state, (b) relatively stable over time (minutes rather than seconds), and (c) a modulator of input stimuli such that the same stimulus experienced in different states results in nonlinear, state-specific output responses (30). Thus, for example, the facial reaction to a heel-lance stimulus delivered while a newborn is asleep is not the same as that seen when the infant is awake and alert (31).

In Wolff's classification (30), the crying state is described as follows:

> Cry vocalizations are the essential defining criterion; they may vary in intensity from persistent whimpering to loud screaming. Vigorous cry vocalizations are accompanied by diffuse motor activity or a rigid posture of the trunk in partial extension. During vigorous crying, resistance of the limbs to passive movement is high; the face is contorted into a cry grimace and may be flushed bright red. Except during the early stages, patterns of respiration are subordinate to crying.

Fussing, in contrast, is conceptualized as a state transition characterized by intermittent vocalizations and less intense and nonrhythmic motor activity (30). Fussing is often a transition to (or from) the state of waking activity, characterized by bursts of generalized motor activity and open eyes. Occasional moaning, grunting, or whimpering can occur in this state, but it is always unsustained.

Considering crying in light of the concept of infant state may help to explain some of the commonly reported phenomena attributed to colic. First, Wolff's description of the vocalizations, motor behavior, facial expression, and vascular reactivity that characterize crying as a self-organizing state in normal infants closely parallels the clusters of behaviors that are recognized as typical of colic. Colic infants would be distinctive only insofar as they are "in" that behavioral state more than infants without, not because new causes need to be hypothesized to account for it. Because states comprise a "discontinuous" set of behaviors, this discontinuity between the states of crying and fussing may well explain how the crying of colic may be seen as distinct from common fussing and intermittent crying but still be a manifestation of normal behavior. Second, it may help to explain why infants with colic are said to be resistant to soothing interventions. In principle, at least, a soothing stimulus applied to an infant who is fussing or who has just begun to cry (i.e., in whom a crying "state" has not yet been organized) is more likely to be successful in aborting the transition from awake activity to crying than when it is applied to the infant after the crying has become sustained. Third, although the state of crying may be the behavioral manifestation of a noxious (pain) stimulus, it may be equally well established by nonpain stimuli such as hunger or separation, accounting for the nonspecificity of the crying of infants with colic.

In short, the crying of infants with and without colic is similar in pattern and probably similar in representing a self-perpetuating, self-organizing state that has the same (phenotypic) characteristics whether it is induced by pain or nonpain stimuli. However, such crying states may be the "paroxysms" of crying thought of as colic bouts, which, once established, are relatively immune to external intervention. Consequently, the (phenotypic) behavior characteristic of colic probably represents the final common pathway of a variety of contributing influences that may or may not be pain related.

These similarities illustrate how difficult it is to determine whether the syndrome of colic can and should be understood as simply the upper range of the spectrum of crying of normal infants, a distinct crying type or behavior (e.g., a pain cry), or a manifestation of some underlying "disease" (32). The question remains unresolved, although the weight of evidence favors the former. If the phenomena used to define the syndrome are indeed those of the crying state, then any one or all three influences may contribute in any particular infant. An infant with colic may simply be in a crying state more often, but in some cases this may be true because of pain or disease and in some cases (probably most) not.

Finally, although seldom made explicit, the colic syndrome often refers to crying seen as a problem and taken to the physician as a complaint, and not just to the crying characteristics of the infant. Acknowledging this feature has the advantages of reflecting clinical practice by recognizing parental concern as a component of the interaction around colic (33–35). It also implies that no specific amount or quality of crying may be manifest in all infants with colic (36). Both common sense and systematic observation confirm that the cognitive set of the caregiver as well as the characteristics of the cry will affect whether the cry is perceived and interpreted as hunger or sickness (37–41), and this is likely to affect whether crying is brought to the physician. This seems to be confirmed in the few studies comparing infants with colic with nonclinical controls. Parity is not related to the amount or pattern of crying that is considered "excessive," but more firstborns are referred for clinical help, presumably reflecting the anxiety associated with the firstborn infant (5). In addition, in a significant subgroup of infants referred for "colic," the crying behavior is in all respects similar to nonreferred control infants, except that crying that occurs after meals is perceived as "sick" sounding (6). Interestingly, this interpretation of postmeal crying has been shown to be related to acoustic differences in the cries of infants with colic after a meal (15). Understanding colic as a complaint brings the problems closer to the reality of clinical problem solving concerning crying behavior in the first few months of life.

COLIC AS A PAIN SYNDROME

There could be no better illustration of how much there is still to learn about the nature of pain in infants than to try to justify the inclusion of colic in this volume, i.e., to demonstrate that colic is a pain syndrome of infancy. In recent years, it has become increasingly clear that all infants, even those born prematurely, are capable of mounting a behavioral and physiologic stress response to tissue damage (42) and, in this sense at least, they are sensitive to pain. However, the capacity for pain experience does not imply that the colic syndrome is a manifestation of pain on the part of the infant.

There are three important reasons for this. First, because infants with colic are preverbal, our understanding of whether they are in pain can only be inferential, and it is limited to indirect evidence via behavioral and physiologic measures. Second, reasonable inferences that pain is being experienced might nevertheless be possible if there were specific or pathognomonic relationships between behavioral and/or physiologic responses and known noxious stimuli. Although there is increasing evidence that there are vocal, facial, motoric, and physiologic features that are "characteristic" responses to noxious stimuli (31,43–45), these features are also seen in nonpain stress situations and therefore are not specific to pain experience (46,47). Third, almost all our understanding of infant pain behavior derives from responses to procedures in which the pain is acute and the timing and nature of the noxious stimuli are known. In sharp contrast, the behavior typical of colic is recurrent, the crying bouts paroxysmal, and the nature of the stimulus (or stimuli) unknown. Consequently, even if there was a specific behavioral/physiologic response to acute pain stimuli (a "pain signature"), it is not clear that it would generalize to the phenomenology of colic.

Three types of evidence could be taken as support for the interpretation that infants with colic are experiencing pain. The first is phenomenologic evidence that some behavior or physiologic marker that is other than, rather than just more of, the behavior seen in highly aroused normal infants is specific to colic and to recognizable pain experiences. In principle, such evidence might be obtainable from techniques such as acoustic analyses of infant cries (48), facial analyses (31,49,50), and cerebral imaging techniques (51), but no such convincing evidence of these kinds is available to date. The few studies to date of acoustic analyses of cries of infants with and without colic do not permit a clear conclusion on the specificity of acoustic features or their possible relationship to pain experiences (14–16).

The second is evidence that colic results from disease processes, especially if these disease processes were known to be painful or associated with inflammation. The evidence for and against organic disease processes underlying colic has been the subject of several reviews (4,22,23,52,53). Unfortunately, much of the evidence is subject to potentially serious methodologic biases and cannot be generalized to all infants with colic. However, a conservative summary of the evidence to date might be that (a) relative to the overall prevalence of colic of 16% to 40% (17,54,55), colic ascribable to nongastrointestinal disease is rare, and the crying pattern is often atypical (22,56); (b) based on diet trials primarily, there is reasonable indication that protein intolerance accounts for some cases of colic (57–63), but the mechanism remains obscure, the crying improvement attributable to protein is only modest, and it is unlikely that this cause accounts for more than a small proportion of all infants with colic (4,59); and (c) there is weak evidence concerning the likely role of incomplete carbohydrate absorption as a cause of colic (19,20,64–67) and no evidence to date that modifying intestinal gas thought to be implicated in symptom production is effective (20,21,68).

This is not to say that gastrointestinal etiologic factors have been ruled out as causes of, or exacerbations of, otherwise normal developmental processes. Because of the nature of colic symptoms, it is likely that any intra-abdominal pain causes would be visceral, producing crampy, intermittent pain, possibly accompanied by autonomic symptoms arising from noxious stimuli affecting an abdominal viscus. By contrast, parietal pain secondary to noxious stimuli of the parietal peritoneum would typically be exaggerated by movement, the opposite of what is observed in an infant with colic, in whom activity is typically increased (53). However, there are many mechanisms that could be relevant to the production of visceral pain, although none has had sufficient evaluation. Consequently, gastrointestinal pain may yet be demonstrated to be important in colic, despite the current lack of evidence.

A plausible, but as yet undemonstrated, integrative hypothesis for the processes underlying colic phenomenology is that colic behavior reflects visceral hypersensitivity to otherwise innocuous intestinal stimuli, where the hypersensitivity is owing to developmental processes and minor insults that alter afferent mechanisms or changes in the excitability of central neurons onto which these afferents project. *Hyperalgesia* refers to a reduced pain threshold and/or a greater or longer duration of response to a painful stimulus that could be the mechanism for the hypersensitivity. *Allodynia* refers to painful or discomforting experiences owing to stimuli that do not normally produce pain or discomfort. In the context of colic, this might occur if intestinal distention, reflux of gastric contents, or changes in motility that would not normally be painful or discomforting were sensed as such.

Afferent hypersensitivity occurs when changes in the sensitivity of primary afferent neurons develop as noxious stimuli that "alter the gain" of the afferent system through the action of chemical mediators that might be activated by inflammation or repeated noxious procedures (69,70). This altered sensitivity may change the sensory information transmitted to secondary, dorsal horn neurons, or it may affect reflex loops that regulate a variety of functions of the enteric nervous and gut effector cell systems, including motility, secretion, and blood flow. Afferent hypersensitivity can also be owing to central hyperexcitability in dorsal horn cells. It is this central hyperexcitability that would most likely be responsible for allodynia. There is considerable interest in how such processes might be implicated in gastrointestinal pain syndromes such as nonulcer dyspepsia, recurrent abdominal pain, and irritable bowel syndrome in older children and adults. These processes could be activated even in young infants. Indeed, the normal developmental progression of neuronal growth and connectivity is consistent with these mechanisms being implicated. In general, excitatory pathways mature early and continue to mature postnatally. Inhibitory influences develop later on. Both local inhibitory interneuronal connections in the substantia gelatinosa and the functional development of descending inhibition from the brainstem are all postnatal events, at least in the rat and probably in humans (71).

These mechanisms could be relevant to understanding the pathogenesis of colic for a number of reasons. First, they are plausible mechanisms for understanding how such apparent discomfort can be expressed in the absence of detectable signs of disease, as is the case for the vast majority of infants with colic. Second, visceral hyperalgesia and allodynia may persist long after the initial stimulus has gone but can still be transient (72). This is consistent with the current evidence that colic does not have persistent effects on health and development after the colic has resolved (56). Third, descending cortical modulation is considered to play an important role in governing the excitability of dorsal horn neurons, especially in regard to pain perception (69,73). This modulation inhibits excitatory tone so that, in its absence, resting activity and responses to various sensory inputs to spinal dorsal horn neurons are increased. Fourth, central hypersensitivity can persist beyond the initiating stimulus (such as inflammation or repetitive noxious stimulation) and can be associated with reduction in thresholds and increases in the receptive field size of the dorsal horn neurons, allowing otherwise innocuous stimuli to excite previously unexcitable nociceptive pathways.

These mechanisms may help to explain why such a wide variety of apparently disparate factors (such as protein intolerance, gas, motility differences) that have been implicated in colic might cause discomfort without any one of them being wholly responsible for the behavioral manifestations of the syndrome. Of specific interest for infants in general, but for those with colic especially, is that the maturation of the inhibitory systems is delayed relative to the functional maturity of the afferent systems (72,74,75). Until these inhibitory systems are fully in place, infants may be predisposed to being more sensitive to otherwise innocuous stimuli. The evening clustering of symptoms could be a function of the relatively increased density of sensory input to centrally hyperexcitable neurons during daylight hours. The decline in crying behavior typical of the developmental course of colic syndrome could be a function of the modulation of sensory input by the increasing maturity of local inhibition owing to interneuronal synaptogenesis in the spinal cord and of the descending inhibitory systems from the brainstem and cortex as the infant matures. Although much less is known about the maturation of cortical pain systems, the relative delay of inhibitory connections compared with excitatory ones appears to be a general pattern there as well (71).

The third type of evidence that would support the interpretation that infants with colic are experiencing pain is simply the fact that it is perceived as such by their caretakers. This social evidence makes no claims about the experience of the infant *per se* but rather recognizes the fact that the signals are often taken to indicate a pain experience of the infant. Whether the caretakers are responding to indicators of sensory pain or emotional distress (or both) remains unknown, and it is not completely understood which behavioral indicators that the caretakers are using to make the assessment (37,50,76–78).

Despite these limitations, the perception that the infant with colic is in pain is widespread. Being in pain or having a pain facies is explicitly identified as a feature of colic by approximately 25% of the authors on the subject (79). Parents of infants who present to their physician with "colic" differ from parents of matched controls in rating their infants' cries as more "sick" sounding, regardless of the amount of crying (6). This perception is no doubt highly relevant to the anxiety produced in caretakers. Consequently, colic appears to function as a pain syndrome, whether or not the infant is in fact experiencing pain.

MANAGEMENT

In principle, a thorough understanding of the condition provides rational guidelines for specific therapy and management. Colic, however, remains complex and unclear. Of course, therapy can be shown to be effective without any clear understanding of the problem because effective therapies do not necessarily indicate anything about cause or pathophysiology. However, with the exception of dicyclomine (80,81), there is no well-designed reproducible evidence of any therapeutic modality in other than small select groups of infants (4). The role of therapeutic formula changes for presumed cow's milk protein intolerance has the most support, but the number of infants for whom that is relevant and how to select them remain controversial (52,62,82–84). Consequently, the likelihood of defining specific therapies is small, and management remains difficult and uncertain for most infants.

In the absence of well-defined mechanisms, a potential approach may be organized in terms of the target behaviors of the intervention. There are two basic elements: one is the infant's behavior; the other is the caregiver's tolerance for the behavior. Both the crying and the caregiver's tolerance can change over time. Thus, for example, as previously described, the crying tends to increase and then decrease as the infant gets older. Similarly, caregiver tolerance may diminish as, for example, in a mother with postpartum depression. Effective management entails being sensitive to both.

There is no necessary and sufficient amount of crying that will determine whether an infant is seen as having colic (6,36). This will depend on the amount of crying in conjunction with the caregiver's tolerance. Tolerance can depend on a number of factors, including but not restricted to whether the mother is emotionally labile, whether the in-laws are pressuring the mother, other demands on her time, the health of the relationship of the mother and father, and so on. Furthermore, both the infant's and caregiver's behavior may interact to further change both infant behavior and caregiver tolerance. Thus, for example, Tronick and Gianino (85) argue that maternal depression might disrupt the normal "external" regulatory function that maternal responding typically provides for infants in the early postnatal months. In its absence, infants may increase self-directed behaviors (including crying) that reduce their engagement with the external environment and/or reflect their negative emotional state. As previously mentioned, depression may directly reduce maternal tolerance. However, the increased crying may also evoke egoistic, self-protective behavior in the caregiver (37), further reducing the likelihood of appropriate responding and reducing caregiver tolerance. Conversely, the increased crying may increase the caregiver's altruistic caring behavior, improving appropriate contingent responding and improving tolerance. In short, infant crying and caregiver tolerance are only the surface characteristics used to illustrate how the clinical concern can be generated. Both may be affected by mother–infant interactions that mutually exacerbate or diminish the likelihood of a clinical complaint.

TREATMENTS DIRECTED AT REDUCING INFANT CRYING

Medications

Although many medications have been tried, only dicyclomine hydrochloride has been studied systematically and found to be helpful in appropriately designed trials (80,81). However, colic has been removed as an indication for its use because of anecdotal reports of potentially dangerous side effects

(86,87). The other medications commonly used are combinations of alcohol, phenobarbital, and/or anticholinergics, but there is no systematic evidence for their efficacy (88,89). "Gripe water" is the most popular over-the-counter preparation; its active ingredients are sodium bicarbonate and alcohol. It has been speculated that its mechanism of action is the increased production of gastric gas through contact with gastric acid, thereby stimulating burping (18). Despite its popularity, its efficacy remains untested. To date, there are no controlled trials in which known analgesics have been shown to be effective.

Nutritional Treatments

Nutritional treatments have been the traditional first line of defense when colic is diagnosed. They are often suggested as a "therapeutic trial" and may "work" because the trial is started just about the time that crying would otherwise resolve. In a recent meta-analysis (62), the authors argued that the evidence supported the strategy of a formula change to remove cow's milk protein from the diet. However, this interpretation of the evidence has been challenged on methodologic grounds (52,84), and the issue remains unresolved. The challenge is to know which of the infants presenting with colic may benefit from a therapeutic trial and which may not. Gormally and Barr (22) have suggested that there are four clinical clues that may increase the likelihood that organic disease in general and cow's milk protein in particular may be implicated. They are infants (a) whose crying is described as "high pitched," who regularly arch their back during crying bouts and whose crying does not manifest a diurnal pattern; (b) for whom crying is not the only concern, i.e., there is also associated increased frequency of regurgitation of feeds, vomiting, diarrhea, or a positive physical examination; (c) in whom there is a late-onset increase in the third month after a switch from breast to formula feeding owing to cow's milk protein intolerance; and (d) whose crying persists beyond the third, and especially the fourth, month of life. It remains the case that the evidence that dietary changes are useful is true only for small, select groups of infants with colic, the size of the effect is modest, and the findings are unlikely to generalize to most infants with colic (4,23).

In breast-fed infants, colic is usually presumed to be secondary to "insufficient milk," for which a switch from formula is recommended. However, there is no evidence that breast-fed infants cry more or have more colic than formula-fed infants (54,90–92). One reason that a switch to formula might appear to work is that crying gets redistributed during the day (more in the morning and less in the evening), even though the overall 24-hour crying remains the same (91). A second option is to restrict intake of milk products in the mother because cow's milk proteins can be passed in breast milk (60,92). Impressive evidence for a positive effect was found in a small, select subgroup of infants in one study (58), but similar effectiveness was not confirmed in another (93).

Although not systematically studied, formula changes are most likely to be helpful in the subgroup of infants with manifestations other than crying, such as visible gastrointestinal peristalsis after cow's milk ingestion, weight loss, persistent regurgitation, or diarrhea (94). A therapeutic trial of formula change may also be indicated in refractory cases in which other options have failed. However, changing formula for its placebo effect is not indicated and has the negative effect of increasing maternal perception of infant vulnerability (95).

Behavioral Treatments

In general, behavioral treatments that work capitalize on the responsiveness of infants to constant, rhythmic stimulation, which may include auditory stimulation or movement of the infant. Noncommercial examples include background music, motor sounds from a washing machine, aquarium sounds (96), and rides in a car or stroller. Similar effects are obtained from a variety of technical substitutes available commercially. Such treatments are typically effective only while they are being used, with little effect after cessation of the intervention.

TREATMENTS DIRECTED AT INCREASING CAREGIVER TOLERANCE

Patient Information

There are probably few things that produce frustration and anxiety more effectively than the persistence, and especially the increase, of a behavior seen as indicating pain or hunger despite all attempts at "good mothering." Three types of information are important. The first concerns the typical course of crying (both in infants with and without colic) in the first 3 months, including its increase until 2 months and the evening clustering. Because it is commonly known as "3-month colic," it is also important to underline that colic may persist into the fourth and fifth months in 30% of infants. The second concerns identification of the caretaker's primary anxiety, usually that the infant is hungry, sick, or in pain. Understanding the crying does not necessarily entail that these consequences can be eliminated. Convergent evidence against hunger and disease can be obtained from the history and physical examination. Assurance that the infant is not in pain is impossible to demonstrate with confidence, although understanding that there are other possibilities and the elimination of disease entities reduce the likelihood that pain is implicated. New findings have increased the evidence that pain is unlikely to be responsible for the crying. One is the finding that, during a physical examination, infants with colic cried about twice as much as infants without, but there were no significant differences in heart rate, vagal tone (a measure of parasympathetic influence), or salivary cortisol (97). A second is the finding that, in all the follow-up studies to date, infants with colic do not fare any less well on any physical, behavioral, or temperamental outcome than infants without, assuming otherwise intact families (56).

The third informational task is to address some common misconceptions. Although much remains unknown, several assumptions from the cultural and medical lore are probably better classified as "misconceptions" than facts.

1. Neither crying nor colic is more common in breast- or formula-fed infants.
2. By performing "sham" diaper changes, Wolff (98) showed that wet diapers were not a sufficient cause of infant crying.
3. The concept that not responding to crying infants (in the first 3 months of life) prevents them from being "spoiled" has not been demonstrated. Furthermore, it is inconsistent with anthropologic evidence from other cultures in which immediate response to crying signals is virtually universal (99–101). As a treatment, withholding responses is both difficult and ineffective (102).
4. The belief that changing formulae is effective is out of proportion to the evidence supporting it.
5. There is no evidence that a "switch" from breast-feeding to formula is necessary or helpful in normally growing infants with colic.
6. Although affective disorders such as postpartum depression may affect infant behavior, colic also occurs in infants of parents without any affective distress in the postpartum period.

INFORMATION ABOUT WHAT NOT TO DO

Information about what not to do is as important as information about what to do. The single most serious consequence of crying that exceeds caregiver tolerance is shaken baby syndrome. Every parent should be counseled about the importance of never shaking their infant, no matter how long or how hard the infant cries. Although parents should be generally counseled to be responsive, it should be unambiguously clear that they should never shake their infant but rather put the infant down in a safe place and walk away until the frustration level subsides.

PROVISION OF RESPITE

A straightforward logistic adjustment that improves caretaker tolerance is provision of some degree of respite from the crying. The burden is usually asymmetrically borne by the mother; shared participation by the father is most helpful. Simply sharing nighttime feeding is worthwhile because maternal sleep deprivation is virtually universal. The crying often makes parents unwilling to leave the infant with other caretakers, fearing that they are "needed" by their infant. However, permitting the infant to be cared for by other family members or a baby-sitter is helpful, even for brief periods.

Caretaker As Co-investigator

Making the parents active co-investigators in a meaningful way in the detection of potential disease helps reduce anxiety. Keeping a parental diary (103) is helpful because it can provide critical information to evaluate the crying (104). The pattern on any particular day is likely to be highly variable, but an atypical pattern of crying across a week may raise the suspicion of disease. Diary records of formula intake are quite accurate (19). With daily records of weight, they can help screen for disease or inadequate nutrition. Furthermore, the act of recording crying often helps the caretaker to see that, despite impressions, the infant is not "crying all of the time."

Treatment for Affective Disturbance

Increased symptoms of maternal reactive depression are present in mothers of infants who present with "colic" (105,106). Whatever the causal direction, supportive intervention for the mother is indicated if postpartum depression is clinically significant.

TREATMENT AIMED AT CHANGING CARETAKER–INFANT INTERACTION

Crying in normal infants can be changed by modifications in caretaker–infant interaction, including carrying and rocking, immediate responsivity to infant signals, and shorter interfeed intervals (25,107–111). The strongest evidence is available for carrying and holding. In a randomized, controlled trial, increased carrying reduced the crying of noncolicky infants by 43% at 6 weeks of age or by 54% during the evening hours (25). The evidence is less strong, however, for infants with colic. In a parallel study in infants with established colic who were already being carried 4 hours a day, increasing carrying by 50% was no more effective than typical pediatric advice (25). In a small randomized, controlled trial, infants whose parents were closely followed by their pediatrician reduced their crying more quickly than those given formula changes, but the groups were small (112). However, new behavioral intervention trials with positive results are continuing to be reported in infants who, although not necessarily meeting the criteria for colic, are nevertheless irritable and cry a lot (52,84). Most emphasize sensitive and flexible contingent responsivity to infants and infant signals.

PREVENTION

With the exception of medications and feeding changes, the strategies relevant to modifying infant crying and caretaker tolerance are potentially more useful for prevention than for therapy. In the study of Barr and Hunziker of healthy infants, for example, only 16% of the infants whose parents increased their carrying time at 4 weeks subsequently met Wessel's criteria for colic, whereas 36% of the control infants did (25,34). Similarly, !Kung San mothers whose caretaking practice from birth includes a variety of features that might be predicted to be soothing have infants whose crying is similar to that of Western infants in pattern and frequency, but the duration is only approximately half as long (28) . However, recommending increased carrying from birth did not seem to be effective in one study (113). These findings imply that anticipatory guidance directed at encouraging more flexibility in caretaking behavior and anticipating parental concerns may have an important role in prevention, although more than increased carrying may be required.

SUMMARY

Many of the characteristics of the crying that is the criterion behavior of colic syndrome predispose to its being seen as a pain syndrome. These include its tendency to increase despite adequate caretaking, the prolonged crying bouts resistant to usual interventions, and the facial features, body posture, and vascular changes. However, independent evidence that colic is a manifestation of pain is lacking. The phenotypic similarities with, and lack of distinguishing features from, infants highly aroused but not in pain produce a "pain perplex" toward which caregiver tolerance and clinician response may vary, depending on their assumptions and significance.

In the face of such uncertainty, principles of management include attention to both the behavior of concern and the perception of the behavior. Whether or not pain is being experienced, measures that reduce distress in the infant, in the caretaker, or in the interaction are warranted, as they would be in any well-defined pain syndrome. Although demonstrated therapies are few, the syndrome is amenable to increasingly systematic investigation and well-controlled studies. When this pain perplex is untangled, we will understand much more about pain in infants.

REFERENCES

1. Little W, Fowler NO, Coupey S. *The shorter Oxford English dictionary on historical principles*, 3rd ed. Oxford: Clarendon Press, 1973.
2. Wessel MA, Cobb JC, Jackson EB, et al. Paroxysmal fussing in infancy, sometimes called "colic." *Pediatrics* 1954;14:421–434.
3. Illingworth RS. "Three months' colic." *Arch Dis Child* 1954;29:165–174.
4. Barr RG. Colic and gas. In: Walker WA, Durie PR, Hamilton JR, et al., eds. *Pediatric gastrointestinal disease*, 3rd ed. Hamilton, ON: BC Decker, 2000: 116–128.
5. St. James-Roberts I, Conroy S, Wilsher K. Clinical, developmental and social aspects of infant crying and colic. *Early Dev Parent* 1995;4:177–189.
6. Barr RG, Rotman A, Yaremko J, et al. The crying of infants with colic: a controlled empirical description. *Pediatrics* 1992;90:14–21.
7. St. James-Roberts I, Conroy S, Wilsher K. Bases for maternal perceptions of infant crying and colic behaviour. *Arch Dis Child* 1996;75:375–384.
8. Barr RG. Crying in context. *Early Dev Parent* 1995; 4:157–159.
9. Papousek M. Persistent crying, parenting and infant mental health. In: Fitzgerald HE, Osofsky JD, eds. *WAIMH handbook of infant mental health*, 4th ed., East Lansing, MI: World Association for Infant Mental Health, 1999.
10. Papousek M, von Hofacker N. Persistent crying in early infancy: a non-trivial condition of risk for the developing mother-infant relationship. *Child Care Health Dev* 1998;24:395–424.
11. Barr RG. Excessive crying. In: Sameroff AJ, Lewis M, Miller SM, eds. *Handbook of developmental psychopathology*, 2nd ed. New York: Kluwer Academic/Plenum Press, 2000:327–350
12. Lester BM, Boukydis CFZ, Garcia-Coll CT, et al. Symposium on infantile colic: introduction. *Infant Ment Health J* 1990;11:320–333.
13. Barr RG. Normality: a clinically useless concept; the case of infant crying and colic. *J Dev Behav Pediatr* 1993;14:264–270.
14. Lester BM, Boukydis CFZ, Garcia-Coll CT, et al. Infantile colic: acoustic cry characteristics, maternal perception of cry, and temperament. *Infant Behav Dev* 1992;15:15–26.
15. Zeskind PS, Barr RG. Acoustic characteristics of naturally occurring cries of infants with "colic." *Child Dev* 1997;68:394–403.
16. St. James-Roberts I. What is distinct about infants' "colic" cries? *Arch Dis Child* 1999;80:56–62.
17. Stahlberg M-R. Infantile colic: occurrence and risk factors. *Eur J Pediatr* 1984;143:108–111.
18. Levin S. Gripe water. *South Afr Med J* 1968;42: 753–757.
19. Barr RG, Wooldridge JA, Hanley J. Effects of formula change on intestinal hydrogen production and crying and fussing behavior. *J Dev Behav Pediatr* 1991;12: 248–253.
20. Miller JJ, McVeagh P, Fleet GH, et al. Effect of yeast lactase enzyme on "colic" in infants fed human milk. *J Pediatr* 1990;117:261–263.
21. Metcalf TJ, Irons TG, Sher LD, et al. Simethicone in the treatment of infant colic: a randomized placebo-controlled, multicenter trial. *Pediatrics* 1994;94: 29–34.
22. Gormally SM, Barr RG. Of clinical pies and clinical clues: proposal for a clinical approach to complaints of early crying and colic. *Ambul Child Health* 1997;3: 137–153.
23. Miller AR, Barr RG. Infantile colic: is it a gut issue? *Pediatr Clin North Am* 1991;38:1407–1423.
24. Brazelton TB. Crying in infancy. *Pediatrics* 1962; 29:579–588.
25. Hunziker UA, Barr RG. Increased carrying reduces infant crying: a randomized controlled trial. *Pediatrics* 1986;77:641–648.
26. Barr RG. The normal crying curve: what do we really know? *Dev Med Child Neurol* 1990;32:356–362.
27. St. James-Roberts I, Halil T. Infant crying patterns in

the first year: normal community and clinical findings. *J Child Psychol Psychiatry* 1991;32:951–968.

28. Barr RG, Konner M, Bakeman R, et al. Crying in !Kung infants: a test of the cultural specificity hypothesis. *Dev Med Child Neurol* 19911 33:601–610.
29. Barr RG, Paterson JA, McMartin LM, et al. "What is colic?": a test of the early difficult temperament hypothesis. *Pediatr Res Suppl* 2000;47:23a.
30. Wolff PH. *The development of behavioral states and the expression of emotions in early infancy: new proposals for investigation*. Chicago: University of Chicago Press, 1987.
31. Grunau RVE, Craig KD. Pain expression in neonates: facial action and cry. *Pain* 1987;28:395–410.
32. Barr RG. The "colic" enigma: prolonged episodes of a normal predisposition to cry. *Infant Ment Health J* 1990;11:340–348.
33. Geertsma MA, Hyams JS. The dilemma of infantile colic: distributing cry viewed in the context of communication and interpretation. In: Lester BM, Newman J, Pedersen F, eds. *Social and biological aspects of infant crying*. New York: Plenum, 1991.
34. Barr RG, McMullan SJ, Spiess H, et al. Carrying as colic "therapy": a randomized controlled trial. *Pediatrics* 1991;87:623–630.
35. St. James-Roberts I. Infant crying and its impact on parents. In: Barr RG, St. James-Roberts I, Keefe MR, et al., eds. *New evidence on unexplained early infant crying: its origins, nature and management*. New Brunswick, NJ: Johnson & Johnson Pediatric Institute, 2001:5–24.
36. Barr RG. Recasting a clinical enigma: the problem of early infant crying. In: Zelazo PH, Barr RG, eds. *Challenges to developmental paradigms*. Mahwah, NJ: Lawrence Erlbaum Associates, 1989:43–64.
37. Murray AD. Infant crying as an elicitor of parental behavior: an examination of two models. *Psychol Bull* 1979;86:191–215.
38. Bernal J. Crying during the first ten days of life. *Dev Med Child Neurol* 1972;14:362–372.
39. Bisping R, Steingrueber HJ, Oltmann M, et al. Adults tolerance of cries: an experimental investigation of acoustic features. *Child Dev* 1990;61:1218–1229.
40. Donovan WL, Leavitt LA. Simulating conditions of learned helplessness: the effects of interventions and attributions. *Child Dev* 1985;56:594–603.
41. Donovan WL, Leavitt LA, Walsh RO. Maternal self-efficacy: illusory control and its effect on susceptibility to learned helplessness. *Child Dev* 1990;61: 1638–1647.
42. Anand KJS, Hickey PR. Pain and its effects in the human neonate and fetus. *N Engl J Med* 1987;317:1321–1347.
43. Izard CE, Hembree EA, Hembree RR. Infants' emotional expressions to acute pain: developmental changes and stability of individual differences. *Dev Psychol* 1987;23:105–113.
44. Johnston CC, Strada ME. Acute pain response in infants: a multidimensional description. *Pain* 1986;24: 373–382.
45. Owens ME, Todt EH. Pain in infancy: neonatal reaction to heel lance. *Pain* 1984;20:77–86.
46. Barr RG. Pain experience in children: developmental and clinical characteristics. In: Wall PD, Melzack R, eds. *Textbook of pain*, 3rd ed. London: Churchill-Livingstone, 1994:739–764.
47. McGrath PA. *Pain in children: nature, assessment and treatment*. New York: Guilford Press, 1990.
48. Golub HL, Corwin MJ. A physioacoustic model of the infant cry. In: Lester BM, Boukydis CFZ, eds. *Infant crying: theoretical and research perspectives*. New York: Plenum Press, 1985:59–82
49. Grunau RVE, Johnston CC, Craig KD. Neonatal facial and cry responses to invasive and non-invasive procedures. *Pain* 1990;42:295–305.
50. Craig KD, Gilbert-MacLeod CA, Lilley CM. Crying as an indicator of pain in infants. In: Barr RG, Hopkins B, Green JA, eds. *Crying as a sign, a symptom, and a signal: clinical, emotional and developmental aspects of infant and toddler crying*. London: Mac Keith Press, 2000:23–40.
51. Talbot JD, Marrett S, Evans AC, et al. Multiple representations of pain in human cerebral cortex. *Science* 1991; 251:1355–1358.
52. Wolke D. The treatment of problem crying behavior. In: St. James-Roberts I, Harris G, Messer D, eds. *Infant crying, feeding and sleeping: development, problems and treatments*. New York: Harvester-Wheatsheef, 1993:47–79.
53. Geertsma MA, Hyams JS. Colic—a pain syndrome of infancy? *Pediatr Clin North Am* 1989;36:905–919.
54. Hide DW, Guyer BM. Prevalence of infantile colic. *Arch Dis Child* 1982;57:559–560.
55. Canivet C, Hagander B, Jakobsson I, et al. Infantile colic—less common than previously estimated? *Acta Paediatr* 1996;85:454–458.
56. Lehtonen L, Gormally SM, Barr RG. Clinical pies for etiology and outcome in infants presenting with early increased crying. In: Barr RG, Hopkins B, Green J, eds. *Crying as a sign, a symptom, and a signal: clinical, emotional, and developmental aspects of infant and toddler crying*. London: Mac Keith Press, 2000:67–95.
57. Lothe L, Lindberg T. Cow's milk whey protein elicits symptoms of infantile colic in colicky formula-fed infants: a double-blind crossover study. *Pediatrics* 1989; 83:262–266.
58. Jakobsson I, Lindberg T. Cow's milk proteins cause infantile colic in breast-fed infants: a double-blind crossover study. *Pediatrics* 1983;71:268–271.
59. Forsyth BWC. Colic and the effect of changing formulas: a double-blind, multiple-crossover study. *J Pediatr* 1989;115:521–526.
60. Clyne PS, Kulczycki A. Human breast milk contains bovine IgG. Relationship to infant colic? *Pediatrics* 1991;87:439–444.
61. Estep DC, Kulczycki A Jr. Treatment of infant colic with amino acid-based infant formula: a preliminary study. *Acta Paediatr* 2000;89:22–27.
62. Lucassen PLBJ, Assendelft WJJ, Gubbels JW, et al. Effectiveness of treatments for infantile colic: systematic review. *BMJ* 1998;316:1563–1569.
63. Lucassen PLBJ, Assendelft WJJ, Gubbels JW, et al. Infantile colic: crying time reduction with a whey hydrolysate: a double-blinded, randomized, placebo-controlled trial. *Pediatrics* 2000;106:1349–1354.
64. Hyams JS, Geertsma A, Etienne NL, et al. Colonic hydrogen production in infants with colic. *J Pediatr* 1989;115:592–594.
65. Miller JJ, McVeagh P, Fleet GH, et al. Breath hydrogen excretion in infants with colic. *Arch Dis Child* 1989; 64:725–729.

66. Moore DJ, Robb TA, Davidson GP. Breath hydrogen response to milk containing lactose in colicky and noncolicky infants. *J Pediatr* 1988;113:979–984.
67. Kearney PJ, Malone AJ, Hayes T, et al. A trial of lactase in the management of infant colic. *J Hum Nutr Diet* 1998;11:281–285.
68. Danielsson B, Hwang CP. Treatment of infantile colic with surface active substance (Simethicone). *Acta Paediatr Scand* 1985;74:446–450.
69. Mayer EA, Gebhart GF. Basic and clinical aspects of visceral hyperalgesia. *Gastroenterology* 1994;107: 271–293.
70. Fitzgerald M, Millard C, McIntosh N. Cutaneous hypersensitivity following peripheral tissue damage in newborn infants and its reversal with topical anaesthesia. *Pain* 1989;39:31–36.
71. Fitzgerald M. Neurobiology of fetal and neonatal pain. In: Melzack R, Wall PD, eds. *Textbook of pain*, 3rd ed. Edinburgh: Churchill-Livingstone, 1994:153–163.
72. Fitzgerald M, Anand KJS. Developmental neuroanatomy and neurophysiology of pain. In: Schechter NL, Berde CB, Yaster M, eds. *Pain in infants, children, and adolescents*. Baltimore: Williams & Wilkins, 1993:11–31.
73. Owens CM, Zhang D, Willis WD. Changes in the response states of primate spinothalamic cells caused by mechanical damage of the skin or activation of descending controls. *J Neurophysiol* 1992;67:1509–1527.
74. Fitzgerald M. Development of pain mechanisms. *Br Med Bull* 1991;47:667–675.
75. Fitzgerald M, Koltzenburg M. The functional development of descending inhibitory pathways in the dorsolateral funiculus of the newborn rat spinal cord. *Dev Brain Res* 1986;24:261–270.
76. Hadjistavropoulos HD, Craig KD, Grunau RVE, et al. Judging pain in infants: behavioural, contextual, and developmental determinants. *Pain* 1997;72:319–324.
77. Gustafson GW, Green JA. On the importance of fundamental frequency and other acoustic features in cry perception and infant development. *Child Dev* 1989; 60:772—780.
78. Gustafson GE, Wood RM, Green JA. Can we hear the causes of infants' crying? In: Barr RG, Hopkins B, Green JA, eds. *Crying as a sign, a symptom, and a signal: clinical, emotional and developmental aspects of infant and toddler crying*. London: Mac Keith Press, 2000:8–22.
79. Barr RG. Colic and gas. In: Walker WA, Durie PR, Hamilton JR, et al., eds. *Pediatric gastrointestinal disease: pathophysiology, diagnosis and management*. Burlington, VT: BC Decker, 1991:55–61.
80. Weissbluth M. Dicyclomine in infantile colic. *J Pediatr* 1984;105:503–504.
81. Illingworth RS. Evening colic in infants: a double blind trial of dicyclomine hydrochloride. *Lancet* 1959; 2:1119–1120.
82. Lucassen PLBJ, Assendelft WJJ, Gubbels JW, et al. Infantile colic: crying time reduction with a whey hydrolysate: a double-blind, randomized, placebo-controlled trial. *Pediatrics* 2000;106:1349–1354.
83. Wolke D, Meyer R. The colic debate. *Pediatrics* 1995; 96:165–166.
84. Wolke D. Behavioral treatment of prolonged crying: evaluation, methods and a proposal. In: Barr RG, St. James-Roberts I, Keefe MR, et al., eds. *New evidence on unexplained early infant crying: its origins, nature and management*. Miami: Warner Brothers Publications, 2001:187–207.
85. Tronick EZ, Gianino AF Jr. The transmission of maternal disturbance to the infant. In: Tronick ES, Field T, eds. *Maternal depression and infant disturbance: new direction for child development*, 34th ed. San Francisco: Jossey-Bass, 1986:5–11.
86. Williams J, Watkin-Jones R. Dicyclomine: worrying symptoms associated with its use in some small babies. *BMJ* 1984;288:901.
87. Edwards PD, Spoudeas H, Shribman S. Dicyclomine in colic [letter]. *BMJ* 1984;288:1230.
88. O'Donovan JC, Bradstock AS. The failure of conventional drug therapy in the management of infantile colic. *Am J Dis Child* 1979;133:999–1001.
89. Robinson LA, Brown AL. Colic: pharmaceutic and medical intervention. *Pediatr Nurs* 1979;5:61–64.
90. Thomas DW, McGilligan K, Eisenberg LD, et al. Infantile colic and type of milk feeding. *Am J Dis Child* 1987;141:451–453.
91. Barr RG, Kramer MS, Pless IB, et al. Feeding and temperament as determinants of early infant cry/fuss behaviour. *Pediatrics* 1989;84:514–521.
92. Jakobsson I, Lindberg T, Benediktsson B, et al. Dietary bovine beta-lactoglobulin is transferred to human milk. *Acta Paediatr Scand* 1985;74:342–345.
93. Evans RW, Fergusson DM, Allardyce RA, et al. Maternal diet and infantile colic in breast-fed infants. *Lancet* 1981;1:1340–1342.
94. Gormally S. Clinical clues to organic etiologies in infants with colic. In: Barr RG, St. James-Roberts I, Keefe MR, et al., eds. *New evidence on unexplained early infant crying: its origins, nature and management*. New Brunswick, NJ: Johnson & Johnson Pediatric Institute, 2001:133–148.
95. Forsyth BWC, Canny PF. Perceptions of vulnerability 3 1/2 years after problems of feeding and crying behavior in early infancy. *Pediatrics* 1991;88:757–763.
96. Peña SL. How we cured colic. *McCall's* May 1991: 63–64.
97. White BP, Gunnar MR, Larson MC, et al. Behavioral and physiological responsivity, sleep and patterns of daily cortisol production in infants with and without colic. *Chil Dev* 2000;71:862–877.
98. Wolff PH. The natural history of crying and other vocalizations in early infancy. In: Foss BM, ed. *Determinants of infant behavior*. London: Methuen, 1969: 81–108.
99. Bakeman R, Adamson LB, Konner M, et al. Sequential analyses of !Kung infant communication: inducing and recruiting. In: Amsel E, Renninger KA, eds. *Change and development: issues of theory, method, and application*. Mahwah, NJ: Lawrence Erlbaum Associates, 1997:173–192.
100. Konner M J. Maternal care, infant behavior and development among the !Kung. In: Lee RB, DeVore I, eds. Kalahari hunter-gatherers, studies of the !Kung San and their neighbors. Cambridge: Harvard University Press, 1976:218–245.
101. Lozoff B, Brittenham G. Infant care: cache or carry. *J Pediatr* 1979;95:478–483.
102. Taubman B. Clinical trial of the treatment of colic by modification of parent-infant interaction. *Pediatrics* 1984;74:998–1003.

103. Barr RG, Kramer MS, Leduc DG, et al. Parental diary of infant cry and fuss behaviour. *Arch Dis Child* 1988; 63:380–387.
104. Hill DJ, Menahem S, Hudson I, et al. Charting infant distress: an aid to defining colic. *J Pediatr* 1992;121: 755–758.
105. Miller AR, Barr RG, Eaton WO. Crying and motor behavior of six-week-old infants and postpartum maternal mood. *Pediatrics* 1993;92:551–558.
106. Murray L, Cooper P. The impact of irritable infant behavior on maternal mental state: a longitudinal study and a treatment trial. In: Barr RG, St. James-Roberts I, Keefe MR, et al., eds. *New evidence on unexplained early infant crying: its origins, nature and management.* New Brunswick, NJ: Johnson & Johnson Pediatric Institute, 2001:149–164.
107. Barr RG, Elias MF. Nursing interval and maternal responsivity: effect on early infant crying. *Pediatrics* 1988;81:529–536.
108. Bell SM, Ainsworth DS. Infant crying and maternal responsiveness. *Child Dev* 1972;43:1171–1190.
109. Sander LW, Stechler G, Burns P, et al. Early mother-infant interaction and 24-hour patterns of anxiety and sleep. *J Am Acad Child Psychiatry* 1970;9:103–123.
110. Gordon T, Foss BM. The role of stimulation in the delay of onset of crying in the newborn infant. *Q J Exp Psychol* 1966;18:79–81.
111. Ourth L, Brown KB. Inadequate mothering and disturbance in the neonatal period. *Child Dev* 1961;32: 287–295.
112. Taubman B. Parental counselling compared with elimination of cow's milk or soy milk protein for the treatment of infant colic syndrome: a randomized trial. *Pediatrics* 1988;81:756–761.
113. St. James-Roberts I, Hurry J, Bowyer J, et al. Supplementary carrying compared with advice to increase responsive parenting as interventions to prevent persistent crying. *Pediatrics* 1995;95:381–388.

43

Facial Pain in Children and Adolescents

Nalton F. Ferraro

ACUTE AND CHRONIC FACIAL PAIN

Overview

This chapter deals with both acute and chronic facial pain in children and adolescents. Headache is presented in another chapter, but there is a definite relationship between headache and facial pain. The child often complains of both. In the evaluation of a child with facial pain, it is important to think regionally, with an awareness of the pain referral patterns that exist.

For simplicity's sake, pain from various structures is considered separately (e.g., teeth, jaws, paranasal sinus, ears, temporomandibular joint (TMJ), nasopharynx, oropharynx, eyes, and periorbital areas). A regional approach is then discussed. The diagnosis can be straightforward; for example, a child can point to a carious tooth and state that this is the tooth that aches. The diagnosis can be difficult; the ear pain in a teenager may be from a carious but impacted lower wisdom tooth. So when a particular facial region hurts, the anatomy of the region and the referral pattern of pain must be considered. A seasoned examiner can still be humbled from time to time because of the number, complexity, and "shared innervation" of the structures of the head and face.

The diagnosis and management of pain syndromes and chronic pain in the face carry with them the same "anatomic burdens" that acute pain does but now with the additional complexities of chronic pain.

The child with chronic facial pain may present weeks or months after the onset of pain. Multiple diagnostic tests and workups may have preceded, and many practitioners may have been consulted. Conversely, the child or teenager may have been cared for initially for an acute problem, but the usual predictable responses do not occur. The patient does not get better in the usual time period. One then faces a chronic pain problem, and, even in retrospect, the caretaker cannot define the transition zone from acute pain to chronic pain. It often takes a "stepping back" for a new look at the problem. The patient and family, of course, must be part of this stepping back and reorienting. This reorientation must be done with sensitivity and tact by all involved and particularly by the primary practitioner. Surgeons and dentists, by nature of their practices, must be particularly aware of this phenomenon. Their orientation is often toward mechanical causes of pain, and if a mechanical cause is not found, the problem may be discounted.

For example, an endodontist treats a patient with a bad toothache from a tooth that has an unequivocally inflamed pulp. Root canal treatment is accomplished, but the patient continues to have pain. Antibiotics and narcotics are continued for 2 to 3 weeks or longer, but the toothache continues. The other teeth are examined carefully during this period; the root canal filling is removed from the tooth, but the pain continues. Diagnostic local anesthetic blocks appear to help. A decision is finally made to remove the tooth. The patient has continuing, severe postextraction pain. Narcotics have now been used for more than a month. The endodontist and oral surgeon suggest that a neuralgia might be the diagnosis, and the patient is sent to a neurologist. The patient has an evaluation including magnetic resonance imaging (MRI) of the brain and base of the skull; no pathology is noted. The pain is not consistent with one of the "classic" neuralgias.

There is a clear danger here of undermining whatever remaining confidence the patient and family has or of making the family defensive indeed. This happens if the reorientation is too abrupt, if the primary practitioner paints a black-and-white picture between physical causes of pain and psychologic causes of pain. The patient will come away thinking that the practitioner thinks that "this pain is all in my head." The patient will vacillate between agreeing with this conclusion at times to being defensive and angry because he is "not believed."

It takes experience and patience to help a patient at this time. Even if the primary practitioner does not understand the subtleties of modern pain theory, it must be understood that pain is a complex phenomenon. One must recognize the characteristics of chronic pain, the important psychologic manifestations, the risk factors in the patient that compound the pain and its perception, and the "emotional and physical consequences of persistent severe pain" (1).

It is perfectly consistent to work up a patient for an occult base of skull tumor that might be the cause of facial pain while providing or referring the patient for psychologic support or other therapies to help deal with the consequences of pain or factors that may be exacerbating it. Bonica (2) states that "pain is always subjective." Practitioners must not paint a black-and-white picture of pain and its causes. If MRI of the brain and skull base does not reveal a tumor, this is important. It, however, does not absolve the observed anatomic structures from participation in the production of pain. It just means that the limits of resolution of our "looking glass" into the human body have been reached. Reminding the patient of this is itself beneficial.

With experience comes a good sense of the typical course of the acute diseases and injuries that we see and of the operations and procedures that we perform. While allowing for natural variations among people, we must keep a keen eye out for warning signs that pain is becoming chronic, with its attendant behavioral changes. Early intervention may prevent much suffering.

OROFACIAL STRUCTURES AND PAIN

Teeth and Supporting Structures

Dentistry and Pain

Pain and anxiety have been associated with both dental disease and dental treatment. Toothache can be excruciating, but the dental profession has long been in the forefront of the management of dental pain and anxiety. In the 1840s, Horace Wells and William T. G. Morton founded general anesthesia. Wells, a dentist, used nitrous oxide, and Morton, a physician and dentist, used ether for surgical procedures (3). The introduction of intravenous barbiturates in the 1930s led to the techniques of intravenous general anesthesia for ambulatory oral surgery. Victor Goldman and Stanley Drummond-Jackson in England and Adrian Hubbell in the United States were pioneers in this work (3). Local anesthetics have become a mainstay in dental practice. In this section, the various types of dental pain in children and adolescents are described.

Pertinent Dental and Oral Anatomy

The innervation of the oral mucosa is regionally specialized, and patterns differ in lip, cheek, tongue, gingiva, and palate. Innervation is extensive and includes free nerve endings, Merkel-receptor complexes, and chemosensory corpuscles in the epithelium. Subepithelial receptors include mechanosensory corpuscles, Ruffini-like receptors, and free nerve endings (4).

There are rich free nerve endings at the epithelial junction of the gingiva to the tooth. Within the periodontal ligament are mechanoreceptors and free nerve endings, especially in the inferior (apical) one-third of the root (4). The mechanoreceptors are ex-

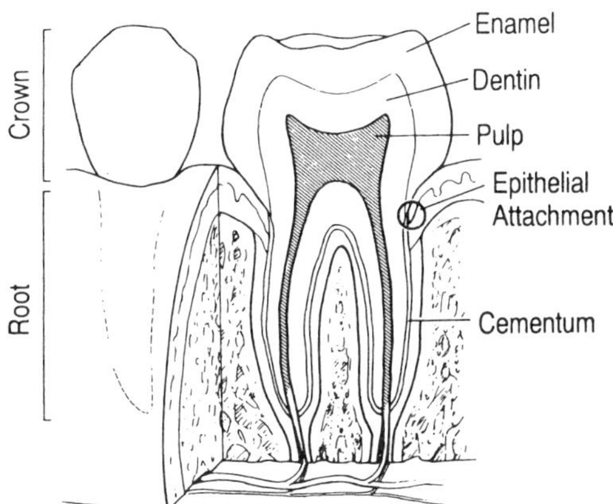

FIGURE 43.1. The tooth. There is an epithelial attachment of hemidesmosomes that encircles the tooth separating the oral environment from the alveolar bone and periodontal ligament. Both the periodontal ligament, which "attaches" the tooth to the alveolar bone, and the pulp are highly innervated.

ceedingly important and sensitive; a dental restoration that is a fraction of a millimeter too high can be discerned.

The pulp of the tooth is innervated by unmyelinated c fibers and very small myelinated fibers, and there are free nerve endings into the dentin. Recall that the enamel is the hard outer layer of the tooth crown; the root is covered by the softer cementum. The middle layer of the tooth is dentin, and the pulp chamber and pulp canal are innermost (Fig. 43.1). Electrical stimulation studies of human teeth have been performed (5,6) and demonstrate that the most sensitive fibers conduct with small intensity stimuli that produce a "prepain" stimulus (4,5). At higher intensities, a sharp pain is felt, and, at the high intensities, a dull ache is perceived. There is fluid within the dentinal tubules (the structural element of dentin), and this fluid can conduct thermal, osmotic, and mechanical stimuli to the nerve endings deep within the dentin and pulp. A break in the enamel makes transmission to the dentin easier. Inflammatory products (substance P, histamine, bradykinin, prostaglandins, and serotonin) have additional affects on the c fibers once inflammation begins.

Toothache

Early Toothache (Fig. 43.2A)

The first sensation noted in a carious tooth can be sensitivity to sweets (presumably from osmotic effect on the dentinal tubules) and to cold drinks (thermal effect on the dentinal fluids). The sharp pain that is felt is strictly lim-

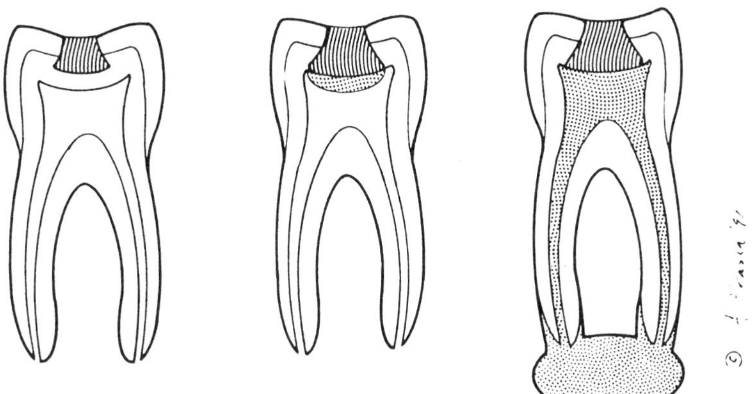

FIGURE 43.2. A: Caries (the breakdown of tooth structure by bacterial action) represented by the hatched area has involved the dentin. **B:** The pulp has now become involved with caries, and there will be pulpal inflammation and necrosis. **C:** The pulp is infected and necrotic, and the periapical area of the alveolar bone can contain an abscess.

ited and disappears after the stimulus is removed from the tooth. The cold- or sweet-sensitive tooth can usually be treated with removal of caries and placement of a restoration. At this time, the pain can be localized to the offending tooth.

Irreversible Pulpitis (Fig. 43.2B)

If untreated, the pain will progress. Thermal stimulation will provide sharp, sometimes excruciating pain that will continue after the stimulus is removed for minutes to hours. The pain will also occur spontaneously, sometimes awakening the patient from sleep. At this time, the pain can become diffuse. An upper molar can initiate pain that involves the whole hemimaxilla, into the retro-orbital area and extending into the anterotemporal area. All the teeth on the affected side can be involved in what becomes an unrelenting, throbbing pain. An upper anterior tooth can refer pain to the eye and orbit.

A lower molar inflamed to this degree can also cause a diffuse pain that will involve all the lower teeth, the ear, and the posterior temporal region (Fig. 43.3). The patient soon cannot localize the pain to the upper or lower arch. The patient paces, cradles the head, takes large doses of proprietary analgesics but gains no relief. The younger child will cry and scream inconsolably.

The pulp at this point is irreversibly inflamed. There can be microabscesses within the pulp, and necrosis begins. The pulp is within a rigid structure, and edema leads to ischemia and pulpal necrosis. In a multirooted tooth, one pulp canal may have intensely in-

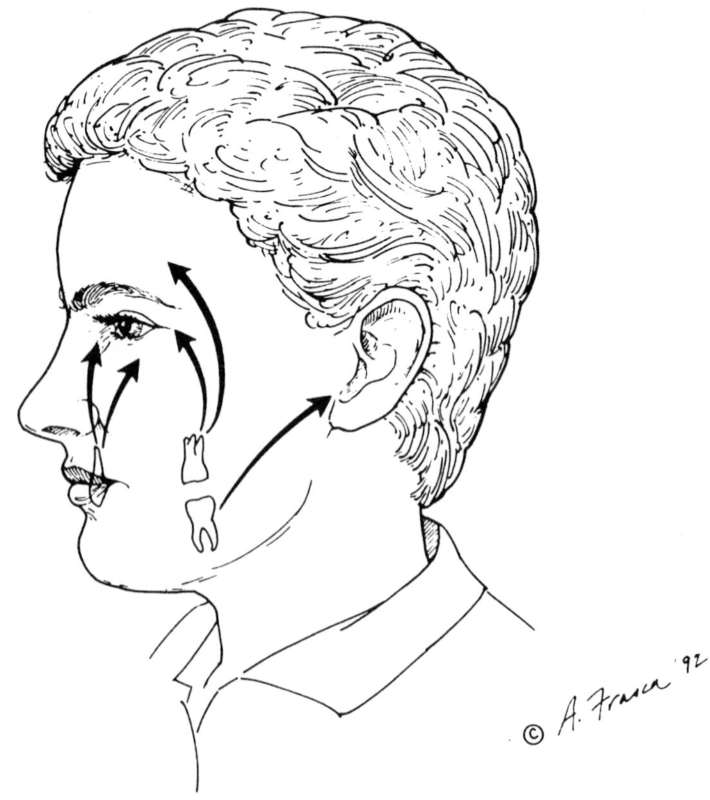

FIGURE 43.3. Referral and radiating pain patterns from an upper anterior tooth, upper molar, and lower molar.

flamed pulp and another canal can have totally necrotic pulp (4).

If the tooth is not treated, this intense pain may continue for days with occasional abatement. In some patients, cold will bring relief. This is usually discovered accidentally as the patient takes some water with pain medicine. Seeing a drawn and exhausted patient in the emergency department holding a container of ice water reinforces the terrible reputation of toothache.

The patient and the dentist may not be able to localize the involved tooth. The tooth may not be sensitive to percussion or palpation; there may be no facial swelling.

The toothache that becomes spontaneous and continuous indicates a pulp that is irreversibly inflamed. A simple restoration cannot be done; the tooth must have the pulp removed (root canal therapy) or be extracted.

Periapical Abscess (Fig. 43.2C)

If treatment is not received, the toothache may spontaneously remit after the pulp is necrotic. The periapical area of the tooth becomes the next area of activity. This periapical area contains both free nerve endings and mechanoreceptors; pain from inflammation and sepsis in this area can be provoked by tapping on the tooth. This tenderness to percussion can develop while the intense pulpal pain is ongoing. Conversely, weeks or months may pass before the tooth becomes tender to palpation and percussion, or the tooth may never become symptomatic again after the pulpal toothache subsides. The sensitivity of the periodontal/periapical innervation is sometimes dramatically underscored. Even a noninfected tooth that is being occlusally traumatized can become exquisitely tender. A 10-year-old boy presented to the emergency department in agony with left facial pain and headache. He required parenteral narcotics, and an emergency head computed tomography scan was obtained, which was negative. The cause of his pain was a tooth that had been elevated in its socket by an orthodontic device. He traumatized this tooth every time he bit down. The appliance was removed, and the patient was pain free in 12 hours.

An abscess or granuloma can develop in this periapical-alveolar bone region (4). Osteolysis with a periapical radiolucency may be seen on radiographs. This situation can result in an acute abscess with a tooth that is elevated in its socket because of edema in the periapical region. Such a tooth then begins to throb, sometimes agonizingly so, and the tooth is easily identifiable because it is exquisitely tender to percussion. The patient will not chew or allow the teeth to occlude. The danger here is that the suppurative process at the periapical area can track through the alveolar bone and perforate into the subperiosteal space. From this space, the infection can track into various anatomic spaces of the head and neck and cause facial or pharyngeal swelling. These spaces include the vestibular spaces, submandibular space, parapharyngeal spaces, buccal space, orbital area, paranasal sinuses, and the large veins of the head extending intracranially. Odontogenic infections are beyond the scope of this chapter, but it is critical to note the complete spectrum of events that begin with caries in a tooth.

Having described a classic progression of a toothache, the classic case is not the only presentation. A patient may have a carious tooth with a periapical radiolucency but not recall a toothache. If a toothache is recalled, it is not as dramatic as the pulpal toothache described above. Variations in presentation exist.

Toothache in Children

With this foundation in the classic progression of a toothache, the differences in children can now be noted. Deciduous teeth rarely produce the intense toothache described; why this is so is not known. Children can have primary molars that have nonvital pulps and report no pain (7). The child with neglected primary dentition can first present with a swollen face. On close questioning, a history of pain can be elicited from the parents, but parents who are not dentally aware may dismiss the pain's importance when it subsides.

The other major difference is that the pulp in deciduous teeth can be more forgiving than that in fully developed permanent teeth. Developing permanent teeth also have reduced sensitivity. Incomplete development of the sensory innervation is said to be the reason for this experimental and clinical finding (4). These exceptions aside, the child and adolescent can be subject to toothache and odontogenic abscess in its various forms.

Periodontal Pain

The periodontium includes the supporting structures of the tooth, gingiva, gingival epithelial attachment to the tooth, and periodontal ligament that "suspends" the tooth in its socket by linking the alveolar bone to the cementum with ligamentous fibers. Recall that the periodontal ligament includes blood vessels and various nerve fibers, including free nerve endings and mechanoreceptors.

Acute Necrotizing Ulcerative Gingivitis (Trench Mouth, Vincent Infection) and Recurrent Aphthous Stomatitis

Acute Necrotizing Ulcerative Gingivitis

Acute necrotizing ulcerative gingivitis is a painful gingival infection that results in ulceration and necrosis of the dental gingival papillae, the formation of a pseudomembrane covering the ulcerated gingiva. Lymphadenopathy, fever, malaise, and anorexia are associated. The putative pathogens are spirochetes and fusiform bacilli (8). The pain can be intense, and good pain management is part of the early care of these patients. The incidence of acute necrotizing ulcerative gingivitis is decreasing in industrialized nations, but it certainly is not rare in teenagers. In underdeveloped countries, it is common and affects children younger than 10 years of age. Factors that predispose children to acute necrotizing ulcerative gingivitis include malnutrition, emotional stress, lack of sleep, and debilitating systemic illnesses (8).

Recurrent Aphthous Stomatitis (Canker Sores)

Young patients can have recurrent oral ulceration (canker sores). These lesions can appear singly or in clusters. They have a necrotic center with an erythematous halo involving multiple mucosal sites. Canker sores are exquisitely tender and of unknown origin. They can appear at times of physical or emotional stress. Differential diagnosis includes Behçet syndrome, herpetic lesions, allergic stomatitis, and (rarely) pemphigus or mucous membrane pemphigoid, and erythema multiforme. Treatment is symptomatic, and various remedies are provided in the section on stomatitis secondary to chemotherapy for cancer.

Pericoronitis (Fig. 43.4)

The flap of gingiva that covers a partially erupted tooth is prone to infection; this is pericoronitis. Food, oral debris, and anaerobic bacteria collect under the gingival flap and cause a soft-tissue infection with edema of the tissue flap (9). If an opposing tooth is present, the swollen gingival flap is now traumatized by the opposing tooth. Pericoronitis is most common at lower third molar sites. Treatment includes oral rinses, antibiotics, removal of the impinging opposing wisdom tooth, and removal of the lower wisdom tooth when the infection subsides. Pericoronitis from lower wisdom teeth can be trivial or can develop into a life-threatening infection. The anatomic proximity of the parapharyngeal space makes wisdom tooth pericoronitis potentially dangerous. The midteens to early 20s is the peak age period for wisdom tooth pericoronitis. Although full-blown pericoronitis is painful, it does not present any diagnostic dilemmas.

This discussion of pericoronitis is important background for related but more subtle issues. The possibility of pain from impacted teeth, especially the third molar, is a recurrent theme. In fact, a wisdom tooth that is apparently covered by gingiva can become carious and develop a toothache. There can be a tiny opening in the gingival covering of an im-

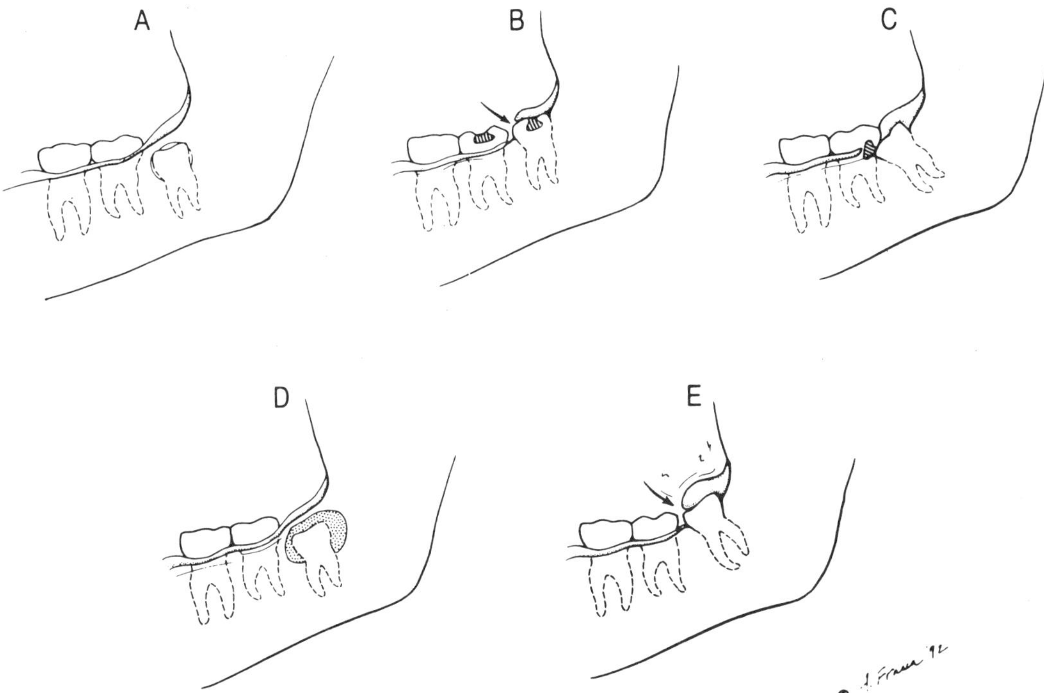

FIGURE 43.4. A: A totally impacted lower wisdom tooth without oral communication. **B:** A soft tissue–covered wisdom tooth that can become carious because it communicates with the oral environment and is impossible to clean. **C:** A tipped impacted wisdom tooth that has caused caries in or damage to the second molar tooth. **D:** A totally impacted tooth with an associated dentigerous cyst. **E:** Pericoronitis. The soft-tissue flap (operculum) covering a partially impacted tooth can become infected often with anaerobic bacteria. The flap swells and can then be traumatized by an opposing tooth. Pericoronitis can extend and become a life-threatening parapharyngeal infection.

pacted tooth. This opening can allow substrate and caries-causing bacteria to colonize the tooth; caries then develops in a tooth that is basically not visible in the mouth. Severe pain has been noted in this circumstance, and only careful radiographs of the impacted tooth can shed light on a diagnostic dilemma. The author has seen young teenagers treated for otitis and TMJ pain when the cause was pulpal pain from a carious wisdom tooth.

Fully Impacted Tooth

The converse situation involves a totally impacted wisdom tooth that does not communicate with the oral cavity. One must assume that these teeth are not the cause of facial pain. If fully impacted teeth were the cause of facial pain, then one could expect unusual facial pain patterns in most children from infancy through the late teens because the jaws are filled with impacted teeth through childhood. These pain patterns are, however, not seen. Anecdotes perpetuate the relationship of impacted wisdom teeth and facial pain. They are based on the cases in which wisdom teeth are removed for facial pain that has eluded diagnosis and the pain abates.

Teeth that are fully impacted and radiographically normal should not be considered the cause of vague facial pain for an important reason: Attention will be turned from more fruitful diagnostic paths; important pathology may be missed. The prophylactic removal of wisdom teeth has pros and cons, and there is disagreement in the oral and maxillofacial surgical profession on this matter. Debate about indications for prophylactic removal is beyond the scope and concern of this chapter, but the caveat remains. Fully impacted wisdom teeth are rarely the cause of facial pain.

Nose and Paranasal Sinuses

Sinusitis and Pain

The pain from sinus disease is closely related to dental pain. After the maxillary sinus is formed and aerated after age 6 years, acute sinusitis can present as midfacial pain with painful maxillary teeth that are tender to percussion. The pain can radiate to the orbit and the anterior temporal region, which is in the V2 dermatome. Periapical dental infections can (rarely) cause sinusitis by perforation of the antral lining with the septic process or the sinusitis may be of independent origin with pain referred to the teeth.

The other paranasal sinuses can also be involved with periorbital, frontal, and cheek pain. Signs such as tenderness to palpation, pain with bending the head, swelling, erythema, and pus visualized intranasally (especially at the middle meatus) should be sought (10).

Pain Referral Patterns from Nose and Paranasal Sinuses

A very interesting collection of diagrams is provided by Stevenson (11) regarding work performed by Harold Wolff and associates. These diagrams map the location of facial pain after electrical stimulation of various nasal and paranasal structures. Stimulation of the inferior turbinate caused pain in the upper teeth and along the cheek in the V1 to V3 distribution. Superior turbinate stimulation resulted in pain along the nose and medial orbit. Middle turbinate stimulation caused pain in the middle part of the cheek from the preauricular area to the nasolabial region. Stimulation of the maxillary sinus ostium caused pain that extended from the infraorbital region up to the temporal region. Superior nasal cavity stimulation elicited periorbital pain and pain in the canine and bicuspid teeth. Sphenoidal sinus stimulation resulted in pain at the top of the head. Maxillary sinus stimulation elicited pain in the upper teeth and the periorbital region. Emotional conflict resulted in nasal hypersecretion pain in the midface, the preauricular region, and into the frontal region (Fig. 43.5).

Clinical examination and radiographic studies can help in the diagnosis of acute sinusitis. Although acute sinusitis does not present in children as flagrantly as it does in adults (12), patients older than 10 years of age are more likely to show an adult pattern. Children 2 to 6 years of age often show posterior nasal obstruction with adenoid blockage. Patients younger than the age of 2 years have a picture indistinguishable from viral upper respiratory infection. Milmoe (12) stresses that when the diagnosis of sinusitis is considered, one must look for symptoms and signs of nasal congestion, allergies, snoring, quality of the rhinorrhea, odor, coughing, eye discomfort, visual dysfunction, and dental pain.

Nasal Obstruction

Nasal congestion and obstruction can result from several important problems in addition to chronic sinusitis. These include adenoid hyperplasia, allergic rhinitis, chronic hypertrophic rhinitis, nasal polyposis, and deviated nasal septum. A list of congenital malformations and tumors that result in nasal obstruction includes encephalocele, various craniofacial deformities, dermoids, craniopharyngiomas, teratomas, posterior choanal stenosis, and nasoalveolar and nasopharyngeal cysts (13). One must be very cautious when there is unilateral sinusitis or nasal obstruction because foreign bodies or tumors must be considered.

Chronic Sinusitis and Pain

The important lessons here are (a) sinusitis must be considered when there is facial pain

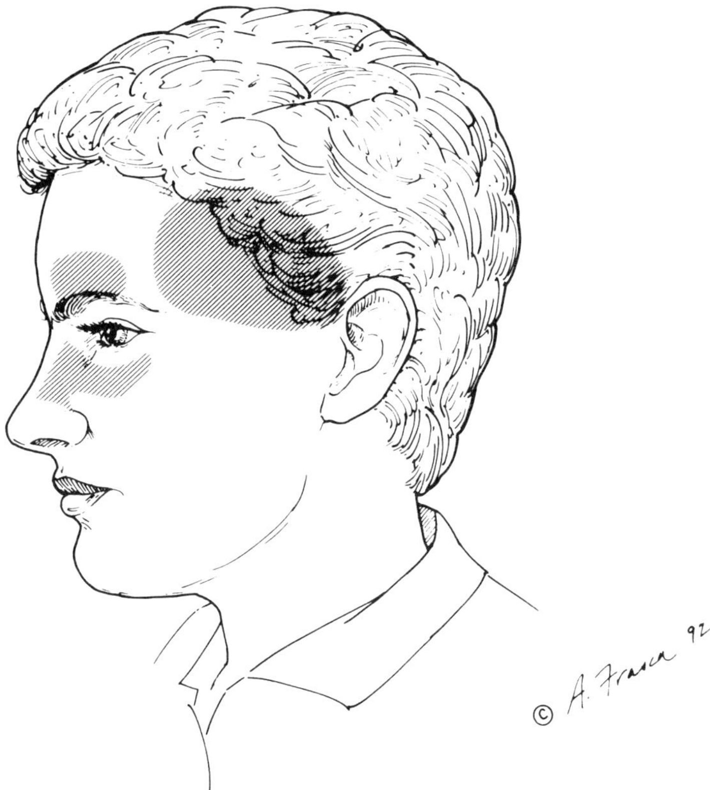

FIGURE 43.5. This is only one example of a pain pattern that can be secondary to a nasal or antral lesion. Referral patterns are listed in detail in the text.

in a child; (b) it is important to search for symptoms and signs that are related, e.g., nasal obstruction and the others listed above; (c) unilateral sinusitis and pain raises a red flag in regard to causes; (d) sinusitis cannot be a "dumping ground" diagnosis (a parent very often decides that the cause of the child's facial pain is "sinusitis"); and (e) appropriate referral to an otorhinolaryngologist should be made in a timely fashion.

Milmoe (12) states that "chronic sinusitis in children has become a popular band wagon in the past several years with much medical therapy and now even more surgical therapy being espoused." Chronic sinusitis is an important diagnosis, but it should be a well-considered diagnosis based on clinical and radiographic data. Its relationship to facial pain must be determined on a case-by-case basis.

Preauricular and Ear Region Pain

Ear pain and preauricular pain are very common in childhood. Otitis media is probably the most common diagnosis that is made in pediatric practice associated with ear pain. The febrile child crying and pulling at an ear is a classic pediatric image. These acute earaches are generally diagnosed and treated in a straightforward manner. Hayden and Schwartz (14) graded clinically the severity of otalgia associated with acute otitis media with effusion by questioning the parent and/or child. Pain was severe in 42% and more likely to be associated with redness of the tympanic membrane. Pain was more likely to be absent in children younger than 2 years of age (14,15). Sometimes the ear pain may not be from middle ear disease. This can be quite confusing when a child has a long history of otitis media; subsequent bouts of ear pain are quickly determined to be related to ear disease, but this may not be the case.

Temporomandibular Joint and Ear Pain

Temporomandibular joint pain and myofascial pain can present as ear pain. In the chronic pain section, this area of overlap is covered very thoroughly. In any case, when there is acute ear pain, the ear must be examined and ear disease ruled out before considering the other causes.

The diagnosis of otitis externa is made by inspection of the ear canal and the finding that traction on the pinna or tragus is painful. Acute TMJ tenderness can be elicited by pressure or traction on the tragus but not on the pinna.

Salivary Glands

The differential diagnosis of pain in the ear/preauricular region must also include salivary gland disease. The area of the parotid gland must be palpated, searching for swelling. Recall that the superior pole of the gland is at the level of the tragus, and its bulk is inferior, hugging the posterior border of the mandibular ramus. Buccal and submandibular swellings can be misdiagnosed as parotitis because of an unfamiliarity with the anatomy. There are lymph nodes within the parotid gland, and lymphadenitis can also be misdiagnosed as a primary parotitis. Gentle palpation of the gland while inspecting intraorally with good lighting is important. One can see whether there is any salivary flow at the Stensen duct and whether it is clear, cloudy, or frankly purulent. Recurrent parotitis of bacterial origin is an entity recognized in children (16,17).

Intermittent submandibular pain with swelling can be the result of intermittent obstruction of the submandibular salivary gland, often from sialolithiasis. The submandibular gland is easily palpated bimanually with the gloved index finger in the floor of the mouth and the finger pads of the other hand on the skin of the submandibular region. The submandibular (Wharton) duct can be examined at its ostium behind the lower anterior teeth while the gland is gently palpated; salivary flow can be observed (17).

Ear and Pharyngeal Relationship

Pain in the ear canal/preauricular area may also be the first sign of tumor in the otomastoid, retromandibular/infratemporal fossa area. A high index of suspicion and thorough pursuit of persistent complaints of pain are important (18). We have also observed sclerosing osteomyelitis of the mandible present with preauricular and ramus pain (9). Pharyngeal processes and tonsillar processes can also refer pain to the ear.

Eye and Periorbital Structures, Ocular Pathology, and Pain

Previous sections noted that the teeth, sinuses, and nasal structures can refer pain to the eye and orbit. Headaches can frequently refer pain to the eyes. It is important to state that "without obvious ocular pathology, the eye itself is rarely responsible for pain and discomfort" (19). Carlow (19) notes also that refraction disorders and muscle imbalance have been overemphasized as a cause of ocular headache. In addition, eyestrain headache should not be associated with nausea and vomiting. It is common for parents who have a child with a headache or facial pain to be concerned about the eyes as a cause. The parents often relate that they have already taken the child for an eye examination to see whether glasses or a new lens prescription is needed.

The eye must be examined in both acute and chronic facial pain that involves the orbital/frontal regions. In acute pain, the search is for the acute ocular pathology that Carlow (19) mentions. Acute angle-closure glaucoma can cause severe ocular pain that radiates over the entire head. The eye findings are dramatic: blurred vision, marked photophobia, mid-dilated pupil, a steamy cornea, and a tender eye.

A steamy or hazy cornea is an important sign of congenital glaucoma that may be the result of ocular anomalies, congenital rubella, or vascular malformations (20). Epiphora may be the earliest sign in these infants, but pain is not. More problematic is open-angle glaucoma; a low-grade headache can be present for some time before decreased vision is noted (19). A pediatric group at risk is children with vascular malformation in the trigeminal distribution (Sturge–Weber syndrome). The children at risk for glaucoma are those with malformation in V1 or V1 and V2 distribution (21). All these children should be checked for glaucoma by an ophthalmology service regularly, and headache must raise the issues of glaucoma or a problem developing intracranially because of intracranial vascular malformation.

Ocular and Periorbital Neoplasms

Ocular neoplasms are usually not associated with headache or eye pain, but metastatic orbital neoplasms that erode the bony orbital walls can cause pain in the ophthalmic trigeminal division; nasopharyngeal carcinomas can do this. Tumor invasion of structures innervated by the ophthalmic division of the trigeminal nerve can cause referred pain in the eye and periorbital area (19). These include structures in the cavernous sinus, cerebellar tentorium, falx cerebri, cribriform plate, and sphenoid wing. A supraclinoid aneurysm can cause retro-orbital pain that can proceed to third nerve paresis (19).

Mention must be made of Raeder paratrigeminal syndrome, which involves ocular pain and is divided into migrainous and symptomatic varieties. A discussion of the relationship of Raeder syndrome with other headache syndromes and discussion of migrainous Raeder syndrome are beyond the scope of this chapter (22). One can think of symptomatic Raeder syndrome as unilateral ocular pain with loss of sensation over V1. Tumors of the middle cranial fossa and parasellar region and those invading from the base of the skull can result in such a pattern of pain and decreased sensation. Many of the soft-tissue sarcomas of the head and neck that spread to the base of the skull can invade this parasellar area. A simple test such as the corneal reflex would be of vital importance here.

The preceding sections include a regional survey of the face from the standpoint of pain and acute disease. This is a springboard to discuss facial pain syndromes, chronic facial pain, and management. The area of TMJ pain and myofascial pain is best covered in the section on chronic pain.

Local Anesthesia

Standard Local Anesthetics and Vasoconstrictors

The cornerstone of modern dental/oral surgical treatment is local anesthesia and its adept administration. Standard textbooks devote considerable space to the subject of local anesthesia, and whole volumes are devoted to the topic (23).

The standard local anesthetic in dentistry continues to be 2% lidocaine with a vasoconstrictor, generally epinephrine in a 1:100,000 concentration. There are many other options available. Attempts to decrease the concentration of lidocaine are problematic. One such study demonstrated the effectiveness of a 1% lidocaine compound compared with 2% lidocaine, but this held true only for very minor procedures in children (24).

Vasoconstrictors

The use of vasoconstrictors is also important to prevent the rapid dissipation of the local anesthetic, with decreased local effectiveness and increased blood levels of local anesthetic, and also to provide a "dry" field, which is important in most oral surgical, periodontal, and restorative procedures. The arbitrary restriction of the use of epinephrine in local anesthetics in patients with cardiac disease may in fact have a paradoxical effect. If the depth of local anesthesia is not profound and the procedure is difficult because of local bleeding and a lack of vasoconstriction, the net sympathetic activity in the patient may be much greater than if adequate local anesthesia has been established. Increasing sedation to make up for inadequate local anesthesia is a slippery slope indeed.

A recent study attempted to differentiate the extent to which surgical stress and the epinephrine in the local anesthetic solutions influence serum catecholamines, cyclic adenosine 3′,5′-monophosphate, and potassium levels and contribute to changes in cardiohemodynamic parameters (25).

Four milliliters of 4% articaine hydrochloride with two different epinephrine doses was injected into patients before the removal of impacted mandibular third molars. The study was well structured. The results demonstrate that the amount of epinephrine absorbed from the intraoral injection site predominantly determined the serum epinephrine concentration. In this study, the anesthetic-induced increase in the serum epinephrine concentration did not correlate with changes in the cardiohemodynamic parameters. The serum cyclic adenosine 3′,5′-monophosphate levels correlated with serum epinephrine levels; the serum potassium levels remained unchanged. Using a randomized, double-blind crossover design, it became obvious that the surgical stress caused by third molar removal was strong enough to induce changes in the systemic norepinephrine level at the time of tooth extraction only when the 1:200,000 epinephrine solution was used. In contrast, the serum norepinephrine concentration was not detectable when the 1:100,000 epinephrine solution was used. The conclusion of the study is that depth of anesthesia and freedom from pain in third molar removal were linked to the epinephrine concentration in the local anesthetic solution.

If epinephrine is truly contraindicated in a patient, then phenylephrine in a 1:2,500 concentration can be used with the local anesthetic. The α-adrenergic effect will be provided without any β effect (23).

Techniques of Administration

Great care is given to the actual administration of the local anesthetic. Topical anesthetic can first be applied to the mucosa. Lidocaine-prilocaine cream (EMLA) has been used orally with success (26,27).

Diversion and counterirritant tactics are used, such as vigorously shaking the cheek during injection and/or pressing very firmly on the mucosa (particularly the palate) with a blunt instrument at the time of the injection. The patient can be concentrating on a leg lift in the dental chair during the injection; keeping the foot 6 in. off the chair is an excellent diversion. Having the patient use a portable cassette player with headphones and the patient's favorite music is another excellent diversion.

The concept of field anesthesia is also important: anesthetizing a small field first and then giving subsequent injections within that field. All the teeth in a quadrant can be anesthetized with the patient feeling a barely perceptible single "pinch" posteriorly. The injections are then carried anteriorly but always keeping the needle within the anesthetized zone. Such techniques take time and patience but pay dividends in patient comfort. Blocks of deeper nerves can be given painlessly by advancing the needle through an "anesthetized zone."

Analgesic Strategies for Dental and Oral Surgery

Multiple strategies can be used to deal with the physically and emotionally traumatic aspects of the surgical procedures. These include operative sedation, solid carefully administered local anesthesia, and bupivacaine blocks at the end of the procedure to provide a few hours of continued relief (28,29). In some anatomic locations, local anesthetic pumps can be placed for 1 to 5 days. Stryker Corporation manufactures one such pump that is mechanical (spring driven) and uses an inline filter valve to regulate flow. Unfortunately, it is difficult to technically place catheters at some sites, such as oral sites. Postoperative medications include narcotic analgesia in sufficient doses with acetaminophen, addition of a nonsteroidal anti-inflammatory drug (NSAID) (e.g., ibuprofen), and the use of an anxiolytic drug that provides some antiemetic effect (e.g., hydroxyzine). Local therapy with ice, elevation of the head, and good oral hygiene also improve comfort. A telephone call from the nurse or surgeon in the evening of the procedure also has a calming beneficial effect. The combination of many small aspects of care is synergistic in decreasing pain and enhancing comfort.

There are reports of many novel approaches to this end. These include the use of a preparation of rapid- and slow-release NSAIDs, diclofenac (Voltaren) to treat postoperative pain and the use of aprotinin in the postextraction dental sockets. Aprotinin is a bovine-derived polypeptide that inhibits the activation of some chemical mediators of acute inflammation (30).

New agents, of course, must be compared with currently used drugs. A study comparing glucamethacin, an analogue of indomethacin, with aspirin and placebo in the relief of pain after the removal of wisdom teeth demonstrated that glucamethacin was not better than placebo in the relief of postoperative pain (31). Another recent study compared four common oral analgesics to treat the postoperative pain of impacted wisdom tooth removal. Acetylsalicylic acid; ibuprofen; a combination of paracetamol, codeine, and caffeine; and dihydrocodeine were compared. They all had equal analgesic efficacy except for dihydrocodeine. Dihydrocodeine alone was found to be a poor analgesic in this pain model (32). For the outpatient then, the combination of narcotic, acetaminophen, and NSAID is rational (33).

A recent study demonstrated that patients can remember quite accurately their pain perceptions 3 years after impacted tooth removal. This is counter to other studies that find that pain memory is short-lived (34). The surgery is a significant event for the patient.

Four Important Points in the Management of Acute Pain Illustrated by Clinical Situations

Four special situations in the management of acute pain from oral conditions can be encountered in the general pediatric hospital. These situations, which highlight several important points, are as follow:

The severely ill patient. The anxious patient who has severe congenital cardiac disease and requires significant oral surgery (e.g., the removal of a symptomatic impacted wisdom tooth). A combination of intravenous sedation, solid local anesthesia, frequent reassurance, and good postoperative pain control will allow successful treatment without a general anesthetic. In some instances, the general anesthetic is preferable. Good interdisciplinary communication is needed.

Airway compromise and analgesia. The patient who has had significant craniomaxillofacial surgery and has relative swelling in the airway, maxillomandibular fixation, and multiple painful bone graft donor sites illustrates a case in which there may be a concern about giving too much narcotic analgesic when the airway may be tenuous. Our approach here is to keep the patient in the intensive care unit on a continuous or intermittent intravenous narcotic; when stable, the patient is transferred to the ward. Intravenous patient-controlled analgesia is continued on the ward and a NSAID is added. A transition is then made to an oral narcotic and acetaminophen elixir and a NSAID. The patient has excellent safe analgesia without the risk of over- or underdosing with intramuscular boluses.

Analgesia and pulmonary toilet. The patient with cystic fibrosis who requires significant oral surgery (e.g., removal of impacted symptomatic wisdom teeth) is prepared first with a pulmonary clean out. The operation can usually be done with intravenous sedation, solid local anesthesia, and a calm, reassuring manner. The patient can be given bupivacaine blocks at the end of the surgical procedure for prolonged analgesia. The postoperative analgesia is very important in this group of patients so that they can continue with their vigorous pulmonary toilet. If severe jaw pain prevents good coughing and respiratory effort, then a cycle of atelectasis and retained secretions in the lungs begins. We can enable the patient to continue with vigorous chest PT during the most painful postoperative period by the use of patient-controlled analgesia and intermittent bupivacaine blocks. This can be continued until the jaw pain becomes negligible.

Topical medication and the mucosa. The pediatric patient with cancer undergoing chemotherapy and/or radiotherapy presents another important point. The management of cancer pain is covered in another chapter, but the oral ulceration and mucositis that these patients can have is often helped by topical means. Several formulations in the literature have demonstrated effectiveness in pain relief for mucositis. These include sucralfate suspension, diphenhydramine syrup plus kaolin pectin (35), prostaglandin E_2 lozenges (Prostin E2) (36), and various topical anesthetics. This is a reminder not to minimize the importance of topical formulations for pain relief in the oral cavity.

FACIAL PAIN SYNDROMES

Of the various well-described facial pain syndromes of the adult, only a few are noted in children and adolescents. The most common in our center is TMJ pain dysfunction/myofascial pain dysfunction (MPD). This overlaps with tension headache and at times with migraine-like headache and is discussed in a subsequent section.

Neuralgias

Neuralgias are quite rare in children. Consider for the sake of comparison just two recognized cranial neuralgias: trigeminal neuralgia (tic douloureux) and glossopharyngeal neuralgia. Trigeminal neuralgia is by far the more common. Heyck (22) cites statistics that indicate trigeminal neuralgia is 60 to 200 times more common than glossopharyngeal neuralgia. In 336 cases of tic douloureux seen in an 18-year period at the Zurich Neurosurgical Clinic, nine patients were younger than 20 years of age, with the youngest being 12 years old. Glossopharyngeal neuralgia is exceedingly rare in children and adolescents.

A brief description of these two classic neuralgias will help to place other neuralgias and atypical facial neuralgias within a frame of reference.

Trigeminal Neuralgia

Trigeminal neuralgia is most common in the second and third trigeminal divisions and usually unilaterally. The pain comes in attacks that are brief, lancinating, and excruciating. This "lightning-like" pain can occur in the upper or lower lips, chin, cheek, or ear. The name tic douloureux refers to the tic-like muscle contraction of the face because of the paroxysm of pain. The paroxysms can be grouped, and the intervals are usually pain free, although a background of dull, more constant pain can develop. There is often a trigger zone that will set off the painful paroxysm. The stimuli on the trigger zone can be slight (e.g., a very light touch or cold breeze against the skin).

A discussion of the cause of trigeminal neuralgia is beyond the scope of this chapter. Dental, osseous, and neural theories have been espoused. Of interest are the clinical observations of Dandy and Cushing in the earlier part of the century that the intracranial vessels tend to sag in old age (22). Janetta, using this observation, explored a new approach of decompression of the trigeminal nerves at the root entry zone by lifting sagging vessels off the nerves, speculating that these sagging vessels were etiologic. Results have been good (37). This hypothesis would explain the extreme rarity of cases in children and adolescents. If trigeminal neuralgia presents in young patients, multiple sclerosis must be considered (22). There is a report of neurovascular compression of the trigeminal and glossopharyngeal nerves with pain in three children (38).

Glossopharyngeal Neuralgia

Glossopharyngeal neuralgia is characterized by unilateral, usually intense pain in the posterior tongue, pharyngeal wall, and tonsil that radiates to the ear. The pain can last a few to many seconds. Swallowing or touching the pharynx can trigger attacks. There has been a vagal phenomenon associated with the pain; events from bradycardia to cardiac arrest have been described.

Eagle Syndrome

An elongated styloid process and calcified stylohyoid ligament have been incriminated by Eagle as causing a glossopharyngeal-like neuralgia (Eagle syndrome), especially when the neck is turned (10). There may be some substance in this because surgical removal of the styloid and calcified ligament has produced relief of pain (39). The very important caution here is that elongated styloid and calcified stylohyoid ligament are quite common. Using 30 mm as normal styloid length, a study of 1,771 panoramic radiographs of the jaws revealed 319 elongated styloid processes. Only eight patients in this study had symptoms, some minor, consistent with Eagle syndrome (40). The styloid can be elongated in the radiograph of adolescents; one must not conclude that pharyngeal, ear, or neck pain is owing to the elongated styloid process without a thorough workup for other causes.

Cluster Headache and Sphenopalatine Neuralgia

Sphenopalatine Neuralgia

A very confusing area concerns so-called sphenopalatine neuralgia (22). Sluder described pain in the maxilla, orbit, ear, and even into the neck and shoulder. It was mainly observed in middle-age women. Eagle, a student of Sluder's elaborated on this neuralgia (22). Sluder thought that the neuralgia involved the sphenopalatine ganglion because of observed nasal (parasympathetic) irritation symptoms such as rhinorrhea, stuffiness, lacrimation, and facial erythema. Many surgical approaches to the sphenopalatine ganglion have been espoused (41,42).

Cluster Headache

It is probable that some of the patients described by Sluder and Eagle experienced migraine, cervical pain, or, particularly, cluster headache. In fact, many authors include sphenopalatine neuralgias with cluster headache (10). Cluster headache is usually severe, unilateral, and located around the forehead, orbit, maxilla, zygoma, and temporal regions. It may feel like a toothache at times. The patient is restless because of the pain and, in contrast to the patient with migraine, paces incessantly like a toothache patient. An attack can last from 10 to 30 minutes (usually) or 2 hours (rarely). Sweating of the face, flushing, and ipsilateral lacrimation, conjunctival injection, stuffiness, and rhinorrhea are classic associated signs (22,43). Sluder's patients had these nasal symptoms and can be placed in a cluster headache category. Two types of cluster headache have been described: upper type with radiation to the forehead and lower-half headache with radiation to cheek and maxilla. Another characteristic feature of cluster headache is the recurrence of a number of separate attacks during a 24-hour period. The duration of the period of the disease is the range of 10 days to 8 months (22). Recurrence can be annual. The full cluster pattern described is a classic pattern. The cluster headache is much more common in men; a significant difference when compared with patients with sphenopalatine neuralgia. Cluster headache is much less common than migraine headache (50:1). Cluster headache has been noted from ages 10 to 60 years, but it is rare in children. Barlow (44) treated four children (ages 7, 8, 11, and 15 years) of 300 patients with cluster headache.

To Split or to Lump

It is the author's opinion that splitting midfacial neuralgia into a number of different diagnoses such as Sluder neuralgia, sphenopalatine neuralgia, vidian neuralgia, and lower-half headache and making the group separate from cluster headache is exceedingly confusing and may have no good basis in fact. If the pain meets the criteria for cluster headache; it should be classified as cluster headache. If it does not, it may be best to classify the pain pattern as an atypical neuralgia after searching for other causes.

Trigeminal Herpes Zoster

Shingles of the trigeminal distribution can present in children. Dysesthesia or neuralgia can precede the appearance of red papules by a few days. Vesicles develop from the papules, and the distribution of these vesicles in the trigeminal dermatome distribution becomes quite obvious. Fever, pain, tenderness, and successive crops of vesicles can appear for days to weeks. The pain can be excruciating. A particular danger of shingles in the V1, distribution is involvement of the cornea. The author has observed prodrome of tingling pain along the dorsum of the nose to its tip for 3 days before the appearance of papules and vesicles in the V1 dermatome in a teenager.

Immunosuppressed states must be considered when any patient presents with shingles, but the appearance of zoster in childhood is prevalent when the primary chicken pox infection is *in utero* or within the first 6 months of life. Symptomatic care and aggressive pain management are a cornerstone of treatment. Acyclovir can also be used (45). Injury to the roots of lower posterior teeth has been reported in a 15 year old who had had V3 shingles at 7 years of age (10).

Ramsay–Hunt Syndrome

Ramsay–Hunt syndrome is a zoster infection of the sensory and motor branches of the facial nerve; the eighth nerve can also be affected. The patient has deafness, vertigo, facial paralysis, and herpetic vesicular eruption of portions of the ear, ear canal, mastoid, and sometimes the anterior tongue, (chorda, tympani), soft palate, and pharyngeal wall (10).

Postherpetic Neuralgia

Neuralgia that remains after a herpes zoster reactivation can be excruciatingly painful. There is always a concern that prolonged postherpetic neuralgia will develop after shingles; this appears to be a function of age, with older patients more at risk.

Occult Tumors And Infections

The burden is ever present to search for occult tumor or infection when a child or adolescent presents with facial pain that does not have an obvious cause. The following is a group of ominous clinical presentations that may signify tumor or infection either intracranially or extracranially.

Trotter Syndrome

A tumor in the infratemporal fossa or nasopharyngeal wall can present with numbness and/or pain in the V3 distribution, headache, ipsilateral decreased hearing acuity, otitis, a feeling of a blocked ear, soft palatal edema, bulging of the ipsilateral palatine tonsil, and deflection of the soft palate to the opposite side. This is Trotter syndrome (46).

Jugular Foramen Mass

A jugular foramen mass can present with many of the symptoms and signs listed above. In addition, there can be decreased gag reflex, elevation of the palate to the contralateral side with phonation, and hoarseness or decreased voice volume because of the involvement of the ninth and tenth cranial nerves. The author has observed hypoglossal nerve involvement with a nasopharyngeal carcinoma metastatic to the jugular and hypoglossal foramina in a 14-year-old patient.

Sphenoid and Infratemporal Fossae Masses

Tumor involving the greater wing of the sphenoid can result in pain and paresthesia in the mandible, lip, and chin by involvement of V3 near the foramen ovale. Mahan and Alling (10) describe eosinophilic granuloma in a 15-year-old girl presenting in this way. Interestingly, this patient's diagnosis was obscured by an abscessed lower second molar. Tumor primary or metastatic to locations along the course of the trigeminal nerve can present with pain and/or paresthesia of the chin or lips; sometimes numbness without pain is noted. The author has observed this in young patients: Hodgkin lymphoma at the mandibular lingula presenting as lower lip and chin numbness and Ewing sarcoma involving the mandibular ramus presenting as TMJ pain and lip and chin numbness.

Cerebellopontine Angle Masses

Cerebellopontine angle tumors can also present with facial symptoms. The acoustic neuroma usually has eighth cranial nerve involvement, but a case illustration demonstrates that other presentations are possible. A 15-year-old patient was scheduled for removal of all four third molars because she had some mild discomfort at the upper left third molar. She also noted pain and tingling in her left cheek. Fortunately, an admission physical examination by an astute house officer documented decreased sensation in left V2, and V3, and a bedside whispered hearing test demonstrated a marked decreased acuity in the left ear. Workup revealed a large cerebellopontine angle tumor that was finally diagnosed as an acoustic neuroma. A recent study examined the issue of cerebellopontine angle tumor and facial pain (47).

Other Masses and Temporal Pain

Multifocal schwannoma of the masseteric nerve presented with unilateral temporal headache (48); another report described metastatic lesions to the TMJ from breast adenocarcinoma presenting as TMJ pain (49). These reports demonstrate the importance of having a high index of suspicion for occult tumors.

Importance of Numbness

The cases above illustrate a striking pattern in regard to the presentation of numbness, tingling, or "novocaine-like" feeling in the face. Reports of such symptoms cannot be ignored; a workup including full examination and imaging studies must be carried out to rule out mass or infiltrative lesions.

Second Tumors

An oncologic group of great concern includes children and teenagers who have had treatment for a pediatric malignancy of the head and neck. There is a possibility of the development of a second malignancy, often in the field of radiation. A patient with the retinoblastoma oncogene who has been successfully treated for retinoblastoma must be followed particularly closely for development of a sarcoma in the head and neck.

Headache and facial pain in these children must be treated very seriously. Two case histories underscore this point. A teenager had a history of malignant hemangiopericytoma of the left mandibular region that was treated 10 years previously with surgery, radiation, and chemotherapy. He had no evidence of recurrence over this period. During a workup for a secondary facial reconstructive procedure, he complained of left temporal headache. Evaluation revealed undifferentiated sarcoma at the base of the skull in the infratemporal fossa. A teenager who had been treated for retinoblastoma as an infant presented with maxillary pain. A workup revealed an osteosarcoma of the maxilla. A recent case report describes rhabdomyosarcoma arising in the masseter muscle in a 12 year old who had been treated for retinoblastoma as a baby (50).

Posttraumatic Neuralgia and Causalgia

Injuries to peripheral sensory nerves, blood vessels, and sympathetic nerves of the face occur in children for many reasons. In a sense, removal of a tooth results in an avulsive injury to a number of c fibers at the root apex. The inferior alveolar nerve and the lingual nerve can be injured in the removal of lower wisdom teeth. Facial injuries can result in nerve injury. The infraorbital nerve can be injured during zygoma fractures, orbital blow-out fractures, and maxillary wall fractures. The supraorbital. nerve can be injured with blows to the superior orbital ridge and forehead. The inferior alveolar nerve is at risk with a fracture of the mandibular body and angle.

Many of the facial osteotomies that can be performed in modern craniomaxillofacial surgery involve manipulation, stretching, and "bruising" of at least the epineurium of many trigeminal sensory branches. In tumor surgery of the jaws and face, it is necessary at times to section the infraorbital nerve, inferior alveolar nerve, or whole trigeminal divisions. Despite these multiple opportunities for injury, posttraumatic neuralgia, causalgia, or anesthesia dolorosa are exceedingly rare in children. This is fortunate indeed because the posttraumatic pain syndromes can be refractory and severely debilitating to the patient (22).

Atypical Facial Neuralgia and Atypical Odontalgia

This category can become a large unwieldy basket for the group whose histories and presentations do not fit one of the other more defined categories of facial pain. It is a legitimate category, but its use must be preceded by a thorough search for other more specific diagnoses. In atypical facial pain, the pain may have different characteristics at different times and cross trigeminal dermatomes and the midline. The patient may state that there is a trigger point and demonstrate it by touching it or allowing the examiner to touch it, a maneuver that the patient with tic douloureux would not allow.

In atypical odontalgia, the pain arises from a tooth or group of teeth, but standard dental tests do not reveal odontogenic pathology: no periapical radiolucencies, no caries, no evidence of tooth fracture or of pulp inflammation. This patient is at risk of having multiple endodontic treatments and multiple extractions with no significant pain relief. The feedback from diagnostic local anesthetic blocks may be confusing because the pain may disappear after an individual tooth is blocked, incriminating that tooth.

The atypical facial neuralgias and odontalgias are chronic and idiopathic and do not involve pain in the muscles or TMJ. If the pain is in the muscles of mastication or TMJ, the diagnoses of MPD and/or TMJ pain dysfunction are more appropriate. Harris uses the term facial arthromyalgia to encompass MPD and TMJ presentations (51). (A subsequent section elaborates on these entities thoroughly.)

The psychogenic nature of many of these facial pains is now quite clear (51). Stressful life events or neuroses are quite common in this patient group; 33% of the patients of Feinmann and Harris met criteria for depression. Severe psychopathology can exist but was uncommon in this group of adult patients.

Atypical Facial Pain in Children

It is not entirely clear, but atypical facial pain in children may indicate proportionately more psychopathology than for adults. In two studies at The Children's Hospital, Boston, the incidence of primary psychopathology in patients with facial pain was 35% for pediatric patients and 6.25% for adults (52,53). Another study placed the incidence of primary psychopathology at 25% for children between 7 and 16 years of age (54). Depression was seen most frequently. Traumatic events in childhood and chronic pain are recognized (55).

A specific type of atypical causalgia that presents with burning tongue (glossodynia) is a disease of older women primarily and would be exceedingly rare in children. The author has treated a 9-year-old boy with a burning tongue that appeared to fall into an atypical pain category. Close inspection with magnification revealed tiny red papules at the tongue tip. Biopsy showed a psoriasiform pattern. Further examination revealed "callus-like" lesions of the fingertips. The diagnosis of psoriasis was made; the patient has improved with 1% hydrocortisone cream to the tongue tip. Burning tongue should also provoke a workup for vitamin B and iron deficiencies and candidiasis. If these are negative and no specific nutritional replacement therapy or antifungal therapy is indicated, tricyclic antidepressants are very helpful.

Treatment of the Various Facial Neuralgias

As has been stressed before in this chapter, specific causes must be sought and treated as necessary. Are there any occult masses or infection? From the very beginning, the signs of chronic pain and psychologic stress must be sought; it is perfectly consistent to search for occult masses and help the patient to get psychologic relief from the pain and its circumstances simultaneously. It is not an either/or phenomenon; it is not a matter of ruling out all "real" causes and then suggesting a "psychiatrist" to the parents. The family dynamics, the stressed lives of the parents, the child's emotional state, the missed school days, and the depression must be addressed at the outset.

Drugs

Carbamazepine and Phenytoin

Carbamazepine is dramatically successful in classic tic douloureux. Heyck (22) states that carbamazepine rendered all previous drugs obsolete. The standard adult dose is 600 to 800 mg per day in three to four divided doses. For children, the dose is 15 to 25 mg/kg per day in three to four divided doses. The dose must be gradually built up to these levels over a couple of weeks (56). Pretreatment and monthly complete blood count with platelet count and liver function tests must be obtained while the patient is on carbamazepine. Aplastic anemia has been reported with carbamazepine but very rarely; elevation of liver enzymes has also been reported. Although carbamazepine is the classic drug treatment, gabapentin has become the drug of choice for many because of its lower side effect profile.

In the atypical neuralgias and odontalgias, carbamazepine and gabapentin are not as efficacious but are worth trials. The author treated an 8-year-old patient with carbamazepine for atypical facial pain with modest improvement.

Antidepressants

Tricyclic antidepressants and now the selective serotonin reuptake inhibitors have a definite place in the treatment of facial pain (51). Atypical facial neuralgia and odontalgia respond better to the antidepressants than to the antiseizure medicines. Imipramine has been used most in pediatric practice, and the drug is started at a low level (0.5 mg/kg per day) given as a bedtime dose. An electrocardiogram is obtained pretreatment, and the presence of anticholinergic signs is monitored. The author has not used tricyclic antidepressants for facial pain in patients younger than 12 years of age.

Topical Agents

For postherpetic neuralgia, 0.025% capsaicin topical cream can be applied to the skin or lips. Pretreatment with topical anesthetic may be needed during the first applications to prevent the pain that can be associated with the first few capsaicin treatments (10). The author has used capsaicin with some effect in posttraumatic neuralgia. Lidocaine ointment and dyclonine liquid have also been used on the oral mucosa to gain relief from neuralgic pain involving the gingiva, buccal mucosa, and tongue.

Local Anesthesia

Local anesthetic blocks can be used to help gain relief when there has been a particularly severe exacerbation of pain. The injections can also be given in a series of four or five injections over a 14-day period to try to break a pain cycle. Trigger points in muscles can be injected (57,58). Scar tissue can be injected as well as peripheral nerves. Local anesthetic injection can sometimes provide dramatic relief exceeding the practitioner's expectations. The author has seen dramatic relief for chronic temporal pain that developed after right temporal craniotomy for arteriovenous malformation in a teenager. The locus of pain may have been a scar within the temporal muscle. Dramatic relief of left angle of the mandible pain at the insertion of the stylomandibular ligament was provided with a series of local anesthetic injections. The pain developed after a high cervical surgical approach to the carotid artery.

Physical Therapy

Physical therapy treatments include ultrasonography, ice, heat, and transcutaneous electrical nerve stimulation. In my experience, facial neuralgias are refractory to physical therapy methods compared with myogenic pain, which is readily responsive. The one exception, of course, is transcutaneous electrical nerve stimulation. Some persistence with transcutaneous electrical nerve stimulation and experimenting with electrode placement are important before a decision is made that it is not efficacious. For the face, voltage settings must be started at very low levels; children who feel they have been "shocked" may want nothing more to do with the transcutaneous electrical nerve stimulation unit. Transcutaneous steroidal and local anesthetic iontophoresis has also been used successfully for postherpetic neuralgia (59).

Behavioral Medicine

Biofeedback and behavioral medicine techniques can be very helpful; the patient can learn to avoid the behaviors that exacerbate pain. These therapies are extremely helpful with MPD and TMJ pain syndromes.

Comprehensive Care

Comprehensive pain clinic referral is important to ensure that all potential avenues of therapy are investigated. Treatment of psychologic and family dynamic problems is paramount and requires sensitive integration into the plan. Treatment of concomitant depression, for example, would be crucial to the overall success of the pain treatment program.

Despite the thorough workup of a pain problem and the initiation of a good, solid therapeutic program, patients may remain resistant because of the seemingly insurmountable walls that they feel surrounding them. Both teenagers and younger children can experience this and not be able to verbalize it. One child with facial pain had missed almost 2 months of school in the seventh grade. The physical, psychologic, and family dynamics were complex, but what frightened the child the most was going back to school and facing 2 months of course work and make-up examinations. The child felt that she was in a deep pit and could not envision escape. Working out a plan that would reintegrate the patient with her class without daunting or frightening demands was imperative. She understood that her classwork would require extra effort, but, importantly, she also understood that her predicament was appreciated. She figuratively and literally breathed a sigh of relief after the scholastic plan was discussed with her. She started to improve from that day.

There must be commitment to an interdisciplinary, interactive approach to these patients, and it must extend beyond the family and involve school teachers and other school officials.

Neurolytic Lesions and Decompression Operations for Pain Control

The decision to produce a neurolytic lesion in a child or adolescent child is one that should be made only after great interdisciplinary circumspection. It must be considered a major step. If a case can be made to interrupt a peripheral sensory nerve, some procedures may have theoretic advantages in children. Neurolysis has been accomplished with alcohol injection, glycerol, streptomycin, cryotherapy, well-modulated heat by radio frequency thermocoagulation, and simple neurectomy.

Streptomycin Lidocaine Injections and Cryotherapy

Two techniques that may be the least objectionable for children are cryotherapy and streptomycin/lidocaine injection (60–62). Both techniques have demonstrated efficacy in reducing pain with good preservation of touch. Regeneration of nerve fibers has been a criticism of the two techniques in adults; repeat treatments are required some months later (63). This actually may be a benefit in young people—the possibility of full recovery of the peripheral nerve. However, one must always approach neurolytic lesions as irreversible, and trials of local anesthetic injections must be performed first to show efficacy and to demonstrate that the patient can tolerate the sensory change.

Radiofrequency Lesions

Gregg et al. (64) have used radiofrequency lesions peripherally and have shown that radiofrequency lesions are selective for small myelinated and unmyelinated fibers (64). Technically, radiofrequency lesions are more difficult to perform than cryotherapy lesions or lidocaine/streptomycin injections. Cryotherapy does require an open approach or radiologic guidance, the probe must be placed immediately on the nerve, and the nerve is frozen in three cycles (60,63). Alternatively, radiofrequency lesions can be performed at the gasserian ganglion percutaneously via the foramen ovale. This is the technique described by Sweet and Wepsic (65). Experience in children is exceedingly limited.

Peripheral Nerve Decompression

Decompression may be useful if there is evidence of constriction of a bony canal, especially after injury, associated with pain and/or sensory changes. The inferior alveolar canal and the infraorbital canal and foramen are two structures prone to injury with facial bone fractures. Excision of neuromas and repair of nerves or nerve grafts can be performed in an attempt to gain relief of pain thought to be secondary to nerve injury.

Other Procedures

Multiple neurosurgical procedures have been described for pain relief. The experience in children is very limited, as is the case for peripheral lesions. The Janetta decompression procedure was described earlier for tic douloureux.

When palliation of pain because of head and neck cancer is required, the various procedures mentioned can be considered. In addition, intrathecal narcotics can be provided via a lumbar catheter and implantable subcutaneous drug delivery pump in patients who fail oral narcotic pain management and an alternative to intravenous narcotics is needed (66). Local anesthetic delivery via catheter and pump can also be considered, as noted earlier.

MYOFASCIAL PAIN DYSFUNCTION OF THE FACE AND TEMPOROMANDIBULAR JOINT PAIN DYSFUNCTION

Many names have been used for the pain and dysfunction discussed in this section: MPD syndrome, TMJ pain dysfunction syndrome, facial arthromyalgia, and craniomandibular syndrome. Many patients simply state that they think they have TMJ.

There are variations in the definitions and there are advocates for each name, but basically there are two related processes that must be discussed. The first involves pain in the facial muscles, especially the muscles of mastication (Figs. 43.6, 43.7, and 43.8). These muscles can have high resting tone, can be in spasm, and may be tender. An important, but not invariable, part of this picture is muscle hyperfunction or parafunction. This includes daytime or nocturnal bruxism (grinding of teeth), daytime or nocturnal clenching of the jaws, habitual side-to-side jaw movements that serve no function, incessant gum chewing or fingernail biting, and even the playing of musical instruments (67). The second process involves internal derangement of the TMJ.

Temporomandibular Joint Anatomy

Before discussing internal derangement, the normal joint and its functions must be described. The TMJ is a diarthrodial joint with a mandibular condyle that fits into a glenoid fossa at the base of the skull. The posterior limit of the joint is the auditory canal; anteriorly there is a convex eminence. The condyle slides over this eminence. Interposed between the condyle and the glenoid fossa is a fibrocartilage disc that is attached anteromedially to the lateral pterygoid muscle in most cases, although there is debate about this (68). A posterior attachment consists of a superior and inferior layer of elastin. The central portion of the posterior attachment contains areolar connective tissue with sinusoids and nerve tissue within it. The posterior attachment is quite vascular, whereas the disc proper is avascular.

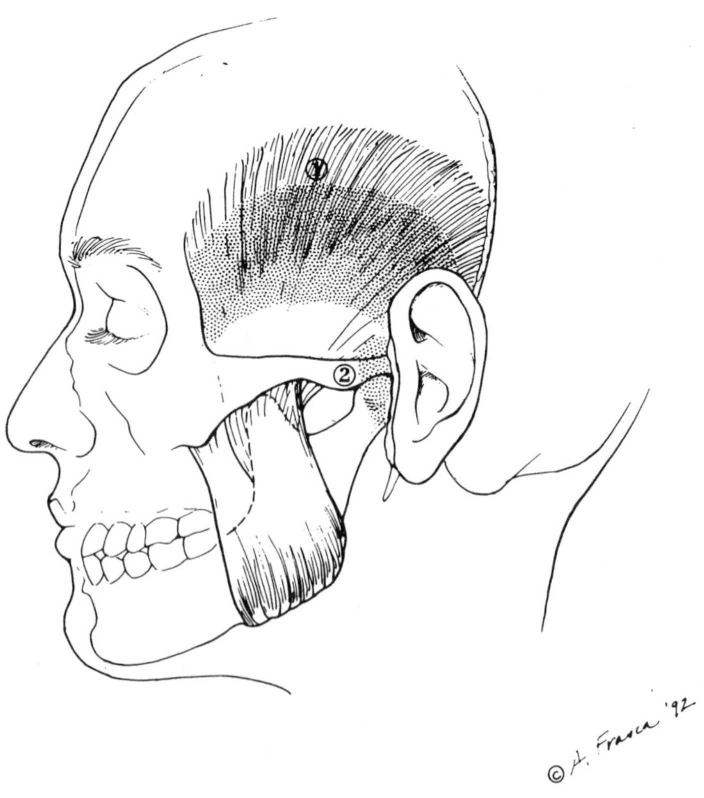

FIGURE 43.6. Myofascial pain dysfunction. *1*, Pain and tenderness in the belly of the temporalis muscle. *2*, There is often associated tenderness and pain in the preauricular area.

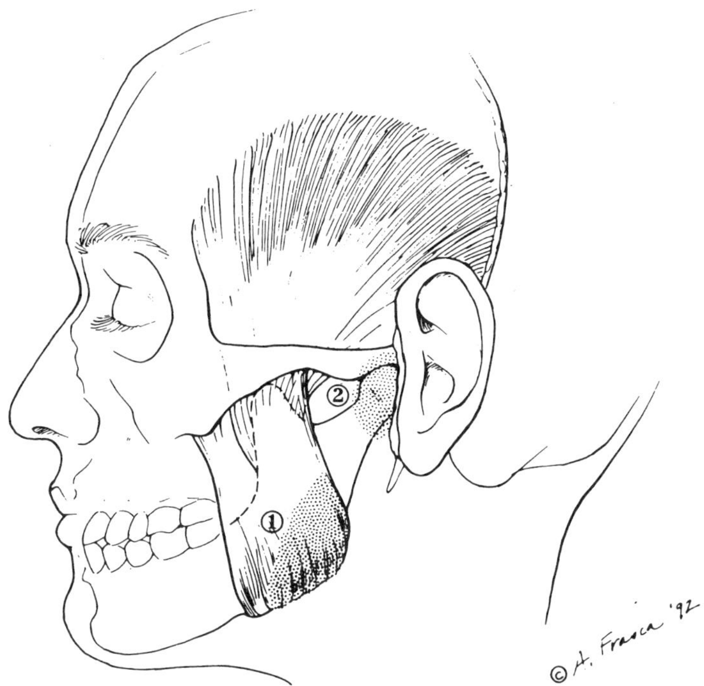

FIGURE 43.7. Myofascial pain dysfunction. *1*, Another common area of pain and tenderness is the insertion of the masseter muscle on the mandibular angle. *2*, There can also be associated preauricular pain and tenderness.

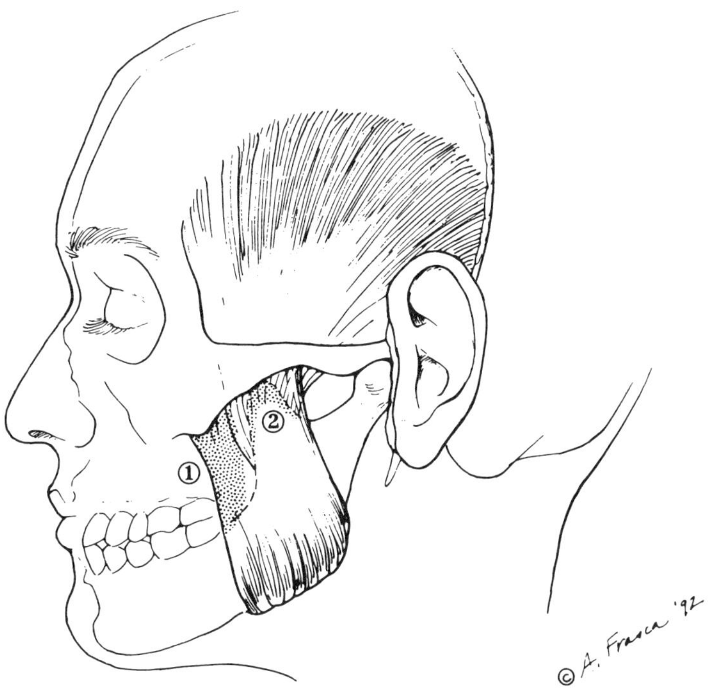

FIGURE 43.8. Myofascial pain dysfunction. From an oral approach, tenderness can be elicited along (*1*) the anterior border of the masseter and (*2*) temporalis insertion on the coronoid process of the mandible.

The posterior attachment attaches to the posterior capsule of the TMJ, which in turn adheres to the anterior wall of the bony and cartilaginous auditory canal. The TMJ capsule is quite complete except at the anteromedial aspect where the lateral pterygoid muscle exits. The articular eminence is covered by fibrocartilage. The fibrocartilage is thickest on the posterior slope of the articular eminence and at its apex and on the anterosuperior pole of the condyle—the "working" parts of the joint. The disc divides the joint space into an upper and lower compartment. Synovial cells are found mainly on the posterior attachment (68).

Jaw Opening (Fig. 43.9)

There are two distinct motions for jaw opening. The condyle first rotates on its own axis. The disc sits over the condyle like a bonnet and the condyle rotates in relation to the disc. The condyle then is pulled anteriorly down the slope of the articular eminence by the contracting lateral pterygoid muscle. Rotation generally opens the jaw 25 mm (interincisal distance), and the forward translation of the condyle on the eminence allows a full opening of 45 mm. As the condyle slides down the eminence, the disc rides with it like a bonnet on a head. This rotation and transla-

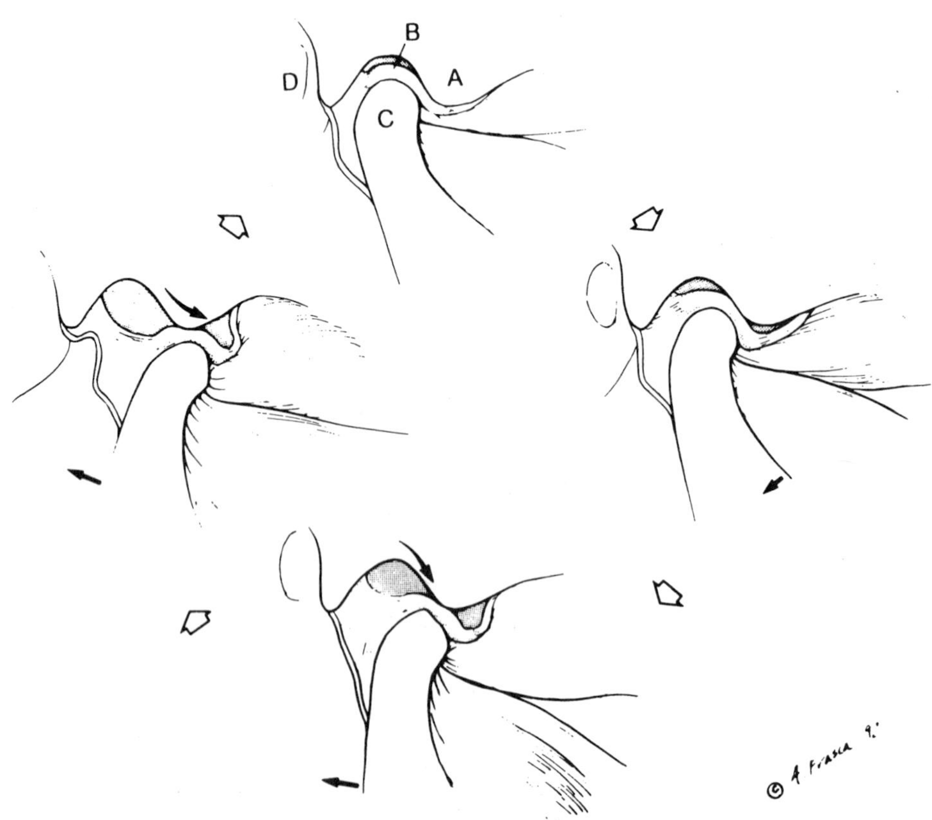

FIGURE 43.9. The temporomandibular joint. *A*, articular eminence; *B*, meniscus (disc); *C*, condyle; *D*, auditory meatus. This clockwise sequence demonstrates the condyle's initial rotation with jaw opening. The condyle then translates down the articular eminence for full opening. The meniscus remains as a cap covering the condyle.

tion are generally inaudible to nearby observers, and it occurs smoothly.

Masticatory Muscles

The closing muscles of the jaws are paired and include the temporalis muscles, masseters, and medial pterygoids. The posterior fibers of the temporalis muscles provide some mandibular retraction, but this is a minimal movement in the human joint. The opening muscles of the jaw include the paired lateral pterygoids, anterior bellies of the digastric muscles, geniohyoid, and mylohyoid muscles. Gravity also plays a role as do the muscles of facial expression.

Differential contraction of the lateral pterygoid muscles allows lateral jaw excursion. If the left lateral pterygoid muscle contracts and the right one does not, the jaw pulls to the right. If the lateral pterygoid muscles contract in tandem without any condylar rotation, the jaw protrudes in the midline without opening.

Internal Derangements of the Temporomandibular Joint

Anterior Displacement with Reduction (Fig. 43.10)

Internal derangements of the TMJ have been noted in medical literature since the

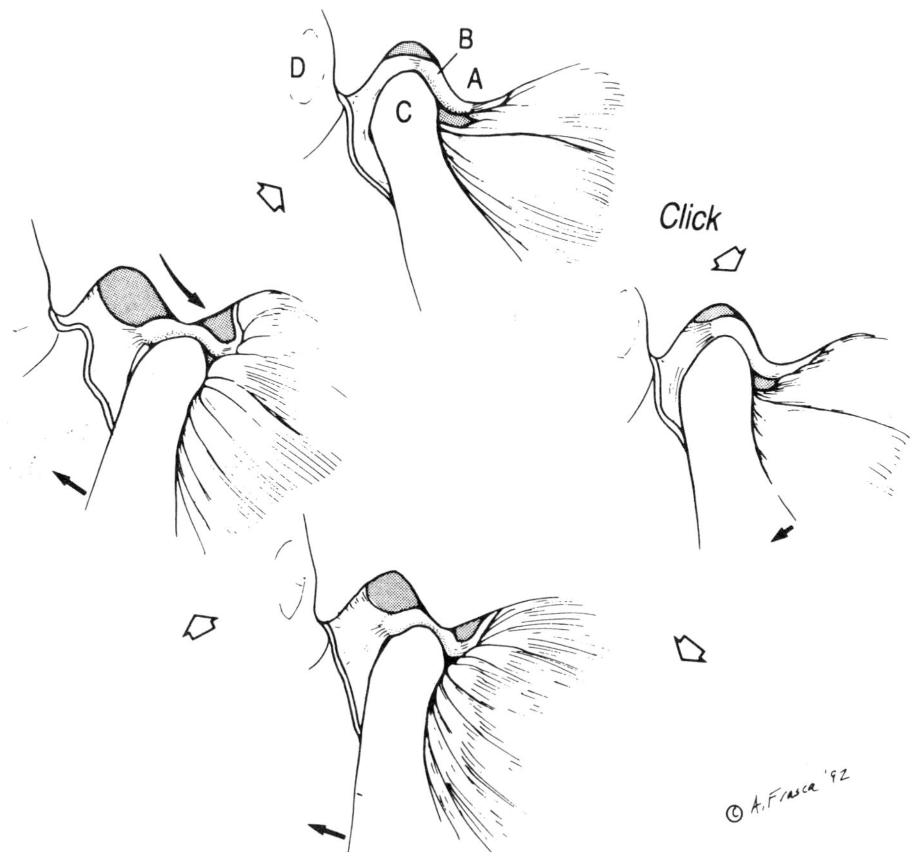

FIGURE 43.10. Anterior displacement of the temporomandibular joint disc with reduction. When the jaw is closed and the condyle is in the glenoid fossa, the disc is anteriorly displaced. As the jaw opens and the condyle begins to translate, the disc clicks back into a normal position. As the condyle comes back into the fossa, the disc "clicks" back out of normal position. *A–D* as defined in Fig. 43.9 legend.

nineteenth century (69,70). The name denotes a malrelationship between the condyle and the disc. The earliest derangement is anterior displacement of the meniscus with reduction. The meniscus is displaced anteriorly in relation to the condyle; as the jaw opens and squeezes against the disc, there is a "click," the condyle squeezes under the disc into a normal relationship, and the opening movement is completed. As the jaw closes, there is a reciprocal click and the meniscus "pops" anteriorly to the condyle again. This anterior displacement of the meniscus with reduction can be painless or painful, intermittent or continuous over a number of years.

Closed Lock

Episodes of closed lock may then develop. The starting point is the same, with the disc anteriorly displaced in relation to the condyle, but as jaw opening occurs, a blockage develops. The condyle can rotate, but as it starts to translate, the condyle does not "click" under the disc (71). The patient may have to massage the jaw or manipulate it to get it open. This closed-lock episode can last from seconds to hours before the disc reduces.

Anterior Displacement Without Reduction (Fig. 43.11)

The internal derangement can then progress to a permanent lock position. At this time, the condyle does not get by the displaced disc. The disc does not slip back into its normal position on the condyle. The patient can only rotate and open to approximately the 25-mm range.

There is one hypothesis that the disc may lock out in a vacuum seal mechanism against the fossa and then cannot move. This is akin to a rubber suction cup being attached to a wall and then an attempt is made to slide it against the wall. This hypothesis is promoted because when the joint spaces are lavaged at the time of arthroscopy, the closed lock can be relieved (72). There is no definite evidence, however, that lavage results in disc reduction. Aside from this possible acute mechanism, the displaced disc undergoes chronic changes. It loses its disc shape and becomes rounder; the amount of cartilage in it increases. The posterior attachment loses the inherent elasticity that helps to hold the disc in place posteriorly. The anteriorly displaced disc without reduction can be associated with significant pain and jaw limitation. Jaw opening will increase as the posterior attachment stretches and pain may decrease.

Perforation and Degenerative Joint Disease

The stretched meniscus and posterior attachment can perforate. A tear in the disc correlates very well with the clinical sign of joint crepitus (73). It is suspected that degenerative joint disease (DJD) is initiated after perforation; there is also the possibility that occasionally a roughened condyle can initiate the perforation (68).

Cause

There is no unified explanation for the cause of internal derangements and DJD. At times, there is an obvious initiating factor, such as a condylar fracture. This, however, is the exception. Our studies demonstrate that 50% of a large group of young military patients with internal derangements date the derangement from a traumatic episode; the trauma in this group of more than 100 patients did not include fracture. The trauma ranged from motor vehicle accidents with blows to the mandible; other blows to the jaw during sports, play, assaults, or altercations; wide opening of the jaw for dental work; or intubation. Many of the patients had predating clicks that became symptomatic after the trauma. This group comprised patients who developed chronic problems. They should be differentiated from patients who have an injury and develop TMJ pain that is often called traumatic capsulitis. These patients will respond to soft diet, analgesics, jaw rest, and physical therapy; their recoveries are full.

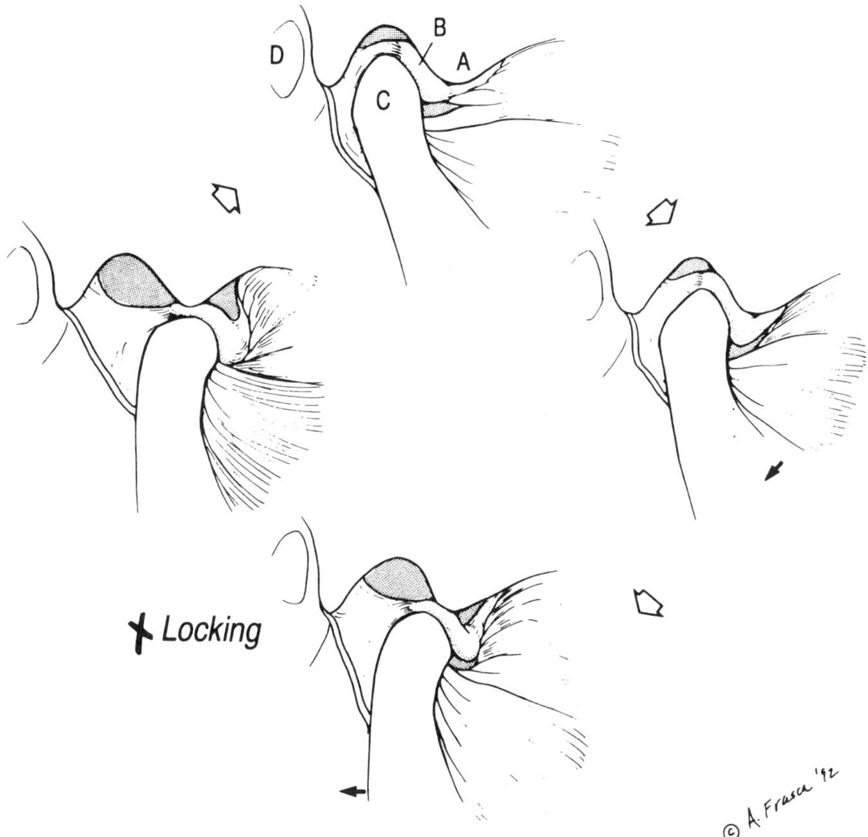

FIGURE 43.11. Anterior displacement of the temporomandibular joint disc without reduction. The disc is anteriorly displaced; as the condyle begins to translate forward, it is stopped by the displaced disc, and translation cannot continue. This is termed *closed lock. A–D* as defined in Fig. 43.9 legend.

Fifty percent of the patients, however, gave no trauma history. Theories regarding the cause of internal derangements include muscle hyperfunction (especially the lateral pterygoid), parafunctional habits, anatomic peculiarities within the TMJ, gender predilection (female patients > > male patients), and malocclusions. Orthodontics has been credited with both causing and curing internal derangements.

Importance Of The Internal Derangement

A pivotal question must be asked whenever a patient with facial pain is discovered to have an internal derangement: how important a contributor is the internal derangement to the overall pain problem? A well-done MRI study demonstrates the importance of this question. Fifty-seven asymptomatic volunteers with no history of TMJ problems or treatment underwent MRI. Eighteen patients had joint abnormalities (30 affected joints); this is 26% of the examined joints. Twenty-three joints showed disc displacement with reduction, seven joints showed disc displacement without reduction, and three joints had evidence of DJD (74). Another study demonstrated that 50 patients with symptoms and signs of unilateral disc displacement had the displacement confirmed arthrographically in all 50 symptomatic joints. Disc displacement was discovered in 30 of the asymptomatic joints. By the end of a 5-year follow-up, pain had developed in 57% of the asymptomatic joints (75).

Sometimes the pain is very localized and specific—a sharp preauricular pain with clicking at every opening movement. In such a case, the internal derangement's importance is probably evident (Fig. 43.12). At times, however, the pain is diffuse, involving other areas of the face (Fig. 43.13). The importance of an internal derangement in such a patient is not quite so clear. This, briefly, is the diagnostic dilemma when such patients are evaluated.

Overzealousness has been noted in the occlusal and surgical management of patients with internal derangements. Extensive occlusal equilibrations and occlusal rehabilitations have been espoused, when the literature on cause and efficacy is very mixed indeed. Likewise, a period of aggressive surgical management of patients (including teenagers) with internal derangements ensued in the decade of the late 1970s to the late 1980s.

Myofascial Pain Dysfunction and Internal Derangements

The link between MPD and internal derangements is not completely worked out, but most patients have features of both entities. The author regards the MPD syndrome the more global problem, and the internal derangements may very well be secondary to muscle hyperfunction. Laslo Schwartz (76) wrote about stress-related muscle hyperactivity more than 30 years ago and included a psychiatrist in his interdisciplinary group. The important link between stress and muscle hyperfunction has been well documented in electromyographic studies (77,78). Studies have linked stressful activity with bruxing and clenching of the jaws. Very often the patient is aware of this behavior, and the patient or parents will recognize high-stress traits.

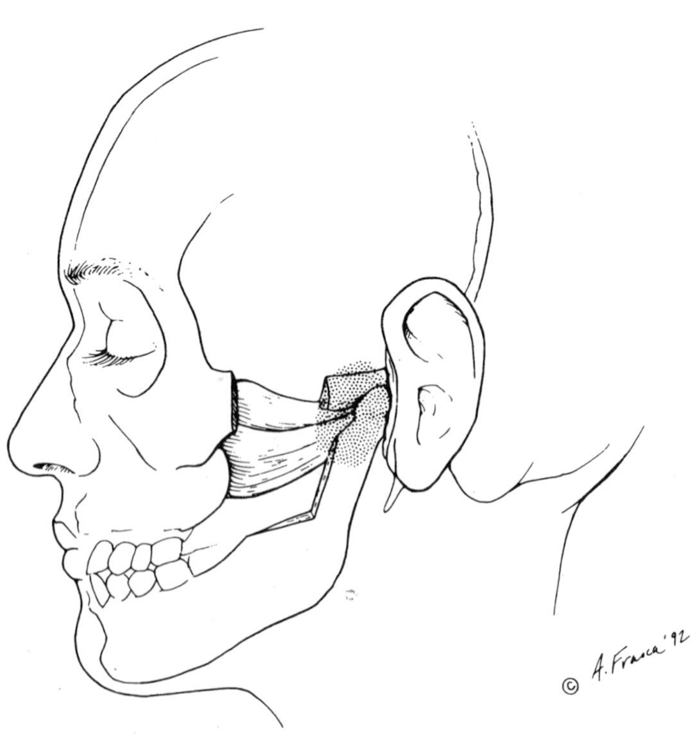

FIGURE 43.12. An internal derangement can have quite specific preauricular pain and tenderness (*stippled area*).

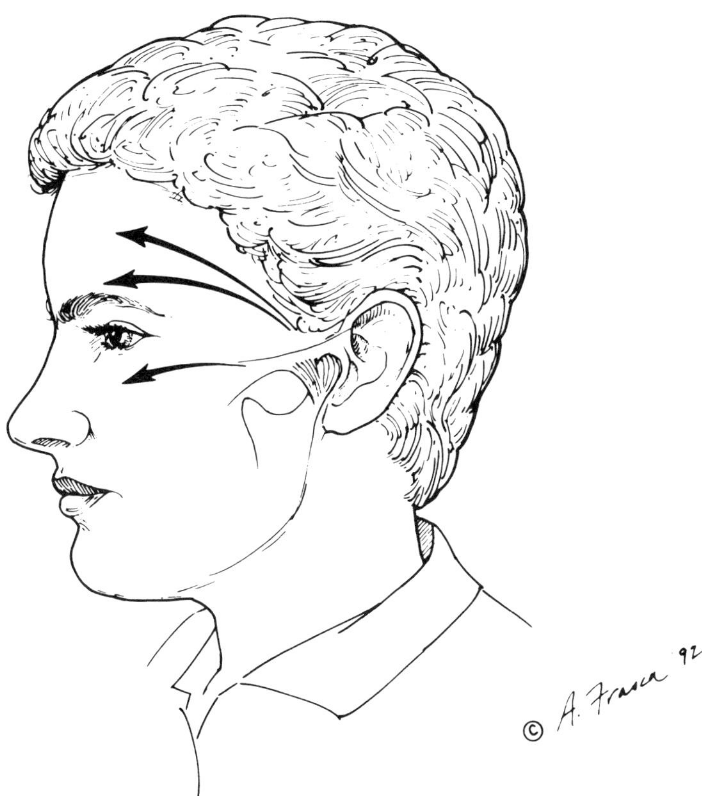

FIGURE 43.13. Internal derangements can also be associated with myofascial pain dysfunction, giving a more diffuse pain pattern.

Occlusion

Interestingly, the link between malocclusion and muscle of mastication hyperactivity is not as clear. It had been postulated that interferences in the occlusion would trigger muscle hyperactivity, but this does not appear to be the case (78). A study by Goodman et al. (79) demonstrated that mock occlusal equilibration had a placebo effect. The teeth were adjusted with a drill and bur, but it was mock equilibration because the occlusal surfaces of the teeth were not touched, and therefore no change in the occlusion was made. In this study, 16 of 25 patients with MPD responded to mock equilibration. Sixty-four percent reported a total or nearly total remission of their symptoms.

A study by Huber and Hall (80) was conducted to demonstrate whether there was a definite relationship between occlusion, occlusal interferences, TMJ disorders, and masticatory muscle pain. A sample of 217 women and 217 men who were symptom free was studied. The presence of occlusal disharmonies was quite striking. There was a centric relation to centric occlusion condylar slide in 48% of the women and 49% of the men. Nonworking contacts were present in 32% and 35%, respectively. Posterior working disclusive contacts were present in 13% and 15%, respectively. Deviation on opening was noted in 45% and 50%, respectively. TMJ sounds could be heard or palpated in 51% and 52%, respectively, and a maximal incisor opening of less than 37 mm was noted in 5%. There was no gender difference in the prevalence of occlusal discrepancies. The conclusion that occlusal interferences are not central to TMJ dysfunction is supported by three lines of evidence: (a) a relatively high prevalence of occlusal discrepancies in a symptom-free population cannot be ignored; (b) there is a lack of gender difference in the prevalence of occlusal discrepancies, although women exhibit a much higher (9:1) prevalence of TMJ dysfunction (M. Beehner and N. F. Ferraro, unpublished data); and (c) there is also a lack of association between occlusal discrepancies and some common signs of TMJ dysfunction such as clicking and jaw deviation.

Egermark-Eriksson et al. (81) reported on a group of 238 patients with malocclusion and craniomandibular disorder. Five years previously they had reported on 402 children in three age groups (7, 11, and 15 years old) and were now looking at these children at ages 12, 16, and 20 years. They found weak correlations between signs and symptoms of craniomandibular disorders and various morphologic malocclusions. No single occlusal factor was of major importance in the development of craniomandibular disorders. Fifteen percent of the 20-year-old patients had received orthodontic treatment, but TMJ dysfunction and pain was no greater than in the 20-year-old patients who had not received orthodontic treatment.

In sharp contrast to the studies that show minimal influence of the occlusion on MPD and TMJ pain dysfunction is a study that endorses the efficacy of occlusal equilibration (82). In this study, 53 patients with MPD were treated. The common occlusal element was lack of anterior guidance with molar interferences in excursive jaw movements. The aim of treatment was to remove any centric relation–centric occlusion slides, remove posterior interferences, and establish anterior guidance. Forty-four patients reported complete pain relief at the second treatment appointment, and six reported complete relief at the third appointment. On follow-up, 46 patients reported no recurrence. The longest follow-up was 4 years, but the range and average follow-up were not provided. Fifty-five percent of patients had had orthodontic treatment. The occlusal factors that the authors had singled out as important and treated are the very factors that Huber and Hall (80) indicated are unimportant as causative factors for MPD and TMJ pain syndromes.

Orthodontics, Orthognathic Surgery, and Temporomandibular Joint Disorders

An excellent review article by Reynders (83) looks at 91 articles published between 1966 and 1988 that discuss the association between orthodontic and temporomandibular disorders. Only six were sample studies, the rest were anecdotal case reports or editorials. Four of the sample studies found no relationship between orthodontics and temporomandibular disorders. The other two studies demonstrated that in some patients orthodontic treatment improved TM disorders. Both of these studies, however, had design flaws regarding controls.

Orthognathic surgery to reposition the jaws because of dentofacial deformities and malocclusions can be done for several indications: better dental relationships for chewing (e.g., closing an open bite), relief of potentially damaging dental relationships (e.g., deep bite with lower incisors occluding into the palate), esthetic improvement of facial proportions, and improvement of the airway (e.g., mandibular advancement). The most tenuous indication is the treatment of MPD and TMJ pain and dysfunction (84).

An occasional study attempts to relate reduction in TMJ pain dysfunction to the surgical correction of dentofacial deformities. A study from Sweden, unfortunately uncontrolled, investigated TMJ dysfunction before and after mandibular osteotomies. Half the patients listed TMJ symptoms as their reasons for seeking surgery. The authors claim that surgery decreased muscle pain and headache. Of 14 patients who had reported recurrent headaches preoperatively, six became headache free and another five reported decreased frequency. Surgery did not improve mandibular mobility, TMJ function, TMJ pain, or pain on movements (85).

At our institution, a firm approach has been taken that orthodontics and orthognathic surgery are not offered for the primary indication of treating TMJ pain and dysfunction. Patients with TMJ symptoms are not denied treatment if there are other indications. It is important, however, that they are informed about the lack of data supporting orthodontics and jaw-repositioning operations for TMJ pain relief.

Bruxism

Bruxism is an interesting phenomenon that has been tied to both life stresses and occlusion. It can be observed in babies as soon as the primary teeth erupt. The incidence of nocturnal bruxism in children is 12% to 15%. Its extremely destructive, uninhibited side can be seen when a patient with head injury is decorticate.

Tooth contact during sleep is very common and takes two forms: a single episode of muscle activity referred to as clenching and rhythmic contraction of the muscles referred to as bruxism. It is not clear whether clenching and bruxism are jaw activities with different causes or are the same phenomenon. The duration of nocturnal bruxing events is quite variable. There is uncertainty as to the number, duration, and strength of bruxing events that will result in muscle pain. There must be great host variability (86). Christensen (87) has shown that pain in the masseter muscle occurs after a 20- to 60-second clench. The relationship of bruxism, clenching, and masticatory muscle pain is not clearly worked out, but there is evidence accumulating that defines a relationship (88).

Rapid Eye Movement Sleep and Bruxism

An interesting view of myofascial pain and bruxism has been elucidated in a polysomnographic study (89). Patients with severe MPD symptoms attributed to nocturnal bruxism were compared with a sleep group that did not have facial pain but were noted to have bruxism on polysomnogram. Because the MPD group consisted of young women with depression, a control group of nine female depressed patients reporting insomnia was included. Although this was a small retrospective study, three results were noteworthy. First, the overall level of bruxism between the sleep group and the MPD group did not differ significantly, although the MPD group had more bruxism episodes and more bruxism seconds per minute of rapid eye movement (REM) sleep Second, general body movement accompanied bruxism in all groups regardless of sleep stage relationship. In 75% to 85% of patients with bruxism, there was anterior tibialis activity (a disturbance of sleep). Third, the control depressed female group showed little bruxism overall; three of the four subjects with bruxism had more REM sleep than stage 2 sleep. In the MPD group, more REM bruxism was the pattern. This study must be confirmed by larger prospective studies, but the relationship of bruxism to facial pain and REM sleep is intriguing, and there are implications for treatment by manipulating REM sleep pharmacologically (e.g., tricyclic antidepressants).

Bruxism: Central Control

A Japanese study recorded polysomnograms of eight male tooth grinders and included audio recordings of tooth-grinding activity. The authors concluded that the bruxism that they heard was often preceded by a K complex on electroencephalography and lightening of sleep stage. Fifty-seven incidents of tooth grinding were recorded during REM sleep. They were short in duration without exception and never observed during eye-movement bursts. During the eye movement bursts, the arousal threshold was higher than in the ocular-quiescent phase of REM sleep.

Heart rate was always elevated during bruxism events. The authors postulate that bruxism is a peripheral manifestation of the central events occurring during arousal. Hypothesizing further, the authors note that dopamine-containing neurons are responsible for arousal and may be important in tooth grinding. The authors were able to induce tooth grinding in their subjects with sonic stimuli. They also note a patient with Parkinson disease who began tooth grinding when given dihydroxyphenylalanine, the precursor of dopamine (90).

Bruxism and Emotional State

Whether the bruxing in the Japanese study is different from the facial pain-associated bruxism is not clear. Whether there is a psychologic or emotional drive to bruxism has not been worked out. In an excellent 1978 review article on TMJ pain affliction, the authors note a bruxism–emotional state link (91). In response to this review in a letter to the editor, Reding (92) noted that his study failed to show significant psychologic and personality differences between 30 bruxers and 30 matched controls using mental health histories, Minnesota Multiphasic Personality Inventory, and Cornell Medical Index. This author's opinion is that there is a distinct subgroup of bruxers and clenchers that have an emotionally driven process that produces pain. This is in keeping with the findings of the REM/bruxism study cited above.

Bruxism and Occlusion

There is a school of thought that supports the occlusal causes of bruxism. In one study, 34 patients with severe bruxism were studied electromyographically and clinically before and after occlusal adjustment. The author concludes that an occlusal interference between centric relation and centric occlusion is the most common occlusal factor resulting in bruxism. Occlusal adjustment eliminated bruxism in all 34 patients (93). The evidence for the occlusal causes of bruxism is rather scant, although centrally controlled and emotionally driven bruxism is receiving much attention.

Myofascial Pain Dysfunction and Temporomandibular Joint Pain Symptoms and Signs in Children and Adolescents

Adolescents

In one Scandinavian study, 285 17-year-old adolescents were examined; masticatory muscle tenderness was observed in 41%, and 22% had a clicking TMJ (94,95). A Japanese study examined 145 children of junior high school age and 429 children of senior high school age for 3 years (96). The authors noted an incidence of TMJ dysfunction that increased from 10% to 16% in 3 years in the junior group. The incidence increased from 12% to 31% over 3 years in the senior high school group. Over the 3-year period, 31% of the juniors and 39% of the seniors had some sign of TMJ dysfunction. These signs are generally mild. A study of 1,018 12-year-old children demonstrated that almost half of the patients had symptoms or signs of craniomandibular disorders but that only a very small minority required treatment (97).

Young Children

A study of 3- to 5-year-old children showed that 41% had an oral parafunctional habit such as thumb sucking, finger biting, or tooth grinding. In addition, 22% complained of earache, 7% complained of headache, 5% exhibited TMJ clicking, 5% exhibited muscle tenderness, 20% exhibited irregular condylar movements, 11% exhibited deviation of the jaw on opening, and 26% had tooth wear (98).

Infants

TMJ noise has even been noted in infants. The clicking on jaw opening or sucking in infants is probably owing to the condyle sliding out of a shallow, immature glenoid fossa (99; N. F. Ferraro, unpublished data). There is one report of TMJ pain in a 17-month-old boy (100).

The conclusion from these data is that if one looks carefully enough, TMJ clicking, occasional masticatory muscle pain, and jaw deviation on opening are quite common. The group that comes to the attention of practitioners are the children who have limited jaw opening or who complain of jaw or masticatory muscle pain, especially when school attendance is affected by repeated episodes of jaw pain. It is from this group that Pillemer et al. (54) produced their study showing a significant degree of emotional distress. At this time, it is reasonable to state that children can have both MPD symptoms and signs of internal derangement.

Myofascial Pain Dysfunction and Headache

These children can also present with headache. The association between MPD/TMJ pain dysfunction syndrome and tension headache is quite solid (101). Approximately 75% of children will have experienced headache by 15 years of age. Weekly headaches occur in more than 15% of 10 to 17 year olds, and half the time they are tension headaches (102). There has also been an association made between migraine headache and TMJ pain dysfunction syndrome (103). One study notes that in 100 consecutive headache clinic patients, 14 young women met the criteria for TMJ pain dysfunction syndrome. The authors state that these patients resemble patients with pure tension headache, but associated symptoms are different (101).

The children with MPD/TMJ pain dysfunction are often serious students with excellent school grades. There may be a positive history of daytime clenching or bruxing, especially when concentrating or when under emotional stress. The parents may report nocturnal tooth grinding, and wear facets on teeth can be seen. The diagnosis of nocturnal bruxing or clenching is sometimes difficult to make without a sleep study. We rely on parents' or siblings' histories, wear facets on teeth or on acrylic night guards, and morning pain and stiffness. Clenching can leave few telltale signs: no noise or no facets or wear patterns on splints; morning pain may be the only clue. The occlusion in our patients ranges from normal mixed dentition to normal permanent dentition to significant malocclusion. Our clinic's bias agrees with the many studies that downplay the effect of the occlusion on the production of facial pain.

Temporomandibular Joint Pain Dysfunction and the Ear

Often, patients who have had recurrent treatment for otitis and continue to complain of ear pain, despite no evidence on examination of acute ear disease, are then referred for evaluation of the TMJ and masticatory system. The ear and TMJ share the same embryologic origins, and there is some shared innervation via the auriculotemporali sensory nerve. For years authors have tried to relate otologic and TMJ symptoms anatomically and functionally. Costen (104), in the 1930s, hypothesized that TMJ symptoms and otologic symptoms such as vertigo, tinnitus, and otalgia were produced when the posterior teeth were lost and the condyle was posteriorly repositioned against the auditory canal. TMJ syndrome is sometimes called Costen syndrome, even today. How the TMJ causes otologic symptoms was never explained, but hypotheses continue to appear in the literature (105,106). Claims are made about the treatment of TMJ symptoms resulting in the relief of otologic symptoms such as vertigo and tinnitus (107). More work in this area is needed. The safest approach is never to assume that vertigo, tinnitus, otalgia, or blocked ear are a result of TMJ disorder unless the otologic vestibular workup is complete (108).

In addition to the ear, the examiner must make sure that there is no other occult pathology at the base of the skull, in the infratemporal fossa, or in the parotid gland and no osseous disease within the mandible (e.g., Garré osteomyelitis).

Imaging of the Temporomandibular Joint

MRI is now the preferred way to image the TMJ in the parasagittal plane (109). It demonstrates internal derangements, except for perforations, very well, and it does a reasonable job of imaging the condyle itself. If greater bony detail is needed (e.g., in DJD), a computed tomography scan must be obtained. Arthrogram with injected contrast medium into the lower joint space is the only imaging technique that consistently defines disc perforations (110,111). Plain radiographs of the TMJ are always obtained in patients who have complaints consistent with MPD or TMJ pain dysfunction syndrome to ensure that no gross lesions of DJD or bony destruction are being missed. MRI is ordered if there is confusion regarding the diagnosis, if a baseline (e.g., before orthodontic therapy or orthognathic surgery in a symptomatic patient) is needed, or if significant splint or invasive treatment is contemplated. Others, however, recommend MRI evaluation for all children with clicking and locking because they believe that degenerative changes can occur (109). These same investigators imaged 150 symptomatic children older than 5 years of age (131 girls and 19 boys, ages 7 to 16 years) using tomography, arthrography, computed tomography, and MRI. DJD was noted in 37% of joints and internal derangements in 85% of joints. Four patients had ankylosis.

Treatment of Myofascial Pain Dysfunction and Temporomandibular Joint Pain Dysfunction

Our treatment in general focuses mainly on the myofascial pain, muscle-related hyperactivity, stress-related components, and, to a lesser extent, on the internal derangement itself. The goals of treatment include diminishing behavior that is noxious to the muscles and the TMJ (e.g., stress-related clenching); decreasing the frequency, duration, and intensity of pain episodes; providing support and counseling about stress reduction and other psychologic concerns; and providing a functional and adequate, if not entirely normal, jaw opening. No specific effort is made to reduce a displaced disc except in some very limited circumstances. Generally, the word cure is not used because recurrences are commonplace and teaching the patient to deal with these episodes is realistic.

Special Consideration for Rheumatoid Disease and Other Systemic Diseases

Children with rheumatoid diseases, especially juvenile rheumatoid arthritis, can have TMJ pain. They can show the common signs of internal derangement: clicking, locking, and preauricular tenderness, and thus be very similar to the much more common patient without rheumatoid disease.

Three sequelae to rheumatoid disease set this group of patients apart. Often there will be significant joint crepitus and/or some retardation of mandibular growth with resultant retrognathia. Less frequently, there can be significant loss of joint structure and vertical height, with resultant backward rotation of the mandible and open-bite deformity. Severe jaw hypomobility can result.

It is extremely unusual for TMJ pain and inflammation to be the first presentation of undiagnosed juvenile rheumatoid arthritis. In a study at The Children's Hospital, Boston, one of 37 patients with juvenile rheumatoid arthritis had TMJ symptoms as one of the first manifestations of the disease, but within 5 years, 50% of the children had developed some TMJ symptoms and signs (17; N. F. Ferraro, unpublished data).

These patients have their anti-inflammatory medicines monitored by the rheumatologist. Other treatment modalities are helpful, including physical therapy for the TMJ and muscles and biofeedback if there are associated muscular hyperfunction habits. The retrognathia can be treated with orthodontics and orthognathic surgery. Before undertaking orthognathic surgery, the inflammatory portion of the disease must be under control (17). Infrequently, the TMJ must be reconstructed. The author's choice has been autogenous reconstruction with costochondral bone graft and temporalis myofascial flap.

Other rheumatoid diseases in which TMJ pain has been noted is scleroderma and psoriasis. In the differential diagnosis of tenderness in the TMJ/temporal region, one must also include temporal (giant cell) arteritis in elderly patients, but this diagnosis has not been made in children. Other systemic diseases in which TMJ pain has been noted include Crohn disease with TMJ arthritis, Ehlers–Danlos syndrome with painful TMJ dislocations (112), and myasthenia gravis (113). Several authors have noted the association of craniomandibular disease and joint hypermobility even when the diagnosis of Ehlers–Danlos syndrome cannot be made (114).

Treatment Options

Treatments for MPD and TMJ pain dysfunction syndromes include soft diet, medicines, home and formal physical therapy, bite splint therapy, muscle and joint injections, biofeedback, behavioral medicine, stress-reduction training, and psychologic counseling and treatment. In children, arthroscopy is not of proven efficacy, but experience has been established in adults. TMJ arthroplasty and reconstruction are rarely indicated for pain in children but must be discussed because rare indications for open-joint procedures in the teenage years do exist.

Medicines

Nonsteroidal Anti-inflammatory Drugs

NSAIDs continue to be a standby for the pain of MPD and TMJ pain dysfunction syndromes. One study, unfortunately uncontrolled, demonstrated that 90% of a small group of patients with MPD responded to ibuprofen (115). Another study, however, compared piroxicam (NSAID), acetaminophen, and placebo for TMJ pain. Symptoms and signs in all groups improved significantly over time, and pain relief was not significantly different among groups (116). Our group still considers the NSAIDs the first line of treatment for MPD/TMJ pain dysfunction syndromes unless there is a contraindication.

Muscle Relaxants

Muscle relaxant drugs are a varied group. Cyclobenzaprine (Flexeril), a tricyclic antidepressant analogue, methocarbamol (Robaxin), a carbonate derivative of guaifenesin, and baclofen, a chlorophenyl derivative, have all been used as antispasticity and muscle relaxant drugs. Although they work at the spinal cord level, their efficacy for facial pain has not been consistent (117). Baclofen can also be formulated as a topical agent.

The benzodiazepines have been used for MPD of the masticatory muscles and for bruxism, and they have good efficacy in the short term. A double-blind study with clonazepam and placebo taken orally demonstrated that clonazepam relieved MPD symptoms much better than placebo in adults. The clonazepam dose was started at 0.25 mg every 4 hours and increased by intervals to a 1-mg maximal daily dose if needed (118). Diazepam decreases bruxism when taken before sleep (119). Because of the risk of psychologic dependence, the benzodiazepines have been used only rarely for children in our clinic.

Tricyclic Antidepressants

The tricyclic antidepressants have been used with good result in the MPD group of patients, even if depression is not a major part of the pain syndrome. (The tricyclic antidepressants were discussed more fully in the neuralgia section of the chapter.)

Temporomandibular Joint Injections

Another drug that has given relief in the short term for articular pain is intra-articular injections of corticosteroids. Intra-articular injections, however, can produce significant degenerative change, such as the destruction of articular cartilage (120). As a result, the author sparingly uses intra-articular corticosteroid injections. Local anesthetic injections (1% lidocaine) into tender masticatory muscles, especially at trigger points, can decrease

MPD symptoms after a single injection or a series of injections over 1 to 2 weeks (57,58). Intra-articular injection of sodium hyaluronates is quite straightforward. This has proven efficacious in trials (120–122).

Other Drugs

Neutral amino acids (L-tryptophan, D-phenylalanine) have been reported anecdotally to decrease facial pain. This, however, is unproven treatment and has not been used in our institution (120). Tryptophan has also been tried to decrease nocturnal bruxism, and, compared with placebo, it was not effective. Intra-articular morphine has not helped (123).

Physical Therapy

Physical therapy has proven effectiveness in decreasing pain and improving jaw function in MPD and TMJ pain dysfunction syndromes. This can be as simple as ice and heat treatment to the facial muscles self-administered or administered by a family member. Adherence to a soft diet is a temporary physical measure that can help decrease pain.

Formal physical therapy includes the use of postural exercises, gentle range-of-motion exercises, ultrasonography to the masticatory muscles and TMJ, cold and heat therapy to the muscles (especially with stretching of the muscles), cryotherapy for acute tenderness, massage for the muscles of the head and neck, and TENS for acute and chronic pain in the TMJ and for MPD syndrome (124–127).

Iontophoresis

Two techniques are available that can help topical pharmacologic agents (e.g., corticosteroids) penetrate the skin: phonophoresis and iontophoresis. A double-blind study of transcutaneous iontophoresis with local anesthetic and then corticosteroid demonstrated relief in postherpetic neuralgia (59).

Manipulation

If there is an internal derangement with anterior displacement of the disc without reduction and limited opening, the jaw should not be manipulated open beyond the most comfortable opening. Forcing the mouth open risks further damage to the disc and posterior attachment. Closed manipulation of the jaw to reduce a displaced disc is seldom efficacious in the author's opinion (N. F. Ferraro, unpublished data). There is a school of practice supporting closed manipulation of the mandible to reduce displaced discs (128). What is often forgotten, however, is that by the time a disc displaces without reduction, it has undergone permanent morphologic change in many cases. Lysis and lavage of the TMJ via arthrocentesis with and without the addition of hyaluronate has proven to be quite beneficial in decreasing TMJ pain and improving opening in joints with internal derangement (122).

Splint Therapy

Dental splint therapy is a well-regarded and time-tested treatment for MPD and TMJ pain dysfunction syndromes. There are many splint variations, but for the sake of simplicity, two classes of bite splints (occlusal wafers, night guards) are discussed. The first is the flat-plane splint that can be made of hard or soft material and can be made to fit on the upper or lower teeth and provides a flat surface for the opposing teeth to glide on so there will not be traumatic side-to-side dental cusp interferences during grinding. It changes the resting length of the masticatory muscles fibers and neutralizes whatever malocclusion there might be. For these reasons, it can reduce the symptoms in MPD and TMJ pain dysfunction syndromes. Importantly, hard acrylic splints may decrease nocturnal bruxism (86). Whether the splint is maxillary or mandibular does not seem to matter. A study demonstrated that both groups of patients with TMJ pain improved (129). Our clinic uses a hard, flat-plane splint that may decrease bruxism and avoids soft splints that can increase bruxism. Most of our splints are fabricated for the maxilla. The second splint type is the repositioning splint that tries to position the condyle into a different relationship with the disc. The literature regarding the ability of these splints to cause the reduction of displaced discs is mixed, but symptomatic relief can often be achieved. A full discussion of these splints is beyond the scope of this chapter.

Behavioral Techniques, Biofeedback Techniques, Psychologic Therapy

Electromyographic biofeedback has become extremely important in the treatment of patients with MPD and TMJ pain dysfunction syndrome. The ability to relax tense and contracted muscles is something that the patient can carry away to be used when needed. Stress-reduction therapy and relaxation training are important parts of this modality also. Excellent results have been noted in muscle contraction headache and MPD syndrome (130). Behavioral therapies to gain control of noxious oral habits such as clenching and abnormal tongue and jaw movements are also important and efficacious (78).

There are patients who will require psychologic and psychiatric therapies to deal with depression, neuroses, and anxieties. The rarer individual who has one of the serious somatoform disorders associated with facial pain will need significant psychologic/psychiatric involvement as will patients who have dependence disorders.

Botulinum Toxin

Botulinum toxin type A relaxes the muscles by blocking at the neuromuscular junction. It has many uses now, including the cosmetic reduction of wrinkles. Injection into spastic masticatory muscles is proving to be safe and efficacious (131).

Temporomandibular Joint Arthroscopy

Arthroscopy is available for the diagnosis and treatment of intracapsular disorders including internal derangements of the TMJ and intracapsular adhesion. Via the arthroscope, the upper joint space can be lavaged, adhesions can be lysed, and drugs such as steroid or sodium hyaluronate can be injected. Improvement in pain and maximal opening has been quite good (132,133), although the ability to actually anatomically reposition the disc is not good (134). TMJ arthroscopy requires general anesthesia and carries risks that are similar to open-joint procedures and some complications that are unique to arthroscopy. Lavage alone can be performed for internal derangement with improved opening and decreased pain (135,136).

Temporomandibular Joint Surgery

Open TMJ operations for internal derangement and TMJ pain dysfunction have been performed for more than 100 years (69,70), but there has been a large increase in surgical activity over the past 20 years (71). The author is loathe to operate on the joint of a child or teenager for internal derangement.

Adults who are well screened can have a good result with internal derangement surgery, with improvement of jaw function and decreased pain. If there is a significant muscular hyperfunction problem, it must be addressed and treated or the surgical result will be poor. The patient's expectations must also be realistic.

Operations include repositioning of a displaced meniscus, meniscectomy if the disc is irreparable, condyloplasty if the condyle has significant DJD, and eminence reduction. If a meniscectomy is performed, the meniscus can be reconstructed with a temporalis myofascial flap. Alloplastic meniscus substitutes, including Teflon, silastic, and Proplast have fared poorly with fragmentation, regional lymphadenitis, and foreign body reaction (137,138). Except for silastic, which can be used as a temporary replacement (139), they are no longer used.

There is no evidence that surgery for internal derangement has a prophylactic benefit, i.e., decreases the rate or incidence of TMJ degeneration. As a result, we have always advised our patients that if they are coping and functioning, there is no place for surgery, even in the face of an internal derangement. An article by Wilkes (139) that includes long-term follow-up of adult patients who have had internal derangement and did not have surgery notes that the patient who did not have surgery had more DJD of the TMJ. More studies and substantiation are needed.

A patient with juvenile rheumatoid arthritis will rarely come to total joint reconstruction. If it is needed, we have opted for autogenous reconstruction with costochondral grafts and temporalis myofascial flaps. Alloplasts have been avoided. Occasionally, a young patient with Ehlers–Danlos syndrome needs to have an operation for painful, continual TMJ dislocations. Either a tethering operation with Mersilene tape to hold the condyle in the glenoid fossa or an eminectomy to prevent the condyle from locking out of the fossa can be performed.

The metal-on-metal Christensen total TMJ replacement appears to be quite safe and has established a track record of use (140).

CONCLUSION

This chapter presents an overview of facial pain ranging from acute dental, sinus, and ear pain to more chronic pain syndromes. Weight is given to the MPD and TMJ pain dysfunction syndromes because of the frequency of occurrence in children.

The principles stressed for diagnosing and treating facial pain are (a) know the anatomy, (b) have a low threshold to investigate for occult lesions, (c) consider all the factors that are contributing to a patient's pain (physical, emotional, and social), and (d) make use of an interdisciplinary group for the best patient care.

ACKNOWLEDGMENT

I am forever grateful to Aujah Fairbain for her remarkable work and to Marilou Stockton and Maureen Podolski.

REFERENCES

1. Bonica JJ. History of pain concepts and therapies. In: Bonica JJ, ed. *The management of pain*, 2nd ed. Philadelphia: Lea & Febiger, 1990:2–15.
2. Bonica JJ. Definitions and taxonomy of pain. In: Bonica JJ, ed. *The management of pain*, 2nd ed. Philadelphia: Lea & Febiger, 1990:18.
3. Malamed SF. *Sedation: a guide to patient management*, 2nd ed. St. Louis: CV Mosby, 1989.
4. Burgess JA, Byers MR, Dworkin SF. Pain of dental and intraoral origin. In: Bonica JJ, ed. *The management of pain*, 2nd ed. Philadelphia: Lea & Febiger, 1990:746–758.
5. Azerad J, Woda A. Sensations evoked by bipolar intrapulpal stimulation. *Pain* 1977;4:145–152.
6. Narhi M. The characteristics of intradental sensory units and their responses to stimulation. *J Dent Res* 1985;64:564–571.
7. Kennedy DB, Kapala JT. The dental pulp: biologic principles of protection and treatment. In: Braham RL, Morns ME, eds. *Textbook of pediatric dentistry*. Philadelphia: BC Decker 1988:492–498.
8. Armitage GC. Periodontal diseases of children. In: Braham RL, Morris ME, eds. *Textbook of pediatric dentistry*. Philadelphia: BC Decker, 1988:235–252.
9. Killey HC, Seward GR, Kay LW. *An outline of oral surgery, part 1*. Bristol: John Wright & Sons, 1975: 120–123.
10. Mahan PE, Alling CC III. *Facial pain*, 3rd ed. Philadelphia: Lea & Febiger, 1991:311–322.
11. Stevenson DD. Allergy, atopy, nasal disease, and headache. In: Dalessio DJ, ed. *Wolff's headache and other head pain*, 5th ed. New York: Oxford University Press, 1987:220–229.
12. Milmoe GJ. Sinusitis: acute, chronic, and complications. In: Healy GB, ed. *Common problems in pediatric otolaryngology*. Chicago: Year Book, 1990:209–215.
13. Brodsky L. Nasal obstruction in childhood. In: Healy GB, ed. *Common problems in pediatric otolaryngology*. Chicago: Year Book, 1990:157–164.
14. Hayden GF, Schwartz RH. Characteristics of earache among children with acute otitis media. *Am J Dis Child* 1985;139:721–723.
15. Barr RG. Pain in children In: Wall PD, Melzack R, eds. *Textbook of pain*, 2nd ed. New York: Churchill-Livingstone, 1989:575.
16. Gates GA. Salivary gland disease in children. In: Healy GB, ed. *Common problems in pediatric otolaryngology*. Chicago: Year Book, 1990:289–295.
17. Kaban LB. *Pediatric oral and maxillofacial surgery*. Philadelphia: WB Saunders, 1990:195–207.
18. Malins TJ, Farrow A. Facial pain due to occult parotid adenoid cystic carcinoma. *J Oral Maxillofac Surg* 1991;49:1127–1129.
19. Carlow TJ. Headache and the eye. In: Dalessio DJ, ed. *Wolff''s headache and other head pain*. New York: Oxford University Press, 1987:304–320.
20. Avery ME. Corneal opacities at birth. In: Avery ME, First LIZ, eds. *Pediatric medicine*. Baltimore: Williams & Wilkins, 1989:1218–1219.
21. Mulliken JB, Young AE. Vascular birthmarks. Philadelphia: WB Saunders, 1988:177–178.
22. Heyck H. *Headache and facial pain*. Chicago: Year Book, 1981:125–126.

23. Malamed SF. *Handbook of local anesthesia*, 3rd ed. St. Louis: Mosby Year Book, 1990.
24. Wilson TG, Primosch RE, Melamed B, et al. Clinical effectiveness of 1% and 2% lidocaine in young pediatric dental patients. *Pediatr Dent* 1990;12:353–359.
25. Knodd-Kohler E, Knoller M, Brandt K, et al. Cardiohemodynamic and serum catecholamine response to surgical removal of impacted mandibular third molars under local anesthesia. *J Oral Maxillofac Surg* 1991; 49:957–962.
26. McMillan AS, Walshaw D, Meechan JG. The efficacy of EMLA and 5% lignocaine gel for anesthesia of human gingival mucosa. *Br J Oral Maxillofac Surg* 2000; 38:58–62.
27. Tulga F, Mutlu Z. Four types of topical anesthetic agents: evaluation of clinical effectiveness. *J Clin Pediatr Dent* 1999;23:217–220.
28. Chapman PJ, Ganendran A. Prolonged analgesia following preoperative bupivacaine neural blockade for oral surgery performed under general anesthesia. *J Oral Maxillofac Surg* 1987;45:233–235.
29. Bouloux GF, Punnia-Moorthy A. Bupivacaine versus lidocaine for third molar surgery: a double blind, randomized, crossover study. *J Oral Maxillofac Surg* 1999;57:510–515.
30. Brennan PA, Gardiner GT, McHugh J. A double blind clinical trial to assess the value of aprotinin in third molar surgery. *Br J Oral Maxillofac Surg* 1991;29: 176–179.
31. Gallardo F, Carstens M, Ayarza M. Analgesic and anti-inflammatory effects of glucamethacin (a nonsteroidal anti-inflammatory analgesic) after the removal of impacted third molars. *Oral Surg Oral Med Oral Pathol* 1990;69:157–160.
32. Habib S, Matthews RW, Scully C, et al. A study of the comparative efficacy of four common analgesics in the control of postsurgical dental pain. *Oral Surg Oral Med Oral Pathol* 1990;70:559–563.
33. Dionne RA. Additive analgesic effects of oxycodone and ibuprofen in the oral surgery model. *J Oral Maxillofac Surg* 1999;57:673–679.
34. Sisk AL, Grover B, Steflik DE. Long term memory of acute postsurgical pain. *J Oral Maxillofac Surg* 1991; 49:353–358.
35. Barker G, Loftus L, Cuddy P, et al. The effects of sucralfate suspension and diphenhydramine syrup plus kaolin-pectin on radiotherapy-induced mucositis. *Oral Surg Oral Med Oral Pathol* 1991;71:288–293.
36. Porteder H, Rausch E, Kment G, et al. Local prostaglandin E in patients with oral malignancies undergoing chemo and radiotherapy. *J Craniomaxillofac Surg* 1988;16:371–374.
37. Janetta PG. Microsurgical approach to the trigeminal nerve. *Prog Neurol Surg* 1976;7:180–200.
38. Childs AM, Meaney JF, Ferrier CD, et al. Neurovascular compression of trigeminal and glossopharyngeal nerve: three case reports. *Arch Dis Child* 2000;82:311–315.
39. Massey EW, Massey J. Elongated styloid process (Eagle's syndrome) causing hemicrania. *Headache* 1979;19:339–344.
40. Sivers JE, Johnson GK. Diagnosis of Eagle's syndrome. *Oral Surg Oral Med Oral Pathol* 1985;59: 575–577.
41. Eagle WW. Sphenopalatine ganglion neuralgia. *Arch Otolaryngol* 1942;35:66.
42. Cook N. Cryosurgery of migraine. *Headache* 1973;12: 143–150.
43. Zakrzweska JM. Cluster headache: review of literature. *Br J Oral Maxillofac Surg* 2001;39:103–114.
44. Barlow CF. *Headaches and migraine in childhood.* Philadelphia: JB Lippincott, 1984.
45. Huang AS. Perspectives in virology. In: Avery ME, First LR, eds. *Pediatric medicine*. Baltimore: Williams & Wilkins, 1989:1039.
46. Lee KJ, Lee KE. Syndromes and eponyms In: Lee KJ, ed. *Essential otolaryngology*, 4th ed. New York: Medical Examination Publishing Company, 1987:675.
47. Nguyen M, Maciewicz R, Bouckoms A, et al. Facial pain symptoms in patients with cerebellopontine angle tumors. *Clin J Pain* 1986;2:3.
48. Ishikawa T, Murakami K, Yasui R, et al. A multifocal schwannoma of the masseteric nerve causing hemicrania. *Oral Surg Oral Med Oral Pathol* 1991;71: 329–332.
49. Webster K. Adenocarcinoma metastatic to the mandibular condyle. *J Craniomaxillofac Surg* 1988;16: 230–232.
50. Chemello PD, Neldon CL, Tomich CE, et al. Embryonal rhabdomyosarcoma arising in the masseter muscle as a second malignant neoplasm. *J Oral Maxillofac Surg* 1988;46.899–895.
51. Feinmann C, Harris M. Psychogenic facial pain. Part II: management and prognosis. *Br Dent J* 1984;156: 165–168.
52. Belfer ML, Kaban LB. Temporomandibular joint dysfunction with facial pain in children. *Pediatrics* 1982; 69:564–567.
53. Kaban LB, Belfer ML. Temporomandibular joint dysfunction: an occasional manifestation of serious psychopathology. *J Oral Surg* 1981;39:742–746.
54. Pillemer FG, Masek BJ, Kaban LB. Temporomandibular joint dysfunction and facial pain in children: an approach to diagnosis and treatment. *Pediatrics* 1987;80:565–570.
55. Goldberg RT, Pachas WN, Keith D. Relationship between traumatic events in childhood and chronic pain. *Disabil Rehabil* 1999;21:23–30.
56. Knoben JE, Anderson PO. *Handbook of clinical drug data*, 6th ed. Hamilton: Drug Intelligence Publications, 1988:564.
57. Travell JG, Simons DG. *Myofascial pain and dysfunction: the trigger point manual.* Baltimore: Williams & Wilkins, 1983.
58. Bonica JJ. Local anaesthesia and regional blocks. In: Wall PD, Melzack R, eds. *Textbook of pain*, 2nd ed. Edinburgh: Churchill-Livingstone, 1989:724–743.
59. Gangarosa LP, Mahan PE, Ciarlone AE. Pharmacologic management of temporomandibular joint disorders and chronic head and neck pain. *J Craniomandib Pract* 1991;9:335–336.
60. Zakrzewska JM, Nally FF, Flint SR. Cryotherapy in the management of paroxysmal trigeminal neuralgia. *J Maxillofac Surg* 1986:14:5–7.
61. Sokolovic M, Todorovic L, Stajcic Z, et al. Peripheral streptomycin/lidocaine injections in the treatment of idiopathic trigeminal neuralgia. *J Maxillofac Surg* 1986;14:8–9.
62. Stajcic Z, Juniper RP, Todorovic L. Peripheral streptomycin/lidocaine injections versus lidocaine alone in the treatment of idiopathic trigeminal neuralgia. A

double blind controlled trial. *J Craniomaxillofac Surg* 1990,18:243–246.
63. Juniper RP. Trigeminal neuralgia-treatment of the third division by radiologically controlled cryo blockade of the inferior dental nerve at the mandibular lingula: a study of 31 cases. *Br J Oral Maxillofac Surg* 1991;29: 154–158.
64. Gregg JM, Banerjee T, Ghia JN, et al. Radiofrequency thermoneurolysis of peripheral nerves for control of trigeminal neuralgia. *Pain* 1978;5:231–243.
65. Sweet WH, Wepsic JG. Controlled thermocoagulation of trigeminal ganglion and rootlets for differential destruction of pain fibres. Part 1: trigeminal neuralgia. *J Neurosurg* 1974;40:143–156.
66. Andersen PE, Cohen JI, Everts EC, et al. Intrathecal narcotics for relief of pain from head and neck cancer. *Arch Otolaryngol Head Neck Surg* 1991;117: 1277–1280.
67. Bryant GW. Myofascial pain dysfunction and viola playing. *Br Dent J* 1989;166:335–336.
68. Hylander WL. Functional anatomy. In: Sarnat BG, Laskin DM, eds. *The temporomandibular joint: a biological basis for clinical practice*. 4th ed. Philadelphia: WB Saunders, 1992:60–92.
69. Annandale T. On displacement of the interarticular cartilage of the lower jaw and its treatment by operation. *Lancet* 1887;1:411.
70. Wakeley CG. The causation and treatment of displaced mandibular cartilage. *Lancet* 1929;2:543–545.
71. McCarty WL, Farrar WB. Surgery for internal derangements of the temporomandibular joint. *J Prosthet Dent* 1979;42:191–196.
72. Nitzan D, Dolwick MF. An alternative explanation for the genesis of closed-lock symptoms in the internal derangement process. *J Oral Maxillofac Surg* 1991;49: 810–815.
73. Graham CS, Ferraro NF, Simms DA. Perforations of the temporomandibular joint meniscus: arthrographic, surgical and clinical findings. *J Oral Maxillofac Surg* 1984;42:35–38.
74. Hatala MP, Westesson P-L, Tallents RH, et al. TMJ disc displacement in asymptomatic volunteers detected by MR imaging. *J Dent Res* 1991;70:278.
75. Isberg A, Stenstrom B, Isacsson G. Frequency of bilateral joint disc displacement in patients with unilateral symptoms: a 5-year follow-up of the asymptomatic joint. *Dentomaxillofac Radiol* 1991;20:73–76.
76. Schwartz L. *Disorders of the temporomandibular joint*. Philadelphia: WB Saunders, 1959:45–54.
77. Rugh JD, Solberg WK. Psychological implications in temporomandibular pain and dysfunction. In: Zarb GA, Carlsson GE, eds. *Temporomandibular joint function and dysfunction*. Copenhagen: Munksgaard, 1979: 239–268.
78. Rugh JD. Behavioral therapy for temporomandibular disorders. *Curr Opin Dent* 1991;1:497–502.
79. Goodman P, Greene CS, Laskin DM. Response of patients with myofascial pain-dysfunction syndrome to mock equilibration. *J Am Dent Assoc* 1976;92: 755–758.
80. Huber MA, Hall EH. A comparison of the signs of temporomandibular joint dysfunction and occlusal discrepancies in the symptom-free population of men and women. *Oral Surg Oral Med Oral Pathol* 1990;70: 180–183.
81. Egermark-Eriksson I, Carlsson GE, Magnusson T, et al. A longitudinal study on malocclusion in relation to signs and symptoms of cranio-mandibular disorders in children and adolescents. *Eur J Orthod* 1990;12: 399–407.
82. Kerstein RB, Farrell S. Treatment of myofascial pain-dysfunction syndrome with occlusal equilibration. *J Prosthet Dent* 1990;63:695–700.
83. Reynders RM. Orthodontics and temporomandibular disorders: a review of the literature (1966–1988). *Am J Orthod Dentofacial Orthop* 1990;97:463–471.
84. Kobayashi T, Honma K, Izumi K, et al. TMJ syndromes and disc displacement in patients with mandibular prognathism. *Br J Oral Maxillofac Surg* 1999; 37:455–459.
85. Magnusson T, Ahlborg G, Finne K, et al. Changes in temporomandibular joint pain dysfunction after surgical correction of dentofacial anomalies. *Int J Oral Maxillofac Surg* 1986;15:707–714.
86. Okeson JP. Bruxing events and sleep. *TMJ Update* 1986;4:109–112.
87. Christensen LV. Facial pain and internal pressure of masseter muscle in experimental bruxism in man. *Arch Oral Biol* 1971;16:1021–1031.
88. Widmalm SE, Christionasen RL, Gunn SM. Oral parafunctions as temporomandibular disorder risk factors in children. *Cranio* 1995;13:242–246.
89. Ware JC, Rugh JD. Destructive bruxism: sleep stage relationship. *Sleep* 1988;11:172–181.
90. Satoh T, Harada Y. Tooth-grinding during sleep as an arousal reaction. *Experientia* 1971;27:785–786.
91. Guralnick W, Kaban LB, Merrill RG. Temporomandibular-joint afflictions. *N Engl J Med* 1978;299: 959.
92. Reding GR. Letter to the editor. *N Engl J Med* 1978; 299:123–129
93. Ramfjord SP. Bruxism, a clinical and electromyographic study. *J Am Dent Assoc* 1961;62:21–43.
94. Wianman A, Agerberg G. Mandibular dysfunction in adolescents. I. Prevalence of symptoms. *Acta Odontol Scand* 1986;44:47–54.
95. Wianman A, Agerberg G. Mandibular dysfunction in adolescents. I. Prevalence of signs. *Acta Odontol Scand* 1986;44:55–62.
96. Ohno H, Morinushi T, Ohno K, et al. A longitudinal study on individual fluctuation of signs in accordance with TMJ dysfunction syndrome in adolescents. *Jpn J Pedodont* 1989;27:64–73(abst).
97. Mohlin B, Pilley JR, Shaw WC. A survey of craniomandibular disorders in 1000 12-year-olds. Study design and baseline data in a follow-up study. *Eur J Orthod* 1991;13:111–123.
98. Bernal M, Tsamtsouris A. Signs and symptoms of temporomandibular joint dysfunction in 3 to 5 year old children. *J Pedod* 1986;10:127–140.
99. Razook SJ, Gotcher JE Jr, Bays RA. Temporomandibular joint noises in infants: review of the literature and report of cases. *Oral Surg Oral Med Oral Pathol* 1989;67:658–664.
100. Franklin D, Smith RJ, Catlin FL, et al. Temporomandibular joint dysfunction in infancy. *Int J Pediatr Otorhinolaryngol* 1986;12:99–104.
101. Reik L Jr, Hale M. The temporomandibular joint pain dysfunction syndrome: a frequent cause of headache. *J Headache* 1981;21:151–156.

102. Smith MS, Womack WM, Chen ACN. Intrinsic patient variables and outcome in the behavioral treatment of recurrent pediatric headache. In: Tyler DC, Krane EJ, eds. *Advances in pain research and therapy: pediatric pain, vol 15*. New York: Raven Press, 1990:305–311.
103. Watts P, Peet K, Juniper R. Migraine and the temporomandibular joint: the final answer? *Br Dent J* 1986; 161:170–173.
104. Costen JB. A syndrome of ear and sinus symptoms dependent upon disturbed function of the temporomandibular joint. *Ann Otol Rhinolaryngol* 1934;43: 1–15.
105. Malkin DP. The role of TMJ dysfunction in the etiology of middle ear disease. *Int J Orthod* 1987;25: 20–21.
106. Myers LJ. Possible inflammatory pathways relating temporomandibular joint dysfunction to otic symptoms. *Cranio* 1988;6:64–70.
107. Williamson EH. The interrelationship of internal derangements of the temporomandibular joint, headache, vertigo, and tinnitus: a survey of 25 patients. *J Craniomandib Pract* 1990;8:301–306.
108. Gagnon P. Temporo-mandibular joint pain dysfunction syndrome in children. *J Otolaryngol* 1978;7: 549–555(abst).
109. Sanchez-Woodworth RE, Katzberg RW, Tallents RH, et al. Radiographic assessment of temporomandibular joint pain and dysfunction in the pediatric age group. *ASDC J Dent Child* 1988;55:278.
110. Helms CA, Katzberg MC, Dolwick MF, et al. Arthrotomographic diagnosis of meniscus perforations in the temporomandibular joint. *Br J Radiol* 1980;53: 283–285.
111. Dolwick MF, Katzberg, Helms CA, et al. Arthrotomographic evaluation of the temporomandibular joint. *J Oral Surg* 1979;37:793–799.
112. Sacks H, Zelig D, Schabes G. Recurrent temporomandibular joint subluxation and facial ecchymosis leading to diagnosis of Ehlers-Danlos syndrome: a report of surgical management and review of the literature. *J Oral Maxillofac Surg* 1990;48:641–647.
113. Lloyd JM, Mitchell RG. Myasthenia gravis as a cause of facial pain. *Oral Surg Oral Med Oral Pathol* 1988; 66:45–46.
114. Buckingham RB, Braun T, Harinstein DA, et al. Temporomandibular joint dysfunction syndrome: a close association with systemic joint laxity (the hypermobile joint syndrome). *Oral Surg Oral Med Oral Pathol* 1991;72:514–519.
115. Buxbaum JD, Parente FJ, Myslinski NR. Ibuprofen an effective treatment for myofascial pain dysfunction. *Pain Manage* 1987;1:27.
116. Gordon SM, Montgomery MT, Jones DL. Comparative efficacy of piroxicam, acetaminophen and placebo for temporomandibular pain. *J Dent Res* 1991;70:329(abst).
117. Bouckoms AJ, Keith DA. Pharmacologic treatment for chronic facial pain. *Curr Opin Dent* 1991;1:480–484.
118. Harkins S, Linford J, Cohen J, et al. Administration of clonazepam in the treatment of TMD and associated pain: a double blind pilot study. *J Craniomandib Disord Facial Oral Pain* 1991;5:179–186.
119. Rugh JD, Davis SE. Temporomandibular disorders: psychological and behavioral aspects. In: Samat BG, Laskin DM, eds. *The temporomandibular joint*, 4th ed. Philadelphia: WB Saunders, 1992:338.
120. Kopp S, Wenneberg B, Haraldson T, et al. The short-term effect of intra-articular injections of sodium hyaluronate and corticosteroid on temporomandibular joint pain and dysfunction. *J Oral Maxillofac Surg* 1985;43:429–435.
121. McCain JP, Balazs EA, de la Rua H. Preliminary studies on the use of a viscoelastic solution in arthroscopic surgery of the temporomandibular joint. *J Oral Maxillofac Surg* 1989;47:1161–1168.
122. Millinger G. Neutral amino acid therapy for the management of chronic pain. *Cranio* 1986;4: 157–163.
123. Etzel KR, Stockstill JW, Rugh JD, et al. Tryptophan supplementation for nocturnal bruxism: a report of negative results. *J Craniomandib Disord* 1991;5: 115–120.
124. Sturdivant J, Fricton JR. Physical therapy for temporomandibular disorders and orofacial pain. *Curr Opin Dent* 1991;1:485–496.
125. Clark GT, Adachi NY, Dornan MR. Physical medicine procedures affect temporomandibular disorders: a review. *J Am Dent Assoc* 1990;121:151–162.
126. Kirk WS, Calabrese DK. Clinical evaluation of physical therapy in the management of internal derangement of the temporomandibular joint. *J Oral Maxillofac Surg* 1989;47:113–119.
127. Bremerich A, Wiegel W, Thein T, et al. Transcutaneous electric nerve stimulation (TENS) in the therapy of chronic facial pain. Preliminary report. *J Craniomaxillofac Surg* 1988;16:379–381.
128. Harkins SJ, Marteney JL, Cueva L. A simple technique for the distraction and mobilization of the temporomandibular joint condyle in nonreducing disc derangements. *J Prosthet Dent* 1987;58:623–625.
129. Schumann S, Nohr A, Hagen B, et al. Comparative efficacy of maxillar and mandibular splints for TMD pain. *J Dent Res* 1991;70:441(abst).
130. Masek BJ, Russo DC, Varni JW. Behavioral approaches to the management of chronic pain in children. *Pediatr Clin North Am* 1984;31:1113–1131.
131. Freund B, Schwartz M, Symington JM. Botulinum toxin: new treatment for temporomandibular disorders. *Br J Oral Maxillofac Surg* 2000;38:466–472.
132. Perrott DH, Alborzi A, Kaban LB, et al. A prospective evaluation of the effectiveness of temporomandibular joint arthroscopy. *J Oral Maxillofac Surg* 1990;48: 1029–1032.
133. White RD. Retrospective analysis of 100 consecutive surgical arthroscopies of the temporomandibular joint. *J Oral Maxillofac Surg* 1989;47:1014–1021.
134. Montgomery MT, Van Sickels JE, Harms SE, et al. Arthroscopic TMJ surgery: effects on signs, symptoms, and disc position. *J Oral Maxillofac Surg* 1989; 47:1263–1271.
135. Indresano AT. Surgical arthroscopy as the preferred treatment for internal derangements of the temporomandibular joint. *J Oral Maxillofac Surg* 2001;59: 308–312.
136. White RD. Part II: arthroscopic lysis and lavage as the preferred treatment for internal derangement of the temporomandibular joint. *J Oral Maxillofac Surg* 2001;59:313–316.
137. Wagner JD, Mosby EL. Assessment of Proplast-Teflon disc replacements. *J Oral Maxillofac Surg* 1990;48: 1140–1144.

138. Rooney TP, Haug RH, Toor AH, et al. Rapid condylar degeneration after glenoid fossa prosthesis insertion: report of three cases. *J Oral Maxillofac Surg* 1988;46: 240–246.
139. Wilkes CH. Surgical treatment of internal derangements of the temporomandibular joint: a long-term study. *Arch Otolaryngol Head Neck Surg* 1991;117: 64–72.
140. Garrett WR, Abbey RA, Christensen RW. Temporomandibular joint reconstruction with a custom total temporomandibular joint prosthesis: use in the multiply operated patient. *Surg Technol Int VI* 1997;4:347–354.

44

Pain Management for the Critically Ill Child in the Pediatric Intensive Care Unit

Joseph D. Tobias

Several factors may be responsible for the pain experienced by children in the pediatric intensive care unit (PICU). Although acute pain can be directly related to the underlying medical illness or traumatic event, several other factors may be responsible for the emotional pain, anxiety, and distress experienced during the PICU experience. Separation from parents, disruption of the day–night cycle, the presence of unfamiliar people, the continuous noise of imposing machines and monitoring devices, fear of death, and loss of self-control can all lead to feelings of fear, pain, hopelessness, and emotional distress. Additionally, therapies aimed at controlling the primary illness may result in additional pain. Dressing changes for burns, the presence of an endotracheal tube, or placement of central venous or arterial cannulae and other invasive procedures all affect the patient in the PICU. Although open communication, reassurance, and parental presence may alleviate or prevent some of these problems, pharmacologic intervention is frequently necessary to control pain and emotional distress.

Although the importance of aggressive sedation and pain control for the patient in the PICU cannot be overemphasized, the use of such agents should not proceed without appropriate caution and preparation (Table 44.1). The PICU provides the optimal environment for monitoring a patient's cardiorespiratory status. Because any of the agents reviewed in this chapter can have significant deleterious effects, monitoring the patient's cardiorespiratory status, in accordance with the guidelines of the American Academy of Pediatrics, is suggested (1).

Physiologic causes of agitation such as hypoxemia, hypercarbia, and cerebral hypoperfusion from a low cardiac output state must be excluded. Identification of the cause of the distress can be used to guide the selection of the most appropriate agent. Ongoing tissue injury and the presence of pain require the use of analgesic agents, whereas emotional distress and anxiety may be more appropriately treated with anxiolytic agents. Variability that may influence the choice of agents is also pre-

TABLE 44.1. *Preparation for pediatric intensive care unit sedation*

1. Rule out treatable causes of agitation
   a. hypoxia
   b. hypercarbia
   c. cerebral hypoperfusion
   d. bladder distention
   e. surgical lesion, necrotic bowel
2. Identify cause of pain or agitation to guide appropriate selection of agent or agents
3. Monitoring according to the standards suggested by the American Academy of Pediatrics
4. Decision points
   a. agent to be used
   b. route of administration (intravenous, inhalation, subcutaneous, oral, neuraxial)
   c. mode of administration (intermittent bolus, continuous infusion, or patient-controlled delivery)
5. Titrate the dose based on the patient's clinical response
6. Observe for adverse effects
7. Monitor response using formalized pain/sedation scales
8. Observe for signs of tolerance and continue to increase dose as needed

sent when considering the length of time during which sedation or analgesia is required. Sedation and analgesia may be needed for less than 15 minutes for an invasive procedure, for 1 to 2 hours during magnetic resonance imaging, or for days or weeks during mechanical ventilation or after acute traumatic injuries. When selecting an agent, the half-life and its duration of effect need to be considered. Short-acting drugs that provide rapid recovery may be considered for brief procedures, whereas longer acting agents or continuous infusions of short-acting agents are used for longer procedures.

Unfortunately, few studies have evaluated the pharmacokinetics and pharmacodynamic properties of analgesic and sedative drugs in critically ill patients in general and in children in particular (2–4). Most pharmacokinetic studies are performed in healthy adult volunteers or postoperative patients and then extrapolated to the critical care population. Unstable patients can present significant differences with regard to end-organ function, cardiorespiratory stability, volume of distribution, and metabolic processes. The variability of the patient in the PICU can also include drug–drug interactions, end-organ (hepatic, renal) failure, malnutrition, and low plasma proteins with altered drug binding as well as changes in uptake (of particular concern when using the nonintravenous route), distribution (owing to alterations in cardiac output), and volume of distribution. Although there are no clear guidelines to identify each of these problems and their eventual effects on the specific analgesic or sedative agent used, all should be considered when selecting a specific drug, the dose, and the route of administration.

When providing sedation and analgesia for the patient in the PICU, three basic choices must be made: (a) the agent to be used, (b) the route of administration, and (c) the mode of administration. Several agents have been used for sedation in the intensive care unit (ICU) setting (Table 44.2). Despite experience with all these agents, none can be expected to be effective in all patients or meet the criteria of the ideal agent (Table 44.3). When caring for children in the PICU, physicians should attempt to become skilled in using several agents. Such flexibility allows one to switch from one agent to another when the first-line drug is either ineffective or leads to adverse effects. When initiating a sedation/analgesia regimen, monitoring the response to the therapy is equally important. This may involve the use of formal pain/sedation scoring systems by the nursing staff that can be assessed with the other routine vital signs at specific intervals. This monitoring should be an ongoing process so that the doses are increased as needed over time when tolerance develops. Equally as important is monitoring the patient for adverse effects related to the introduction of sedative/analgesic agents.

TABLE 44.2. *Possible agents for sedation in the pediatric intensive care unit*

Inhalational anesthetic agents
Nitrous oxide
Benzodiazepines
Opioids
Phenothiazines
Butyrophenones
Antihistamines
Chloral hydrate
Etomidate
Ketamine
Barbiturates
Propofol
Clonidine/dexmedetomidine

TABLE 44.3. *Properties of the ideal agent for pediatric intensive care unit sedation*

Rapid onset
Easy to titrate by intravenous infusion
Predictable duration of activity
No active metabolites
Effects dissipate rapidly when agent is discontinued
Multiple options for route of delivery
Limited effects on cardiorespiratory function
Limited adverse effect profile
Effects and duration not altered by renal or hepatic disease
No interference with effect or metabolism by other drugs
Wide therapeutic index
Cost effective
Slow development of tolerance

Because of the diversity of the population in the PICU and the indications for these agents, it is impossible to formulate a "cookbook" with strict guidelines for the drugs to be used and the doses required for sedation and analgesia. These drugs are not dosed on a per-kilogram basis like other medications such as antibiotics. The dosing recommendations are merely suggested starting doses with the actual amount titrated up or down to achieve the desired level of sedation or analgesia while avoiding adverse effects. Katz and Kelly (5) demonstrated the interpatient variability of the PICU population. When evaluating the infusion rates of fentanyl required to provide sedation during mechanical ventilation in neonates and infants, they noted variability ranging from 0.47 to 10.3 μg/kg per hour.

Options for the route of delivery in the patient in the PICU have expanded. In most patients, the intravenous route is chosen; however, in some situations, alternative, nonintravenous routes may become necessary. Drug incompatibilities may preclude intravenous administration in patients with limited intravenous access. With specific drugs, alternative routes of delivery may be employed (Table 44.4). Additionally, when specific agents are chosen, they may allow delivery via only one route. For example, chloral hydrate requires oral or rectal administration, isoflurane requires inhalation administration, and propofol requires intravenous administration. Other agents such as midazolam provide several options for the route of delivery (Table 44.5), although the nonintravenous route may not be optimal for repeated administration and also negates to some extent a rapid titration to the desired level of sedation.

TABLE 44.4. *Routes of delivery for sedativeanalgesic agents*

Intravenous
Intramuscular
Subcutaneous
Oral
Transmucosal
Buccal
Nasal
Rectal
Sublingual
Transdermal
Inhalation

TABLE 44.5. *Suggested dosing guidelines for midazolam administration*

Route	Dose (mg/kg)	Maximal dose (mg)	Ref.
Oral	0.5–0.7	20	24,25
Rectal	1.0	20	24
Nasal	0.2–0.4	10	26,27
Sublingual	0.2	10	26
Intravenous	0.03–0.05	2	21–23
Intramuscular	0.05	5	20
Subcutaneous	Same as intravenous	—	28

With intravenous administration, the dose can be repeated every 3 to 5 minutes and titrated to effect. The onset time of the alternative routes varies from 5 to 10 minutes with nasal and sublingual administration 20 to 30 minutes with oral and rectal administration.

The third variable is the mode of administration. Options include continuous administration, intermittent dosing, or patient-controlled techniques. Although longer acting agents may be used by intermittent bolus administration, when the need for sedation/analgesia is prolonged, short-acting agents are usually best administered by a continuous infusion to maintain a steady-state serum concentration, thereby providing an ongoing effect. Another alternative that has gained popularity for the delivery of analgesic agents is a patient-activated device known as patient-controlled analgesia. The use of patient-activated devices may also be considered for the delivery of sedative and anxiolytic agents, thereby allowing patients some control over their level of sedation. The initial clinical studies in the operating room setting where patient-controlled delivery of sedative agents is used during brief surgical procedures have demonstrated results similar to those of studies using patient-controlled analgesia; patients report an increased level of satisfaction with a decreased requirement for sedative or analgesic agents.

Despite the difficulties of providing sedation and analgesia to the patient in the PICU, the benefits of such care are extraordinary.

Aside from the obvious humanitarian concerns, clinical studies have demonstrated improvements in morbidity and mortality rates with effective analgesic regimens after cardiovascular surgery for congenital heart disease in neonates and infants (6,7). Although it may not be possible to extrapolate these benefits to the entire PICU population, effective sedation may provide benefits under other circumstances. Sedation during mechanical ventilation has become increasingly important with newer modalities of mechanical ventilation such as permissive hypercapnia, reverse inspiratory:expiratory (I:E) ratio ventilation, and high-frequency techniques. Sedation may serve as a therapeutic tool to treat intracranial hypertension or to modulate pulmonary vascular resistance in patients at risk of pulmonary hypertension.

AGENTS FOR SEDATION

In the current clinical setting, opioids and benzodiazepines remain the most frequently used agents for sedation (8). Several alternatives are available including the inhalational anesthetic agents, nitrous oxide, ketamine, propofol, the phenothiazines, the butyrophenones, and the barbiturates. These alternative agents are most commonly chosen when opioids and benzodiazepines, either alone or in combination, are ineffective or associated with significant adverse physiologic effects.

Despite some inherent problems, there remains a large wealth of clinical experience demonstrating the efficacy and safety of the benzodiazepines and opioids. Before the widespread acceptance and application to clinical practice, careful evaluation of new agents is required. Lessons learned from the past with agents such as etomidate emphasize the importance of such concepts. After its introduction into clinical practice, etomidate appeared to be a beneficial agent for ICU sedation because of its lack of adverse effects on cardiovascular function. However, when used by continuous infusion for prolonged sedation in the ICU population, increased mortality occurred related to its depressant effects on adrenocortical function and the inhibition of cortisol production (9). Despite this, etomidate, because of its lack of effects on cardiovascular function and its beneficial effects on the cerebral metabolic rate for oxygen ($CMRO_2$) resulting in a lowering of intracranial pressure (ICP), remains a useful agent for providing sedation/anesthesia during endotracheal intubation in the patient with increased ICP or altered cardiovascular function. In this setting, etomidate is used as a single dose of 0.2 to 0.3 mg/kg along with a neuromuscular blocking agent (10,11). Other associated adverse effects are pain on injection, myoclonic movements, and nausea/vomiting.

Inhalational Anesthetic Agents

The inhalational anesthetic agents (halothane, isoflurane, desflurane, enflurane, and sevoflurane) are used every day to provide amnesia and analgesia during surgical procedures. Despite limited use in the United States, some centers in Europe have significant experience with these agents for providing sedation in adult patients in the ICU (12,13). To date, there are no reports concerning the administration of the two newer inhalational anesthetic agents sevoflurane, desflurane for sedation in the ICU. Although the other three agents (halothane, enflurane, and isoflurane) have all been used in an ICU setting, because of specific considerations, only isoflurane remains in common clinical use for sedation in the ICU. Problems with halothane include a direct negative inotropic effect, arrhythmogenic properties especially in the setting of increased catecholamines or when used in conjunction with other medications (aminophylline), and hepatitis, related to an immunologic reaction directed against the oxidative metabolite, trifluoroacetic acid (14,15). Although the latter problem has been reported with the other inhalation agents including isoflurane, its incidence is much lower with isoflurane because of its limited metabolism (0.2%) compared with that of halothane (15% to 20%). These issues may relate not only to the patient but also to other health care providers who work in the area that may be contaminated with these inhalational agents (see below for further discussion regarding the issue of scavenging exhaled gases). Concerns with enflurane include a similar negative inotropic effect and the release of fluoride during metabolism. Although only 2% of enflurane is metabolized, its content of fluoride is high enough that, with a 2% metabolism rate, serum fluoride concentrations can increase with prolonged administration. Fluoride concentrations greater than 50 μmol/L can result in direct nephrotoxicity with a decreased glomerular filtration rate and renal tubular resistance to vasopressin with nephrogenic diabetes insipidus. The newer agent sevoflurane undergoes significant metabolism (3% to 5%), and prolonged administration can result in elevated serum fluoride concentrations.

The primary hemodynamic effect of isoflurane is peripheral vasodilation. The latter decreases afterload, thereby increasing cardiac output as opposed to the decrease in cardiac output that occurs with either halothane or enflurane. Reflex tachycardia can increase myocardial oxygen demand and lead to an imbalance in the myocardial oxygen delivery/demand ratio in susceptible patients. Although its existence and clinical significance have been questioned, coronary steal is at least a theoretic concern in patients with fixed stenosis of a coronary artery. Because of these concerns, isoflurane should be used cautiously in patients at risk for myocardial ischemia or in those who are unable to tolerate tachycardia and a decrease in systemic vascular resistance.

Clinical experience with these agents demonstrates particular characteristics that may be beneficial for sedation in the ICU including rapid onset, rapid awakening on discontinuation, and ease of control of the depth of sedation. Additionally, these agents are administered through the respiratory system, thus eliminating the need for mixing infusions and intravenous administration. However, logistic problems may limit their usefulness outside the operating room. Regulations may restrict those who are allowed to adjust the inspired concentration of the agent. Depending on the hospital's policy, the nursing staff may not be permitted to alter the vaporizer setting. Alterations in the inspired concentration may need to be made by physicians or even members of the anesthesiology staff, thereby increasing the manpower issues of this form of sedation. When administered in the operating room, the exhaled gases are collected and channeled out of the room. Because ICU ventilators do not routinely scavenge exhaled gases, effective scavenging devices must be connected to ICU ventilators to prevent environmental pollution. Delivery of these agents requires specialized equipment including vaporizers and monitors to measure the end-tidal (exhaled) concentration of the drug. Although it may be possible to move an anesthesia machine into the ICU, most anesthesia machine ventilators have limited capabilities, making their use difficult or impossible in patients with significant alterations in pulmonary resistance and compliance. Therefore, most ICUs that rely on this form of sedation use an ICU ventilator with a vaporizer attached to it. These ventilators can be modified to deliver the inhalational anesthetic agent and to permit scavenging of the exhaled agent.

Additional concerns with the inhalational anesthetic agents include their potential as a triggering agent for malignant hyperthermia, cost issues, effects on ICP, and alterations of the metabolism of other medications. In addition to the cost of the specialized equipment for delivering and monitoring the agent, the average daily cost for isoflurane can range from $50 to 150 per day depending on the inspired concentration, the size of the patient, and the minute flow through the ventilator. Regardless of the agent used, cerebral vasodilation may occur, resulting in an increase in ICP. The degree of cerebral vasodilation is least with isoflurane and can be partially prevented by hyperventilation to a P_aCO_2 of 25 to 30 torr (16,17). With the availability of other agents (see below), many of which have beneficial effects on the $CMRO_2$ and ICP, the inhalational anesthetic agents cannot be recommended for continuous sedation in patients with altered intracranial compliance. The inhalational agents alter the metabolism of lidocaine, β-adrenergic blocking agents, benzodiazepines, local anesthetics, and other agents administered in the PICU setting (18).

Perhaps the greatest issue with the inhalational anesthetic agents is that there remains limited reported clinical experience with their use for prolonged sedation in the PICU population. Arnold et al. (19) administered isoflurane for sedation during mechanical ventilation to ten patients ranging in age from 3 weeks to 19 years old (19). Effective sedation was achieved in all patients without adverse effects on end-organ function. The highest fluoride concentration was 26.1 μmol/L, and no evidence of renal toxicity was noted.

Benzodiazepines

In many institutions, benzodiazepines remain the most commonly used agents for sedation in the PICU. The benzodiazepines act through the facilitation of the inhibitory neurotransmitter γ-aminobutyric acid (GABA). Binding of the benzodiazepine molecule to the α subunit of the GABA receptor facilitates binding of the GABA molecule to the β subunit, resulting in increased chloride conduction across the neuronal membrane and neuronal hyperpolarization. These agents have no intrinsic analgesic properties, and the concomitant administration of an opioid is necessary in situations requiring analgesia.

Currently, the three benzodiazepines in common clinical use in the United States for sedation of children in the ICU include diazepam, midazolam, and lorazepam. For many years, diazepam was the agent of choice for sedation in both pediatric and adult ICUs. Its high lipid solubility results in a rapid onset of action. Because of its low solubility in water, it is administered in a solution of propylene glycol that, when administered through a peripheral intravenous site, can cause pain on injection and thrombophlebitis. A newer formulation of diazepam eliminates the propylene glycol diluent and delivers diazepam in a lipid base, thereby alleviating the discomfort associated with its intravenous administration. A significant issue with diazepam is the presence of several active metabolites including oxazepam and *n*-desmethyldiazepam, which have elimination half-lives that far exceed that of the parent compound. After repeated administration over several days, these metabolites can accumulate and result in prolonged sedation and delayed awakening when the drug is discontinued. Because of this problem, diazepam is not generally considered an ideal agent for prolonged use in the patient in the PICU.

Midazolam is an imidazobenzodiazepine with a rapid onset of action and a short elimination half-life (20). Because of its short half-life, midazolam is generally administered by a continuous infusion except for brief procedures. Several clinical trials have demonstrated the efficacy of continuous midazolam infusions for sedation in the PICU in doses ranging from 0.05 to 0.2 mg/kg per hour (21,22). Midazolam has recently been approved by the U.S. Food and Drug Administration (FDA) for use by continuous infusion for sedation in the ICU.

Rosen and Rosen (23) reported their retrospective experience with midazolam infusions for sedation during mechanical ventilation in 55 pediatric patients. Midazolam was administered as a bolus dose of 0.25 mg/kg followed by a continuous infusion of 0.4 to 4 mcg/kg per minute. Midazolam provided effective sedation in all patients without significant hemodynamic effects. They did note that midazolam became ineffective in one patient after the institution of extracorporeal membrane oxygenation and related this to data showing that midazolam binds to the surface of the membrane oxygenator.

An additional benefit of midazolam is the availability of several alternative routes of delivery when intravenous administration is not practical. Although intravenous administration is generally preferable in the patient in the PICU, several investigators have described novel routes of delivery for midazolam including oral, rectal, transmucosal (nasal, rectal, sublingual), and subcutaneous (24–28).

Owing to limited absorption, except for subcutaneous administration, increased doses are required for these alternative routes of delivery (Table 44.5). These alternative routes, although rarely indicated and generally not practical for ongoing sedation in the PICU, may have some role for one-time sedation for brief diagnostic/invasive procedures. A significant drawback of nonintravenous administration is the need to use the intravenous preparation of midazolam, which contains the preservative benzyl alcohol. Benzyl alcohol can cause significant discomfort when applied to mucous membranes. Until recently, the intravenous preparation was also used for oral administration, which necessitated mixing the medication in a solution aimed at masking its flavor. Roche Pharmaceuticals has marketed an oral preparation of midazolam that does not contain benzyl alcohol and may eliminate some of the problems of oral administration. An additional problem with any of the nonintravenous routes is the limitation of the ability to titrate the dose to effect. Because of the delayed onset of activity of 10 to 20 minutes depending on the route, one must depend on the one dose to provide effective sedation.

Some medications or underlying conditions may potentiate the effects of midazolam either through alterations in metabolism or decreases in protein binding. Midazolam is metabolized by the P-450 system of the liver. Drug interactions with other pharmacologic agents (cimetidine and anticonvulsants) or hepatic dysfunction can alter midazolam pharmacokinetics. Alterations in protein binding with increases in the free fraction may also occur with heparin administration and hepatic/renal dysfunction (29,30).

Additional issues must also be considered with the use of midazolam in the patient in the PICU. Previously, price had been a concern, with acquisition costs ranging from $50 to 100 per day in a 20-kg patient requiring an infusion of 0.1 to 0.2 mg/kg per hour. However, with the recent introduction of generic forms, acquisition costs have markedly decreased. Recent studies have suggested that after prolonged administration, the accumulation of the parent compound and an active metabolite may result in a prolonged effect (31). Problems of tolerance, physical dependency, and withdrawal are discussed later in this chapter.

Lorazepam is a water-soluble benzodiazepine that may find some role in sedation in the PICU. Although midazolam's short half-life necessitates its administration by continuous infusion, lorazepam's duration of action is longer, allowing its administration either by continuous infusion or intermittent on-demand dosing. An additional difference of lorazepam compared with midazolam is its metabolism by glucuronyl transferase and not the P-450 system. Medications known to alter the P-450 system (anticonvulsants, rifampin, cimetidine) have no effect on the pharmacokinetics of lorazepam. In patients with advanced liver disease, phase II reactions (glucuronyl transferase) are better preserved than phase I reactions (P-450 system). Therefore, even in patients with advanced liver dysfunction, the pharmacokinetics of lorazepam remain unchanged. Additionally, lorazepam has no active metabolites.

Pohlman et al. (32) compared lorazepam with midazolam for sedation in 20 adult patients in the ICU. The mean infusion rate (milligram per kilogram per hour) at the time of achieving adequate sedation was 0.06 with lorazepam and 0.15 with midazolam. The maximal and mean infusion rates (milligram per kilogram per hour) for the entire study period were 0.1/0.06 for lorazepam and 0.29/0.24 for midazolam. The number of infusion rate adjustments per day was 1.9 for lorazepam and 3.6 for midazolam. The mean time to return to baseline mental status was 261 minutes with lorazepam and 1,815 minutes with midazolam. Three of six surviving patients in the midazolam group required longer than 24 hours to return to their baseline mental status as opposed to all seven in the lorazepam group returning in less than 12 hours. The investigators reported a potency ratio of lorazepam to midazolam of 2.5:1 to achieve the initial sedation, 2.9:1 at the point of maximal infusion rate and 4:1 overall during the study.

Similar efficacy in sedating adult patients in the ICU with lorazepam was reported by Dundee et al. (33). A prospective, open-label investigation was performed in 25 ICU patients. Lorazepam in a dose of 4 mg was administered at a 4- to 6-hour interval. Lorazepam provided effective sedation without significant adverse effects. Cardiac output was measured in nine patients after lorazepam administration. No significant change in the hemodynamic profile was noted.

To date, there are limited published data concerning lorazepam for sedation of the patient in the PICU. Lugo et al. (34) described the use of enteral lorazepam to decrease the need for intravenous midazolam and thereby decrease costs during mechanical ventilation in 30 infants and children. The midazolam infusion was continued until the requirements were stable for 24 hours. The enteral lorazepam dose was one-sixth the total daily intravenous midazolam dose. Lorazepam was administered every 4 to 6 hours. The midazolam infusion was then titrated to provide the desired level of sedation. The dose of midazolam was significantly reduced on day 1. By day 3, the midazolam infusion was discontinued in 24 of 30 patients. In the remaining six patients, although the midazolam could not be discontinued, the daily infusion requirements were reduced by 52%. Overall, midazolam use was decreased by 52%, resulting in a projected savings of more than $40,000 for the 30 patients. Oral administration of lorazepam has also been reported by Tobias et al. (35) for the treatment/prevention of withdrawal after prolonged administration of intravenous benzodiazepines in the patient in the PICU (see below).

A more recent issue centering on lorazepam relates not to the compound itself but rather to propylene glycol, the diluent used in the intravenous formulations (36,37). These problems highlight the importance of taking into account not only the compound itself but also the carrier vehicle and diluents when considering potential toxicities (see below for a discussion of problems related to the intralipid carrier for propofol). Anecdotal case reports have described the occurrence of propylene glycol toxicity with high-dose or prolonged infusions of lorazepam. These toxicities were manifested by metabolic acidosis, renal failure/insufficiency, and an elevated osmolar gap (36,37). Because of such concerns, calculation of the propylene glycol infusion rate and periodic measurement of the osmolar gap should be considered during high-dose or prolonged lorazepam infusions.

The benzodiazepines are generally well tolerated and have limited effects on cardiorespiratory function, especially when used as monotherapy. However, some situations may arise that necessitate a reversal agent. Flumazenil is a GABA antagonist, marketed as a reversal agent for the benzodiazepines. After administration of flumazenil, reversal of midazolam sedation was observed in 14 of 15 patients in the ICU (38). However, because the half-life of flumazenil is less than that of midazolam and its metabolites, resedation occurred in seven of the patients. Therefore, continued observation of patients is necessary when flumazenil is used to reverse life-threatening adverse effects. With increased clinical use, additional adverse effects of flumazenil have been reported. Seizures may occur owing to the antagonistic effects of flumazenil at the GABA receptor, especially in patients receiving long-term treatment with benzodiazepines or those exposed to other medications that are known to lower the seizure threshold (39). Therefore, flumazenil is not suggested for use in the patient in the PICU who has been chronically receiving benzodiazepines. The issues of tolerance, physical dependency, and withdrawal related to the benzodiazepines are discussed at the end of this chapter.

Ketamine

Introduced into clinical use in 1965 (40), ketamine is an intravenous anesthetic agent that is chemically related to phencyclidine. A unique attribute of ketamine, making it particularly attractive for sedation of the patient in the PICU, is the provision of both amnesia and analgesia. The currently available preparation of ketamine is a racemic mixture of the two optical (+, –) isomers; however, initial trials are underway with the isolated isomer form (see below). Metabolism occurs primarily by hepatic *N*-demethylation to norketamine, which is further metabolized via hydroxylation pathways with subsequent urinary excretion. Norketamine retains approximately one-third of the analgesic and sedative properties of the parent compound. Because ketamine is primarily dependent on hepatic metabolism, doses should be reduced in patients with hepatic dysfunction. Additionally, owing to the renal excretion of norketamine, dose adjustments may also be required in patients with renal dysfunction.

Beneficial properties of ketamine include preservation of cardiovascular function and limited effects on respiratory mechanics in most patients. These latter properties make it an effective agent for the provision of amnesia and analgesia during brief, painful, invasive procedures in the spontaneously breathing patient (41). It remains a frequently used agent for procedures such as central line placement, bone marrow biopsy, or burn dressing changes. For such purposes, it is administered as incremental, intermittent bolus doses (0.5 to 1 mg/kg) and titrated to effect. It is often combined with an antisialagogue such as glycopyrrolate to prevent salivation and a benzodiazepine to limit the occurrence of emergence phenomena.

In most clinical situations, ketamine administration results in a dose-related increase in heart rate and blood pressure that are mediated through a sympathetic nervous system response and the release of endogenous catecholamines (42). The release of endogenous catecholamines accounts for ketamine's actions as a bronchodilator and makes it a particularly attractive agent for patients with status asthmaticus. The indirect sympathomimetic effects from endogenous catecholamine release generally overshadow ketamine's direct negative inotropic properties and maintain blood pressure and heart rate. However, hypotension may occur in patients with diminished myocardial contractility (43,44). In these patients, it is postulated that ketamine's direct negative inotropic properties predominate because the endogenous catecholamine stores have been depleted by stress or chronic illness.

An additional issue of concern with ketamine, especially in patients with congenital heart disease, is its effect on pulmonary vascular resistance (PVR). This issue remains controversial because varying results have been reported in the literature. An increase in PVR has been reported in adults and avoidance of ketamine has been recommended by some clinicians in patients with pulmonary hypertension (45). However, these initial studies were performed during spontaneous ventilation, and the alterations in PVR may have been related to increases in P_aCO_2 and not the direct effects of ketamine on the pulmonary vasculature. After ketamine administration to spontaneously breathing infants with congenital heart disease, Morray et al. (46) noted statistically significant increases in pulmonary artery pressure (from a mean of 20.6 to 22.8 mm Hg) and increases in PVR. However, one has to consider whether there is any clinical significance to a mean increase in the PVR of 2.2 mm Hg. Hickey et al. (47) found no change in PVR in intubated infants with minimal ventilatory support (four breaths per minute and an F_IO_2 of 0.4). The latter study included 14 patients, seven with normal and seven with elevated baseline PVR. Pending further investigations, ketamine should be used cautiously in patients with pulmonary hypertension, especially during spontaneous ventilation.

Functional residual capacity, minute ventilation, and tidal volume remain unchanged after ketamine administration (48), whereas other investigators have demonstrated improved pulmonary compliance, decreased resistance, and prevention of bronchospasm (49). These effects on respiratory mechanics have also been at least partially attributed to the release of endogenous catecholamines. Although minute ventilation is generally maintained, elevations of P_aCO_2 and a rightward shift of the CO_2 response curve have been reported (50). Controversy remains concerning ketamine's effects on protective airway reflexes (51). Although clinical use and experimental studies suggest that airway reflexes are maintained, aspiration and laryngospasm have been reported after ketamine in spontaneously breathing patients without a protected airway (52). An additional effect that may affect airway patency is increased oral secretions. The concomitant administration of an antisialagogue such as atropine or glycopyrrolate is recommended because ketamine increases salivary and bronchial gland secretion through stimulation of central cholinergic receptors. In higher doses or in severely compromised patients, ketamine can cause apnea, which again emphasizes that all sedative/analgesic agents, especially when administered to critically ill patients, should be administered only in a controlled environment with appropriate monitoring.

Ketamine increases ICP and therefore should be avoided in patients with altered intracranial compliance (53,54). Ketamine's effects on ICP result from direct cerebral vasodilation, mediated through central cholinergic receptors and are not secondary to alterations in cerebral metabolic rate or changes in P_aCO_2 (55,56). Another issue of some controversy related to the central nervous system (CNS) regarding ketamine is its use in patients at risk of or with an underlying seizure disorder. Electroencephalographic recordings during ketamine administration demonstrate increased frequency and amplitude and occasional paroxysmal or seizure activity (57,58). However, no clinical evidence of seizure activity has been reported with ketamine administration. Furthermore, ketamine has been found to possess anticonvulsant activity in laboratory animals (59,60) and has even been suggested as treatment for refractory status epilepticus in clinical practice (61).

The adverse effect related to ketamine that receives the most attention is the occurrence of emergence phenomena or hallucinations. Emergence phenomena are dose related, occurring more commonly in older patients. Their incidence can be decreased by the preadministration of a benzodiazepine (62). It is postulated that emergence phenomena result from the alteration of auditory and visual relays in the inferior colliculus and the medial geniculate nucleus leading to the misinterpretation of visual and auditory stimuli (62). The administration of a benzodiazepine (lorazepam or midazolam) 5 minutes before the administration of ketamine is generally effective in preventing emergence phenomena and allows the use of ketamine even in older patients. For years, ketamine has been available for clinical use as a racemic mixture of the two optical isomers. More recently, the single enantiomer form [S or (+)] has been released (outside the United States) for clinical use (63). It has been suggested that the isolated (+) enantiomer has fewer of the psychomimetic effects. Future clinical trials are needed to address this issue.

There remains limited reported clinical experience with the use of ketamine for sedation of the patient in the PICU. Tobias et al. (64) reported their anecdotal experience with the use of ketamine infusions for sedation in five patients in the PICU, four of whom experienced adverse cardiorespiratory effects following the administration of benzodiazepines and/or opioids. Hartvig et al. (65) reported their experience with the use of a ketamine infusion to provide sedation and analgesia after cardiac surgery in ten pediatric patients ranging in age from 1 week to 30 months. Five patients received ketamine in a dose of 1 mg/kg per hour, and the other five received 2 mg/kg per hour. Both groups received supplemental as-needed doses of midazolam. The mean plasma clearance of ketamine was 0.94 ± 0.22 L/kg per hour with an elimination half-life of 3.1 ± 1.6 hours. Norketamine demonstrated an elimination half-life of 6.0 ± 1.8 hours. The two groups had similar and acceptable levels of sedation.

Most likely related to its limited use, there are currently no reports describing withdrawal issues with ketamine. However, when used for repeated procedures over time, tolerance to the effects of ketamine has been reported (66), suggesting that if tolerance develops, physical dependence will also and withdrawal can occur if its administration is abruptly discontinued after prolonged administration.

Because of its favorable effects on cardiorespiratory function, ketamine may be quite useful in patients who require sedation during mechanical ventilation yet develop myocardial depression with opioids or benzodiazepines (64). Another setting in which ketamine may be useful is the provision of sedation with the preservation of spontaneous ventilation that may be required when using noninvasive ventilation techniques. Dosing regimens for ketamine infusions include a bolus dose of 1 to 2 mg/kg followed by a continuous infusion of 1 mg/kg per hour, titrated up or down as necessary. The infusion can be supplemented with as-needed doses of midazolam to provide a steady baseline level of sedation and prevent emergence phenomena. Another option is to combine ketamine and midazolam in a single solution (10 mg/mL ketamine and 1 mg/mL midazolam). The infusion is then started at 0.1 mL/kg per hour, which provides 1 mg/kg per hour ketamine and 0.1 mg/kg per hour midazolam. Ketamine is also a useful agent to provide sedation and analgesia during the performance of painful invasive procedures, especially in spontaneously breathing patients. For this purpose, an anticholinergic agent (5 μg/kg glycopyrrolate) and midazolam (0.03 to 0.05 mg/kg) are administered intravenously followed by incremental boluses of ketamine (0.5 mg/kg) every 1 to 2 minutes as needed. As with midazolam, several alternative routes of delivery exist for ketamine. These alternative routes of delivery (oral, nasal, and rectal) have generally been used for one-time dosing of the agent for sedation during a procedure and have a limited role for ongoing sedation of the patient in the PICU.

Propofol

Propofol is classified as an intravenous anesthetic agent of the alkyl phenol family. Because it is classified as an intravenous anesthetic agent, there is ongoing controversy in many institutions (as there is with ketamine) as to who should be allowed to administer these medications. Can they be administered by any physician or only by an anesthesiologist? What about PICU physicians? Because there are no hard data to support either side, further discussion of this issue will not be provided. However, the minimal requirements for the use of any of the sedative and analgesic agents reviewed in this chapter are the ability to monitor and support cardiorespiratory function and provide support including bag-mask ventilation as needed.

Propofol's chemical structure is distinct from that of the barbiturates and other commonly used intravenous anesthetic agents (67). Propofol shares a similar mechanism of action with the benzodiazepines and the barbiturates in that it facilitates the binding of the inhibitory neurotransmitter GABA to specific membrane-bound receptors that increase chloride conductance resulting in neuronal hyperpolarization. However, its recognition binding site is distinctly different from that of the barbiturates or benzodiazepines. Like the barbiturates, it can be categorized as a sedative/amnestic agent that possesses no analgesic properties. Therefore, it is recommended that it be combined with an opioid infusion in patients requiring analgesia. After its introduction into anesthesia practice, its pharmacodynamic profile including a rapid onset, rapid recovery time, and lack of active metabolites made it a logical choice for evaluation as an agent for sedation in the ICU (68,69). When compared with midazolam for sedation in adult patients, propofol has been shown to provide shorter recovery times, improved titration efficiency, and reduced posthypnotic obtundation with faster weaning from mechanical ventilation (70).

In addition to its favorable properties with regard to sedation, propofol has beneficial effects on CNS dynamics including a decreased $CMRO_2$ with reflex cerebral vasoconstriction and lowering of ICP (71). The latter effect is much the same as that seen with the barbiturates and etomidate. These latter effects suggest that propofol may be an effective and beneficial agent for sedation in patients with altered intracranial compliance. The preliminary laboratory and clinical experience with propofol has demonstrated its potential as a therapeutic agent in regulating CNS dynamics and controlling ICP. Nimkoff et al. (72) evaluated the effects of propofol, methohexital, and ketamine on the cerebral perfusion pressure (CPP) and ICP in a feline model of cytotoxic and vasogenic cerebral edema. Vasogenic cerebral edema was induced by inflation of an intracranial balloon, whereas cytotoxic cerebral edema was caused by an acute reduction in blood osmolarity using hemofiltration. Propofol lowered ICP and maintained CPP in vasogenic cerebral edema but had no effect on cytotoxic cerebral edema. The authors postulated that the loss of autoregulatory function with diffuse cytotoxic edema uncouples $CMRO_2$ from cerebral blood flow and therefore eliminated propofol's efficacy.

Watts et al. (73) evaluated the effects of propofol and hyperventilation on ICP and somatosensory evoked potentials in a rabbit model of intracranial hypertension (73). After inflation of an intracranial balloon to increase ICP to 26 ± 2 mm Hg and produce a 50% or more reduction in somatosensory evoked potentials, the animals were randomized to group 1 (propofol followed by hyperventilation) or group 2 (hyperventilation followed by propofol). The ICP decrease was significantly greater in group 1 (final ICP: 12 ± 2 mm Hg versus 16 ± 5 mm Hg, $p = 0.008$). When comparing propofol with hyperventilation, propofol resulted in a greater ICP decrease (16 ± 2 mm Hg with propofol versus 21 ± 5 mm Hg with hyperventilation, $p = 0.007$). When propofol was administered first, there was a significant increase in the amplitude of the somatosensory evoked potentials. The mean arterial pressure (MAP) was maintained at baseline levels by the infusion of phenylephrine. More phenylephrine ($p < 0.02$) was required to maintain the MAP with propofol than with hyperventilation.

Despite these encouraging animal studies, the review of the literature concerning propofol in humans provides conflicting results, especially in regard to its efficacy in controlling ICP. Although several studies demonstrate a decrease in ICP, propofol's cardiovascular effects with a lowering of the MAP can result in a decrease in CPP. The decreased CPP leads to reflex cerebral vasodilation to maintain cerebral blood flow. The cerebral vasodilation increases cerebral blood volume, which can increase ICP in patients with altered intracranial compliance. This effect may result in an increase in ICP that negates the decrease in ICP related to the decrease in $CMRO_2$ induced by propofol.

Herregods et al. (74) evaluated the effects of propofol (2 mg/kg) administered over 90 seconds on ICP and MAP in six adults with an ICP greater than 25 mm Hg. Mean ICP decreased from 25 ± 3 to 11 ± 4 mm Hg ($p < 0.05$). However, they also noted a decrease in the MAP and consequently a decrease in CPP from 92 ± 8 mm Hg to a low of 50 ± 7 mm Hg. CPP was less than 50 mm Hg in four of six patients. No vasoconstrictor agent was administered to maintain the MAP.

Similar results were obtained by Pinaud et al. (75) during their evaluation of the effects of propofol on cerebral blood flow, ICP, CPP, and cerebral arteriovenous oxygen content difference in ten adults with traumatic brain injury. Although propofol decreased ICP (11.3 ± 2.6 to 9.2 ± 2.5 mm Hg, $p < 0.001$), there was also a decrease in MAP that resulted in an overall decrease in CPP from 82 ± 14 mm Hg to 59 ± 7 mm Hg ($p < 0.01$). Other investigators of patients with traumatic brain injury (76) or during cerebral aneurysm surgery (77) have noted similar effects of propofol on ICP and the MAP with an overall lowering of CPP owing to the greater decrease in the MAP than ICP.

Farling et al. (78) reported their experience with propofol for sedation in ten adult patients with closed head injuries. Propofol was administered as a continuous infusion of 2 to 4 mg/kg per hour for 24 hours. Additional therapy for increased ICP included mannitol and hyperventilation. The mean rate of propofol infusion was 2.88 mg/kg per hour. There was a statistically significant decrease in the mean ICP of 2.1 mm Hg achieved at 2 hours after the start of the propofol infusion. No decrease in the MAP was noted. CPP increased during the 24-hour study period, and the difference was statistically significant at the 24-hour point (CPP increase of 9.8 mm Hg, $p = 0.028$). The authors concluded that propofol was a suitable agent for sedation in patients with head injury requiring mechanical ventilation.

Spitzfadden et al. (79) reported their experience with the use of propofol to provide sedation and control ICP in two adolescents. Dopamine was used to maintain the MAP and CPP. Propofol resulted in adequate sedation and control of ICP. When compared with barbiturates, the usual time-honored therapy for pharmacologic control of ICP, the authors suggested that a significant advantage of propofol was a much more rapid awakening. The latter effect may be evident after prolonged (≥48 hours) administration of barbiturates.

Also of importance with propofol is the accumulating evidence concerning its beneficial effects in patients at risk of airway reactivity. Eames et al. (80) randomized 77 patients to receive propofol (2.5 mg/kg), etomidate (0.4 mg/kg), or thiopental (5 mg/kg) for anesthetic induction. After tracheal intubation, respiratory resistance was significantly less with propofol compared with either etomidate or thiopental. Pizov et al. (81) randomized asthmatic or nonasthmatic patients to anesthetic induction with 5 mg/kg thiopental/thiamylal, 1.5 mg/kg methohexital, or 2.5 mg/kg propofol. In asthmatic patients, the incidence of wheezing heard with auscultation after endotracheal intubation by a blinded observer was 45% with thiopental/thiamylal, 26% with methohexital, and 0% with propofol. In nonasthmatic patients, the incidence of wheezing was 16% with thiopental/thiamylal and 3% with propofol.

Propfol's beneficial effects on airway reactivity are further supported by animal studies. Chih-Chung et al. (82) demonstrated that propofol attenuates carbachol-induced airway constriction in canine tracheal smooth muscle. The mechanism involves a decrease of inositol phosphate accumulation and a decrease of intracellular calcium availability. The latter results from a decrease in release from intracellular stores and a decrease in transmembrane movement. Pedersen et al. (83) demonstrated that propofol was more effective in preventing bronchoconstriction to several provocative agents in an isolated guinea pig trachea smooth muscle model.

With its increased use for sedation and anesthetic induction in the ICU, some adverse effects have been reported with propofol (Table 44.6). As mentioned previously, propofol's cardiovascular effects are similar to those of the barbiturates including peripheral vasodilation and negative inotropic properties (84). These effects are particularly prominent after bolus administration. Although tolerated by patients with adequate cardiovascular function, these effects may have detrimental physiologic effects in patients with compromised cardiovascular function. Tritapepe et al. (85) demonstrated that the administration of calcium chloride (10 mg/kg) prevented the deleterious cardiovascular effects of propofol during anesthetic induction in patients undergoing coronary artery bypass grafting.

In addition to the negative inotropic properties, central vagal tone may be augmented leading to bradycardia (86) or asystole. Cardiac slowing may be particularly apparent when propofol is combined with other med-

TABLE 44.6. *Adverse effects described with propofol*

Hypotension
Negative inotropic effects
Vasodilation
Bradycardia
Neurologic sequelae
Opisthotonic posturing
Seizure-like activity
Myoclonus
Anaphylactoid reactions
Metabolic acidosis and cardiac failure
Pain on injection
Bacterial contamination of solution
Hyperlipidemia
Potential for depletion of trace elements (zinc)

ications known to alter cardiac chronotropic function such as fentanyl and/or succinylcholine (87). Although the relative bradycardia is generally considered a beneficial effect in patients at risk of myocardial ischemia, it may be detrimental in patients with a fixed stroke volume in whom cardiac output is heart rate dependent.

Neurologic manifestations including opisthotonic posturing, myoclonic movements (especially in children), and seizure-like activity have been reported with propofol (88–90). The movement disorders seen with propofol administration have been attributed to its effects (antagonism) at glycine receptors in subcortical structures. Although some of the initial reports suggested actual seizure activity, these concerns have most likely been overemphasized. There remains no true electroencephalographic evidence of seizure with the abnormal movements seen with propofol administration. Hewitt et al. (91) evaluated the effects of propofol and thiopental on the surface electroencephalograms of 20 patients undergoing temporal lobe surgery. No difference in the rate of discharge or extension of the irritative zone was seen when comparing thiopental with propofol. Furthermore, propofol has been used to treat status epilepticus and is included in algorithms as recommended therapy of patients with refractory status epilepticus (92,93).

In children, significant issues with propofol for prolonged sedation in the PICU setting are reports of metabolic acidosis, brady-dysrhythmias, and fatal cardiac failure (94,95). The initial report of Parke et al. (94) included five children with respiratory infections and respiratory failure who were receiving relatively high doses of as much as 13.6 mg/kg per hour. Bray (96) reviewed the medical literature on 18 children with suspected propofol infusion syndrome. Risk factors for the syndrome included propofol administration for more than 48 hours or doses greater than 4 mg/kg per hour. However, several children received doses greater than 4 mg/kg per hour for longer than 48 hours, suggesting that factors other than dose and duration may be necessary for development of the syndrome. Other associated factors included age; 13 of the 18 patients were 4 years of age or younger, and only one of 18 was more than 10 years of age. As with the initial report of Parke et al. (94), there may be an association of respiratory tract infections in the cause of the syndrome because 82% of the reported cases have been in children with such infections. Since the review of Bray (96), the syndrome has been reported in a 17-year-old patient (97) and more recently in a cohort of adult patients with head injury (98). In addition to the cardiovascular manifestations, other features have included metabolic acidosis, lipemic serum, hepatomegaly, and muscle involvement with rhabdomyolysis and hyperkalemia. Suggestions for treatment include discontinuation of the propofol and symptomatic treatment of cardiovascular dysfunction. In patients with rhabdomyolysis and renal failure, hemodialysis has been used (97). Although hemodialysis has been effective in the management of these patients, it is unknown whether its only effect is in the management of the renal dysfunction or whether it may also have a therapeutic effect through the removal of a suspected toxic metabolite. Recent work has shed some light on a potential mechanism for the so-called propofol infusion syndrome. Using a guinea pig cardiomyocyte preparation, Schenkman and Yan (99) demonstrated that propofol either impairs oxygen utilization or inhibits electron flow along the mitochondrial electron transport chain. Wolf et al. (100) provide further evidence for disruption of mitochondrial function as the cause of propofol infusion syndrome. They report a 2-year-old boy who developed propofol infusion syndrome. Biochemical analysis of their patient revealed an increased concentration of malonylcarnitine, which results in inhibition of the transport protein necessary to the transport of long-chain fatty acids into the mitochondria and an increase in the concentration of C_5-acylcarnitine indicative of inhibition of the respiratory chain at complex II. Also of note was their decision to institute hemofiltration with the recognition of the syndrome and reversal of the problems and recovery in their patient. As the evidence mounts that propofol may interfere with mitochondrial function and oxidative phosphorylation, the similarity of propofol infusion syndrome with primary involvement of cardiac and skeletal muscle with lactic acidosis and the clinical presentations of patients with inborn errors of metabolism known as mitochondrial myopathies becomes remarkably similar.

With increasing information concerning this problem, caution is suggested with the administration of propofol by continuous infusion in the patient in the PICU in doses exceeding 4 mg/kg per hour or for longer than 48 hours. If propofol is administered in this setting, intermittent analysis of acid base status and creatinine phosphokinase (evaluating for rhabdomyolysis) is suggested. If a base deficit is noted with an increasing serum lactate, immediate discontinuation of the propofol infusion is recommended. Immediate discontinuation of the propofol infusion with the first signs of developing lactic acidosis may allow spontaneous resolution of the problem (79), whereas other authors have suggested the use of hemodialysis (97) or hemofiltration (100).

Despite these reports and the author's contention that propofol should not be used for prolonged sedation of the patient in the PICU unless there are associated CNS issues (e.g., increased ICP), this belief is not unanimously embraced by the medical community. There remain reports of the safe and successful use of propofol for sedation in the PICU setting (101,102). Considering the above-mentioned beneficial properties of rapid awakening, propofol has played a role in providing short-term sedation in younger patients and for more prolonged use in older patients. However, all this must be considered in context of the "Dear Health Care Provider" letter issued in March 2001 from AstraZeneca (Wilmington, DE), the manufacturers of Diprivan, one of the two commercially available propofol preparations. The letter refers to the FDA's review of a new clinical trial in which propofol was being compared with other agents used for sedation in the PICU. The study comprised a total of 327 patients who were randomized to receive propofol or other sedative agents. During the trial or the 28-day follow-up period, there were 12 (11%) deaths in the 2% propofol group, nine (8%) in the 1% propofol group, and four (4%) in the standard sedation group. Although careful review failed to show a specific pattern to the causes of death, there was enough concern that the company issued a letter stating: "propofol is currently not approved for sedation in pediatric ICU patients in the United States and should not be used for this purpose."

One area in which propofol has seen greater use is for short-term sedation for procedures or imaging studies that require immobilization in the patient in the PICU (103). For such purposes, the propofol infusion is initiated in the PICU in a tracheally intubated and mechanically ventilated patient. The patient is then transported from the PICU to the radiology department for the procedure. After the procedure is completed and the patient returned to the PICU, the propofol infusion is discontinued. An area of controversy is who accompanies and monitors the patient during transport. Can this be performed by a respiratory therapist and a PICU nurse or should a physician accompany the patient? If propofol is used, does this require an anesthesiologist or a PICU physician? The debate and discussions will continue concerning such issues and because there are no scientific data to definitely support any side, future studies and ongoing quality assurance programs are needed to provide additional data.

In our PICU, patients receiving short-term infusions of benzodiazepines and/or opioids who have not developed physical dependency and therefore do not require tapering to prevent withdrawal (see below) are frequently transitioned to 4 to 6 hours of propofol before extubation. The latter avoids problems related to the context-sensitive half-time of short-acting agents such as fentanyl or midazolam. Although these agents have short half-lives when administered by bolus administration, with prolonged infusions, their half-lives increase (i.e., context-sensitive half-time) and therefore patients may have prolonged sedation even after the infusion is discontinued. This problem is not seen with propofol or remifentanil (see below).

In the PICU setting when sedation is required, most patients are endotracheally intubated, receiving mechanical ventilation. However, the respiratory depressant effects of propofol should not be overlooked. Although propofol has become a popular agent for deep sedation of the spontaneously breathing patient, reports demonstrate a relatively high incidence of respiratory effects including hypoventilation, upper airway obstruction, and apnea (103). As with any sedative agent, some degree hypoventilation is likely to occur in all patients breathing spontaneously, thereby resulting in hypercarbia and its obvious deleterious effects on ICP and CPP. Despite these potential deleterious effects on respiratory function, as mentioned previously in this section, laboratory and clinical studies suggest that propofol may be advantageous when instrumenting the airway of patients with reactive airway disease.

Additional problems with propofol relate to its delivery in a lipid emulsion (the same lipid preparation that is used in parenteral hyperalimentation solutions otherwise known as intralipid). There have been rare reports of anaphylactoid reactions, which may be more likely in patients with a history of egg allergy (104).

Pain on injection is commonly seen with propofol administration through a peripheral infusion site. Variable success in decreasing the incidence of pain has been reported with various maneuvers including the preadministration of lidocaine, mixing the lidocaine and propofol in a single solution, diluting the concentration of the propofol, or cooling it before bolus administration. Another alternative is the administration of a small dose of ketamine (0.5 mg/kg) before the administration of propofol (105). Because propofol has limited analgesic properties, ketamine and propofol can be administered together to take advantage of the analgesia provided by ketamine and the rapid recovery with propofol. This combination can be used for brief invasive procedures or for sedation in the ICU. For these purposes, the two solutions can be administered separately or ketamine can be added to the propofol solution to result in a mixture containing 3 to 5 mg/mL ketamine and 10 mg/mL propofol. For brief procedures, incremental doses of 0.1 mL/kg of the mixed solution can be administered, resulting in the delivery of 0.3 to 0.5 mg/kg ketamine and 1 mg/kg propofol.

Unlike other medications used for continuous sedation, the initial production of propofol did not contain preservatives. Laboratory investigations have demonstrated that the lipid emulsion will serve as a suitable culture media for bacteria (106). Systemic bacteremia and postoperative wound infections have been linked to extrinsically contaminated propofol (107). A modification of the initial preparation by AstraZeneca Pharmaceuticals, manufacturer of the original form of propofol, included the addition of disodium ethylenediaminetetraacetic acid as a preservative, which may limit the risk of bacterial contamination and growth. However, strict aseptic technique is still recommended. Opened, but unused vials, should be disposed of promptly and not saved for later use. Our current policy in the PICU is to change the vial and tubing every 12 hours during continuous infusions. An additional theoretic problem with disodium ethylenediaminetetraacetic acid is the chelation and depletion from the body of essential trace minerals such as zinc. Although there are no formal studies to demonstrate that this is a problem, concerns related to this issue are outlined in the manufacturer's package insert.

A generic preparation of propofol, manufactured by Baxter Pharmaceuticals, is also available. This latter preparation contains sodium metabisulfite as a preservative. There remains some controversy over the possible association of sodium metabisulfite with allergic reactions, especially in patients with asthma and other atopic conditions. However, several other commonly used medications contain sodium metabisulfite, and there have been no reports of problems with these medications. Additionally, the evaluation by the FDA concluded that these two preparations were equivalent. More recently, concern has been raised that the two formulations are different in their compatibility with other medications. In our ICU, we frequently administer propofol with parenteral nutrition and several other medications including vasoactive and sedative agents. Trissel (108) provided preliminary information that the compatibility of various medications is different with the two propofol preparations. Because this is an extremely important issue for pediatric patients in whom intravenous access may be limited, future studies are needed to further define this issue.

Additional problems related to the high lipid content of the solution have included hypertriglyceridemia (109,110). A case report suggests the anecdotal association of high-dose propofol infusion with an increasing P_{aCO_2} during mechanical ventilation (110). The authors report a patient who required as much as 200 µg/kg per minute of propofol to maintain an adequate level of sedation, resulting in a total caloric intake of 4,500 calories/day (53% from the lipid in the propofol diluent). The P_{aCO_2} increased from 67 mm Hg to a maximal value of 78 mm Hg despite increasing the minute ventilation from 11 to 13 L per minute. The lipid content of propofol should be taken into consideration when calculating the patient's day caloric intake. A propofol infusion of 2 mg/kg per hour provides approximately 0.5 g/kg per day of fat. In an attempt to eliminate or lessen such problems, a 2% solution of propofol is currently undergoing clinical trials (111). Although the issues related to increased triglycerides may be eliminated with the 2% solution, preliminary data suggest that there may be some alteration in propofol's bioavailability because there seems to be an increased dose requirement when the 2% solution is used compared with the 1% solution (112).

Barbiturates

The barbiturates are one of the oldest class of agents used for sedation in the ICU. As with many of the agents described, their effects on cardiorespiratory function are dose dependent. In healthy patients, sedative doses can be expected to have limited effects on cardiovascular function, respiratory drive, and airway protective reflexes, whereas larger doses, especially in patients with cardiorespiratory compromise, can produce respiratory depression, apnea, or hypotension. The cardiorespiratory effects are additive with other agents such as opioids. Hypotension with barbiturates results from both peripheral vasodilation and a direct negative inotropic effect.

The barbiturates can be classified according to their duration of activity. Short-acting agents include methohexital, thiopental, and thiamylal. These agents have a duration of action of 5 to 10 minutes and are usually used by intravenous bolus administration for brief procedures such as endotracheal intubation. When a more prolonged effect is needed, a continuous infusion may be used to maintain constant plasma levels; however, when this is done, the offset time is also markedly prolonged and dependent on the duration of the infusion. Longer acting agents with half-lives of 6 to 12 hours include pentobarbital and phenobarbital.

Beneficial physiologic effects of the barbiturates include a decrease of the $CMRO_2$ with a reduction in cerebral blood flow, cerebral vasoconstriction, and a decrease in ICP (113,114). The barbiturates are potent anticonvulsants and may be used to treat status epilepticus unresponsive to other agents (115,116). Although still controversial, animal studies suggest that they may provide some degree of cerebral protection during periods of cerebral hypoxia or hypoperfusion (117,118).

Although the barbiturates are used most commonly for their therapeutic effects (as anticonvulsants or to decrease ICP), these agents may be an effective alternative for providing sedation of the patient in the PICU when the usual combination of benzodiazepines and opioids, either alone or in combination, fail to provide adequate sedation (119). Tobias (120) recently reported a retrospective evaluation of pentobarbital use for sedation in 50 children in a PICU. The 50 patients ranged in age from 1 month to 14 years and in weight from 3.1 to 56 kg. All required sedation during mechanical ventilation. Before switching to pentobarbital, the level of sedation was inadequate despite midazolam doses of 0.4 mg/kg per hour, fentanyl doses of 10 μg/kg per hour, and morphine doses of 100 μg/kg per hour. The duration of pentobarbital infusion ranged from 2 to 37 days (median, 4 days) in doses ranging from 1 to 6 mg/kg per hour (median, 2 mg/kg per hour). Twelve patients also received an ongoing opioid infusion for longer than 48 hours after starting the pentobarbital infusion to control pain related to a surgical procedure or an acute medical illness. There was an increase in pentobarbital infusion requirements over time. In the 14 patients who received pentobarbital for 5 days or more, the requirements increased from 1.2 mg/kg per hour on day 1 to 3.4 mg/kg per hour on day 5. No significant adverse effects related to pentobarbital were noted.

One particularly difficult situation is the provision of sedation during extracorporeal membrane oxygenation (extracorporeal membrane oxygenation). Although fentanyl is the most commonly used agent, clinical experience has demonstrated the rapid development of tolerance and the need for dose escalations as high as 30 to 50 μg/kg per hour. Pentobarbital may be an effective alternative to more conventional agents in sedating pediatric patients during extracorporeal membrane oxygenation (119,120). The barbiturates have also been efficacious is providing sedation, anxiolysis, and comfort measures during the end stages of terminal malignancies (121).

Because all barbiturates have negative inotropic effects, they should be used cautiously in patients with cardiovascular dysfunction. The risks of adverse cardiovascular effects can be limited by slow administration (over 5 minutes) of the bolus doses. Another problem that may limit their use is that the solution is alkaline, thus making it incompatible with other medications and parenteral alimentation solutions. Therefore, the barbiturates should be administered separately from other medications. Local erythema and thrombophlebitis can occur with subcutaneous infiltration. Despite such problems, pentobarbital may be effective when benzodiazepine/opioid combinations become ineffective. For sedation in the PICU, a loading dose of pentobarbital (1 to 2 mg/kg) is followed by a continuous infusion of 1 to 2 mg/kg per hour. The bolus dose can be repeated and the infusion can be increased as needed.

Opioids

Although generally used for analgesia, opioids also possess sedative properties and are often chosen as a first- or second-line agent for sedation for the patient in the PICU. Clinical experience suggests that the opioids may be more efficacious in neonates and infants. The latter may relate to the well-developed endogenous opioid and receptor system of the neonate. Even with high-dose fentanyl (50 to 75 μg/kg) techniques commonly used during repair of congenital heart defects, opioids provide analgesia but not amnesia. Additional agents are suggested when amnesia is desired (the older infant or child who is receiving a neuromuscular blocking agent).

Despite their widespread use, there is limited information concerning the optimal opioid for sedation in the PICU or postoperative analgesia. In the patient with compromised cardiovascular status or at risk of pulmonary hypertension such as an infant with a large preoperative systemic to pulmonary shunt, the synthetic opioids (fentanyl, sufentanil) provide cardiovascular stability, beneficial effects on pulmonary vascular resistance, and blunting of the sympathetic stress. Because of their prompt redistribution and resultant short plasma half-lives after a bolus administration, synthetic opioids are generally administered by a continuous infusion to maintain plasma concentrations adequate to provide analgesia. When comparing the different synthetic opioids (fentanyl, sufentanil, alfentanil, remifentanil), there does not seem to be an inherent advantage with regard to any one of these agents. However, fentanyl is the least expensive of the synthetic opioids. Although fentanyl, sufentanil, and alfentanil, like other opioids, are dependent on hepatic metabolism, remifentanil is metabolized by nonspecific esterases in the plasma with a resultant clinical half-life of 5 of 10 minutes. Because of its short half-life (5 to 10 minutes) and duration of effect even after 12 to 24 hours of continuous infusion, it may be a useful agent for providing a deep level of sedation and allowing a rapid dissipation of its effects when the infusion is discontinued. To date, there is limited information concerning the use of remifentanil in the PICU population. Tobias (122) reported anecdotal experience in four patients who required a deep level of sedation for endotracheal intubation for 12 to 24 hours. Issues with remifentanil include the rapid development of tolerance and cost, thus limiting its application for more prolonged administration (longer than 12 to 24 hours).

Two caveats regarding any of the synthetic opioids are their effects on ICP and the occurrence of chest wall rigidity. Although still controversial, recent evidence suggests that the synthetic opioids may secondarily increase ICP in patients with altered intracranial compliance. Sperry et al. (123) noted a moderate decrease in the MAP that, when combined with the increase in ICP, further decreased CPP. The mechanism underlying the effect on ICP is thought to be a reflex cerebral vasodilation in response to the decrease in the MAP (124). If the MAP is maintained by the administration of a direct-acting vasoconstrictor, no change in ICP is noted.

Another possible deleterious effect described with the synthetic opioids is chest wall rigidity (125,126). Although Pokela et al. (125) noted significant decreases in compliance and oxygen saturation in four infants receiving alfentanil and concluded that these agents should not be used without concomitant neuromuscular blockade, chest wall rigidity does not routinely occur in all patients receiving synthetic opioids. Irazuzta et al. (127) demonstrated improved compliance of the respiratory system in neonates and infants receiving fentanyl for sedation during mechanical ventilation. The incidence of chest wall rigidity is related to the dose and rate of administration. It is a centrally mediated, idiosyncratic reaction that, when severe, can interfere with effective respiratory function. Chest wall rigidity can be reversed with naloxone or interrupted with neuromuscular blocking agents.

Other opioids such as morphine are an acceptable and less expensive alternative in patients with normal cardiovascular function. Morphine causes some venodilation and thus may decrease blood pressure in hypovolemic patients. However, for most patients, morphine is an effective opioid for sedation and analgesia. Lynn et al. (128) demonstrated that morphine infusions of 10 to 30 μg/kg per hour resulted in serum concentrations of 10 to 22 ng/mL and provided effective analgesia and sedation during mechanical ventilation after surgery for congenital heart disease, without impairing the ability to wean mechanical ventilatory support. Quinn et al. (129) showed that morphine infusions blunted the sympathetic response and reduced epinephrine levels in neonates requiring endotracheal intubation and mechanical ventilation for hyaline membrane disease.

Alternative opioids to morphine include hydromorphone, meperidine, and methadone. To date, there is little or no information concerning the use of these agents for sedation of the patient in the PICU. However, there is ample information concerning use of these agents in the management of acute pain. Hydromorphone may be advantageous when adverse effects related to histamine release such as pruritus occur with morphine (130). The equipotent dose of hydromorphone can be determined by considering the potency ratio of the two opioids with hydromorphone five to seven times as potent as morphine (Table 44.7).

TABLE 44.7. *Potency and half-life of opioids*

Agent	Potency	Half-life (hr)
Morphine	1	2–3
Meperidine	0.1	2–3
Hydromorphone	5	2–4
Methadone	1[a]	12–24
Fentanyl	100	0.3–0.5
Sufentanil	1,000	0.2–0.4
Alfentanil	20	0.2–0.3
Remifentanil	100	0.1

[a]The potency ratio of morphine to methadone has recently been questioned by several studies in patients with chronic pain of various causes (163,164). Part of this effect may result from methadone's effects as an *N*-methyl-D-aspartate receptor antagonist (162).

Issues with meperidine that preclude its use in the PICU include a relatively high incidence of adverse CNS effects including dysphoria, agitation, and seizures (131). CNS toxicity (including seizures) results from the accumulation of normeperidine after hepatic *N*-demethylation of the parent compound. Normeperidine has a long half-life (15 to 20 hours) and is dependent on renal excretion. High or toxic levels are more likely in the setting of renal insufficiency with the coadministration of drugs such as phenobarbital that stimulate hepatic microsomal enzymes and with large doses (more than 2 g per day in an adult). The latter issue becomes problematic in the patient who is receiving long-term treatment with opioids in whom dose escalations are needed to provide effective analgesia. Because of these considerations and because meperidine offers no particular advantage over other opioids, morphine and fentanyl are commonly used as first-line agents.

Another opioid occasionally used in the treatment of acute pain is methadone. Methadone's half-life is 12 to 24 hours with a potency previously considered to be approximately equivalent to that of morphine. (The potency ratio of morphine to methadone has recently been questioned; see below for a more thorough discussion of this subject.) Therefore, a single dose of methadone results in a prolonged serum concentration and thus a prolonged duration of action without the need for a continuous infusion. Berde et al. (132) evaluated the efficacy of methadone for postoperative analgesia in children 3 to 7 years of age. Children who received methadone (0.2 mg/kg after the induction of anesthesia) had lower pain scores and required fewer doses of supplemental opioid analgesics over the next 36 hours. Although limited experience exists with the use of methadone in children, its longer duration of action offers some advantages over the intermittent administration of agents with shorter half-lives. Oral methadone may also be used to slowly taper opioid therapy in patients who have developed tolerance after prolonged opioid administration (see below).

Although the intravenous route is generally chosen for the patient in the PICU, some situations such as limited intravenous access and drug incompatibilities may preclude or interfere with intravenous administration. The subcutaneous administration of several different opioids may be possible. Although most experience with subcutaneous opioid infusions has been in the patient with terminal cancer (133), Bruera et al. (134) reported their experience with subcutaneous infusions of opioids in the adult ICU population. Opioids were administered by either intermittent subcutaneous dosing or by continuous infusion to 13 patients for 60 patient-days. The infusions were delivered via a 25-gauge butterfly needle inserted subcutaneously in the subclavicular area or the anterior abdominal wall. No infectious complications were noted, and the insertion site was changed only three times because of local problems such as erythema. The authors expressed a theoretic concern over possible delays in onset of activity or decreased absorption in patients with decreased peripheral perfusion, although they noted no such problems in their patients. The subcutaneous route is also a possible alternative in the patient in the PICU in whom drug incompatibilities limit the intravenous route or during the recovery period when a slow taper of the opioid infusion is necessary to prevent withdrawal (see below) (28,135). In either circumstance, the technique is the same. Concentrated solutions of opioids/sedatives are used so that the total volume is limited to 3 mL per hour or less. The subcutaneous infusion is started at the same time that the intravenous infusion is discontinued. Either a standard 22-gauge Angiocath or a butterfly needle can be used. Before placement, the tubing and needle are flushed with the opioid solution and after sterile preparation of the area, the needle is inserted subcutaneously and covered with a bioocclusive dressing. The same infusion pumps that are used for intravenous drug administration can be used for subcutaneous administration. The pressure limit may need to be adjusted to allow subcutaneous administration. Several different opioids are suitable for subcutaneous administration including morphine, hydromorphone, and fentanyl. Methadone can cause significant tissue reaction with erythema and is not recommended for subcutaneous administration.

Miscellaneous Agents

Anecdotal experiences with varying degrees of success have been reported with several other agents or combinations of agents (Table 44.8). Phenothiazines and butyrophenones are considered the major tranquilizers and are generally used in the treatment of psychiatric disturbances or for their antiemetic properties. Neither of these classes of agents has found great popularity as sedatives in the PICU. Of the many agents available, haloperidol appears to the most frequently chosen of this class for sedation of adults in the ICU. Although not approved by the FDA for intravenous administration, there is an abundance of clinical experience with its use by this route. Riker et al. (136) reported their experience with haloperidol by continuous intravenous infusion (range, 3 to 25 mg per hour) for sedation in eight adult patients in the ICU. The authors cited many benefits of haloperidol including rapid onset, minimal respiratory depression, and no active metabolites. Adverse effects associated with the butyrophenones and phenothiazines include hypotension related to α blockade and peripheral vasodilation, dystonic and extrapyramidal effects, lowering of the seizure threshold, and, in rare cases, neuroleptic malignant syndrome. Of even greater concern in the patient in the ICU are the possible effects on the cardiovascular system that have been previously reported with haloperidol including cardiac arrest and torsade de pointes. In the study of Riker et al. (136), cardiac events included atrial dysrhythmias, prolongation of the QT interval, and ventricular tachycardia in one patient. Alterations in repolarization induced by this class of agent may be particularly dangerous in patients with altered sympathetic function associated with fever, pain, or the stresses of an acute illness.

TABLE 44.8. *Miscellaneous agents for intensive care unit sedation*

Phenothiazines
Butyrophenones
Chloral hydrate
Antihistamines
α_2-adrenergic agonists
Clonidine
Dexmedetomidine

Health care providers may be more familiar with the use phenothiazines in the pediatric population in combination with other agents in a formulation known as the DPT (Demerol, Phenergan, and Thorazine). The latter is commonly used for invasive procedures. Although this formulation has achieved success, the combination of these agents may result in prolonged sedation and the risk of respiratory depression and apnea (137). If such combinations are used, careful and prolonged postprocedure monitoring is suggested.

Although diphenhydramine is most commonly used for its antihistamine effects to treat pruritus or as an antiemetic, the associated sedative properties may be beneficial in the patient in the PICU. Although there is a limited role for the phenothiazines, butyrophenones, and antihistamines for sedation of the patient in the PICU, they may be useful in the spontaneously breathing patient in whom a sedative agent is required (the toddler with bronchiolitis or status asthmaticus). In such situations, diphenhydramine (0.5 mg/kg intravenously every 4 to 6 hours) or droperidol (10 to 20 μg/kg every 4 to 6 hours) may be an effective agent for sedation with limited effects on respiratory function. When administered individually, these agents have limited effects on respiratory function; however, when combined with other agents such as opioids or benzodiazepines, they may further potentiate respiratory depression.

Chloral hydrate, a sedative-hypnotic agent, is metabolized in the liver to its active form, trichloroethanol, which has a half-life of 8 to 12 hours. Because there is no parenteral formulation, oral or rectal administration is necessary, which may result in a slow onset of action of as long as 20 minutes, thus limiting its utility in controlling the acutely agitated patient in the PICU. Repeated administration can lead to the accumulation of active metabolites and prolonged sedation that may persist after its discontinuation. Its use is not recommended for infants younger than 3 months of age or in patients with hepatic dysfunction. Additionally, the active metabolite trichloroethanol is related to the halogenated hydrocarbons and has been associated with the occurrence of ventricular arrhythmias especially in patients at risk for such problems (tricyclic antidepressant ingestions) (138, 139).

Clonidine, a centrally acting α_2 agonist that decreases central sympathetic outflow, was initially introduced for the treatment of hypertension with more recent clinical experience demonstrating its efficacy as a premedicant for the operating room (140,141). Beneficial physiologic effects of the α_2 agonists include sedation, anxiolysis, decreased anesthetic requirements, cardiovascular stability, and the potentiation of opiate-induced analgesia (142). In addition to its sedative properties, clonidine and the other α_2-adrenergic agonists possess intrinsic analgesic effects that are thought to be mediated at the spinal level (dorsal horn) through the interaction with specific adrenergic receptors. Activation of presynaptic receptors (first-order neurons) results in the decreased release of the nociceptive transmitter substance P, whereas postsynaptic activation decreases the rate of depolarization of second-order neurons. To date, clonidine for sedation in the ICU has appeared only as anecdotal case reports (143).

More recently, dexmedetomidine has been released for clinical use. Like clonidine, it is a centrally acting, α_2-adrenergic agonist and shares the same clinical properties of clonidine. However, it possesses an affinity of eight times that of clonidine for the α_2 receptor, a differential α_1 to α_2 agonism of 1:1,600 and a half-life of 2 hours, which is approximately fourfold shorter than clonidine. Dexmedetomidine is currently approved by the FDA for short-term (24 hours or less) sedation of adult patients during mechanical ventilation. Venn et al. (144) compared the effects of dexmedetomidine with those of placebo in 119 adult patients who required mechanical ventilation after cardiac and general surgical procedures. Dexmedetomidine was administered as a bolus of 1 μg/kg followed by a infusion of 0.2 to 0.7 μg/kg per hour. Patients who received dexmedetomidine required 80% less midazolam and 50% less morphine. Eighteen of the 66 patients who received dexmedetomidine experienced hypotension (MAP <60 mm Hg or a greater than 30% decrease from baseline) or bradycardia (heart rate less than 50 beats per minute). The cardiovascular changes were noted during the administration of the bolus dose in 11 of the 18 patients. This resulted in the interruption of the infusion in three patients and a withdrawal from the study of three others.

Hall et al. (145) evaluated the analgesic, sedative, and cardiovascular effects of two infusion rates of dexmedetomidine (0.2 and 0.6 μg/kg per hour) in healthy, adult volunteers. Both dexmedetomidine infusion rates resulted in significant sedation, reduction of pain to the cold pressor test, and impairment of memory and psychometric performance. They also noted small, but clinically significant decreases in the MAP and heart rate, although no patient developed bradycardia or hypotension.

Although the clinical use of the α_2-agonists in the pediatric population is currently limited, their beneficial physiologic properties suggest their potential for future use both as sedatives and analgesics in the patient in the PICU. To date, there are no reports of the use of dexmedetomidine for sedation of the patient in the PICU; however, we would anticipate such trials and evaluations in the not too distant future.

PHYSICAL DEPENDENCY, TOLERANCE, AND WITHDRAWAL

With increased attention to the need for providing appropriate sedation and analgesia to the patient in the PICU, there has been increased use of sedative/analgesic agents in this group of patients. Along with the increased use are new issues that must be addressed and treated including tolerance, physical dependency, and withdrawal phenomena. Effective management schemes to treat these problems and methods to delay or prevent them are needed so that these newly recognized issues do not limit the appropriate use of sedative and analgesic agents in the patient in the PICU. Tolerance is a decrease in a drug's effect over time or the need to increase the dose to achieve the same effect. Tolerance is related to changes at or distal to the receptor. The plasma concentration of the drug remains constant while the effect is decreased. The magnitude of tolerance that can occur is illustrated by our report of a 16-year-old, 52-kg boy requiring mechanical ventilation for 5 weeks (146). Sedation was provided by the continuous infusions of lorazepam and fentanyl. Progressive tolerance resulted in the need to intermittently increase the fentanyl infusion to a maximum of 3,500 μg per hour (67.3 μg/kg per hour) or 70 mL per hour of fentanyl (50 μg/mL) at the end of the 5-week period. Because of the large volume of fluid required to administer the fentanyl, the sedation regimen was changed to sufentanil. The patient eventually made a full recovery and was discharged home on an oral methadone taper (see below).

Withdrawal includes the physical signs and symptoms that manifest when a sedative/analgesic agent is abruptly discontinued in a patient who is physically tolerant. The symptomatology of withdrawal varies from patient to patient and may be affected by several factors including the agent involved, the age of the patient, the patient's cognitive state, and associated medical conditions. Physiologic (physical) dependence is the need to continue a sedative or analgesic agent to prevent withdrawal. Psychologic dependence is the need for a substance because of its euphoric effects. Addiction includes (a) a complex pattern of behaviors characterized by the repetitive, compulsive use of a substance, (b) antisocial or criminal behavior to obtain the drug, and (c) a high incidence of relapse after treatment. Psychologic dependency and addiction are rare after the appropriate use of sedative/analgesic agents (147,148). With the widespread use of different agents, tolerance and withdrawal have been reported with several of the agents used for sedation in the ICU. Although the initial reports involved tolerance to opioids (149,150), an increased awareness of the problem has led to reports of tolerance and withdrawal with benzodiazepines (151, 152), barbiturates (35,153,154), propofol (155), and the inhalational anesthetic agent isoflurane (156,157).

Effective treatment strategies to deal with physical dependency and related problems require the accurate identification and recognition of withdrawal symptoms. Ongoing or associated conditions that manifest similar clinical signs and symptoms as withdrawal should be ruled out before assuming that the patient's symptoms are the result of withdrawal. In the patient in the PICU, these associated conditions may include CNS insults or infections, ICU psychosis, metabolic abnormalities, hypoxia, hypercarbia, and cerebral hypoperfusion from alterations in cardiac output, and cerebrovascular disease.

The time to the onset of withdrawal symptoms may vary depending on the half-life of the agent and its active metabolites. The latter may be several times longer than the parent compound. The signs and symptoms of sedative/analgesic agent withdrawal can be grouped broadly into three classes: (a) CNS activation, (b) gastrointestinal disturbances, and (c) sympathetic hyperactivity. CNS manifestations include irritability, increased wakefulness, tremulousness, hyperactive deep tendon reflexes, clonus, inability to concentrate, frequent yawning, sneezing, delirium, and hypertonicity. In neonates and infants, additional signs of CNS stimulation include a high-pitched cry and an exaggerated Moro reflex. Seizures have been reported with withdrawal from opioids, benzodiazepines, barbiturates, propofol, and the inhalational anesthetic agents. Visual and auditory hallucinations have been described with opioid, benzodiazepine, barbiturate, and inhalational anesthetic withdrawal.

Gastrointestinal manifestations of withdrawal may be especially prominent in neonates and infants. The only manifestation of opioid/sedative agent withdrawal may be feeding intolerance with vomiting, diarrhea, uncoordinated suck and swallow, or persistent residuals with tube feedings. Because these gastrointestinal manifestations may be subtle, they are often attributed to other problems and not withdrawal. Activation of the sympathetic nervous system (tachycardia, hypertension, diaphoresis, and tachypnea) can be a prominent finding of withdrawal from sedative/analgesic agents. Additional signs and symptoms of sympathetic hyperactivity include nasal stuffiness and fever.

The first step in the treatment of patients with dependency and tolerance is identification of the at-risk group and the development of appropriate scoring systems to identify and grade the signs and symptoms of withdrawal. Identifying the risk factors associated with the development of withdrawal allows identification of the at-risk group. Katz et al. (158) evaluated the factors that could be used to identify the at-risk group in 23 infants and children 1 week to 22 months of age who received fentanyl by continuous infusion for sedation. When there was no longer a need for sedation, the fentanyl infusion was decreased by 50% every 24 hours times two and then discontinued. Withdrawal was assessed using a neonatal scoring system described by Finnegan et al. (159). Withdrawal behavior was observed in 13 of 23 patients (57%). The total fentanyl dose and the duration of the infusion correlated with the risk of withdrawal, whereas the maximal fentanyl infusion rate did not. A total fentanyl dose of 1.5 mg/kg or more or a duration of infusion of 5 days or longer was associated with a 50% incidence of withdrawal, whereas a total fentanyl dose of 2.5 mg/kg or more or a duration of infusion of 9 days or longer was associated with a 100% incidence of withdrawal. Similar results were reported by Arnold et al. (156) who noted a correlation of both total dose (>1.6 mg/kg) and duration of administration (>5 days) with the incidence of withdrawal.

Arnold et al. (156) also noted that the total dose administered may be a risk factor for patients receiving sedation using the inhalation anesthetic agent isoflurane. Withdrawal occurred only in patients who had received more than 70 minimum alveolar concentration (MAC)-hours of isoflurane. There are limited data concerning the duration of administration and total dose of benzodiazepines and barbiturates that place patients at high risk of withdrawal symptoms. Fonsmark et al. (153) noted an increased incidence of withdrawal with a total dose of midazolam of 60 mg/kg or more and a total dose of pentobarbital of 25 mg/kg or more.

Regardless of the agent(s) used for sedation, once the decision is made to start weaning the infusion, the patient should be monitored for signs and symptoms of withdrawal. A scoring system is useful to provide a way to quantify the patient's symptoms and assess the need for treatment. Problems with currently available scoring systems are predominantly twofold: (a) they were developed to assess neonatal behavior in infants of drug-addicted mothers and (b) they were developed to assess opioid withdrawal. Several different scoring systems have now been developed. These are outlined in the review of Anand and Arnold (160).

The mainstay of therapy to prevent withdrawal is slowly weaning the sedative/analgesic infusions. This can be done rapidly

(10% to 15% every 6 to 8 hours) in patients who have been receiving these agents for brief periods (less than 3 to 5 days). After prolonged administration, the weaning process may require 2 to 4 weeks to prevent withdrawal symptoms. It may not be possible to decrease the infusion rate in 10% increments when patients are receiving high doses such as fentanyl 20 to 50 μg/kg per hour. In such circumstances, it may be necessary to decrease the rate by as little as 1 μg/kg per hour every 12 hours. Although the weaning process can be accomplished by slowing decreasing the intravenous infusion rate, this requires intravenous access, hospitalization, and, at times, continued monitoring in the ICU. Two options may be considered to facilitate patient care: subcutaneous or oral administration.

If it is decided that tapering the infusion can be accomplished within a reasonable period that will not delay hospital discharge, the patient may be considered a candidate for subcutaneous administration (28). In general, these patients require moderate doses of fentanyl (5 to 10 μg/kg per hour), often in conjunction with midazolam (0.1 to 0.3 mg/kg per hour). Switching to subcutaneous administration allows the removal of central venous access and eliminates the need to maintain peripheral intravenous access. Both fentanyl and midazolam can be effectively administered via the subcutaneous route and the infusions slowly tapered to prevent withdrawal symptoms. The techniques of administration are the same as those described previously when using fentanyl or other opioids by the subcutaneous route for acute pain management/sedation.

When prolonged administration of opioids or other sedative agents is necessary, switching to oral administration of long-acting agents may allow earlier hospital discharge. Although our initial report (150) concerning methadone use for such problems suggested a starting dose of 0.1 mg/kg every 12 hours, the three patients in the cohort were receiving low fentanyl infusion rates and therefore higher doses of methadone were not needed. The subsequent clinical experience indicates that higher doses may be needed depending on the dose of fentanyl (161). Because this problem has become more commonplace, several authors have offered their suggestions for weaning from opioids. The author's current practice is outlined in the following section.

The conversion from intravenous fentanyl to oral methadone accounts for the difference in the potency of the two drugs (fentanyl: methadone = 100:1), the difference in the half-life (fentanyl:methadone = 1:75 to 100), and the oral bioavailability of methadone (75% to 80%). A patient weighing 10 kg who is receiving 10 μg/kg per hour of fentanyl receives 2.4 mg fentanyl per day. Because the difference in potency (100:1) is offset by the difference in half-life (1:100), the total daily dose of methadone equals the total daily dose of fentanyl. Increasing the dose to compensate for the decreased oral bioavailability of methadone (75% to 80%) is generally not necessary to prevent withdrawal symptoms. Cross-tolerance of opioids is not 100%, so that switching from one opioid to another may result in a decrease in the total dose required of the new opioid when calculated on a standard potency ratio. This issue of cross-tolerance relates to many factors, one of which may be the varying potency of opioids as antagonists at the *N*-methyl-D-aspartate receptor (162). Part of the incomplete cross-tolerance when switching to methadone (a lower methadone dose is needed than that based on the suggested equipotent ratios) may relate to methadone's effects at the *N*-methyl-D-aspartate receptor (162).

The starting oral methadone dose is equivalent to the total daily intravenous fentanyl dose (in this case, 2.4 mg per day). The conversion factors are illustrated in Table 44.9. The oral dosing of methadone is started with an every-12-hour dosing regimen. The fentanyl infusion is decreased by 50% after the second oral dose of methadone, by 50% after the third dose, and then discontinued after the fourth dose. Symptoms of opioid withdrawal are graded according to a standardized neonatal opioid withdrawal scale and treated as necessary with rescue doses of morphine (0.05

TABLE 44.9. *Conversion from intravenous fentanyl to oral methadone*

Potency (fentanyl:methadone)	100:1
Half-life (fentanyl:methadone)	1:75–100
Oral bioavailability (methadone)	75–80%

A 10-kg patient is receiving a fentanyl infusion of 10 μg/kg/hr. The total daily fentanyl dose is 2.4 mg daily

1. The starting dose of methadone is 2.4 mg daily divided into an every-12-hour dose.
2. After the second oral dose of methadone, the intravenous fentanyl infusion is decreased by 50% (i.e., to 5 μg/kg per hour).
3. After the third oral dose, the intravenous fentanyl infusion is decreased by 50% (i.e., to 2.5 μg/kg per hour).
4. After the fourth oral dose, the intravenous fentanyl infusion is discontinued.

mg/kg per dose). The morphine requirement over a 24-hour period is added to the next day's methadone dose. Additional rescue doses of morphine are administered during the next 72-hour period, but no change is made in the methadone dose for the next 72 hours. This allows the new methadone dose to achieve a steady-state serum concentration. If excessive sedation occurs, one methadone dose is held and the dose decreased by 10% to 20%. The oral methadone dose is then tapered once a week either in the hospital or as an outpatient after a follow-up telephone call to ensure that the infant or child is doing well. The dose is decreased by 20% of the initial dose so that the oral dose is gradually decreased and discontinued after a 5-week period. It must be stressed that the suggested guidelines listed in Table 44.9 are based on clinical experience and the currently available literature. There is significant debate concerning the potency ratios of morphine and methadone (163,164) suggesting the time-honored 1:1 is not correct and that methadone may be five to ten times as potent as morphine. However, many of these studies do not factor in the half-life differences between the two drugs, which must be addressed with repeated dosing.

Because of the stigma attached to methadone use, discussions with and explanations to the parents are necessary to outline why methadone is being used and to explain the differences between addiction and physical dependency. Because of these issues as well as familiarity with long-acting morphine preparations (MS Contin), which are used in the treatment of children with chronic cancer-related pain, some physicians prefer to use the latter agent. Based on potency and half-life, the dosing of methadone and morphine are similar. Morphine is available only in tablets that cannot be crushed so that administration may be more difficult in younger patients. Methadone, conversely, is available in a liquid formulation. Delayed-release preparations are also available for oxycodone and hydromorphone; however, to date, their use has been limited to the management of acute and chronic pain with no information concerning their use in the treatment or prevention of opioid withdrawal.

Several other agents, both opioid and nonopioid, have been suggested for the treatment and prevention of opioid withdrawal. Mixtures of opioid alkaloids such as paregoric and tincture of opium were the first agents used to treat opioid withdrawal in infants of drug-addicted mothers. Paregoric is no longer recommended in neonates and infants because of concerns of the toxicity of its other components (CNS effects from camphor and cardiovascular manifestations of benzoic acid). Tincture of opium is still used to treat opioid withdrawal in neonates of drug-addicted mothers (160). Because of its short half-life, repeated administration at 4-hour intervals may be necessary.

In addition to opioids, nonopioid agents including benzodiazepines and barbiturates have been used to treat opioid withdrawal. In the author's opinion, this is less than optimal because it seems to make physiologic sense when dealing with the problems of tolerance and dependence to replace the missing agent rather than treat the resulting symptoms. Their only role appears to be in the treatment of seizures that rarely occur with opioid/sedative agent withdrawal.

Clonidine has also been used to treat opioid withdrawal in both neonates and adults. α_2-Adrenergic receptors partially mediate their pharmacologic actions through activation of the same potassium channel as opioid receptors. Owing to clonidine's prolonged duration of action (12 to 18 hours), once- or twice-daily dosing is possible. Clonidine is also available as a patch for transdermal administration. Starting doses range from 3 to 5 μg/kg per day. Adverse effects from clonidine include sedation, bradycardia, and hypotension. Although the use of clonidine is becoming more widespread in pediatric anesthesia, there is limited clinical experience with its use in the treatment of opioid withdrawal. Further information is needed to define more clearly the efficacy and safety of this agent as well as its role in treating opioid withdrawal in the patient in the PICU.

As with many other aspects of tolerance and dependency, most of the information concerning treatment strategies involves the opioids with less information and clinical experience with the benzodiazepines and barbiturates. The subcutaneous administration of midazolam, as previously described (28), is a viable option, although it does require ongoing hospitalization and perhaps continued ICU admission. As with the opioids, longer acting equivalents are available for both the benzodiazepines and barbiturates with agents such as lorazepam and phenobarbital. Experience with such practices is limited. The following information is given as a rough guideline in transitioning from intravenous to oral medications. Owing to limited clinical experience, such transitions are probably best accomplished in the ICU setting. For benzodiazepine tolerance, lorazepam may be preferred over diazepam because the latter agent has active metabolites with variable half-lives and durations of action. As with the conversion from fentanyl to methadone, the conversion from midazolam to lorazepam should account for differences in potency (1:2 to 3) and half-life (1:6) between midazolam and lorazepam as well as the decrease in bioavailability (60% to 70%) with oral administration (Table 44.10). In the sedation of adult patients in an ICU, Pohlman et al. (32) noted an initial/mean/maximal dose of intravenous lorazepam of 0.06/0.06/0.1 mg/kg per hour compared with intravenous midazolam at 0.15/0.24/0.29 mg/kg per hour resulting in potency ratios of 2.5/4/3. Lugo et al. (34) reported a potency ratio of 1:6 when switching from intravenous midazolam to oral lorazepam, so that they calculated the total daily dose of intravenous midazolam and administered one-sixth of that dose as enteral lorazepam.

TABLE 44.10. *Conversion from intravenous midazolam to oral lorazepam*

Potency (midazolam:lorazepam)	1:2
Half-life (midazolam:lorazepam)	1:3–6
Oral bioavailability (lorazepam)	60–70%

A 10-kg patient is receiving a midazolam infusion of 0.3 mg/kg/hr. The total daily midazolam dose is 72 mg. An equivalent daily dose of lorazepam is 72 divided by 6 to 12, which is 6 to 12 mg daily.

1. The starting dose of lorazepam is 6 to 12 mg daily, divided into doses every 4 to 6 hours.
2. After the second oral dose of lorazepam, the intravenous midazolam infusion is decreased by 50% (i.e., to 0.15 mg/kg per hour).
3. After the third oral dose, the intravenous midazolam infusion is decreased by 50% (i.e., to 0.075 mg/kg per hour).
4. After the fourth oral dose, the intravenous midazolam infusion is discontinued.

Several other agents have been evaluated in the adult population for the treatment of benzodiazepine withdrawal including propranolol, carbamazepine, phenobarbital, and clonidine. There is no information concerning the use of these agents in children.

Barbiturate tolerance presents problems similar to those with benzodiazepine tolerance in that there is limited information to suggest and evaluate treatment options. With the increased use of opioids and benzodiazepines, the use of barbiturates for prolonged sedation of the patient in the PICU has declined. Barbiturates are generally second- or third-line choices when the benzodiazepines and/or opioids fail. As with other agents, prolonged use can result in tolerance and withdrawal if these agents are abruptly discontinued. Initially when faced with this problem, pentobarbital was used for oral administration (35). Because of pentobarbital's short half-life, an every-6-hour dosing regimen may be necessary. More recently, we have found that phenobarbital can be used instead of pentobarbital (J.D. Tobias, unpublished data 1998–2001). This provides easy oral administration because phenobarbital is available as an elixir and as tablets and allows an every-12-hour dosing regimen. Our technique involves the use of intravenous phenobarbital substituted for intravenous pentobarbital followed by a transition to oral phenobarbital administration. Because the combination of pentobarbital and phenobarbital may result in significant respiratory depression, this process is accomplished while the patient is still receiving mechanical ventilation. The pentobarbital infusion is discontinued. Six hours later, 50% of the phenobarbital loading dose is administered (Table 44.11). The total loading dose of phenobarbital is administered in two increments separated by 6 hours followed 6 hours later by the maintenance dose. The loading dose and maintenance dose are based on the current pentobarbital infusion rates. These are preliminary data and future studies are needed to determine the efficacy of this regimen.

The heightened awareness of the need for aggressive sedation and pain management of the patient in the PICU has resulted in new issues: tolerance, physical dependency, and withdrawal phenomena. Laboratory investigations have begun to determine the cellular mechanisms of tolerance and dependency with some suggestions of ways to delay their development. Although the initial work is promising, the applications of these techniques into the clinical realm are not yet practical. For now, components in the management of these problems start with the observation for signs/symptoms of withdrawal when the decision is made to decrease the sedative/analgesic agent. Formal scoring systems can be used to document withdrawal symptoms. Rapid weaning and discontinuation of sedative/analgesics in patients who have received these agents for more than 3 to 5 days will generally result in withdrawal. A rapid wean may occur in an effort to get patients extubated and discharged from the ICU when bed availability becomes an issue. Additionally, a rapid wean may occur with the thought that these agents must be discontinued before extubation. Even in patients receiving a high dose of opioids or other agents, mechanical ventilation can be weaned and spontaneous ventilation resumed. Because the weaning process has occurred while these agents are infusing, there is no need to discontinue them before extubation. Our practice is to decrease these agents by 10% to 20% before extubation and then wean as outlined previously.

Treatment options for withdrawal generally rely on agents of the same class. When sedative and analgesic agents have been administered for 5 to 7 days or less, the infusions can be weaned rapidly (10% to 15% every 6 to 8 hours). If a more prolonged weaning regimen is necessary, subcutaneous administration may eliminate the need for intravenous access. When a more prolonged weaning regimen will be necessary, switching to longer acting oral agents should be considered. This can include Morphine or methadone for opioids, lorazepam for benzodiazepines, and phenobarbital for the barbiturates. When switching from intravenous to oral medications, careful monitoring of cardiorespiratory status is suggested. The initial switch is probably best accomplished in the PICU setting. Ongoing education of the parents, patients, and nursing staff is mandatory concerning the differences between tolerance, physical dependency, and addiction.

TABLE 44.11. *Conversion from intravenous pentobarbital to oral phenobarbital*

Pentobarbital infusion (mg/kg/hr)	Phenobarbital loading dose (mg/kg)
1–2	8
2–3	15
3–4	20

The pentobarbital infusion is discontinued. Six hours later, half of the loading dose is infused over 1 hour followed by the remaining half of the loading dose 6 hours later. This is followed in 6 hours by the first of the every-12-hour maintenance dose. The maintenance dose should equal one-third of the initial loading dose. Once the patient is stabilized on the intravenous phenobarbital regimen, the same dose is administered orally and then weaned 10% to 20% every week.

SUMMARY

Because of the diversity of patients and clinical scenarios presenting in the PICU, a "cookbook" approach to sedation and analgesia is impossible. Health care workers involved in the care of these patients should be experienced with several different medications and routes of administration to ensure adequate sedation and analgesia in this diverse patient population. Initial choices for amnesia/sedation may include the continuous infusion of a benzodiazepine. Lorazepam offers a cost-effective alternative to midazolam and eliminates the concerns regarding metabolism by the P-450 system or the presence of active metabolites. A combination of oral lorazepam with intravenous midazolam has been suggested as a cost-saving measure. In situations requiring analgesia, an opioid either by continuous infusion or a patient-controlled analgesia device can be used. Although fentanyl is frequently chosen as the first-line opioid, morphine is an acceptable and cost-effective alternative for patients with stable cardiovascular function. The synthetic opioids are recommended for neonates, especially after cardiac surgical procedures and those at risk for pulmonary hypertension. In this setting, the use of the synthetic opioids may decrease postoperative morbidity and mortality and modulate the deleterious effects of pain and the stress response on the pulmonary vasculature.

When the above agents fail to be effective or are associated with adverse effects, alternatives include ketamine or pentobarbital. Ketamine may be useful for the patient with hemodynamic instability or increased airway reactivity as a component of their disease process. Pentobarbital may be effective when the combination of benzodiazepines and opioids fails to provide the desired level of sedation. Propofol has gained great favor in the adult population as a means of providing deep sedation while allowing rapid awakening. Similar beneficial properties are achieved in the pediatric patient; however, concerns over propofol infusion syndrome may limit the use of this agent in the younger pediatric aged patient. Suggested starting guidelines for dosing of sedative and analgesic agents are listed in Table 44.12.

TABLE 44.12. *Suggested guidelines for dosing of sedative and analgesic agents*

Agent	Dose	Comments
Fentanyl	2–3 μg/kg/hr	Modulates stress response and pulmonary vascular resistance
Morphine	10–30 μg/kg/hr	Inexpensive, venodilation
Midazolam	0.05–0.15 mg/kg/hr	Abundant clinical experience, expensive, P450 metabolism
Lorazepam	0.025–0.05 mg/kg/hr	Limited clinical experience, inexpensive; metabolism: glucuronyl transferase
Ketamine	1–2 mg/kg/hr	Endogenous catecholamine release, bronchodilation, cardiovascular stability, can be mixed 10:1 with midazolam
Pentobarbital	1–2 mg/kg/hr	Alternative to benzodiazepine/opioid, incompatible with other medications, vasodilation/negative inotropic effects
Propofol	1–3 mg/kg/hr	Possible occurrence of propofol infusion syndrome when used for prolonged administration to patients younger than 10 years of age; rapid awakening, high lipid content of solution
Remifentanil	0.5 μg/kg/min	Cardiorespiratory effects similar to other synthetic opioids, rapid development of tolerance and cost may limit application except for limited periods (less than 12–24 hr), rapid dissipation of effects when infusion is discontinued
Dexmedetomidine	0.25–0.5 μg/kg/hr	U.S. Food and Drug Administration–approved for short-term (24 hr) sedation in adults; clinical trials in children ongoing as of July 2002

These infusion rates represent suggestions for starting doses. The infusion should be supplemented with as-needed bolus doses to provide the desired level of baseline sedation. In patients requiring frequent bolus doses, the infusion rate should be increased by 10% to 20%. If patients require no bolus doses and are excessively sedated, the infusion rate should be decreased by 10% to 20%.

In addition to the agent chosen, important decisions regarding the administration of the drug include the mode of administration. Regardless of the agent used, a stable level of sedation is generally best achieved with a continuous infusion supplemented with as-needed doses. Patients requiring frequent bolus doses should have the baseline infusion rate increased. As the infusion rate is increased, the bolus doses should be increased to equal the hourly rate. When sedative and/or analgesic agents are administered for a prolonged period of time, strategies should be implemented to prevent withdrawal syndromes. This may include a gradual tapering of the infusion rate or switching to oral or subcutaneous administration.

REFERENCES

1. The Committee on Drugs of the American Academy of Pediatrics. Guidelines for monitoring and management of pediatric patients during and after sedation for diagnostic and therapeutic procedures. *Pediatrics* 1992;89: 1110–1115.
2. Volles DF, McGory R. Pharmacokinetic considerations. *Crit Care Clin* 1999;15:55–57.
3. Buck ML, Blumer JL. Opioids and other analgesics: adverse effects in the intensive care unit. *Crit Care Clin* 1991;7:615–637.
4. Reed MD, Blumer JL. Therapeutic drug monitoring in the pediatric intensive care unit. *Pediatr Clin North Am* 1994;41:1227–1243.
5. Katz R, Kelly HW. Pharmacokinetics of continuous infusions of fentanyl in critically ill children. *Crit Care Med* 1993;21:995–1000.
6. Anand KJS, Hansen DD, Hickey PR. Hormonal-metabolic stress responses in neonates undergoing cardiac surgery. *Anesthesiology* 1990;73:661–670.
7. Anand KJS, Hickey PR. Halothane-morphine compared with high-dose sufentanil for anesthesia and postoperative analgesia in neonatal cardiac surgery. *N Engl J Med* 1992;326:1–9.
8. Hansen-Flaschen JH, Brazinsky S, Basile C, et al. Use of sedating drugs and neuromuscular blocking agents in patients requiring mechanical ventilation for respiratory failure. *JAMA* 1991;266:2870–2875.
9. Wagner RL, White PF, Kan PB, et al. Inhibition of adrenal steroidogenesis by the anesthetic etomidate. *N Engl J Med* 1984;310:1415–1421.
10. Tobias JD. Airway management in the pediatric trauma patient. *J Intensive Care Med* 1998;13:1–14.
11. Tobias JD. Etomidate: applications in pediatric anesthesia and critical care. *J Intensive Care Med* 1997;12: 324–326.
12. Kong KL, Willatts SM, Prys-Roberts C. Isoflurane compared with midazolam for sedation in the intensive care unit. *BMJ* 1989;298:1277–1280.
13. Breheny FX, Kendall PA. Use of isoflurane for sedation in intensive care. *Crit Care Med* 1992;20: 1062–1064.
14. Satoh H, Gillette JR, Takemura T, et al. Investigation of the immunological basis of halothane-induced hepatotoxicity. *Adv Exp Med Biol* 1986;197:657–773.
15. Kenna JG, Neuberger J, Williams R. Evidence for expression in human liver of halothane-induced neoantigens recognized by antibodies in sera from patients with halothane hepatitis. *Hepatology* 1988;8: 1635–1641.
16. Adams RW, Cucchiara RF, Gronert GA, et al. Isoflurane and cerebrospinal fluid pressure in neurosurgical patients. *Anesthesiology* 1981;54:97–99.
17. Drummond JC, Todd MM, Scheller MS, et al. A comparison of the direct cerebral vasodilating potencies of halothane and isoflurane in the New Zealand white rabbit. *Anesthesiology* 1986;65:462–467.
18. Reilly CS, Wood AJJ, Koshakji RP, et al. The effect of halothane on drug disposition: contribution of changes in intrinsic drug metabolizing capacity and hepatic blood flow. *Anesthesiology* 1985;63:70–76.
19. Arnold JH, Truog RD, Rice SA. Prolonged administration of isoflurane to pediatric patients during mechanical ventilation. *Anesth Analg* 1993;76:520–526.
20. Reves JG, Fragan RJ, Vinik R, et al. Midazolam: pharmacology and uses. *Anesthesiology* 1985;62:310–317.
21. Lloyd-Thomas AR, Booker PD. Infusion of midazolam in paediatric patients after cardiac surgery. *Br J Anaesth* 1986;58:1109–1115.
22. Silvasi DL, Rosen DA, Rosen KR. Continuous intravenous midazolam infusion for sedation in the pediatric intensive care unit. *Anesth Analg* 1988;67:286–288.
23. Rosen DA, Rosen KR. Midazolam for sedation in the paediatric intensive care unit. *Intensive Care Med* 1991;17:S15–S19.
24. Beebe DS, Belani KG, Chang P, et al. Effectiveness of preoperative sedation with rectal midazolam, ketamine, or their combination in young children. *Anesth Analg* 1992;75:880–884.
25. McMillan CO, Spahr-Schopfer IA, Sikich N, et al. Premedication of children with oral midazolam. *Can J Anaesth* 1992;39:545–550.
26. Karl HW, Rosenberger JL, Larach MG, et al. Transmucosal administration of midazolam for premedication of pediatric patients: comparison of the nasal and sublingual routes. *Anesthesiology* 1993;78:885–891.
27. Theroux MC, West DW, Cordry DH, et al. Efficacy of midazolam in facilitating suturing of lacerations in preschool children in the emergency department. *Pediatrics* 1993;91:624–627.
28. Tobias JD. Subcutaneous administration of fentanyl and midazolam to prevent withdrawal following prolonged sedation in children. *Crit Care Med* 1999;27: 2262–2265.
29. Trouvin JH, Farinotti R, Haberer JP, et al. Pharmacokinetics of midazolam in anesthetized cirrhotic patients. *Br J Anaesth* 1988;60:762–767.
30. Vinik HR, Reves JG, Greenblatt DJ, et al. The pharmacokinetics of midazolam in chronic renal failure patients. *Anesthesiology* 1983;59:390–394.
31. Oldenhorf H, Jong M, Steenhock A, et al. Clinical pharmacokinetics of midazolam in intensive care patients: a wide interpatient variability? *Clin Pharmacol Ther* 1988;43:262–269.

32. Pohlman AS, Simpson KP, Hall JCB. Continuous intravenous infusions of lorazepam versus midazolam for sedation during mechanical ventilatory support: a prospective, randomized study. *Crit Care Med* 1994; 22:1241–1247.
33. Dundee JW, Johnston HM, Gray RC. Lorazepam as a sedative-amnestic in an intensive care unit. *Curr Med Res Opin* 1976;4:290–295.
34. Lugo RA, Chester EA, Cash J, et al. A cost analysis of enterally administered lorazepam in the pediatric intensive care unit. *Crit Care Med* 1999;27:417–421.
35. Tobias JD, Deshpande JK, Gregory DF. Outpatient therapy of iatrogenic drug dependency following prolonged sedation in the pediatric intensive care unit. *Intensive Care Med* 1994;20:504–507.
36. Arbour R, Esparis B. Osmolar gap acidosis in a 60 year old man treated for hypoxemic respiratory failure. *Chest* 2000;118:545–546.
37. Reynolds HN, Teiken P, Regan ME, et al. Hyperlactatemia, increased osmolar gap, renal dysfunction during continuous lorazepam infusion. *Crit Care Med* 2000;28:1631–1634.
38. Breheny FX. Reversal of midazolam sedation with flumazenil. *Crit Care Med* 1992;20:736–739.
39. McDuffee A, Tobias JD. Seizure following flumazenil administration in a child. *Pediatr Emerg Care* 1995; 11:186–187.
40. Domino EF, Chodoff P, Corssen G. Pharmacologic effects of CI-581, a new dissociative anesthetic in man. *Clin Pharmacol Ther* 1965;6:279–291.
41. Tobias JD. End-tidal carbon dioxide monitoring during sedation with a combination of midazolam and ketamine for children undergoing painful, invasive procedures. *Pediatr Emerg Care* 1999;15:173–175.
42. Chernow B, Laker R, Creuss D, et al. Plasma, urine, and cerebrospinal fluid catecholamine concentrations during and after ketamine sedation. *Crit Care Med* 1982;10:600–603.
43. Wayman K, Shoemaker WC, Lippmann M. Cardiovascular effects of anesthetic induction with ketamine. *Anesth Analg* 1980;59:355–358.
44. Spotoft H, Korshin JD, Sorensen MB, et al. The cardiovascular effects of ketamine used for induction of anesthesia in patients with valvular heart disease. *Can Anaesth Soc J* 1979;26:463–467.
45. Gooding JM, Dimick AR, Travakoli M, et al. A physiologic analysis of cardiopulmonary responses to ketamine anesthesia in non-cardiac patients. *Anesth Analg* 1977;56:813–816.
46. Morray JP, Lynn AM, Stamm SJ, et al. Hemodynamic effects of ketamine in children with congenital heart disease. *Anesth Analg* 1984;63:895–899.
47. Hickey PR, Hansen DD, Cramolini GM, et al. Pulmonary and systemic hemodynamic responses to ketamine in infants with normal and elevated pulmonary vascular resistance. *Anesthesiology* 1985;62:287–293.
48. Mankikian B, Cantineau JP, Sartene R, et al. Ventilatory and chest wall mechanics during ketamine anesthesia in humans. *Anesthesiology* 1986;65:492–499.
49. Hirshman CA, Downes H, Farbood A, et al. Ketamine block of bronchospasm in experimental canine asthma. *Br J Anaesth* 1979;51:713–718.
50. Bourke DL, Malit LA, Smith TC. Respiratory interactions of ketamine and morphine. *Anesthesiology* 1987; 66:153–156.
51. Lanning CF, Harmel MH. Ketamine anesthesia. *Annu Rev Med* 1975;26:137–141.
52. Taylor PA, Towey RM. Depression of laryngeal reflexes during ketamine administration. *BMJ* 1971;2:688–689.
53. Shapiro HM, Wyte SR, Harris AB. Ketamine anesthesia in patients with intracranial pathology. *Br J Anaesth* 1972;44:1200–1204.
54. Gardner AE, Dannemiller FJ, Dean D. Intracranial cerebrospinal fluid pressure in man during ketamine anesthesia. *Anesth Analg* 1972:51:741–745.
55. Reicher D, Bhalla P, Rubinstein EH. Cholinergic cerebral vasodilator effects of ketamine in rabbits. *Stroke* 1987;18:445–449.
56. Oren RE, Rasool NA, Rubinstein EH. Effect of ketamine on cerebral cortical blood flow and metabolism in rabbits. *Stroke* 1987;18:445–444.
57. Rosen I, Hagerdal M. Electroencephalographic study of children during ketamine anesthesia. *Acta Anaesth Scand* 1976;20:32–39.
58. Manohar S, Maxwell D, Winters WD. Development of EEG seizure activity during and after chronic ketamine administration in the rat. *Neuropharmacology* 1972;11:819–826.
59. Bourn WM, Yang DJ, Davisson JN. Effect of ketamine enantiomers on sound-induced convulsions in epilepsy prone rats. *Pharm Res Commun* 1983;15:815–824.
60. Veliskova J, Velisek L, Mares P, et al. Ketamine suppresses both bicuculline and picrotoxin induced generalized tonic clonic seizures during ontogenesis. *Pharm Biochem Behav* 1990;37:667–674.
61. Sheth RD, Gidal BE. Refractory status epilepticus: response to ketamine. *Neurology* 1998;51:1765–1766.
62. White PR, Way WL, Trevor AJ. Ketamine—its pharmacology and therapeutic uses. *Anesthesiology* 1982; 56:119–136.
63. Haeseler G, Zuzan O, Kohn G, et al. Anaesthesia with midazolam and S-(+) ketamine in spontaneously breathing paediatric patients during magnetic resonance imaging. *Paediatr Anaesth* 2000;10:513–519.
64. Tobias JD, Martin LD, Wetzel RC. Ketamine by continuous infusion for sedation in the pediatric intensive care unit. *Crit Care Med* 1990;18:819–821.
65. Hartvig P, Larsson E, Joachimsson PO. Postoperative analgesia and sedation following pediatric cardiac surgery using a constant infusion of ketamine. *J Cardiothorac Vasc Anesth* 1993;7:148–153.
66. Byer DE, Gould AB. Development of tolerance to ketamine in an infant undergoing repeated anesthesia. *Anesthesiology* 1981;54:255–256.
67. Sebel PS, Lowdon JD. Propofol: a new intravenous anesthetic. *Anesthesiology* 1989;71:260–277.
68. Harris CE, Grounds RM, Murray AM, et al. Propofol for long-term sedation in the intensive care unit. A comparison with papaveretum and midazolam. *Anaesthesia* 1990;45:366–372.
69. Beller JP, Pottecher T, Lugnier A, et al. Prolonged sedation with propofol in ICU patients: recovery and blood concentration changes during periodic interruption in infusion. *Br J Anaesth* 1988;61:583–588.
70. Ronan KP, Gallagher TJ, George B, et al. Comparison of propofol and midazolam for sedation in intensive care unit patients. *Crit Care Med* 1995;23:286–293.
71. Hemelrijck JV, Fitch W, Mattheussen M, et al. Effect of propofol on cerebral circulation and autoregulation in the baboon. *Anesth Analg* 1990;71:49–54.

72. Nimkoff L, Quinn C, Silver P, et al. The effects of intravenous anesthetic agents on intracranial pressure and cerebral perfusion pressure in two feline models of brain edema. *J Crit Care* 1997;12:132–136.
73. Watts ADJ, Eliasziw M, Gelb AW. Propofol and hyperventilation for the treatment of increased intracranial pressure in rabbits. *Anesth Analg* 1998;87:564–568.
74. Herregods L, Verbeke J, Rolly G, et al. Effect of propofol on elevated intracranial pressure. Preliminary results. *Anaesthesia* 1988;43[Suppl]:107–109.
75. Pinaud M, Lelausque J, Chetanneau A, et al. Effects of propofol on cerebral hemodynamics and metabolism in patients with brain trauma. *Anesthesiology* 1990;73:404–409.
76. Mangez JF, Menguy E, Roux P. Sedation par propofol a debit constant chez le traumatise cranien. Resultats preliminaires. *Ann Fr Anesth Reanim* 1987;6:336–337.
77. Ravussin P, Guinard JP, Ralley F, et al. Effect of propofol on cerebrospinal fluid pressure and cerebral perfusion pressure in patients undergoing craniotomy. *Anaesthesia* 1988;43[Suppl]:107–-109.
78. Farling PA, Johnston JR, Coppel DL. Propofol infusion for sedation of patients with head injury in intensive care. *Anaesthesia* 1989;44:222–226.
79. Spitzfadden AC, Jimenez DF, Tobias JD. Propofol for sedation and control of intracranial pressure in children. *Pediatr Neurosurg* 1999;31:194–200.
80. Eames WO, Rooke GA, Sai-Chuen R, et al. Comparison of the effects of etomidate, propofol, and thiopental on respiratory resistance after tracheal intubation. *Anesthesiology* 1996;84:1307–1311.
81. Pizov R, Brown RH, Weiss YS, et al. Wheezing during induction of general anesthesia in patients with and without asthma. A randomized, blinded trial. *Anesthesiology* 1995;82:1111–1116.
82. Chih-Chung L, Ming-Hwang S, Tan PPC, et al. Mechanisms underlying the inhibitory effect of propofol on the contraction of canine airway smooth muscle. *Anesthesiology* 1999;91:750–759.
83. Pedersen CM, Thirstrup S, Nielsen-Kudsk JE. Smooth muscle relaxant effects of propofol and ketamine in isolated guinea-pig tracheas. *Eur J Pharmacol* 1993; 238:75–80.
84. Brussel T, Theissen JL, Vigfusson G, et al. Hemodynamic and cardiodynamic effects of propofol and etomidate: negative inotropic properties of propofol. *Anesth Analg* 1989;69:35–40.
85. Tritapepe L, Voci P, Marino P, et al. Calcium chloride minimizes the hemodynamic effects of propofol in patients undergoing coronary artery bypass grafting. *J Cardiothorac Vasc Anes* 1999;13:150–153.
86. Sochala C, Van Deenen D, De Ville A, et al. Heart block following propofol in a child. *Paediatr Anaesth* 1999;9:349–351.
87. Egan TD, Brock-Utne JG. Asystole and anesthesia induction with a fentanyl, propofol, and succinylcholine sequence. *Anesth Analg* 1991;73:818–820.
88. Trotter C, Serpell MG. Neurological sequelae in children after prolonged propofol infusions. *Anaesthesia* 1992;47:340–342.
89. Saunders PRI, Harris MNE. Opisthotonic posturing and other unusual neurological sequelae after outpatient anesthesia. *Anaesthesia* 1992;47:552–557.
90. Finley GA, MacManus B, Sampson SE, et al. Delayed seizures following sedation with propofol. *Can J Anaesth* 1993;40:863–865.
91. Hewitt PB, Chu DLK, Polkey CE, et al. Effect of propofol on the electrocorticogram in epileptic patients undergoing cortical resection. *Br J Anaesth* 1999;82:199–202.
92. McBurney JW, Teiken PJ, Moon MR. Propofol for treating status epilepticus. *J Epilepsy* 1994;7:21–22.
93. Lowenstein DH, Alldredge BK. Status epilepticus. *N Engl J Med* 1998;338:970–976.
94. Parke TJ, Stevens JE, Rice ASC, et al. Metabolic acidosis and fatal myocardial failure after propofol infusion in children: five case reports. *BMJ* 1992;305:613–616.
95. Strickland RA, Murray MJ. Fatal metabolic acidosis in a pediatric patient receiving an infusion of propofol in the intensive care unit: is there a relationship? *Crit Care Med* 1995;23:405–409.
96. Bray RJ. Propofol infusion syndrome in children. *Paediatr Anaesth* 1998;8:491–499.
97. Hanna JP, Ramundo ML. Rhabdomyolysis and hypoxia associated with prolonged propofol infusion. *Neurology* 19998;50:301–303.
98. Cremer OL, Moons KG, Bouman EA, et al. Long-term propofol infusion and cardiac failure in adult head-injured patients. *Lancet* 2000;357:117–118.
99. Schenkman KA, Yan S. Propofol impairment of mitochondrial respiration in isolated perfused guinea pig hearts determined by reflectance spectroscopy. *Crit Care Med* 2000;28:172–177.
100. Wolf A, Weir P, Segar P, et al. Impaired fatty acid oxidation in propofol infusion syndrome. *Lancet* 2001; 357:606–607.
101. Reed MD, Yamashita TS, Marz CM, et al. A pharmacokinetically based propofol dosing strategy for sedation of the critically ill, mechanically ventilated pediatric patient. *Crit Care Med* 1996;24:1473–1481.
102. Norreslet J, Wahlgreen C. Propofol infusion for sedation of children. *Crit Care Med* 1990;18:890–892.
103. Hertzog JH, Campbell JK, Dalton HJ, et al. Propofol anesthesia for invasive procedures in ambulatory and hospitalized children: experience in the pediatric intensive care unit. *Pediatrics* 1999;103:E30.
104. Laxenaire MC, Mata-Bermejo E, Moneret-Vautrin DA, et al. Life-threatening anaphylactoid reactions to propofol. *Anesthesiology* 1992;77:275–280.
105. Tobias JD. Prevention of pain associated with the administration of propofol in children: lidocaine versus ketamine. *Am J Anesthesiol* 1996;23:231–232.
106. Sosis MB, Braverman B. Growth of *Staphylococcus aureus* in four intravenous anesthetics. *Anesth Analg* 1993;77:766–768.
107. Postsurgical infections associated with extrinsically contaminated intravenous anesthetic agent—California, Illinois, Maine, and Michigan, 1990. *MMWR* 1990;39:426–427, 433.
108. Trissel LA. Drug compatibility differences with propofol injectable emulsion products. *Crit Care Med* 2001;29:466–468.
109. Gottardis M, Khunl-Brady KS, Koller W, et al. Effect of prolonged sedation with propofol on serum triglyceride and cholesterol concentrations. *Br J Anaesth* 1989;62:393–396.
110. Valente JF, Anderson GL, Branson RD, et al. Disadvantages of prolonged propofol sedation in the critical care unit. *Crit Care Med* 1994;22:710–712.
111. Camps AS, Sanchez-Izquierdo Riera JA, Vazquez DT, et al. Midazolam and 2% propofol in long-term sedation of traumatized, critically ill patients: efficacy and

safety comparison. *Crit Care Med* 2000;28: 3612–3619.
112. Barrientos-Vega R, Sanchez-Soria M, Morales-Garcia C, et al. Pharmacoeconomic assessment of propofol 2% used for prolonged sedation. *Crit Care Med* 2001;29:317–322.
113. Astrup J, Sorensen PM, Sorensen HR. Inhibition of cerebral oxygen and glucose consumption in the dog by hypothermia, pentobarbital and lidocaine. *Anesthesiology* 1981;55:263–268.
114. Cormio M, Gopinath SP, Valadka A, et al. Cerebral hemodynamic effects of pentobarbital coma in head-injured patients. *J Neurotrauma* 1999;16:927–936.
115. Krishnamurthy KB, Drislane FW. Depth of EEG suppression and outcome in barbiturate anesthetic treatment for refractory status epilepticus. *Epilepsia* 1999; 40:759–762.
116. Holmes GL, Riviello JJ Jr. Midazolam and pentobarbital for refractory status epilepticus. *Pediatr Neurol* 1999;20:259–264.
117. Ishimaru H, Takahashi A, Ikarashi Y, et al. Effects of MK-801 and pentobarbital on cholinergic terminal damage and delayed neuronal death in the ischemic gerbil hippocampus. *Brain Res Bull* 1997;43:81–85.
118. Morimoto Y, Morimoto Y, Nishihira J, et al. Pentobarbital inhibits apoptosis in neuronal cells. *Crit Care Med* 2000;28:1899–1904.
119. Tobias JD, Deshpande JK, Pietsch JB, et al. Pentobarbital sedation in the pediatric intensive care unit patient. *South Med J* 1995;88:290–294.
120. Tobias JD. Pentobarbital for sedation during mechanical ventilation in the pediatric ICU patient. *J Intensive Care Med* 2000;15:115–120.
121. Collins JJ, Grier HE, Kinney HC, et al. Control of severe pain in children with terminal malignancy. *J Pediatr* 1995;126:653–657.
122. Tobias JD. Remifentanil: applications in the pediatric ICU population. *Am J Pain Manage* 1998;8:114–117.
123. Sperry RJ, Bailey PL, Reuchman MV, et al. Fentanyl and sufentanil increase intracranial pressure in head trauma patients. *Anesthesiology* 1992;77:416–420.
124. Milde LN, Milde JH, Gallagher WJ. Effects of sufentanil on cerebral circulation and metabolism in dogs. *Anesth Analg* 1990;70:138–146.
125. Pokela ML, Ryhanen PT, Koivisto ME, et al. Alfentanil-induced rigidity in newborn infants. *Anesth Analg* 1992;75:252–257.
126. Glick C, Evans OB, Parks BR. Muscle rigidity due to fentanyl infusion in the pediatric patient. *South Med J* 1996;89:1119–1120.
127. Irazuzta J, Pascucci R, Perlman N, et al. Effects of fentanyl administration on respiratory system compliance in infants. *Crit Care Med* 1993;21:1001–1004.
128. Lynn AM, Opheim KE, Tyler DC. Morphine infusion after pediatric cardiac surgery. *Crit Care Med* 1984; 12:863–866.
129. Quinn MW, Wild J, Dean HG, et al. Randomised double-blind controlled trial of effect of morphine on catecholamine concentrations in ventilated preterm babies. *Lancet* 1993;342:324–327.
130. Rosow CE, Moss J, Philbin DM, et al. Histamine release during morphine and fentanyl anesthesia. *Anesthesiology* 1982;56:93–96.
131. Shochet RB, Murray GB. Neuropsychiatric toxicity of meperidine. *J Intensive Care Med* 1988;3:246–252.
132. Berde CB, Beyer JE, Bournaki MC, et al. Comparison of morphine and methadone for prevention of postoperative pain in children. *J Pediatr* 1991;119:136–141.
133. Bruera E, Brenneis C, Michaud M, et al. Use of the subcutaneous route for the administration of narcotics in patients with cancer pain. *Cancer* 1988;62: 407–411.
134. Bruera E, Gibney N, Stollery D, Marcushamer S. Use of the subcutaneous route of administration of morphine in the intensive care unit. *J Pain Symptom Manage* 1991;6:263–265.
135. Tobias JD, O'Connor TA. Subcutaneous administration of fentanyl for sedation during mechanical ventilation in an infant. *Am J Pain Manage* 1996;6: 115–117.
136. Riker RR, Fraser GL, Cox PM. Continuous infusions of haloperidol controls agitation in critically ill patients. *Crit Care Med* 1994;22:433–440.
137. Nahata MC, Clotz MA, Krogg EA. Adverse effects of meperidine, promethazine, and chlorpromazine for sedation in pediatric patients. *Clin Pediatr* 1985;24: 558–560.
138. Rokicki W. Cardiac arrhythmia in a child after the usual dose of chloral hydrate. *Pediatr Cardiol* 1996; 17:419–420.
139. Seger D, Schwartz G. Chloral hydrate: a dangerous sedative for overdose patients? *Pediatr Emerg Care* 1994;10:349–350.
140. Maze MM, Tranquilli W. Alpha-2 agonists: defining the role in clinical anesthesia. *Anesthesiology* 1991; 74:581–591.
141. Mikawa K, Maekawa N, Nishina K, et al. Efficacy of oral clonidine premedication in children. *Anesthesiology* 1993;79:926–931.
142. De Kock MF, Pichon G, Scholtes JL. Intraoperative clonidine enhances postoperative morphine patient-controlled analgesia. *Can J Anaesth* 1992;39:537–544.
143. Bohrer H, Bach A, Layer M, et al. Clonidine as a sedative adjunct in intensive care. *Intensive Care Med* 1990;16:265–266.
144. Venn RM, Bradshaw CJ, Spencer R, et al. Preliminary experience of dexmedetomidine, a novel agent for postoperative sedation in the intensive care unit. *Anaesthesia* 1999;54:1136–1142.
145. Hall JE, Uhrich TD, Barney JA, et al. Sedative, amnestic, and analgesic properties of small-dose dexmedetomidine infusions. *Anesth Analg* 2000;90:699–705.
146. Tobias JD. Fentanyl for sedation in the pediatric intensive care unit: dealing with the problems. *J Pharm Care Pain Symptom Control* 1996;4:21–32.
147. Newman RG. The need to redefine "addiction." *N Engl J Med* 1983;308:1096–1098.
148. Porter J, Jick J. Addiction rare in patients treated with narcotics [Letter]. *N Engl J Med* 1980;302:123.
149. Arnold JH, Truog RD, Orav EJ, et al. Tolerance and dependence in neonates sedated with fentanyl during extracorporeal membrane oxygenation. *Anesthesiology* 1990;73:1136–1140.
150. Tobias JD, Schleien CL, Haun SE. Methadone as treatment for iatrogenic opioid dependency in pediatric intensive care unit patients. *Crit Care Med* 1990;18: 1292–1293.
151. Sury MRJ, Billingham I, Russell GN, et al. Acute benzodiazepine withdrawal syndrome after midazolam infusions in children. *Crit Care Med* 1989;17:301–302.
152. van Engelen BGM, Gimbrere JS, Booy LH. Benzodiazepine withdrawal reaction in two children following

discontinuation of sedation with midazolam. *Ann Pharmacother* 1993;27:579–581.

153. Fonsmark L. Rasmussen YH, Carl P. Occurrence of withdrawal in critically ill sedated children. *Crit Care Med* 1999;27:196–199.
154. Cammarano WB, Pittet JF, Weitz S, et al. Acute withdrawal syndrome related to the administration of analgesic and sedative medications in adult intensive care unit patients. *Crit Care Med* 1998;26:676–684.
155. Au J, Walker S, Scott DHT. Withdrawal syndrome after propofol infusion. *Anaesthesia* 1991;46:238–239.
156. Arnold JH, Truog RD, Rice SA. Prolonged administration of isoflurane to pediatric patients during mechanical ventilation. *Anesth Analg* 1993;76:520–526.
157. Smith RA, Winter PM, Smith M, et al. Tolerance to and dependence on inhalational anesthetic agents. *Anesthesiology* 1979;50:505–509.
158. Katz R, Kelly W, Hsi A. Prospective study on the occurrence of withdrawal in critically ill children who receive fentanyl by continuous infusion. *Crit Care Med* 1994;22:763–767.
159. Finnegan LP, Kron RE, Connaughton JF Jr, et al. A scoring system for evaluation and treatment of the neonatal abstinence syndrome: a new clinical and research tool. In: Morselli PL, Garattini S, Sereni F, eds. *Basic and therapeutic aspects of perinatal pharmacology*. New York: Raven Press, 1975:139–152.
160. Anand KJS, Arnold JH. Opioid tolerance and dependence in infants and children. *Crit Care Med* 1994;22: 334–342.
161. Tobias JD. Outpatient therapy of iatrogenic opioid dependency following prolonged sedation in the pediatric intensive care unit. *J Intensive Care Med* 1996; 11:284–287.
162. Gorman AL, Elliott KJ, Inturrisis CE. The d- and l-isomers of methadone bind to the non-competitive site on the N-methyl-d-aspartate (NMDA) receptor in rat forebrain and spinal cord. *Neurosci Lett* 1997; 223:5–8.
163. Ripamonti C, Groff L, Brunelli C, et al. Switching from morphine to oral methadone in treating cancer pain: what is the equianalgesic dose ratio? *J Clin Oncol* 1998;16:3216–3221.
164. Lawlor PG, Turner KS, Hanson J, et al. Dose ratio between morphine and methadone in patients with cancer pain. *Cancer* 1998;82:1167–1173.

45

Pain-Associated Disability Syndrome

Brenda Bursch, Michael H. Joseph, and Lonnie K. Zeltzer

Children in chronic pain experience varying amounts of disability, from none to severe. The amount of tissue damage sustained by the child and perceived severity may be independent of the degree of disability experienced by the child (1). Biologic, psychologic, social, cultural, and developmental factors each can influence pain-related functioning. Disability, in turn, can contribute to the development of secondary and/or increased pain because of abnormal body posturing and prolonged inactivity.

Traditionally, disability and pain in excess of what would be expected given the amount of tissue pathology have been considered psychogenic. Children and families are frequently informed that the pain has no physiologic basis, with the suggestion that the child is fabricating or exaggerating pain or is psychologically disturbed.

As most medical professionals have observed, however, maintaining the organic versus nonorganic dichotomy can be harmful, by leading either to unnecessary tests, procedures, and medical treatments or, conversely, to a therapeutically detrimental lack of empathy. In fact, because all pain is associated with neurosensory changes, it is physical, and because attention, memory, and arousal influence all pain, it is psychologic, too.

DEFINITION OF PAIN-ASSOCIATED DISABILITY SYNDROME

Pain-associated disability syndrome (PADS) describes a subset of patients with chronic pain with common and severe difficulties in functioning, regardless of the location or cause of their pain (2). It is a model of disability that can help the clinician shift focus to a rehabilitation model of care while avoiding dichotomization of the pain as physical or psychologic. Rather, it is assumed that all pain is physically mediated with biologic, psychologic, and social factors maintaining it (3).

Patients with PADS experience a downward spiral of increasing disability and pain for which acute symptom-focused assessment and treatment strategies have not led to acceptable resolution. This syndrome can affect anyone experiencing chronic pain. In fact, children with somatic symptoms of any sort can fall into a dangerous downward spiral of disability. Once the downward spiral begins, a multifactorial chronic illness model, which also addresses contextual factors, must often be adopted to ensure that comprehensive and appropriate assessment and treatment plans are adopted.

Disability in the above definition refers to school absenteeism and/or severe restriction of functioning in other activities. To meet the criteria for PADS, the severe disability has to have been present for at least 2 months. The initial pain could be caused by a specific identifiable illness or injury, a systemic virus, a developmental challenge, and/or a psychosocial stressor. Often it is not possible to identify the trigger. The time frame for development of PADS varies dramatically.

THEORETIC UNDERPINNINGS

From a social cognitive theory framework, one could hypothesize that one way that disability develops is when a significant life event, physical stressor, or developmental challenge is more than at-risk children can manage given their coping skills. The children's sense of inefficacy results in the appraisal of extreme stress and renders them somatically vulnerable. A somatic symptom (such as pain) allows retreat to a dependent role and possible avoidance of the perceived stressor. Because retreat from a perceived stressor prohibits mastery over the challenge and serves to strengthen inefficacy beliefs, a progressively declining course ensues with decreasing functioning, increasing distress, and increasing vulnerability to emotional and physical impairment. Well-meaning and concerned family members and health care providers may perpetuate the downward spiral of pain and disability by fostering the dependent role and/or by contributing to the stress of the child. Owing to the somatic presentation of pain, however, many reasonable parents question a behavioral or psychiatric diagnosis, especially if they feel blamed for the disorder. Finally, no one is inclined to follow treatment recommendations unless they believe that the recommendations will work and that they are able to follow them.

Research supports this conceptual framework because it reveals that children with severe and persistent pain often have inadequate coping responses and perceive themselves to have little control over their pain (4,5). The type of coping strategy used has been shown to influence pain and functioning, with more active coping strategies increasing the child's sense of control and more passive strategies leading to withdrawal, inactivity, and increased pain (6,7).

Perceived coping inefficacy has been linked to high ratings of subjective distress, autonomic arousal, and plasma catecholamine secretion (8,9). Other research has demonstrated that exposure to physical stressors with the ability to control them has no adverse physiologic effects, but exposure to the same stressors without such control impairs cellular components of the immune system (10). Conversely, there is some evidence to suggest that stress that occurs while increasing one's coping efficacy enhances immune function (11).

Parental behaviors that have been linked to pain and disability in their children include sympathy and attention for symptoms, external help seeking, strong emotional responses, modeling of symptoms, and support for task avoidance (12–15). Cognitive-behavioral treatment interventions with children and their families have resulted in decreased pain and disability (16–19).

CLINICAL EVALUATION

Among children and adolescents who meet criteria for PADS, an extensive evaluation is typically indicated to develop a comprehensive treatment plan that best targets the biologic, psychologic, and social factors that are maintaining the pain and disability. Whenever possible, conducting a concurrent medical and psychosocial evaluation is suggested to reinforce the importance of the biopsychosocial model, regardless of the cause of the symptoms. Including all family members in the evaluation is highly recommended because siblings are often the best source of information.

An extended interview helps to determine whether additional medical or psychologic assessment is indicated. For example, if significant physical findings that have not been previously addressed are identified, referral to the appropriate subspecialist might be indicated for a more thorough evaluation. Additionally, there are numerous common problems experienced by patients with chronic pain that may require intellectual, academic, or psychologic testing to identify.

Based on our clinical population of patients with PADS, subtle social problem-solving skills deficits appear to be relatively common in this population (20), and occasionally intelligence testing (together with other developmental data gathered during the clinical interview) results in the diagnosis of a pervasive developmental disorder. If the child is academically delayed or has a previously unsuspected learning disorder, school can be a significant source of stress, even if the child does not report it as such (21,22). This is especially true among those children who strongly identify with being a good student, attempt to maintain high grades, or experience strong internal or external pressure to achieve. Expressive language disorder is another easily overlooked disorder that has been associated with chronic pain (21). Because of the time and expense associated with psychologic testing, however, such recommendations might be reserved for children who appear to be experiencing an alarming progression of PADS, are already significantly disabled, or have been treatment resistant using an intensive, integrated rehabilitation approach to treatment.

A thorough evaluation might include the following domains of questions:

Clinical Interview, Self-Report Measures, and Observations of Pain Behavior

- Onset and development of the current pain problem
- Results of previous evaluations and treatment attempts (including home remedies and alternative/complementary therapies)
- Locations of pain over the entire body
- Intensity of the pain at different times and under differing circumstances
- Pain quality, duration, variability, predictability
- Exacerbating and alleviating factors
- Impact of pain on the patient's daily life
- Other sensations and symptoms that accompany the pain
- Thoughts and behaviors associated with the pain
- The perceived cause of the pain and beliefs about what will and will not help the pain
- Coping responses and ability to tolerate the pain
- How the pain has affected the lives of family members
- Congruity between verbal reports of pain and chronic pain behavior
- Intensity and types of emotion displayed by the patient and family
- Roles held by various family members and who speaks about which topics
- How family members react to symptoms displayed by the child during the interview
- Any unusual behavior or use of language during the interview
- Child and family history of all significant somatic and emotional symptoms and diagnoses
- Baseline functioning of the child and of each family member
- Birth and early childhood history and developmental milestones of the child
- History of school absenteeism and school performance, including academic difficulties and/or challenges, friends, bullies, teachers, examinations, grades, classes, and academic aspirations
- Social history of family, especially significant (positive and negative) life events, including things such as changes at school or in living arrangements or witnessing or direct experience of physical or sexual assault, a robbery, death, or injury
- Depression; panic; anxiety, worries, or fears related to separation from parents, academic achievement or examinations, social situations, or school; obsessive-compulsive traits; posttraumatic stress; eating disorders; enuresis or encopresis
- Parents' emotional functioning, marital stress, coping skills, and problem-solving behaviors
- Parental behaviors: excessive sympathy and attention for pain symptoms, external help-seeking, strong emotional responses, modeling of symptoms, and/or support for task avoidance

Physical Examination

- General appearance (weight, posture, gait, sick versus healthy appearing)
- Emotional state (mental status examination)
- Vital signs (height, weight, blood pressure, heart rate, respiratory rate, temperature)
- Complete physical examination, including a thorough neurologic examination, as well as particular assessment for muscle spasms, trigger points, and areas of somatic sensitivity to light touch

Psychologic and Academic Testing (Optional But Sometimes Helpful)

- Coping style
- Social problem-solving skills
- Cognitive deficits
- Relative strengths and weaknesses in various domains of intellectual functioning
- Gaps in general knowledge, academic delays
- Learning disorders
- Communication disorders

APPROACH TO TREATMENT

Specific treatment strategies follow directly from data gathered in the assessment. A range of options may be considered, including pharmacologic, psychologic, behavioral, and physical interventions. Most important, a rehabilitation approach is strongly recommended as an alternative to the acute pain model of care. Within a rehabilitation model, pain is accepted as a symptom that may or may not go away. Instead, the focus turns to improving independent functioning and to skills building designed to improve coping and self-efficacy. This means that functioning, rather than pain, is tracked to determine whether progress is being made. In fact, inquiry about pain is contraindicated once the treatment phase has begun. The rationale behind this approach is that asking about pain causes the patient to scan his or her body for somatic cues, thus reinforcing somatic hypervigilance. As functioning, coping skills, and self-efficacy improve, pain and/or the distress related to the pain often remits.

Central to a successful approach to treatment is the integration of the various targeted interventions into a consistent and cohesive package. All professionals involved in the case must first agree on (a) what constitutes completion of the evaluation, (b) what language/words to use to describe the problem and plan, and (c) what interventions should be included in a comprehensive biopsychosocial plan.

Deciding When to Stop Evaluating

The family and treatment team often share anxiety about missing a diagnosis that would be easily remedied with medication or surgery alone. This fear is especially strong when the patient or family exhibits significant distress about the pain and/or disability, and a rehabilitation approach seems too slow or difficult. The treatment team must believe that a reasonable evaluation has been completed so they can refrain from unnecessary assessment that detracts from rehabilitation and continues to focus the family on finding a magic bullet. Once the treatment team can agree that enough information is available to construct a treatment plan, it is important that this decision be clearly communicated to the family and that no further evaluation be conducted. The team's comfort with the available information and treatment plan, if communicated clearly, will often reduce anxiety in the family, thus reducing doctor shopping and requests for continued medical testing.

Conceptual Framework and Language

The biopsychosocial model of chronic pain is an abstract and complicated model, even to most medical professionals. Confusion can be kept to a minimum if each professional working with the family uses the same language/words to describe both the problem and the plan. One advantage of using a rehabilitation model is that most people are already familiar with the concepts and language associated with either physical therapy or some other kind of rehabilitation.

For some parents to believe that treatment interventions will benefit their child, it is important for them to understand what is known about the mind/body link and how interventions target this link. When explaining the PADS problem to the family, it is usually important to initially focus on the pain symptoms and pain mechanisms to reassure them that the pain is real and that it makes sense from a neurophysiologic framework. Specifically, it might be helpful for the family to understand that ongoing nociception can result in a sensitization of the peripheral and central nervous systems that produces neuroanatomic, neurochemical, and neurophysiologic changes, often described as alterations in neural chemicals and signaling. Next, it is important to explain how the interacting biologic and psychologic systems in the child, as well as the systems in the social environment of the child, all influence pain and disability. The role of memory and attention in reinforcing chronic pain may be included in this portion of the education. It is important to explicitly state that neither the patient nor the family is to blame for the pain and disability but that there are things they can do to reverse the downward disabling spiral. Even if parents have difficulty remembering the specifics of how the mind and body interact, the physiologic explanation for the previously unexplainable pain could be sustaining throughout treatment.

The clinician should then present the specific treatment goals of the rehabilitation plan, provide treatment options and rationale for each option, and promote active problem solving by requesting that the family decide which treatment options to follow.

Ongoing education, review of the diagnoses, repeated description of the rationale for the treatment approach, reminders to track functioning rather than pain as an indication of progress, and frequent reassurance that all is proceeding in an expected manner are usually required by families as they progress through the treatment plan.

Specific Interventions

A multimodal approach is recommended over a single sequential treatment approach. Interventions should address possible underlying pain mechanisms, specific symptoms, and disability. In general, treatment goals focus on increasing independent functioning (daily living, academic, social, physical activities); remediation of specific symptoms, deficits, or problems revealed in the assessment; enhancing communication, especially of distress, with peers and family members; and facilitating more adaptive problem-solving skills.

Treatment techniques designed to address possible underlying pain mechanisms and specific symptoms include cognitive-behavioral strategies (e.g., psychotherapy, hypnosis, biofeedback), behavioral techniques, family interventions, physical interventions (e.g., massage, acupuncture, transcutaneous electrical nerve stimulation, physical therapy, occupational therapy), and pharmacologic interventions. In general, interventions that promote active coping are preferred to those that require passive dependence. Evidence-based treatments should be recommended whenever possible.

Most pediatric patients who have functional chronic pain and are on opioids, and their families, report that the opioids are not particularly helpful for pain control. Because they also interfere with restorative sleep and are potentially addictive, most families are open to changing medications. Some patients, however, are quite anxious and resistant to an opioid wean. Such patients can often successfully wean if their anxiety symptoms are addressed with appropriate medications and/or psychotherapy. Medications that reduce general central nervous system irritability and/or that target identified symptoms, such as anxiety, should first be slowly introduced (examples include low-dose tricyclic antidepressants, selective serotonin reuptake inhibitors, anticonvulsants, muscle relaxants, and low-dose phenothiazines). As these medications come to level, it is recommended that the opioid be weaned extremely slowly, often as slow as 10% every fourth day. Often, a low-dose phenothiazine, such as thioridazine, can be effective for breakthrough pain and distress. Benzodiazepines are generally not recommended because they often elicit paradoxical reactions in children and interfere with restorative sleep. If quality restorative sleep is well addressed (e.g., with a low-dose tricyclic antidepressant such as amitriptyline or with trazodone), the child will typically have more ability to cope during the day.

Family interventions can be extensive and are sometimes more important than the patient interventions. They include helping family members to understand the nature of the pain condition (including relevant medical, cognitive, behavioral and/or psychologic contributions), facilitating acceptance of a rehabilitation approach, elucidating biopsychosocial factors that likely contribute to the pain syndrome, altering family patterns that inadvertently maintain or exacerbate the pain syndrome, helping parents to cope with their own and the child's distress during the rehabilitation process, and developing a plan to ensure adequate support for self-management of symptoms and independent functioning.

Example of a Feedback Session

We learned a number of things about Amy, have an idea about what is going on, and have a number of treatment recommendations that we believe can help her. First, it is important for you to know that we have seen and successfully treated a large number of other patients who have had the same medical course as Amy, so we feel confident in our assessment and treatment approach.

We believe, as you do, that it is likely that the stomach flu Amy had 4 months ago started her pain and vomiting. Although our bodies usually stop feeling pain and nausea after the initial illness subsides, Amy's body did not. Her body is still activated to feel these things even though her viral illness and intestinal inflammation are now gone. This persistence in pain and nausea likely happened because her body is still sending her brain neurochemical and neuroelectrical messages that her brain identifies as pain and nausea, and her brain is currently unable to shut these messages down. We believe that her medical tests failed to show the problem because the initial illness is gone and the tests do not measure these neurosignals that occur in the central nervous system.

To treat the problem, Amy's brain needs to help normalize the neurochemical messages from her body that activate the feelings of pain and nausea. There are two goals in treating this kind of problem: (a) to enhance the normal functioning of the sensory signal system so that there is a balance between sensory signaling to the brain and central control of these signals and (b) to help the neural system in the body to be generally less activated or sensitive. These goals are achieved by helping Amy act normally even though she does not feel well, by engaging in therapies to normalize the functioning of her central nervous system, and by addressing any other challenges in her life that might be keeping her body activated or simply adding stress to her body making it harder to recover.

Functioning normally is extremely difficult when you do not feel well and when it is not how we were taught to act when we have pain or are sick. Nevertheless, it is important with chronic pain to try to not let it interfere with normal functioning. Not only do those who lose functioning tend to do worse over time, but functioning can actually help your body start to work more normally again. Functioning normally means attending school, socializing, doing homework, sleeping a normal sleep pattern, eating normally, and getting some form of regular exercise.

Therapies we are recommending today to normalize the functioning of Amy's central nervous system include medications, acupuncture, and hypnotherapy. All the medications that we use to treat chronic pain were originally developed to treat something else such as depression, anxiety, and/or seizures. This is because these medications affect the neurochemical signaling in the central nervous system. They are not addictive and do not adversely interfere with normal sleep patterns. Acupuncture is a traditional Chinese medicine modality that increases the body's own pain control chemicals and is also thought to help to get the body in balance through increasing the flow of life energy. Hypnotherapy is used to alter the attentional focus related to the perceptions of pain and nausea. It also promotes relaxation.

We also learned that, although Amy never recognized that she had anxiety, her episodes of symptoms that include her heart racing and her hands sweating in some situations are symptoms of panic attacks. Changing schools this year probably also added stress to her body, as did the recent death of the family dog. Because these last two events do not appear to be ongoing stressors at this time, our recommendations focus on her pain and disability and on her panic attacks.

Based on our experience and assessment of Amy, our individualized treatment recommendations for Amy include participation in individual psychotherapy to help Amy learn how to better identify when she is anxious and to use behavioral-cognitive techniques to better manage her symptoms of panic. If issues related to changing schools or to the death of your dog surface, these might also be addressed in the therapy setting.

If the family expresses confusion about or resistance to the biopsychosocial treatment approach, it is sometimes helpful to give a more common example of a similar model.

When someone has a heart attack, we often do not know all the biologic, psychologic, and social factors that came together in that one moment to cause the heart attack. However, research has shown us that to make someone healthier and to help them avoid another heart attack, they should engage in a rehabilitation program that includes medication, physical therapy, stress management, dietary restrictions, and lifestyle changes. Although it is doubtful that the argument one had earlier in the day, yesterday's hamburger, or not engaging in aerobic exercise could be said to be "the" cause of the heart attack, each of these factors might have contributed to it. Regardless, if they did contribute or not, changing these risk factors will reduce one's risk of reoccurrence.

COMMON OBSTACLES TO REHABILITATION

The most significant obstacle can be reluctance to adopt a rehabilitation model. It is sometimes difficult to dispel the strong belief that a medication alone or surgery is the only thing that will help. This belief is often accompanied and exacerbated by the perceived absence of meaningful psychosocial stressors or problems other than the pain or the inability to understand how life stressors could be related to a biologic process. Additionally, there may be an intense fear of causing harm or pain to the child by pushing too hard (especially when fears remain that the medical team missed an injury or disease). Finally, the family may have difficulty tolerating the emotional distress of the child and their own distress during rehabilitation.

The treatment team must be able to contain the family's distress as well as their own distress during assessment and rehabilitation. Evaluating progress by tracking functioning in very small increments, rather than by monitoring pain, often helps contain anxiety. Weekly appointments with families are usually needed during the treatment phase, and telephone contacts between appointments are often required at first. Just as the goal of the child's treatment plan is to increase independent functioning, the goal of the family's treatment plan is to increase their ability to respond appropriately and independently to challenges. If all goes well, the family's dependence on the medical team will lessen as they learn how to take responsibility for the rehabilitation program. Close team work, a high level of communication among team members, planning for the common challenges, and monitoring for team contributions to the problem help rehabilitation progress as smoothly as possible.

Inpatient rehabilitation should be considered if the child is extremely disabled, if the child has been on opioids for a significant period of time and requires weaning, if the family is expected to have difficulty following the outpatient treatment recommendations, and/or if outpatient rehabilitation (as outlined above) has failed. Generally speaking, it is recommended that outpatient rehabilitation be attempted first.

CONCLUSIONS

PADS is a term designed to enable clinicians to efficiently describe a sub-set of chronic pain patients with common and severe difficulties in functioning, regardless of the location or etiology of their pain. Once a downward spiral of pain and disability begins, a multimodal chronic illness model, which also addresses contextual factors, is recommended to ensure that comprehensive and appropriate assessment and treatment plans are adopted. General treatment goals include increasing independent functioning; remediating specific symptoms, deficits, or problems revealed in a comprehensive biopsychosocial assessment; enhancing effective communication; and facilitating more active problem solving skills. Depending on the results of the assessment, treatment might include a combination of cognitive strategies, behavioral techniques, family interventions, physical interventions, and pharmacological interventions.

REFERENCES

1. Melzack R, Wall PD. Pain mechanisms: a new theory. *Science* 1965;150:971–979.
2. Bursch B, Walco GA, Zeltzer L. Clinical assessment and management of chronic pain and pain-associated disability syndrome. *J Dev Behav Pediatr* 1998;19: 45–53.
3. Zeltzer L, Bursch B, Walco GA. Pain responsiveness and chronic pain: a psychobiological perspective. *J Dev Behav Pediatr* 1997;18:413–422.
4. Branson SM, Craig KD. Children's spontaneous strategies for coping with pain: a review of the literature. *Can J Behav Sci* 1988;20:402–412.
5. Dunn-Geier B, McGrath PJ, Rourke,BP, et al. Adolescent chronic pain: the ability to cope. *Pain* 1986;26: 23–32.
6. Flor H, Birbaumer N, Rudy DC. The psychobiology of chronic pain. *Adv Behav Res Ther* 1990;12:47–84.
7. Siegel LJ, Smith KE. Children's strategies for coping with pain. *Pediatrician* 1989;16:110–118.
8. Bandura A, Reese L, Adams NE. Microanalysis of action and fear arousal as a function of differential levels of perceived self-efficacy. *J Pers Soc Psychol* 1982;43: 5–21.
9. Bandura A, Taylor CB, Williams SL, et al. Catecholamine secretion as a function of perceived coping self-efficacy. *J Consult Clin Psychol* 1985;53:406–414.
10. Maier SF, Laudenslager ML, Ryan SM. Stressor controllability, immune function, and endogenous opiates. In: Brush FR, Overmier JB, eds. *Affect, conditioning, and cognition: essays on the determinants of behavior*. Hillsdale, NJ: Lawrence Erlbaum Associates, 1985.
11. Wiedenfeld SA, O'Leary A, Bandura A, et al. Impact of perceived self-efficacy in coping with stressors on immune function. *J Pers Soc Psychol* 1990;59:1082–1094.
12. Fordyce WE. *Behavioral methods for chronic pain and illness*. St. Louis: Mosby, 1976.
13. Payne B, Norfleet MA. Chronic pain and the family. *Pain* 1986;26:1–22.
14. Philips HC. Avoidance behavior and its role in sustaining chronic pain. *Behav Res Ther* 1987;25:273–279.
15. Whitehead WE, Busch CM, Heller BR, et al. Social learning influences on menstrual symptoms and illness behavior. *Health Psychol* 1986;5:13–23.
16. Beames L, Sanders MR, Bor W. The role of parent training in the cognitive behavioral treatment of children's headaches. *Behav Psychother* 1992;20:167–180.
17. Finney JW, Lemanek KL, Cataldo MF, et al. Pediatric psychology in primary health care: Brief targeted therapy for recurrent abdominal pain. *Behav Ther* 1989;20: 283–291.
18. Sanders MR, Rebgetz M, Morrison MM, et al. Cognitive-behavioral treatment of recurrent nonspecific abdominal pain in children: an analysis of generalization, and maintenance side effects. *J Consult Clin Psychol* 1989;57:294–300.
19. Sanders MR, Shepherd RW, Cleghorn G, et al. The treatment of recurrent abdominal pain in children: a controlled comparison of cognitive-behavioral family intervention and standard pediatric care. *J Consult Clin Psychol* 1994;62:306–314.
20. Bursch B. Evaluation and development of a strategy for psychological intervention for chronic pain. In: Lonnie Zeltzer, Chair. *Psychological approaches to pediatric pain management*. Invited symposium at the Fourth International Symposium on Pediatric Pain, Helsinki, Finland, 1997.
21. Zeltzer LK, Bursch B. Psychological management of pediatric functional disorders, *J Pediatr Gastroenterol Nutr* 2001;32:S40–S41.
22. Shapiro EG, Rosenfeld AA. *The somatizing child: diagnosis and treatment of conversion and somatization disorders*. New York: Springer-Verlag, 1987.

Appendix/Formulary

APPENDIX TABLE 1. *Oral dosing guidelines for commonly used nonopioid analgesics*

Drug	Dose (mg/kg) (<60 kg)	Dose (mg) (>60 kg)	Interval (hr)	Daily maximal dose (mg/kg) (<60 kg)	Daily maximal dose (mg) (>60 kg)
Acetaminophen	10–15	650–1,000	4	100[a]	4,000
Ibuprofen	6–10	400–600[b]	6	40[b,c]	2,400[b]
Naproxen	5–6[b]	250–375[b]	12	24[b,c]	1,000[b]
Aspirin[d]	10–15[b,d]	650–1,000[b]	4	80[b,c,d]	3,600[b]
Rofecoxib[c,e]	0.6	25	24	0.6	50[e]

[a]Maximal daily doses for acetaminophen should be reduced to 80 mg/kg for infants, 60 mg/kg for term neonates, and 45 mg/kg for preterm neonates 32–36 weeks postconceptional age.

[b]Higher doses may be used in selected cases for treatment of rheumatologic conditions in children.

[c]Dosing guidelines for neonates and infants have not been established.

[d]Aspirin carries a risk of provoking Reye syndrome in infants and children. If other analgesics are available, aspirin use should be restricted to indications for which antiplatelet or anti-inflammatory effect is required rather than as a routine analgesic or antipyretic in neonates, infants, or children. Dosing guidelines for aspirin in neonates have not been established.

[e]Rofecoxib guidelines are based on very limited pharmacokinetic data presented only in abstract form. These guidelines should be regarded as provisional. Although the standard adult dose is 25 mg once daily, short-term use of 50 mg has appeared safe in adult perioperative studies.

APPENDIX TABLE 2. *Opioid analgesic initial dose guidelines*

Drug	Equianalgesic doses		Usual starting intravenous or subcutaneous doses and intervals		Parenteral/oral dose ratio	Usual starting oral doses and intervals	
	Parenteral	Oral	Child <50 kg	Child >50 kg		Child <50 kg	Child >50 kg
Codeine	120 mg	200 mg	N/R	N/R	1:2	0.5–1 mg/kg every 3–4 hr	30–60 mg every 3–4 hr
Morphine	10 mg	30 mg (long term) 60 mg (single dose)	Bolus: 0.1 mg/kg every 2–4 hr Infusion: 0.03 mg/kg/hr	Bolus: 5–8-mg every 2–4 hr Infusion: 1.5 mg/hr	1:3 (long term) 1:6 (single dose)	Immediate release: 0.3 mg/kg every 3–4 hr Sustained release: 20–35 kg: 10–15 mg every 8–12 hr; 35–50 kg: 15–30 mg every 8–12 hr	Immediate release: 15–20 mg every 3–4 hr Sustained release: 30–45 mg every 8–12 hr
Oxycodone	N/A	15–20 mg	N/A	N/A	N/A	0.1–0.2 mg/kg every 3–4 hr	5–10 mg every 3–4 hr
Methadone[a]	10 mg	10–20 mg	0.1 mg/kg every 4–8 hr	5–8 mg every 4–hr	1:1.5–1:2	0.1–0.2 mg/kg every 4–8 hr	5–10 mg every 4–8 hr
Fentanyl	100 μg (0.1 mg)	N/A	Bolus: 0.5–1 μg every 1–2 hr Infusion: 0.5–2 μg/kg/hr	Bolus: 25–50 μg/kg every 1–2 hr Infusion: 25–100 μg/hr	N/A	N/A	N/A
Hydromorphone	1.5–2 mg	6–8 mg	Bolus: 0.02 mg every 2–4 hr Infusion: 0.006 mg/kg/hr	Bolus: 1 mg every 2–4 hr Infusion: 0.3 mg/hr	1:4	0.04–0.08 mg/kg every 3–4 hr	2–4 mg every 3–4 hr
Meperidine[b] (pethidine)	75–100 mg	300 mg	Bolus: 0.8–1 mg/kg every 2–3 hr	Bolus: 50–75 mg every 2–3 hr	1:4	2–3 mg/kg every 3–4 hr	100–150 mg every 3–4 hr

Doses refer to patients older than 6 months of age. In infants younger than 6 months, initial doses per kilogram should begin at approximately 25% of the doses per kilogram recommended here. Higher doses are often required for patients receiving mechanical ventilation. All doses are approximate and should be adjusted according to clinical circumstances.

[a]Methadone requires additional vigilance because it can accumulate and produce delayed sedation. If sedation occurs, doses should be withheld until sedation resolves. Thereafter, doses should be substantially reduced and/or the dosing interval should be extended to 8 to 12 hours.

[b]Meperidine should generally be avoided if other opioids are available, especially with long-term use, because its metabolite can cause seizures.

N/R, not recommended; N/A, not available.

APPENDIX TABLE 3. *Sample titration procedures for medications commonly used for neuropathic pain*

1. Slow titration (e.g., ambulatory outpatients who are attending school or work)

	<50 kg	>50 kg
a. Nortriptyline or amitriptyline	obtain baseline ECG	
Days 1–4	0.2 mg/kg q.h.s.	10 mg q.h.s.
Days 5–8	0.4 mg/kg q.h.s	20 mg q.h.s.

increase as tolerated every 4 to 6 days until
   i. good analgesia or
   ii. limiting side effects or
   iii. dosing reaches 1 mg/kg/d (<50 kg) or 50 mg (>50 mg)
   iv. if condition iii, consider measuring plasma concentration and ECG before further dose escalation. Consider twice-daily dosing (25% in morning, 75% in evening).

b. Gabapentin

	<50 kg	>50 kg
Days 1–2	2 mg/kg q.h.s.	100 mg q.h.s.
Days 3–4	2 mg/kg b.i.d.	100 mg b.i.d.
Days 4–6	2 mg/kg t.i.d.	100 mg t.i.d.
Days 7–9	2, 2, 4 mg/kg (t.i.d. schedule)	100, 100, 200 mg

increase as tolerated every 3 days (with 50% of daily dose in the evening) until
   i. good analgesia
   ii. limiting side effects
   iii. dosing reaches 60 mg/kg daily (<50 kg) or 3 g daily (>50 kg)

2. Rapid Titration (e.g., nonambulatory patients with widely metastatic cancer)
   a. Tricyclics: begin at 0.2 mg/kg (10 mg for >50 kg) and titrate up every 1 to 2 days in steps according to the slow titration regimen
   b. Gabapentin: begin at 6 mg/kg b.i.d. (300 mg b.i.d. for >50 kg) for 1 to 2 days, 6 mg/kg t.i.d. (300 mg t.i.d. for >50 kg) for 1 to 2 days, 6 mg/kg morning and midday, 12 mg/kg q.h.s. (300, 300, 600 mg for >50 kg) for 1 to 2 days, and increase as tolerated to 60 mg/kg daily (3 g/d for >50 kg) over 5 to 10 days.

ECG, electrocardiogram; q.h.s., once daily at bedtime; b.i.d., twice daily; t.i.d., three times daily.

Subject Index

Note: Page numbers followed by f indicate figures; those followed by t indicate tables

C

M